Aesthetic Plastic Surgery

Principles and Techniques

Aesthetic Plastic Surgery

Principles and Techniques

Edited by

Paule Regnault, M.D., F.R.C.S.(C)
Formerly, Professeur Agrégé de Clinique, University of Montreal Faculty of Medicine; formerly, Chief of Service, Hôpital Saint-Luc, Montreal

Rollin K. Daniel, M.D., F.R.C.S.(C)
Professor of Surgery, McGill University Faculty of Medicine; Chief of Plastic Surgery, Royal Victoria Hospital, Montreal

Little, Brown and Company
Boston/Toronto

To my daughter, Dr. Nicole Beccat-Latourelle, who could have become an excellent plastic surgeon but chose psychiatry instead; to the memory of my teacher, Dr. Suzanne Noël, the first woman aesthetic surgeon, who fought for both aesthetic surgery and professional women; and to the future of aesthetic surgery, which rests with the younger generation of plastic surgeons.

P. R.

To my wife and colleague, Beatrix Tirkanits, M.D.

R. K. D.

First Edition

Library of Congress Catalog Card No. 83-82935

ISBN 0-316-73851-4

Printed in the United States of America

Cover design by Curtis & Company

EB

Contents

Contributing Authors *ix*
Preface *xi*
Acknowledgments *xiii*

I. Basic Principles

1. *History of the Development of Aesthetic Surgery* 3
Blair O. Rogers

2. *Aesthetic Surgery: Basic Principles* 31
Robert M. Goldwyn

3. *Design and Management of An Aesthetic Surgeon's Office and Surgery Suite* 45
Ray A. Elliott

4. *Drugs for Outpatient Surgery* 75
Howard L. Gordon

5. *Clinical Photography for Aesthetic Plastic Surgery* 83
Daniel C. Morello

II. Rhinoplasty

6. *Septorhinoplasty* 101
Paule Regnault and Rollin K. Daniel

7. *Aesthetic Rhinoplasty of the Nasal Tip* 173
George C. Peck

8. *Posttraumatic Nasal Deformities* 183
Guy Jost

9. *Secondary Rhinoplasty* 201
Rodolphe Meyer and Ulrich K. Kesselring

III. Facial Procedures

10. *Aesthetic Procedures on the Chin* 221
S. Anthony Wolfe

11. *Otoplasty* 245
Ray A. Elliott

12. *Aesthetic Surgery of the Malar Region* 275
Ulrich T. Hinderer and Juan del Rio Legarreta

13. *Eyelids, Periorbital Region, and Forehead-Lift* 287
Paule Regnault and Rollin K. Daniel

Blepharoplasty 288
James W. Smith and Fredric Newman

14. *Blepharoplasty* 325
Melvin Spira

15. *Advanced Blepharoplasty* 347
Richard J. Siegel

IV. Face-Lift

16. *Rhytidectomy* 371
Paule Regnault and Rollin K. Daniel

17. *Superficial Fascia Rhytidectomy* 421
Mark L. Lemmon

18. *The Male Aging Face* 449
Eugene H. Courtiss

19. *Chemical Face Peeling* 463
Thomas J. Baker and Howard L. Gordon

20. *Ancillary Facial Procedures* 483

Surgical Rejuvenation of the Lips 484
Rodolphe Meyer and Ulrich K. Kesselring

Collagen: A Complement to the Surgeon 489
Hale Tolleth

Comparison of Techniques 494
Paule Regnault

V. Breast Surgery

21. *Breast Reduction* 499
Paule Regnault and Rollin K. Daniel

Inferior Pedicle Technique 522
Robert M. Goldwyn and Eugene H. Courtiss

22. *Breast Ptosis* 539
Paule Regnault and Rollin K. Daniel

23. *Breast Augmentation* 559
Paule Regnault and Rollin K. Daniel

Periareolar Approach 569
James W. Smith and John E. Sherman

Axillary Approach 572
Rex Peterson

24. *Breast Asymmetry and Deformities* 595
Paule Regnault and Rollin K. Daniel

VI. Body Contouring

25. *Abdominoplasty* 617
Paule Regnault and Rollin K. Daniel

26. *Lower Extremity* 655
Paule Regnault and Rollin K. Daniel

27. *Suction Lipectomy* 679

Basic Principles and Indications of Liposuction 679
Paule Regnault

Body Sculpturing with Suction-Assisted Lipectomy 681
Ulrich K. Kesselring and Rodolphe Meyer

Collapsing Surgery and Body Sculpturing 686
Pierre F. Fournier and Yves-Gerard Illouz

28. *Upper Extremity* 693
Paule Regnault and Rollin K. Daniel

29. *Massive Weight Loss* 705
Paule Regnault and Rollin K. Daniel

Appendix 721

Index 725

Contributing Authors

Thomas J. Baker, M.D.
Assistant Clinical Professor of Surgery (Plastic), University of Miami School of Medicine; Senior Attending Surgeon, Plastic and Reconstructive Surgery, Miami Mercy Hospital, Miami

Eugene H. Courtiss, M.D.
Associate Clinical Professor, Boston University School of Medicine, Boston; Chief, Division of Plastic Surgery, Newton-Wellesley Hospital, Newton Lower Falls, Massachusetts

Rollin K. Daniel, M.D., F.R.C.S.(C)
Professor of Surgery, McGill University Faculty of Medicine; Chief of Plastic Surgery, Royal Victoria Hospital, Montreal

Juan del Rio Legarreta, M.D.
Associate Surgeon, Clínica Mirasierra, Madrid

Ray A. Elliott, Jr., M.D., F.A.C.S.
Associate Clinical Professor of Surgery (Plastic), Albany Medical College of Union University; Attending Plastic Surgeon and Head, Subdivision of Plastic Surgery, Albany Memorial Hospital, Albany

Pierre F. Fournier, M.D.
Private Practice, Aesthetic Plastic Surgery, Paris

Robert M. Goldwyn, M.D.
Clinical Professor of Surgery, Harvard Medical School; Head, Division of Plastic Surgery, Beth Israel Hospital, Boston

Howard L. Gordon, M.D.
Assistant Clinical Professor of Surgery (Plastic), University of Miami School of Medicine; Senior Attending Surgeon, Plastic and Reconstructive Surgery, Miami Mercy Hospital, Miami

Ulrich T. Hinderer, M.D.
Director, Clínica Mirasierra de Cirugía Plástica Estética, Madrid

Yves-Gerard Illouz, M.D.
Chief Surgeon, Department of Plastic Surgery, Victor-Masse Hospital; Plastic Surgeon, Spontini Clinic, Paris

Guy Jost, M.D.
Professor, Collège de Médecine des Hôpitaux de Paris; Chief, Department of Plastic Surgery, Hôpital Lariboisiere, Paris

Ulrich K. Kesselring, M.D., F.M.H.
Centre de Chirurgie Plastique, Lausanne, Switzerland

Mark L. Lemmon, M.D.
Clinical Associate Professor, Plastic Surgery, University of Texas Southwestern Medical School at Dallas; Attending Surgeon, Plastic Surgery, Gaston Episcopal Hospital, Dallas

Rodolphe Meyer, M.D.
Privat Docent, Faculty of Medicine, University of Lausanne; Associate Surgeon, Centre Hospitalier Universitaire Vaudois Plastic Surgery, Centre de Chirurgie Plastique, Lausanne, Switzerland

Daniel C. Morello, M.D., F.A.C.S.
Attending Plastic Surgeon, White Plains Hospital Medical Center, White Plains, New York; Clinical Assistant Professor of Surgery (Plastic), The Institute of Reconstructive Plastic Surgery, New York University Medical Center, New York

Fredric Newman, M.D.
Assistant Attending Surgeon, Department of Plastic Surgery, White Plains Hospital Medical Center; Assistant Attending Surgeon, Department of Plastic Surgery, St. Agnes Hospital, White Plains, New York

George C. Peck, M.D.
Associate Clinical Professor of Surgery (Plastic), Columbia University College of Physicians and Surgeons, New York; Chief, Plastic Surgery Section, Beth Israel Hospital, Passaic, New York; Staff, St. Barnabas Hospital, Livingston, New York; Staff, Columbia-Presbyterian Medical Center, New York

Rex Peterson, M.D.
Director, Phoenix Plastic Surgery Residency; Chief of Plastic Surgery, Arizona Children's Hospital, Good Samaritan Hospital, and Maricopa County General Hospital, Phoenix

Paule Regnault, M.D., F.R.C.S.
Formerly, Professeur Agrégé de Clinique, University of Montreal Faculty of Medicine; formerly, Chief of Service, Hôpital Saint-Luc, Montreal

Blair O. Rogers, M.D., F.A.C.S., P.C.
Associate Professor of Clinical Surgery (Plastic), New York University Medical Center; Attending Surgeon, Department of Plastic Surgery, Manhattan Eye, Ear and Throat Hospital, New York

John E. Sherman, M.D.
Associate Attending Surgeon, Cabrini Medical Center; Associate Attending Surgeon, Division of Plastic Surgery, Memorial Sloan-Kettering Cancer Center, New York

Richard Siegel, M.D.
Plastic Surgeon, Kaiser Permanente Medical Group, Honolulu

James W. Smith, M.D.
Clinical Associate Professor of Surgery, Cornell University Medical College; Associate Attending Surgeon, Department of Surgery (Division of Plastic Surgery), The New York Hospital–Cornell Medical Center, New York

Melvin Spira, M.D.
Professor and Head, Division of Plastic Surgery, Baylor College of Medicine, Houston

Hale Tolleth, M.D.
Attending Plastic Surgeon, Mount Diablo Hospital Medical Center, Concord, California

S. Anthony Wolfe, M.D.
Associate Clinical Professor of Plastic Surgery, University of Miami School of Medicine, Miami

Preface

Throughout their training, most residents are taught aesthetic surgery in the operating room and are rarely exposed to the critical decision-making process in the consulting room. After assisting on several different techniques, they choose one method and try to master it before completing their training. Subsequently, in the initial years of practice, aesthetic cases are few, and attainment of good results with minimal complications is the goal. With increasing volume, the single perfected technique is applied to a wide variety of cases, often producing a large number of acceptable results but few that are truly excellent and some that are disastrous. The problem is not poor surgical execution but rather inadequate evaluation of the deformity, a limited surgical repertoire, and lack of awareness of how to avoid complications.

This text is an attempt to help solve this deficiency by providing a firm foundation for the young aesthetic plastic surgeon. The emphasis is on analysis and classification of common cosmetic deformities, which will allow selection of the optimal operative procedure, of which surgical principles and potential pitfalls are detailed. We have eschewed the single-surgeon format in favor of a multi-authored text. Aesthetic surgery is too diverse and too great a challenge for one individual to summarize it all. Each of the authors is an acknowledged expert and practicing aesthetic surgeon who has undergone the same transformation from a broad-based training in plastic and reconstructive surgery to a gradual concentration in aesthetic surgery. It is required that the reader have an understanding and the experience with basic aesthetic procedures before attempting to apply the described operations to a specific patient. This text is neither a primer nor a cookbook for the uninitiated, but rather a stimulus for those seeking better results and happier patients.

Part I begins with the history of aesthetic plastic surgery, emphasizing its broad base and diverse origin. The fundamental principles of how to manage patients seeking aesthetic surgery throughout the perioperative period is discussed, stressing the surgeon's responsibilities. Next, the detailed advanced planning required before establishing the ideal aesthetic surgeon's office is reviewed, followed by the various anesthetic regimens used for ambulatory surgery. It concludes with a chapter on medical photography, an essential record for judging postoperative results.

Part II is an attempt to explain the rhinoplasty operation in four chapters rather than four volumes. The basics of the procedure are reviewed followed by an in-depth discussion of the refinements that allow attainment of the optimal aesthetic result. Two problem areas—the deviated nose and secondary rhinoplasty—are then discussed and highly innovative solutions are offered by masters whose experiences number in the thousands.

Part III looks at certain facial regions that have often been considered "ancillary procedures" by some surgeons but not by most patients. A highly provocative approach to mentoplasty is demonstrated with superb results, followed by a multifaceted approach to otoplasty that confirms the need for reflection rather than reaction to a given deformity. The chapter on malar augmentation shows how an additional procedure can often "maximize" the desired goal. As detailed in the next three chapters, recent advances have led to a better understanding of the interrelationship of the eyelids, periorbital region, and upper third of the face. Blepharoplasty, an operation of millimeters, is discussed from the vantage of the "complete approach" followed by the ultimate pursuit of excellence—the advanced blepharoplasty.

Part IV reflects the total approach to facial deformity that has evolved in the past decade. The chapter on rhytidectomy offers the essentials while its companion on the subfascial rhytidectomy details beautifully the anatomy and concepts of altering the face's fascial foundation. It culminates in a broad view of rejuvenating the entire cervicofacial region with convincing evidence that these deformities are now not only better corrected but also for a longer time period. The specific problems of a separate subgroup, the male patient, are analyzed and modifications enunciated. Completion of facial rejuvenation often requires additional steps. Chemical peeling is a widely practiced art whose applications and cautions are candidly presented. Specific excisions in the periorbital area and documented experience with collagen injection therapy are reviewed followed by a comparison of the various techniques available.

Part V simplifies the plethora of procedures available for breast surgery. The fundamentals of breast reduction are summarized and two basic procedures are offered—the B-technique and the inferior pedicle technique. A graded approach to the problem of breast ptosis is described followed by an analysis of methodology in breast augmentation with emphasis on management of complications. Mastery of all these techniques is then applied in solving the complexities of breast asymmetries and nipple-areolar deformities. Throughout these chapters, the emphasis is on fundamental principles and selection of the optimal procedure based on careful preoperative analysis.

Part VI extends aesthetic principles to body sculpturing. Abdominal wall deformities are divided into the refined abdominoplasty and the equally challenging abdominal lipectomy. Lipectomy of the lower extremity is presented as a continuum of excisions and additive procedures, which fits the operation to the deformity rather than the more common Draconian solution. The new localized lipectomy techniques of suction and curettage are described by their originators whose experience is measured in years rather than months. New approaches to lipectomy of the upper extremity and the deformities of massive weight loss offer dramatic solutions to these often ignored problems.

Although some experienced surgeons may find the text burdensome and state that little is truly new, we hope that the younger surgeon will benefit from a sense of where to begin rather than end, principles rather than procedures, and selection rather than execution. For this book reflects our own experience, the master's pursuit of perfection over three decades and the neophyte's desire to understand.

P. R.
R. K. D.

Acknowledgments

In any multiauthored text, it is the contributors who determine the final quality of the work. We are most appreciative to our coauthors who were committed to the premise that the principles of aesthetic surgery can be taught, and that excellence is attained by selection of individualized operations for each patient. Currently, gestation of a book from inception to delivery exceeds 3 years. Throughout this period, support is required from numerous individuals. This text would have been impossible without the secretarial assistance of the following: Faye Weber, who found every patient as well as the preoperative photographs; Genevieve Holding, who mastered the Cominco Z-80 microprocessor with all of its word-processing accoutrements; Dorothy Carruthers, who provided essential organization at critical moments; as well as Monique Bedard and Micheline Charlebois, whose bilingual capabilities were most appreciated.

Both editors are grateful to Dorothy Irwin, whose clear, concise artwork graces these pages plus the professional results of the medical photographers of the Royal Victoria Hospital (Edith Boltz, Jerry Hodgson, Alan Forster, and Julius Szelei). The cover illustration was originally conceived by Judy Smith, whose creative talents as a medical artist were combined with her spousal knowledge of plastic surgery. At Little, Brown, Fred Belliveau had the vision to see the need for a multiauthored text on aesthetic surgery; Curtis Vouwie served as expediter of numerous labor pains; and Susan Pioli was the midwife who guided this book on its day-to-day course from inception to delivery. We are most grateful for their assistance.

NOTICE

The indications and dosages of all drugs in this book have been recommended in the medical literature and conform to the practices of the general medical community. The medications described do not necessarily have specific approval by the Food and Drug Administration for use in the diseases and dosages for which they are recommended. The package insert for each drug should be consulted for use and dosage as approved by the FDA. Because standards for usage change, it is advisable to keep abreast of revised recommendations, particularly those concerning new drugs.

I. Basic Principles

1. History of the Development of Aesthetic Surgery

Blair O. Rogers

Do you set down your name in the scroll of youth, that are written down old with all the characters of age? Have you not a moist eye, a dry hand, a yellow cheek, a white beard, a decreasing leg, an increasing belly? Is not your voice broken, your wind short, your chin double, your wit single, and every part about you blasted with antiquity? And will you yet call yourself young?
Shakespeare, *Henry IV,* Part II, Act 1, Scene 2

Yellow cheeks, double chins, pendulous abdomens — the despised signs of aging — form an unwelcome contrast to the smooth physiognomy of youth and are easily removed by modern aesthetic operations. Shakespeare in the famous reference to aging found in *Henry IV* [143] described all too accurately for posterity those bodily changes that daily bring the suffering patient to the office of modern aesthetic surgeons. When did corrective or "aesthetic" or "cosmetic" surgery have its very first beginnings?

This type of surgery is relatively recent in the overall history of plastic and reconstructive surgery. Its origins began in the nineteenth century, but the major leap forward in its development took place in the early 1900s.

Considering the scope and definition of aesthetic surgery as we know it today [1], we can probably trace the overall concepts of aesthetic plastic surgery directly, indirectly, or even tangentially to one man in particular, the famous Berlin surgeon Johann F. Dieffenbach (1792–1847) (Fig. 1-1) [22, 31, 135]. He, more than any of his contemporaries in the mid-nineteenth century, was concerned not only with the aesthetic results he obtained as a pioneer in nasal reconstruction (Fig. 1-2) [135], but with the challenges in altering the form of misshapen noses (Figs. 1-3 and 1-4) [132]. With an interest in aesthetically improving the appearance of a nose that was not necessarily a reconstructed nose, such as the surgical narrowing of thick nostril walls, Dieffenbach, for example, advised cutting out small punch-shaped pieces of skin and cartilage, thus reducing the nostril thickness by the tension of the closure of the skin defects. Dieffenbach also externally removed a vertical and horizontal piece of skin and subcutaneous tissue bilaterally for the aesthetic reduction in the size of an overly large nose (Fig. 1-3). Another of his methods for raising a flattened or depressed nasal tip through an external incisional approach for an improved aesthetic result can be seen in Figure 1-4.

The use of external incisions for any and all nasal corrective (aesthetic) or reconstructive surgery was routine in the mid-nineteenth century [132], and any thought of a completely intranasal approach for aesthetic surgery of the nose seems to have escaped the surgeons of that era and

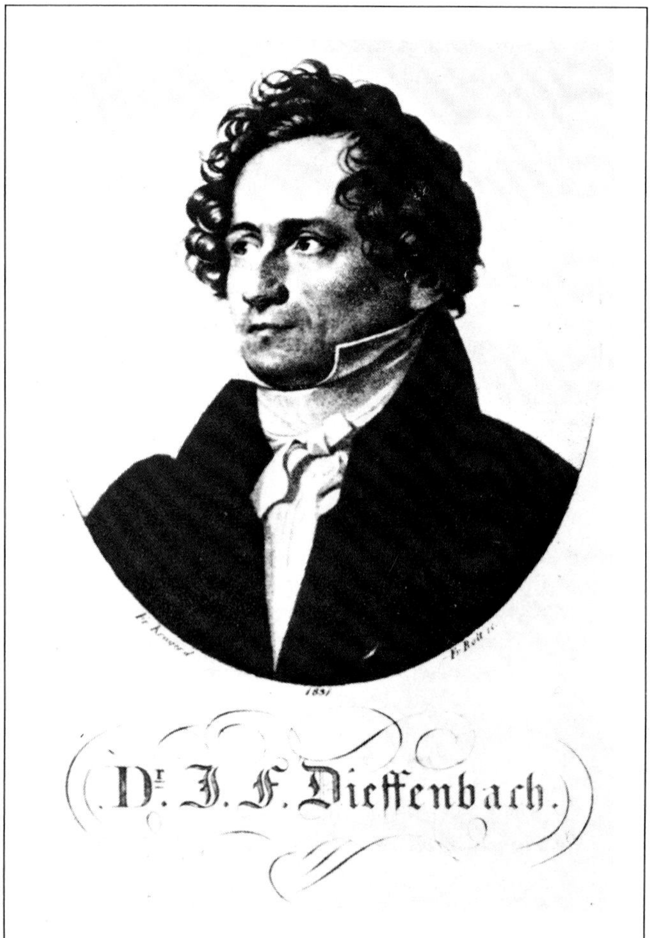

Figure 1-1. Johann Friedrich Dieffenbach (1792–1847). (Courtesy of V. J. Bernback, M.D.)

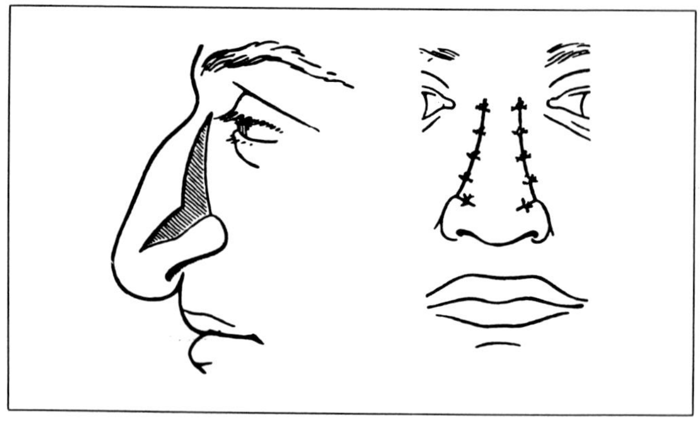

Figure 1-3. Dieffenbach's method of using external excisions to reduce the size of an overly large, hooked, drooping nose. (From J. S. Davis, *Plastic Surgery: Its Principles and Practice.* Philadelphia: Blakiston, 1919.)

Figure 1-2

A. Dr. H., a 36-year-old Silesian whose nose was of the type that ". . . spread disgust and horror wherever [it] appear[s]," the defect caused by syphilitic destruction.
B. The scalp was not used because the forehead was high enough to form the entire flap. Appearance of the patient 3 days postoperatively.
C. The postoperative appearance after smaller revisions. Dieffenbach stated, "If I might estimate my success by the gratitude of my patient, I should be fully justified in supposing I had formed a nose not unworthy of a Pythian Apollo." (From B. O. Rogers, Nasal reconstruction 150 years ago: Aesthetic and other problems *Aesthetic Plast. Surg.* 5:283, 1981.

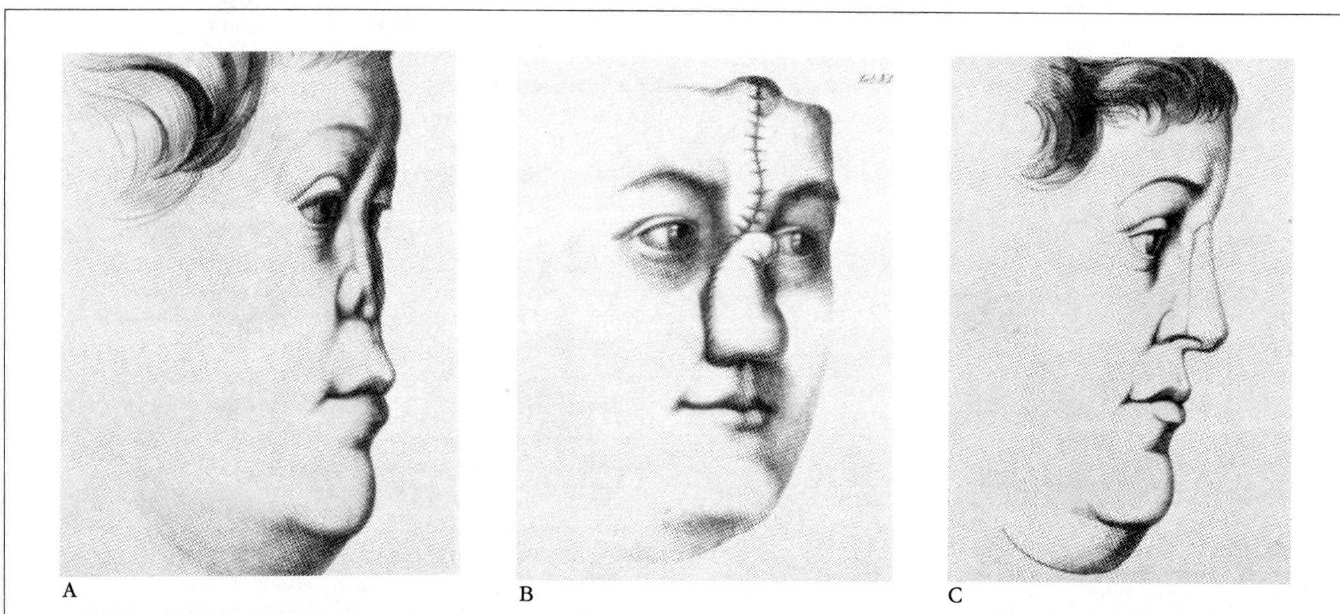

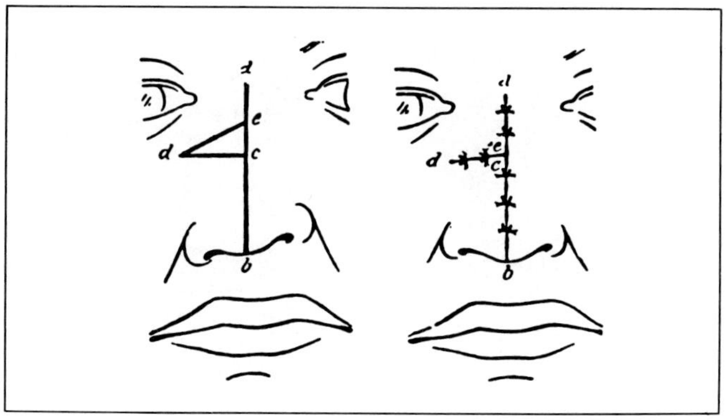

Figure 1-4. Dieffenbach's method of using external excisions to raise a flattened or depressed nasal tip. (From J. S. Davis, *Plastic Surgery: Its Principles and Practice.* Philadelphia: Blakiston, 1919.)

did not have its origin until 1887 when a paper written by a Rochester, New York, otolaryngologist, John Orlando Roe, first appeared in the medical literature [118]. At this point, with our first mention of Dieffenbach and Roe, it must be emphasized that the development of corrective (aesthetic) surgery cannot, and should not, be strictly divorced from the history of reconstructive plastic surgery. Even today one is reminded daily how interwoven these two types of surgery are and always have been! A quote from Gillies and Millard's classic textbook [30] is appropriate here:

> A great percentage of private practice is beauty surgery. It is here that perfection is a necessity. Reconstructive surgery is an attempt to return to normal; cosmetic surgery is an attempt to surpass the normal. No man is a plastic surgeon unless he becomes adept at both. Many never do and are a menace. It is easier to reduce than produce, but in plastic surgery it is nearly always necessary to remold after reduction. Thus anyone can cut off a bit of nose or breast, but not so many can turn out a satisfying result.

Readers who wish to refer to more comprehensive reviews of the history of each body section that has been dealt with from an aesthetic plastic surgical standpoint will find the following review papers of great interest and help:

1. Abdominoplasty—by Regnault [115]
2. Breast plasty—by Lalardrie and Mouly [59]
3. Ear plasty—by Davis and Hernandez [19]
4. Eyelid plasty—by Stephenson [146]
5. Facial plasty (face-lifting)—by Gonzalez-Ulloa [32]
6. Nasal plasty—by McDowell [69, 70]; Rogers [132, 135]
7. Thigh and buttocks plasty—by Grazer and Klingbeil [33]; Rogers [133]

In order to show the gradual development of aesthetic plastic surgery as a historical narrative, this chapter will deal with individual "medical firsts" on a strictly chronologic basis with certain milestones cited from decade to decade as they occur rather than under separate subheadings such as otoplasty or eyelid plasty. Those who wish to follow the year-by-year development of aesthetic plastic surgery of only one portion of the body are referred to the review articles previously listed.

THE LATE NINETEENTH CENTURY

Aesthetic plastic surgery seemed to suddenly occupy the minds of more surgeons than the few giants such as Dieffenbach in the last two decades of the nineteenth century. Unless medical historians can find in the literature earlier attempts at aesthetic correction of the protruding ear, the first true correction of this deformity was performed in 1881 by Edward Talbot Ely, a young otolaryngologic surgeon who described for the first time in the medical literature "An Operation for Prominence of the Auricles" [24]. Ely was the first to recognize the need for excising and removing a piece of the conchal cartilage, in addition to the skin excision, to obtain a more acceptable, permanent change in the positioning of the protruding ear [24]. The patient on whom he operated and reported his surgery in the Manhattan Eye, Ear and Throat Hospital *Annual Report* in addition to his article in the *Archives of Otolaryngology* [24] can be seen in Figure 1-5.

Figure 1-5. Postoperative illustration of the first patient operated on by Ely in 1881 for correction of protruding ears, the right ear showing the operative improvement. (From E. T. Ely, An operation for prominence of the auricles. *Arch. Otolaryngol.* 10:97, 1881; also in *Plast. Reconstr. Surg.* 42:582, 1968.)

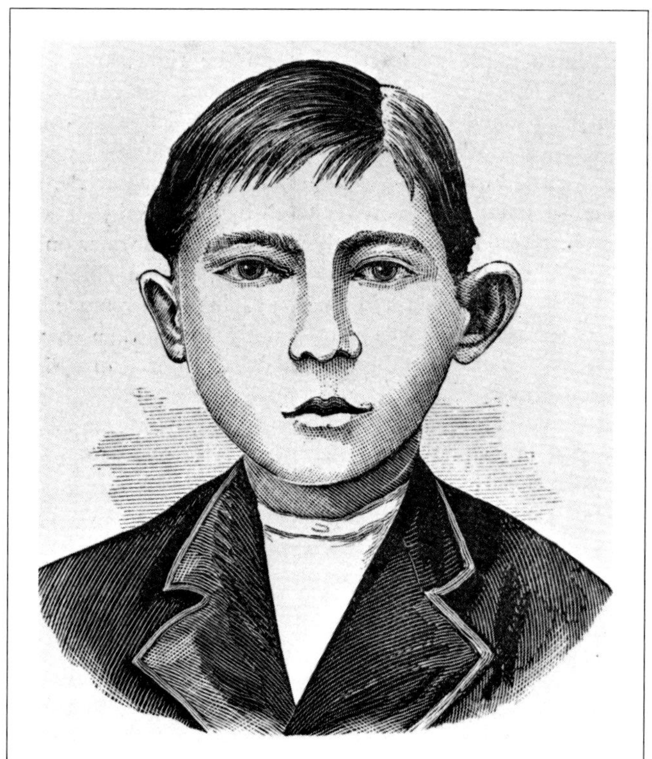

One year later, Theodore Gaillard Thomas reported in the February 21, 1882, *Transactions of the New York Obstetrical Society* what can probably be considered the earliest surgical technique of an aesthetic approach to the excision of benign breast tissue and tumors varying in size ". . . from that of a hen's egg to that of a duck's egg, or a little larger" [147]. He used an incision in the submammary fold for the resection of a glandular benign tumor from the posterior part of the mammary gland. This technique was employed 25 years later by Morestin and Guinard [104] and refined an additional 18 years later by the Swiss surgeon de Quervain, who in 1925, well in advance of his time, performed a subtotal mammectomy leaving only a small retroareolar glandular stump [21].

The age of corrective aesthetic rhinoplasty began in 1887, when John Orlando Roe (1848–1915) (Fig. 1-6) described an intranasal operation confined to the tip of a so-called pug nose. In "The Deformity Termed Pug Nose and Its Correction by a Simple Operation" [118], he described not the external excisions of unsightly tissue that had previously been reported by Dieffenbach and a few other surgeons in the years following Dieffenbach's report, but instead, for the first time, an intranasal operation confined, however, to the tip of the nose. Figure 1-7 shows a woman preoperatively and postoperatively with the improvement obtained after his operation for the pug nose deformity.

Figure 1-6. John Orlando Roe (1848–1915), father of aesthetic rhinoplasty. (From M. H. Cottle, John Orlando Roe: Pioneer in modern rhinoplasty. *Arch. Otolaryngol.* 80:22, 1964.)

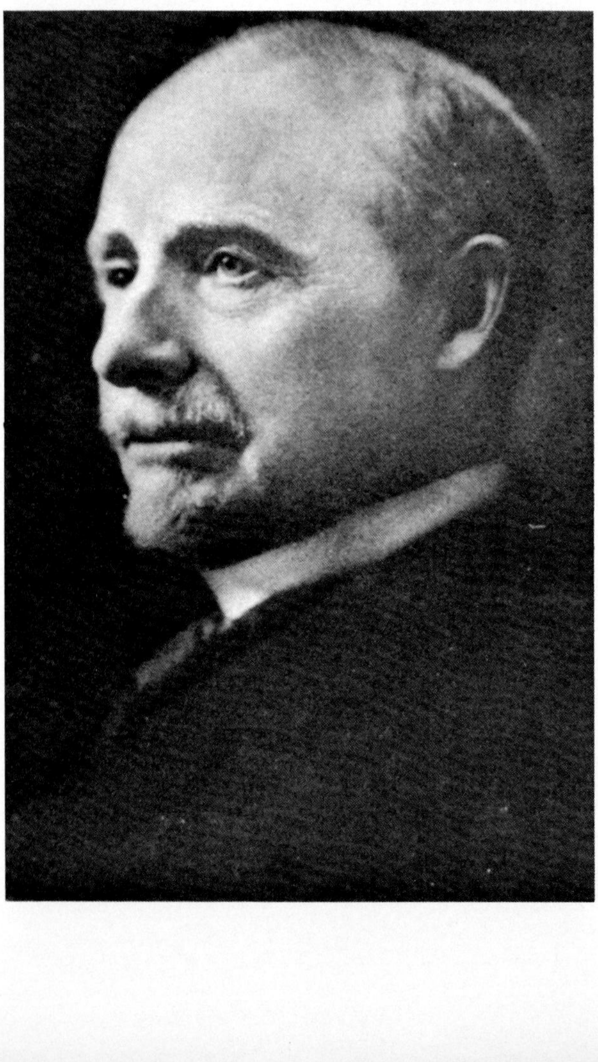

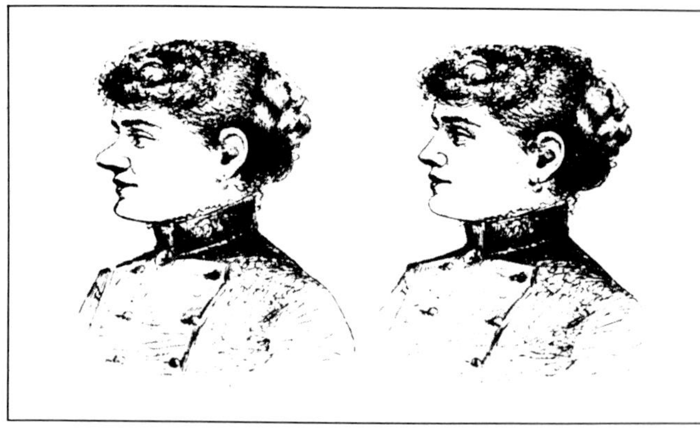

Figure 1-7. Illustration showing a patient preoperatively and postoperatively in Roe's first article in 1887, for correction of a pug nose. (From J. O. Roe, The deformity termed pug nose and its correction by a simple operation. *Med. Rec.* 31:621, 1887; also in *Plast. Reconstr. Surg.* 45:78, 1970.)

His publication in 1891 of another paper, "The Correction of Angular Deformities of the Nose by a Subcutaneous Operation," was more truly the medical first [119] since it described corrective rhinoplasty of the *entire* nose in which the nose was reduced in size throughout because of a prominent bony and cartilaginous hump and profile. A more detailed chronologic survey of the development of aesthetic and corrective rhinoplasty just before the age of Roe and immediately after the introduction of his contributions [118–126] can be read in an article by Rogers included in an international symposium on aesthetic plastic surgery of the nose [132].

Roe's second paper in 1891 reporting his intranasal subcutaneous approach to aesthetic rhinoplasty was written 7 years before Jacques Joseph reported similar success in aesthetic rhinoplasty using external incisions [119]. There is no doubt on the part of medical historians today that these two papers of 1887 and 1891 established Roe as the originator of corrective or cosmetic rhinoplasty, despite Joseph's claim to the title. In all fairness to Joseph, however, who came on the scene in 1898, and because of his accomplishments, no one disagrees when modern historians call him the overall father of corrective aesthetic rhinoplasty.

In 1892 Robert F. Weir (1838–1927) of New York City, a contemporary of Roe who had previously worked as Gordon Buck's assistant, described a new operation; using intranasal incisions, he stabilized newly fractured nasal bones in a more medial position by means of steel needles inserted transversely through the entire nose and held in place with clamps on either side of the nose [154]. In this tedious case, his use of crescent-shaped incisions at the base of the alar nasae to reduce the width of the base and lower the nasal apex was described for the first time.

Vincenz V. Czerny of Heidelberg in 1895 used the upper lateral cartilages cut partially free from the septum, turned medially and upward as flaps from the lateral walls on septal hinges, and sutured back to back on themselves to elevate the dorsum of a saddle nose [16, 68]. This technique with many variations has been reported in subsequent decades by authors who have all too frequently thought their operation original without checking this older literature.

In 1895, the first probable augmentation mammaplasty was also performed by Czerny. He replaced the breast substance lost by the excision of a breast adenoma by successfully transplanting a lipoma taken from the patient's back [17].

In later years, after the work of Erich Lexer of Berlin [61] in 1925 and Raymond Passot of Paris [110] in 1930, the use of fat transplantation for building up deformities of the breast became commonplace, with the fat tissue taken primarily from the buttocks or the abdomen donor sites.

In 1898 Jacques Joseph of Berlin (Fig. 1-8), whose life was indeed a fascinating one [105], excised externally an inverted V-shaped segment along the nasal dorsum through the skin, bone, cartilage, and mucosal lining and the entire thickness of the nasal alae, and removed a wedge from the lower part of the septum to shorten and reduce an overly conspicuous nose all in one single operation [4, 41]. Figure 1-9 shows the preoperative and postoperative photographs of the "28-year-old landowner" on whom Joseph performed this operation. A second paper published in 1902 [42], noted that he had then performed 10 such cosmetic operations but was *still* using external skin incisions and excisions through which he removed the hump and shortened the nose. By 1904, whereas Roe *reported* continued successes in America using intranasal incisions, Joseph [43] admitted that he had finally come around to using this method instead of his previously employed external skin incisions, and by that year he had performed 43 operations. In another operation in 1904 [44], Joseph described for the first time his external clamps and his right angle nasal saws, and in 1905 he reported [45] that he had operated on 100 patients requiring corrective rhinoplasty.

Figure 1-8. Professor Jacques Joseph of Berlin as seen in a photograph published in *Revue de Chirurgie Structure,* vol. 4, 1934.

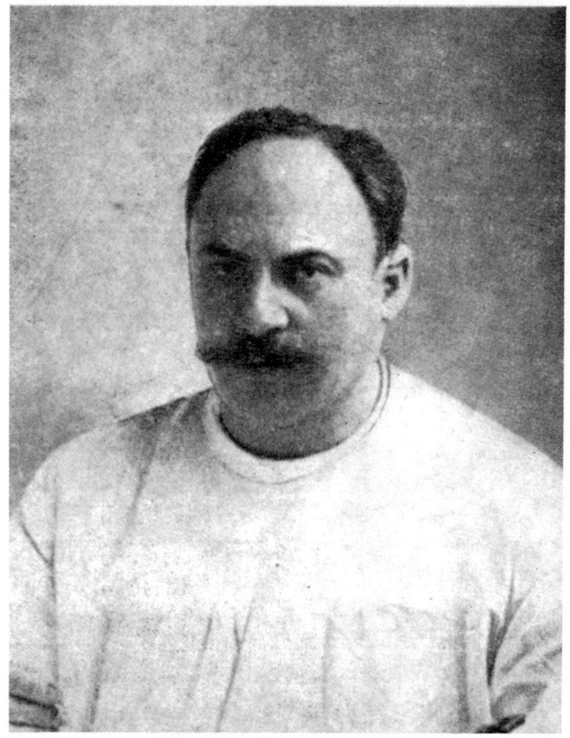

Figure 1-9. Preoperative and postoperative photographs of the "28-year-old landowner" on whom Joseph performed his first rhinoplasty with external excision. (From J. Joseph, Ueber die operative Verkleinerung einer Nase [Rhinomiosis]. *Berl. Klin. Wochenschr.* 40 : 882, 1898; also in *Plast. Reconstr. Surg.* 45 : 78, 1970.)

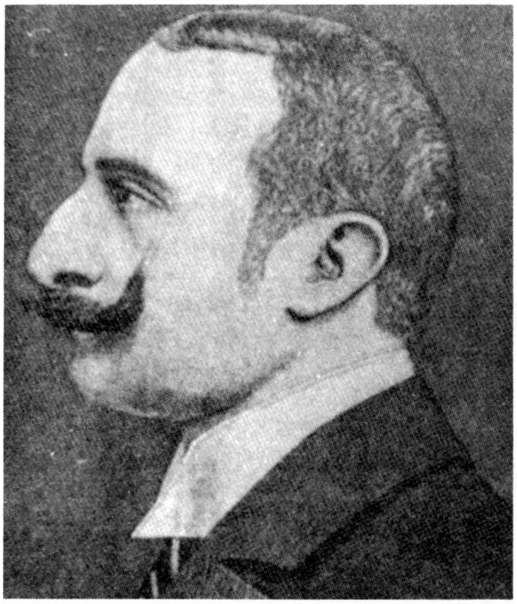

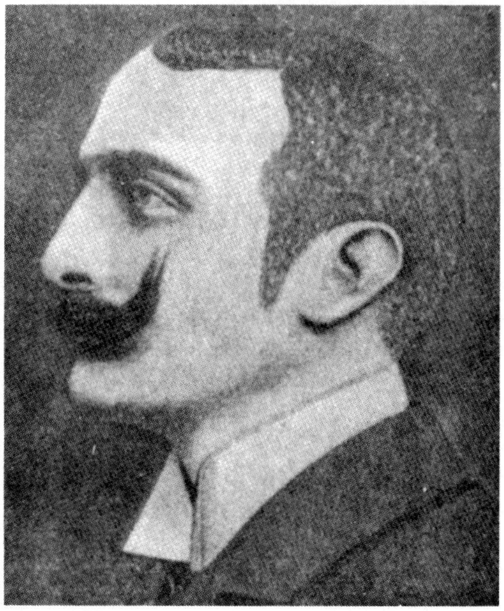

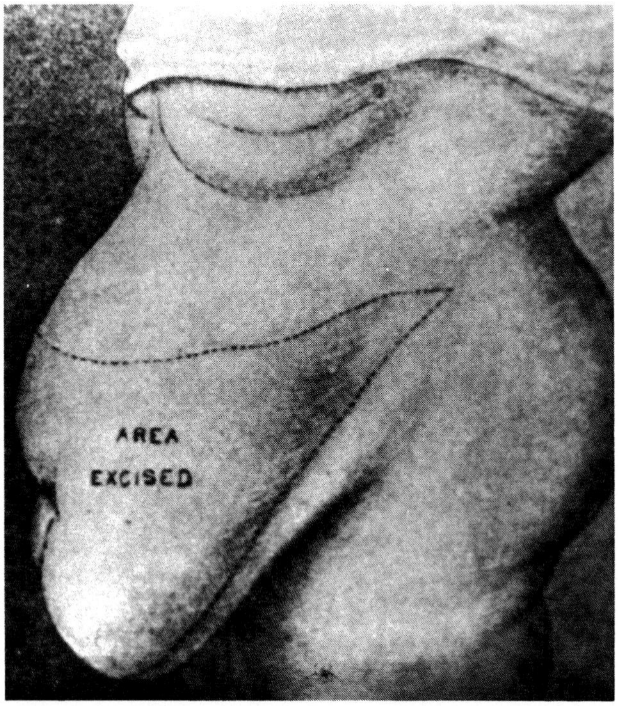

Figure 1-10. First illustration in the medical literature of the surgery to be performed on a woman with a large pendulous abdominal panniculus. (From L. Peters, Resection of the pendulous, fat abdominal wall in cases of extreme obesity. *Ann. Surg.* 33:299, 1901.)

At the very end of the nineteenth century, in 1899, the famous Howard A. Kelly [55] of Johns Hopkins Hospital and University in Baltimore, Maryland, was the first to describe an aesthetic operation for the removal of an unsightly abdominal panniculus.

Two years later in 1901 Peters of Baltimore [113] was given permission by Kelly to describe this operation in more detail. Peters's article included the first illustration in the medical literature of the pendulous abdomen operated on by Kelly (Fig. 1-10). In a subsequent article in 1910 [56], Kelly, a very colorful writer indeed, described a typical patient with this deformity. "A woman who is hampered with this bolster or hammock laden with fat is always unwieldly in appearance, protuberant and waddling in gait, awkwardly balanced, and as a rule short of breath." He depicted the operation as an excision of a wedge of fat and skin ". . . extending from one flank across into the other, down to the deep fascia, much as one would cut a huge slice lengthwise out of a watermelon."

THE TWENTIETH CENTURY

Although numerous papers describing reconstructive ophthalmic plastic surgery were written from the time of von Graefe [128] in 1818 and onward, especially papers describing excess skin folds of the eyelids first published by Mackenzie in 1830 and others who advised excision of the excess skin alone, the true aesthetic surgery of baggy or excessively wrinkled eyelids did not develop until the early 1900s. The earliest attempts to remove excess skin only can be traced to Charles Conrad Miller who, in 1906, wrote his first exclusively aesthetic surgery article on the excision of "bag-like folds of eyelid skin" [74]. One year later in another article there appeared probably the first photograph in medical history illustrating the lower eyelid incisions required for removal of a crescent of wrinkled skin (Fig. 1-11) [82]. Miller's career in cosmetic surgery, as he preferred to call it, was, therefore, already well under way [71–101, 129].

In 1907 Miller published the first book in medical history [78] written on cosmetic surgery (Fig. 1-12), and a second, slightly enlarged edition appeared in 1908 [95]. From 1907 onward, Miller contributed to the literature a host of other articles on cosmetic surgery subjects. He had already shown interest in cosmetic correction of the hump nose in 1906 [73], in correction of crow's-feet in 1907 (Fig. 1-13) [76], in reducing fullness of the lower lip (Fig. 1-14), and can be assumed to have experimented with paraffin injections for several years before the publication of his unfortunate book on this subject in 1908 [94].

Miller's publication of a book on clinical use of injected paraffin was the outgrowth of numerous clinical tests of paraffin injections by certain dubious surgeons. This technique had been introduced in 1900 by Gersuny who described the injection of vaseline for the correction of facial defects [24]. Vaseline injections were soon discarded because of unfavorable results and especially because of complications, including severe local tissue reactions and distant emboli with some instances of fatal pulmonary emboli.

In 1902 Eckstein described the injection of low-melting paraffin [23]. For approximately the next 20 years or more, many physicians unfortunately injected paraffin with immediately good results, as seen in Fig. 1-15, which shows a patient injected for the treatment of a nasal deformity by a surgeon on the staff of the Manhattan Eye, Ear and Throat Hospital in 1904. Paraffin injections were finally discarded after many years of trial, however, because of local paraffinoma formation and distant complications including

Figure 1-11. The line of incision for removal of a crescent of skin to correct excess "bagging," folding, or wrinkling of the eyelid skin. (From C. C. Miller and F. Miller, Folds, bags, and wrinkles of the skin about the eyes and their eradication by simple surgical methods. *Med. Brief* 35:540, 1907.)

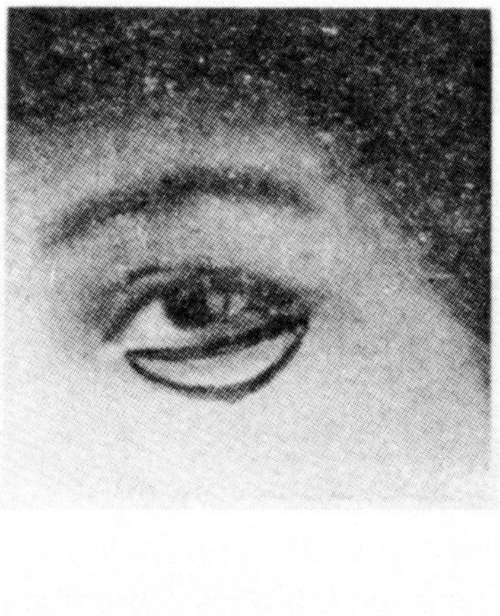

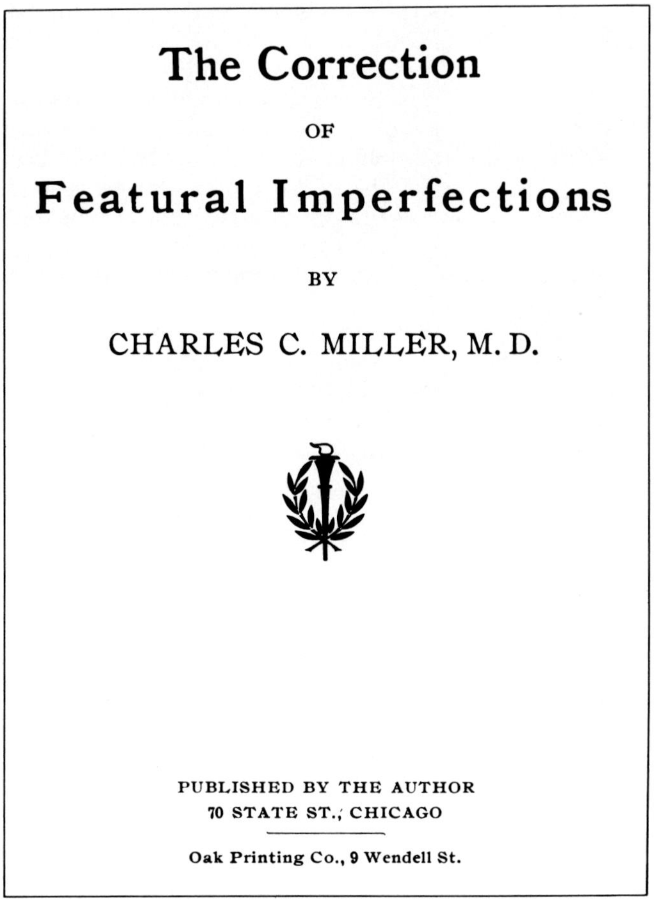

The Correction

OF

Featural Imperfections

BY

CHARLES C. MILLER, M. D.

PUBLISHED BY THE AUTHOR
70 STATE ST., CHICAGO

Oak Printing Co., 9 Wendell St.

Figure 1-12. Title page of Charles C. Miller's first book on cosmetic surgery, published in 1907. (From C. C. Miller, *The Correction of Featural Imperfections*. Chicago: Oak Printing, 1907.)

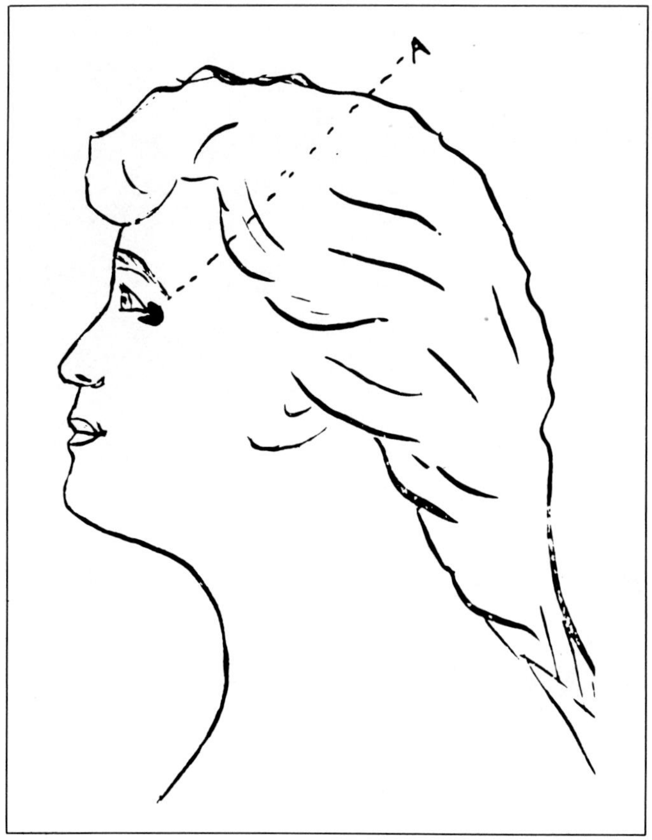

Figure 1-13. Area to be excised for the correction of crow's-feet. (From C. C. Miller, *The Correction of Featural Imperfections* [2nd ed.]. Chicago: Oak Printing, 1908.)

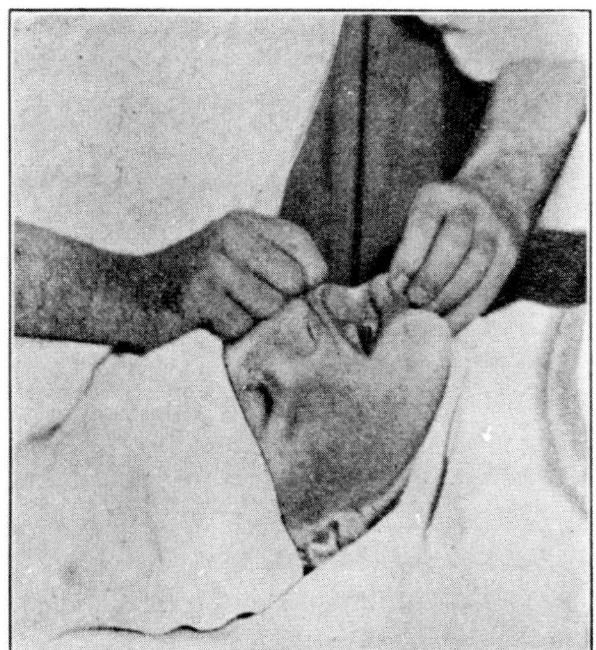

Figure 1-14. A lozenge-shaped area of mucosa from inside the lip, excised for correction of eversion or fullness of the lower lip. (From C. C. Miller, *The Correction of Featural Imperfections* [2nd ed.]. Chicago: Oak Printing, 1908.)

thrombosis, phlebitis, pulmonary emboli, and infarction. Injections of vaseline and paraffin in the first two decades of the twentieth century served as one of the major drawbacks of this era, delaying the more rapid and accepted development of corrective cosmetic surgery in general, and corrective nasoplastic surgery in particular, because all too frequently good cosmetic surgeons such as Frederick Strange Kolle (1871–1929) were also susceptible to the blandishments of quick results obtainable through paraffin injections.

Chronologically, the second author in medical history to describe cosmetic surgery was Kolle (Fig. 1-16), a German-born American who practiced plastic and cosmetic surgery in New York City. In 1911 Kolle published a book entitled *Plastic and Cosmetic Surgery* [58]. This large tome consisted of 511 pages and 522 illustrations, among which were some of the first photographs of a patient before and after the surgical correction of protruding ears (Fig. 1-17). One of Kolle's most interesting contributions was his description of his treatment of wrinkled eyelids, with illustrations of his methods of correction (Fig. 1-18). Miller's operation on the eyelids was less refined, but both men attacked the problem from approximately the same primitive standpoint.

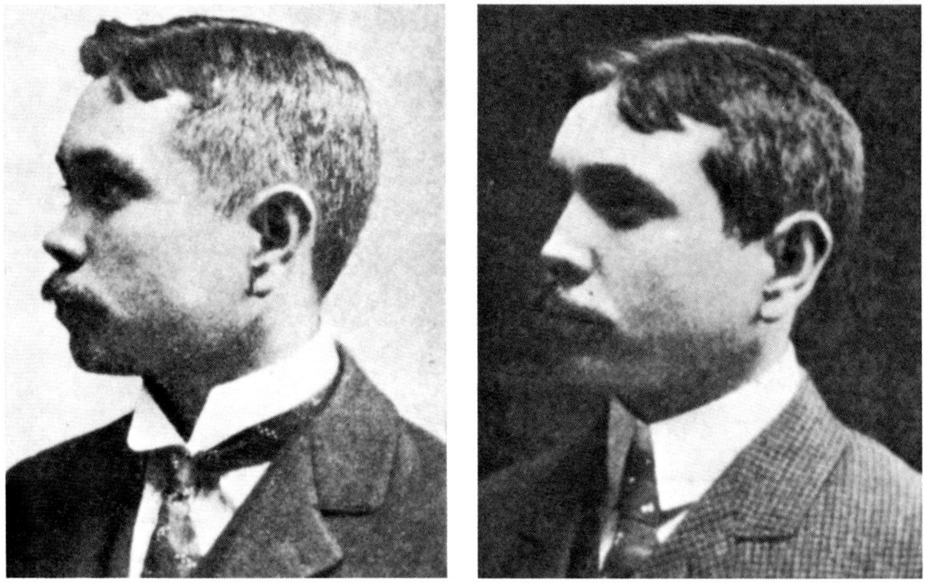

Figure 1-15. Photographs preoperatively *(left)* and after paraffin injection *(right)* to correct a nasal deformity. (From *Annual Reports* of Manhattan Eye, Ear and Throat Hospital, 1904.)

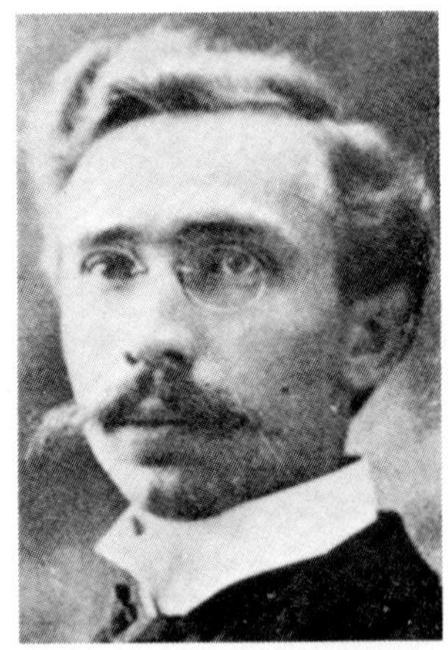

Figure 1-16. Portrait of the German-born American cosmetic surgeon, Frederick Strange Kolle. (From E. R. N. Grigg, *The Trail of the Impossible Light.* Springfield, Ill.: Thomas, 1965.)

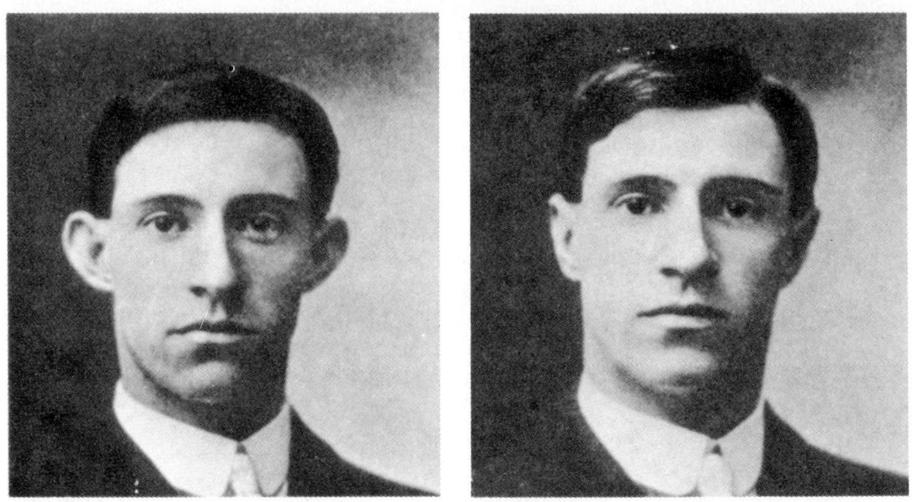

Figure 1-17. Correction of protruding ears, preoperative and postoperative photographs. (From F. S. Kolle, *Plastic and Cosmetic Surgery.* New York: Appleton, 1911.)

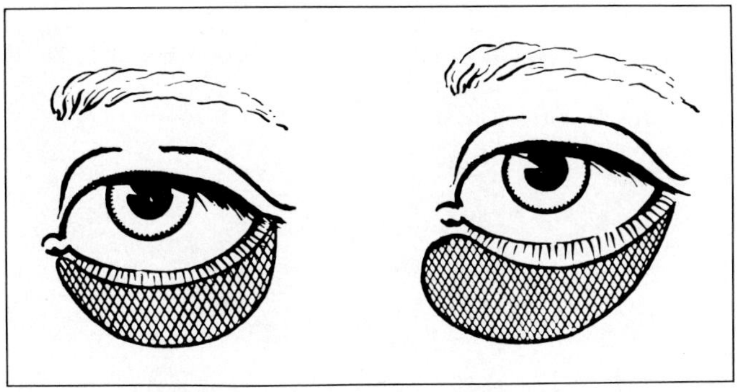

Figure 1-18. Shape of incisions in lower eyelids for removal of loose tissue causing eyelid wrinkles. (From F. S. Kolle, *Plastic and Cosmetic Surgery.* New York: Appleton, 1911.)

In his book, Kolle showed his readers the use of wedge excisions to narrow the alar base, his excisions to reduce and narrow a boxed nasal tip, his method to correct an overly retroussé nose (Fig. 1-19) and a hooked nasal tip, his external excision of redundant columella tissue to correct a hooked elongated nasal tip, and his lateral external incisions on the nose for various other reduction procedures. Unfortunately he had become victimized by the vogue of injecting paraffin and recommended it rather highly in a book [57] on this subject. According to him, paraffin injections were developed partially as a replacement for the objectionable metallic and bony implants. These implants were often unsuccessful in an age in which protective antibiotic therapy was not yet available to those surgeons who had the amazing courage to perform such elective surgery without worrying about the consequences.

After Joseph [46] recommended the insertion of transplants through an intranasal incision rather than a glabellar incision, the controversy over the relative merits of the use of ivory, bone, or cartilage was soon resolved with the majority of surgeons utilizing either fresh cartilage transplants, iliac bone grafts, or tibial bone grafts.

In 1912, one year after the publication of Kolle's book, Eugen Holländer (1867–1932) of Berlin, a pupil of the famous James Israel, contributed a chapter entitled "Cosmetic Surgery" to a volume edited by M. Joseph. At one time he wrote, "as a victim of the art of feminine persuasion," he removed isolated pieces of skin at the margins of the hairline and in the natural aging skin folds of a woman to "freshen up" her wrinkles and drooping cheeks [36]. He did not state in this chapter the year he had performed this operation nor did he illustrate or describe any further surgical details of this single operation. After 1912 he devoted himself largely to writing several outstanding books that dealt primarily with medicine and surgery as depicted in paintings, illustrations, caricatures, and satire in the entire historic period from ancient Greece up to his time. One of Holländer's most famous books, *Medicine in Classical Paintings,* was first published in 1903 [35].

In the year of his death in 1932, probably aware of the increasing number of articles appearing in the surgical literature dealing with face-lifting techniques, and using

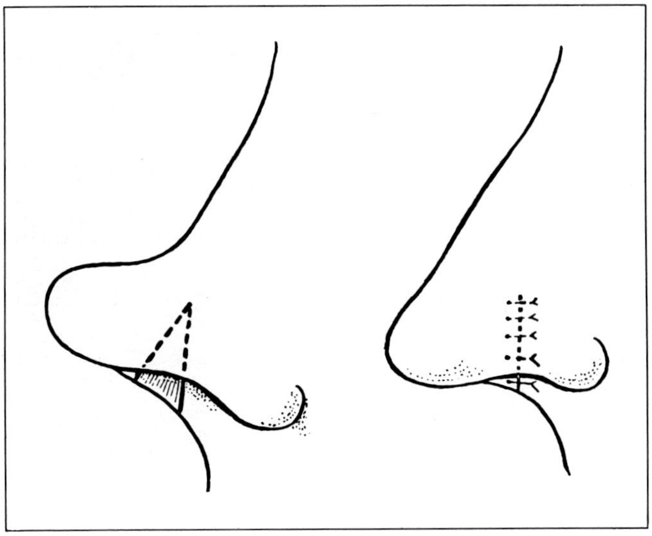

Figure 1-19. Surgical correction of an overly retroussé nose by intranasal and intercolumellar excision of tissue. (From F. S. Kolle, *Plastic and Cosmetic Surgery.* New York: Appleton, 1911.)

obvious surgical hindsight, Holländer wrote that it was actually in 1901 that he was sought by a Polish aristocrat who wished to have a face-lift performed [38]. Until 1901, according to Holländer, this operation was completely unknown.

The next surgeon on the scene, who similarly relied on surgical hindsight many years later, was Erich Lexer (1867–1937). In 1931 Lexer stated that he had not heard of any previous surgical attempts at face-lifting when he performed such an operation on an actress in 1906. Lexer stated in his typical dogmatic fashion, "a single attempt [at this surgery] was successful!" [63].

In Lexer's face-lift operation, as he described it *in 1931,* isolated S-shaped incisions of skin were made in the temporal region in front of and behind the ear, and elliptic excisions were made in the forehead or frontal region (Fig. 1-20). After excising the redundant skin, Lexer anchored the subcutaneous sutures behind the ear to the periosteum of the mastoid region. According to Lexer, it was clear from the very beginning that because of the elasticity of the facial skin a mere simple closure of small skin excisions performed in his day by many so-called cosmetic surgeons, without undermining of the wound defects, resulted in only a short-lived success. Therefore, he decided even in his first case in 1906 not to be content with a simple approximation of the wound edges, but through the use of deep sutures to anchor the edges of the skin flaps to the temporalis fascia. The cutting off of little "spindles" of skin, he said derisively, had little or only short-lived success.

With the end of World War I in 1918, surgeons who may have had an interest in cosmetic surgery before or at the beginning of the war, and who had put their interest aside because of the wartime need for their reconstructive surgical services began publishing articles that had probably lain unwritten during the war years. The most important of these—the first article illustrating fully the multiple small

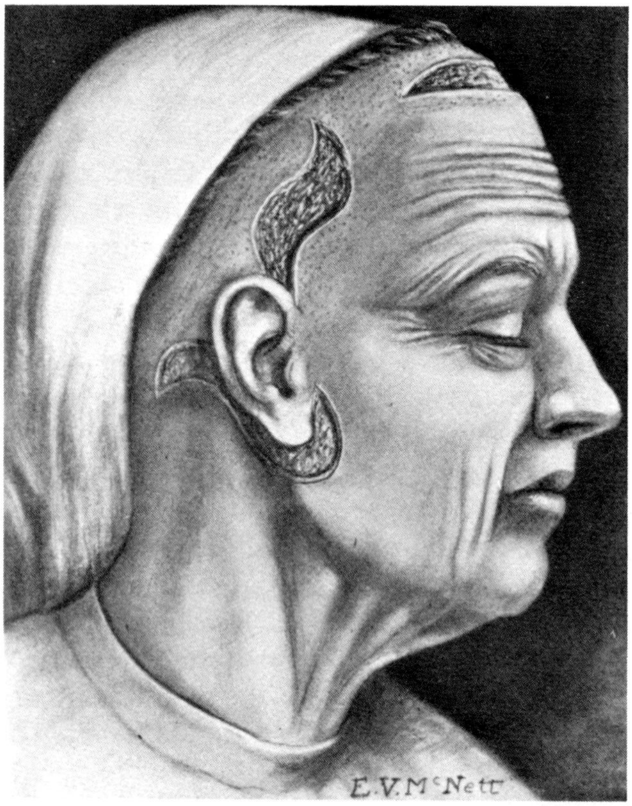

Figure 1-20. Artist's adaptation of Figure 1290 in Lexer's *Die Gesamte Wiederherstellungschirurgie.* (From H. May, *Reconstructive and Reparative Surgery.* Philadelphia: Davis, 1947. P. 146.)

elliptic or ovoid excisions of skin that were then being employed (similar to the minilifts of today)—appeared in the May 12, 1919, issue of *La Presse Médicale* (Fig. 1-21). It was written by Raymond Passot (1886–1933) [108], a pupil of Hippolyte Morestin [136]. In order to obtain an upward or a lateral suspensory tension on various facial wrinkles, Passot excised small pieces of skin in separate areas of the forehead at the scalp hairline, or adjacent to the pretemporal areas, and in the preauricular region adjacent to the attachment of the ear lobule [108, 109].

In addition, the diagram included in Passot's first 1919 article demonstrates that he was also concerned with the "double chin" problem, and he described, perhaps for the first time, an attempt at its correction by the removal of a long ellipse of skin either next to or just below the hyoid, together with its underlying fatty tissue.

In the two articles published in 1919, Passot left no doubt that a certain professor (Samuel-Jean? Pozzi), who may have been one of his teachers, had obtained a nearly perfect operative result in one woman whose face Passot had "retouched" or slightly improved in a subsequent operation. His friend de Martel was successful in three cases performed in cooperation with a colleague, Mlle. Pertat (Madame Noël), and Morestin himself had apparently attempted this type of surgical correction of facial

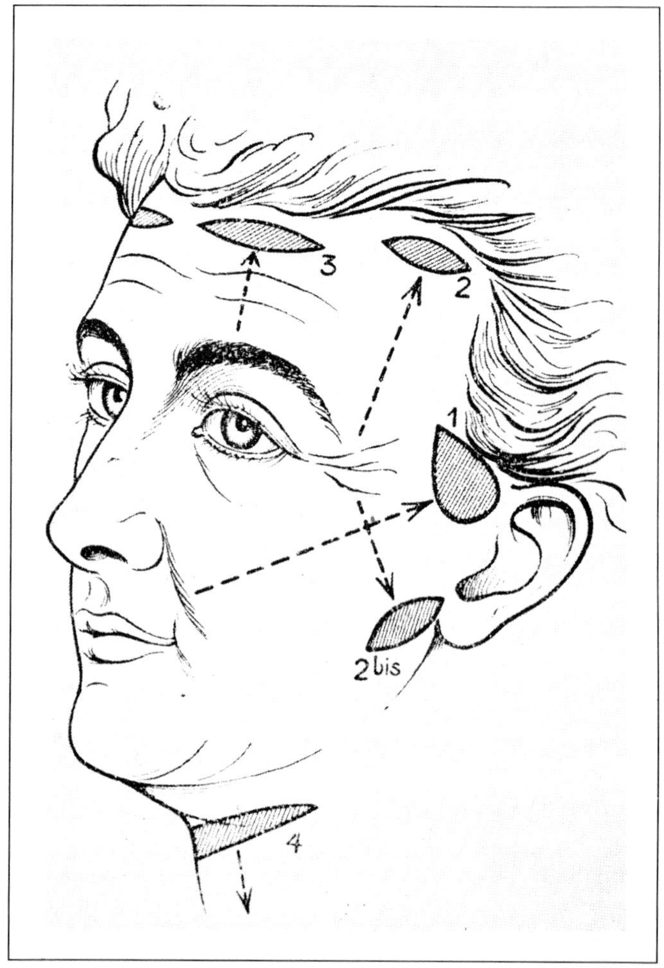

Figure 1-21. Different types of small skin excisions necessary for correction of facial wrinkles. (From R. Passot, La chirurgie esthétique des rides du visage. *Presse Méd.* 27:258, 1919; and La correction chirurgicale des rides du visage. *Bull. Acad. Natl. Med.* 82:112, 1919.)

wrinkles by means of some technique unexplained at that time. Morestin, a moody, talented man totally dedicated to his work, died at the age of 49; his death left a great void in French plastic surgery for many decades to come [136]. Passot took his own life at the age of 47, thus further depriving French plastic surgery of his considerable skill and originality.

One month after the publication of Passot's pioneering article [109], at the annual meeting of the Alumni Association of the University of Oregon's Medical School in Portland in late June 1919, Adalbert G. Bettman (1883–1964) of the same city was probably the first in medical literature to demonstrate to his audience before-and-after photographs of a truly complete face-lift operation [6]. These photographs were subsequently published in an article in *Northwest Medicine* in August 1920 (Figs. 1-22 and 1-23). Although Bettman spoke of removing from the temporal and preauricular regions isolated small pieces of skin varying from the size of a dime to that of a half dollar, Figure VIII in his 1920 article (Fig. 1-22) showed for the

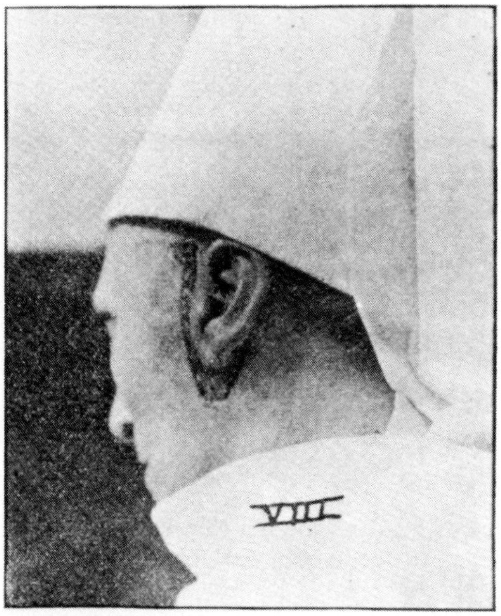

Figure 1-22. First photographic illustration in the medical literature of complete preauricular and postauricular incision employed for the face-lift operation as we know it today. (From A. G. Bettman, Plastic and cosmetic surgery of the face. *Northwest Med.* 19:205, 1920.)

"first time" in medical history a very long, continuous incision extending up into the temporal region, down along the preauricular region, and under and behind the ear lobule. This is essentially the same preauricular and postauricular incision used today in the many modified versions in both shape and extent of what we now call the typical face-lift operation. Thus, for all intents and purposes, in assigning medical firsts from the standpoint of actual publication in the literature, we should treat Bettman as the "father" of the total face-lift operation.

Five months after Passot's first article, in May 1919, Julien Bourguet of Paris similarly described the use of small crescent-shaped, angular, or gendarme-hat–shaped incisions to correct forehead wrinkles, crow's-feet, and neck wrinkles, respectively [10]. These descriptions were published in October 1919, but the drawings illustrating Bourguet's technique, which were part of his Academy of Medicine lecture, were not included in the published version of his paper. Considering the morale and the psychologic suffering of persons with wrinkles, Bourguet was perhaps one of the first to point out that although men with nasal deformities suffer as much as women because of the aesthetics of an unpleasant nose, they are indifferent to or much less concerned with facial wrinkles than women are. He believed that the skin of men usually

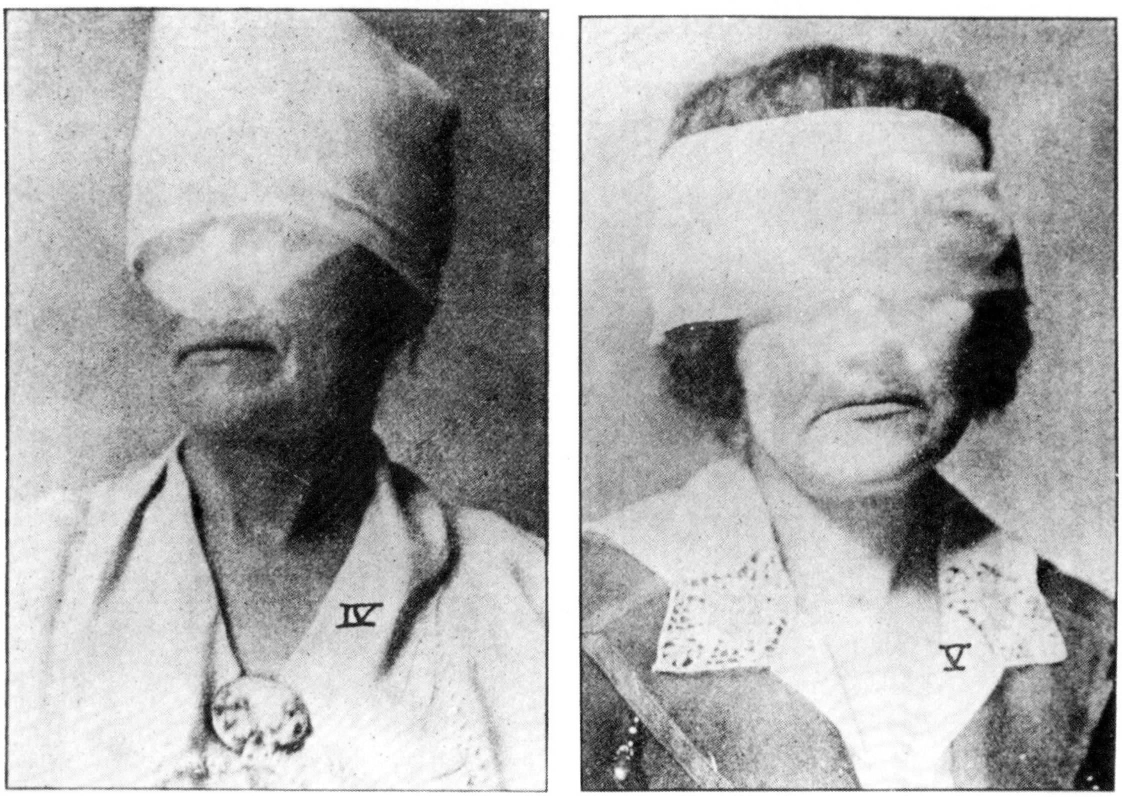

Figure 1-23. First photographic illustration (1920) in the medical literature of complete face-lift operation as we know it today. Preoperative *(left)* and postoperative *(right)*. (From A. G. Bettman, Plastic and cosmetic surgery of the face. *Northwest Med.* 19:205, 1920.)

remained more firm and better preserved with aging than the skin of women [10].

At the end of World War I, John Staige Davis, like many men trained in general surgery, writing in his classic 1919 textbook of plastic surgery [18], had an attitude about cosmetic or aesthetic surgery that left a good deal to be desired. Even as late as 1919, he had not yet adopted Roe's submucosal intranasal approach in corrective nasoplasty and still used the outdated external excisional approach.

He unfortunately described the few corrective aesthetic operations in his book as "secondary rhinoplastic operations." His condescending attitude toward corrective rhinoplastic surgery can be seen in his use of the words ". . . simply to improve appearance." In the few pages devoted to this corrective aesthetic surgery, the illustrations included he had chiefly borrowed from the work of Kolle [58], which had been written 8 years earlier.

In 1921, Jacques Joseph (1865–1934) of Berlin, also using surgical hindsight as did Holländer and Lexer, reminded his readers that he too had performed an operation as far back as 1912 for correction of the redundant aging cheek tissues of a 48-year-old woman [50]. Thus, a series of events, recalled only with surgical hindsight by their authors, has been passed down in the medical literature. These events in the gradual development of face-lifting as a surgical procedure are attributable to three men: Holländer (1901), Lexer (1906), and Joseph (1912). Each of these German surgeons told his readers years after the fact that he had performed the face-lifting operation many years and even decades previously [38, 50, 63]. But to be truly fair, from the standpoint of medical history, it should be emphasized that in actual date of publication, some of the earliest descriptions in the literature for the surgical correction of areas of facial wrinkling must, without doubt, be credited first to Miller [74, 76–78, 80–82, 95] from 1906 to 1909, second to Kolle [58] in 1911, and third to Bettman [6] in 1919, all of them Americans.

To Joseph in 1921, however, belongs the credit for being the second surgeon after Bettman [50] to publish before and after photographs of the results of a face-lift operation (Fig. 1-24). In truth, his photographic results seem to be superior to Bettman's, and, surprisingly enough, Bettman's actual incision, described 2 years earlier, seems to be almost identical to that described in Joseph's 1921 article. A decade later, the results of his face-lift surgery showed a definite improvement as well as a more elegant sophistication in achieving a "normal" postoperative appearance [54].

In 1922 Victor Frühwald of Vienna, impressed by Joseph's paper (1921), operated on a 29-year-old woman who had exceptionally deep nasolabial folds and whose mouth drooped at the corners [28]. Frühwald modified Joseph's incision line at its uppermost temporal margin. For the horsehair sutures Joseph had used in closing the skin he substituted subcutaneous catgut and silk in order to reduce the scarcely visible scar that otherwise appears behind the ear.

In 1922, again in *Northwest Medicine,* another American, F. A. Booth of Seattle, Washington, published his technique for correcting facial sagging with the use of a face-lift incision essentially similar to that described by Joseph and by Bettman several years earlier [9]. In addition, Booth presented a new variation, quite practical, for correcting the double chin (Fig. 1-25).

Figure 1-24. Right side of patient's face has already been corrected by face-lift procedure; left side is as yet uncorrected, showing the advantages of the "lifting" operation itself. (From J. Joseph, Hangewangenplastik (melomioplastik). *Dtsch. Med. Wochenschr.* 47:287, 1921.)

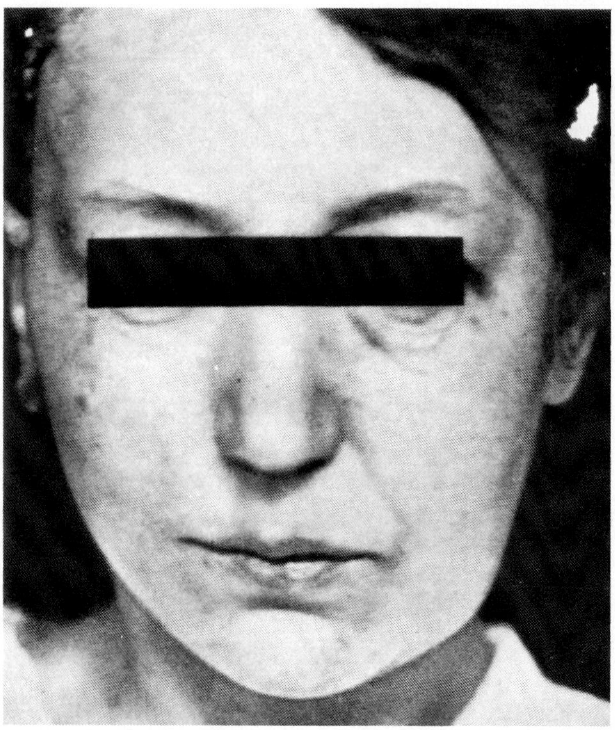

Figure 1-25. (Left) Curved-line incision under the chin for removal of a double chin; *dotted area* demonstrates amount of dissection and undermining for removal of excessive fat. *(Right)* The amount of excised submental skin, with retention mattress sutures inserted to obliterate the "dead space," thus correcting the double chin. (From F. A. Booth, Cosmetic surgery of the face, neck and breast. *Northwest Med.* 21:170, 1922.)

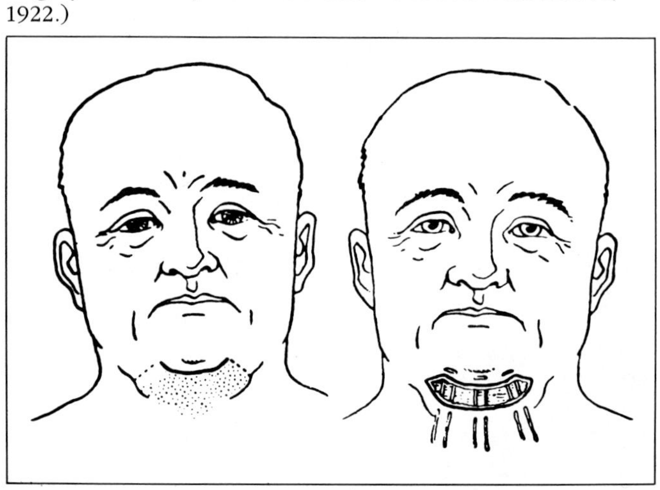

Also in 1922, Max Thorek of Chicago reported for the first time his method of plastic reconstruction of hypertrophied breasts with reduction mammaplasty and, most interestingly, the free transplantation of the nipple. The results were excellent [148].

According to Lalardrie and Mouly [59], the first reduction mammaplasty worthy of the name was performed by Aubert in Marseille and described by him in 1923. Since it dealt with the attempt to combine reduction mammaplasty with nipple transposition, it was another milestone in the history of mammaplasty. As emphasized by the aforementioned authors, "The site and the volume of the glandular resection could be varied, but nipple transposition called for more or less extensive undermining between skin and gland. Failures of glandular reductions in the region of the nipple were soon to draw attention to the importance of taking due account of vascularization" [59].

Five years after his 1919 article [10], in November 1924, Bourguet was probably the first to describe the technique for the excisional correction of pockets of herniated periorbital fat (bags) of the eyelid region [11], and in 1925 he also was probably the first in medical history to publish before and after photographs of patients [12] who had undergone this cosmetic blepharoplastic operation (Figs. 1-26 and 1-27) as well as the double chin corrective procedure (Fig. 1-28). Rather than incising the eyelid skin, Bourguet approached these fat herniations through the mucosa of the conjunctival cul-de-sac of the lower eyelid [12]. Several catgut sutures were used to close the fibrous sac or capsule that usually surrounds the fatty herniated masses.

Despite the innumerable small incisions Miller recommended [101] making in the eyelid skin, as illustrated and

Figure 1-26. First photograph in the medical literature of before-and-after results of the correction of bags in the lower eyelids. (From J. Bourguet, Chirurgie esthétique de la face: Les nez concaves, les rides et les "poches" sous les yeux. *Arch. Prov. Chir.* 28:293, 1925.)

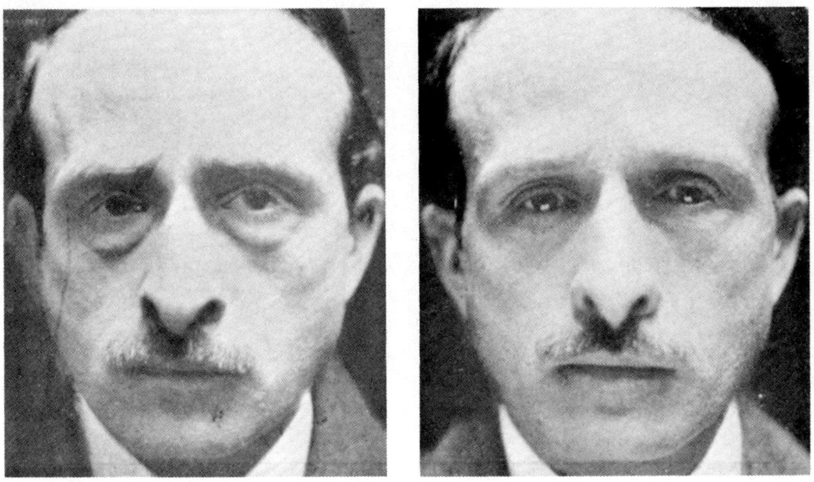

Figure 1-27. (Left) Preoperative and *(right)* postoperative results of another surgical correction of bags of the eyelids. (From J. Bourguet, Chirurgie esthétique de la face: Les nez concaves, les rides et les "poches" sous les yeux. *Arch. Prov. Chir.* 28:293, 1925.)

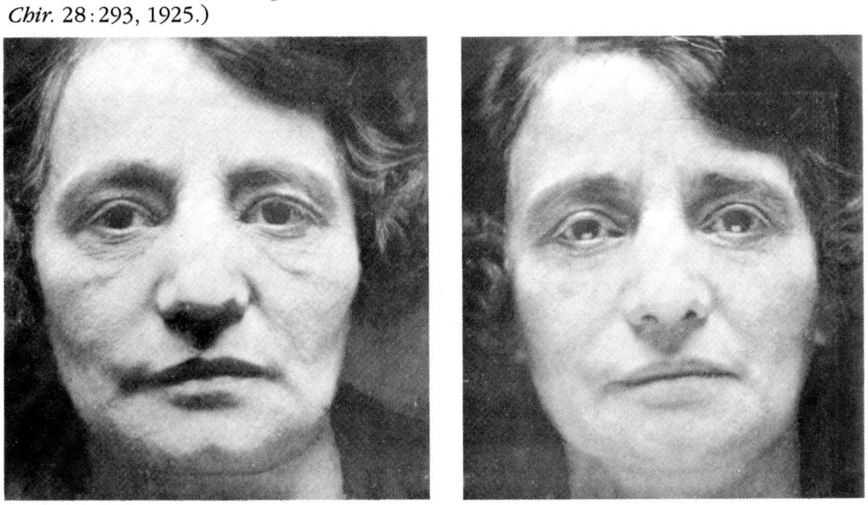

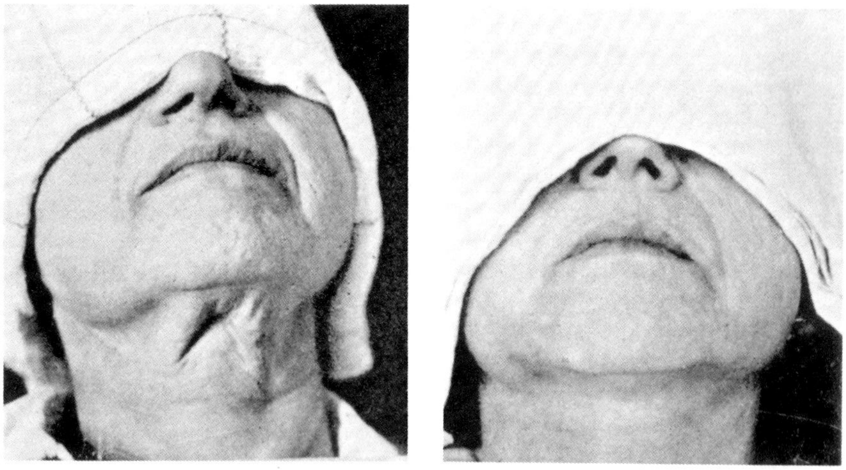

Figure 1-28. First photographs in the medical literature of before-and-after results of the correction of the double chin. (From J. Bourguet, Chirurgie esthétique de la face: Les nez concaves, les rides et les "poches" sous les yeux. *Arch. Prov. Chir.* 28:293, 1925.)

described in his expanded 1925 book on cosmetic surgery, he never included any before-and-after photographs in his book nor did he mention the role of periorbital fat herniation as one of the glaring deformities in many patients who complain of "aging eyelids" (Fig. 1-29).

In this same year, 1925, Erich Lexer [62], 3 years after Thorek's article [148], also reported a reduction mammaplasty with free transplantation of the nipple. Lexer's interest in both reduction mammaplasty and augmentation were revealed in an outstanding article he also wrote on fat transplantation in 1925 [61].

J. Eastman Sheehan, a flamboyant and frequently disliked but innovative plastic surgeon from New York City, wrote probably the first book specifically devoted to corrective nasal plastic surgery in 1925. His *Plastic Surgery of the Nose* [144] was followed by other excellent pioneering textbooks on corrective nasal surgery by Joseph [54] in 1928 to 1931, by Sanvenero-Rosselli [139] in 1931, by Safian [138] in 1935, by Maliniac [65] in 1947, by Seltzer [142] in 1949, by Brown and McDowell [13] in 1951, by Denecke and Meyer [20] in 1967, by Fomon and Bell [27] in 1970, and by Sheen [145] in 1978.

Another fascinating man in the early history of American cosmetic surgery was Harold Napier Lyons Hunt (1882–1954) of New York City [40]. In 1926, the same year that Madame Noël's famous book appeared [106], Hunt's *Plastic Surgery of the Head, Face and Neck* was published [40]. Hunt not only described face-lifting operations, but was probably the very first to describe forehead- or brow-lifting operations with a complete coronal incision (Fig. 1-30), as well as his own procedures for correcting a double chin. He was another prolific writer whose interests ranged beyond plastic surgery. Actually, after 1926, Hunt's interests in the latter field declined considerably, because he devoted himself chiefly to treating impotence by the transplantation of ram and sheep glands [39].

In this brief review of the early development of aesthetic or cosmetic surgery of the facial region, it is almost mandatory to refer to one of the most remarkable people and the first woman in the history of aesthetic surgery. An early pioneer in the development of face-lifting and eyelid plasty techniques was Madame le Dr. A. (Suzanne) Noël (Fig. 1-31) [129–131], whose book *La Chirurgie Esthétique: Son Rôle Social* appeared in 1926 [106]. A German translation appeared 6 years later [107]. Chronologically, hers was the sixth medical book devoted almost solely to cosmetic surgery published in the early twentieth century, after those of Miller [78, 95], Kolle [58], and Hunt [40].

Dr. Noël, known throughout Paris as well as most of Europe as "Madame Noël" (Fig. 1-31), stated that her interest in the field of cosmetic surgery began in the year 1912, when one of the great French actresses returned from America after a triumphal tour [106]. All the newspapers remarked that "by means of a practical operation performed on the scalp, she had regained a surprising degree of youthfulness." Thus, some type of face-lifting procedure was already being performed in America at least as early as 1912 by a surgeon or surgeons not identified. Finally she met the actress whose regained youthfulness had been so widely reported. The woman explained to Noël what had been done during her visit to the United States; her operation did not in any manner resemble the type of procedure Noël was contemplating. Many of the lines in the upper part of her face had been reduced by the simple excision of scalp tissue from an incision that ran from one ear to the other. Closure of the defect in the scalp exerted a favorable upward tension on the skin of the face, the forehead, and the crow's-feet region without modifying the appearance of the lower margins of the face.

World War I interrupted her interest in cosmetic surgery and it was not until 1916 that she renewed her work with her usual ardor. Her cosmetic surgery book published 10 years later in 1926 was the only one of the five previously mentioned that included numerous photographs—59 preoperative and postoperative photographs showing the results of her skillful surgery. Among the subjects described in detail in this book containing 11 operative

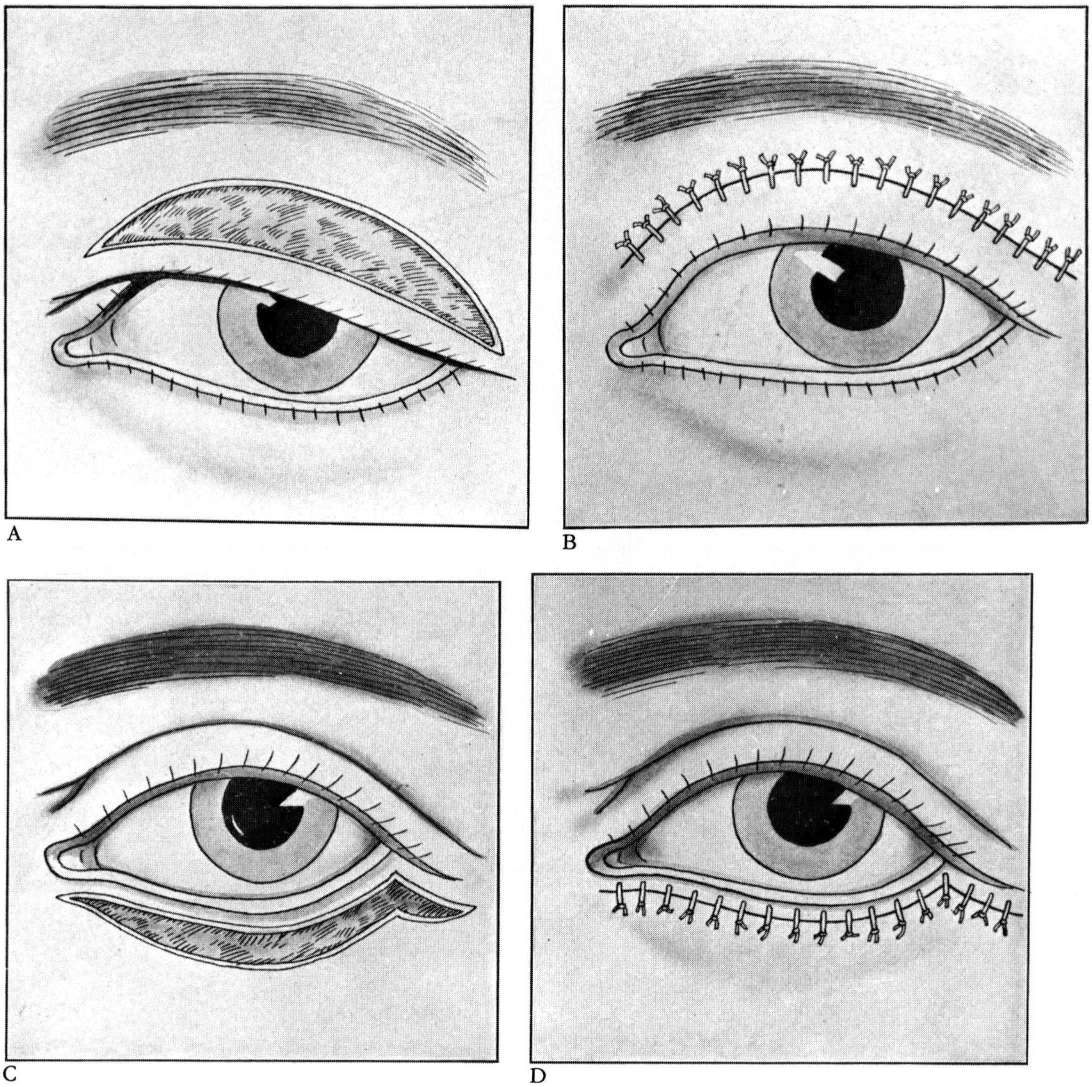

Figure 1-29
A. Method of excising fold of redundant upper eyelid skin.
B. Postoperative result.
C. Modification in the shape of removal of excess wrinkled skin of lower eyelid by employing a "wedge" at the lateral canthal region to prevent eversion or ectropion following cosmetic blepharoplasty.
D. Postoperative result. (From C. C. Miller, *Cosmetic Surgery: The Correction of Featural Imperfections.* Philadelphia: Davis, 1925.)

illustrations and 51 photographs of technique for surgical correction are baggy and wrinkled eyelids (Figs. 1-32–1-34); facial (Figs. 1-35 and 1-36), forehead, and neck wrinkles; and double chins. Also discussed are correction of redundant neck skin by massive excision of skin and scalp tissue in the nape of the neck and in the suboccipital scalp region; the excision of large nevi (hairy and otherwise) of the breast, neck, and postauricular regions; the correction of keloidal burn scars of the neck, of flabby tissues of the arms of aging women, and of protruding ears; and the excision of forearm tattoos. As one can see from perusing her text, Noël was a versatile surgeon. Moreover, she wrote in a charming, warm, and thoroughly womanly fashion, as attested to in the fascinating article written about her recently by Paule Regnault [116], one of her pupils.

At this point in the historical narrative, let us consider the gentle smile on the face of a patient who has just undergone a face-lift operation performed under local anesthesia in Noël's office. The patient has put her handsome bonnet on, is ready to go home, and is calmly drinking a cup of coffee (Figs. 1-35 and 1-36). Perhaps her happy, confident, and pleased expression is symbolic of the attitude of most patients who, since those early years of our specialty more than half a century ago, have undergone aesthetic plastic surgery with all of the postoperative physical, psychologic, and social improvements that are the most rewarding aspects of this most delightful and satisfying branch of the overall practice of plastic and reconstructive surgery.

In a relatively little read, thin book on cosmetic surgery, a German surgeon, Schörcher, traces the operation for a thigh-lifting to Kelly, Madame Noël, and Thorek [140].

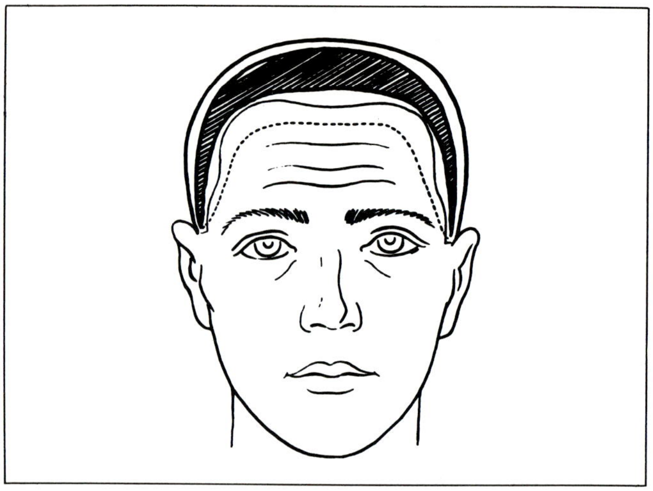

Figure 1-30. The first description in the medical literature of an incision behind the hairline extending from one temporal region to the other, with hair-bearing skin as much as one-half to three-fourths of an inch wide at the midline excised to correct horizontal frown lines. (From H. L. Hunt, *Plastic Surgery of the Head, Face and Neck.* Philadelphia: Lea & Febiger, 1926.)

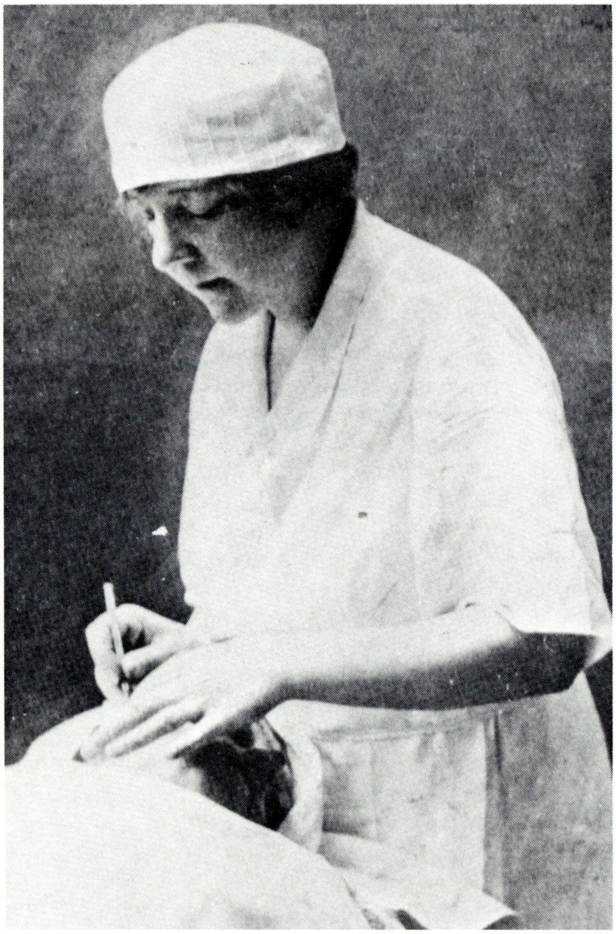

Figure 1-31. Dr. Suzanne Noël, as photographed in 1936, the world's first female cosmetic plastic surgeon. (From G. Robin, Dr. Suzanne Noël. In *Dictionnaire National des Contemporains* (vol. 1). Paris: La Jeunesse, 1936. P. 461.)

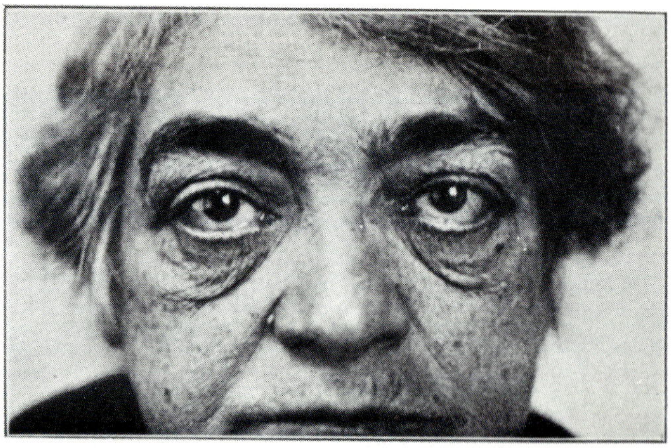

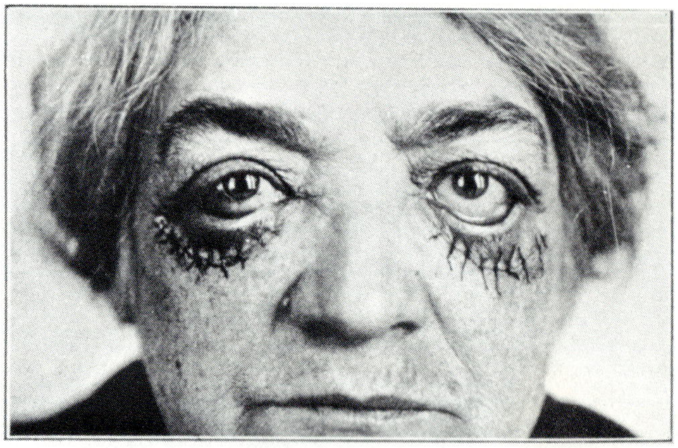

Figure 1-32. (Above) One of Dr. Noël's patients prior to excision of bags and wrinkles of lower eyelid skin. *(Below)* Patient immediately after operation with operative sutures in place, eyes open. (From A. Noël, *La Chirurgie Esthétique: Son Rôle Social.* Paris: Masson, 1926.)

However, a search of the literature of these three well-known personalities reveals that at the most the three surgeons either described or were merely said to have performed local excision of collections of fatty tissue of the thigh and buttocks in a relatively limited manner, confining themselves to the localized excision of fat without any specific concern for the sites of the rather small excisions and scars. Kelly only suggested simple direct excision of localized fatty thigh masses without illustrating his results. The same can be said for Thorek, known better to most of us for his early contributions to abdominoplasty and breast plasty.

Regnault wrote an excellent biography on the work and life of Madame Noël [116], stating that in the amazing cosmetic surgery performed by Madame Noël in the 1920s and 1930s "she seldom had complications, although the methods of preparation and asepsis were not as strict as they are now. Once she scrubbed with her watch on her wrist for a minor operation and told me, 'Don't worry, this watch is very good'. The reader will notice in Fig. 1-34, Madame Noël operating in her office without a mask, without surgical gloves, and without any cap on her frizzy 1920s hairdo. It is interesting in view of the remarkably few complications that Madame Noël had in her surgery in

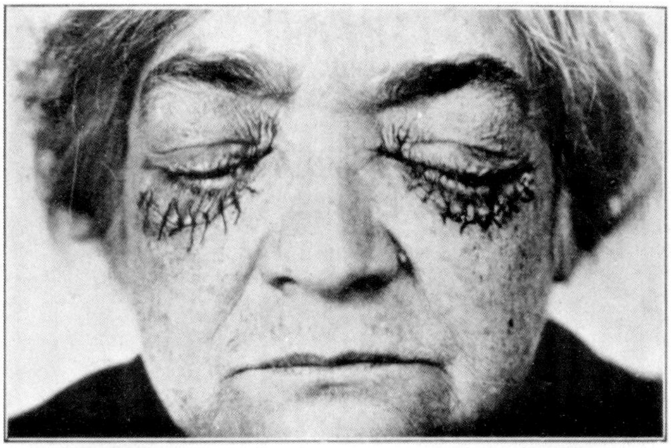

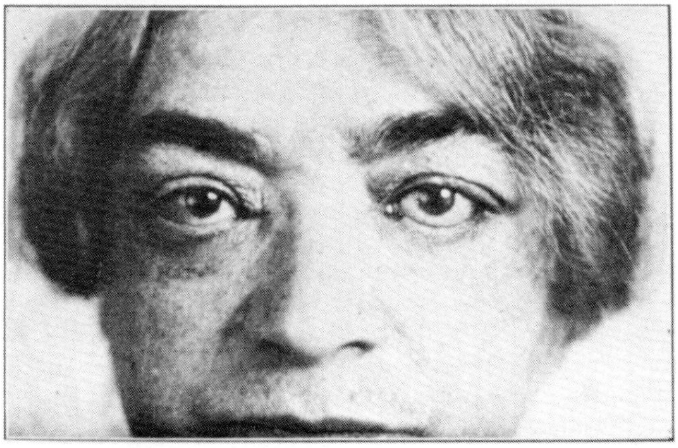

Figure 1-33. Same patient as in Figure 1-32. *(Above)* Operative sutures in place with eyes closed. *(Below)* Results 15 days postoperative. (From A. Noël, *La Chirurgie Esthétique: Son Rôle Social.* Paris: Masson, 1926.)

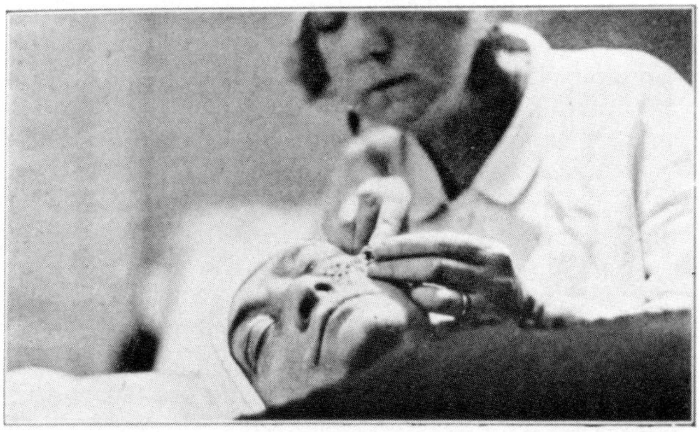

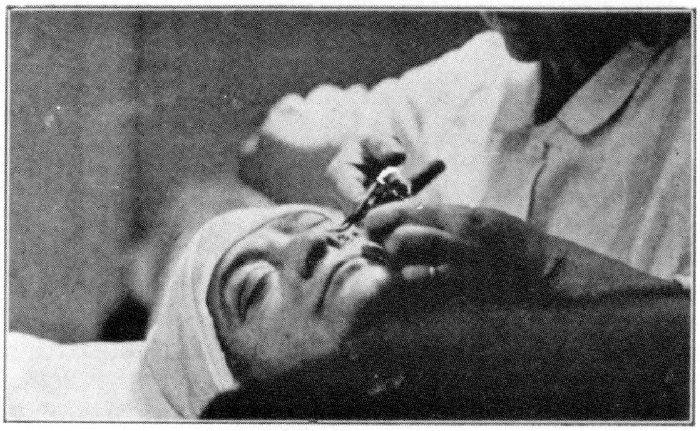

Figure 1-34. Dr. Noël operating on a female patient for bags of the eyelids. Note the absence of any facial mask or surgical gloves. (From A. Noël, *La Chirurgie Esthétique: Son Rôle Social.* Paris: Masson, 1926.)

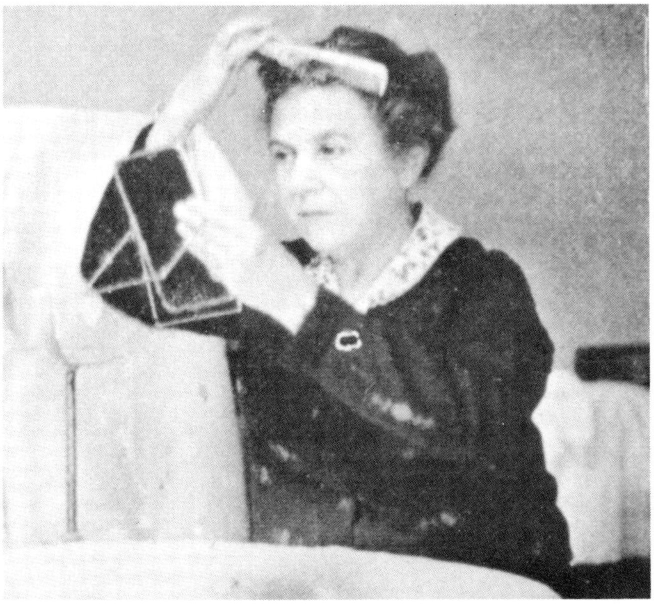

Figure 1-35. A patient combs her hair preparing to go home following a temporal face-lift in Dr. Noël's office. (From A. Noël, *La Chirurgie Esthétique: Son Rôle Social.* Paris: Masson, 1926.)

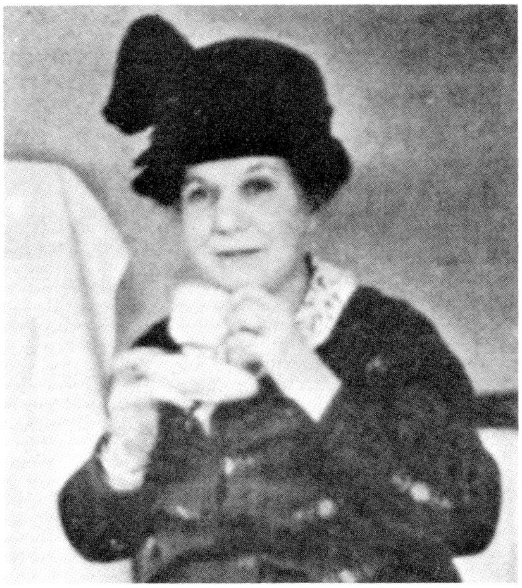

Figure 1-36. Middle-aged patient at the end of a face-lift operation performed under local anesthesia in Dr. Noël's office, with her bonnet on, ready to go home, and calmly drinking a cup of coffee. (From A. Noël, *La Chirurgie Esthétique: Son Rôle Social.* Paris: Masson, 1926.)

these decades long before the use of antibiotics, that, as Regnault puts it, "On a few occasions I assisted her with operations that were very bold for the time. One of these was a complete fat excision of the legs . . . the leg defatting, with wide undermining, was a catastrophe with extensive necrosis of the skin. This case was of concern to her for a considerable length of time."

In the gradual development of reduction mammaplasty surgeons became dissatisfied with mere glandular excision, which reduced the volume of the gland but in which the form and shape of the breast suffered. The need to reconstruct a harmoniously proportioned glandular stump in the form of a small mammary gland created the first attempts at glandular remodeling after the resection itself, and the two names most famous in these surgical advances were Biesenberger and Schwarzmann of Vienna.

In 1928 and 1930, Biesenberger published two articles in succession. The first described "a new method of mammaplastic" with a good series of illustrations demonstrating his reduction technique that combined nipple transposition with remodeling of the gland itself [7].

In the second article, the first photographs of the operation itself and of postoperative results were published (Figs. 1-37 and 1-38). Biesenberger resected the outer glandular segment of the breast by a long S-shaped incision going from the upper to the lower pole of the gland and performed a modeling of the gland in such a way that the upper concave part and the lower convex parts of the glandular section were brought together. Schwarzmann performed a similar glandular resection, which has since borne his name, consisted essentially of incorporating a periareolar deepithelialization [141]. These two surgeons thus initiated a new phase in mammary plastic surgery, the significance of which was to provide a vascular security of the nipple despite undermining between the skin and the gland that enabled subsequent surgeons to increase the volume of glandular resections. Following the reports of Lexer [61] dealing with augmentation of the breast with fat transplants and by Passot [110, 111] in 1930 and 1931 dealing with fat transplants as well as *greffe graisseuse épiploïque,* the use of fat transplantation became more frequent, most of the fatty tissue being taken from abdominal or buttocks donor sites.

In 1931 Flesch-Thebesius and Weisheimer [26] were probably the first to publish preoperative and postoperative photos of an abdominoplasty since Kelly [56] and were the first to describe after Kelly a horizontal excisional removal of the lower part of the abdominal adiposity as well as the umbilicus without any undermining [26].

Passot [111] in 1931 described a lower horizontal crescentic excision with defatting up to the umbilicus, and he also suggested using a local circular periumbilical excision for the first time. The umbilicus was incised in a horizontal "marquise cut" shape and located in a horizontal incision in the upper flap.

In the same publication [111], *Chirurgie Esthétique Pure,* Passot also described his reduction mammaplasty technique (Fig. 1-39), which he first reported in 1925, and included several impressive clinical results.

Despite the use of fat transplants by numerous surgeons, a high degree of resorption of the transplant was encountered. Therefore, Berson [5] in 1944 proposed for the first time the use of dermal fat transplants, which Peer [112] recommended should be of the largest possible volume because even with these a certain amount of resorption could be expected. A number of well-known plastic surgeons of the time utilized dermal fat fascial transplants, but gradually enthusiasm for them fell off; the epiploic free transplants described by Passot did not weather the test of time.

Although in 1930 Schwarzman [141] suggested the use of glass balls as prosthetic inclusions for breast augmentation and this procedure prevailed for years up to and including Thorek's recommendation as late as 1942 for their use "in certain cases," only with the introduction of plastics toward the end of World War II did surgeons come to realize that these might be the solution to most breast

Figure 1-37
A. Fatty breast hypertrophy and ptosis in a 28-year-old woman.
B. Two months after the operation. (From H. Biesenberger, Eine neue Methode der Mammaplastik. *Zentralbl. Chir.* 48:2971, 1930.)

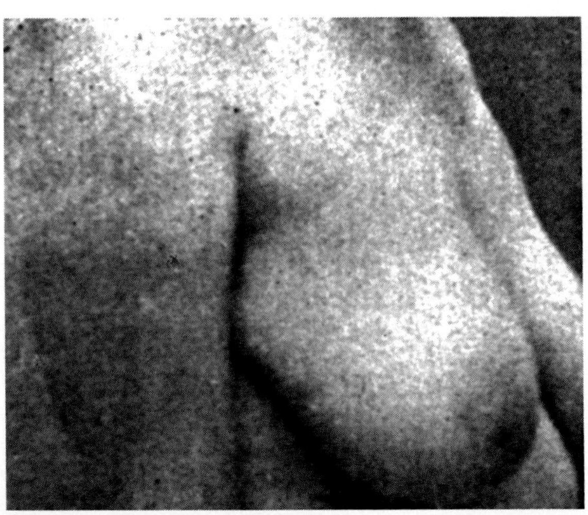

A

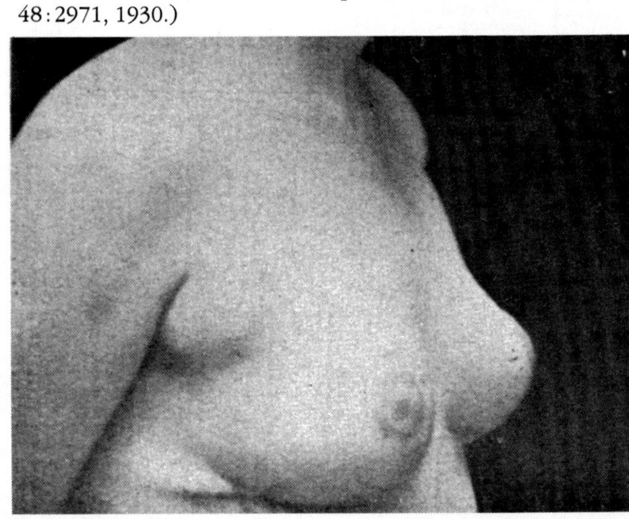

B

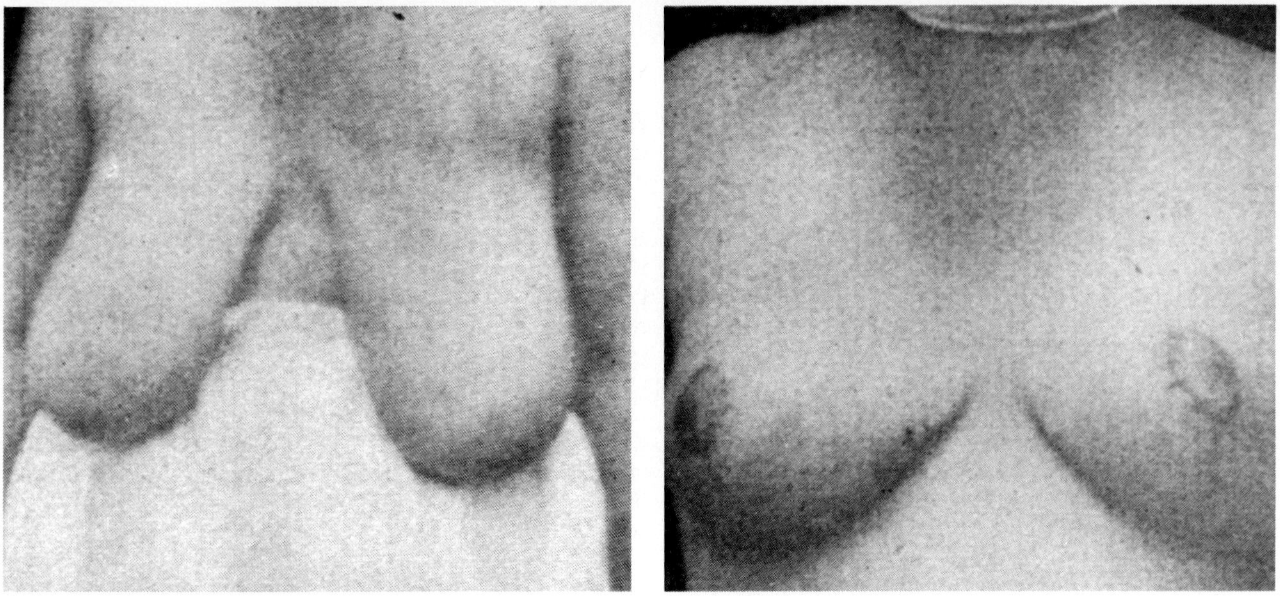

A B

Figure 1-38
A. Hypertrophied ptotic breasts in a 29-year-old woman.
B. Three months after the operation. (From H. Biesenberger, Eine neue Methode der Mammaplastik. *Zentralbl. Chir.* 48:2971, 1930.)

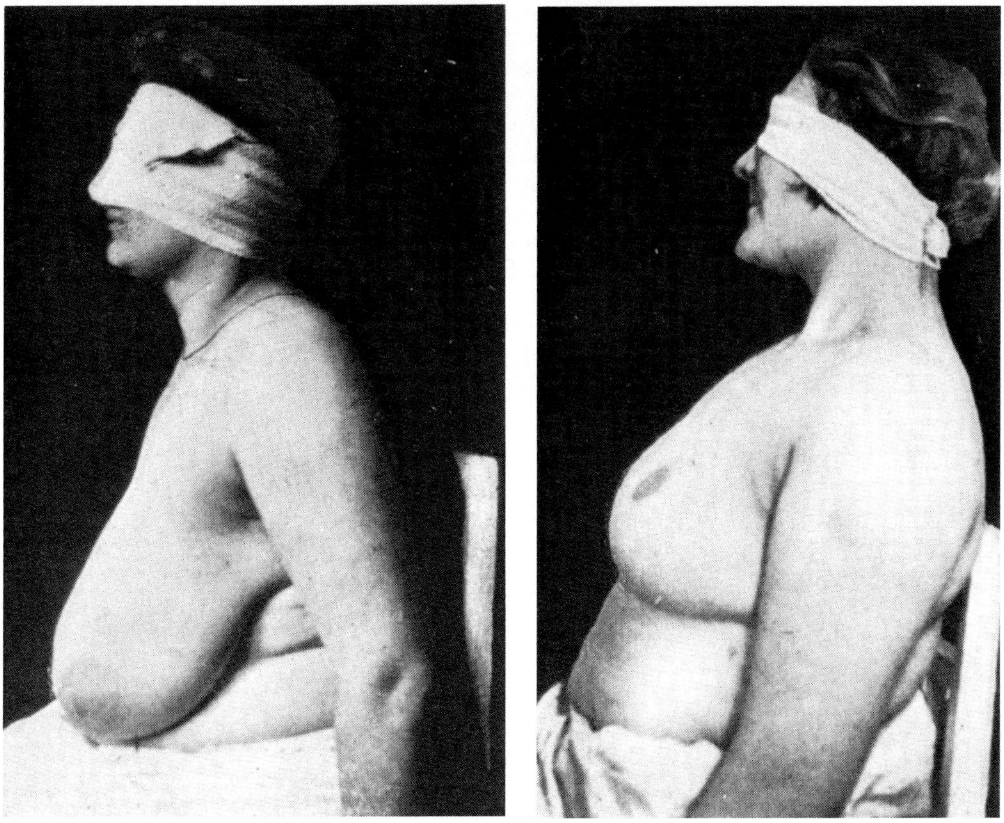

A B

Figure 1-39
A. Large redundant ptotic hypertrophied breasts.
B. Postoperative result as reported by Passot. (From R. Passot, *Chirurgie Esthétique Pure [Technique et Résultats].* Paris: G. Doin, 1931.)

augmentation problems. After World War II, according to Lalardrie and Mouly [59], Levine and Hurst were probably the first to use plastic materials in augmentation breast surgery. Since their introduction, the history of augmentation surgery includes the—at times successful and more frequently unsuccessful—use of ivalon, polistan, etheron, hydron, and silicones and silastics in subsequent years, the latter giving the most satisfactory results and affording the patient "a natural feel to the touch."

The operation to improve lipodystrophy or to correct redundant skin and fat of the thigh and buttocks, known as the "thigh-lift," was first performed and described by John Lewis, Jr., of Atlanta, Georgia, in 1956 [60]. Lewis, whose patients were male, was concerned less with a beautiful cosmetic appearance than with the correction of the obesity itself. Lewis developed and reported a procedure that resulted in a satisfactory degree of improvement with less visible scarring than followed the theoretical procedures outlined in his paper and could be performed in one stage with a prompt healing of the wound edges. His incision started in the inguinal region just below the anterior iliac spine (Fig. 1-40) and traveled along the inguinal regional across the medial aspect of the thigh to the posterior medial aspect of the thigh, high against the buttock, then went down the posterior medial aspect of the thigh to a point just proximal to the knee. Elevation of the skin was accomplished by excising tissue below this incision and pulling the skin upward to close it again in the inguinal region and also by excising a wide ellipse of skin and fatty tissue from the posterior medial aspect of the thigh and closing this incision at the most inconspicuous location.

The first photographs of female patients who had undergone this procedure (Fig. 1-41) did not appear until the article written by Farina and colleagues in 1960 [25]. In contrast to Lewis's excessively obese male patients with redundant flabby skin of the thighs and legs, these female patients suffered from specific fat deposits in the trochanteric region, creating the so-called riding trousers shape deformity, which was first given its name and described in detail by these authors. Their report included illustrations and a description of their laterally placed deep fusiform incision (Fig. 1-42), which they emphasized must be carried deep to the aponeurotic layers. They also showed how the redundant trochanteric fatty tissue was drawn upward and the excess removed in the region of the iliac crest by a backward oblique extension of the incision running into the high region of the iliac crest to improve the aesthetic aspect of the drooping buttocks to make them look higher. But they did not describe the actual details of surgery as Lewis had done 3 years earlier.

In the early 1960s, I was approached by a patient who was trying to keep her husband still interested in her

Figure 1-40. First illustration in the medical literature of the thigh-lift operation as described by Lewis in 1956. (From J. H. Lewis, Jr., The thigh lift. *J. Int. Coll. Surg.* 27:330, 1957.)

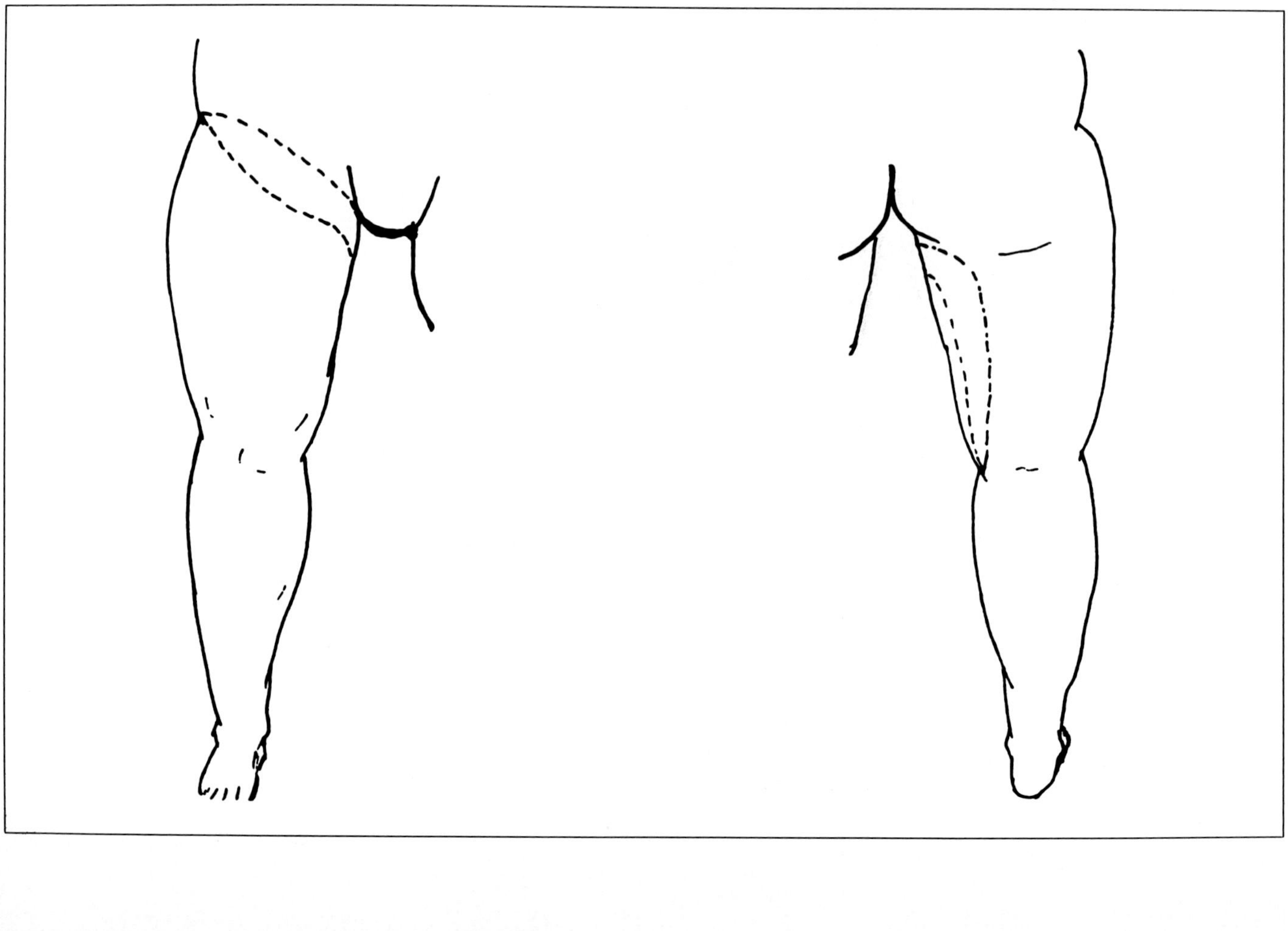

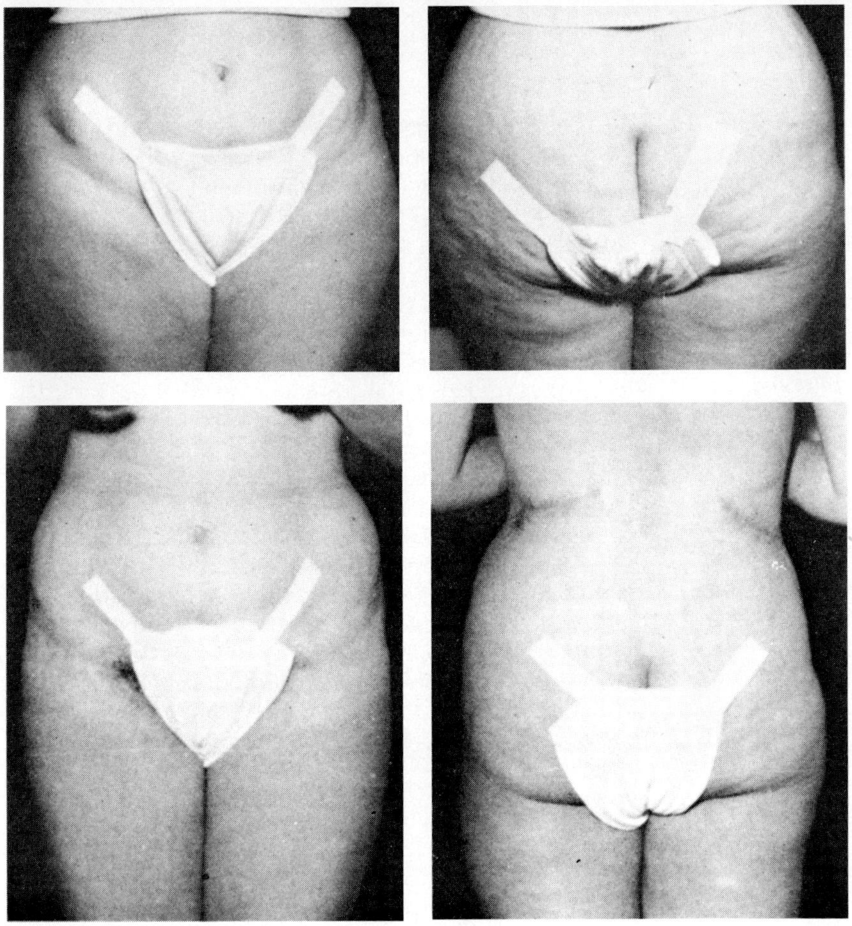

Figure 1-41. First photographs in the medical literature of the results of a correction of trochanteric lipodystrophy in a female by Farina, et al. in 1960. (From R. Farina, et al., Riding trousers like type of pelvicrural lipodystrophy [trochanteric lipomatoses]. *Br. J. Plast. Surg.* 13:174, 1960.)

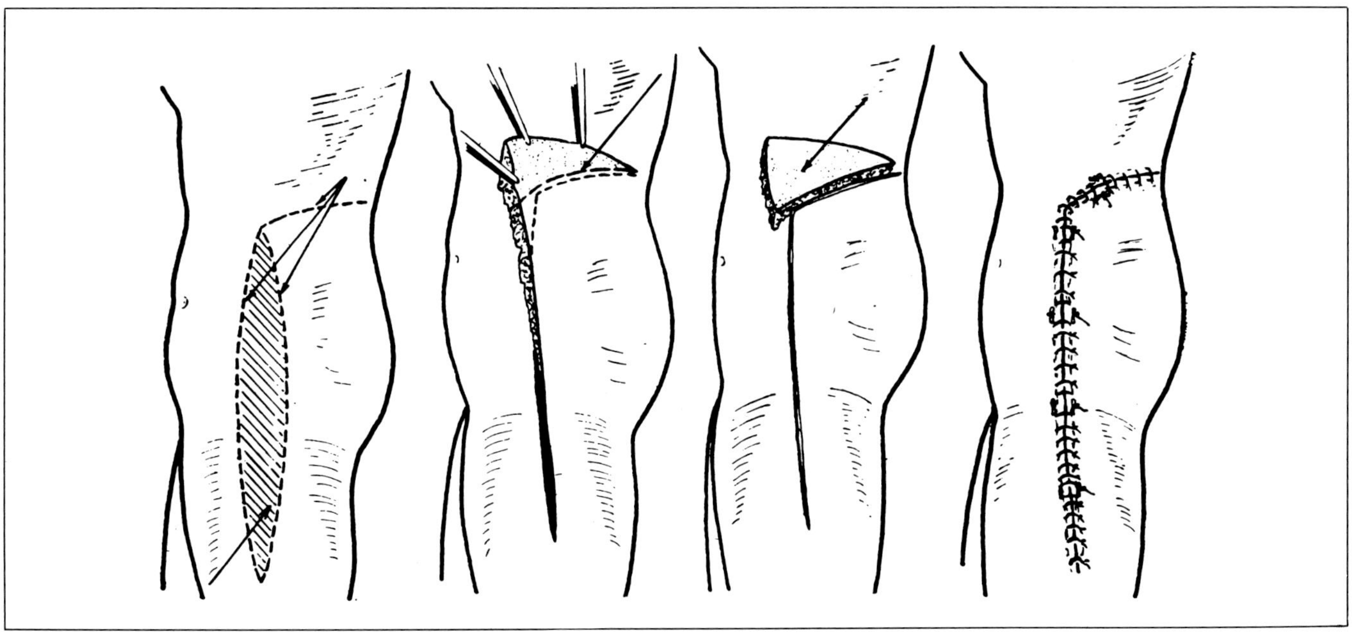

Figure 1-42. Illustrations of the long vertical elliptic incision utilized by Farina, et al. for the correction of trochanteric lipodystrophy. (From R. Farina, et al., Riding trousers like type of pelvicrural lipodystrophy [trochanteric lipomatoses]. *Br. J. Plast. Surg.* 13:174, 1960.)

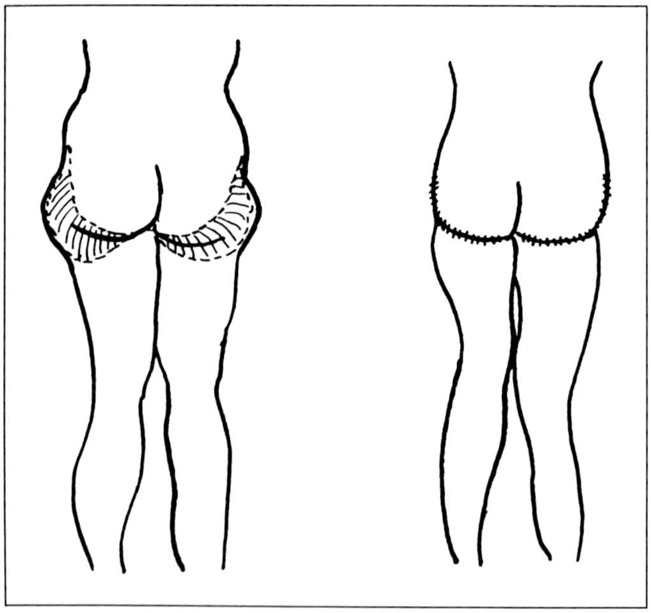

Figure 1-43. Original illustrations by Rogers of first patient treated for trochanteric lipodystrophy, with incisions differing from those previously described by Lewis, and Farina, et al.

sexually. He was a wandering fellow who was philandering more and more. She requested that I try to slim down her buttocks and thigh regions [133]. At one time she had weighed 220 lb. and the loss of weight had left slightly dimpled redundant tissue of her lower body, which today has been inaptly called "cellulite." No amount of exercise or any type of dietary regimen was able to reduce her heavy thighs, both medially and laterally, and her husband found her body increasingly unattractive. I looked in the then available plastic surgery literature to see whether there had been any previous thigh-lifts of a cosmetic nature and found only the two aforementioned articles of Lewis and Farina et al.

My only objection to both of these papers was that the scars left by the operation would not be acceptable to a woman who was trying to keep her husband from looking on her body with any further revulsion and who specifically wanted the scars hidden within her bathing suit line. Finding nothing else in the literature at the time, I tried to devise an operation that would keep the scars of a thigh-lift operation in the bathing suit area. Therefore, using the drawing (depicted in Fig. 1-43) I had made to illustrate the contemplated technique, I performed the operation on this patient with successful results (Fig. 1-44). The reader will see from the incisions made and from the amount of tissue excised that this 1961 operation was identical to an operation reported 3 years later by Pitanguy in *Plastic and Reconstructive Surgery* in 1964 [114]. As a young surgeon just 5 years in private practice, I believed in 1961 that my operation was a rather bold and even risky type of extensive surgery, since this type of incision had never been done by anyone else. In our demonstration clinics at Manhattan Eye, Ear and Throat Hospital, Dr. Converse, my chief, was anxious for me to show this

Figure 1-44

A. Preoperative and B, postoperative photographs of a patient with severe trochanteric lipodystrophy operated on by Rogers according to the technique shown in Figure 1-43. (From B. O. Rogers, Historical Development of Gluteal Trochanteric Lipectomy. Paper delivered at the XIth Instructional Course of the International Society of Aesthetic Plastic Surgery, Lausanne, June 28–July 1, 1978, and the XVth Instructional Course of the International Society of Aesthetic Plastic Surgery, South African Association of Plastic Surgeons, Bophuthatswana, October 23–24, 1980. In press.)

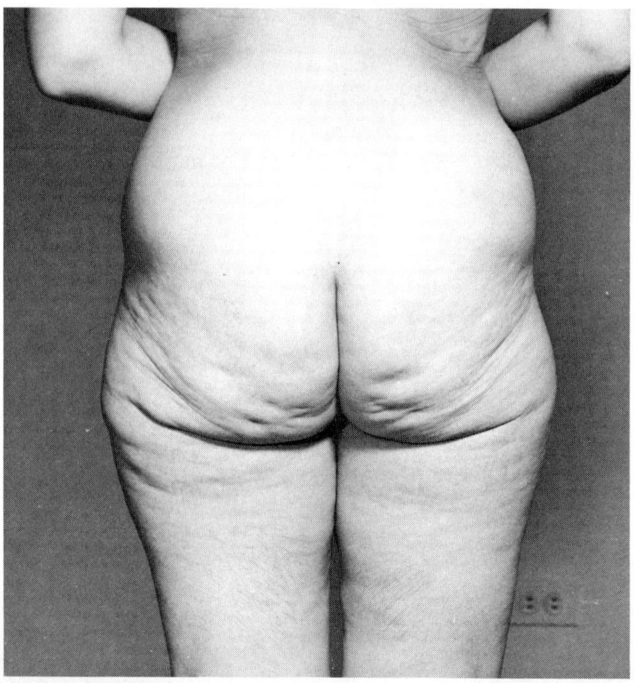

A

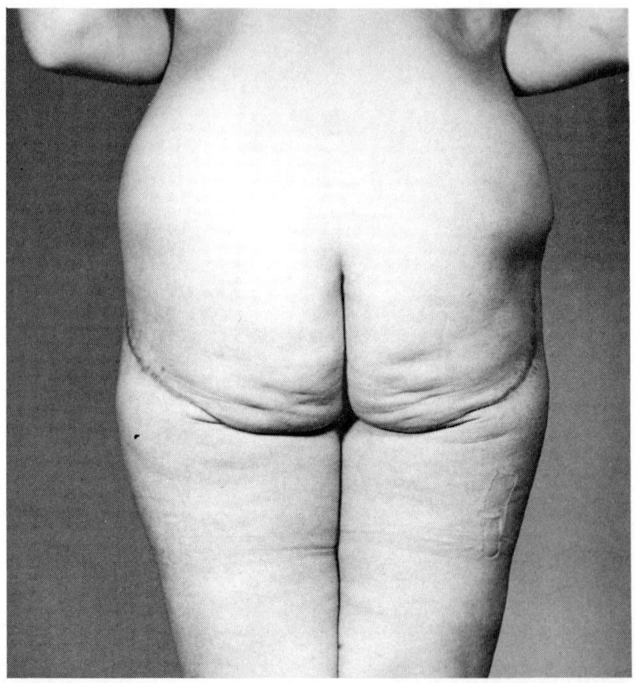

B

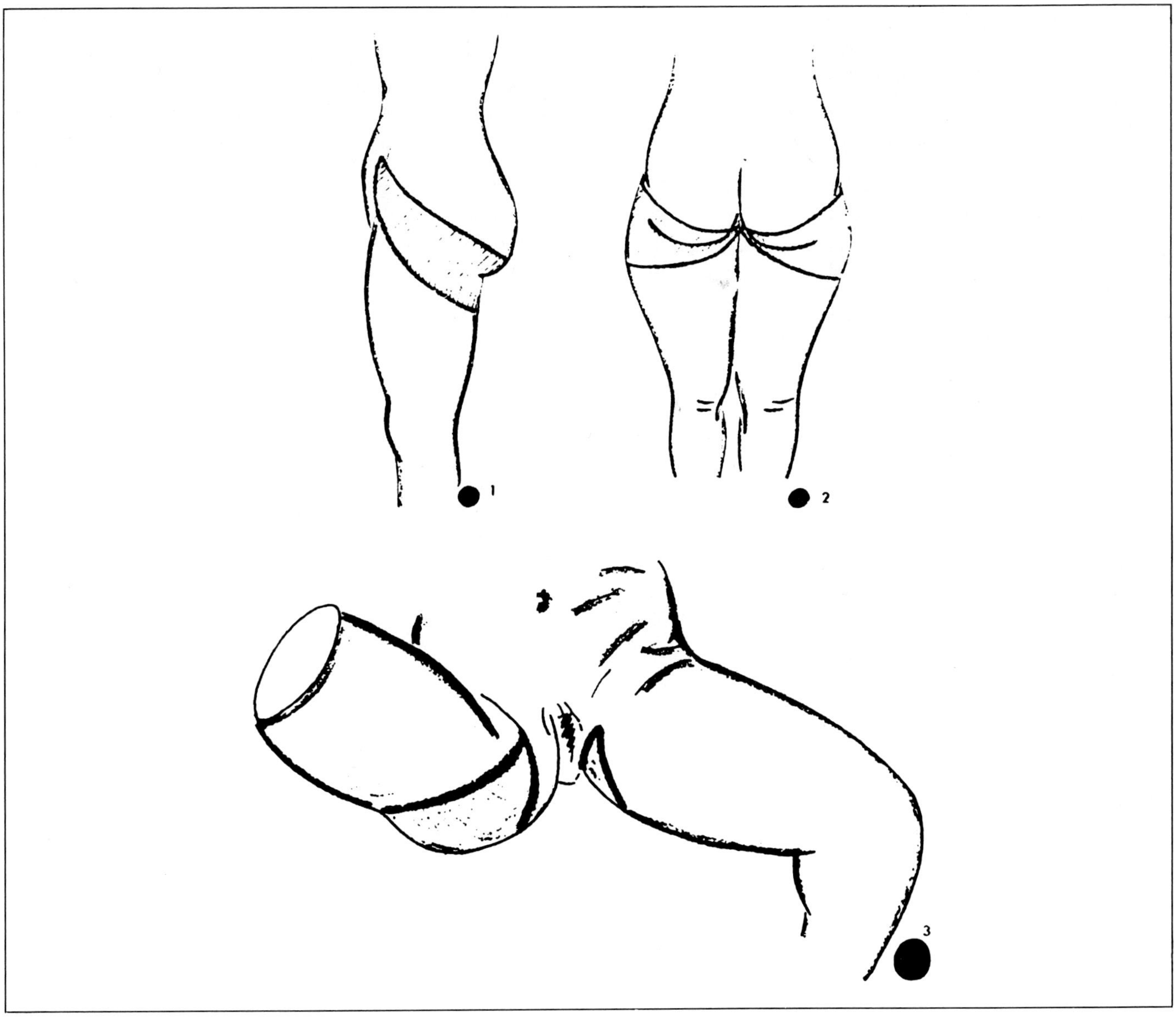

Figure 1-45. Illustrations of the thigh-lift operation as first published in Pitanguy's 1964 article. (From I. Pitanguy, Trochanteric lipodystrophy. *Plast. Reconstr. Surg.* 34 : 280, 1964.)

operation to visitors as an example of the other types of surgery we were introducing and performing at our institute. In 1962 Pitanguy visited our hospital and was interested in the operation and the incisions I had used. He questioned me at length about the success of the procedure and how the patient was handled, and made drawings of my operation.

In the subsequent 3 years I tried to persuade other patients in New York City to have the thigh-lift operation performed, but it was neither a proven nor an acceptable operation, and few were willing to undergo such extensive and relatively untried surgery. I was slowly gathering several more cases over these intervening years until I could write a paper of my own describing my variation of the thigh-lift procedure, which had been stimulated by the articles of Lewis and Farina et al. [25, 60].

It therefore came as a rather unpleasant surprise 3 years later when Dr. Converse, my chief, came in one day to the clinic and waved a copy of the September 1964 issue of *Plastic and Reconstructive Surgery* under my nose and said, "I told you to write up that case." When I saw the operation described by Pitanguy [114], I was somewhat dismayed and annoyed at the same time. If there is anything to be learned from this, it is: surgical literary conservatism and hesitancy to publish what one thinks is a new technique until one can report numerous cases is rather foolish. I now strongly advocate that if any plastic surgeon believes he or she has performed a truly "new" and worthwhile operation not seen in published literature, it should be sent posthaste to the editors of *Aesthetic Plastic Surgery, Annals of Plastic Surgery,* the *British Journal of Plastic Surgery,* or *Plastic and Reconstructive Surgery,* and surely it should receive prompt attention.

In 1964, Pitanguy introduced his technique with his illustrations for the operation (note the similarities to my

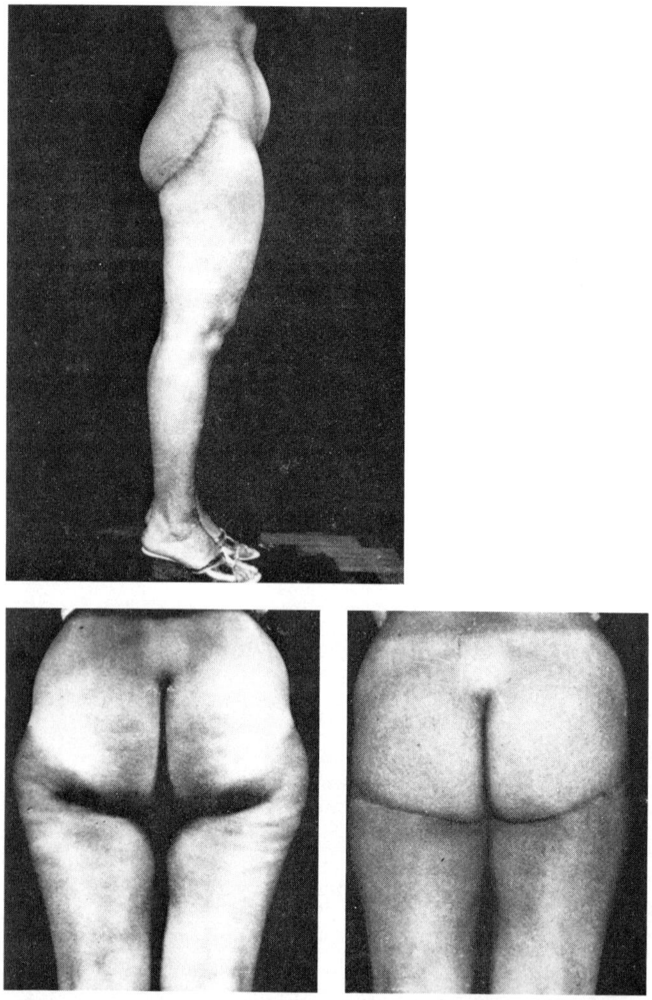

Figure 1-46. Photographs from Pitanguy's 1964 article showing preoperative appearance and postoperative results in patient following the thigh-lift. (From I. Pitanguy, Trochanteric lipodystrophy. *Plast. Reconstr. Surg.* 34:280, 1964.)

own drawings) (Fig. 1-45), and thus he started with his inestimable charm to draw the attention of the surgical world to the aesthetic feasibility of such an operation [114]. His aesthetic results in the two cases published were elegant (Fig. 1-46). Thus, in one bold stroke, according to a respected Brazilian contemporary plastic surgeon of Pitanguy's, "his publishing his technique opened a new door to bring even more plastic surgery patients to our specialty." He emphasized the need to place the incisions high up and deep in the gluteal folds, and since his 1964 paper only a dozen or more articles have appeared describing variations in the technique of thigh-lifting [33].

I leave the rest of the historical account of the development of aesthetic plastic surgery to be described in more detail by the individual authors of each chapter of this book. However, it would be remiss not to urge once again that the reader remember some of the names referred to in this chapter. They perhaps will have a subliminal effect on the reader and might at some time, during an academic examination or a friendly dialogue in the operating room, be brought once again into present day conversation to remind the reader of our audacious, bold, and imaginative forebears.

These physicians never knowingly intended to create the subspecialty of what is now known as aesthetic plastic surgery. In our continuing respect for them, let us once more repeat their names in alphabetical order: Bettman, Biesenberger, Bourguet, Czerny, Dieffenbach, Ely, Joseph, Kelly, Kolle, Lewis, Lexer, Miller, Morestin, Noël, Passot, Roe, Thomas, and Thorek. Other names may come to light in the future through the help of some, or hopefully many, medical historians who undoubtedly will appear on the scene.

REFERENCES

1. Aufricht, G. Philosophy of cosmetic surgery. *Plast. Reconstr. Surg.* 20:397, 1957.
2. Aufricht, G. The development of plastic surgery in the United States. *Plast. Reconstr. Surg.* 1:3, 1946.
3. Aufricht, G. Symposium on corrective rhinoplasty. *Plast. Reconstr. Surg.* 28:241, 1961.
4. Aufricht, G. Commentary on the paper: Operative reduction on the size of a nose (rhinomyosis) by Jacques Joseph. *Plast. Reconstr. Surg.* 46:181, 1970.
5. Berson, M. I. Derma-fat-fascia transplants used in building up the breasts. *Surgery* 15:451, 1945.
6. Bettman, A. G. Plastic and cosmetic surgery of the face. *Northwest Med.* 19:205, 1920.
7. Biesenberger, H. Eine neue Methode der Mammaplastik. *Zentralbl. Chir.* No. 38: p. 2382, 1928.
8. Biesenberger, H. Eine neue Methode der Mammaplastik. *Zentralbl. Chir.* No. 48: p. 2971, 1930.
9. Booth, F. A. Cosmetic surgery of the face, neck and breast. *Northwest Med.* 21:170, 1922.
10. Bourguet, J. II: La disparition chirurgicale des rides et plis du visage. *Bull. Acad. Natl. Méd.* (Paris) 82:183, 1919.
11. Bourguet, J. V. Les hernies graisseuses de l'orbite: Notre traitement chirurgical. *Bull. Acad. Natl. Méd.* (Paris) 92:1270, 1924.
12. Bourguet, J. Chirurgie esthétique de la face: Les nez concaves, les rides et les "poches" sous les yeux. *Arch. Prov. Chir.* 28:293, 1925.
13. Brown, J. B., and McDowell, F. *Plastic Surgery of the Nose* (3rd ed.). Springfield, Ill.: Thomas, 1951.
14. Converse, J. M. Commentary on Roe's "pug nose" operation and Roe's life. *Plast. Reconstr. Surg.* 45:82, 1970.
15. Cottle, M. H. John Orlando Roe: Pioneer in modern rhinoplasty. *Arch. Otolaryngol.* 80:22, 1964.
16. Czerny V. V. Korrektur der Sattelnase durch Bildung eines Nasenrückens aus dem knorplig-knöchernen Seitendache der Nase. *Chir. Kongr. Verhanol.* 2:214, 1895.
17. Czerny V. V. Plastischer Ersatz der Brustdrüse durch ein Lipom. *Zentralbl. Chir.* 27:72, 1895.
18. Davis, J. S. *Plastic Surgery: Its Principles and Practice.* Philadelphia: P. Blakiston, 1919.
19. Davis, J. E., and Hernandez, H. H. History of the aesthetic surgery of the ear. *Aesthetic Plast. Surg.* 2:75, 1978.
20. Denecke, H. J., and Meyer, R. *Plastic Surgery of the Head and Neck. Vol. 1: Corrective and Reconstructive Rhinoplasty.* New York; Springer, 1967.
21. de Quervain, F. Zur operativen Behandlung der Hängebrust. *Zentralbl. Chir.* 43:2423, 1925.

22. Dieffenbach, J. F. *Die operative Chirurgie.* Leipzig; F. A. Brockhaus, 1845.
23. Eckstein, H. Ueber subkutane und submukose Hartparaffinprothesen. *Dtsch. Med. Wochenschr.* 28:573, 1902.
24. Ely, E. T. An operation for prominence of the auricles. *Arch. Otolaryngol.* 10:97, 1881; also in *Plast. Reconstr. Surg.* 42:582, 1968.
25. Farina, R., Baroudi, R., Golcman, B., and de Castro, O. Riding trousers like type of pelvicrural lipodystrophy (trochanteric lipomatoses). *Br. J. Plast. Surg.* 13:174, 1960.
26. Flesch-Thebesius, M., and Weisheimer, K. Die Operation des Hängebauches. *Chirurgie* 3:841, 1931.
27. Fomon, S., and Bell, J. *Rhinoplasty—New Concepts: Evaluation and Application.* Springfield, Ill.: Thomas, 1970.
28. Frühwald, V. Über einen Fall von Hängewange behoben durch eine Modifikation der Joseph'schen Operation. *Wien. Med. Wochenschr.* 33:1336, 1922.
29. Gersuny, R. Ueber eine subcutane Prothese. *Z. Heilkd.* 1:199, 1900.
30. Gillies, H. D., and Millard, D. R., Jr. *The Principles and Art of Plastic Surgery.* Boston: Little, Brown, 1957.
31. Goldwyn, R. M. Johann Friedrich Dieffenbach (1794–1847). *Plast. Reconstr. Surg.* 42:18, 1968.
32. Gonzalez-Ulloa, M. The history of rhytidectomy. *Aesthetic Plast. Surg.* 4:1, 1980.
33. Grazer, F. M., and Klingbeil, J. R. *Body Image: A Surgical Perspective.* St. Louis: Mosby, 1980.
34. Grigg, E. R. N. *The Trail of the Impossible Light.* Springfield, Ill.: Thomas, 1965.
35. Holländer, E. *Die Medizin in der klassischen Malerei.* Stuttgart: F. Enke, 1903.
36. Holländer, E. XVII. Die kosmetische Chirurgie. In M. Joseph (ed.), *Handbuch der Kosmetik.* Leipzig: Verlag von Veit, 1912. P. 688.
37. Holländer, E. *Die kosmetische Chirurgie.* Leipzig: Vexit, 1922. Pp. 708–710.
38. Holländer, E. Plastische (Kosmetische) Operation: Kritische Darstellung ihres gegenwärtigen Standes. In G. Klemperer and F. Klemperer (eds.), *Neue Deutsche Klinik, Vol. 9.* Berlin: Urban and Schwarzenberg, 1932. Pp. 1–17.
39. Hunt, H. L. New theory of the function of the prostate deduced from gland transplantation in physicians. *Endocrinology* 9:479, 1925.
40. Hunt, H. L. *Plastic Surgery of the Head, Face and Neck.* Philadelphia: Lea & Febiger, 1926.
41. Joseph, J. Ueber die operative Verkleinerung einer Nase (rhinomiosis). *Berl. Klin. Wochenschr.* 40:882, 1898; also in *Plast. Reconstr. Surg.* 46:178, 1970.
42. Joseph, J. Ueber einige weitere Nasenverkleinerungen. *Berl. Klin. Wochenschr.* P. 851, 1902.
43. Joseph, J. Nasenverkleinerungen. *Dtsch. Med. Wochenschr.* 30:1095, 1904.
44. Joseph, J. Intranasale Nasenhöckerabtragung. *Berl. Klin. Wochenschr.* P. 650, 1904.
45. Joseph, J. Weiteres über Nasenverkleinerungen. *Münch. Med. Wochenschr.* 52:1489, 1905.
46. Joseph, J. Beiträge zur Rhinoplastik. *Berl. Klin. Wochenschr.* 44:470, 1907.
47. Joseph, J. Nasenkorrekturen. *Ver. Dtsch. Ges. Naturforschr. Ärzte* (Königsberg) Pt. 2, Vol. 2, sec. 2, p. 340, 1910.
48. Joseph, J. Beiträge zur totalen Rhinoplastik. *Münch. Med. Wochenschr.* 51:705, 1914.
49. Joseph, J. Zur Gesichtplastik mit besonderer Berücksichtigung der Nasenplastik. *Dtsch. Med. Wochenschr.* P. 35, 1919.
50. Joseph, J. Hängewangenplastik (Melomioplastik). *Dtsch. Med. Wochenschr.* 47:287, 1921.
51. Joseph, J. Beiträge zur totalen und partiellen Rhinoneoplastik nebst einem Vorschlage zur freien Hautüberpflanzung. *Klin. Wochenschr.* 14:678, 1922.
52. Joseph, J. In Katz and Blumenfeld (eds.), *Handbuch der speziellen Chirurgie.* Leipzig: Verlag von Curt Kabitzsch, 1922.
53. Joseph, J. Verbesserung meiner Hängewangenplastik (Melomioplastik). *Dtsch. Med. Wochenschr.* 54:567, 1928.
54. Joseph, J. *Nasenplastik und sonstige Gesichtsplastik nebst einem Anhang über Mammaplastik.* Leipzig: Verlag von Curt Kabitzsch, 1928–1931.
55. Kelly, H. A. Case 3. Excessive growth of fat. *Johns Hopkins Hospital Bulletin* No. 103, p. 197, 1899.
56. Kelly, H. A. Excision of the fat of the abdominal wall: Lipectomy. *Surg. Gynecol. Obstet.* 11:229, 1910.
57. Kolle, F. S. *Subcutaneous Hydrocarbon Prostheses.* New York: The Grafton Press, 1908.
58. Kolle, F. S. *Plastic and Cosmetic Surgery.* New York: D. Appleton and Co., 1911.
59. Lalardrie, J. P., and Mouly, R. History of mammaplasty. *Aesthetic Plast. Surg.* 2:167, 1978.
60. Lewis, J. H., Jr. The thigh lift. *J. Int. Coll. Surg.* 27:330, 1957.
61. Lexer, E. Zwanzig Jahre Transplantationsforschung in Chirurgie. *Arch. klin. Chir.* 138:251, 1925.
62. Lexer, E. Zur Operation der mammahypertrophie und der Hängebrust. *Dtsch. Med. Wochenschr.* 51:26, 1925.
63. Lexer, E. *Die gesamte Wiederherstellungschirurgie, Vol. 2.* Leipzig; J. A. Barth, 1931. P. 548.
64. Linhart, W. Beiträge zur Rhinoplastik. *Würzb. Med. Z.* 1:37, 1860.
65. Maliniac, J. W. *Rhinoplasty and Restoration of Facial Contour.* Philadelphia: Davis, 1947.
66. May, H. *Reconstructive and Reparative Surgery.* Philadelphia: Davis, 1947. P. 146.
67. May, H. Erich Lexer: A biographical sketch. *Plast. Reconstr. Surg.* 29:141, 1962.
68. McDowell, F. (ed.). *The Source Book of Plastic Surgery.* Baltimore: Williams & Wilkins, 1977.
69. McDowell, F. History of rhinoplasty. *Aesthetic Plast. Surg.* 1:321, 1978.
70. McDowell, F., Vallone, J. A., and Brown, J. B. Bibliography and historical note on plastic surgery of the nose. *Plast. Reconstr. Surg.* 10:149, 1952.
71. Miller, C. C. Practical elective surgery for the general practitioner. *Wis. Med. Recorder* 8:274, 313, 349, 1905.
72. Miller, C. C. The surgical reduction of the nasal tip of excessive length. *Ala. Med. J.* 19:620, 1906.
73. Miller, C. C. Surgical treatment of the hump nose. *Med. Brief* 34:160, 1906.
74. Miller, C. C. The excision of bag-like folds of skin from the region about the eyes. *Med. Brief* 34:648, 1906.
75. Miller, C. C. Outstanding alae nasi. *Am. J. Dermatol. Genitourin. Dis.* 11:286, 1907.
76. Miller, C. C. Semilunar excision of the skin at the outer canthus for the eradication of "crow's feet." *Am. J. Dermatol. Genitourin. Dis.* 11:483, 1907.
77. Miller, C. C. Subcutaneous section of the facial muscles to eradicate expression lines. *Am. J. Surg.* 21:235, 1907.
78. Miller, C. C. *The Correction of Featural Imperfections.* Chicago: Oak Printing Co., 1907.
79. Miller, C. C. The surgical treatment of excessively thick and everted lips. *Cincinnati Lancet Clinic* 98:303, 1907.
80. Miller, C. C. The eradication by surgical means of the nasolabial line. *Ther. Gaz.* (Detroit) 23:676, 1907.
81. Miller, C. C. Cosmetic surgery of the face. *Int. J. Surg.* 20:311, 1907.

82. Miller, C. C., and Miller, F. Folds, bags and wrinkles of the skin about the eyes and their eradication by simple surgical methods. *Med. Brief* 35:540, 1907.
83. Miller, C. C. The nasal tip as a factor in marring the appearance of the face. *Milwaukee Med. J.* 15:277, 1907.
84. Miller, C. C. The dimple surgically produced. *Mobile Med. Surg. J.* 11:1–3, 1907.
85. Miller, C. C. Subcutaneous division of the fibers of the orbicularis muscle for overcoming "crow's feet." *Med. Times* (New York) 35:207, 1907.
86. Miller, C C. The correction of inverted lips by surgery. *Med. Bull.* (Phila.) 29:288, 1907.
87. Miller, C. C. The proper surgical treatment of the nose with the bulbous tip. *Med. Council* (Phila.) 12:273, 1907.
88. Miller, C. C. External canthotomy and section of the fibers of the orbicularis palpebrarum for minimizing "crow's feet." *St. Louis Clin.* 20:213, 1907.
89. Miller, C. C. The reduction of the tip tilted nose. *Med. Fort.* (St. Louis) 32:309, 1907.
90. Miller, C. C. The surgical reduction of the excessively large ear. *Med. Fort.* (St. Louis) 32:354, 1907.
91. Miller, C. C. Hypertrophy and elongation of the nasal tip and its surgical treatment. *Toledo Med. Surg. Rep.* 33:405, 1907.
92. Miller, C. C. The surgical treatment of excessively thick lips. *Va. Med. Semi-monthly* 12:249, 1907–1908.
93. Miller, C. C. The surgical correction of the excessively thick lip and the markedly everted lip. *Va. Med. Semi-monthly* 12:300, 1907–1908.
94. Miller, C. C. *The Care of Rupture by Paraffin Injections.* Chicago: Oak Printing Co., 1908.
95. Miller, C. C. *The Correction of Featural Imperfections.* (2nd ed.). Chicago: Oak Printing Co., 1908.
96. Miller, C. C. Triangular excisions of the mucosa for operation for down turning of the angles of the mouth. *Med. Council* (Phila.) 13:123, 1908.
97. Miller, C. C. Displacement of the nasal tip as a means of altering the appearance of the face. *Med. Brief* (St. Louis) 36:570, 1908.
98. Miller C. C. The most rapid, effective and least bloody method of turbinal removal. *Med. Fort.* (St. Louis) 34:491, 1908.
99. Miller, C. C. The surgical reduction of the nose of excessive length. *Wis. Med. Recorder* 11:217, 1908.
100. Miller, C. C. The limitations and use of paraffin in cosmetic surgery. *Wis. Med. Recorder* 11:277, 1908.
101. Miller, C. C. *Cosmetic Surgery: The Correction of Featural Imperfections.* Philadelphia: Davis, 1925.
102. Monks, G. H. Correction, by operation, of some nasal deformities and disfigurements. *Boston Med. Surg. J.* 139:262, 1898; also in *Plast. Reconstr. Surg.* 48:485, 1971.
103. Morestin, H. La réduction granduelle des difformités tégumentaires. (Translated by John Marquis Converse.) *Plast. Reconstr. Surg.* 42:163, 1968, with commentary by Dr. Converse on p. 172.
104. Morestin, H., and Guinard, A. Hypertrophie mammaire traitée par la résection discoïde. *Bull. Soc. Chir.* (Paris) 33:649, 1907.
105. Natvig, P. Some aspects of the character and personality of Jacques Joseph. *Plast. Reconstr. Surg.* 47:452, 1971.
106. Noël, A. *La Chirurgie Esthétique: Son Rôle Social.* Paris: Masson, 1926.
107. Noël, A. *Die ästhetische Chirurgie und ihre soziale Bedeutung.* Leipzig: Johann Ambrosius Barth, 1932.
108. Passot, R. La chirurgie esthétique des rides du visages. *Presse Méd.* 27:258, 1919.
109. Passot, R. II. La correction chirurgicale des rides du visage. *Bull. Acad. Natl. Méd.* 82:112, 1919.
110. Passot, R. Atrophie mammaire: Réfection esthétique par la greffe graisseuse épiploïque. *Presse Méd.* 37:627, 1930.
111. Passot, R. *Chirurgie Esthétique Pure (Technique et Résultats).* Paris: G. Doin, 1931.
112. Peer, L. A. A loss of weight and volume in human fat grafts. *Plast. Reconstr. Surg.* 5:217, 1950.
113. Peters, L. Resection of the pendulous, fat abdominal wall in cases of extreme obesity. *Ann. Surg.* 33:299, 1901.
114. Pitanguy, I. Trochanteric lipodystrophy. *Plast. Reconstr. Surg.* 34:280, 1964.
115. Regnault, P. The history of abdominal dermolipectomy. *Aesthetic Plast. Surg.* 2:113, 1978.
116. Regnault, P., and Stephenson, K. L. Dr. Suzanne Noël: The first woman to do esthetic surgery. *Plast. Reconstr. Surg.* 48:133, 1971.
117. Robin, G. Dr. Suzanne Noël. In *Dictionnaire National des Contemporains, Vol. 1.* Paris: La Jeunesse, 1936. P. 461.
118. Roe, J. O. The deformity termed pug nose and its correction by a simple operation. *Med. Rec.* 31:621, 1887; also in *Plast. Reconstr. Surg.* 45:78, 1970.
119. Roe, J. O. The correction of angular deformities of the nose by a subcutaneous operation. *Med. Rec.* 40:57, 1891.
120. Roe, J. O. Correction of depressed and saddle back deformities of nose by operations performed subcutaneously without aid of metallic or other artificial supports. *Med. Rec.* 51:798, 1897.
121. Roe, J. O. Case of fracture and depression of anterior wall of maxillary antrum, with restoration of depressed wall. *Trans. Am. Laryngol. Assoc.* P. 203, 1898.
122. Roe, J. O. Correction of nasal deformities by subcutaneous operations. *Am. Med. Quart.* 1:56, 1899.
123. Roe, J. O. New operation for restoration of columna and anterior portion of nasal septum. *Trans. Am. Laryngol. Assoc.* P. 221, 1902.
124. Roe, J. O. Removal of obstructions and cicatricial contractions of nose by plastic method. *Trans. Am. Laryngol. Assoc.* P. 257, 1903.
125. Roe, J. O. The correction of nasal deformities. *Laryngoscope* 18:782, 1908.
126. Roe, J. O. Nasal deformity as cause of nasal obstruction corrected by subcutaneous method. *Trans. Am. Laryngol. Assoc.* P. 285, 1915.
127. Rogers, B. O. Ely's 1881 operation for correction of protruding ears: A medical "first." *Plast. Reconstr. Surg.* 42:584, 1968.
128. Rogers, B. O. Carl Ferdinand von Graefe (1787–1840). *Plast. Reconstr. Surg.* 46:554, 1970.
129. Rogers, B. O. A chronologic history of cosmetic surgery. *Bull. N.Y. Acad. Med.* 47:265, 1971.
130. Rogers, B. O. A brief history of cosmetic surgery. *Surg. Clin. North Am.* 51:265, 1971.
131. Rogers, B. O. The development of aesthetic plastic surgery: A history. *Aesthetic Plast. Surg.* 1:3, 1976.
132. Rogers, B. O. Early Historical Development of Corrective Rhinoplasty. In R. D. Millard, Jr. (ed.), *Symposium on Corrective Rhinoplasty.* St. Louis: Mosby, 1976. P. 18.
133. Rogers, B. O. Historical Development of Gluteal Trochanteric Lipectomy. Paper delivered at the XIth Instructional Course of the International Society of Aesthetic Plastic Surgery, Lausanne, June 28–July 1, 1978 and the XVth Instructional Course of the International Society of Aesthetic Plastic Surgery, South African Association of Plastic Surgeons, Bophuthatswana, October 23–24, 1980. In press.
134. Rogers, B. O. Julius von Szymanowski (1829–1868): His

life and contributions to plastic surgery. *Plast. Reconstr. Surg.* 64:465, 1979.

135. Rogers, B. O. Nasal reconstruction 150 years ago: Aesthetic and other problems. *Aesthetic Plast. Surg.* 5:283, 1981.
136. Rogers, B. O. Hippolyte Morestin (1869–1919): Part I: A brief biography. *Aesthetic Plast. Surg.* 6:141, 1982.
137. Rousset. Thèse sur la Rhinoplastie. Thèse de Paris, 1828. Cited by C. Nelaton, and L. Ombrédanne. La Rhinoplastie. Paris: G. Steinheil, 1904.
138. Safian, J. *Corrective Rhinoplastic Surgery.* New York: Paul B. Hoeber, 1935.
139. Sanvenero-Rosselli, G. *Chirurgia Plastica del Naso.* Rome: Luigi Pozzi, 1931.
140. Schörcher, F. *Kosmetische Operationen.* München: J. F. Lehmanns Verlag, 1955.
141. Schwarzman, E. Die Technik der Mammaplastik. *Chirurg.* 2:932, 1930.
142. Seltzer, A. P. *Plastic Surgery of the Nose.* Philadelphia: Lippincott, 1949.
143. Shakespeare, W. The second part of Henrie the fourth, continuing to his death. . . . London: printed by V. S. for Andrew Wise and William Aspley, 1600, Act I, Sc. 2, line 204.
144. Sheehan, J. E. *Plastic Surgery of the Nose.* New York: Paul Hoeber Co., 1925.
145. Sheen, J. H. *Aesthetic Rhinoplasty.* St. Louis: Mosby, 1978.
146. Stephenson, K. L. The history of blepharoplasty to correct blepharochalasis. *Aesthetic Plast. Surg.* 1:177, 1977.
147. Thomas, T. G. On the removal of benign tumors of the mamma without mutilation of the organ. *Trans. N.Y. Obstet. Soc.* Pp. 76–80, Feb. 21, 1882.
148. Thorek, M. Possibilities in reconstruction of the human form. *N.Y. Med. J. Rec.* 116:572, 1922.
149. Thorek, M. Plastic reconstruction of the female breasts and abdomen. *Am. J. Surg.* 43:268, 1939.
150. Thorek, M. *Plastic Surgery of the Breast and Abdominal Wall.* Springfield, Ill.: Thomas, 1942.
151. Vernon, S. Umbilical transplantation upward and abdominal contouring in lipectomy. *Am. J. Surg.* 94:490, 1957.
152. von Szymanowski, J. *Handbuch der operativen Chirurgie.* Braunschweig, Germany: F. Vieweg u. Sohn, 1870.
153. Weinhold, S. Bauchdeckenplastik. *Zentralbl. f. Gynäk.* No. 38, p. 1332, 1909.
154. Weir, R. F. On restoring sunken noses. *N.Y. Med. J.* 56:449, 1892.

2. Aesthetic Surgery: Basic Principles

Robert M. Goldwyn

A unique feature of aesthetic surgery is the confusion about its name and definition as well as its spelling. Many plastic surgeons prefer the word *aesthetic* to *cosmetic* in order to avoid the connotations of makeup and beauty parlors. Aside from purposes of literary style, placing an *a* before esthetic serves also to upgrade the image by conferring on it a classic lineage. This apologetic stance is seen also in another common practice: using more impressive names for procedures usually called *face-lift (rhytidectomy)* or *eyelidplasty (blepharoplasty), nose job* or *nasal surgery (rhinoplasty).* Like any fledgling, aesthetic surgery has had to fight for its place within the medical establishment. In many ways, its growth and development is similar to that of psychiatry where the need for it preceded by many decades its acceptance by the older embedded specialties.

Some surgeons choose to call cosmetic or aesthetic surgery the surgery of appearance or body-image surgery to imply more than bringing about only superficial changes. The definition of cosmetic surgery by the American Society of Plastic and Reconstructive Surgeons is as follows:

> Cosmetic surgery shall be defined as that surgery which is done to review or change the texture, configuration, or relationship with contiguous structures of any feature of the human body which would be considered by the average observer to be within the broad range of "normal" and acceptable variation for age and ethnic origin, and in addition is performed for a condition which is judged by competent medical opinion to be without potential for jeopardy to physical or mental health [1].

This attempt to provide something useful to insurance companies, which must decide whether or not to defray costs, is awkward, albeit valiant. Where beauty ends and function, anatomic and psychologic, begins has been the subject of controversy and an arena for inconsistency for millennia. As an example, is it simply "aesthetic" to rebuild a missing breast? For several years some insurance companies would not pay for breast reconstruction but would for restoring a nose deformed by cancer and its treatment. Yet the ability to smell and breathe remains essentially unchanged after the reconstruction.

The concern with appearance is not a peripheral matter for most human beings [9, 17, 21, 22, 29]. Every society has a standard of beauty, a hierarchy of values pertaining to what is pleasing or ugly to the eye. Admittedly, there is great variation among societies, but within each culture, standards of attractiveness are not ambiguous. Furthermore, evidence for the need to embellish our bodies can be found among our earliest traces. This urge has taken different forms: using makeup, styling hair, scarifying flesh, distorting lips and earlobes, binding feet, and performing circumcision, the last being an example of modifying the body in order to confer group identity and solidarity. Today's patient coming for cosmetic surgery also has in mind the group to which he or she wishes or does not wish to belong. Although motivations for the surgery of appearance may not be expressed or may be articulated in terms of personal goals, they nevertheless must be judged also in their social and cultural context [21, 22].

We tend to regard cosmetic surgery as a phenomenon of technically advanced societies. Indeed, cosmetic procedures require some measure of economic adequacy; however, we should not forget that subsistent societies, even in crisis, such as war, engage in body modification.

The dichotomy between appearance and function, between vanity and modesty, has had reverberations throughout recorded history. While the Scriptures admonish against "vanity," they contain also many passages extolling human beauty. No society can live on dessert alone, but none seems able to survive on just bread. The proper mixture becomes the challenge since the need for both has long been demonstrated. How society decides rationally or irrationally at any particular time what is "useful" and what is not or how it apportions its resources necessarily affects its members and their views on aesthetic surgery. The increasing popularity of aesthetic surgery throughout most of the world indicates its need and its greater acceptance and availability. The effect is cyclic: Demand increases supply, and supply augments demand.

SPECIAL CHARACTERISTICS OF AESTHETIC SURGERY

Enhancement

An important characteristic of aesthetic surgery is that the patient considers the result of the operation an enhancement, not a loss as is usual after other procedures, such as cholecystectomy or hysterectomy. The benefits are objective as well as subjective. A person who is better looking becomes more socially desirable. The importance of physical beauty has been generally downplayed, particularly by intellectuals in our democratic society, whose shibboleth is that by hard work everyone can achieve equality. Reluctance among some social psychologists and psychiatrists to recognize the pivotal significance of physical beauty is surprisingly inconsistent because our society, for example, touts fashion models and athletes. Good physical attributes are important not just in those specialized roles. Walster and associates [29] found that physical attractiveness was the most important personal characteristic influencing how much one is liked in a man-woman dating situation. Especially for the woman, good looks are the passport to popularity and upward mobility. The confluence of beauty, wealth, and power is a universal phenomenon. Literally, it pays to be beautiful.

Kalick [17] conducted an experiment in which subjects viewed preoperative and postoperative photographs. Individuals pictured postoperatively were judged to have more desirable personalities, to be better potential marriage partners, and to have happier lives than the same persons photographed before operation. Since all the impressions were from photographs, actual personality was not a factor in the study. Kalick's findings and those of other researchers suggest that aesthetic surgery may have a stronger social impact on patients' lives than had been assumed. The "enhancement" of appearance from the operative procedure is not only in the mind of the patient but also in the minds of those around him or her. These beneficial effects are found not only in a dating situation but also in an occupational setting. Some executives, in fact, have credited their rise to a cosmetic procedure. Whether or not the operation itself directly accomplished this by changing their appearance is difficult to know. Perhaps it was the fact that because they felt better about themselves they were able to project themselves more favorably.

Elective Nature of the Surgery

Unlike almost every other surgical situation, operating for aesthetic reasons is totally elective, more so even than in other areas of plastic surgery, where the objective is to restore (reimplantation) or replace (by means of a flap or skin graft) a missing part. For the aesthetic surgical patient, survival is rarely the issue. He or she is usually in good health and willing to risk it in order to achieve a better self-image. The plastic surgeon, in fact, makes well patients ill in order to make them feel better—about themselves.

Because patients are usually well and the proposed procedure is seldom life-threatening, the prognosis in terms of morbidity and mortality is excellent. Anticipated pain is minimal; complicated ancillary procedures and prolonged nursing are unnecessary.

The fact that an aesthetic operation is elective allows the patient and the surgeon time to decide. The patient can obtain additional consultations and frequently does. The surgeon need not feel forced into operating as he or she might otherwise, in an emergency.

Guilt and Embarrassment

It is not unusual for a patient seeking an aesthetic procedure to feel guilty about wanting it. He or she as well as family or friends might consider this step "frivolous." Frequently, such a patient will apologize for "taking your valuable time" or being in the office or in the hospital when "other patients need you more and are much sicker."

A patient, especially if older, who is to have a cosmetic operation may receive little or no emotional support from loved ones, unlike patients with life-threatening disease, who are cajoled and even forced to go to the doctor. Family physicians, also, may try to thwart the cosmetic patient. Often a patient tells the plastic surgeon not to write to his or her internist because "he would never approve."

Finances

For the cosmetic patient, going it alone as a modus operandi applies also to financial aspects. Insurance plans generally do not cover so-called cosmetic surgery and many will not defray the expenses of treating a complication. Prepayment to the surgeon and the hospital is customary for aesthetic operations, unlike most other areas of medicine, except, perhaps, for orthodontia.

Rapid Recovery and Little Regression

Most aesthetic operations are not prolonged and dangerous. Most can be done under local anesthesia, with or without intravenous supplementation, and commonly on an outpatient basis. Even when general anesthesia is used, patients regain consciousness quickly and are often discharged the same day or the next. Contact with the environment, therefore, is almost constant. Because rapid recovery is the rule, they usually are back to work early. For the cosmetic patient there is little incentive for secondary gain by delaying the resumption of normal activities. In fact, most patients do not want anyone to know that they are having a face-lift or a blepharoplasty, for example. Because they expect to return soon to normal, any complication becomes harder to surmount; it strains the doctor-patient relationship because emotionally it was unexpected, even though the patient was told that it could happen.

Minimizing the Surgical Reality

In the relationship between the surgeon and the aesthetic patient, there are features and pressures that lead each to minimize the surgical reality [7, 12]. The patient has usually read or heard that an aesthetic operation is relatively simple. Most articles in the lay press would give the impression that complications are unusual and that an excellent result is customary. When the surgeon tries to tell the patient about possible complications, the patient may be primed not to hear or not to remember them. If the patient truly expected, for example, ectropion, infection, or blindness from a blepharoplasty, he or she would never have it done. The surgeon, by doing the procedure under local anesthesia on an ambulatory basis, may perpetuate the notion that this is not "real surgery," which usually, in the patient's mind, involves general anesthesia and at least a few days or a week in the hospital, with the implication of a greater likelihood of serious complications and longer recuperation.

Sometimes the surgeon reinforces the patient's conception that the surgery is "only skin deep." Questions about the patient's past medical history may be superficial and the physical examination may be only regional—that is, inspection of the nose only if a rhinoplasty is to be done. A few patients have seemed surprised when I asked them details about their health. One of them said, "I just want to have my eyes done and you are questioning me like my internist." This kind of patient is not ready to think of a possible complication. Should it occur, despite her being well informed, in words and in writing, she will be astonished and even angry since such an event was not in her life plan. The fact that aesthetic surgery may be done in a doctor's office is convenient for the patient but may also add to his or her misconception that it is not truly an operation, which most patients usually associate with a hospital setting.

Sometimes the words describing the procedure add to the fantasy. For example, *tummy-tuck* is used for an abdominoplasty. If judged by the name alone, what could possibly go wrong with a tummy-tuck? If, however, the operation were routinely termed *abdominal surgery to remove excess skin and tighten loose muscles,* it would have a different and more realistic connotation.

Preponderance of Women

Another distinctive feature of aesthetic surgery is that at least 85 to 90 percent of patients are women [15]. The reasons are not anatomic, as in gynecology, but cultural and personal. That most surgeons performing cosmetic surgery are men is also an important fact. Our culture places a higher value on the attractive appearance of women than on that of men; and many women, deprived of the many sources of gratification available to men, have learned to use and value their bodies, consciously and unconsciously, to please themselves and others. This behavior is rewarded, perpetuated, and reinforced throughout their lives by such acts as using makeup, adopting hair and clothing styles, and keeping "young and trim."

As a father of two daughters, I found it unsettling to read on occasion the magazines geared for teenaged girls. Almost every issue in its entirety was devoted to attracting boys and to enhancing physical features. Rare was an article on professional careers or social issues. From childhood, women feel obliged to change or maintain their bodies to promote pleasure for others and consequently for themselves. Aiding them in the battle for beauty is the plastic surgeon along with the many other agencies and resources within the culture. Usually a man, as noted, the plastic surgeon does not think it strange for a woman to enhance her appearance through an operation. What we now accept as part of our culture may change with the rise of feminism. However, there is no indication yet that plastic surgical procedures have decreased in relative frequency.

Happiness as an Objective

Aesthetic surgery involves the elusive objective of "happiness." Results of psychotherapy are also judged in terms of that hard-to-define (and to acquire) mental state, whereas in most of medicine the efficacy of therapy is ordinarily measured in decreased pain or increased function. It would be unusual to ask a patient after a cholecystectomy to assess his degree of "happiness" or "unhappiness." Patient satisfaction in aesthetic surgery becomes as important as patient morbidity and survival in other contexts of medicine. For this reason, an operation's results, if measured by the wobbly yardstick of happiness, become hard to assess. If a patient is not happier after a face-lift, for example, she may feel that the operation was a failure even though it was a success from a technical standpoint.

THE INITIAL CONSULTATION

Doctor-Patient Relationship

The phrase *doctor-patient relationship* has become almost a cliché but it still denotes a special interaction [8, 16, 23]. Although it has been called a "two-party contract," it contains much that is noncontractual—intangibles that cannot be guaranteed in any legal agreement between two people. Indeed, the confusion in the doctor-patient interchange relates to these impalpable but critical components of concern and compassion [24–26]. Patients want more than having a service performed.

Much has been written about what happens when a patient and a doctor meet for the first time. For purposes here, it is important to emphasize that although the initial consultation may bring together two people who have never known each other before, the scene was set long ago. Into that meeting each carries an established personality with behavior patterns evolved from innumerable responses to countless stimuli; each has had thousands of social interactions—for the patient, some probably also of a medical nature. The doctor too has no doubt been a patient on more than one occasion. The patient and the doctor will behave in a way that each perceives as the proper role of being the doctor or being the patient—roles culturally defined and traditionally taught.

In theory the patient and the doctor could interact in infinite ways but in reality they do not. While there are unpredictable variations, there is always a predictable theme. In all cultures, the ones who are ill have a responsibility to help themselves get better with guidance from the healers, who are the physicians in our society [19, 27, 28]. Sickness is allowed under most circumstances, but it is not praised or perpetuated since no society could function effectively or survive if most of its members were unable to perform their tasks. For the doctor, the privileges and power that he or she may have are not without responsibilities. Physicians should be available and are expected to utilize maximally their skills to help the patient. They are also expected to behave with concern, compassion, dignity, and honesty. Furthermore, the physician is not supposed to exploit the patient, sexually, financially, or in any other way. In a world with so much mistrust, it is reassuring and even surprising to see how patients will reveal confidences, allow examination (and even photographs) of parts of the body not usually seen by strangers, and trust their lives to a person previously unknown to them except by name; sometimes, as in emergencies, even that is unknown. The fact that patient and doctor today can usually establish a satisfying relationship is not due wholly to the actions of each of them. The background is centuries old, and the relationship has lasted because it has fulfilled the needs of untold numbers of patients and physicians. The modern doctor and patient are the beneficiaries of an ancient legacy. By the same reasoning, a betrayal or a breach in the relationship between the patient and doctor of our day will have repercussions beyond those two specific individuals.

THE SETTING

Another important factor of the initial consultation is the setting: a private office, a private clinic, a clinic at a teaching hospital. Wherever the initial interaction takes place, the physician should remember that the patient—isolated from his or her usual environment—is on your turf. If a member of the family accompanies the patient, the physician may get some idea of the family dynamics but only at a distance and only partially. The most common location for the first contact between a surgeon and a patient seeking aesthetic surgery is a private office. During the time the patient is waiting, he or she is consciously and unconsciously forming an impression of the office and the surgeon. In reality, the physician is the office. The way it is furnished, decorated, equipped, and managed is an extension of the physician. Even the reading material is pertinent. Some surgeons who wish to give the impression that their clientele is sophisticated and wealthy are likely to subscribe to *Vogue* and *Réalités* rather than *Popular Mechanics* or *Baseball Digest.* The intended slant is toward upper-class women. Doctors may view this as a plus in their relationship with patients, but some patients may wonder whether they will be financially exploited if the ambience is lavish and stylish. Other patients, however, may feel reassured and comfortable because the doctor seems to understand their kind of people. Most patients expect at least that their doctor's office be clean, orderly, and attractive. Decor differs with geography, and what may appear modern in Beverly Hills might seem distasteful in Boston.

More important than how the office is decorated is how the doctor reacts to the patient. Qualities that most human beings appreciate are those that they like or should like in themselves: honesty, concern, and competence. That doctors vary in how they interact with patients is not surprising because of the wide range of personalities among human beings. Some are overtly warm; others, visibly cold and remote. While it may be possible to learn how to manage the negative aspects of one's personality, it would be too much to expect that at age 35 or older a surgeon could do an emotional somersault. More than that, it is not necessary since different physicians attract different patients. However, there is an irreducible minimum of manners and empathy below which a physician should not descend. The worst behavior is an uncaring attitude. The patient may make allowances for a doctor's being brisk, hurried, and harried but generally will not excuse a blatant lack of concern and sympathy [5, 6]. The patient does not want to feel like an intruder or a penitent. Keeping someone waiting excessively, without apologizing, or not listening, or accepting telephone interruptions, or signing or reading letters, or forgetting the patient's name is the mark of an inconsiderate human being. It accurately reflects a lack of esteem for the person in front of you.

Writing about a house call Osler once made, a neighbor wrote, "In a room full of discordant elements, he entered and saw only his patient and his patient's greatest need, and instantly the atmosphere was charged with kindly vitality. Everyone felt that the situation was under control . . . the moment Sir William gave you was yours . . . becoming wholly and entirely a part of the fabric of your life . . . he is one of those who have great possessions, gave all that he had" [18].

In addition to a caring attitude on the part of the doctor, the patient rightfully expects it from the staff. A hostile secretary or an unfeeling nurse does much to impede the relationship between the patient and the physician. The patient correctly concludes that the doctor who has such employees must sanction their actions.

Who accompanies the patient to the office is significant because it identifies the important human beings in that person's life. I encourage all patients to bring into the consultation whomever they wish. Sometimes the patient will be visibly relieved to have someone with him or her; other times, the offer may be rejected in order to preserve privacy.

THE MEDICAL HISTORY

A physician should never assume the reason for the patient's presence. On occasion a patient has asked, "I suppose you know why I am here?" The easy but dangerous reply to someone with a big nose is "Why, of course, you are here because you wish to have your nose changed," whereas the reality is that the patient has a concern about her prominent ears. This faux pas illustrates the first general admonition: Be a good listener. There is no need to interrupt a patient who is furnishing an adequate history. Sometimes a little forbearance is required of surgeons who pride themselves on their efficient yet inflexible routine, which is more like that of a precinct sergeant questioning a suspect than of a physician eliciting a history from a patient. Of course, when a patient becomes too discursive, the physician should gently lead him or her back to the central issue. But before asking the patient the reason for making the appointment, it is advantageous to put that person at ease. A few general remarks—wrongly demeaned by the term *small talk*—are useful. The patient may realize what the physician is trying to do, but that is no disadvantage since it indicates concern about the patient's feelings. Sometimes one can say to the patient directly, "You seem nervous to be here. That is quite common, but tell me why you are anxious about it." The physician's perception of the patient's discomfort is in itself reassuring, and patients who vent their feelings become more relaxed.

The medical history should be complete, not only with respect to the primary problem but with regard to all aspects of the patient's physical and mental health. Some physicians let patients complete a questionnaire; others have someone in the office to do it; still others perform that function themselves. The objective is to get the information and to be able to follow important leads. For this reason, I would encourage all physicians to take their own histories. I think this is the least one can expect from a doctor, especially one to whom someone is paying top money for services. "Saving time" by taking shortcuts during the initial consultation will probably waste time because of the undesirable consequences of an inexcusable omission.

With regard to the present illness, it is crucial to determine why the patient wants a procedure at this time in his or her life. What psychologic correlates does the patient expect from a physical change? The physician must determine what the person wants and why before telling him or her how to get it.

In the medical history, it is important to know about general health and allergies as well as previous operations and the patient's emotional reaction to those procedures.

The reader might protest my emphasis on completeness, saying that, after all, every physician, like any human being, must conform to the strictures of time. True, but there is no necessity to overschedule oneself to the degree that one cannot adequately evaluate a patient coming for the first time or returning for another visit. Remember that for the patient this appointment is unique although for the physician it may be the twentieth in a busy morning.

Admittedly, some surgeons can relax a patient more and find out more in a half hour than others can in an hour. However, a consultation that is too brief is dangerous and unsatisfying. One of the most common complaints of patients is "He didn't spend enough time with me." Usually, what the patient is bemoaning is that the consultation left him or her emotionally unfulfilled even though the physician during that period might have been able to diagnose accurately and to recommend appropriately. The doctor might argue, "There was no need to spend any more time with her." Whose need? The essence of medicine, its joy as well as its difficulty, is the fact that, as physicians, we do not simply dispense a measured service. If the surgeon views himself as a mechanic, he is truly operating a body shop. Fortunately, or unfortunately, human beings are not insensate vehicles. I once overheard a patient tell a friend that her gynecologist was "a very good surgeon but he is not really like a doctor—you know, you can never talk to him about anything."

PATIENT SELECTION FOR AESTHETIC SURGERY

Some patients should not have cosmetic surgery; their soma or psyche makes them unsuitable. A well-executed procedure will not necessarily produce a happy or satisfied patient [7]. While it is true that if we operated on everyone who came to us we probably would be correct in 90 percent of instances; but that batting average is not high enough. One error can be a disaster not only for the patient but for ourselves. In the practice of medicine, and particularly in performing aesthetic surgery, we have to hit home runs, with perhaps a triple every once in a while. Anything less on a frequent basis would be unacceptable.

Let us consider types of patients for whom an operation might lead to an unhappy outcome [13].

The Patient Who Writes an Excessively Long Letter to Arrange the Initial Consultation

Generally, the letter contains an obsessively described saga of repeated dissatisfaction following multiple treatments of a condition that may or may not be as serious as the patient imagines. Often, the patient may be persisting in complaining about a minor problem that you will probably never solve. Perhaps several surgeons have already attempted to correct the difficulty. This does not mean that you should not see the patient, but you should be aware that the patient may be so perfectionistic that nothing you could accomplish surgically would relieve the anxiety. Commonly, this type of patient will profess great relief at having finally found someone as competent as you. Be wary.

The Rude or "Pushy" Patient

Some patients refuse to accept the next open appointment but insult or try to bypass the secretary to have you see them earlier. They may even have a doctor or friend call you at home at night. It is hard to say no to this kind of patient. If you take him or her out of order, your office staff may protest because you have ignored them unfairly and have been unjust to others on the waiting list. Patients who are distastefully aggressive want to be treated as exceptions, and their great self-entitlement may make them difficult to have as patients, especially if complications ensue.

The Unkempt Patient

While it is true that some patients with a pervasive deformity such as macromastia may "let themselves go," a dirty or slovenly appearance may indicate a severely disturbed personality. Cleanliness is the minimum that one should expect from a patient seeking aesthetic surgery. The Bowery look may prompt you to consider psychiatric referral.

The Patient Who Makes Your Office His or Her Home

If a patient whom you have never met is looking through your books and papers on your desk and calls you by your first name, you should react negatively to this inappropriate intimacy. Patients who act this way wish to be in control by establishing a relationship that is truly unsuitable. Their behavior may indicate underlying anxiety about dependency, which they are trying to overcome by dominating every situation. They attempt to direct their own care. Sometimes it may be necessary to remind the patient that *you* are the surgeon and he or she is the patient. Frequently, the patient acquiesces very easily, almost thankful that you now carry the responsibility.

The Patient Who Praises You Excessively and Denigrates Your Colleagues

This may be the same person who writes an inordinately long letter to arrange the initial consultation. A patient who builds you up is equally capable of cutting you down, just as he or she has done with past physicians. Early in practice, one may fall into the trap because of one's own vulnerability and desire for praise and recognition. Doctors, like all human beings, have difficulty in resisting flattery, even if it is insincere.

The Patient Who Gives a False History

Some patients profess that they have never been to a plastic surgeon, but their questions belie them. While no physician should insist on being the patient's only or first surgeon, one should expect the patient to tell the truth. I have had patients who asked me to "do something about my nose." When I told them I thought the nose looked perfectly adequate, they confessed to having had a rhinoplasty and simply trying to get my judgment on the result.

Some patients give conflicting statements about dates of operations or previous illnesses. Often, these patients have had psychiatric attention and may at present be in therapy. It is wise always to ask whether a patient is receiving any treatment from anyone. Saying "anyone," rather than specifying a physician, eliminates the possibility that the patient will deny being in psychotherapy if he or she is seeing someone other than a psychiatrist, such as a social worker or a psychologist.

Frequently, a person who is a drug addict may seek a procedure in order to obtain more medication now as well as to establish a relationship with a doctor who can be called on for prescriptions later.

The Indecisive or Vague Patient

It is not unusual for a patient to come to you and say, "Take a look at me and tell me what I need." Always resist the temptation to fill in the blanks. You should tell the patient that, since she (or he) has consulted you, it is her responsibility to tell you what she does not like about herself. The patient with an indecisive attitude may have poor self-esteem and may be in the throes of a depression.

An indecisive patient may have a conflict about the operation and may schedule and reschedule her procedure. Instead of getting angry at the patient—a common and understandable reaction of your secretary—it is better to ask that individual why he or she is behaving in this fashion. You might even suggest that such behavior indicates uncertainty about having the operation. On more than one occasion a patient has replied with relief that this was indeed the situation. Your understanding might allow the person to bow out gracefully.

The Patient with Minimal Deformity

The worst combination for a satisfactory surgical result is the patient with maximal concern about a minimal deformity. Since surgery is potentially hazardous, the objective of the procedure should warrant the risks. The patient whose emotional energies are directed toward a minute bump on the nose had better first see a psychiatrist. If, indeed, a rhinoplasty is performed, the patient's dissatisfaction will be focused elsewhere.

The Patient Who Refuses to Cooperate

Some patients may refuse to undress for proper examination or to be photographed or to have certain basic laboratory tests. If their reasons are not cogent, you should refuse to operate on them. Making exceptions will put you and the patient at a disadvantage in getting an optimal result.

A patient may make the reasonable request that a chest x-ray examination, recently done, not be repeated. This is a much different situation from that in which someone demands an unusual departure from a reasonable routine.

The Perfectionistic Patient

I have alluded previously to the kind of individual who wants everything in life, including surgical results, to be "perfect"—every wrinkle gone or "the nose just so." It is usually impossible to satisfy that person because surgery and wound healing are beyond absolute precision and control.

Those who seek the faultless are hard on themselves and others. Instinctively, we plastic surgeons who tend to be perfectionistic can sympathize with anyone wanting an outcome without blemish. The combination, however, of a perfectionistic patient and an obsessive plastic surgeon frequently produces imperfection. We should resist the temptation to accomplish the impossible by viewing ourselves as the patient's savior. The perfectionistic patient is frequently a shopper.

The Shopper

The surgical shopper looks not necessarily for the lowest fee but for the surgeon who will guarantee the result. He or she may be in flux about having a procedure or in doubt about who should do it. Like any shopper, this patient considers surgery a commodity—something to purchase and to return if defective or if the buyer is dissatisfied. Most surgical results are never completely reversible. Do not consider yourself lucky to operate on a person who has finally chosen you after having consulted numerous doctors.

The Plasti-Surgiholic

This patient, usually a woman, is the seeker and bearer of multiple operations. She may recite a list of famous plastic surgeons who have operated on her, hoping that you will chase the carrot. Although relatively young, she may already have had her nose and eyelids done, her breasts augmented, her abdomen tightened—with repeats. Why she has to submit her body to surgery and its attendant pain is a matter for a psychiatrist.

It is easy to get trapped into operating on such a patient to correct a deformity, such as prominent scars, resulting from previous operations. You may delude yourself by thinking that you are doing not an operation but a "touch-up." Your remedial procedure is still surgery, and it will be just one more notch on her ever-expanding belt.

The Acquiescing Patient

A patient wishing an operation to please someone else should be avoided. Usually this is a female, who may be trying to save a deteriorating relationship. Commonly, she says, "My husband has always admired women with large breasts, and he has told me that he would like me to have this operation." Chances are that with or without the procedure the marriage will never be satisfactory [2].

Another acquiescing patient is the adolescent who capitulates to her mother's insistence that she have a rhinoplasty. Again, one should not jump into the fray.

The Paranoid or Depressed Patient

Elective surgery, especially if cosmetic, is best not performed on individuals who are paranoid or depressed. With psychotherapy, that person may become a suitable candidate for operation, but it must be carefully timed with the advice of the therapist, whose clinical judgment hopefully is sound. Although there have been reports of astounding psychologic successes following an aesthetic operation in a severely disturbed individual, these events are rare and unusual. The common sequence is a worsening of the emotional problem. This does not mean that one should not operate on a patient in therapy who is improving and whose concern about an unsightly body feature is reasonable and focused, but one must be very careful (see below).

A depression in a patient does not always involve the loss of a person, as in divorce or death, but may follow the loss of a body part, such as after mastectomy or hysterectomy.

The Patient in Psychotherapy

As mentioned, the fact that someone is in psychotherapy is not by itself a contraindication to aesthetic surgery; in fact, it may be an advantage. It does require, however, that you communicate with the therapist and be certain that the contemplated procedure is correctly timed psychologically. The patient should be informed that you will get in touch with the therapist; a letter is preferable, with a copy to the patient. This openness helps to eliminate ambiguity and the patient's feeling that if surgery is not done the decision was due to collusion, not collaboration, between the therapist and you. Often, the patient has never mentioned to the therapist his or her plans for an operation.

I would never operate on a patient whose therapist is opposed. In my opinion, it is better to refuse when you are uncertain about the patient than to acquiesce to the therapist if you do not feel comfortable with his or her judgment. That attitude perhaps unfairly discriminates against an occasional patient who might go through an operation without difficulty but it also serves to protect you, the surgeon, who must ultimately bear responsibility for having performed the procedure and the patient who may have been harmed by it.

The Male Patient

Although more males now request aesthetic surgery than before, the majority of patients are still female. My experience has been that older males who seek a cosmetic rhinoplasty in the absence of trauma or respiratory obstruction are more likely to have psychologic problems and postoperative dissatisfaction than those who ask for face-lift, blepharoplasty, hair transplantation, otoplasty, dermabrasion, abdominoplasty, scar revision, or the correction of gynecomastia [20]. Perhaps the dissatisfaction is related to their basic problem of sexual identity. This patient may be confused emotionally and intellectually about how masculine or feminine he wants himself and his nose to be. The conflict has practical ramifications for the operation that we perform since the surgeon may be confused in his operative planning by the patient, who is undecided about what he wants for his nose—for example, how long or short it should be. What has just been stated should not lead surgeons to exclude automatically any male patient seeking a rhinoplasty but it should alert them to the possibility that this patient may be made unhappy when the presumed purpose of the procedure was the reverse.

The "Special" Patient (VIP)

The danger with the "special" patient is that surgical judgment may defer to status. The patient may want to be treated as someone different, or you may change your routine because you feel that he or she is "important," as frequently happens when one treats physicians and their families. Departing from your usual regimen increases the likelihood of error. Realistically, no doctor treats everybody the same since we must take into account a patient's personality, intelligence, and background. However, the physician should be treating primarily the patient's problem, not his or her socioeconomic position.

The Patient Whom You Dislike

Fortunately, disagreeable patients are rare. When encountered, they palpably project their bitterness about life, their insatiability, and their hostility. There is no reason to suppose that an operation will transform them magically into fun-loving people. Unlike psychiatrists, whose work is to deal with many unpleasant emotions, such as aggression, surgeons who are doing aesthetic surgery, which is elective, have the opportunity to refuse to operate. This situation is very different from that of the patient who becomes hostile during the course of your treatment—postoperatively. Your responsibility then is to find the cause and hopefully resolve the problem. It is not your duty to become a therapist to an angry patient who comes to your office for the first time to seek cosmetic surgery. Under those circumstances, you might consider referring the patient to a psychiatrist.

When, Why, and How to Say No

Most physicians, who have been trained to say yes to responsibility, find it difficult to say no. But it is easier to say no to some patients than to others. For example, a patient who wants a face-lift but does not have sufficient signs of aging to warrant the operation will understand your reluctance to operate if it is explained to him or her tactfully and fully.

Saying no should also be easier if you do not feel competent to do the operation required by the patient's problem. Nobody should be reluctant to admit that someone else may be better qualified. In most areas of the country there are plastic surgeons nearby who probably have the needed skill. Someone observed, "You make your living by operating and your reputation by not."

Refusing to operate is the only alternative when the patient's health will not permit it. This situation does arise commonly in older patients who want aesthetic surgery but who have, for example, severe hypertension or angina.

It is harder to say no when the patient could benefit anatomically from the operation but because of his or her personality you do not wish to undertake it. To the "perfectionistic" patient, I usually say, "My skills are not such that I can give you what you want. I doubt whether anyone will guarantee that kind of result. Perhaps, however, some other plastic surgeon might be able to do better for you." You could then offer to refer the person to another plastic surgeon, with or without an accompanying letter.

The most difficult circumstance is to refuse an operation to someone whom you truly dislike. As gently as possible, I usually tell the patient, "For some reason, you and I do not have the same vibrations. If I operated on you, I really believe that we would be on different wavelengths. You would be better off with someone else."

Where to Start and Where to Stop

In general, an aesthetic operation should answer a specific need that the patient has expressed. If someone wishes to have a blepharoplasty, he or she should not be talked into having also a face-lift, rhinoplasty, and mentoplasty. Occasionally, however, doing the upper lids alone may make the lower lids worse. This possibility should be pointed out to the patient, but no one should entice or urge the patient into more surgery than he or she wants or is prepared to accept emotionally and intellectually. Projecting one's personality favorably, as all physicians must do in relating to patients, is different from being a salesman.

THE PHYSICAL EXAMINATION

Within this book are chapters devoted specifically to various procedures. The point to be made here is that the regional examination, at least, should be thorough. Too frequently, plastic surgeons schedule a patient for rhinoplasty but have never carefully and meaningfully examined the nose. For these plastic surgeons, and, unfortunately, for their patients, a nose is a nose is a nose. This irresponsible and cavalier attitude engenders disaster. Admittedly, there are types of noses, but within each genus considerable variations occur. A correct physical examination is a necessary prelude to a correct operation. For example, in assessing a patient for a blepharoplasty, one must properly appraise the vision as well as the presence or absence of redundant skin, muscle atrophy, periorbital fat, skin lesions (premalignant or malignant), symmetry of eyebrow, and frontalis action.

The physical examination is not the occasion to save time by being superficial and careless. You do not have to be a cardiologist to take a blood pressure.

Another point to remember is that the patient should be touched gently, not roughly. Furthermore, every patient, especially those of the opposite sex, should be allowed to get undressed and dressed with some privacy. For women patients, I as a man always have a female member of my office staff present when examining breasts, abdomen, or thighs. Unless a photograph is being taken, the patient should be discreetly draped and not left totally uncovered to his or her embarrassment if no medical purpose is being served by nakedness.

The results of the physical examination should be noted in detail in the record.

Photographs

Just as cardiologists take electrocardiograms, plastic surgeons take photographs. Hopefully, the preoperative and postoperative views will be made under the same conditions to show adequately the area of concern. Surgeons, like photographers, differ in what they consider optimal for their purposes. The proof of the apparatus is in the picture. If the photographs consistently come out well, there is less incentive to change one's setup than if their quality is poor.

Showing Photographs

The photographs of a patient are as confidential as the rest of his or her record. They can be used to show the patient the problem and your operative plans. In this regard, some surgeons employ an instant camera to obtain an immediate picture at the time of the initial consultation as a basis for discussion. Having a patient see such a photo is worthwhile. However, showing patients photographs of other patients is a different matter. I do this only if the other patients have given their consent and only to emphasize *not* the superb result but the average or even unfavorable outcome. For example, the patient should understand what the average scars may be following reduction mammaplasty or a typical result from a breast reconstruction or an instance of capsular contracture following augmentation mammoplasty. The photographs are to transmit information so that the patient comprehends the reality of the proposed procedure; they are not for the purpose of talking the patient into having an operation.

THE END OF THE INITIAL CONSULTATION

As in the beginning, there is an art to ending the initial consultation. It should terminate naturally, not abruptly by your unexpectedly standing up and saying, "Well, I think we have covered everything." The use of *we* is offensive and may not be warranted since the patient may still have questions.

Always let patients know that if they have further concerns they may call your office. Questions may arise when the patient discusses the consultation with friends or family. Offer also to see the patient again if his or her spouse or strategic family member or friend wants to be present. The opportunity is usually not taken, but the knowledge that you are available does much to relieve anxiety. Obviously, you should not extend the invitation if you do not intend to honor it.

Some patients will ask whether they can speak to someone who has had a specific procedure, such as a breast reduction or breast reconstruction. I try to discourage this practice primarily because I believe that the patient usually ends up talking to someone who is pleased with the operation—hardly an unbiased sample. Only a person who is happy with the result would offer to talk to a prospective candidate, and only with this kind of patient would a surgeon feel comfortable enough to ask a favor. Another negative about using other patients is that they do have a right to their privacy. Yet in some circumstances, especially with breast reconstruction and reduction, patient-patient contact is helpful. My secretary arranges this and it is usually done by telephone so that neither patient knows the other's last name.

A SECOND VISIT

Generally, in my experience, repeat consultations are infrequent if one spends enough time initially with a patient. But, there are some patients about whom you are uncertain and who are uncertain about you and the operation, in which case another discussion is helpful. Sometimes, however, seeing someone again when you are already wary about accepting that individual as a patient makes eventually saying no even more difficult. There are no definitive rules for every patient and every surgeon and every situation. The main point is to be sure that the patient is as fully informed as possible and that you know him or her sufficiently well to be the surgeon.

INFORMING THE PATIENT

In a chronologic sequence, I take the patient through the contemplated operation. If it is to be a blepharoplasty, I discuss the mechanisms of outpatient surgery (at the hospital), the use of local anesthesia with intravenous supplementation, the expected pain, the length of the procedure, and the fact that someone must drive him or her home; the regimen of bed rest, head elevation, and iced dressings to the eyes for 24 hours; the return visit to the office for suture removal in 3 to 5 days and the expected resumption of normal activities in 10 to 14 days; the need to wait some time for the expected result; the length of time for the ecchymosis and swelling to subside; the inevitability of scars; the possibility of infection, hematoma, blindness in one or both eyes, and even that of dying from the operation. The realities of the procedure as well as the possible complications are not recited in the manner of a tobacco auctioneer. Each is discussed fully with opportunity for questions. In addition, the patient is given written material to ponder. The informed consent goes into detail about possible undesirable sequelae. Surgeons differ in what they tell patients and in their informed consents. In some states or in some areas legal advice is against having any informed consent. The purpose of my remarks here is not to outline a universal practice but to stress the need for adequate communication with the patient about the prospective procedure, including not only what to expect but what can go wrong. Patients are notorious for not remembering most of what is told them and they are particularly likely to forget the unpleasant. It is probably safe to say that few patients are totally informed in the sense that they have been told everything and have remembered everything and have reacted appropriately to everything both intellectually and emotionally.

I never tell a patient that an operation is "minor." As someone once said, "Any operation that is happening to you is major."

If one minimizes the reality of an operation to a patient, then any complication will be much harder to manage. Admittedly, the surgeon must walk the narrow line between informing accurately and discouraging patently. To inform is not to frighten, but to encourage is not to minimize.

The patient who decided against an operation after being informed should not be a cause for mourning. It may be in the patient's best interests not to have the procedure and in yours not to do it. The one that got away should have gotten away!

SCHEDULING FOR OPERATION

Numerous methods exist for scheduling patients for operation. These differ according to where (in the office or hospital) and when (now or later).

Wherever the operation will be performed, the patient must have the proper preoperative and postoperative information.

The patient who is scheduled many months after consultation must be examined before the procedure. If he or she is not ambulatory and has been admitted to the hospital, the surgeon should visit the night before. Some patients feel better coming to the office a few days prior to their procedure in order to talk things over since they may not have seen you for more than 6 months. One should not have an inflexible assembly line approach that is incapable of meeting patients' needs. These are not "demands" but reasonable requests from a person who is risking life and body in the interest of improvement and has paid money to do so.

THE DISSATISFIED PATIENT

The unhappy patient is as much a reality of surgical practice as is the satisfied patient. Although in a minority, the unhappy patient generally has a greater emotional impact, admittedly unpleasant, on the surgeon. The following dos and don'ts apply in dealing with this difficult situation [14].

Know When and Why a Patient Is Dissatisfied

Usually the patient will remove all ambiguity by a strong statement of complaint, but if this is not forthcoming, we should be alert to veiled discontent—a sullenness, an irritability, or some form of passive-aggressive behavior such as not keeping appointments. Before the patient explodes, it may be helpful to say, "You don't seem too happy today. What is troubling you?"

Sometimes patients are more unhappy than reality dictates. They may forget that you told them the tip of the nose would be swollen for several months, and when you remind them of that fact, they are relieved. In other situations, the surgical reality is that they should be upset: nipples too high or asymmetric after reduction mammoplasty.

Admit the Reality of the Problem

A patient will be justifiably infuriated if a surgeon pretends that things are "just fine" when they are not. Not only has the surgeon done a "bad job" (according to the patient), but he or she is "dishonest" as well and thinks "I am a fool." Any error is worse if compounded. It is better to say to a patient whose left breast is bigger than the right after reduction mammoplasty, "Yes, I should have taken more off the left side but I can easily do this on an outpatient basis after things have healed, in 4 or 5 months." This type of acknowledgment also contains a plan.

Establish a Plan

As mentioned, no patient should be left in limbo, especially someone who is unhappy. Structure the situation. If that means obtaining a consultant, then do it. Always be ahead of the patient in thinking of a consultant. Your offer to have someone else evaluate the situation will decrease the patient's anxiety. The patient will think more highly of you for not wanting to hide the problem or denying the patient access to its solution. If you are arranging for a consultant, you may wish to dictate a letter to that person, but send a copy to the patient. In the letter, emphasize that the consultant should say exactly what he or she thinks. Many, if not most, patients suspect that doctors protect each other to the detriment of the patient in their care. Make clear in the letter that you will continue the care of the patient if that is your intention. If it is not, indicate that the consultant is free to assume treatment of the patient. Some patients resent the fact that they have to pay a consultant's fee. I offer to pay it for them. Usually, a colleague is happy to forgo a fee in these difficult situations. You should do the same under similar conditions.

Always Be Available

Dissatisfied patients have the hot line to your office. Under certain circumstances, I have given such patients my home telephone number. Surprisingly, they do not call, but knowing that you care and are not hiding from them relieves their anxiety and helps to maintain the relationship. Resist the temptation to flee. You know how upset you would be if a carpenter did not return to fix something that did not come out properly—especially if you had already paid him for his work.

In addition to speaking to the patients by phone, it is obviously necessary to see them a few times a week and even daily if that is required either medically or emotionally. Sometimes patients who are initially dissatisfied become your most staunch supporters if they have been treated as you would wish to be treated in the same situation.

Occasionally I have said to a distressed patient, "I know that you are probably angry at me, and the tendency of any doctor is to feel defensive about what happened. We both would like not to have to go through this, but I still consider you my responsibility and hopefully you will think of me as a friend. I am sure that together we can overcome this problem if we work with one another and are honest with each other." I see nothing wrong with a doctor's admitting his or her discomfort if that is the reality. Furthermore, such frankness indicates to the patient that you too are upset by what happened and are not "unfeeling" or "cold and remote."

Do Not Add to the Financial Burden

Because most aesthetic operations are not covered by insurance, neither are their complications. Some surgeons feel it necessary to charge a patient for a reoperation or a revision. Their lawyers have advised that not to do so would be an admission of negligence. Perhaps that is the case legally, but I believe each surgeon has to do what makes him or her and the patient comfortable. I prefer not to charge for a secondary procedure that corrects a problem resulting from my first operation. As a specific example, I do not charge for a revision rhinoplasty if I was the initial surgeon. I cannot advocate this practice for everyone, but it suits me and my patients. Since I do not perform office surgery, the patient must still pay hospital costs.

Do Not Increase the Patient's Guilt and Anger

In managing a dissatisfied patient, the surgeon must remember that he or she probably felt guilty in first seeking the operation and now that something has gone wrong feels even guiltier, perhaps interpreting the misfortune as divine retribution for vanity. Friends may say, "I told you so," or something equally soothing such as, "You paid all that money and went through it all to look the way you do?" In addition to guilt, the patient is usually engulfed by depression and anger. Allow the catharsis, unpleasant though it may be. In turn, restrain yourself from retorting in kind because this will make a bad situation worse by adding to the patient's guilt and anger. The objective is to end with a satisfied patient. How one deals with a dissatisfied patient largely determines whether that person will look for legal recourse. My point is that good relations with a patient mean good medicine. Being considerate of a patient's predicament would be expected in any other relationship of value. Why should the ground rules for decent behavior change under surgical circumstances? The fact that caring for a patient, even one who is dissatisfied, makes good medicolegal sense is a bonus but should not be the basis for your actions.

ANOTHER SURGEON'S DISSATISFIED PATIENT

Thus far, the discussion has centered on the patient who is dissatisfied after your operation or treatment. Frequently, we see unhappy patients from other doctors, just as they see some of ours [11].

Do Not Use an Unhappy Patient to Boost Your Own Ego

The fact that a patient is unhappy (as is the surgeon) should not cause secret rejoicing. Medicine has too many vultures. There is always someone, unfortunately, ready and eager to pounce on the victim. An arched eyebrow signifying pretended amazement at what befell the patient; a vicious query, "He did that?"; a low whistle or a muttered "My God"—all are, I am afraid, conscious stratagems (not even unconscious) on the part of some surgeons to harpoon their supposed colleagues. The patient is not helped by such foul play. If you cannot act properly on the basis of decency then do so from fear. Remember, one of the patients you are about to operate on that day or tomorrow might be in the other doctor's office within a few weeks.

It is better to let the patient talk and express emotions, and to determine and record in detail to the best of your ability what happened and what went wrong than to interrupt with a judgmental remark.

Emphasize the Present

The task at hand is to make the patient better or to help the other doctor continue care of the patient. You may say something like this: "I know, Mrs. Edwards, that you are upset and I am sure that your doctor also is sorry that things have worked out this way. However, you should know that we all have problems, and perhaps he is seeing one of my own patients at this moment. Unfortunately, in plastic surgery, as in life, things do go wrong. Now let's see what can be done to help the matter. I am sure the situation can be improved." Usually the patient will allow you to get in touch with his or her surgeon. Sometimes, however, a patient requests that you do not. This is sticky, but the law in my state (Massachusetts) is clear on this matter: The patient's confidentiality takes precedence over collegiality. Nevertheless, you may tell the patient that for you to evaluate him or her properly it is necessary to get as much information as possible and you do not know how this can be done without communicating with that doctor. Under those circumstances the patient may relent.

If we are honest, I am sure we can recall occasions on which we have not reacted most nobly to the patient who has come from another physician. It takes a superhuman effort, sometimes, not to act like a human: to feel more important by leveling somebody else.

The discerning patient will perceive that the doctor who talks ill of a colleague is probably not without blemish himself. Furthermore, this petty internecine combat does considerable harm to our profession.

A consultant who is able to help a patient in trouble also helps a family and a colleague, as well as the colleague's family. There are few situations in medicine that demand greater sense and sensibility but give more satisfaction.

SURGEON, HEAL THYSELF

A good or bad operation is usually due primarily to the efforts of the surgeon. His or her actions are determined by many variables, of which skill is only one. Admittedly, the analysis of a surgeon, especially self-analysis, is difficult and conjectural. However, there are some things that a surgeon may do that set the stage for calamity [10]. Many of these have already been discussed, but a few will be mentioned now for emphasis.

An Incomplete Initial History and a Hasty Physical Examination

A history and physical examination are better left unfinished, to be completed properly at another visit, than rushed through. As emphasized previously, saving time by a superficial evaluation of a patient will ultimately cause more time to be squandered with a worse outcome.

Operating for the Wrong Reasons

The decision to operate should be made for medical reasons, not for ambition, convenience, money, or pride. Most of the errors that I see are due to the surgeon's operating on a marginal problem—when the decision should have been to avoid or postpone operation. Some surgeons who would pass every recertification examination are too quick with the knife. Consequently, they may not screen out a patient who would never have been satisfied with any result. These misguided and potentially dangerous surgeons, fortunately a small minority, act principally in their own self-interest.

Not Referring a Patient or Seeking a Consultation

Periodically, we should assess our own abilities with objectivity. What we are today is not necessarily what we were as residents. For example, some surgeons have not done a microsurgical case for 4 years; why should they begin with one this week? Not all plastic surgeons are capable by training or inclination of performing aesthetic surgery, which has undergone further differentiation so that some are more skilled in rhinoplasty, others in reduction mammoplasty, others in blepharoplasty. I am not advocating that everyone become a one- or two-operation surgeon but I insist that surgeons not undertake procedures for which they have little enthusiasm and moderate talent when they could easily refer the patient. Since aesthetic surgery is elective, the patient does have the time to get optimal care.

Poorly Informing the Patient

I have already emphasized the need for adequately informing a patient. Every surgeon should remember that a patient may dislike the objectively good result if he or she did not comprehend beforehand the pain, time, and costs involved, as well as the nature of the scars and the limitations of the operation. Sometimes the patient did not truly know what the surgeon had in mind for the procedure because the surgeon did not really know. Both become victims of the "schedule now, think later" approach.

A Poorly Planned or Poorly Performed Operation

Although bad preoperative and postoperative management can ruin a good operation, only infrequently can a bad operation be transformed into a good result by bedside attentions.

When the surgeon carries out the procedure in the operating room, it should not be for the first time. The operation should have been done in the mind's eye before, perhaps in the office but certainly in the 12 hours prior to operation, if the case is elective. Ad-libbing may be good for jazz trumpeters but it is not ideal for a surgeon, who should take the time to plan his or her next move, especially when the health of another human being is involved.

A surgeon doing an aesthetic operation should take every precaution against standardizing the procedure. There is a temptation to "do a rhinoplasty." As stated before, we must individualize according to the patient's needs. In breast reduction, for example, each surgeon should have a few techniques that are employed according to the individual case. One operation does not fit all. Furthermore, during the procedure, one must be attentive to the variations required to give a superior result.

If the patient is in satisfactory condition, the operation should not be terminated until it has been done as well as the surgeon can possibly do it. Boredom, fatigue, or the press of a schedule should not compromise standards. A result that looks just fair at operation will generally look worse in the office. A few more minutes can make an important difference. Time spent then is more worthwhile than apologies and explanations later.

During operation, surgeons must be aware of the activities of their team, including those of the anesthesiologist. They should be alert to the vital signs of the patient and possible breaks in aseptic technique. They must know whether the patient is properly protected against pressure necrosis. In short, they should be actively concerned and not passively involved in the operation.

Concluding the Case with the Operation

In reality, the operation is not over until the patient is discharged from the surgeon's care. The cut-and-run technique has no place in surgery. The patient and the patient's problem should not fade from the surgeon's consciousness as soon as the dressing is applied. Careful observation, detailed orders, and clear instructions are obviously critical. Residents are helpful but should not be an excuse for an absent surgeon. It should not be below a surgeon's dignity to remove sutures. In fact, watching how a wound heals may improve the surgeon's technique. There are some surgeons who prefer not to see their patient until a few weeks after operation—until the patient's swelling and ecchymosis have disappeared. While they may soothe a surgeon's mind, it does little for the patient's tranquillity. The relationship between a doctor and a patient requires a doctor. This does not mean that the doctor works alone, but, in my opinion, there is too much of a trend to relegate the functions of a doctor to someone else, all in the name of efficiency. This kind of efficiency is really deficiency. Under such conditions, interaction between doctor and patient is prone to atrophy and disintegration. Doctors who establish systems that protect them from daily small problems will become the targets of large ones. Furthermore, the tendency to "process" patients and to be distant from them erodes the satisfaction of being a doctor. Most of us went into medicine in order to take care of patients, and if we streamline our activities to the exclusion of those we are supposedly to help, what is left?

The Truncated Follow-Up

Surgeons who fail to observe their patients long enough lose a singular opportunity to learn. The temptation is to quit while ahead: to see the patient until he or she looks good, from our point of view, and has no complaints. However, an extended follow-up will allow us to witness many things, some wondrous, others painful, but all instructive. A year later the revised scar that initially looked so disappointing will have improved miraculously. The rhinoplasty that seemed "just perfect" at 6 months may look worse later. If we avoid the long-term result of our efforts, we will never learn properly. We shall subject future patients to the same errors, and with time our standards will decrease along with our reputation and self-esteem. The head in the sand is a survival mechanism for ostriches but not for surgeons.

THE BIONIC SURGEON

An operation is a series of interdigitating sequential acts, whose quality depends on the soma and psyche of the surgeon as well as of the patient. Overworked, overstressed surgeons do themselves little good and may do their patients considerable harm. There is an almost irresistible sequence: Young surgeons with the least experience have more time to spend with the patients and are attentive to every detail. Middle-aged surgeons have a large practice and get a little sloppy; they are willing to have several failures if they can also produce many successes. Old surgeons would like to have more patients, but their referrals are fewer and their skills are not what they were; they run the danger of operating from pride, of reasserting their capability, and of not knowing when to retire. In short, every stage of a surgeon's career has its problems and compensations. Not to recognize the pitfalls is poor living and bad medicine.

In conclusion, aesthetic surgery offers an opportunity for self-actualization on the part of the patient and the surgeon. Technical competence alone, though mandatory, does not ensure success. The surgeon must have also concern, honesty, intuition, judgment, and luck, the last increasing in importance as the other desiderata become neglected. The purpose of this chapter has been to expand the surgeon's awareness so that he or she will assume greater responsibility with more knowledge and, hopefully, will then leave less to chance.

REFERENCES

1. American Society of Plastic and Reconstructive Surgeons, Inc. Official definition of cosmetic and noncosmetic surgery. Written communication, November 1979.
2. Beale, S., Lisper, H. O., and Palm, B. A psychological study of patients seeking augmentation mammoplasty. *Br. J. Psychiatry* 136:133, 1980.
3. Bennett, A. E. (ed.). *Communication Between Doctors and Patients.* London: Oxford University Press, 1976.
4. Bennett, G. *Patients and Their Doctors: The Journey Through Medical Care.* London: Bailliére Rindall, 1979.
5. Bird, B. *Talking with Patients* (2nd ed.). Philadelphia: Lippincott, 1973.
6. Blumgart, H. L. Caring for the patient. *N. Engl. J. Med.* 270:449, 1964.
7. Dicker, R. L., and Syracuse, V. R. *Consultation with a Plastic Surgeon.* Chicago: Nelson-Hall, 1975.

8. Entralgo, P. L. *Doctor and Patient.* New York: McGraw-Hill, 1969.
9. Goin, J. M., and Goin, M. K. *Changing the Body: Psychological Effects of Plastic Surgery.* Baltimore: Williams & Wilkins, 1981.
10. Goldwyn, R. M. Ingredients for Failure. In R. M. Goldwyn (ed.), *The Unfavorable Result in Plastic Surgery: Avoidance and Treatment.* Boston: Little, Brown, 1972. Pp. 2–4.
11. Goldwyn, R. M. The Consultant and the Unfavorable Result. In R. M. Goldwyn (ed.), *The Unfavorable Result in Plastic Surgery: Avoidance and Treatment.* Boston: Little, Brown, 1972. Pp. 5–7.
12. Goldwyn, R. M. High hopes and malpractice. *Arch. Surg.* 111:1042, 1976.
13. Goldwyn, R. M. Patient Selection: The Importance of Being Cautious. In E. H. Courtiss (ed.), *Aesthetic Surgery Trouble: How to Avoid It and How to Treat It.* St. Louis: Mosby, 1978. Pp. 14–16.
14. Goldwyn, R. M. The Dissatisfied Patient. In D. Gowlian and E. H. Courtiss (eds.), *Symposium on Surgery of the Aging Face* (vol. 19). St. Louis: Mosby, 1978. Pp. 81–84.
15. Goldwyn, R. M. The Woman and Esthetic Surgery. In M. T. Norman and C. C. Nadelson (eds.), *The Woman Patient. Medical and Psychological Interfaces* (vol. 1). *Sexual and Reproductive Aspects of Women's Health Care.* New York: Plenum, 1978. Pp. 271–280.
16. Goldwyn, R. M. *The Patient and the Plastic Surgeon.* Boston: Little, Brown, 1981.
17. Kalick, S. M. Aesthetic surgery: How it affects the way patients are perceived by others. *Ann. Plast. Surg.* 2:128, 1979.
18. Karsh, E. The Doctor-Patient Relationship Through the Ages. In W. E. Preece (ed.), *Medical and Health Annual.* New York: Encyclopaedia Britannica, 1977.
19. Lederer, H. D. How the Sick View Their World. In E. G. Jaco (ed.), *Patients, Physicians, and Illness: Sourcebook in Behavioral Science and Medicine.* New York: Free Press, 1958. Pp. 247–256.
20. Leff, L. A Secret of Success: Be Good at Getting Wrinkles Ironed Out. *Wall Street Journal* November 15, 1979.
21. MacGregor, F. C., et al. *Facial Deformities and Plastic Surgery: A Psychological Study.* Springfield, Ill.: Thomas, 1953.
22. MacGregor, F. C. *Transformation and Identity: The Face and Plastic Surgery.* New York: Quadrangle Times Books, 1974.
23. Magraw, R. M. Social and Medical Contracts: Explicit and Implicit. In R. J. Bulger (ed.), *Hippocrates Revisited.* New York: Medcom, 1973. Pp. 148–157.
24. Parsons, T. Social Structure and Dynamic Process: The Case of Modern Medical Practice. In T. Parsons (ed.), *The Social System.* New York: Free Press, 1951. Pp. 428–479.
25. Parsons, T. Definitions of Health and Illness in the Light of American Values and Social Structure. In E. G. Jaco (ed.), *Patients, Physicians and Illness: Sourcebook in Behavioral Science and Medicine.* New York: Free Press, 1958. Pp. 165–187.
26. Parsons, T. The sick role and the role of the physician considered. *Milbank Mem. Fund. Q.* 53:257, 1975.
27. Rosenberg, M. L. *Patients: The Experience of Illness.* Philadelphia: Saunders, 1980.
28. Siegler, M., and Osmond, H. *Patienthood: The Art of Being a Responsible Patient.* New York: Macmillan, 1979.
29. Walster, E., et al. Importance of physical attractiveness in dating behavior. *J. Pers. Soc. Psychol.* 4:508, 1966.

3. Design and Management of An Aesthetic Surgeon's Office and Surgery Suite

Ray A. Elliott

Aesthetic surgery and ambulatory surgery have gained popularity, almost hand in hand, for more than a decade. But the acceptance of ambulatory surgery in an office setting has a much shorter history.

Rapidly rising hospital costs, delayed or uncertain admissions for elective surgery, and patient demand have led to a widespread interest in ambulatory surgery. Freestanding surgical centers, outpatient hospital facilities, and office surgery suites now compete as the settings of choice. With greater acceptance of ambulatory surgery, many informed patients come to prefer the office setting for its greater privacy and convenience.

In exchange for their trust, the surgeon who offers office surgery must assume responsibility for the quality of the facility. Safety, efficiency, and cost containment are of prime importance, and these concerns should be reflected in both design and management. Because the office surgery suite is usually an extension of the basic office, the entire complex deserves consideration as a single unit.

THE BASIC OFFICE

The design and management of the offices of the many aesthetic surgeons where I have had the pleasure to visit have each reflected the individual surgeon's unique vision, taste, and temperament. It is not likely that a single design, decor, and management system will ever be totally acceptable for adoption. There are, however, some basic principles and standards that apply to most offices. A review of these may help the surgeon whose vision still awaits fulfillment.

Choice of Location

The aesthetic surgeon must weigh several factors in choosing the ideal location for his office. The inclusion of a surgical suite introduces additional important considerations.

Selection of a safe and stable neighborhood will protect the investment and obviate later relocation. Patients will appreciate easy access near a major highway and on a well-known street. The availability of public transportation is an added convenience. Proximity to a population center is perhaps less important than the choice of a well-lighted area with adequate parking.

If the office is located near a major hospital equipped to handle emergency admissions, a measure of comfort and safety is added in the event of an emergency in the surgery suite. Ideally, the surgeon would have admitting privileges and could follow his patients. Otherwise, a written

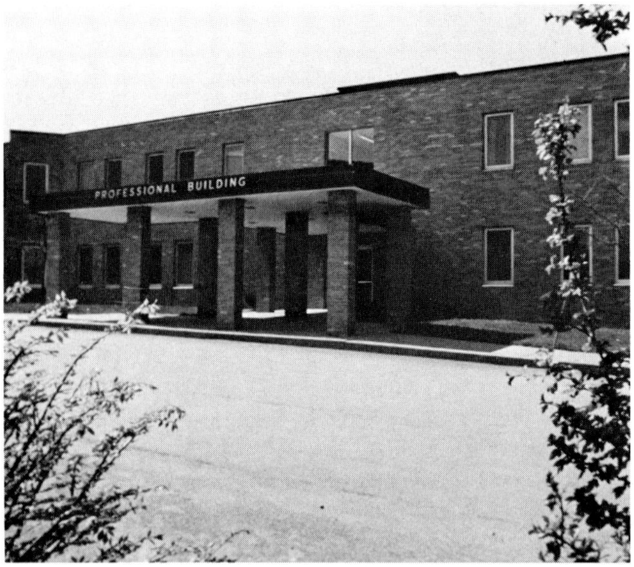

Figure 3-1. A professional building attached to a hospital will provide convenience and a measure of safety for office surgery.

agreement to accept bona fide emergency patients from the office is advisable.

Obviously, it would be convenient to have the office located near a hospital where the surgeon worked regularly. If the surgeon operates in a number of hospitals, one or more may have a professional building (Fig. 3-1). Referral from other doctors in a professional building is one factor to consider, but it must be weighed against the possibility of being identified with one hospital exclusively.

Where hospitals are many miles apart and traditionally serve different populations, the surgeon may consider a satellite office for patient convenience and to attract referrals. The added expense and potential inconvenience to the doctor must be part of the evaluation. Inclusion of a surgery suite in a satellite office is a separate consideration. These decisions must not be based on emotion or ego alone; they must be business decisions.

It is well to remember that the aesthetic surgeon's practice will ultimately depend on the excellence of results and reputation. In time, the majority of patients will be referred by other satisfied patients. Referrals from other physicians are gratifying and are very important for establishing a practice, but referral patterns change and dependency lessens as the practice matures.

Rental Versus Ownership

The ownership of a landmark office complex, complete with operating room suite, on a choice piece of land in a prime location, remains the primary goal of many aesthetic surgeons (Fig. 3-2). Many have realized their dream with fulfillment and pleasure; others would classify the result as a nightmare. Too often it is the financial planning that will make the difference. Not every surgeon has the business acumen or the personal motivation to be an owner with the responsibility for the development and maintenance of a real estate venture. But all surgeons must become business executives to control their destiny and protect their investment, even in a rental situation.

With current mortgage rates and construction costs at an historic high, the capital outlay required for ownership may be out of reach of the new practitioner and will significantly tax the resources of the established surgeon. The inevitable overruns and the expenditures required for furnishings and equipment must be considered. Space rental will be a desirable option in many cases. Ownership of furnishings and equipment should have priority even if capital is short, as this type of leasing is very expensive.

It is important to have expert advice in the preparation and execution of an office lease. The terms and options for renewal are basic concerns. It is also wise to protect any investment in cabinetry and attached fixtures with a lease that permits their removal for sale or subsequent use. We have realized significant savings by removing items that could be incorporated in the design of subsequent suites.

Architect and Contractor

CONSTRUCTION TEAM

The most important member of the team for renovation or construction of a new building, the architect, must be knowledgeable, innovative, and flexible to ensure the best product. This professional will be the unique buffer between you and the contractor, a supplier of refreshing ideas, an informant regarding design and materials options, and hopefully, a friend and troubleshooter when problems arise.

The contractor must have a proved record of quality construction and financial stability, and a reputation for ethical business practice. Fairness, flexibility, and dependability are hallmarks of a quality contractor.

CONTRACTS

The architect and the builder should have separate contracts so that the architect can maintain independence as your representative and project manager. A diligent architect will obviate the need and expense for a separate project manager; an enthusiastic architect will welcome the increased responsibility. All contracts should be scrutinized and approved by your legal and accounting advisers. Mortgaging institutions will also review these documents because of their vested interest.

A guaranteed maximum price (GMP) contract with the builder is usually advisable to establish a basic cost for financial planning. All change orders should be in writing and should receive prior approval by the architect and the owner. Any deviation from this procedure will invite uncontrolled cost overruns.

A contract for "fast-tract" construction is another trap to avoid. In essence this gives the owner and architect the flexibility to make changes and develop details of planning any time in advance of the actual construction of any portion of the project. Unfortunately, this method lacks

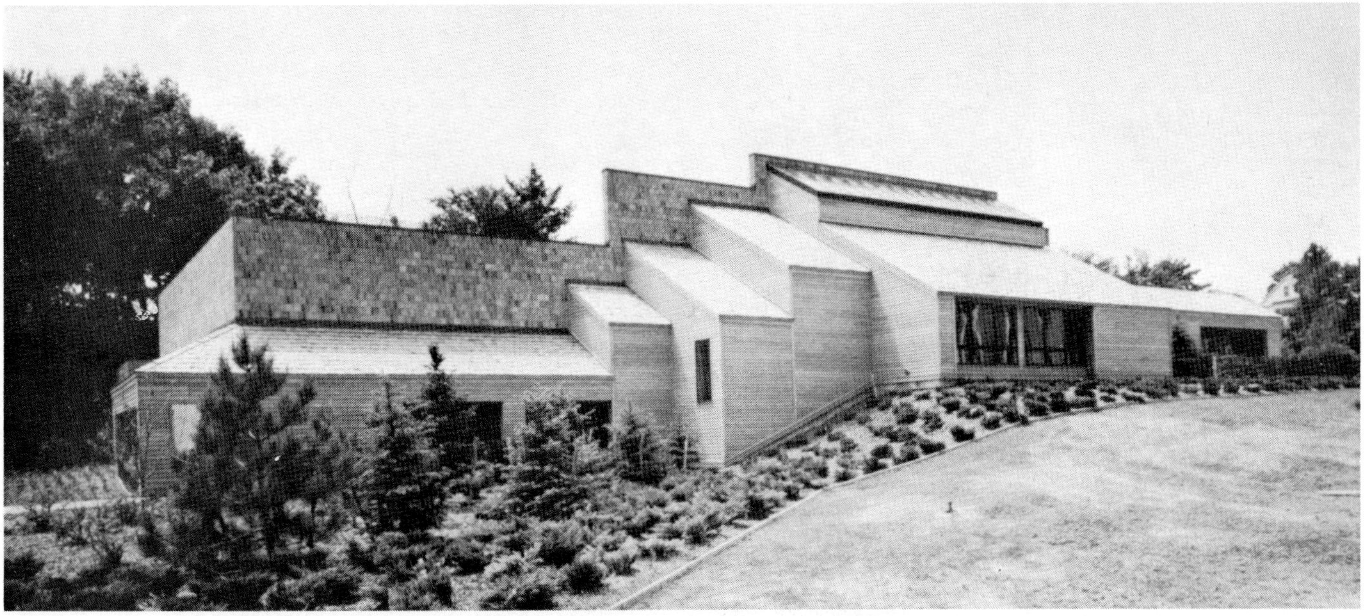

Figure 3-2. Medical building located near several hospitals has 7000 sq ft on each of two levels. Albany Plastic Surgeons Associated offices and surgery suite occupy the upper level. The lower level accommodates a pharmacy, a dentist, an internist specializing in rheumatology, a hand therapy facility, an apartment, storage, utility, and a maintenance shop.

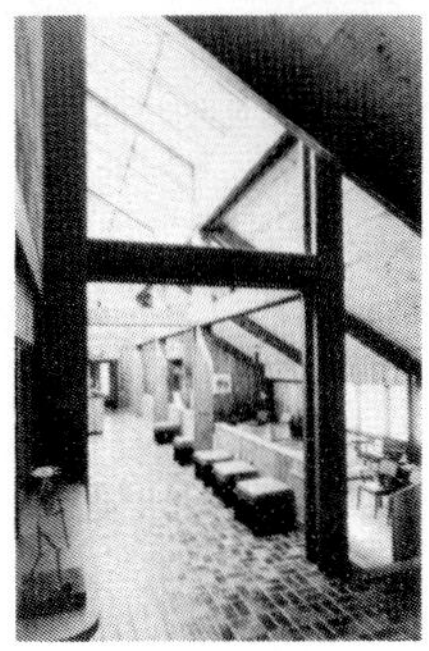

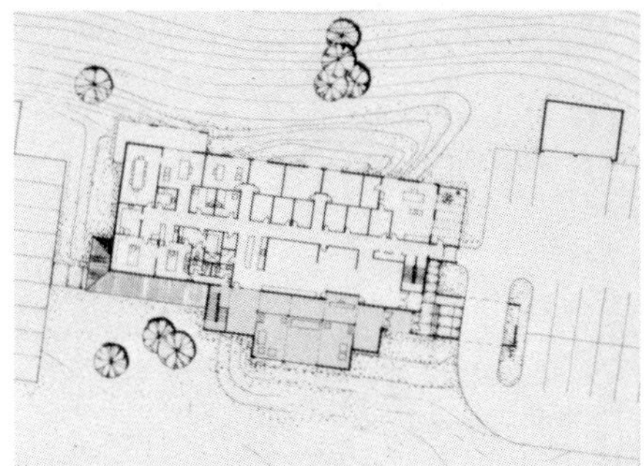

commitment to definite costs, and in reality the project is likely to be quite a bit more expensive because of segmental buying of services and supplies.

Design and Decor

Energy efficiency and low maintenance costs are realistic goals with today's options for design and materials. The architect and contractor should present the options and their relative cost.

With few exceptions, it will be the surgeon who must determine the modules required for his or her type of practice and potential needs for expansion in the future. The capacity of the waiting room, the equipment and furnishings planned for the various areas, the use of the private office for consultations, the number of personnel utilizing the examining rooms, the need for a conference area or a library, and patient photography requirements are examples of variables that will depend on practice habits.

FUNCTIONAL REQUIREMENTS
The functions that must be provided for in the basic office plan include reception, coat storage, waiting, appointment scheduling, consultation, examination, photography, surgery scheduling, business office, bookkeeping, staff lounge, staff coat storage, instrument care, utility, and supply storage. Separate rest rooms for patients and staff will be appreciated by the staff. A library and a conference area should also be considered. It is desirable to have a work area for minor maintenance. This may be combined with the utility, storage, or instrument care area to conserve space. Some architects will avoid the issue, but provision must be made for handling the temporary storage of refuse. The demands of an office surgery suite will make this consideration even more vital.

SPACE REQUIREMENTS
The type, size, and number of rooms required for an office practice will vary with the volume of patients and the individual mode of practice. Some differences are unique to the basic office of a surgeon whose practice is confined to aesthetic surgery. For example, in a practice in which prepayment of surgery fees is nearly routine and third-party payers are seldom involved, one will require a smaller business office than that utilized in a full-spectrum practice.

Examination Rooms. It is always desirable to have at least two examining rooms, but more will increase the efficiency of even the solo practitioner, particularly if the dressings and suture removal are delegated to nurses, as

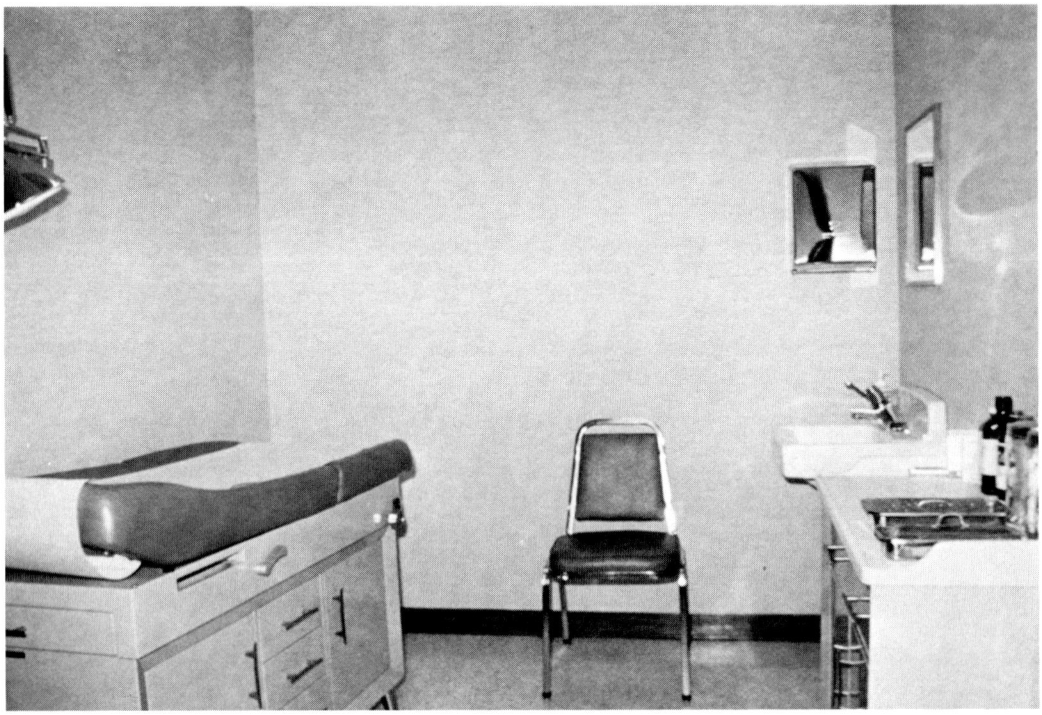

A

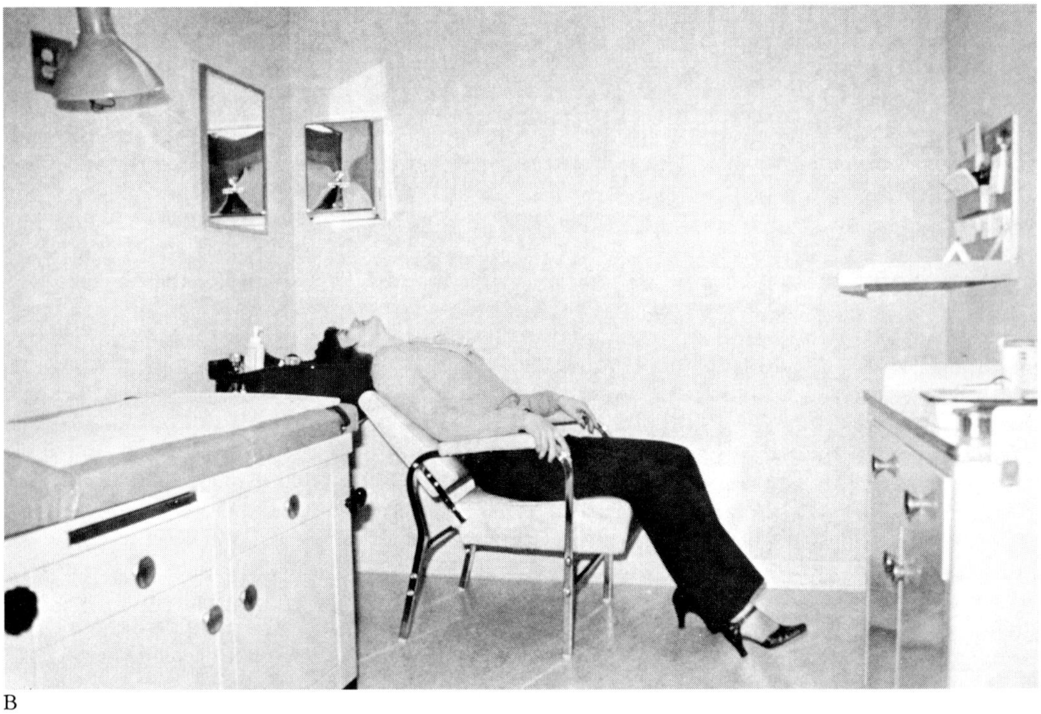

B

Figure 3-3. The average size of an efficient examining room is 8×10 ft.

A. Standard examining room with adjustable table.

B. Examining room with tilt-back chair and notched sink for washing hair.

C. Examining room with adjustable examination and treatment chair.

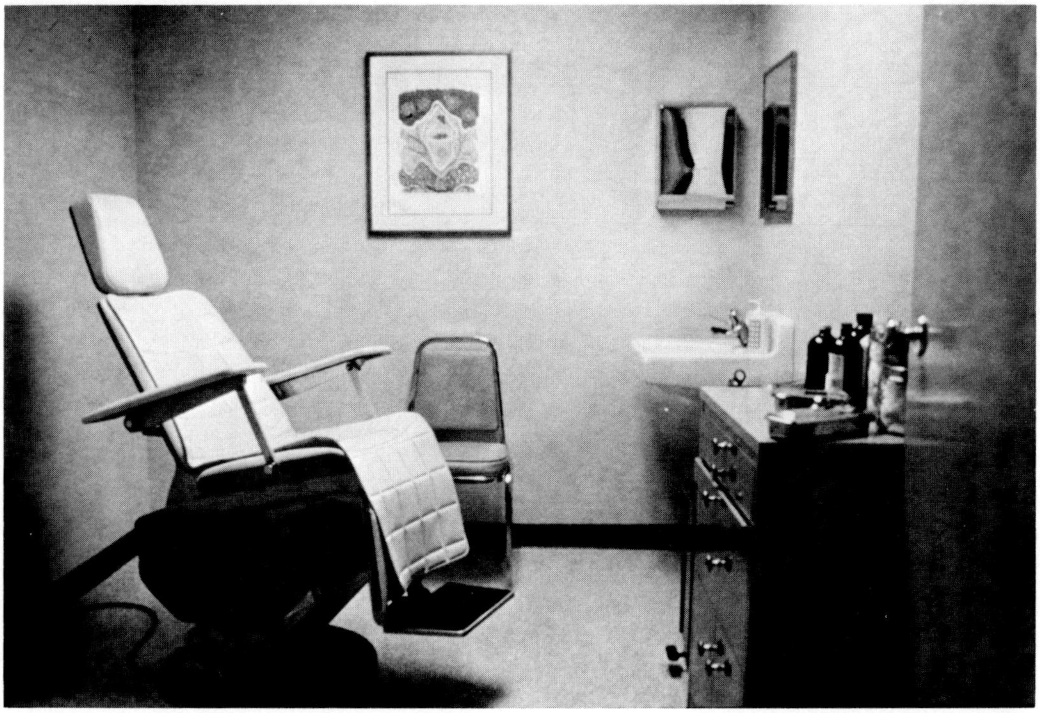

C

they are in many offices (Fig. 3-3). The average size of an efficient examining room is 8 × 10 ft.

Consultation Rooms. The private office of the surgeon should be more spacious if it is to be used for the initial consultation, as this requires seating for the patient and two friends or relatives (Fig. 3-4). The minimum size is 10 × 10 ft, but at least 10 × 12 ft should be planned if possible. Larger private offices will reflect the taste and desire of the surgeon, at proportionately higher cost. If the surgeon elects to delegate the discussion of fees to a member of the staff, a separate, well-appointed, 10- × 10-ft room will be very adequate for this purpose.

Photography. Every aesthetic surgeon will need to provide for photography. Even if the basic task of taking preoperative and postoperative photographs is delegated to a professional studio, an in-office provision is essential if the patient's course is to be documented. A separate inside room with a rheostat lighting control and a uniform background is better than an examining room for taking photographs unless the same requirements can be met. Adequate depth of the room is more important than width, and size will vary with the camera and lights selected and storage requirements.

Multipurpose Rooms. The multipurpose concept in office planning is important as it conserves space in the small office and allows for future expansion in any office. For example, in one of our former offices a photography room doubled as a dressing room, the recovery room became an examining room during regular office hours, and another examining room became a second recovery room for office surgery. In my first office a workroom-library was designed to accommodate an additional partner and eventually served this purpose. In our present office, the conference room–library gains additional use for lecture preparation and projects, and the staff lounge doubles as a food and beverage service area for the occasional conference (Figs. 3-5 and 3-6). Relocation of these two units and the suite entrance door will permit further expansion of the operating suite if needed. An extra storage room has been wired and plumbed as an examination room but could become a holding area if necessary. Advance planning for this kind of flexibility is a logical part of the initial office design.

Circulation and Storage. Perhaps the most common architectural fault encountered in plans that I have reviewed is excessively long hallways. Every square foot of the office figures into the overhead costs, and short hallways increase efficiency. Five-foot-wide hallways are desirable for comfortable traffic flow and maneuvering wheelchairs and stretchers; some busy circulation spaces should be even wider. Adequate storage space is also a frequent deficiency. Base and wall cabinets add useful, convenient storage, but a separate room for bulk storage is also recommended.

TRAFFIC FLOW

Modules and Layout. Once the size, number, and function of modules have been decided on, the pattern of traffic flow requires attention. Only after patient flow has been determined can the architect go to work to put these

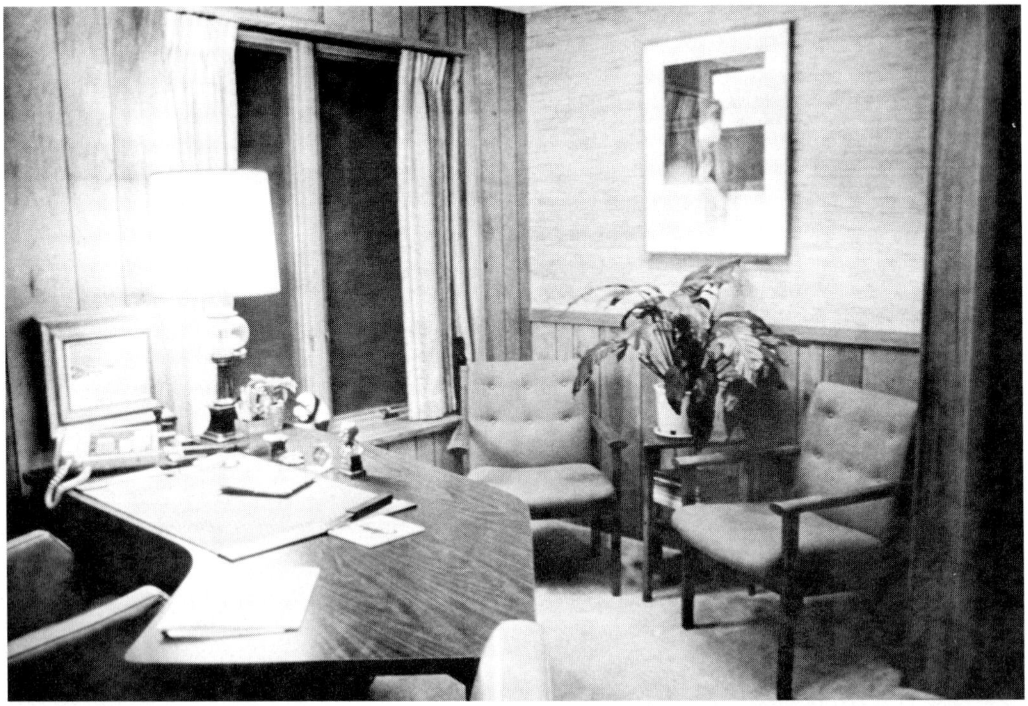

A

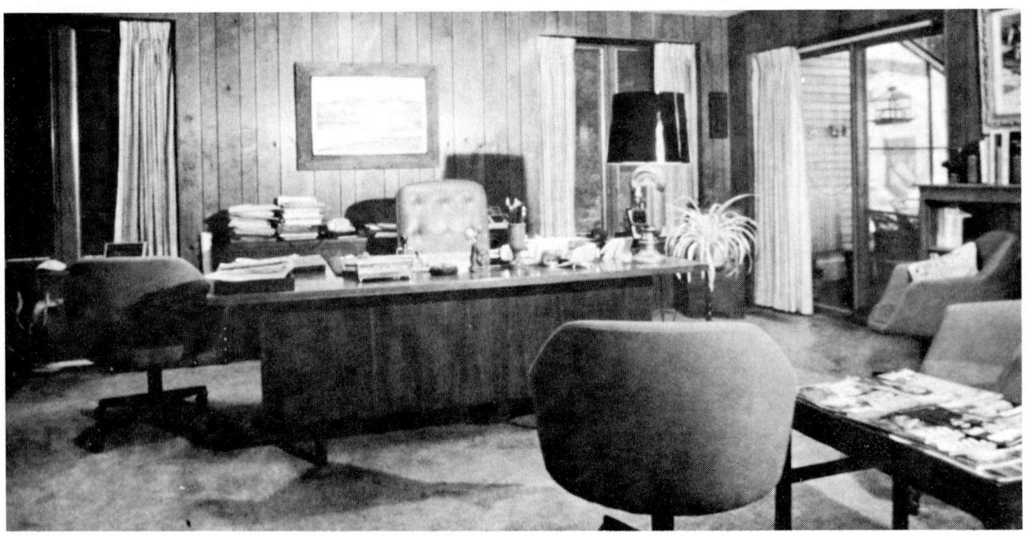

B

Figure 3-4. Consultation room should be at least 10 × 12 ft.
A. Standard size provides seating for patient and two relatives or friends.
B. Larger private office doubles as small conference area and permits conversion to library-conference area if needed (see Fig. 3-5B).

various units into a workable format. Probably a number of layout options and multiple revisions will be offered before the final selection is made. Devotion of the architect and surgeon, working together, will be essential at this stage if costly alterations are to be avoided later. Outlining a patient's route through the office on paper will lead to more efficient planning (Fig. 3-7).

Privacy. It is well to remember that patients will usually prefer privacy when discussing their surgery or their financial matters. Properly arranged circulation space can provide contact with the appropriate staff while maintaining reasonable privacy. Greater privacy can be afforded by interviewing within the business modules if desired, but this contingency must be provided for during planning (Fig. 3-8).

MATERIALS AND DECOR

Decorator. Beautiful and functional offices can be developed with or without the services of a professional decora-

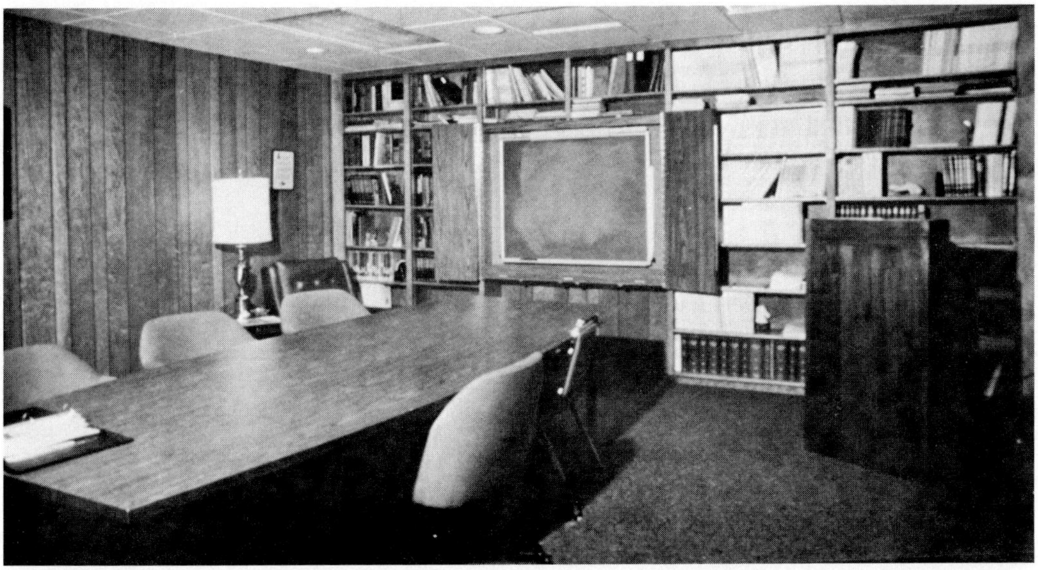

A

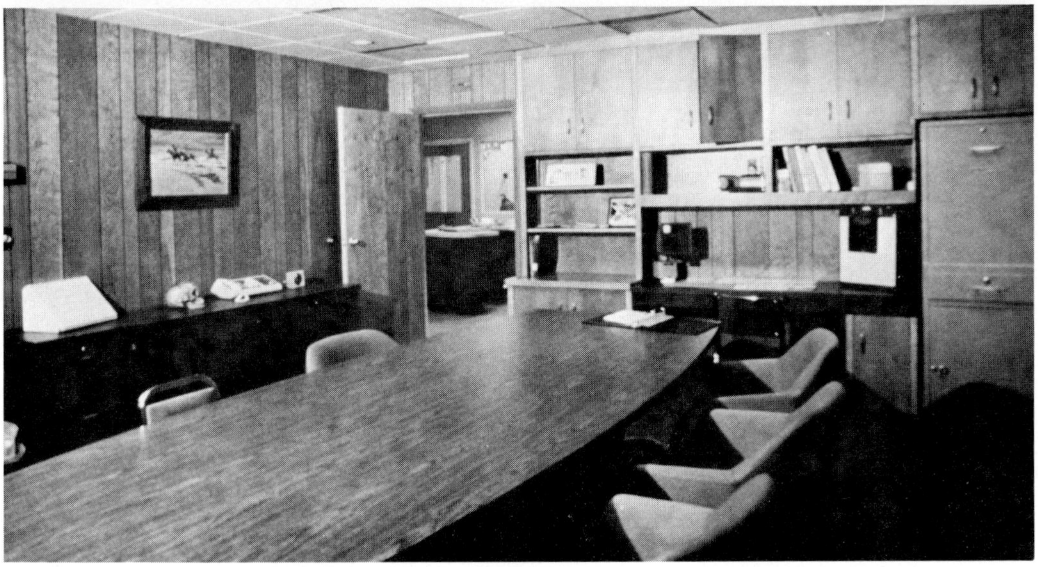

B

Figure 3-5. Multipurpose conference-library-project room.
A. Lecture facilities and library.
B. Lecture preparation and project areas; proximity to surgery suite planned for potential suite expansion.

tor. The office should reflect the personality and taste of the surgeon, and ideally a decorator should be responsible primarily for presentation of the options, arbitration of conflicting opinions, and coordination of the final selections. In some instances the entire project should be delegated, but it is a rare aesthetic surgeon who will lack the ego, taste, and personal concern to be closely involved with his home away from home.

Appearance. The new patient's impression of the surgeon will begin with the appearance of the office complex. The facility should appear professional but at the same time warm and inviting (Fig. 3-9). Expensive decor and furnishings are not automatically tasteful, but quality materials will show and will last. Simple elegance is a reasonable goal. Vinyl seat coverings are durable and easy to maintain and come in all colors. The earth tones have stood the test of time in our office, but I have seen many beautiful offices more starkly modern and bolder in color.

Environment. Today, zoned air conditioning is a basic consideration. Soft background music enriches the atmosphere of the waiting room and circulation areas. The surgeon and the staff may find other areas where music is desired.

Wall Coverings. The architect, builder, or decorator will provide samples of wall coverings and color charts for paint. It is important to select durable materials that can be cleaned easily. Washable vinyl wall coverings are recom-

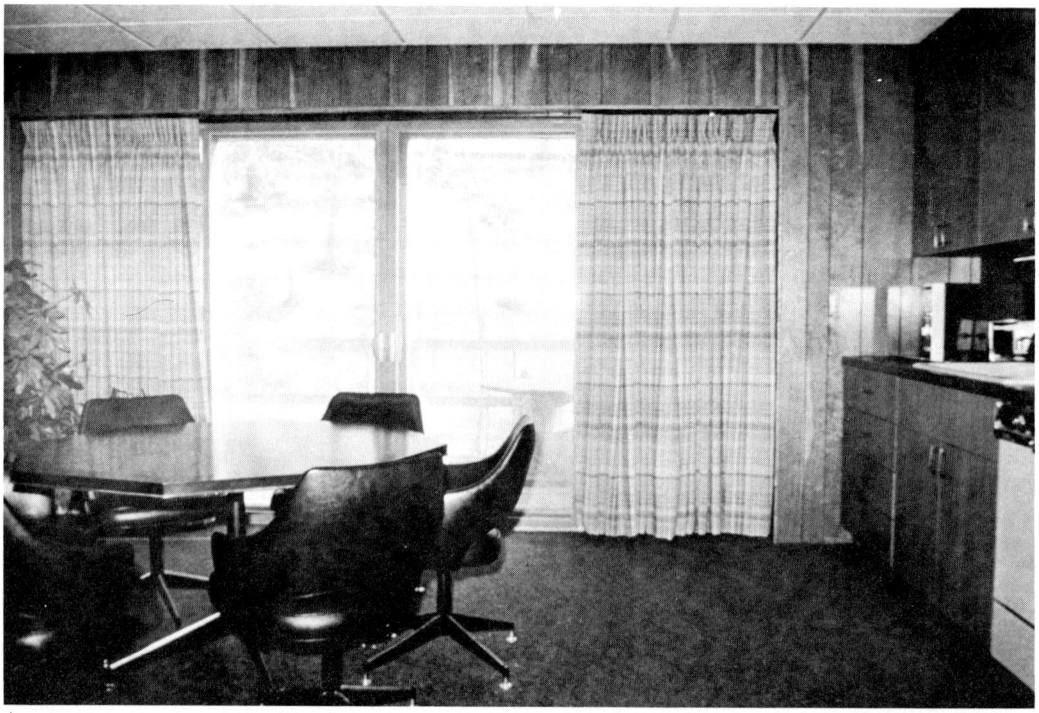

A

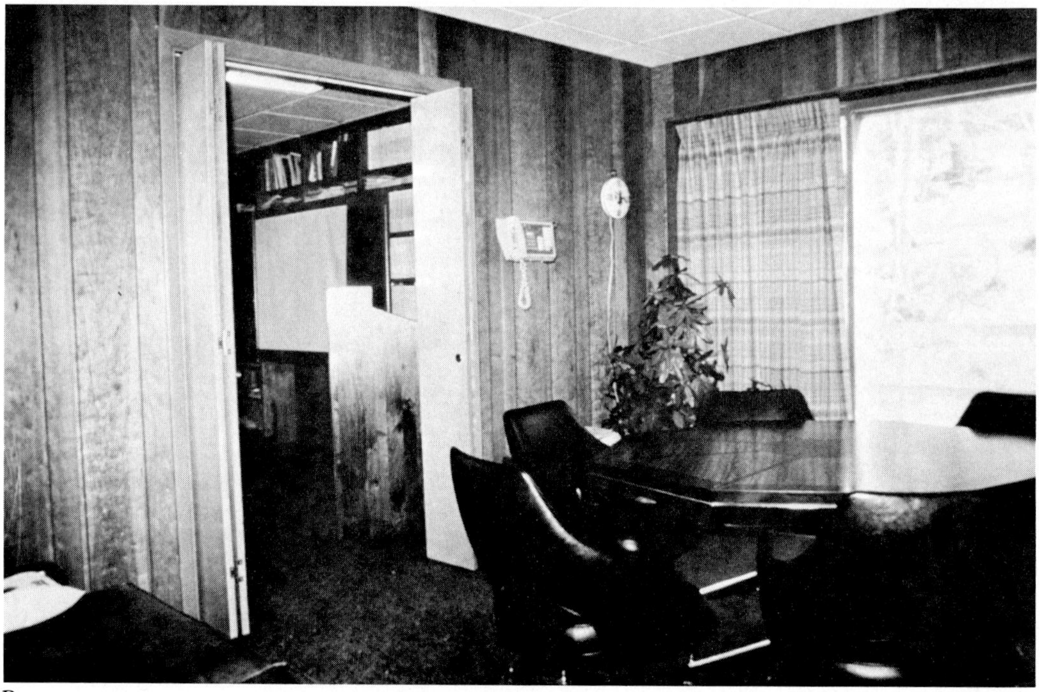

B

Figure 3-6. Multipurpose staff lounge, convertible to enlarge surgery suite.

A. Lounge outfitted for food and beverage service and cleanup; opens onto a back deck.

B. Conference-library entered via bifold doors.

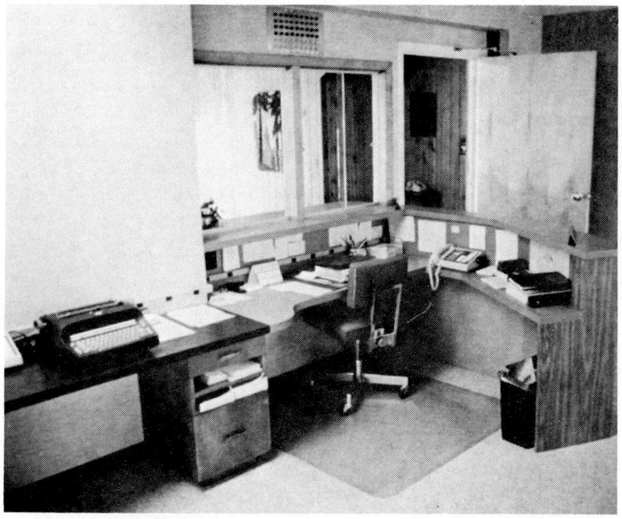

Figure 3-7. Reception desk inside the business module affords privacy. Patients can be interviewed via sliding windows or within the module. The central light system monitor is seen overhead, and the patient telephone is in the background.

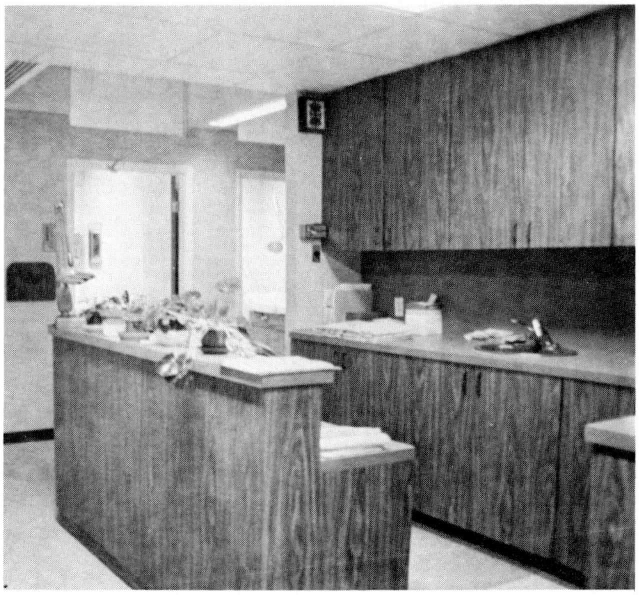

Figure 3-8. The surgery scheduling area is within the clinical suite and has custom-built counter and cabinets. Examining rooms and hallway to two of the recessed private consultation rooms are seen in the background.

mended for the business office, hallways, exam rooms, bathrooms, and operating suite, but the rich warmth of wood may be more appealing for the waiting room, the doctor's offices, and perhaps the library and conference areas. The choices of wood and prefinished wood paneling will satisfy almost every conceivable decor. When mounted over Sheetrock, quarter-inch-thick panels are stable and durable and meet the goal of simple elegance with considerable savings when contrasted with solid wood boards. Insulation provides an inexpensive, effective sound barrier and should be part of the wall construction in all new or renovated offices.

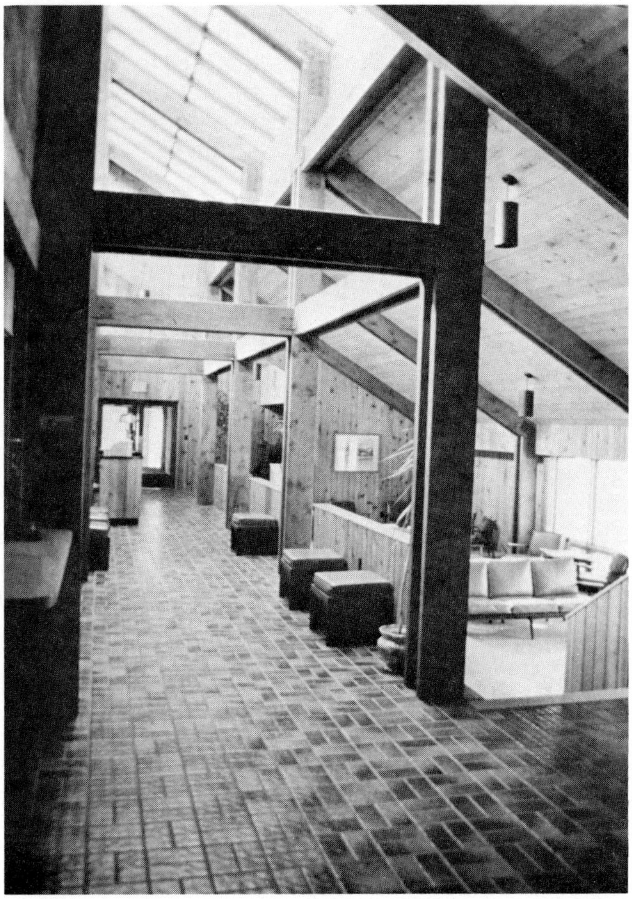

Figure 3-9. Facility should be warm and inviting. Entry door at far center leads patient to front reception desk. New patients complete forms on seats in the skylit entryway. Sunken waiting room and wheelchair landing show on the right and clinical reception counter on the left.

Cabinets and Counters. Cabinets and counter tops of laminated plastic will be durable and easy to maintain. Cabinet shelves can be surfaced and edged with plastic laminate and should be adjustable. A wood-grain pattern on the cabinet and counter face, and lighter solid colors for the tops and shelves provide a pleasant appearance. Counters and cabinets should be of sufficient depth to accommodate necessary functions and supplies. Custom-built units will have an obvious advantage in this regard.

Floor Coverings. Wall-to-wall carpet is recommended for comfort, warmth, and sound control in the waiting room, hallways, business office, library, doctor's offices, and dressing areas; vinyl floor coverings should be used for examining rooms, bathrooms, and the operating room suite. A good grade of tightly woven, short-pile, commercial carpet should be selected, and sheet vinyl will be easier to maintain than individual tiles.

Communications

A telephone and an intercom system satisfy the minimum voice communication requirements of the aesthetic surgeon's office. The addition of a light system or mechanical flags to locate personnel, and the use of color coding will improve efficiency. Standardization of narrative reports, the use of short-form letters, and the use of patient information materials and routing slips will also save time.

TELEPHONE SYSTEMS

Options. Good telephone service is a basic necessity in the professional office. In recent years many options have become available, including the opportunity to own the system. Any of these options will add expense, but careful evaluation of the potential convenience and added efficiency offered by each should lead to a proper business decision. Ownership of a system of 10 or more phones is almost always economically desirable, but only if capital is available for purchase of a quality system from a reliable vendor with a proved record of good service.

Location. Every work area should have easy access to a telephone, but I do not recommend the location of phones in the examination rooms. Telephones should ring only in the business areas during normal office hours; selected phones should have this capability after hours when a staff member is not available to direct the call. We provide a waiting room phone for patients, away from the main traffic areas and controlled by a switch at the receptionist's desk.

Number of Lines. The telephone company will run a busy signal analysis free of charge to help determine the need for extra lines, but two incoming-call rotary lines and an unpublished line for calling out should be the minimum for any busy office. A separate number for bookkeeping can be very helpful. Additional lines will be needed for call-in dictation and monitored security systems.

INTERCOM SYSTEMS

Selection. An office intercommunication system is a necessity. The Executone system has excellent fidelity, but other systems of comparable quality are available in many communities. Investigation of various systems is important. Reliability and prompt service will reduce frustration and downtime.

Features. Hands-off reception of discreet calls is important for the operating surgeon and in the examining rooms, but a handset should be available for privacy on most if not all units. Calls to patient areas certainly should have this feature.

A paging capability is useful for locating specific staff persons when they are away from their usual work stations. The background music speakers used and multiple zones will be helpful in larger offices and can exclude specific areas such as the waiting room or surgical suite.

Combining the intercom system and the telephone is quite feasible with modern technology. Space conservation is obvious, and cost savings can be significant, particularly if the units are purchased.

SIGN-IN AND LOCATOR SYSTEMS

The flow of patients and the location of professional personnel is greatly enhanced by a low-voltage light system. The rapid transfer of telephone calls and messages is enhanced by pinpointing the location of personnel. A similar system for sign-in of doctors and nurses can be monitored throughout the office to identify the presence of these persons. A custom-designed system has unique advantages, but commercial units are also available. Lower-cost mechanical flag indicators, color coded for specific personnel, are an option for examining rooms, but the more sophisticated light systems are preferred. They can be monitored from the specific doctor's office or from any other remote location as desired. Even the solo practitioner will benefit from the added efficiency of these systems.

COLOR CODING

Many efficiencies can be effected by the use of color. It is an aid to both rapid identification and communication.

Name and Year. Perhaps the best-known application of color coding in the modern office is the supplement to alphabetic indices. The colors facilitate chart identification and accurate refiling.

Another common aid is the color and number strip on the edge of the chart, which indicates the year of the most recent office visit. This system helps the staff pull inactive files for separate filing.

Dot Systems. A colored dot code on the exposed surface of the chart can provide ready information regarding the nature or etiology of the condition, financial responsibility, need for special reports, previous collection problems, payment for reports, and identification of important teaching cases, to name a few. The identification of malignancies and multiple illnesses is another valuable application for accurate follow-up care in the busy office. Also, colored dots that identify the charts of patients who have been discharged or reactivated are helpful for refiling in the proper area. The possibilities for dot systems are limited only by the imagination.

Paper Supplies. In a multisurgeon office, the appointment book, surgery schedule systems, and even the chart cover itself may be in color to identify each surgeon. Using colored charts to identify a deformity or its treatment is less rewarding, as many cosmetic surgery patients return for multiple conditions.

In our office the consultation notes, follow-up notes, and operative reports for office surgery are all on different colored paper for easy identification. Pastel colors are the most practical. Internal office action slips and telephone message forms are also colored to clearly identify them and thus speed communication.

INTERNAL COMMUNICATION
A variety of preprinted forms are used for internal communication. Routing slips, action forms, telephone message pads, and surgery scheduling slips are beneficial in every office. Daily production of a surgery schedule, hospital rounds slips, and an appointment list will further increase efficiency in the busy practice.

Route Slips. The use of a patient route slip to identify the service, charges, return appointment, discharge, and need for photographs, x-ray studies, or special tests is basic in most offices. These slips can also be used for routing a patient for surgery scheduling, preoperative counseling, or an interview with the bookkeeper. Numbering the slips serially and retention of a duplicate by the receptionist will add an internal control.

Action Forms. A preprinted, colored form is helpful for routing internal messages and materials. A series of boxes can be designed to check off the action requested, and there is ample room for a brief message on the usual form. Forms are available commercially or can be custom designed.

Telephone Messages. The commonly available forms for telephone messages lack two important features: space for the reply and information about the time, date, and person who replied. Design of a color-coded form with these features is highly recommended. Important messages regarding patient care should be filed in the patient's chart. Our forms have a box to check if the message and reply are to be filed (Fig. 3-10).

Surgery Schedule Forms. Preprinted forms should be completed by the surgeon to indicate the diagnosis, procedure, hospital or office setting, anesthesia, length of procedure, special tests or equipment needed, and advance payment fees, as a minimum. This information will be required by the scheduling person.

Daily Lists. The planned surgery and out-of-office meeting schedule of the surgeon should be available to all key personnel daily. An electronic beeper would then be needed only as a supplement for locating the doctor, thus obviating its use during scheduled events. A daily update of the list and location of hospitalized patients will facilitate rounds by the professional staff, and an indication of the number of new patients and follow-up patients to be seen during scheduled office hours will help the surgeon plan time and pace.

LETTERS AND REPORTS
Short Form Letters. The standardization of letters and reports will speed communication (Fig. 3-11). Fill-in letter forms can be used for reporting the results of consultation, operative findings, pathology, and follow-up status. Another short form letter can be used for referrals, for excuse from activity, and for release to work or school. These forms can be completed by the medical assistant or nursing staff from notations on the patient's chart. Handwritten reports are proofed by the surgeon before being typed and then returned for signature. Regular, rapid, brief reporting of the pertinent facts will make a more favorable impression on the recipients than two-page newsy letters, which take more effort to prepare and to digest, not to mention the greater lag time created by the process.

Message: Telephone ☐ Other ☐

For ______________________ By ______________

Date ____ Time ______________________________

From ____

Of ____

Phone (_____) __________ Ext. _______________

Message _____________________________________

____

____

____

____

____

Reply _______________________________________

____

____

____

____

____

Date of Reply ________ Time _________________

By __________________________ File in Chart ☐

APSA REV. 3-81

Figure 3-10. Message form for documenting both message *and* reply.

Narrative Reports. When narrative reports are indicated because of the complexity of the problem or to meet requests from insurance carriers or attorneys, a basic reporting format will expedite the task in many instances. With modern technology offering second- and third-generation word processing, a standard format and standard paragraphs are adaptable for certain of these reports. Short form letters are inexpensive advertising and may encourage continuing referrals. Narrative reports are much more tedious and expensive to prepare, and their use should be reserved for recipients who are willing to pay for them.

Albany Plastic Surgeons Associated, P.C.
60 Hackett Boulevard
Albany, New York 12209

Ray A. Elliott, Jr., M.D.
James G. Hoehn, M.D.
James A. Edmond, M.D.

Telephone 472-9148
Area Code 518

To: ______________________________ Date: ______________________________

Your patient ______________________________ was examined in our office today

for examination of: ______________________________ ☐ progress report

☐ Accident ______________ ☐ Surgery ______________________________

Impression: ______________________________

Recommendation: ______________________________

____

____

Treatment ☐ scheduled ☐ completed ☐ discussed ______________________________
Present status ☐ maximum improvement ☐ will follow ☐ discharged ______________
☐ working ☐ not working ☐ to work ______________

Thank you for the courtesy of this referral.

______________________________ M.D.

Plastic • Reconstructive • Cosmetic • Hand • Head and Neck Cancer • Maxillofacial • **Surgery**

A

Albany Plastic Surgeons Associated, P.C.
60 Hackett Boulevard
Albany, New York 12209

Ray A. Elliott, Jr., M.D.
James G. Hoehn, M.D.
James A. Edmond, M.D.

Telephone 472-9148
Area Code 518

To: ______________________________ Date: ______________________________

Your patient ______________________________ was seen in consultation

today at ______________________________ Hospital.

Impression: ______________________________

Recommendations: ______________________________

____

____

A full report was recorded in the patient's hospital record. Thank you for the courtesy of this referral.

Copies to: Sincerely,

______________________________ M.D.

Plastic and Reconstructive • Cosmetic • Hand • Head and Neck Cancer Surgery

B

Albany Plastic Surgeons Associated, P.C.
60 Hackett Boulevard
Albany, New York 12209

Ray A. Elliott, Jr., M.D.
James G. Hoehn, M.D.
James A. Edmond, M.D.

Telephone 472-9148
Area Code 518

To: ______________________ Date: ______________________

Your patient ______________________ was treated at: ______________________

Hospital: ______________________ as an ☐ inpatient ☐ outpatient

Findings: ______________________

____

Treatment: ______________________

____

Laboratory report: ______________________

Follow up: ______________________

Thank you for the courtesy of this referral.

______________________ M.D.

Plastic • Reconstructive • Cosmetic • Hand • Head and Neck Cancer • Maxillofacial • Surgery

C

Albany Plastic Surgeons Associated, P.C.
60 Hackett Boulevard
Albany, New York 12209

Ray A. Elliott, Jr., M.D.
James G. Hoehn, M.D.
James A. Edmond, M.D.

Telephone 472-9148
Area Code 518

To: ______________________ Date: ______________________

This is to certify that ______________________

☐ Is/was under our care for ______________________

☐ Should be excused from ______________________ until ______________________

☐ Is/was released to ______________________ effective ______________________

☐ Is/was referred for ______________________

Remarks: ______________________

Sincerely,

______________________ M.D.

Plastic and Reconstructive • Cosmetic • Hand • Head and Neck Cancer Surgery

D

Figure 3-11. Short form letters expedite reporting.
A. Office consultation and follow-up visit report.
B. Hospital consultation report.
C. Surgery and pathology report.
D. Miscellaneous form for referral, excuse, release, etc.

Lengthy reports should be dictated for convenient transcription by the typist. Short letters may be dictated directly to a secretary, but this practice is less efficient. Shorthand has all but disappeared in the modern office.

Personnel, Services, and Advisers

The office personnel, contracted services, and professional advisers are all important to the efficient operation and growth of any business. All will affect the management work load of the surgeon, who must accept the ultimate responsibility.

PERSONNEL TASKS

The tasks that must be performed in the basic office of an aesthetic surgeon include appointment scheduling, reception, monitoring of traffic flow, preparing reports, counseling, wound care, photography, responsibility for inventory and supplies, bookkeeping, making out insurance forms, surgery scheduling, and chart and file maintenance. Other special tasks can be identified, such as travel arrangements, meeting planning, and the preparation of brochures, patient information forms, and manuscripts. The list goes on! Is it any wonder that occasionally things go wrong?—or right?

OFFICE PERSONNEL

The hiring and preservation of qualified personnel will be an important key to an efficient office. Personnel must be pleasant, neat, efficient, skilled, and well paid. A trained employee who cannot perform the tasks for which he or she is hired should be replaced. For the surgeon, the practice must be a business; for the employee, it is a job. Every employee is entitled to adequate training for the peculiarities of the job assigned. There should be a regular periodic review of performance, and an opportunity for advancement in responsibility and reward. Although many of the tasks, even hiring and firing, must be delegated, the ultimate responsibility for office management and efficiency lies with the surgeon. The number of personnel required for the regular completion of daily business will vary greatly, but simply increasing numbers will not compensate for deficiencies in training and quality of performance. For convenience, at least one employee should be a notary.

CONTRACTED SERVICES

Contracted services such as cleaning, maintenance, and trash removal should be carefully screened and their performance judged regularly. The quality of these services will contribute to, or detract from, the operation of the business. The answering service is another area of importance. Courteous, prompt, and professional performance is essential. This service should be considered an extension of your office and a valuable contact with your patients, colleagues, and referral sources.

PROFESSIONAL ADVISERS

Professional advisers will be needed for accounting, insurance, investment, banking, and legal matters. Tax planning, contracts, corporate documents, benefit plans, and investments are but a few of the areas requiring input from one or more of these persons. They must be chosen carefully for their availability, competence, and reputation, then judged by their performance on a regular basis. As members of a team, they must be able to work together and pool their skills for the best product.

Records and Files

THE OFFICE CHART

A concise, organized documentation of the patient's consultation, treatment, and follow-up, combined with the routine information for identification and billing, comprises the basic record. Photographs, telephone messages, consent forms, pathology and operative reports, and correspondence are also filed in the chart along with the processed billing record. The use of color coding has already been discussed.

FILING AND CHART RETRIEVAL

Patient charts should be filed alphabetically. In a busy office there should be a separation of active and inactive files and eventually a third area for very old inactive files.

In addition, each department of the office should maintain a subfile in alphabetic order for ready access of charts being processed for consultation, follow-up, insurance billing, correspondence, lecture preparation, or any other function that requires the entire record. Vertical files with end-tab patient identification have replaced the bulky, inefficient drawer-file systems in most modern offices. It is well to utilize the method for identifying inactive and reactivated charts so that they can be returned to the proper file. Numeric filing requires a cross-file that is clumsy and time-consuming, and it is not recommended.

Insurance

LIABILITY AND CASUALTY

Liability and broad casualty coverage is necessary. Expensive equipment, furnishings, books, art, and supplies should be considered when the limits of the casualty policies are being set. A complete inventory of the office contents will be revealing; a videotape record will be convincing. Both should be kept in a bank safe deposit box, and at least the inventory should be updated regularly.

Personal liability and casualty insurance and the insurance needs for your office are best coordinated and consolidated by a single broker whenever possible. The total premium cost is likely to be less and the advisory and claim service better.

MALPRACTICE

All professional personnel participating in the clinical care of patients should be covered by malpractice insurance. Perhaps the surgeon can make a personal decision for his own coverage, but coverage for the staff should not be arbitrary. Many hospital boards now consider malpractice insurance a requirement for appointment to the staff.

HEALTH AND LIFE
Basic medical-surgical, hospitalization, major medical, dental, disability, and life insurance policies are attractive fringe benefits for keeping key personnel. But experience has shown that they are not a substitute for adequate pay. If life insurance policies are provided, they should be term policies. Ordinary life insurance is much more expensive, and the front-end load makes it a very poor investment. Workers' compensation and basic disability coverage are required by law in most states.

Security

DETERRENTS AND DETECTION
The problem of security exists in any building, and a doctor's office may be a prime target for theft in some communities. Quality doors and locks, secure windows, and good external lighting are basic deterrents to amateur burglars. Internal lighting of areas visible to passersby may also help. Private security patrol for an isolated building is expensive. A modern electronic surveillance system is an excellent alternative. We prefer voice monitoring and the use of a discrete code for each authorized person. Our system provides 24-hour monitoring of smoke detectors and the emergency panic alarms and voice monitoring of the unoccupied office. Temperature extremes can also be detected. Construction plans should deal with security from the beginning.

CONTROLLED SUBSTANCES
State law requires locked storage for narcotics and other substances. A two-level lock system is required in some states. I would recommend unmarked storage for these drugs and their special prescription pads. Unfortunately, problems of pilferage and misuse are not always external; internal control is also needed. The responsibility for inventory, utilization records, and security should be delegated to the supervising nurse, but irregular spot checks are advised.

Emergency Systems

FIRE
Fire is an acute and potentially frightening emergency. This hazard can be diminished in the modern suite, but it cannot be eliminated entirely. The office staff must be drilled in the handling of this event. Notification of the fire department and rapid evacuation of patients and personnel are basic. Directly wired smoke and heat detectors and an alarm system are recommended particularly for remote areas of the office. There must be 24-hour protection, however, for the entire office. A sprinkler system should be considered in a new construction. Lower fire insurance rates will offset some of the cost of these various options.

LIGHTING
Clearly marked exits are required by law. Emergency lighting in the event of a power failure is advised for key locations such as exit hallways. Emergency lighting units contain rechargeable batteries that are on a constant trickle when electric current is flowing. We use these same units for emergency lighting of the operating table and recovery room in lieu of a standby generator or storage battery source. They are efficient and dependable.

THE SURGERY SUITE

Making the Decision

The decision to develop an office surgery facility must be primarily a business decision based on a logical analysis of a number of pertinent factors. The emotional high that might result from the pride of ownership of a personal facility must not take precedence over the realities of a thoughtful business analysis.

ADVANTAGES
Patient. Benefits for the patient include an element of privacy in a pleasant setting, potential decrease in the anxiety inherent in the usual hospital experience, and greater warmth and personalized care from a staff whose training is refined to the special needs of the patient. It is likely that there will be a real saving in operating room charges when compared with the rapidly escalating costs of comparable facilities in a major hospital, where charges are based primarily on time, without regard for the nature of the procedure, and depreciation of very sophisticated equipment is shared by all patients. In the selected instances in which aesthetic surgery (e.g., scar revision) is covered by third-party payers in the hospital setting, the savings for patients and insurance companies will be substantial when these benefits are extended to the lower-cost office setting. Accreditation of office facilities is a major step toward this goal.

Surgeon. The surgeon will benefit by added convenience and better utilization of time. Travel time aside, all surgeons are aware of the valuable time lost between cases in most hospitals. The opportunity to do routine office work between cases is an advantage in our practice. In-office control of the operating room environment, personnel, and equipment is an obvious advantage to the specialist. Since this control carries with it the surgeon's personal responsibility for quality and refinement, some surgeons might consider it a disadvantage.

DISADVANTAGES
Tradition. For decades patients have been conditioned to relate ultimate safety to the hospital setting, and they have learned to expect hospital care for any surgical treatment. The spiraling increase in the general hospital operating room charges created a widespread interest in separate ambulatory facilities, but the costs for outpatient surgery have not been substantially lessened in most hospital units. Reeducation of the patient population regarding use of an office facility for surgery cannot be rushed. The patient must be confident that care and safety of comparable quality can be provided in this unfamiliar setting.

Surgeon. Aesthetic surgeons who perform most, or all, of their surgery in the office will necessarily lose valuable contact with their colleagues and with the hospital. This must be considered a disadvantage, particularly for the surgeon who is new in the community. There is little problem for the surgeon who also maintains a significant practice in the hospital. The lack of overnight facilities for continuing care, and the absence of ancillary support in the event of an emergency or adverse event must also be considered.

Expense. The high initial cost of the office surgery suite and equipment will be followed by significant increases in overhead for personnel, supplies, and maintenance. Once the investment has been made and the magnitude of these additional expenses is clearly evident, the unwary may try to justify them by an increased utilization that is beyond the reasonable requirements of the practice. A careful practice analysis with cautious projections for a changing profile is essential before one embarks on a plan for office surgery.

PRACTICE ANALYSIS

After a careful and serious evaluation of the advantages and disadvantages of performing office surgery, it is logical to analyze the planned or existing practice and its future direction.

Reimbursement. The types of procedures that are performed in the office will vary with community standards, the surgeon's philosophy, patient acceptance, and sophistication of the facility. However, it is reasonable to assume that at the present time, and until third-party payments are made for office facilities, the vast majority of aesthetic surgeons will use the operating suite for elective cases not customarily reimbursed by insurance plans. The operating list would grow rapidly with insurance company support of the office setting for those normally reimbursable cases. As a practical matter, some patients who are aware of the advantages will choose the office facility despite the additional out-of-pocket expense.

The practice analysis must include, then, primarily those cases that would not have reimbursable hospital costs, with a projection of the potential case load that might result from a change in third-party payment policy. Conservative projections will help prevent overdesigning, while multipurpose utilization of space, equipment, and staff, and proper planning will allow for future expansion.

Case Selection. The decision to do a certain type of operation in the office rather than in the hospital will be quite individual, as will be the need for general anesthesia. The surgeon who utilizes an intermediate facility for the postoperative care of detained patients will have more latitude in case selection, and this type of management, strictly speaking, is not ambulatory surgery and will not be considered here. Surgeons who do extensive procedures such as abdominoplasty on an ambulatory basis must be aware of the potential postoperative risks and be prepared to deal with them.

Technically, most of the common aesthetic procedures can be done in the office operating room that is well designed, properly equipped, and staffed by trained personnel. But prudence must be exercised in patient selection. This option should be offered only to patients of nearly zero risk who can be returned to their home environment with reasonable safety. Operations normally performed on an outpatient basis at the hospital, such as minor excisions, scar revisions, and dermabrasions, can clearly be done in the office. With proper selection, patients for nasoplasty, otoplasty, blepharoplasty, breast augmentation, hair plugs, scalp flaps, chin augmentation, limited lipolysis, and segmental rhytidectomy are also among the candidates for office surgery.

Some breast reduction and mastopexy operations may be performed in the office when blood loss and operating time have been considered. A decision to equip for general anesthesia will obviously make it more feasible to include some of these procedures. It is questionable, however, even with general anesthesia, whether one should elect to do abdominoplasty, extensive lipolysis, or thigh- or buttock-lift procedures in the office routinely. These procedures are included by some surgeons. Total rhytidectomy on an ambulatory patient may well become a trend and is already offered in many facilities.

Thus, the list of procedures to be considered in the analysis will be variable. Experience with the safe performance of procedures of magnitude may alter the pattern of utilization in the future. But the type and number of procedures that the surgeon feels can be done on a regular basis is a consideration of the present. Multipurpose usage of the space and of the staff will permit a more orderly approach toward a greater volume of cases. Other considerations, however, must be aired before a discussion of such factors.

PERSONAL ANALYSIS

One of the most important analyses is the possibly painful, objective look at one's own temperament. The planning, building, and maintenance of an office operating suite will demand personal attention if it is to reflect the wishes of the surgeon. Although many of the tasks can be delegated, the constant supervision of, and ultimate responsibility for, the administration of this additional facility with all of its time-consuming realities remains with the surgeon. If the surgeon prefers to avoid detail and would rather operate without responsibility for management of the setting, office surgery will create a conflict.

Of equal or greater concern is the acceptance of a relative isolation from medical colleagues. The quality of surgeons' work is traditionally judged by their peers in a hospital setting. Criticism, justified or not, may be launched against surgeons who avoid this interplay, particularly if they are financially successful. Perhaps, once established in the medical community and at the hospitals, a trend toward a nearly full-time office surgery practice will be less criticized, but an ongoing contact with hospitals and peers will obviate much of the concern and preserve a good reputation, if deserved.

EVALUATION OF THE OPTIONS

It is important to evaluate the options provided by existing facilities in freestanding units and hospitals as to quality of environment, equipment, staff, and management. The availability of the operating room and the convenience and cost to the patient are also of prime importance. The development of an office surgery suite to obtain additional practice income is not by itself a proper motive and may be disappointing as a business decision if cost containment for the patient is an honest goal.

On the other hand, if office surgery is common in the community, this may be a positive influence on the decision. If most aesthetic surgeons offer this alternative, strong consideration of the need to provide office surgery is obvious, and the experience of colleagues should be helpful in the planning. However, if your businesslike analysis of all the factors discussed in this chapter has been thorough and the indications are positive, perhaps your office surgery suite will and should be the first in the community.

PRESENT SPACE AND LOCATION

If a new office is contemplated, the surgery suite can be part of the plan. For offices already situated the addition or relocation of space will require careful study and perhaps professional consultation regarding feasibility.

As previously noted, the location of the office demands special attention beyond the usual concerns for the surgeon's convenience and population density. The safety of office operating is greatly enhanced by a location in reasonable proximity to a hospital that is willing, by staff privilege or written agreement, to accept emergency admissions should the need arise. Obviously staff privilege should be sought in order to permit firsthand monitoring of the patient who requires admission.

Planning the Suite

Once the decision has been made to offer ambulatory office surgery, planning the suite is the next step. Renovation, expansion, and relocation are alternatives.

The basic office facilities for patient management will be available to patients using the surgery suite and need not be duplicated. However, some changes may be necessary for efficient traffic flow, particularly of postoperative patients, and for relative isolation of the suite from the basic office.

SPACE REQUIREMENTS

Although requirements will vary, there is a tendency to be grandiose and to duplicate the familiar hospital facilities. Ingenuity, conservative design, and application of the multipurpose concept can save space and money, yet allow for future expansion.

Efficiency Suite. An efficient surgery suite for local anesthesia cases can be developed within a 300-sq-ft area. The layout for one such facility is shown in Figure 3-12. In this suite the multipurpose concept was applied to minimize overhead and permit better space utilization. The operating room was the only area not employed routinely as part of the basic office, except that its liberal cabinet space was used for storage of examining room supplies. Thus, the cost of *not* operating in the office was decreased significantly.

Separate Suite. If the volume of potential cases is sufficient to justify the expenditure, an isolated surgery suite is ideal (Figs. 3-13, 3-14, and 3-15). The total area requirements will vary with the case load, type of surgery, and number of surgeons operating at one time. General anesthesia will require larger operating, recovery, and storage areas. The volume of cases will influence space allocations for the workrooms and storage areas, and rapid case turnover will affect plans for waiting and changing areas.

Operating and Recovery Rooms. Although smaller areas may suffice, I feel that for local anesthesia cases the main operating room should be at least 250 sq ft, and a minor operating room or recovery room should be at least 160 sq ft. In our present facility, the recovery room also functions as a minor operating room (Fig. 3-13G). The patient flow is quite flexible with this type of plan. It will be discussed further.

Cleanup and Sterilizing. A cleanup room and a separate room for clean storage and sterilization should be planned (Fig. 3-13A). A clean storage and sterilizing room of 100 to 120 sq ft will suffice for the support of most suites, but smaller or larger areas will be determined by the needs of a particular practice. The cleanup room can usually be smaller, again depending on the equipment and storage needs.

Nursing Station and Scrub. The nursing station can be incorporated in the circulation area outside the operating and recovery areas to permit surveillance of these units (Fig. 3-13C). This arrangement is more efficient than use of a separate office. The latter should be considered only in very large suites with a requirement for privacy for the supervisor. Scrub sinks can also be located in the circulation area, with a window view of the operating room (Fig. 3-13B,C). These functions can all be accommodated in 200 sq ft or less.

Change Area. The dressing areas for men and women can be separate, but a single area is adequate for most suites (Fig. 3-13D). Subdivision of this area can provide additional privacy for shower and change. Patient and staff lockers, makeup area, and toilet facilities are part of the unit. Approximately 125 sq ft should be allotted as a minimum for the area.

Waiting Area. Relatives and preoperative patients can use the main waiting room. When premedications have been administered, however, patients will require surveillance. In the event the recovery room is not available, a separate adjacent holding area within the suite may be desired. We obviate this additional overhead by utilizing a portion of the recovery room, but a very busy office surgery schedule

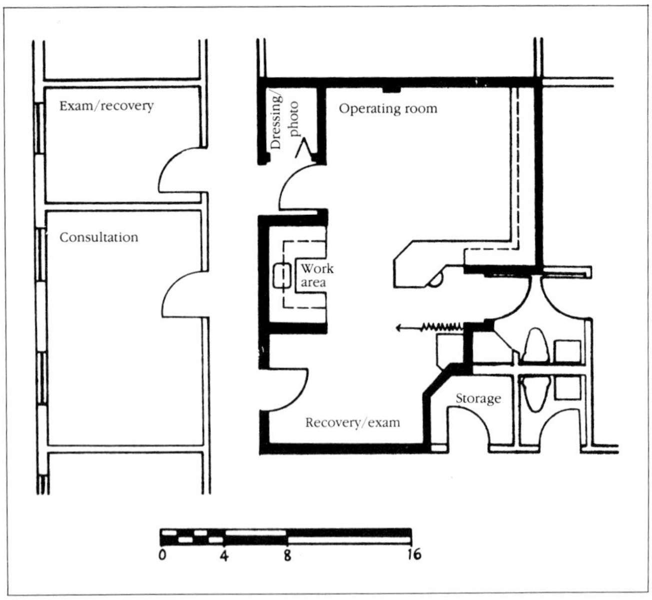

A

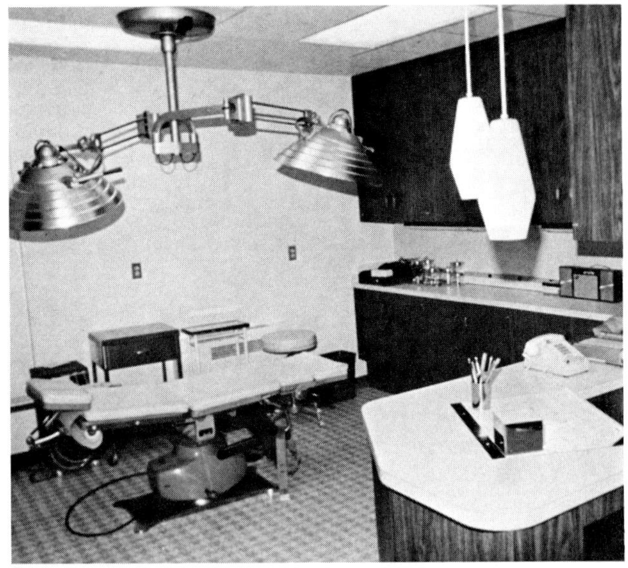

B

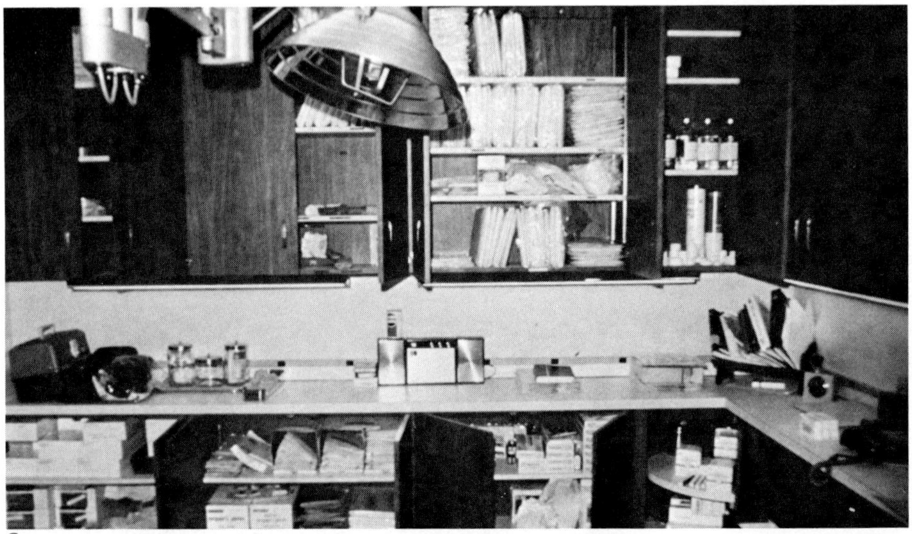

C

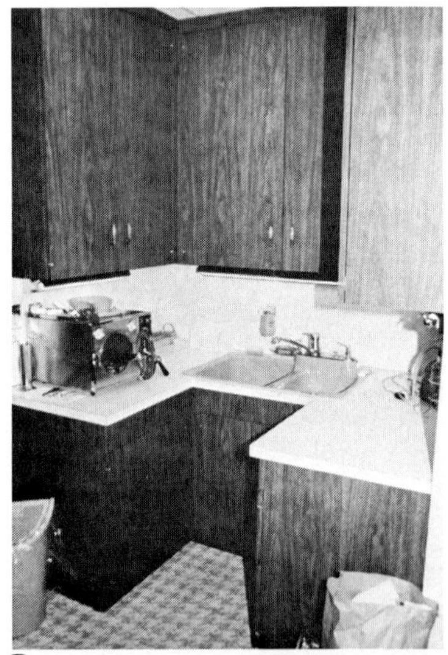

D

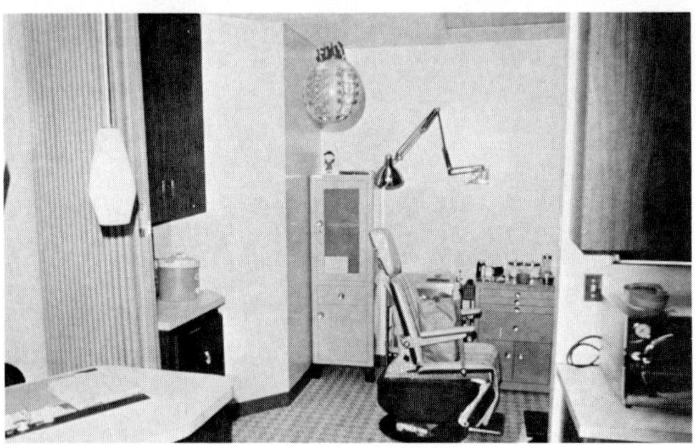

E

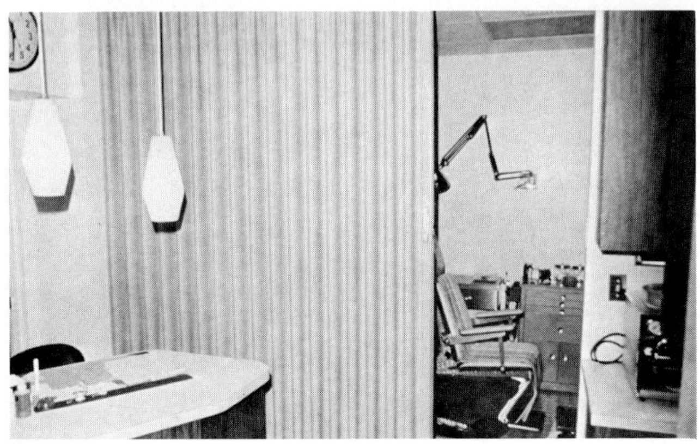

F

Figure 3-12. Compact surgery suite with multipurpose support facilities—initial facility of Albany Plastic Surgeons Associated, P.C.

A. Floor plan.
B. Operating room and nursing station.
C. Liberal counter and cabinet space also stores backup supplies for examining rooms.
D. Work area, scrub sink, and instrument autoclave for entire office.
E. Accordion wall between operating room and recovery area.
F. Recovery area doubles as examination and treatment room during office hours.

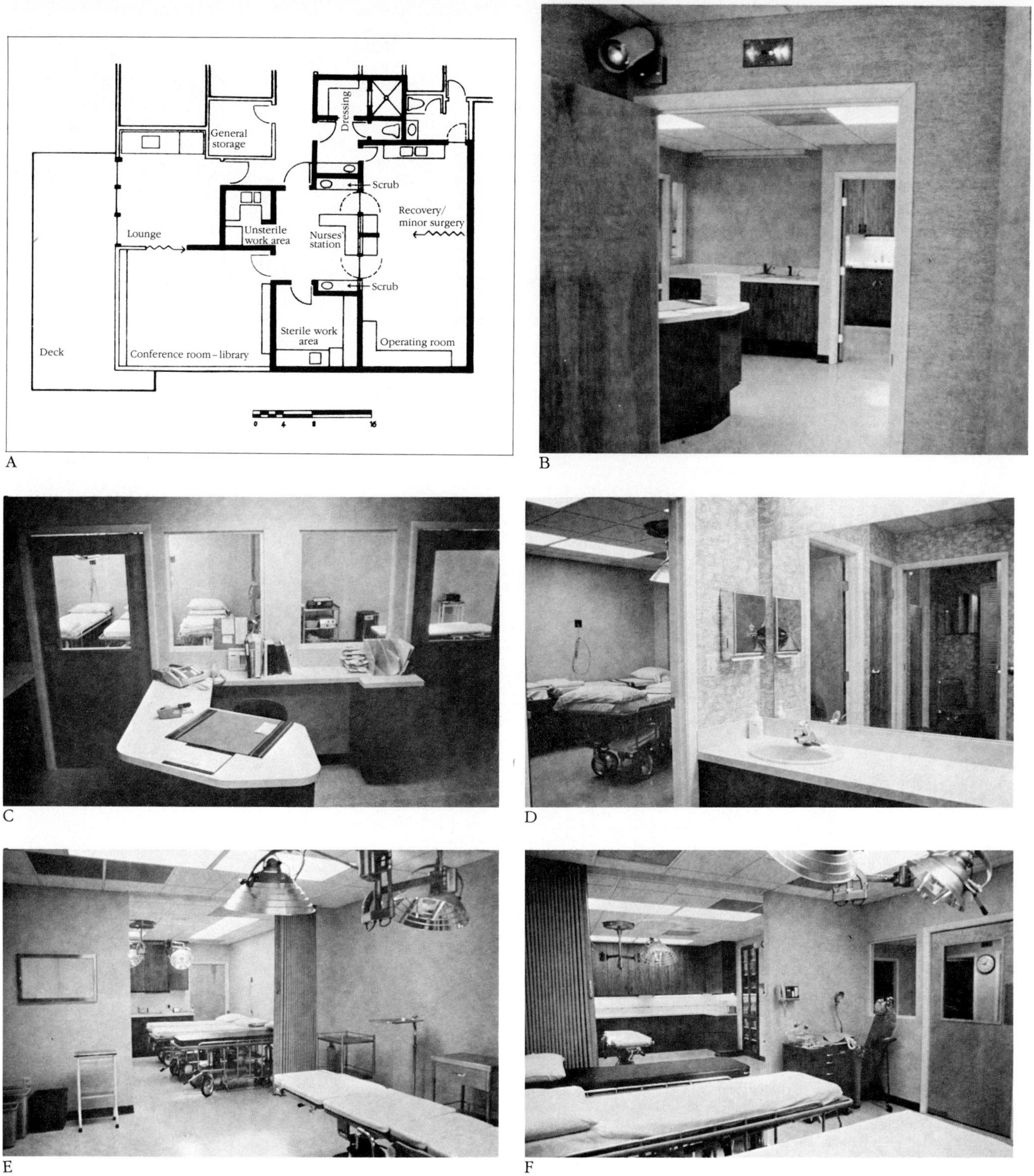

Figure 3-13. Present office surgery suite of Albany Plastic Surgeons Associated, P.C.

A. Floor plan.
B. Entrance showing nursing station, scrub sink, and sterile workroom.
C. Nursing station with view of and access to operating and recovery rooms.
D. Alternative entrance to minor operating room – recovery room via dressing room.
E. Operating room and recovery room joined by an accordion wall.
F. Resuscitation equipment is kept in the recovery room.

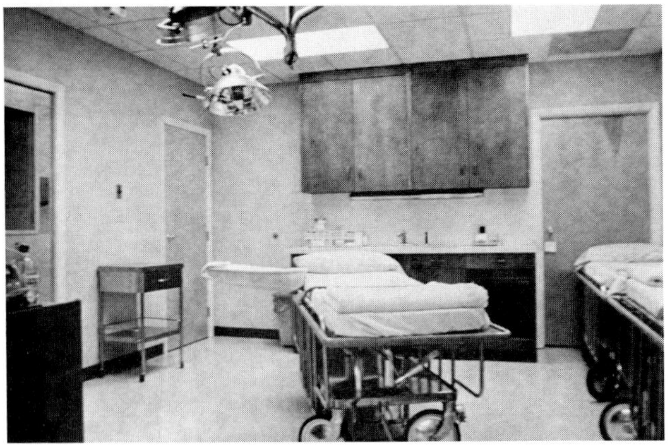

G

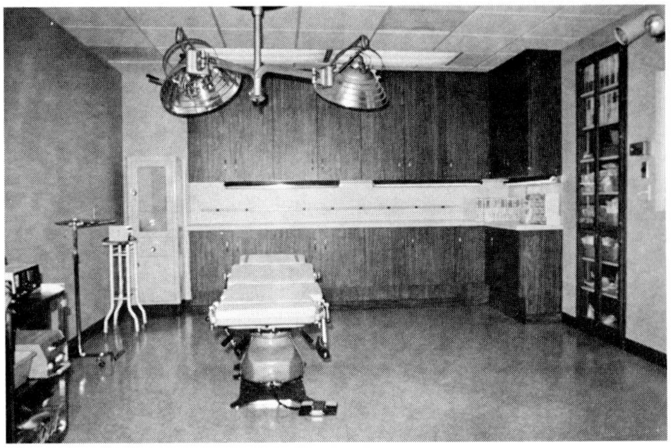

H

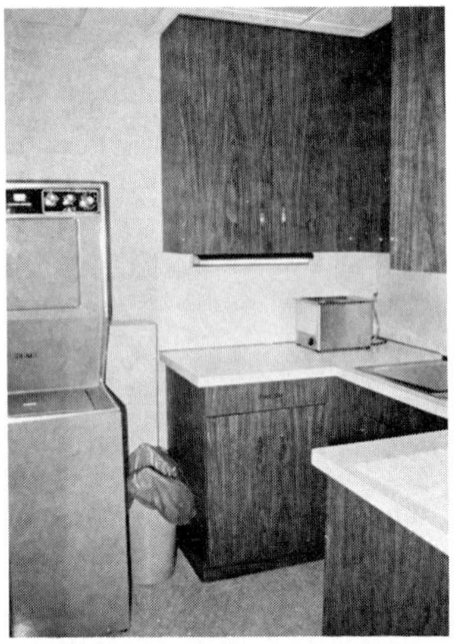

I

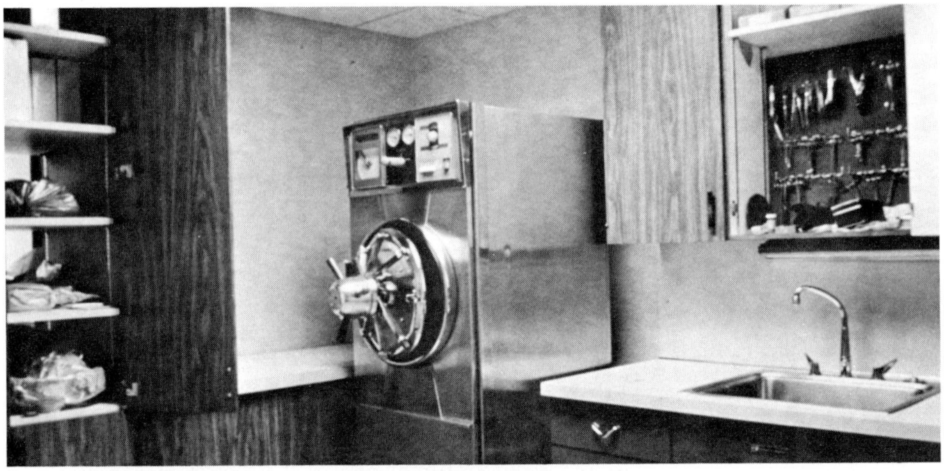

J

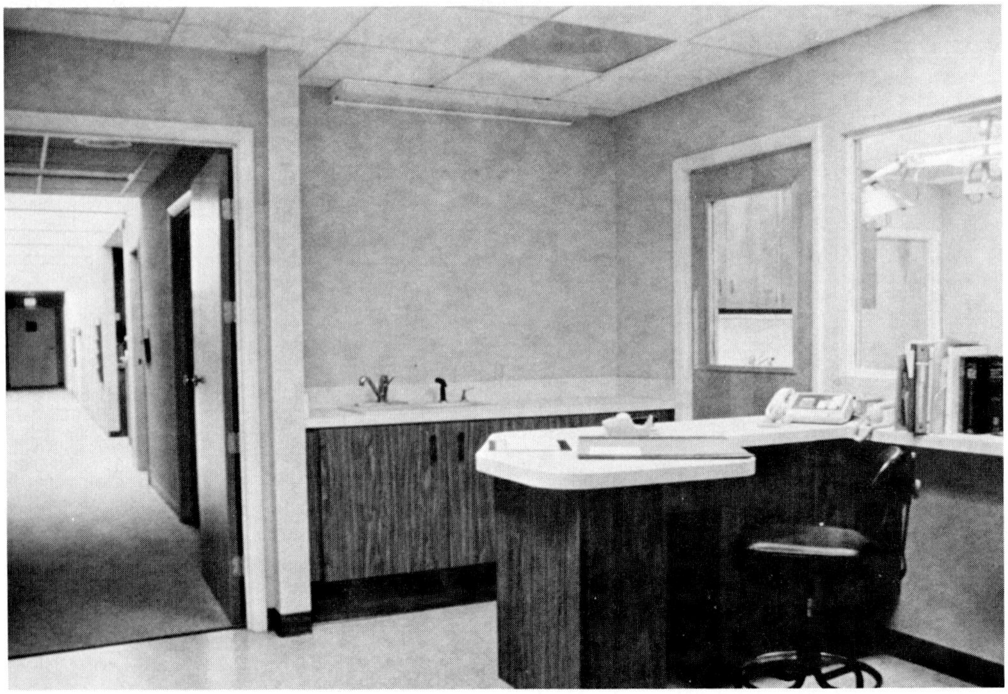

K

Figure 3-13 (continued)

G. Recovery room arranged as a minor operating room.

H. Main operating room with pass-through cabinet to sterile workroom and emergency lighting on right wall.

I. Cleanup room transplanted from former office; counters and cabinets expanded and washer-dryer unit added.

J. Sterile workroom with pass-through cabinet to main operating room.

K. An exit from the surgical suite to the parking lot that obviates passing through the main waiting room is highly recommended. This exit hallway is through the clinical area and leads to a covered loading ramp and driveway.

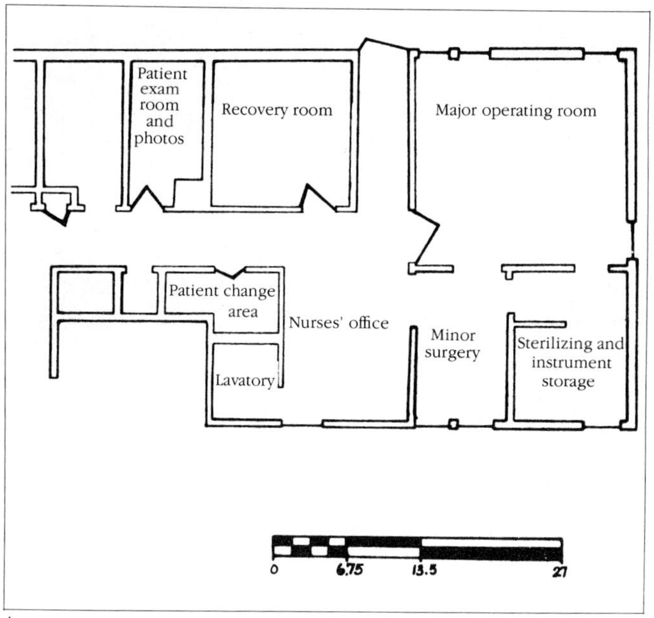

A

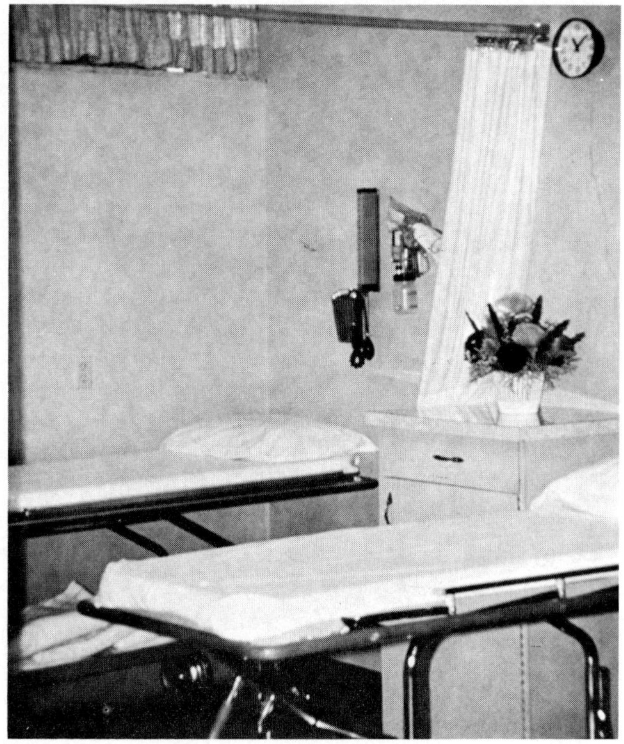
B

Figure 3-14. Office surgery suite of Ohio Plastic Surgeons, Inc., Columbus, Ohio.
A. Floor plan.
B. Recovery room with overhead curtain rails.

can perhaps justify the extra space and personnel. Approximately 100 sq ft should be adequate for this purpose if one stretcher is used; a larger room will be required for multiple patients.

Laboratory. If a laboratory is not part of the basic office, the minimal testing that is required can be accommodated readily in one of the existing areas of the suite. The countertop space, cabinets, and sink in the recovery room make this a logical choice.

Storage. Although base and wall cabinets in each of the described areas provide ready access to supplies used in that area, the large volume of necessary supplies requires a provision for bulk storage. A separate locked stockroom near, but outside of, the suite will accommodate deliveries, provide storage, and help control inventory (Fig. 3-13A). At least 100 sq ft should be planned if possible.

LAYOUT AND TRAFFIC FLOW

Ideally, the surgery suite should be isolated from the normal traffic pattern of the personnel and patients using the basic office. At least the major operating room(s) should be off limits for anyone not properly clothed. Adherence to this protocol is an important part of infection control. A minor operating room used for the treatment of emergencies can be approached in street clothes much like an emergency room at the hospital, if desired.

Patient Flow. Most patients will enter the surgical suite via a dressing area where privacy, lockers, and toilet facilities should be provided (Fig. 3-13D). In a compact suite, this area may open directly into an emergency operating room and will communicate with the recovery room. As previously discussed, the emergency operating room and recovery room may be a single unit with dual function (Fig. 3-13G). It may also be the holding area for premedicated patients and may serve as the examination room and laboratory for preoperative patients on the day of surgery.

All but minor cases should be treated in the major operating room with its stricter protocol. These patients normally go to the recovery room and then return to the dressing area. Ideally, patients should be able to leave the office without passing through the main waiting room and reception area.

The various potential patterns of flow should be tested on paper again and again and the modules rearranged until the desired result is evident. The architect and builder will reward this effort with savings of time and money.

Staff Flow. Properly clothed professional staff will circulate freely throughout the suite. Scrub clothing, caps, masks, and shoe covers are appropriate dress in the major operating room(s). Hands are scrubbed outside of the operating room, preferably where the surgeon can observe the operating room. Chart work, dictation, and records prepared before and after the operation are conveniently completed at the nursing station desk in the same circulation space. The recovering patient can also be observed from this area in our suite (Fig. 3-13C).

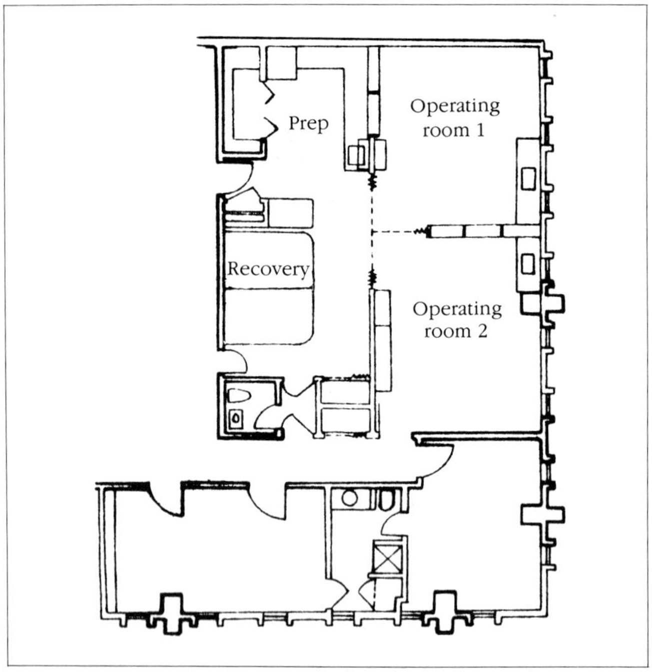

A

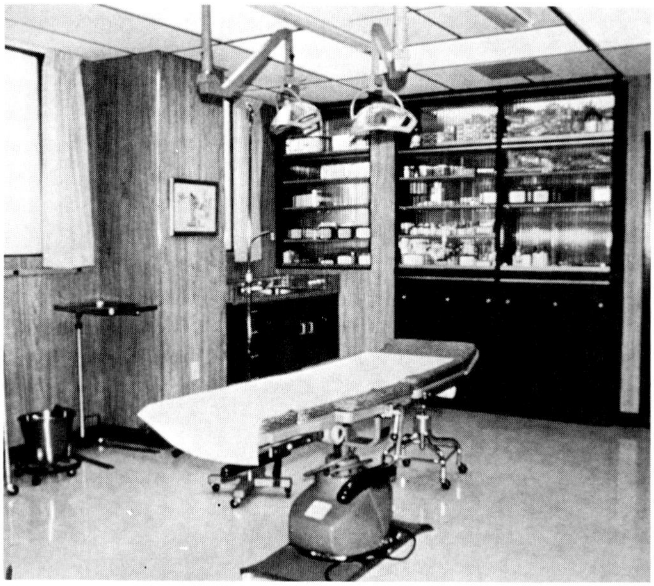

B

Figure 3-15. Office surgery suite of Plastic Surgery Clinic, Inc., Jacksonville, Florida.
A. Floor plan.
B. Operating rooms joined by an accordion door.

Cleanup between cases and at the end of the schedule is facilitated by using a separate room near the operating and recovery rooms. A separate room for clean storage, pack preparation, and sterilization is recommended. Efficiency is maximum if at least some of the storage cabinets in this area are double-sided with glass doors opening into the operating room and solid doors into the sterilization room (Figs. 3-13H,J).

Support Modules. Trash should be bagged between cases and removed to a remote, verminproof holding area between cases or promptly after the schedule is completed. The module designed for receipt and storage of bulk supplies for the surgery suite need not be located inside the suite but should be nearby.

A staff lounge located near the surgery suite will be handy for breaks between operations. A library–conference room located near the suite is convenient for privacy and for reference review by the professional staff. It can also function as an additional waiting area for relatives, friends, or unmedicated patients. These rooms should be outside of the basic office traffic pattern. However, their location near the surgery suite is not only a convenience between cases but, if properly planned, offers flexibility for future expansion of the surgery suite (Fig. 3-13A).

ENVIRONMENT AND DECOR

Most of the suggestions and comments referable to the basic office also apply to the surgery suite. Patient acceptance is a primary consideration. The impact of a clean, professional setting that is at the same time warm and inviting can be a positive factor.

A comfortable waiting area with soft music and current reading materials is a good beginning. The lavatory should be clean and colorful. The dressing area needs privacy, individual lockers for clothing, adequate mirrors, wall-to-wall carpeting, and a soothing decor.

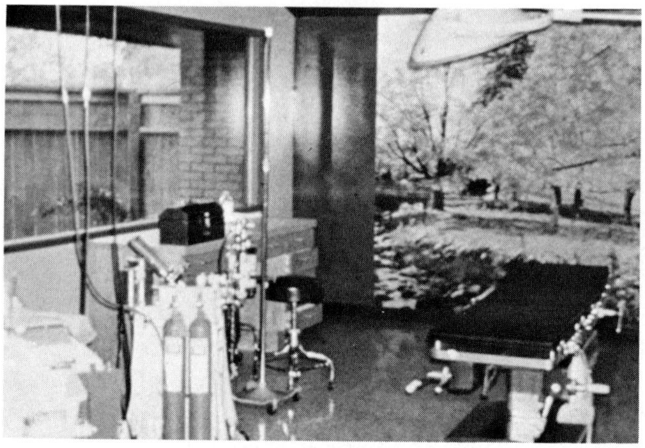

Figure 3-16. Operating room with wall mural and garden view photographed at the Salt Lake Surgical Center, Salt Lake City, Utah.

The operating and recovery rooms, although unmistakably clinical, can also be warm and inviting (Fig. 3-13E–H), in contrast to the Spartan appearance of the usual hospital operating room. Wall coverings of washable paint or vinyl provide flexibility in decor and are just as serviceable as the tiles seen in many hospitals. Wall murals can add a very pleasant effect. A beautiful view can be captured with a picture window as an alternative when available (Fig. 3-16). Cabinets and counters surfaced with plastic laminated inside and out will be durable and easy to clean. Air conditioning and a separate exhaust system are highly recommended for the entire suite; a large sterilizer may require special consideration. Overhead room lighting and separately controlled area lighting over the counters are basic needs. Background music, if desired, should be zone controlled.

Personnel

The person in charge of the surgery suite should be a trained, registered nurse with proved administrative ability. The office operating facility is a minibusiness with major management responsibilities, and the supervisor is the key to its efficiency and quality control. This person should be personable, intelligent, responsible, innovative, and dedicated to the concept of office surgery. The additional personnel for the surgery suite can be registered nurses, licensed practical nurses, physician's assistants, or trained technicians.

The number of persons involved in the delivery of office surgery will vary with layout and volume, but a minimum of two trained persons will be needed for all but the most minor procedures. Complex operations require a scrub nurse and a circulating nurse; a remote recovery area for sedated patients demands a third person. The same persons can obviously be utilized for a variety of tasks in the basic office. In a busy practice there is no problem keeping qualified surgery personnel occupied productively. But, as previously noted in regard to the selection of basic office staff, the mere addition of numbers is not cost-effective. One must hire efficient, qualified, productive individuals to meet defined needs.

Equipment

Quality care demands good equipment. If office surgery is to survive and thrive as a competitive entity, the support equipment must be at least comparable to that of the hospital.

OPERATING ROOM

Instruments. The choice of surgical instruments will reflect the specific needs of the surgeon for efficient completion of the procedures offered and for any potential emergency related to them. Many surgeons already own special instruments for use in the hospital, which obviously do not need to be duplicated. As a standard, the same fine-quality instruments requested in the hospital setting should be made available in the office suite.

Operating Lights. Surgeons almost traditionally complain about operating lights at the hospital. In a private office suite the surgery light source should be carefully researched and chosen by the surgeon. Sterilizable handles are an excellent feature. They should be easy to insert and cuffed to avoid contamination of the operating team. Sterile sleeves to shield fixed handles, and ceiling spotlights that are adjusted with a pole have no place in the modern operating room. Fully adjustable lighting on a flexible extension is most practical, and twin overhead lights are preferred.

Mobile floor lights are not a substitute for overhead lights. The loss of floor space is an important negative factor. The fiberoptic headlight is a much more practical source of supplemental light for office surgery and may be the best primary light for some procedures. Lighted retractors add significant cost and offer little or no advantage over a headlight.

An emergency light source in the event of power failure is a safety feature of importance. A hand-held, battery-operated light is the least expensive. A storage battery or a remote standby gasoline generator may be considered as an alternate source of power if long power failures are common. The storage battery is the better of these two options for most suites. In the rare emergency most surgeons can complete a procedure safely without electrically operated suction apparatus, electrocautery, or monitors; hence, only a light source is mandatory. A reasonable option is the wall-mounted emergency lighting unit, discussed under Emergency Systems for the basic office.

Operating Table. A motorized operating table is a convenient luxury; adjustable height, tilt, and back elevation are necessities. Obviously, the expense varies with features and accessories, but there are some basic needs. The surface pad should be comfortable and easy to clean, and the table should be mobile on a pedestal or rollers. A safety belt and arm restraints are also basic. Arm supports and an ether screen are other options that will be needed in most practices.

An adjustable stretcher may be used as an operating table in a minor operating room and double as a recovery room unit, but most designs are not stable enough for more complex surgery and the bulky undercarriage is a disadvantage to the operating team. Less expensive non-adjustable carts are available for transport and recovery, but adjustability for height and back elevation is worth considering for all units.

While contoured operating chairs are comfortable for head and neck surgery and may be used for some procedures on the anterior torso, most do not flatten enough to permit lateral or prone positions. A unit with modular attachments for the Mayo stand, intravenous pole, and miscellaneous equipment for suction, cautery, and monitoring may be attractive for close quarters, but it is not practical as the only operating table in the usual suite, even if its high cost could be justified.

Special Equipment. Suction, electrocautery, oxygen source, monitoring, and resuscitation equipment is needed in every modern surgery suite.

The suction equipment can be central or portable but must be reliable and easily cleaned. Portable equipment is less expensive than a central system, but the latter eliminates room noise. Adjustable strength is a desirable feature, and a backup unit and an alternative power source should be considered. A reasonably priced portable cabinet unit manufactured by Dri-Clave Corporation provides efficient variable suction via dual hoses that accept standard suction tubing. The availability of two tubes has an obvious advantage.

The aesthetic surgeon will use disposable battery-operated cautery units and sophisticated electrocautery units in the hospital setting. These should also be available in the office operating room. Valley Labs, Electro-Medical Systems, and others manufacture suitable electrocautery units. The decision should be based on practice requirements, cost, and availability of maintenance. The modern solid-state units require little maintenance, but a backup unit or provision for a loaner is still an important consideration. Hyfrecators are not a substitute for cautery; their use should be restricted to the examining room.

Oxygen must be available, even for local anesthesia cases; use will be only occasional, and a portable tank with catheter and masks for adults and children should suffice. When general anesthesia is planned, the anesthesiologist is the logical consultant for more sophisticated equipment needs.

Equipment for monitoring pulse and blood pressure are basic. Instant readout units are quite expensive, but their convenience and accuracy are attractive. For other than the most minor procedures, electrocardiographic (ECG) monitoring is advised. Datascope, Physio-Control, and others offer a full range of features and prices. Battery operation for transport, and permanent tracing capability are recommended. Although telephone telemetry to a hospital-based unit is an option on some equipment, this expensive feature is difficult to justify in the usual office surgery suite.

Resuscitation will require the establishment and maintenance of an airway. A lighted laryngoscope, nasal and oral tubes of various sizes, suction, and oxygen are needed. The Ambu bag and Elder valve are helpful for providing aeration in the emergency situation.

When ECG monitoring is used, a synchronized defibrillator is recommended. Minor ECG changes may simply indicate the need for oxygenation, but in the rare instance in which defibrillation is called for there is no substitute.

Trained personnel, emergency drugs, and reliable equipment ensure the best response to an untoward reaction or emergency situation. An established plan for transfer of the patient to a hospital has already been suggested; it will be required for accreditation.

Miscellaneous Hardware. An inventory of the necessary supporting hardware used in the average operating room will surprise the unwary, and the potential cost is significant. An instrument stand and back table are obvious needs. But not to be overlooked are the intravenous poles, kick buckets, solution basins, stools, and various equipment stands. Many of these are stainless steel, and all are expensive. Other requirements include a step for patients and platforms for the nurse, shorter assistants, and observers.

All items should be selected for safety, durability, and easy maintenance. The materials should resist stains and be readily cleaned. A compromise in quality will become evident in time and may even introduce a hazard.

RECOVERY ROOM

The equipment required for the recovery area will vary with the patient load, type of surgery, and level of sedation. A modern transport stretcher can easily double as a recovery room bed and may even serve as a minor operating room table. The mobile units that are adjustable for height and position, although more expensive than stationary beds, allow the greatest flexibility. When multipurpose utilization of the recovery room is planned for minor or emergency surgery, the ability to clear the floor space becomes very important. Equipment should be mobile or mounted on the wall or ceiling.

Privacy is not essential but can be provided by mobile screens or curtain rails suspended from the ceiling if desired (Fig. 3-14B). There should be good lighting and an emergency call button in each patient area, as well as equipment for monitoring and resuscitation. Portable equipment reduces capital expense. If the room also serves as a minor operating room, the operating lights on flexible arms may be entirely adequate for extra lighting to supplement normal ceiling lights. Ceiling spotlights and wall-mounted extension lights are alternatives. Soft lighting can be provided by the lights mounted under the wall cabinets in the counter work area.

Built-in cabinets for supplies and equipment, a countertop work space, a sink, and a refrigerator will all be practical. The locked cabinet for drugs may be located in this area; the nursing station is an alternative location.

NURSING STATION

A desk and countertop work space will be needed for the nurses. Its location near the operating and recovery rooms will make this a convenient place for record preparation and the dictation of operative notes. Filing space for records, supply catalogs, and other references pertinent to the surgical suite should be included. This work area, separate from the basic office, will add efficiency for suite-related projects. A typewriter may be beneficial, but the other office machines need not be duplicated in the average suite. It is likely that a computer terminal will be part of the modern nursing station in the near future, and a sophisticated word processor may become routine equipment.

WORKROOMS

A cleanup area and a space for preparation of surgical packs and sterilization are needed for support of the operating room. Ideally, they should be separate rooms, but they can be combined in an economy suite. In keeping with the multipurpose concept, these workrooms can also be used as support for the examining rooms.

Cleanup. The cleanup area needs a sink, storage cabinets, and well-lighted counter space as a minimum. A double sink with shallow and deep sections is recommended. An ultrasound cleaner and regular use of instrument lubricants will preserve fine instruments. Provision should be made for the temporary storage of soiled linens and trash. A combination washer-dryer unit is practical in this area. Twenty-four-inch-wide piggyback machines are available and function well for a small suite. Larger units should be accommodated in the plans if disposable drapes are not used. The savings from the laundry of scrub suits, towels, and sheets can be significant.

Sterilization. The sterilization room should have adequate storage space for clean and sterile equipment and supplies. Cabinet depth is particularly important in this area. Liberal countertop space is also needed. This workroom will be an active area in the busy suite.

The autoclave or sterilizer used for surgical packs and instruments must have sufficient capacity and quality for the anticipated needs. A "flash" sterilization cycle will add efficiency. Any additional expense for this feature will be weighed against the expense of duplicating instruments and the inevitable delay if a particular instrument requires sterilization during surgery. There must be provision for the adequate exhaust of steam.

Gas sterilization is relatively slow, but it is ideal for some supplies. Small units or bag-and-cartridge techniques will suffice for most suites.

Cold sterilization in a solution such as Cidex is rapid and convenient. Most hospitals use this technique between cases, particularly for preservation of sharp instruments that may be damaged by steam.

STAFF LOUNGE

The staff lounge shared by the basic office staff will be a convenient break area for the surgical team if located near the suite. A coffee machine, refrigerator-freezer, toaster, microwave oven, disposal, and dishwashing machine can all be justified in the busy office to minimize lost time. Adequate seating and a pleasant environment will be rewarded by staff appreciation and utilization.

Communication

A telephone and intercommunication system should be available in the recovery room and at the nursing station as a minimum. The intercom should be available to the operating team, but telephone communication in the operating room is optional.

The light system developed for the basic office can be extended to the surgical suite, where it will help the office staff locate the surgical team and provide information to the team regarding the office sign-in of other professional personnel.

Patients in the recovery area should each have a call button to summon aid. Additional voice monitoring or television monitoring can be useful in some instances. Heavily sedated patients and those recovering from general anesthesia require constant surveillance by the professional staff.

Supplies

The inventory of supplies for the efficient functioning of an office surgery suite parallels that of a hospital. Surgical supplies, medications, and intravenous solutions must be kept in adequate stock. The storage and disposal problems have already been discussed.

BASIC AND SPECIAL SUPPLIES

An office surgery practice will require a supply of surgical gowns, gloves, towels, drapes, suture material, drains, catheters, sponges, prep solutions, dressings, and intravenous solutions, as well as administration units, just to name a few. Needles, syringes, drugs, ECG pads, patient gowns, shoe covers, scrub suits, hair covers, and masks add to the routine inventory.

Special supplies will vary with the type of surgery. Battery-operated cautery, nerve stimulators, and implantable prostheses are examples of the seemingly never-ending list. The need for cash flow and for storage space is obvious.

DISPOSABLE SUPPLIES

The use of disposable supplies wherever possible is highly recommended both for safety and for maintenance. Most surgeons prefer cloth gowns and drapes in the hospital setting. However, for office surgery, paper supplies are more practical.

The quality of disposable items has been improved greatly in response to the increasing demand. Disposable gloves, needles, shoe covers, masks, and hair covers are used in most hospitals. Disposable cautery, nerve stimulators, catheters, and resuscitation supplies have joined the growing list. Safety and efficiency have created a preference for prepackaged disposable supplies.

Records

Records for an office surgery suite can be less complex than those required at the hospital, but certain records are necessary as a minimum.

PATIENT RECORDS

The patient's surgery records should be an intregral part of the basic office chart. A surgical consent form, photographic permission, preoperative laboratory data, interval history, recent examination, operative note, medication sheet, anesthesia record, recovery room notes, and follow-up data are all included. They may be stapled together for easy reference. Ultimately the pathology report and any other reports relative to the surgery become part of this file. All dictated reports should be signed by the appropriate person, and unusual laboratory reports and all reports of malignancy should be initialed by the surgeon.

SURGERY AND RECOVERY LOGS

The logbook of operations is a permanent record of the activity in the surgery suite. Pertinent data include the patient's name, surgical team, procedures, medications, length of time in the operating room, length of the procedures, and type of anesthesia as a minimum. A record of any drains and complications is also advisable.

The recovery room log can be combined with the surgical log, but a separate log is advised for the busy suite. The name of the supervising person, medications, length of time in the recovery room, and any untoward reactions or complications should be noted.

The length of time in each unit will be helpful in the cost accounting of a specific procedure. The average time for a procedure will help scheduling, and the other data may be useful for a review of the surgical management of patients and for quality control.

MEDICATIONS
Controlled drugs must be accounted for with a strict protocol. The inventory of these drugs should be matched against utilization by patient name and amounts discarded. The signature of the responsible person is mandatory to satisfy most state regulations.

Locked storage is required for controlled substances, as previously noted. The supervising nurse should be responsible for precautions against pilferage and misuse, and occasional spot checks by the surgeon will offer an added deterrent.

All other medications should be stored under the supervision of the senior nurse, with much the same protocol, except for the locked storage. An accurate inventory and utilization log will discourage misuse.

SUPPLIES
A continuous inventory of supplies is required for efficient management. Records of utilization will be mandatory for inventory control. The storage of excessive supplies is expensive. A supply equal to 1.5 to 2.0 times the average amount used between order and receipt will usually suffice for commonly used supplies; rarely used items will require less inventory stock. Unusual quantity discounts may justify a modification of this formula for a specific item.

The inventory records should include the source of the item, a catalog number, the quantity per case, and the cost per case and per unit. Cost accounting for each procedure requires the unit cost, and of course it will be needed for comparison shopping.

EQUIPMENT
An accurate record of all equipment in the suite should be required. The equipment should be labeled to establish ownership, and where appropriate the serial number and model identification should be entered in the log. The source, date of purchase, catalog number, and cost will establish a record for loss and will facilitate replacement.

Brochures, operating instructions, and warranty agreements should be filed for ready reference. The routine maintenance schedule suggested by the manufacturer should be followed and recorded. Other routine maintenance such as scissor sharpening should be recorded, including the vendor, date, and cost. Periodic inspection, testing, and calibration by an outside laboratory is advisable for sophisticated equipment.

MISCELLANEOUS
Federal and state regulatory agencies, third-party payers, and even malpractice and liability insurance carriers are likely to become more involved in the planning, function, and quality control of office surgery suites. The paperwork is certain to increase. Some states already have laws affecting these facilities.

If the facility is rented for use by persons other than partners, the impact of these various agencies and insurance companies must be researched carefully. The regulations and insurance cost may be increased significantly.

Accreditation will mandate most of the described records. Third-party payers will have a particular interest in the cost-accounting records.

Patient Selection and Management

The efficient running of an office surgery facility demands careful patient selection and management. The mechanism for scheduling consultations and office follow-up care already exists in the basic office. Some special considerations are needed for office surgery.

CONSULTATION
The selection of patients for ambulatory surgery is part of the aesthetic surgeon's expertise, after due consideration of the patient's wishes. Medical condition is a prime consideration in any setting, but only low-risk patients should be treated in an office facility.

After feasibility has been determined, preoperative tests, the surgical procedure, anesthesia, postoperative course, options, risks, and cost must all be discussed. The latter is particularly important when fees and operating room charges are payable in advance. These costs must be separated for the patient so that comparisons will be valid and surgical fees do not appear excessive. If experience has determined that the patient's insurance company will cover operating room charges in the hospital and will not cover them in the office setting, this fact must be made known to the patient.

A patient frequently relies on the judgment of the surgeon, but an informed choice can be made only if the reasonable advantages and disadvantages of the office setting are clearly described. When the concept of office surgery is not clearly acceptable to the informed patient, an alternative setting should be selected. Information brochures and instructions, outlining in lay terms the things that are discussed pertinent to specific procedures, are helpful.

An informed consent for surgery and photographic permissions must be signed by the patient or legally responsible person. Since legal consent cannot be obtained from a patient after sedation, delay in the execution of these forms until the day of surgery is not advised. As the forms should be read and the signature witnessed, it is usually more efficient to delegate this task to a qualified member of the office staff rather than to include it in the consultation. The scheduling person is one logical choice. If there is a provision for further counseling by an informed staff member, the patient has an opportunity to review the information learned from the surgeon and any printed material, and to ask additional questions. The consent forms could be signed during that interview.

PATIENT FLOW
All patients for whom sedation is prescribed, and all minors, should be transported by a responsible adult. If the consent forms and charges have been handled in advance, the intake procedure should be brief.

The patient should be greeted by a surgical nurse, who reviews drug sensitivities, laboratory reports, and the interval medical history as a check for any possible contraindication to the planned surgery. All patients are encouraged to use the toilet before changing into a paper gown and disposable slippers. The gown is worn with the opening in the back or front, depending on the planned procedure.

A nurse administers the appropriate medication in the holding area. All medicated patients are observed for untoward reactions and are kept under surveillance. The chart is reviewed and a physical examination is performed by the nurse and reviewed and countersigned by the surgeon.

Patients receiving light premedication can frequently walk to the operating room, but heavily sedated patients will require stretcher transportation. An intravenous line is started on all sedated patients, and the appropriate monitors are applied. Intravenous medications are directed by the surgeon.

Discharge directly from the operating room is routine for minor procedures and may even be feasible after more complicated procedures when the patient is alert. Discharge via the recovery room is common after major operations, particularly those that tend to have early postoperative complications. The period of observation varies, and transportation from the office to a waiting car is normally by wheelchair. The office discharge procedure should be simple.

TELEPHONE FOLLOW-UP

The written instructions given to the patient at the time of discharge should include a telephone number to reach the surgeon or a staff member in the event of an emergency. A valuable personal touch is added by a call to the patient at home to inquire about his or her condition. This call from the surgeon or nurse shows professional concern, offers reassurance, and adds an element of quality to the postoperative care.

Standards and Safeguards

Office surgery is relatively new in some regions of the United States. As with any new concept that offers change from an established practice, criticism may precede acceptance. A variety of standards and safeguards are recommended to meet this challenge and assure quality control.

SUITE DESIGN

Quality materials provide a good beginning. Like the basic office, the surgery suite must be professional in its appearance and, as previously emphasized, warm and inviting. Washable vinyl wall covers, wood-grain cabinets, and solid colors on counters and shelves can be coordinated with vinyl coverings on tables and stools for a special warmth, durability, and easy maintenance. The options are exciting and quite individual. The choice of materials for the suite can give an unmistakably clinical appearance without the Spartan look of most hospital units. Easily cleaned materials are particularly important in the surgery suite if bacterial contamination and infections are to be avoided.

Fire-resistant construction and decor may be supplemented by a sprinkler system if desired. Modern fixtures are efficient and aesthetic, and this safeguard usually results in lower fire insurance rates to help offset the cost. However, most aesthetic surgeons will avoid general anesthesia, and explosive anesthetics should not be permitted. Therefore, the fire hazard related to office surgery is not significant beyond the considerations already addressed for the basic office. Conductive flooring is not needed in the usual suite. All staff members should be familiar with the operation of available fire equipment and be regularly drilled for fire emergency.

Electric outlets should be plentiful to avoid the hazard of extended leads. Utility molding with an outlet every 12 in. in counter areas provides flexibility and obviates exact preplanning for the location of each piece of equipment. Grounded plugs that have been inspected for proper polarity should be used for all equipment.

PATIENT SURVEILLANCE

Surveillance of patients is important for safety. An observation window from the surgeon's scrub area into the operating room is basic. If the nursing station is located in the circulation area with an observation window into the operating rooms and recovery area, additional efficiency and safety are provided. Where the operating room and recovery area are separated by a folding door wall, fewer circulating personnel will be needed to control both areas safely.

EDUCATION

The selection of quality personnel for the surgical suite has already been discussed. There should be policy and procedure manuals for the personnel, with which all should be familiar. Periodic testing of this knowledge is recommended. Each person should also have a written job description, and there should be a regular evaluation of individual performance.

Continuing education should be encouraged. Obtaining new knowledge and preserving previously learned skills will be important to the quality of patient care. All operating personnel should be trained in basic life support (cardiopulmonary resuscitation—CPR) and the indications for its use. They should also be familiar with the equipment and medications used in the treatment of cardiac arrest, respiratory arrest, and anaphylactic emergencies. There should be a written protocol for these emergencies and regular drills for staff refinement.

Although not always possible, hospital privileges for nursing personnel enable the office nurses to assist with surgery and hospital care. This opportunity affords a valuable form of continuing education and a continuity of care that adds prestige to the surgery suite.

TRAFFIC AND DRESS

The admission of persons to the surgery suite should be controlled by the nurse supervisor. Relatives and friends should not be permitted in the operating room.

All persons entering the elective surgery operating room should be properly dressed in an appropriate gown or scrub outfit. During surgery the entire team and any observers must wear scrub suits or dresses, shoe covers, surgical hats, and masks.

Recovery room personnel should observe clean technique, and the use of scrub outfits is optional but suggested. Ideally, everyone working in the suite should change from street clothes, but in this area at least a gown cover is appropriate. These precautions are sufficient for minor emergency surgery in the multipurpose suite.

SAFETY AND SECURITY

Smoking must not be allowed anywhere within the surgery suite. Explosive anesthetic agents must be prohibited, and all volatile or combustible materials need to be properly stored.

Emergency systems and security have already been discussed. The basic systems apply to the surgery suite as well as the main office. Emergency lighting for the operating and recovery room and for marking exits are very important.

Security for patient's clothing and valuables should be less of a problem in the well-managed office than in a hospital, but patients should be encouraged to leave their money, jewelry, and other valuables at home or with the relative or friend who transports them. Individual locked storage or a check-in system for valuables should also be available, as some patients will not be accompanied. Lockers for clothing and valuables will usually suffice, and extra-large keytags will reduce the problem of lost keys. A supply of spare keys in a secure location will obviate inconvenience.

Cost Accounting

Beware! An office surgery suite is not a means for increasing the surgeon's income. It is rather a convenience and luxury for the surgeon and, if properly managed, should provide a savings for the patient. Start-up costs will vary greatly with design and new equipment needs. A range of $15,000 to more than $100,000 can be anticipated, with actual costs depending on the magnitude of the project. An increase in overhead is certain. Careful cost accounting and the prepayment of all charges will minimize the potential loss.

OVERHEAD

The calculation of overhead must include the rent or amortized construction costs, depreciation of equipment, general supplies, payroll costs, insurance, taxes, and utilities. Security, waste removal, maintenance, and record and accounting costs must also be included. Some expenses can be clearly assigned to the surgery suite for accounting purposes while others are best calculated as a percentage of the total office overhead based on the relative area devoted to the suite.

PROCEDURE COST

After the annual overhead has been calculated, actual utilization will be needed to arrive at a per-hour cost. If the direct cost of supplies and the payroll costs are figured separately and added to the fixed overhead expenses, the charges can be related more closely to the procedure. Using average figures for supplies and personnel time will suffice for the calculation of a basic cost for each procedure, to which additional special supply costs can be added. Supply costs must include all shipping charges and taxes. Cost-accounting methods should avoid the arbitrary prorating of charges by time alone that has caused hospital charges for minor procedures to rise out of proportion to the service rendered.

PATIENT'S COST

In a busy suite it will be appropriate to add a factor for profit. Actually, the inventory costs and other hidden expenses are likely to require some such adjustment in charges to ensure a break-even venture.

Until utilization is sufficient to dilute fixed overhead costs, some subsidy for the facility may be in order as part of the reasonable start-up expense. However, the practice of absorbing suite costs in the usual and customary fee for surgery can only lead to a significant reduction in income. I feel that it is mandatory to charge a separate fee for the use of a sophisticated office surgery facility. This charge must be clearly defined for the patient, and, like the surgery fee, it should be paid in advance.

As a practical reference, the charge for the office setting should be less than the hospital charge for a comparable procedure. In a busy office facility that is managed with efficiency, savings for the patient should be significant.

REIMBURSEMENT

If there is a consistent, significant savings in facility costs in the office setting, it seems only a matter of time until insurance carriers accept this alternative for reimbursement for those procedures ordinarily insured. Then an even greater utilization and further reduction of the fixed overhead portion of the charges would be permitted.

Inquiry by the surgeon, followed by an inspection by the insurance carrier, has been the usual route to a successful reimbursement policy. In the future, standardization and accreditation are likely requirements. The third-party payers must be informed regarding the true costs and the facility standards in order to negotiate a proper reimbursement. The need for detailed and accurate cost accounting is obvious.

Accreditation

A program for voluntary inspection and accreditation of office surgery facilities, if properly developed, should be beneficial to the surgeon, the patient, and interested third-party payers. It is one way to develop creditable standards of quality care. The definition of minimum standards and formal recognition of compliance may delay or forestall government intervention while inviting positive consideration by insurance companies.

JCAH

The Joint Commission on Accreditation of Hospitals indicated an interest in the accreditation of office facilities when it formed an Accreditation Council for Ambulatory

Health Care. The pilot program did not meet the need of the majority of offices as only suites used by three or more surgeons were included. Although a number of office facilities were accredited under this program, it failed to gain wide acceptance among aesthetic surgeons.

AAAAPSF

In 1976 the president of the American Society of Plastic and Reconstructive Surgeons, Fred McCoy, M.D., appointed an ad hoc committee to study the feasibility of an accreditation process for office surgery facilities of its members. The author was the chairman of this committee. Dr. McCoy's perception of a need reached fruition with support from the American Society of Aesthetic Plastic Surgeons and under the strong leadership of Charles Vinnick, M.D., and Edward Truppman, M.D., as succeeding chairmen of the permanent ASPRS Committee on Office Surgery. In 1980, the proposed American Association for Accreditation of Ambulatory Plastic Surgery Facilities was awarded a seed grant from ASPRS, and the first Certificates of Accreditation were awarded in October 1981. This has been a giant step forward.

This organization has launched an educational program with the reasonable goal of formalizing minimum standards and has developed a voluntary certification program for compliance. Recertification every 2 years and interim-year reporting are required. Facilities are accredited in one of three categories, which reflect the standards for minor procedures, major operations under local anesthesia, or major surgery with general anesthesia. Variations in category depend on the application request, sophistication of the facility, and confirming evidence from peer inspection.

The AAAAPSF Checklist/Questionnaire is highly recommended as a guide for the current standards for the design and management of a surgery suite.

CONCLUSION

The development of an aesthetic surgeon's office and the incorporation of a surgery suite can take many directions. The design and management of the facility take great effort, but this effort, if properly directed, will be a source of satisfaction and pride for the surgeon and will provide an efficient setting for quality care for the patients. The myriad of details and the variations encountered in such a project could easily fill a textbook, but it is the author's sincere hope that this chapter, with its shortcomings, will offer some help to the surgeon who is embarking on this course.

4. Drugs for Outpatient Surgery

Howard L. Gordon

One of the changes that is taking place in the constantly evolving world of surgery, and in particular the world of plastic surgery, is the current trend toward the use of ambulatory outpatient surgical facilities. The benefits to patients and surgeons are many. They include lower costs to the patient, increased convenience for the surgeon, and greater potential for quality and cost control. Along with these and other benefits comes increased responsibility on the part of the surgeon. In this new setting, the surgeon is no longer surrounded by a team of supporting experts, such as the anesthesiologist, the operating room supervisor, the administrator, the pharmacist, and all the other members of the enormous team that today constitutes a large hospital staff. In the outpatient surgical unit of today the surgeon must assume all the roles in order to make the unit function well and safely.

OBJECTIVES

In the selection of drugs to use before, during, and after surgery, the modern surgeon is faced with what may appear to be a bewildering panoply of medications. Who can possibly keep up with even the new drugs coming on the market each year, much less maintain a mastery of the ones already at hand? This presentation is not intended as a prescription of what to give and what to do; rather, it offers a rational approach to the individual selection of drugs that best suits the combined needs of the patient and the operating surgeon. The general theme of the approach is: Keep it simple—keep it safe.

Let us consider the needs of the patient at the three distinct parts of the surgical journey—before the operation, during the operation, and following the operation.

In the days just prior to the surgery, the patient's needs are primarily related to relief of anxiety and fear. Almost all of us, when confronted by an upcoming surgical procedure, have a variety of fears, some reasonable and some unreasonable, but all real to us. We are often afraid that the anesthetic will not be effective and that we will have pain. We are often afraid that with the stimulus of the pain we will act in a way that is not acceptable. Some of us fear that we will tell "secrets" under the influence of the drugs. Some fear that the operating will begin too soon, that is, before the anesthesia is complete, and others that they will wake before the surgery is finished. Some wonder whether they will wake up at all. All of us have a dread about scarring and mutilation, and, to many, all forms of surgery carry this risk. To some, the word *surgery* carries with it the possibility of finding cancer. There is no doubt

Acknowledgment is made to Dr. Lorne Eltherington, Associate Professor of Clinical Anesthesia, Stanford University Medical Center, for having been my pharmacologic "guru." It was he who first espoused the principle "Keep it simple—keep it safe" discussed here.

that the efforts of the surgeon prior to surgery should be directed toward allaying these and other anxieties by the use of direct communication, primarily verbal. Explaining the procedure in a manner the patient can understand often helps a great deal. It is likewise valuable to give the patient some insight into the thought processes the surgeon uses to arrive at a "game plan."

The mental attitudes of the patient, the surgeon, and the assistants have a profound effect on the course of the procedure. A positive, helpful, and sympathetic attitude can go a long way toward reducing the fears and anxieties of the patient.

To lessen this heavy burden of the prospective patient is a worthwhile goal, not only from the standpoint of sheer compassion, but also because a relaxed, well-rested patient coming to the operating room free of serious anxiety makes the work of the surgeon easier, more pleasant, and safer. Resistance to the drugs being used rises as the anxiety level rises. Toxic levels of drugs may be reached in a situation in which a frightened patient is given more and more medication in an attempt to "control" him or her.

It would seem, therefore, that the only drugs required in the days before surgery are for relief of anxiety and to allow the patient to get adequate sleep.

The needs of the patient just prior to the surgery—for example, when the patient arrives at the outpatient surgical facility on the morning of the surgery—should be looked at carefully. We seem to be captives of tradition and habit in many ways, and, alas, the prescription of medications is no exception. Thus, the custom of giving patients atropine prior to surgery probably relates to the days when ether anesthesia was common and some agent to reduce secretions in the tracheobronchial tree was a lifesaving necessity. How many patients since those days have been exposed to the distressing effects of atropine when there was no necessity for the drug? If abundant secretions occur in the rare instance today, it would seem prudent to treat the problem as it arises. In a similar vein, narcotics have traditionally been given prior to surgery in order to relieve pain and for whatever sedative value they might have. Many patients, however, do not come to the operating room with any pain in the setting currently under discussion. The period of pain relief we are most probably interested in is during the administration of the local anesthetic. It does not seem to make much sense to give a long-acting analgesic when only a few minutes of analgesia are required. Furthermore, the narcotic drugs are poor for relief of anxiety and frequently cause nausea and vomiting. The value of sedation is questionable in any case, for many surgeons prefer a more alert and cooperative patient.

Other reasons for giving medications prior to surgery are to prevent bradycardia, to protect against or reduce central nervous system (CNS) irritability, and to protect against nausea and vomiting. If one makes a rational and safe selection of drugs, as will be outlined and described later, the need for this kind of "protection" will be rare, and in the unusual event that one of these symptoms appears, it can be treated.

The only real need of the average patient prior to surgery is to have fears and anxieties calmed. Liberal doses of tender loving care and judicious use of tranquilizers seem to fit the bill.

During the surgery itself (and we are here speaking only of outpatient plastic surgery under local anesthesia) the only added need is for suppression of the pain that is experienced during the administration of the local anesthetic. Since this takes only a few minutes, reason dictates that the drug used at this time should have a very brief effect. Later, a dissociative drug, ketamine, or a very short-acting narcotic analgesic, fentanyl, will be suggested for this purpose.

So far, we have focused on the needs of the patient prior to and during the surgery. Certainly these have first priority, but there are the needs of the surgeon to consider as well. Most surgeons would agree that a quiet calm patient is easier and safer to operate on. Many would say that they prefer not to have to talk to the patient during surgery, or at least they would rather not have the patient talk to them. They wish to have a sedated patient or even one who is asleep. There is a price to pay for this advantage: The most reliable way of assessing the condition of the sensorium of the patient, the consciousness of the patient, is denied them. Some operators would prefer, as would many patients, that there be virtually complete amnesia for the events during the surgery. On the other hand, many would like to remember something of what goes on if they could be assured of happy memories. Another common need of the surgeon is to have a patient free of nausea and vomiting. The most certain way to avoid these unpleasant, and in special circumstances dangerous, occurrences is to avoid the most common cause, narcotics. Finally, a growing requirement of many surgeons is to have the effects of the drugs wear off quickly so that the patient may be transferred out of the surgical unit. Having a limited recovery bed capacity and a plethora of heavily sedated patients will quickly tax the most efficient of operating crews. Surgeons should have specific goals as to how they wish to work, and in the world of pharmacologic abundance in which we find ourselves, they should be able to tailor a program that suits their individual needs.

AGENTS

Let us consider an arbitrary categorization of the most commonly used drugs in an outpatient surgical setting: analgesics, sedative hypnotics, tranquilizers, anticholinergics, antiadrenergics, local anesthetics, and finally ketamine. We will keep in mind the benefits and drawbacks of each, for there are very few instances in which both are not inherent.

Analgesics

Most of the analgesic drugs used preoperatively are either naturally occurring or synthetic narcotics. In administering drugs such as the narcotics to patients in the setting under discussion (patients who are not in pain, who are waiting to go to the operating room, and who are in reasonably good health), what are we trying to achieve? The most common drugs given—morphine, meperidine (Demerol), hydromorphone (Dilaudid), and alphaprodine (Nisentil)—do change the affect with which the pain is experienced. That is to say, the pain is not removed, but the way it is perceived is changed. That is the benefit intended in giving the narcotic before the surgery. However, these drugs have a half-life of hours to relieve pain that lasts only a few minutes, i.e., during the injection of the local anesthetic. The big disadvantage of the narcotics as preoperative medications is that there are many and severe side effects, such as nausea and vomiting, respiratory depression, and a feeling of dysphoria. For example, when 10 to 15 mg of morphine is administered to normal persons, it produces drowsiness and euphoria in some but anxiety and nausea in others. One combination of drugs commonly used preoperatively is fentanyl (Sublimaze), a potent, very short-acting narcotic, and droperidol, a butyrophenone tranquilizer. The former has a half-life of about one-half hour, the latter a half-life of several hours.

Considering the need, the benefits, and the shortcomings of the narcotics as preoperative medications, it would seem a little like killing a fly with a howitzer to use them. There is no doubt the fly is dead, but the wall is gone.

Sedative Hypnotics

The barbiturates most commonly used preoperatively are probably secobarbital (Seconal) and pentobarbital (Nembutal), with phenobarbital (Luminal) as a distant third. The usual effect desired is a degree of sedation combined with some relief of anxiety. The problem is that the sedative effect far surpasses the anxiety relief. In fact, some patients, particularly the very old and the very young, become agitated under the effect of barbiturates. Another problem is that the dose-response curve is steep. The significance here is that there is a narrow spread between the effective dose and a toxic dose. Other disadvantages of the barbiturates are a longer half-life than desired and the fact that significant respiratory depression occurs. Why, then, the enormous generalized usage? The barbiturates are among those "time-tested" drugs with which most doctors are comfortable. The dosages and the toxic effects are well known. They are effective orally and are inexpensive, and they usually do not produce nausea or vomiting.

The benzodiazepine drugs have recently achieved great popularity as preoperative medications because they offer antianxiety effects without excessive sedation or ataxia. Some of the ones in common usage are diazepam (Valium), chlordiazepoxide hydrochloride (Librium), oxazepam (Serax), lorazepam (Ativan), and flurazepam (Dalmane). The last is largely used as a hypnotic. The others differ only in half-lives, Serax having the shortest (several hours) and Valium the longest (several days). They have anticonvulsant actions, and for this reason are thought by some physicians to offer some protection against CNS toxicity produced by other concomitant drugs. Caution should be exercised in giving these drugs to patients who are taking barbiturates, alcohol, opiates, or other substances that depress the CNS. They are psychologically addictive and are frequently overused.

Antihistamines, such as diphenhydramine (Benadryl) and promethazine (Phenergan), are probably not used often enough as preoperative medications. They have a mild sedative effect that is pleasant in relatively small doses, even in very old or very young patients. There is some anticholinergic effect resulting in a drying of salivary and bronchial secretions. There has been some feeling that Phenergan potentiates narcotics, but it now seems that what potentiation occurs does so more for the sedative than the analgesic effect.

Hydroxyzine (Vistaril, Atarax) are antianxiety agents that also have hypnotic, anticholinergic, and antihistaminic properties. Vistaril is frequently used preoperatively for its action in potentiating the analgesic effects of narcotics.

Other drugs used for their sedative hypnotic activity are ethanol, chloral hydrate, ethchlorvynol (Placidyl), and the piperidinediones (Noludar and Doriden). Chloral hydrate is an old, but useful, drug, particularly in elderly patients or in those having sensitivities or allergies to the barbiturates. Ethanol can be very useful as a sedative hypnotic in alcoholic patients before and during surgery. It is available as a commercially prepared intravenous solution.

Tranquilizers

The tranquilizers, or antianxiety drugs, that are in the benzodiazepine group are listed above in the sedative hypnotic category because of the similarity of their pharmacologic effects to those of the other sedative hypnotics. They are different in that they are less likely to produce tolerance and physical dependence, and they are much safer than the rest of the sedative hypnotics when taken in suicidal doses.

The tranquilizers, or antipsychotic drugs, are represented by the phenothiazines, the thioxanthenes, and the butyrophenones.

PHENOTHIAZINES

The phenothiazines differ one from the other from the standpoint of their potency, extrapyramidal effects, and sedative effects. The piperazines, as represented by prochlorperazine (Compazine), trifluoperazine (Stelazine), and perphenazine (Trilafon), are the most potent of the phenothiazines.

Next in potency of the phenothiazines are the aliphatics, such as chlorpromazine (Thorazine), promazine (Sparine), and triflupromazine (Vesprin). Since chlorpromazine is the prototype of the phenothiazines, its pharmacologic activities and uses will be discussed.

Least in potency of the phenothiazines are the piperidines, as exemplified by thioridazine (Mellaril) and mesoridazine (Serentil). As a group these produce the fewest extrapyramidal effects and the most sedation.

Chlorpromazine was the original and prototypical phenothiazine tranquilizer. It is still a useful drug because of its many and varied activities. It has calming effects helpful in treating anxiety. It also occasionally causes dysphoria and confusion. Long-term usage may produce abnormal muscular movements, blood dyscrasias, cholestatic jaundice, skin reactions, and photosensitivity. Chlorpromazine has some atropinelike effects that manifest themselves by dry mouth, urinary retention, constipation, and blurred vision. There may be rapid and marked hypotension resulting from the parenteral administration of chlorpromazine. It is very effective in the prevention and treatment of nausea and vomiting caused by other chemical agents. Chlorpromazine's hypotensive action may be explained on the basis of a beta-adrenergic vasodilatation. Parenteral administration of small doses (e.g., 2.5 mg) can be made to lower blood pressure during an intraoperative hypertensive episode.

Potencies are compared on a basis of doses that produce the same effect, not according to the sizes of the effects produced by the same dose. Potency alone is much overrated, for the only advantage in using a more potent drug is that a smaller dose need be taken. A more efficacious drug, on the other hand, may accomplish things that are unattainable with a less efficacious drug, regardless of dose.

THIOXANTHENES

The thioxanthenes, exemplified by chlorprothixine (Taractan) and thiothixene (Navane), are similar pharmacologically and chemically to the phenothiazines. Thiothixene is the more potent of the two. These drugs have little use in the outpatient setting. They are primarily employed in long-term therapy with psychotics.

BUTYROPHENONES

The butyrophenones, haloperidol (Haldol) and droperidol, are used primarily in psychiatry and anesthesiology. Droperidol is often used in combination with a narcotic analgesic, fentanyl. The droperidol is a potent tranquilizer and antiemetic with a half-life of several hours, while the fentanyl is a very short-acting narcotic analgesic. The combination of the two is marketed under the trade name Innovar. It produces an anestheticlike state, which has been termed *neuroleptanesthesia.* Fentanyl, like all narcotics, causes severe respiratory depression and, if given too rapidly intravenously, can produce a peculiar increase in the tone of the chest muscles. This "wooden rigidity" can be avoided by administering the drug slowly. There is some question as to the rationality of giving two drugs together whose half-lives are so different, several hours for the droperidol and 30 minutes for the fentanyl.

Anticholinergics

Atropine, scopolamine, and glycopyrrolate (Robinul) are frequently given the patient prior to surgery along with sedatives, narcotics, and tranquilizers. The reasons for the administration of such potent drugs with so many disagreeable side effects have always been said to be to decrease vagal cardiac tone and to reduce secretions in the tracheobronchial tree. They do have these effects, but the necessity for these pharmacologic effects has passed along with the use of secretion-producing irritant anesthetics such as diethyl ether and cyclopropane. The actions of atropine and scopolamine on the cardiovascular system are very similar. The big difference between the two is in their CNS effects. In low, therapeutic doses scopolamine is likely to produce considerable sleepiness and, in certain instances, excitation and even a rather maniacal effect. Atropine does not have this effect in low doses. There is usually some degree of dysphoria, accompanied by dry mouth, tachycardia, blurred vision, and hot and dry skin. If one feels that the use of an anticholinergic is necessary prior to or during the surgery, glycopyrrolate would probably be a better choice, for it does not pass the blood-brain barrier very readily, and the patient is spared many unpleasant and unnecessary side effects.

Antiadrenergics

Antiadrenergics, or adrenergic-blocking agents, are drugs that competitively inhibit the actions of catecholamines on their specific receptors. Norepinephrine (Levophed), epinephrine (Adrenalin), and dopamine are the endogenous catecholamines, and isoproterenol (Isuprel) is a synthetic analog. Adrenergic-blocking agents are classified as alpha- and beta-blocking agents because of the existence of two types of receptors. In the tissues in which both types of receptors are found, such as most blood vessels, alpha stimulation causes contraction and beta stimulation causes relaxation. Conversely, alpha-blocking agents in such a tissue cause dilatation. In organs whose receptors are almost exclusively beta—the heart, for example—the beta blockers oppose the excitatory effects of norepinephrine.

Epinephrine acts on both alpha and beta receptors in the peripheral vascular system. In the presence of an alpha blocker such as phentolamine (Regitine), the effect of epinephrine on the beta receptors would be apparent because of the blockage of the drug's effect on the alpha receptors. The end result would be vasodilatation instead of the usual vasoconstriction in the presence of epinephrine. Phentolamine is used in the diagnosis of pheochromocytoma. Another alpha blocker, tolazoline hydrochloride (Priscoline), causes peripheral vasodilatation by direct relaxant effect on vascular smooth muscle.

The beta-adrenergic-blocking agents competitively inhibit the effects of catecholamines on all beta receptors. The most widespread use of a beta blocker is seen in the enormous popularity of propranolol (Inderal). It is in use for a wide variety of conditions, such as cardiac arrhythmias, angina pectoris, and hypertension. The majority of the effects of propranolol are cardiovascular and include decreased heart rate, decreased myocardial contractility, decreased myocardial oxygen uptake, and decreased blood pressure. It is important to understand the mechanism of action of this particular drug because of its ubiquity. Many patients coming to surgery are taking it on a long-term basis. They should be cautioned to continue the medication during the surgical episode because the abrupt discontinuation of the beta blocker can cause severe hypertension, acute angina, tachyarrhythmias, myocardial infarction, or sudden death. Lesser symptoms may include anxiety, tremor, tachycardia, headache, and malaise.

Certain drug interactions with beta blockers, such as propranolol, are noteworthy. The drug has a tendency to cause hypoglycemia and may interfere with the recovery from hypoglycemia following the administration of insulin. Digitalis-induced bradycardia may be worsened by the effect of propranolol, but the bradycardia responds to treatment with atropine. The hypotensive effects of the phenothiazines are enhanced by propranolol. It is important to know what medications every patient is taking, but particularly in this instance of such a widely used drug.

Local Anesthetics

Local anesthetics are drugs that produce loss of sensation in an area of the body by interfering with nerve conduction. The effects are transient and reversible. They have several types of clinical application: infiltration and block anesthesia, surface anesthesia, spinal anesthesia, epidural and caudal anesthesia, and intravenous anesthesia. For the most part, only infiltration and block anesthesia are considered here.

Local anesthetics prevent both the generation and the transmission of nerve impulse. The main site of action is at the cell membrane. They block conduction by interfering with the increased permeability of the cell membrane to sodium ions that is produced by the depolarization of the membrane. They stabilize the membrane. Most local anesthetics exist as weak bases, which are converted into salts and ionized in solution. Only the ionized form is available for its pharmacologic effect. Therefore, acidity impedes and alkalinity enhances its activity.

Nerve fibers can be classified into three types: A, B, and C fibers. A fibers are the largest and are myelinated, B fibers are smaller and myelinated, and C fibers are the smallest and not myelinated. Local anesthetic drugs depress the smallest and unmyelinated fibers first and the largest and myelinated fibers last. Therefore, the order of loss of function is first pain and then temperature, touch, proprioception, and skeletal muscle tone.

Absorption depends on the site of injection, the vascularity of the depot, the dose, and the presence of a vasoconstrictor in the injected solution. The more vascular the site of injection, the higher the blood level achieved and the sooner the peak of concentration in the blood. For a given site, absorption depends on dose alone, not on the concentration of the solution injected. Local vasoconstriction caused by the use of epinephrine mixed in the anesthetic solution slows absorption, so that more anesthetic is retained longer at the target site. The result is more profound and prolonged anesthesia locally and lower levels of circulating drug at any moment.

Ester-linked local anesthetics, such as procaine (Novocain), chloroprocaine (Nesacaine), and tetracaine (Pontocaine), are hydrolyzed in the plasma and excreted in the urine. Amide-linked local anesthetics, such as lidocaine (Xylocaine), mepivacaine (Carbocaine), prilocaine (Citanest), and bupivacaine (Marcaine), are metabolized in the liver and excreted in the urine. The metabolites are usually less toxic than the parent drugs, with the single exception of prilocaine, the metabolic products of which have been reported to cause methemoglobinemia.

Properties of local anesthetics to be considered in choosing which will be used are potency, duration of action, onset time, and toxicity. One perfect anesthetic does not exist; if it did, everyone would be using it. Each of the popular anesthetics mentioned above has advantages and disadvantages as compared to the others. By far the most widely used local anesthetic today is lidocaine. It has a relatively short time of onset; its duration is satisfactory for most procedures; and, being an amide-linked local as opposed to an ester-linked local, it has very little chance to produce an allergic reaction.

In almost every instance, toxicity to local anesthetic agents is purely a matter of overdose. There are maximum safe doses allowed for each one of the local anesthetics, with and without epinephrine mixed, and these doses should not be exceeded. The signs of impending or early toxic reaction relate to CNS stimulation and are headache, tinnitus, dizziness, blurred vision, slurred speech, nystagmus, and shivering. Note that a patient who is conscious enough to talk can relate these symptoms to the surgeon. In a severe toxic reaction the early CNS stimulation gives way to convulsions and finally to cardiovascular collapse. Prophylaxis of local anesthetic toxicity is primarily dose control, followed by good ventilation, administration of oxygen, and possibly diazepam. The treatment of the acutely toxic state definitely includes the diazepam as the treatment of choice. Good ventilation, administration of oxygen, Trendelenburg position, airway, and even endotracheal intubation should be available. Remember, the convulsion is not the problem. The problem is hypoxia.

Dissociative Anesthetic

Ketamine hydrochloride is a phencyclidine derivative that produces a trancelike state and freedom from pain. This state has been called *dissociative anesthesia.* While the patient given a narcotic analgesic still has the pain but with a different effect, the patient given ketamine actually feels no pain, being "dissociated" from the pain stimulus. The drug can be given intramuscularly or intravenously. We have administered it only intravenously, believing that this route gives more accurate control of the dose and shorter onset of action.

The drug is not a new one. It has found its widest use heretofore in young children having multiple frequent anesthetics for short procedures that required no muscle relaxation, such as burn dressings and debridements. Many tales have been told about postanesthetic psychic problems after ketamine administration. These have ranged from terrifying dreams during the anesthetic to flashbacks and schizophreniclike episodes occurring days or weeks later. In our hands, using what will be referred to as low-dose ketamine, and in combination with diazepam, there has not been a single instance of this type or any other type of unpleasant reaction in more than a thousand cases.

The ketamine is used to provide a pain-free period of 5 to 10 minutes, during which time the local anesthetic can be injected. Most patients have received 15 mg of diazepam by mouth about a half hour before going to the operating room. In the operating room enough diazepam is given intravenously to produce a drowsy state, from which the patient can easily be aroused. Sometimes the additional amount of diazepam is 5 mg and in other instances it may be as much as 20 or 30 mg. Then the ketamine is administered intravenously over the course of a minute or two. The dose has ranged from 0.5 to 1.0 mg/kg. During the dissociative state thus produced, the local is injected, with the patient feeling and remembering nothing. There is usually transient—perhaps 5 or 10 minutes—hypertension and tachycardia. In the rare case in which more local is needed some time later in the procedure, the ketamine is repeated but in a lesser dose —say, one-half of the original dose. We have used this regimen in a variety of types of cases, including rhytidectomies, blepharoplasties, rhinoplasties, augmentation mammoplasties, and mastopexies. The experience of the patients and operating surgeons has been so overwhelmingly favorable that we continue to use and even expand our usage of this technique.

Because ketamine raises the blood pressure and pulse, even transiently, we consider hypertension to be a contraindication to the use of the drug. We also exclude patients who have a history of psychotic disease.

In some patients, the blood pressure remains elevated longer than the arbitrarily set limit of 10 minutes. In this event, a very small amount of chlorpromazine (e.g., 2.5 mg intravenously) usually lowers the blood pressure to normal levels within a few minutes. This is an uncommon situation, but it has occurred. On several occasions, hypersecretion of tenacious mucus from the respiratory tract has necessitated suctioning. These few untoward and easily handled situations are the only problems we have seen in a thousand cases.

The use of diazepam, low-dose ketamine, and local anesthetic has proved to be safe and effective as a drug regimen to be used in cosmetic surgery on an outpatient basis.

Anesthesiologists sometimes criticize the use of ketamine in the manner described. Some of the criticism may stem from experience with the drug in larger doses than are recommended here. Much of the experience that has been characterized as unpleasant or even dangerous may also not have included the concomitant use of diazepam, and the diazepam is essential. There is likewise some controversy about whether the trancelike state that ketamine produces is loss of consciousness in the anesthetic sense. I believe that more communication between anesthesiologist and plastic surgeon will resolve these differences, for there is no doubt in the minds of those of us who have a large experience with this technique that it is worthwhile to pursue.

SPECIFIC REGIMENS

As examples of the application of the principles and experiences accumulated in the years of operating in our outpatient surgical unit, the following specific regimens are submitted. These are not, of course, the only ways to handle these situations. Each surgeon and each patient has individual needs to be satisfied. Tailor the programs to fit your own needs.

Face-Lifts

Most patients who are waiting for their morning of surgery have some degree of anxiety. Much of it can be overcome by reassurance. What anxiety is left can be ameliorated with drugs. A sedative hypnotic such as chloral hydrate (0.5 or 1.0 gm orally) or hydroxyzine (100 mg) can be given one or two nights beforehand. Antianxiety medication for several days before is seldom used but if it is necessary could be diazepam, 5 mg, 2 or 3 times a day.

When the patient arrives at the office on the morning of surgery, 15 mg of diazepam is given by mouth. The patient is then dressed in a hospital-type gown and put to bed. In a drowsy state she or he will later walk to the operating room. After being placed on the operating table, the patient is attached to the electrocardiographic monitor and the blood pressure monitor. A cannula is placed in an antecubital vein, and a slow, continuous drip of Ringer's lactate solution is maintained. Through the intravenous cannula more diazepam is given if necessary, to produce a calm, tranquil affect. Usually the speech is slightly slurred at the optimum level of sedation. If the patient is not hypertensive, ketamine is administered (0.5–1.0 mg/kg) slowly over about 1 minute. If the patient is hypertensive or is a hypertensive under control with medication, we have elected not to use ketamine. In this latter case we would use a short-acting narcotic, such as fentanyl (0.05–0.1 mg). If the rise in blood pressure and pulse that is usually seen with the administration of ketamine lasts longer or is higher than the usual (experience will have to dictate these parameters), a small dose (2.5 mg) of chlorpromazine (Thorazine) intravenously is in order, or nitroglycerin is given sublingually or percutaneously in the form of a paste applied directly to the skin.

Additional diazepam can be given during the operation if the patient becomes anxious. Remember that increasing restlessness and anxiety can be caused by hypoxia or pain, and each of these should be treated specifically.

If a second injection of local anesthetic is necessary later on—say, in a different area from the first—a repeat dose of ketamine can be used. About one-half of the original dose is usually sufficient on this infrequent occasion.

Just before the intravenous cannula is removed prior to taking the patient from the table, we usually give 5 mg prochlorperazine (Compazine) intravenously.

Postoperatively, the patients receive flurazepam (Dalmane) as a sleeping medication for bedtime and propoxyphene (Darvon) for pain relief.

Rhinoplasty

The regimen for rhinoplasty patients is much the same as that outlined for face-lift patients. Since the mean age for this procedure is lower than that for face-lifts, the necessity for antianxiety and sleeping medications prior to the day of surgery is less.

Patients are requested to stop all intranasal medications for at least 6 weeks prior to surgery.

As soon as the ketamine is administered and has taken effect, the nose is packed with gauze saturated with 5% cocaine solution. It is a worthwhile safety precaution to have this solution tinted so that it cannot be visually confused with the local anesthetic solution.

Augmentation Mammoplasty

The drug regimen in augmentation mammoplasty cases is much like that of the face-lift patients. I prefer to use larger doses of the ketamine, perhaps nearer the 1.0 mg/kg of body weight than 0.5 mg/kg. This affords a few more minutes of the pain-free trancelike state produced by the ketamine. During the pain-free period most of the blunt dissection between the breast and the pectoralis muscle or between the pectoralis muscle and the rib cage can be accomplished.

Blepharoplasty

The regimen for blepharoplasty is much the same as that for the face-lift. Since the time required for the injection of the local anesthetic solution in the eyelids is briefer than that needed in the case of augmentation mammoplasty or face-lift, a lesser dose of ketamine is used: 0.5 mg/kg of body weight instead of 1.0 mg/kg.

MONITORING AND SUPPORT SYSTEMS

Monitoring

The technology of monitoring a patient's physiologic condition has reached the point where one can depend on the equipment as a useful and even necessary part of the operating and recovery room equipment. This is not to say that mechanization and electronic gadgetry should be replacements for the personal watchfulness of the surgeon or the anesthetist. It is apparent that constant monitoring of the level of consciousness of the patient is one of the best indices of the general state, and the way to utilize this during surgery is for the patient and surgeon to communicate. If the patient is so heavily sedated that response is not possible, a valuable parameter of monitoring technique is lost.

Trial and error have proved the following equipment valuable in our outpatient surgical unit.

When the patient is placed on the operating table, the monitoring equipment is immediately attached. An automatic apparatus that takes the blood pressure at variable intervals and displays the information in the form of a digital readout display is used. This type of machine can be adjusted to take blood pressure readings at 1-, 2-, or as much as 7-minute intervals. We use the shorter intervals in the beginning and adjust the time to longer intervals during the operation. The same apparatus displays the pulse rate as well.

An electrocardiographic (ECG) monitor is also used in every case. Leads are attached to the patient, disposable adherent pads ensuring adequate contact. The display readout varies from one machine to another. On some machines the display enables one to see several ECG complexes simultaneously; others offer only one at a time. Still others have the capacity to produce a printed record simultaneously. This is valuable in following the progress of an arrhythmic state. Many ECG machines also provide digital pulse readouts.

At this juncture it is necessary to say that all personnel in the outpatient surgical unit should be trained and certified in cardiopulmonary resuscitation (CPR) techniques. Further, at least the physicians in the unit should be trained and certified in advanced CPR techniques. What good is the presence of the monitoring equipment if we are unable to interpret the data and act on them?

Support Systems

Every patient on the operating table in our unit has an intravenous flexible cannula in place (usually in an antecubital fossa vein) delivering fluid (such as Ringer's lactate). Through this system most of the drugs are administered before, during, and often after the surgery. We almost never give intramuscular medications because of the discomfort involved, the risk of local tissue damage, and the unreliability of uptake of intramuscular drugs.

Oxygen is constantly available in the operating rooms and in the recovery rooms. We prefer small portable tanks rather than a central oxygen system. Central systems may have maintenance problems, such as leakage, and putting a central system in an already built surgical unit is expensive and time-consuming. The oxygen is delivered to the patient by mask or nasal cannula, depending on the circumstances.

A suction apparatus is an indispensable part of the support system. Individual and movable units are preferred to the central suction system because of ease of maintenance and reliability factors.

At least one movable cart or table supplied with emergency drugs and resuscitation equipment is a must. It should have various kinds and sizes of airways, laryngoscopes, a means of providing positive pressure breathing assistance (such as an Ambu bag), and defibrillator. All this equipment should be restocked and tested at regular intervals.

CONCLUSION

This has been an overview of some of the more common drugs used and abused in the outpatient surgery setting. It has been suggested that one assume a rational position about drug selection, taking into consideration the needs of the patient and of the surgeon. Our thesis continues to be: Keep it simple—keep it safe.

REFERENCE

1. Elliott, R. A. Organization and Efficient Function of Office Surgery. In R. C. Schultze (ed.), *Ambulatory Surgery.* Philadelphia: Lea & Febiger, 1979.

BIBLIOGRAPHY

AAAAPSF Checklist/Questionnaire for Accreditation of Ambulatory Plastic Surgery Facilities. Route 2, 359 Milwaukee Ave., Half Day, Ill. 60069.

Appendix

CITED EQUIPMENT SUPPLIERS

1. Castle Company, Division of Sybion Corporation, 1777 East Henrietta Road, Rochester, New York 14603. The Castle light, model #L195, has the described features at a reasonable cost.
2. Datascope Corporation, 580 Winters Avenue, Paramus, New Jersey 07652.
3. Dri-Clave Corporation, 54 Kinkel Street, Westbury, New York 11590.
4. Electro-Medical Systems, Inc., 14 Inverness Drive East, Englewood, Colorado 80110.
5. Executone Inc., P.O. Box 1430, Long Island City, New York 11101.
6. Johnson and Johnson, Dental Products Company, 20 Lake Drive, East Windsor, New Jersey 08530.
7. Komtek, Box 11, White Lakes Road, Stanley, New Mexico 87056.
8. Laurel Office Aids, Inc., Bronxville, New York 10708 (Form OA-4).
9. Luxo Lamp Corporation, Monument Park, Port Chester, New York 10573.
10. Physio-Control, 5 Mile Landing, 71 Rowayton Avenue, Rowayton, Connecticut 06853.
11. Puritan-Bennett Corporation, 26 Plaza Drive, Westmont, Illinois 60059.
12. Robershaw Life Support Products, 333 North Euclid Way, Anaheim, California 92803.
13. Tab Products Co., 2690 Hanover Street, Palo Alto, California 94304.
14. Valley Labs, 5411 Western Avenue, Boulder, Colorado 80301.

5. Clinical Photography for Aesthetic Plastic Surgery

Daniel C. Morello

What is the use of a book, thought Alice,
without pictures or conversation?
Lewis Carroll
Alice's Adventures in Wonderland

. . . the plastic surgeon with average photographic
ability for the species . . . would do well to
eliminate as many variables as possible.
F. McDowell
Plast. Reconstr. Surg. 58:214, 1976

The purpose of clinical photography is to document the patient's appearance accurately and in a reproducible fashion. Quality photographic records are essential in the practice of aesthetic plastic surgery. They can guide the planning of surgical procedures, allow valid comparison of the preoperative and postoperative states, and reassure or encourage a patient. In this age of litigation, a photographic record that accurately documents the clinical situation can be equally important.

This chapter is not intended as an all-inclusive review of the subject of clinical photography, but rather as an attempt to delineate features of a personal system that can be adopted by anyone to obtain uniform photographic records simply and easily [4].

CAMERA EQUIPMENT AND FILM

A 35-mm single lens reflex (SLR) camera is preferred. The quality differences among various makes are practically insignificant. Desirable features include interchangeability of screens for the viewfinder, a power winder, and a manual override if the camera has an automatic mode.

The focal length of a lens is the distance (in millimeters) from the effective center of the lens to the film plane, with the distance at infinity. A long focal length lens (100 mm) refracts light at an angle that is greater than that of a shorter focal length lens (50 mm). Thus, a larger image is produced for the same distance setting.

A long focal length lens is best (100–105 mm). I use a 105-mm macrolens as the only lens for my clinical photography. Most SRLs are sold equipped with a 50- or 55-mm lens, as this is useful over a wide range of application. The disadvantage of this lens is that when facial clinical photographs taken with it are compared with those taken with a longer lens, central facial "distortion" is apparent. The effect is more obvious when a photograph made with a 28-mm lens is added for comparison (Fig. 5-1). Normally we view and evaluate patients from a distance of 3 to 5 ft. For a photograph taken with a 50-mm lens to encompass just the head and neck, the focal distance (distance from camera to subject) would be about 15 in. The result is altered visual perspective* when compared to normal—

* *Perspective* is representation of a three-dimensional subject on a plane surface.

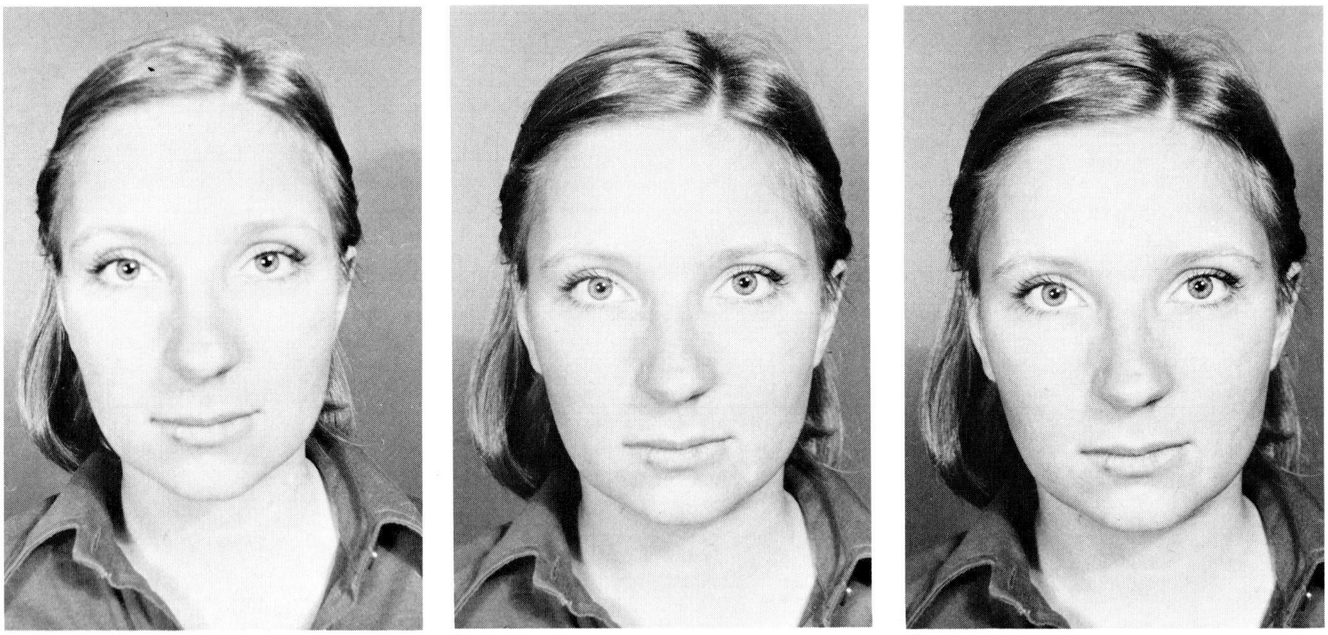

A B C

Figure 5-1. The effect of different focal length lenses on facial photographs.
A. 28 mm
B. 50 mm
C. 105 mm
From D. C. Morello, J. M. Converse, and D. Allen, Making uniform photographic records in plastic surgery. *Plast. Reconstr. Surg.* 59:366, 1977.

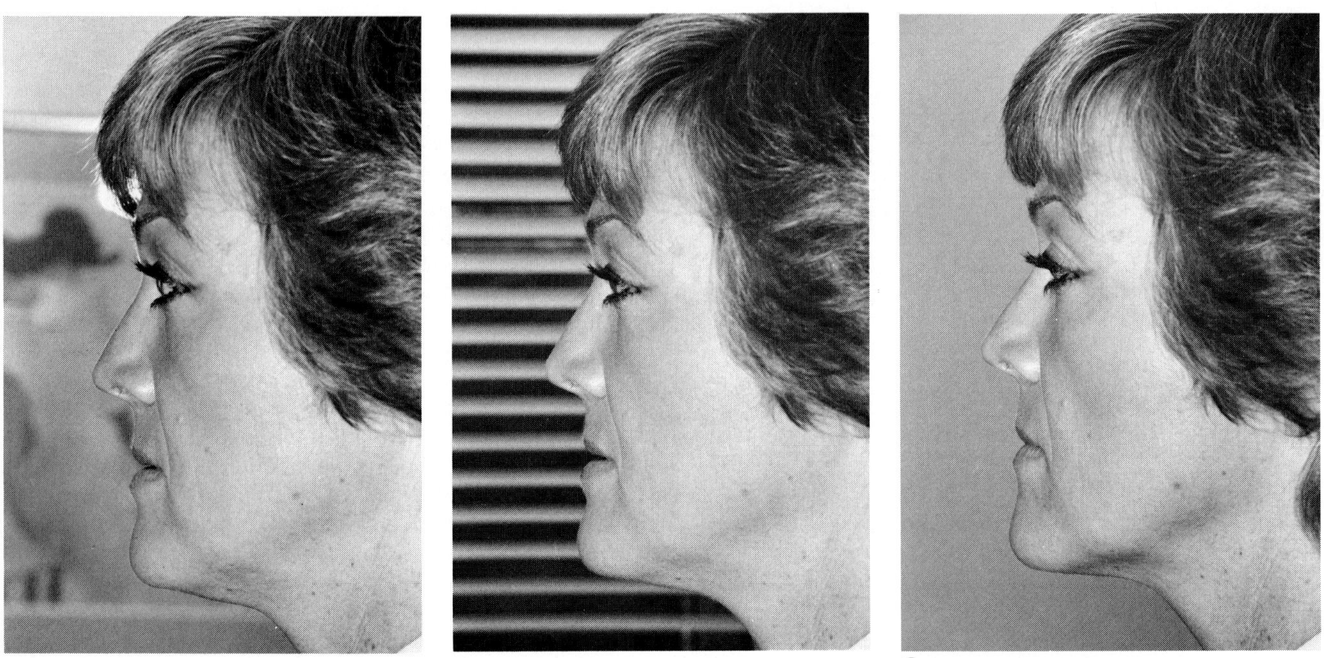

A B C

Figure 5-2
A, B. Distracting effect of cluttered background.
C. Compared with plain background.

commonly thought of as "distortion." However, this altered perspective is not an integral function of the lens but rather is due to the distance between the subject and the lens. It occurs when a subject is photographed at one distance and viewed at another.

Only one lens (105 mm) is required for a broad range of photographs. In some quarters the addition of a 50-mm lens to take full-length photographs is recommended, but I have not found such photographs necessary or desirable.

A plain, nonreflective background provides no distraction and concentrates attention on the subject (Fig. 5-2). The color of the background can affect the result by changing the color nuances of the skin adversely—a black background, for example. Generally, a neutral blue gray color has proved to be best and is suitable for use with either color or black-and-white film. I use Savage Widetone, a nontextured photographic background paper widely available commercially.

My preference is to take slides and have prints (usually color) made as necessary. Kodachrome 64 film (ASA 64) offers good reproducibility of color and natural skin tones. Kodachrome 25 is similar but requires a lower f-stop for a given distance, resulting in less depth of field. The important point is to choose a widely available film and stay with it to minimize variations. Recently I have been using a Polaroid Polaprinter to obtain prints from slides. Either color or black-and-white prints can be made from color slides, and the Polaprinter is convenient, simple to use, and economical.

LIGHTS AND LIGHTING

Modern automatic flash units have sensors that read the amount of light reflected by the subject and shut off the flash at the precise time for correct exposure. They produce relatively consistent illumination and minimize exposure variations. They also allow the use of a single f-stop setting and one shutter speed, eliminating these as potential variables.

Most flash units are compact and can be powered by alkaline or rechargeable batteries. Recycle time (the time for the unit to recharge and be ready to flash again) is a consideration in the selection of a flash unit, less than 10 seconds being desirable. Flash units also have "guide numbers," which indicate their relative power outputs. The guide number (GN) is the product of the f-stop multiplied by the focal distance in feet (GN = f-stop × distance). Thus, a flash with a higher GN will require a higher f-stop at any given distance than a flash with a lower GN. Since depth of field increases as the f-stop increases, a higher GN is desirable when one is choosing between two otherwise similar flash units. A GN of 80 or more (rated for ASA 100) has proved satisfactory. Higher guide numbers are available in larger units, but a balance must be struck.

More sophisticated are the autothyristor flashes. Ordinary automatic flash units use more energy than necessary for most exposures. The proper amount of energy is used for the flash, and the excess is "dumped off" from the capacitor. Instead of wasting this energy, thyristor circuitry conserves it for use in the next flash. Thus, many more flashes are possible from one set of batteries, and the recycle time is shortened since some energy remains in the capacitor. These advantages of autothyristor flashes are significant in terms of convenience. These units are by necessity slightly larger and more costly than other flashes.

"Dedicated" flash units work in conjunction with appropriate cameras to produce correct exposures. They automatically set the correct shutter speed and aperture when used with a compatible camera. The viewfinder of a camera with a dedicated flash will display exposure information (by means of light-emitting diodes) such as a confidence light to indicate correct exposure, a ready signal to indicate when the flash is fully recycled, and the correct shutter speed for synchronization. In most other respects, dedicated units are similar to other automatic flashes.

Most electronic flashes have a "ready light" to indicate when the capacitor is charged. Ordinarily the light glows when the capacitor is only 70 to 80 percent charged. Discharging the flash immediately when the light glows can thus result in variation in light intensity. A useful hint is to allow an additional 50 percent of the recycle time after the ready light glows to ensure full capacitor charge, thus producing consistent light. In the automatic mode, however, correct exposure usually results even if the capacitor is only 75 percent charged (i.e., just when the ready light glows) except with extremes of distance or lens aperture.

Another potential source of illumination error is batteries that are not well charged. A progressive lengthening of the recycle time indicates the need for replacement of batteries.

The color temperature of the flash should balance with the color temperature of the film. For daylight film, this is 5000 to 5500°K. Most electronic flashes are calibrated for this range.

One or more light sources can be used. Double flashes have been recommended by others, but I feel that this arrangement gives no significant advantage over a single flash unit on top of the camera. Further, with double flashes (one on each side of the camera) objectionable background shadowing can occur on lateral and oblique photographs. Double off-camera studio lights, at 45-degree angles from the patient, are recommended by Reeder [6]. They are positioned above head level and thus throw shadows downward so that they do not appear in the background of the photograph (see Studio Lighting). A disadvantage of the on-camera single-flash setup is that when framing an anteroposterior (AP) facial view with the camera held vertically one creates some shadowing on the side of the face and background opposite the side of the flash. This is easily eliminated by adjusting the position of the flash when taking the full-face AP view. Shadowing is not a problem in any other view. A facial series shot using a single on-camera flash is shown in Figure 5-3.

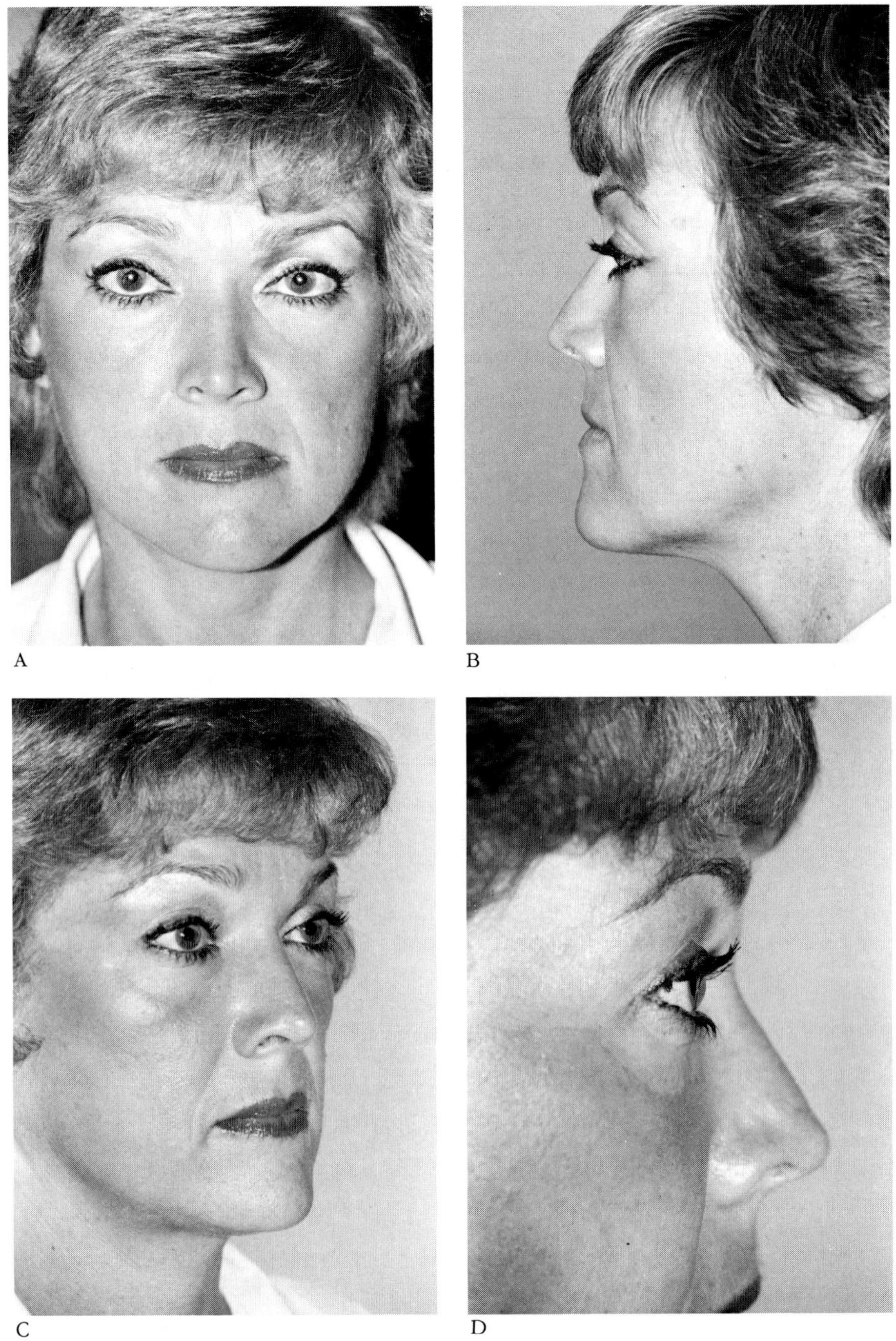

Figure 5-3. Facial series of photographs. The complete series includes the opposite oblique, lateral, and eye lateral, which have been omitted here.

Studio Lighting

A studio setup [5] will allow production of photographic records of the highest quality and accuracy. Such an arrangement is necessarily more expensive, requires its own allotted space, and is more time-consuming and complicated to use. Only persons with a solid commitment to obtaining quality photographic records should take this approach. In a studio setup, with its added complexity, there is much more chance of error.

For studio lighting, a three-light system is used, with two main or fill lights and a third light for background or highlighting. I have used three electronic flash units (Vivitar 252) in off-camera locations. One unit is triggered by means of a cord attached to the camera. The other two are triggered by "slave" units, which are small photocells that connect to a flash via a hot shoe or PC cord. The flash is triggered by the photocell when another flash is fired nearby. Since both light and electricity travel at 186,000 miles/second, the delay between firing the main unit and

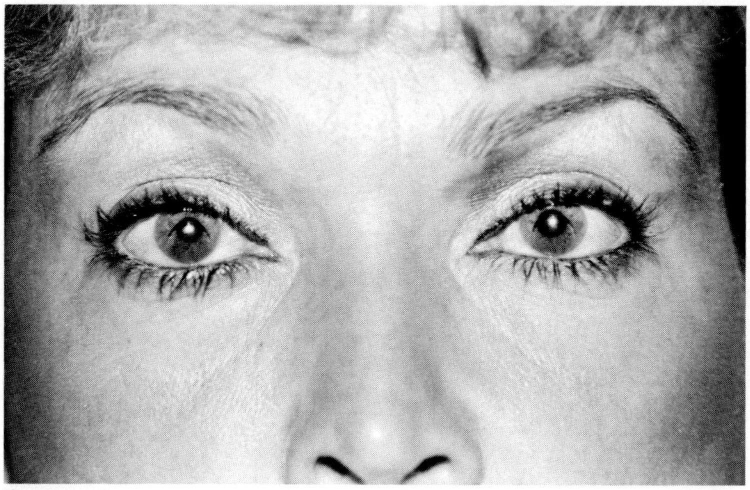
E

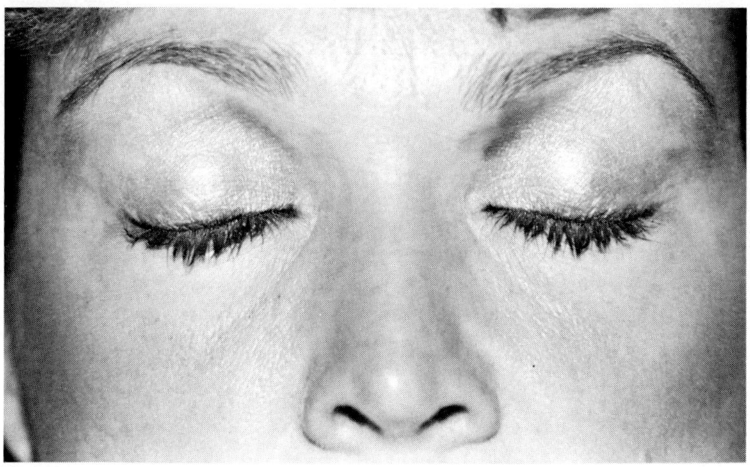
F

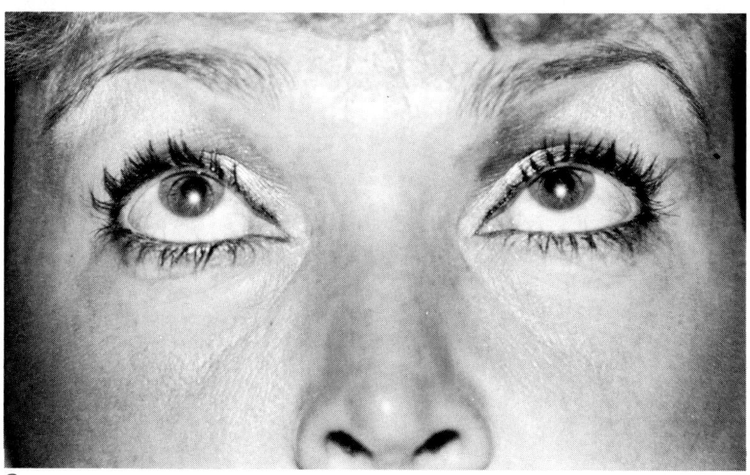
G

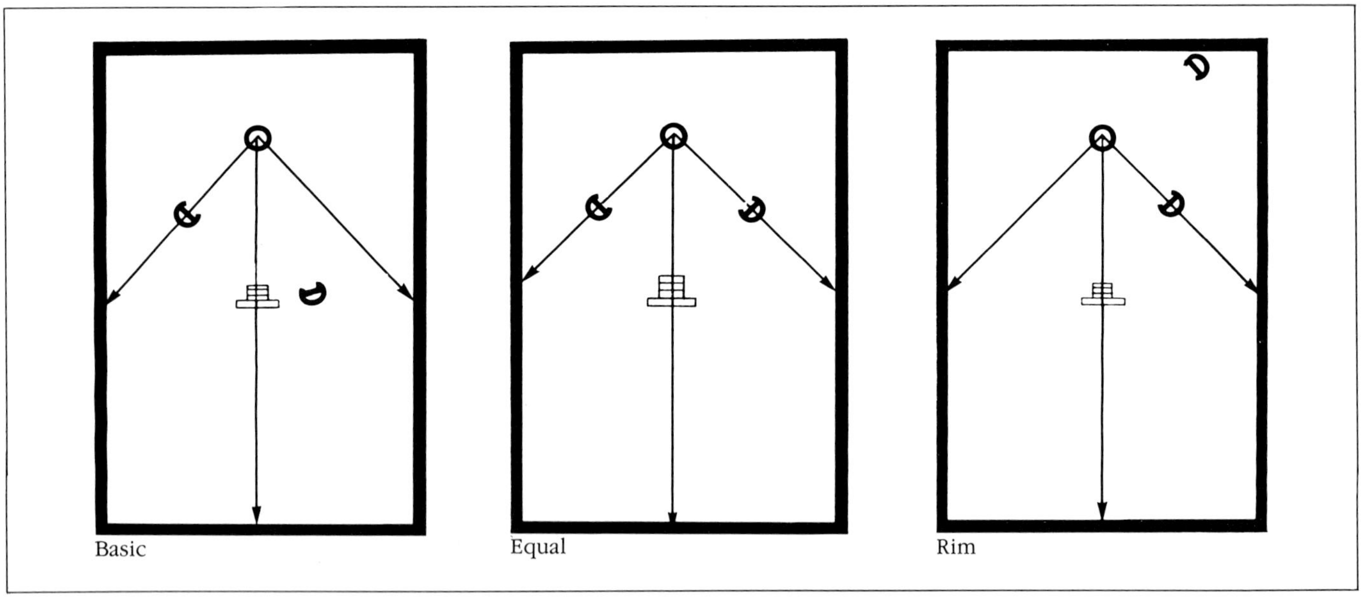

Figure 5-4
A. Basic lighting setup.
B. Equal lighting setup.
C. Rim lighting setup.
From D. C. Morello, J. M. Converse, and D. Allen, Making uniform photographic records in plastic surgery. *Plast. Reconstr. Surg.* 59:366, 1977.

firing the slave unit is insignificant. This system can be accommodated in a 9- × 11-ft room.

A more elaborate but similar system is that designed by John B. Tebbetts, M.D., of Dallas, who uses studio photographic lights suspended from a mobile overhead track system. The lights are AC-powered through a power pack mounted on the wall [7].

Types of Studio Lighting

Basic lighting utilizes a main light source placed 5 ft from the patient at a 45-degree angle to the camera-subject plane (Fig. 5-4A).

A second, "fill" light source is positioned 9 ft from the patient on the other side of the camera. In practical application in a 9- × 11-ft room, the fill light is placed in one corner of the room behind the camera position. Its distance from the patient determines the distance for the main light. A lighting ratio of 3 : 1 is desirable for good demonstration of textures and contours (modeling). Since light intensity varies with the square of the distance, the fill light should be about 1.7 times as far from the patient as the main light to produce a 3 : 1 ratio. Conversely, the main light should be about 0.58 times the distance of the fill light (approximate at 60%). With the fill light at 9 ft and the main light at 5 ft, the ratio is 3.1 : 1.0. A third light is used for the background and produces more visual separation between it and the patient. This "basic" lighting is used for full face, oblique (three-quarter), and torso photographs.

Equal lighting uses a background light with the other two lights equidistant (3–5 ft) and 45 degrees from the patient (Fig. 5-4B). This is used for neck and submental photographs. For otoplasty photographs, the background light can be directed slightly toward the patient to achieve a silhouette effect.

Rim lighting is used for all lateral photographs. The main light is 45 degrees in front of the patient, and the fill light is in a corresponding position behind (Fig. 5-4C). Only these two lights are used. The lighting is thus similar to that of the equal lighting setup, but the camera position is different.

Test exposures must be made through a broad range to determine the correct exposures. The distances for the lights and the correct exposures can be recorded on data cards for reference. Variations will be minimal, however, and the routine is easily memorized.

COMPOSITION AND SHOOTING

I prefer to hand-hold my camera and to photograph with the patient standing. Standard poses are used to ensure reproducibility. Standardization of each view is achieved by utilizing anatomic landmarks in conjunction with the viewfinder grid screen (Fig. 5-5). The central lines on the grid screen are used to line up the midsagittal plane and the Frankfort horizontal (a line from the tragus through the infraorbital rim) on all facial photographs (Figs. 5-6 and 5-7). Since these reference points are always on the same lines of the viewfinder grid, control of composition is achieved. Although at first seemingly complicated, the grid method is quickly learned.

On lateral facial views, the posterior edge of the ear should just be included in the picture (Fig. 5-8). On oblique facial views, the medial canthus and the oral

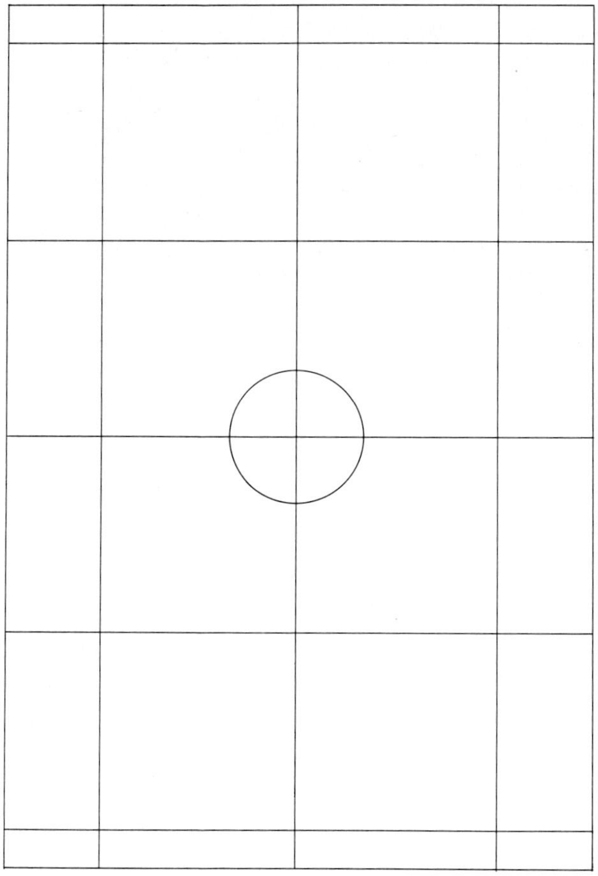

Figure 5-5. Configuration of Canon D grid screen.

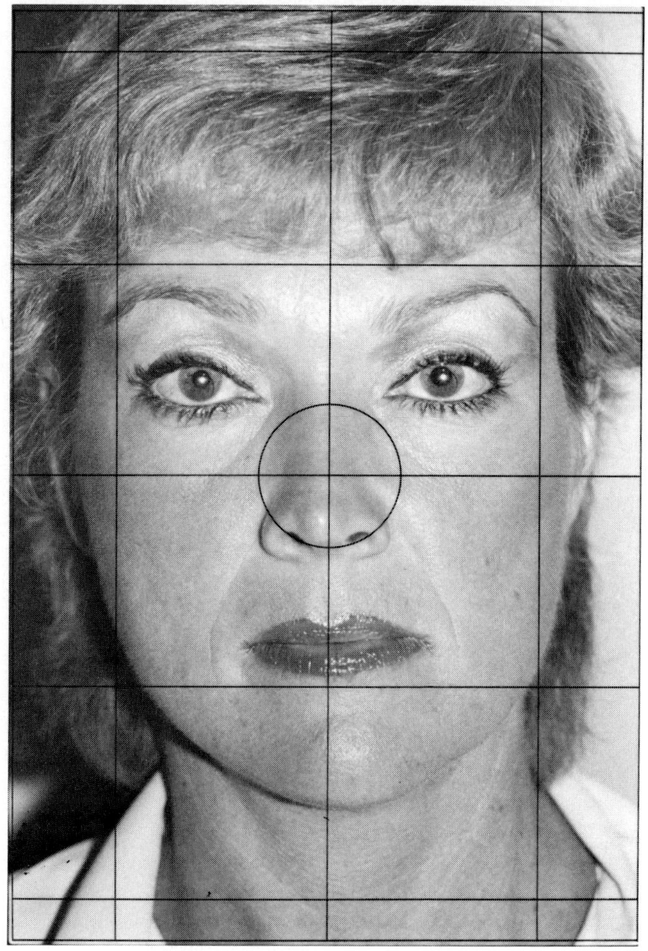

Figure 5-7. Grid screen alignment of frontal facial photograph. Note midsagittal line and Frankfort horizontal.

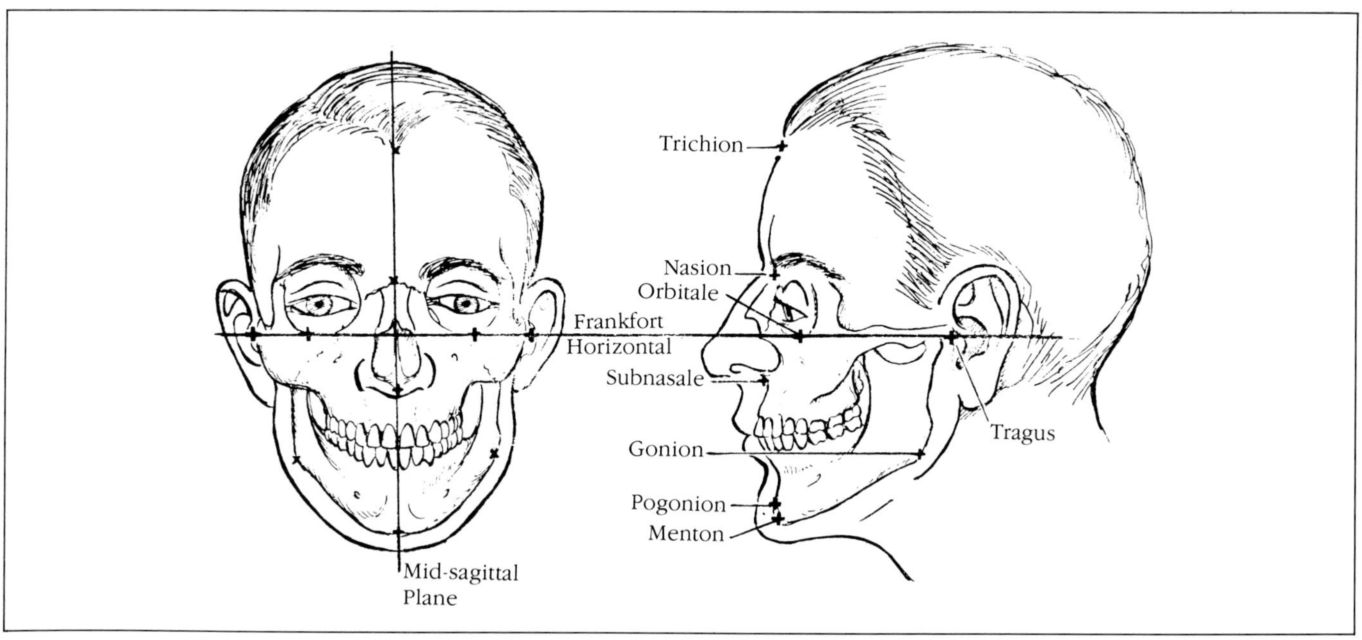

Figure 5-6. Anthropometric points of the face. Note the midsagittal plane and the Frankfort horizontal. From J. M. Converse (ed.), *Reconstructive Plastic Surgery.* Philadelphia: Saunders, 1977.

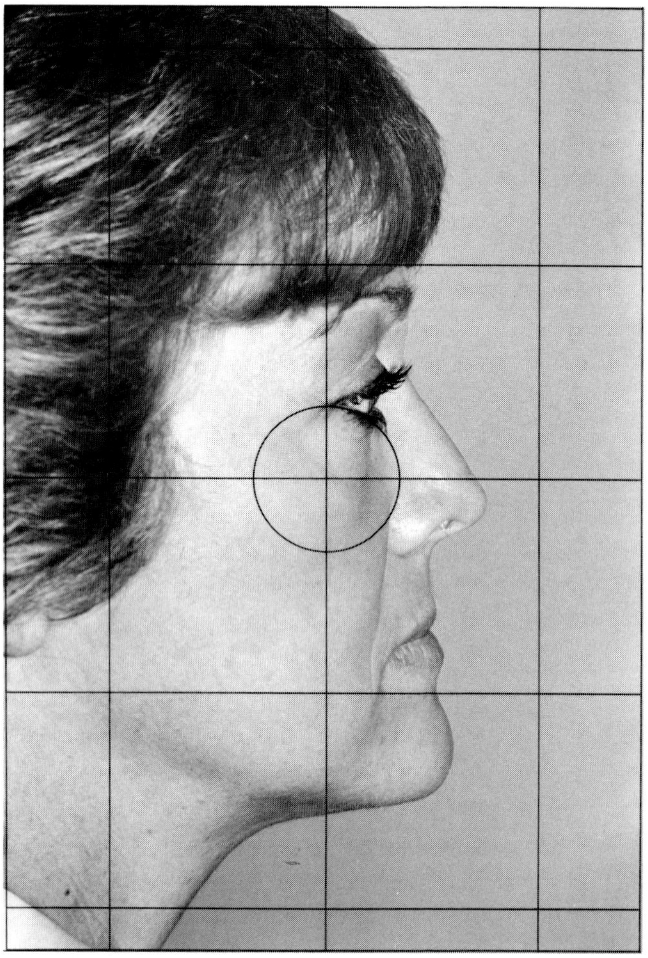

Figure 5-8. Grid alignment on lateral facial photograph. Note Frankfort horizontal; also note that the posterior edge of the ear is used as a framing reference.

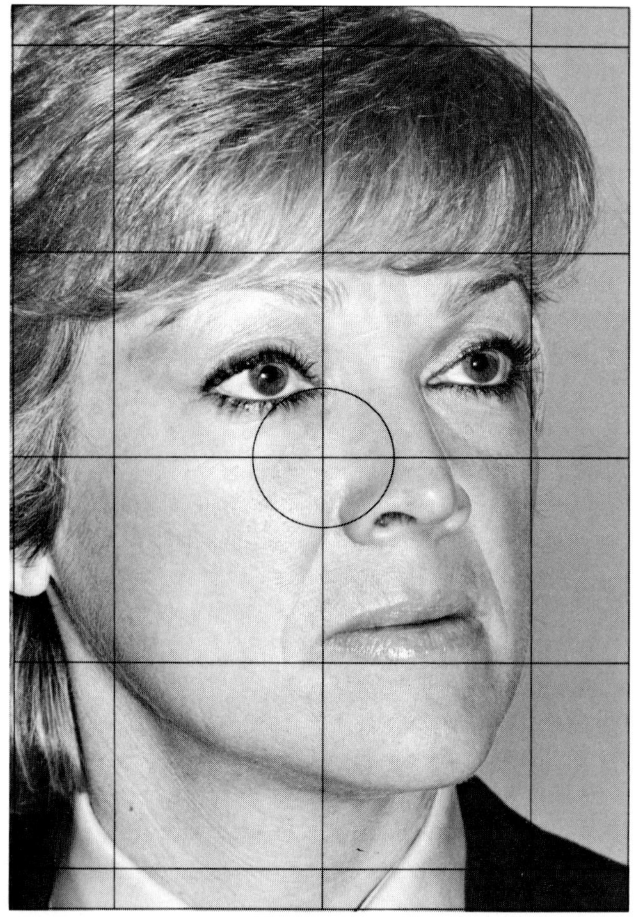

Figure 5-9. Grid alignment for oblique facial photograph. Note Frankfort horizontal; note too that the vertical center grid is lined up with the inner canthus of the eye and the oral commissure.

commissure are aligned with the vertical centerline of the grid, and the Frankfort horizontal is also used (Fig. 5-9). Thus, on all full facial views (AP, lateral, oblique) the Frankfort horizontal is used.

Further standardization of composition is achieved by using anatomic landmarks in conjunction with the grid screen [5]. These landmarks should be relatively stationary both preoperatively and postoperatively. For example, the nipples are not used as reference points in breast photographs since their position may change postoperatively (as in reduction mammoplasty or mastopexy), resulting in a change in composition of the photographs. Similarly, using the nasal dorsum as a reference point in nasal photographs may alter the composition. A chart of various reference points and guidelines for the different photographs is offered in Table 5-1.

A single-distance setting (about 30 in. for a 105-mm lens) is chosen for all frontal, lateral, and oblique views of the head and neck. This corresponds to the 1-m setting on most lenses. When focusing, the photographer moves back and forth through the ideal plane of focus, taking the exposure when sharp focus is obtained. Note that the distance setting is not adjusted for focusing, ensuring uniform composition and reproducibility. Correspondingly, for all closeups another distance setting is selected (15 in. or 0.65 m). This setting is used for eye and ear closeups and for the basal nasal view (Figs. 5-10, 5-11, and 5-12). For all breast, abdomen, and other trunk photographs, a setting of about 6 ft (2 m) is used (Fig. 5-13). Focusing is achieved by moving back and forth with the camera.

The point of focus is also important for standardization. Obviously a variation in the point of focus is more critical in closeups than in photographs taken at longer distances. On all facial oblique and frontal views, including closeups, the focal point is the eyelashes. The exception is the basal nasal view, in which the focal point is the nasal tip (Fig. 5-14). For full facial laterals the focal point is the nasal dorsum, while for closeup eye laterals it is the lashes. Figure 5-15 demonstrates eye lateral closeups with different points of focus. Additional information on focal points is contained in Table 5-1.

Table 5-1. Reference points and guidelines for photographs

Series	View	Lens distance (m)	Framing	Point of focus	Grid landmarks
Facial	AP	1	Vertical	Lashes	FH + midsagittal
	Right oblique	1	Vertical	Nasal dorsum	FH, inner canthus, and oral commissure
	Left oblique	1	Vertical	Nasal dorsum	FH, inner canthus, and oral commissure
	Right lateral	1	Vertical	Nasal dorsum	FH, posterior edge of ear
	Left lateral	1	Vertical	Nasal dorsum	FH, posterior edge of ear
Nasal (add to facial)	Basal nasal	0.65	Horizontal	Nasal tip	Inner canthi and nasal tip
Eyes (add to facial)	AP closeup, open	0.65	Horizontal	Lashes	Inner canthi
	AP closeup, closed	0.65	Horizontal	Lashes	Inner canthi
	AP closeup, up	0.65	Horizontal	Lashes	Inner canthi
	Right lateral closeup	0.65	Horizontal	Lashes	Grid circle on globe
	Left lateral closeup	0.65	Horizontal	Lashes	Grid circle on globe
Ears (add to facial)	Right lateral closeup	0.65	Horizontal	Helical root	Helical root, tragus
	Left lateral closeup	0.65	Horizontal	Helical root	Helical root, tragus
Breast	AP	2	Horizontal	Nipples	Top grid line on shoulders, midsagittal
	Right oblique	2	Vertical	Nipples	Top grid line on shoulders, 45-degree turn
	Left oblique	2	Vertical	Nipples	Top grid line on shoulders, 45-degree turn
	Right lateral	2	Vertical	Nipple	Top grid on shoulder, posterior shoulder
	Left lateral	2	Vertical	Nipple	Top grid on shoulder, posterior shoulder
Abdomen	AP	2	Vertical	Umbilicus	Top grid on shoulder, midsagittal
	Right lateral	2	Vertical	Umbilicus	Top grid on shoulder, posterior shoulder
	Left lateral	2	Vertical	Umbilicus	Top grid on shoulder, posterior shoulder
Buttock/thighs	PA	2	Horizontal	Cleft	Midsagittal, grid center at top of cleft
	Right lateral	2	Vertical	Buttock	Grid center at buttock-thigh junction
	Left lateral	2	Vertical	Buttock	Grid center at buttock-thigh junction

Key: FH = Frankfort horizontal.

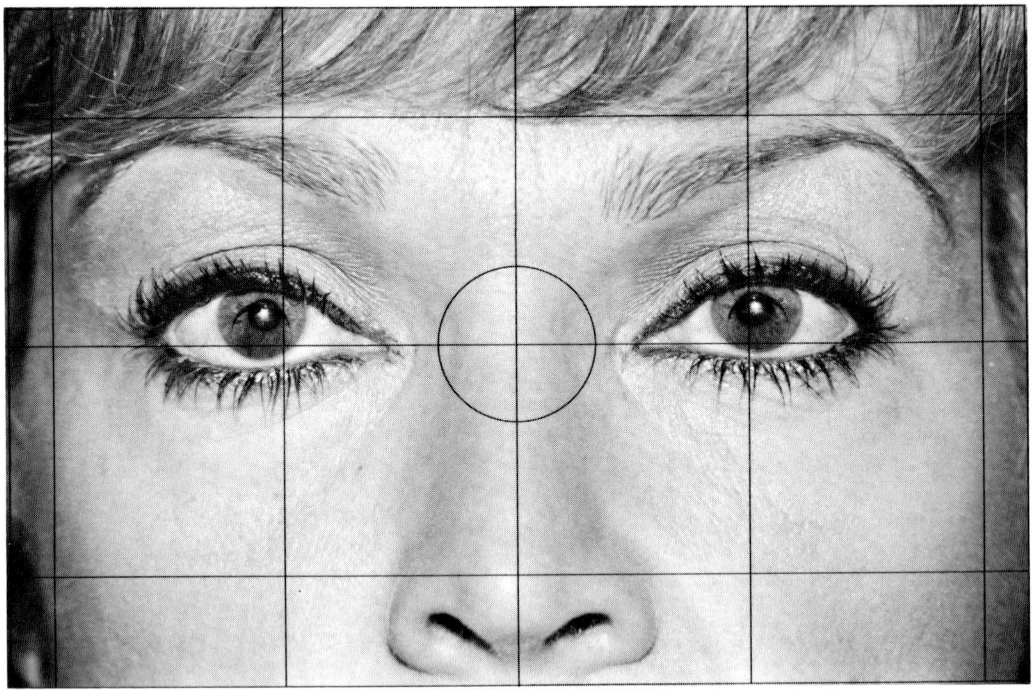

Figure 5-10. Eyes closeup photograph taken at same distance setting as in Figures 5-11 and 5-12. Note alignment of midsagittal plane and of center horizontal grid line through the inner canthi.

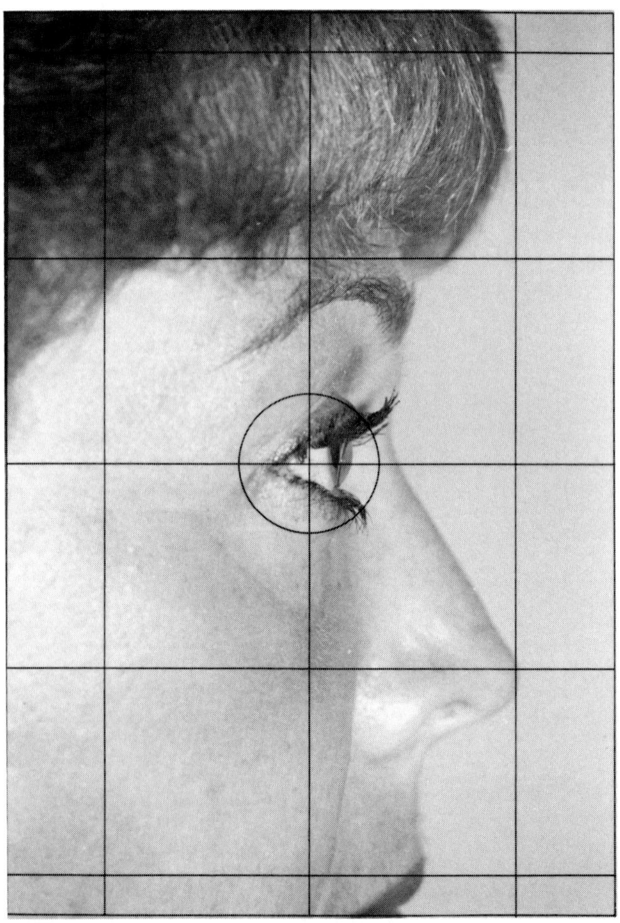

Figure 5-11. Eye lateral closeup with centering of eye on grid screen and proper vertical and horizontal relationships.

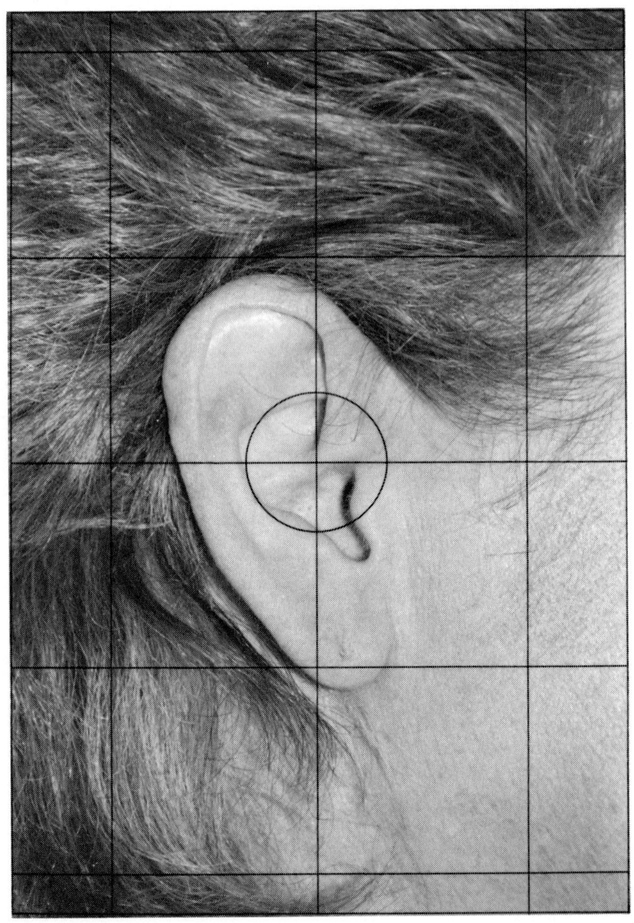

Figure 5-12. Ear closeup with grid centering on helical root and proper vertical and horizontal relationships.

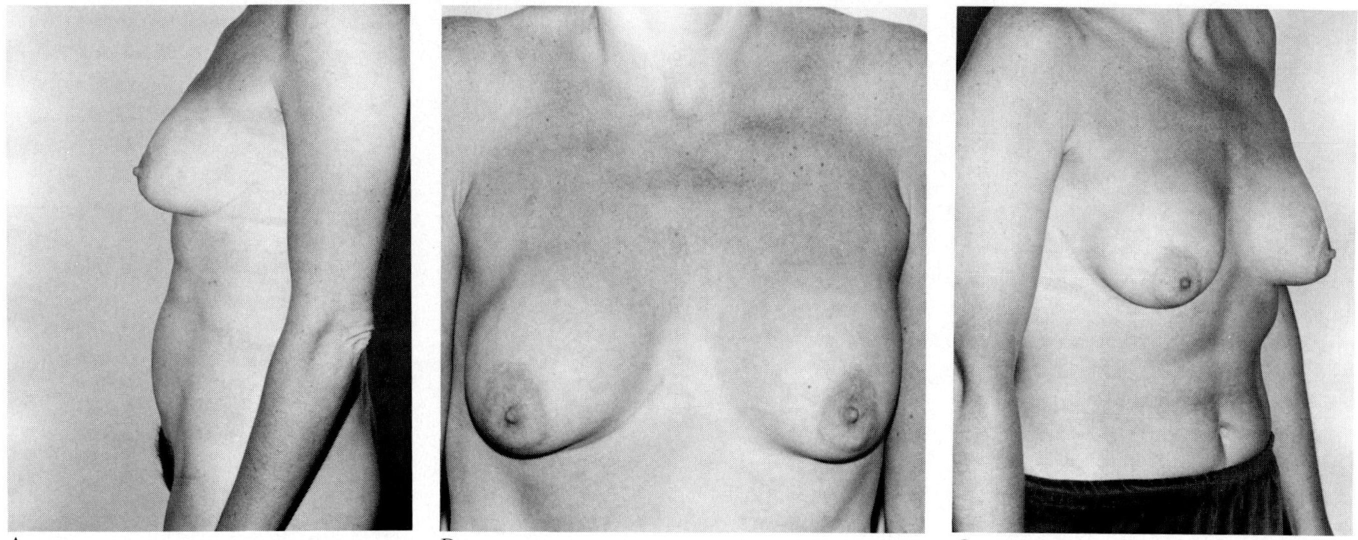

A B C

Figure 5-13. Representative breast and abdominal photographs. These are taken at the same distance setting as is used for buttock and thigh photographs.

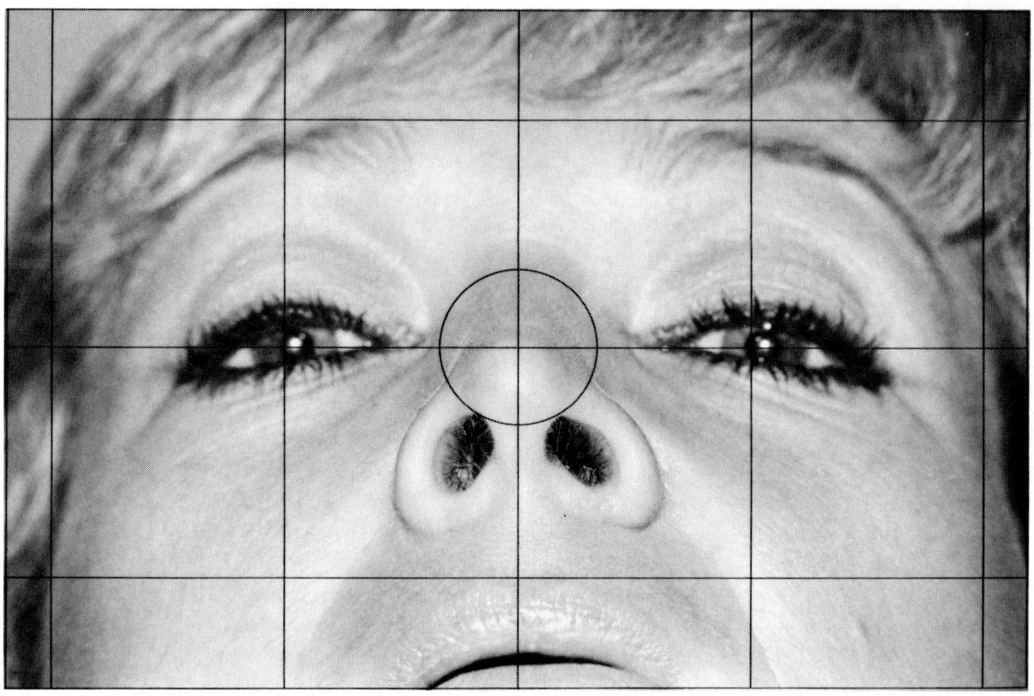

Figure 5-14. Basal nasal closeup, taken at same distance setting as for eyes and ears. Note centering of vertical grid line on columella and alignment of horizontal grid line with nasal tip *and* with inner canthi.

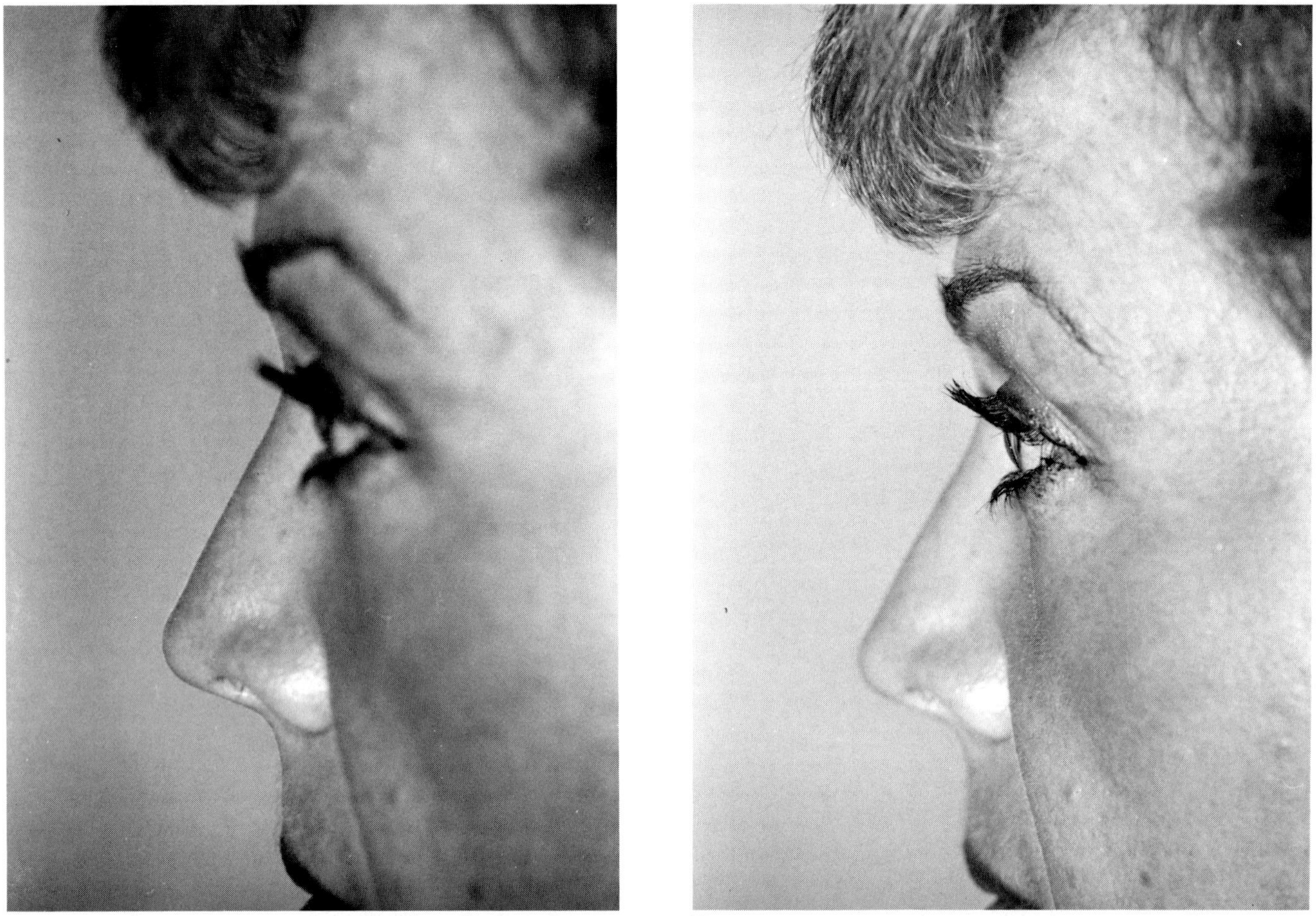

A B

Figure 5-15

A. Eye lateral closeup photographs taken with nose as point of focus.

B. With eyelashes as point of focus.

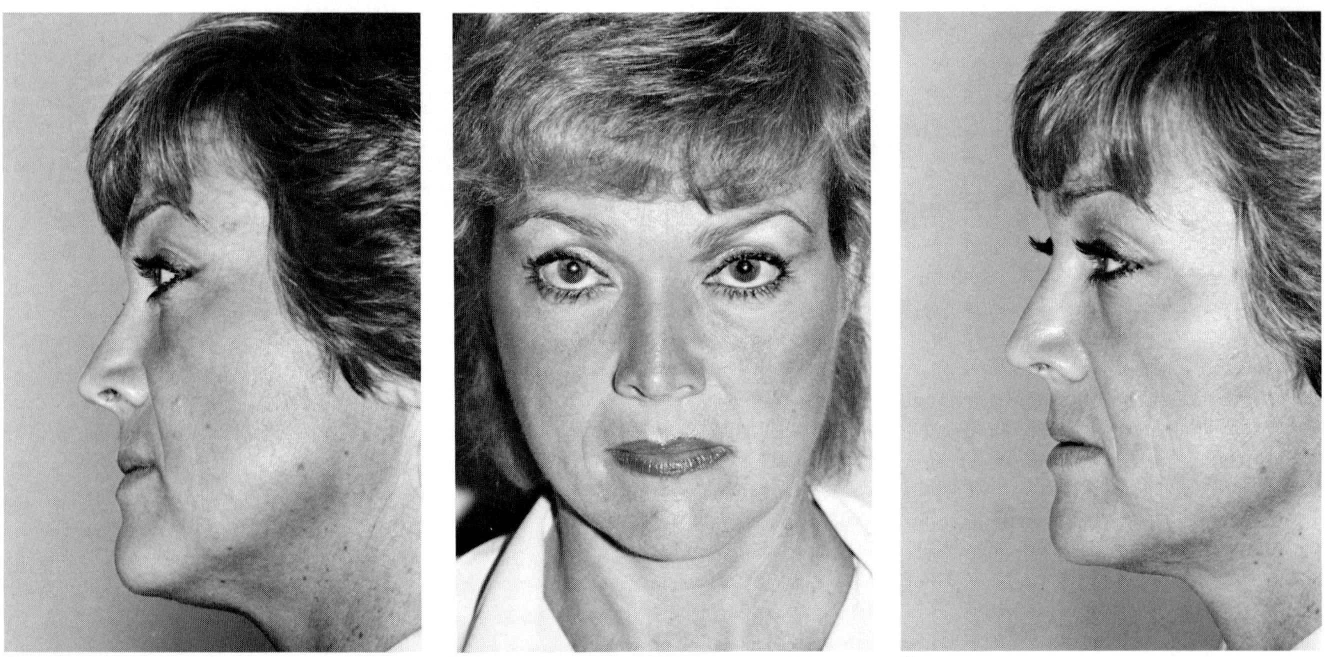

A B C

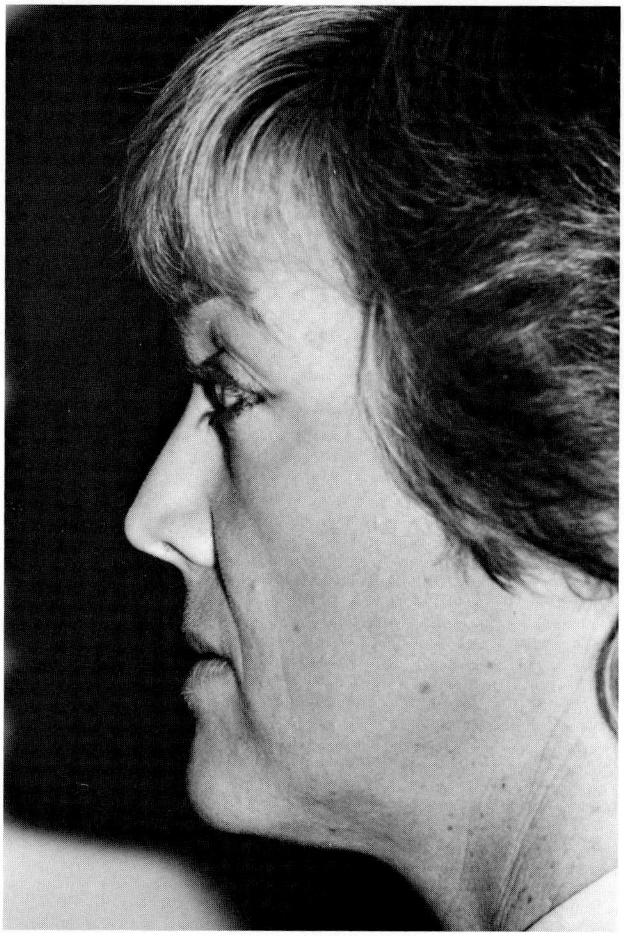

Figure 5-17. Common error. The flash was positioned on the wrong side of the camera.

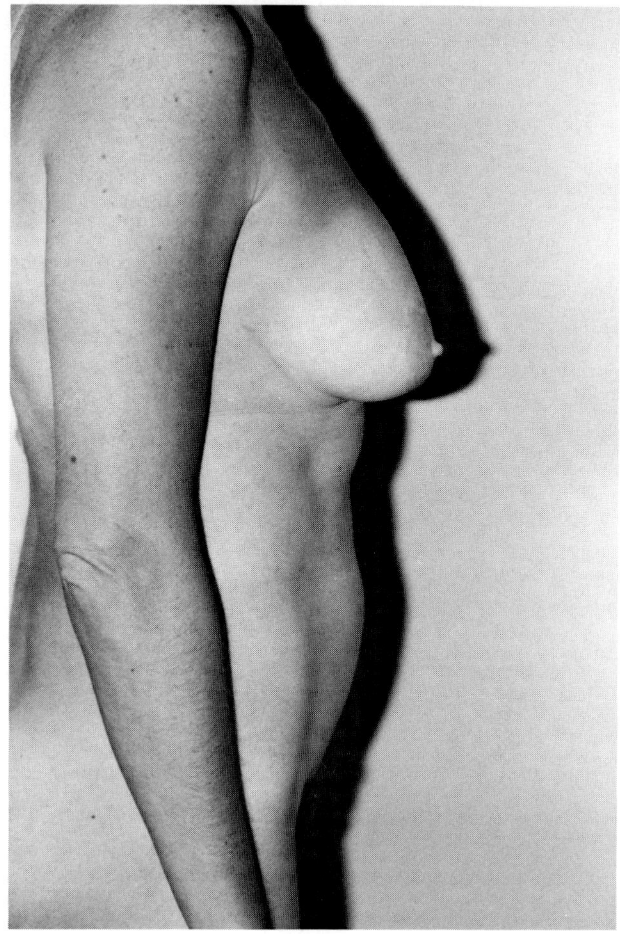

Figure 5-16. Common errors. The first two errors are prevented by using the Frankfort horizontal; the last by proper attention to positioning.

A. The head is tilted away from the camera, giving the appearance of a hanging columella.
B. The face is tilted downward, giving the false impression of scleral show.
C. The head is rotated, showing the opposite side eyelashes and the philtrum.

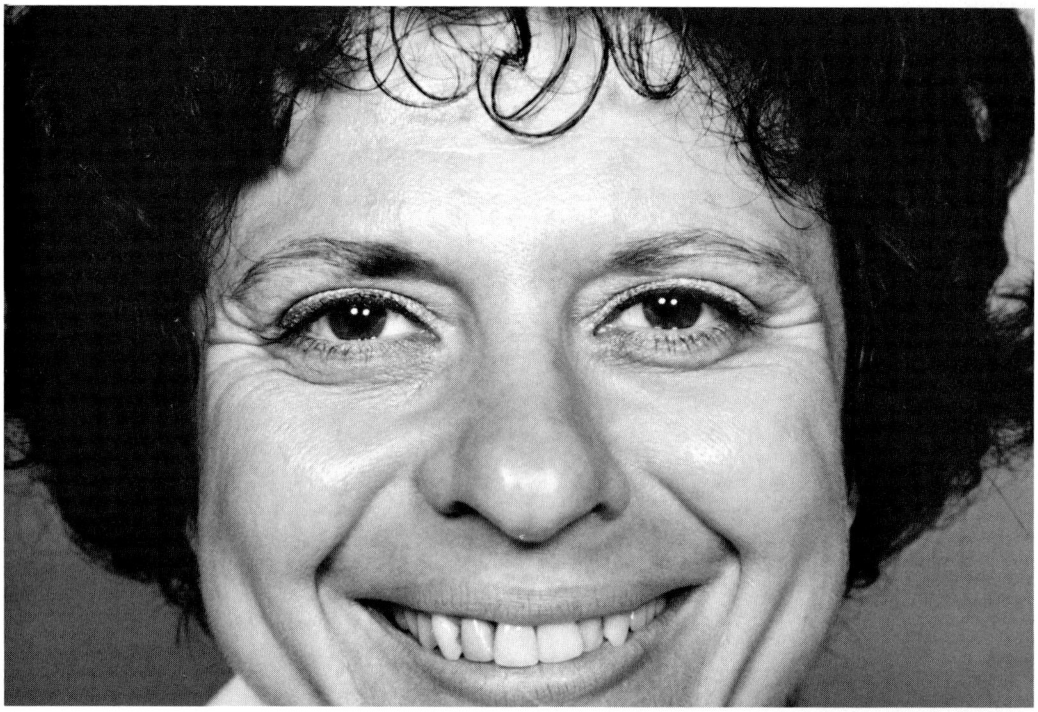

A

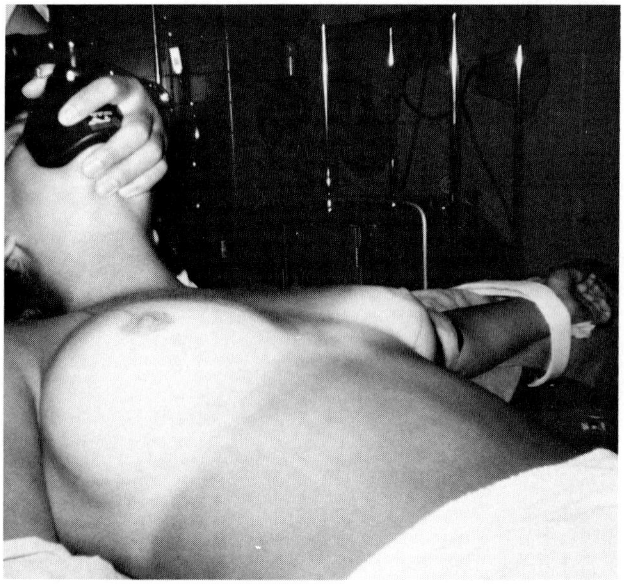

B

Figure 5-18
A. Preoperative nasal photograph with horizontal instead of vertical framing. The nasal tip is out of focus, and the use of a 50-mm lens has resulted in central facial distortion.
B. Preoperative photograph for correction of mammary asymmetry. The asymmetry is obvious only on very close inspection in this view. Preoperative photographs taken with the patient under anesthesia in the operating room have the disadvantages of distortion, cluttered background, and improper positioning.

A series of standard views should be selected for each area of interest and taken in a predetermined sequence. Adherence to this routine each time photographs are taken minimizes chances of error. Errors commonly encountered include poor positioning or grid alignment (Fig. 5-16), shadowing due to incorrect flash position (Fig. 5-17), use of different points of focus, and distracting backgrounds. The plethora of poor illustrations in most journals and texts can be corrected by attention to photographic details (Figs. 5-18, 5-19, and 5-20). The subject of photographic misrepresentation has been reviewed by Dickason and Hanna [2] and by Chappel and Stephenson [1].

THE PATIENT'S RIGHT TO PRIVACY

The patient has a right to have information concerning his or her medical condition and treatment remain secret and not be the subject of publicity [3]:

Clayman vs. Bernstein, 38 PA. D and C, 543, 548 (1940).
While the court appreciates the development of the art of photography generally, and in the medical profession particularly, not only as a means of diagnosis and treatment, but also as a means of instruction, its progress has not yet reached a stage at which physicians have been accorded the right to photograph their patients without their consent, nor has medical jurisprudence recognized the unlimited right of a physician to perform any test, administer any treatment, or perform any operation without the authority of the patient.

The unauthorized taking of pictures of a patient, even those not for publication, can give rise to a cause of legal

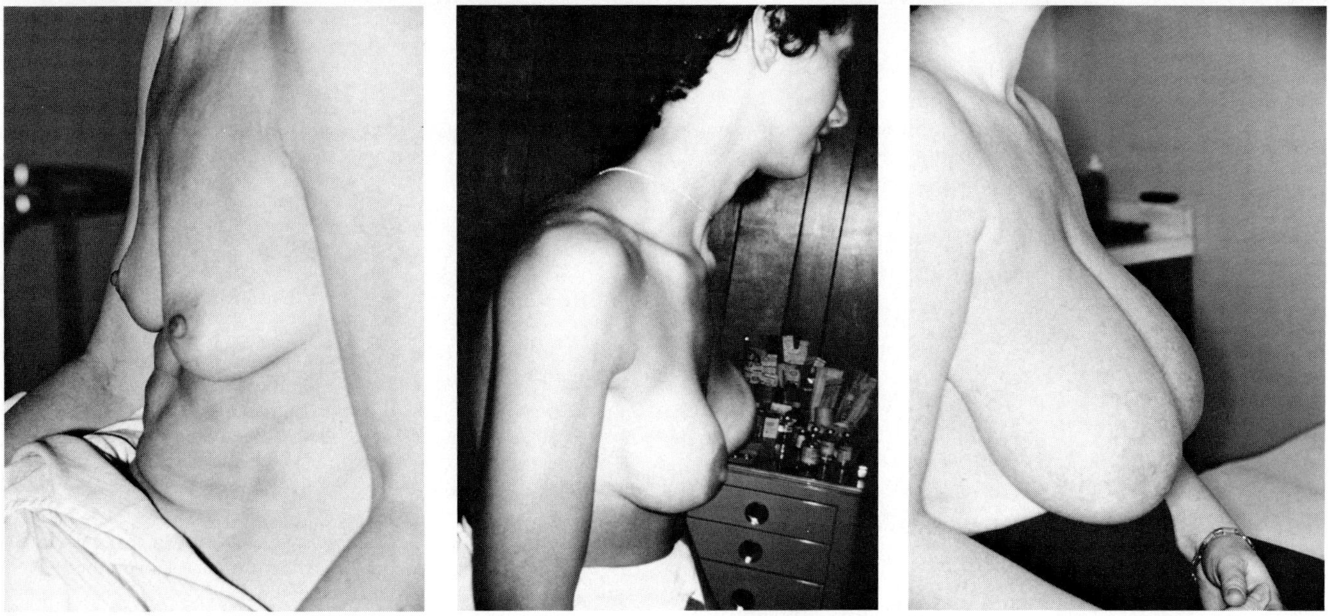

A B C

Figure 5-19

A. Preoperative breast photograph that is neither true lateral nor true oblique. The background, arm position, and sitting position are distracting. The near breast is out of focus.

B. Postoperative augmentation mammoplasty photograph showing poor lighting, rotation, cluttered background, and poor focus.

C. Reduction mammoplasty preoperative photograph with the patient positioned halfway between the lateral and correct oblique positions. Cluttered background, shadowing, sitting posture, and hand positioning make evaluation of the breasts difficult.

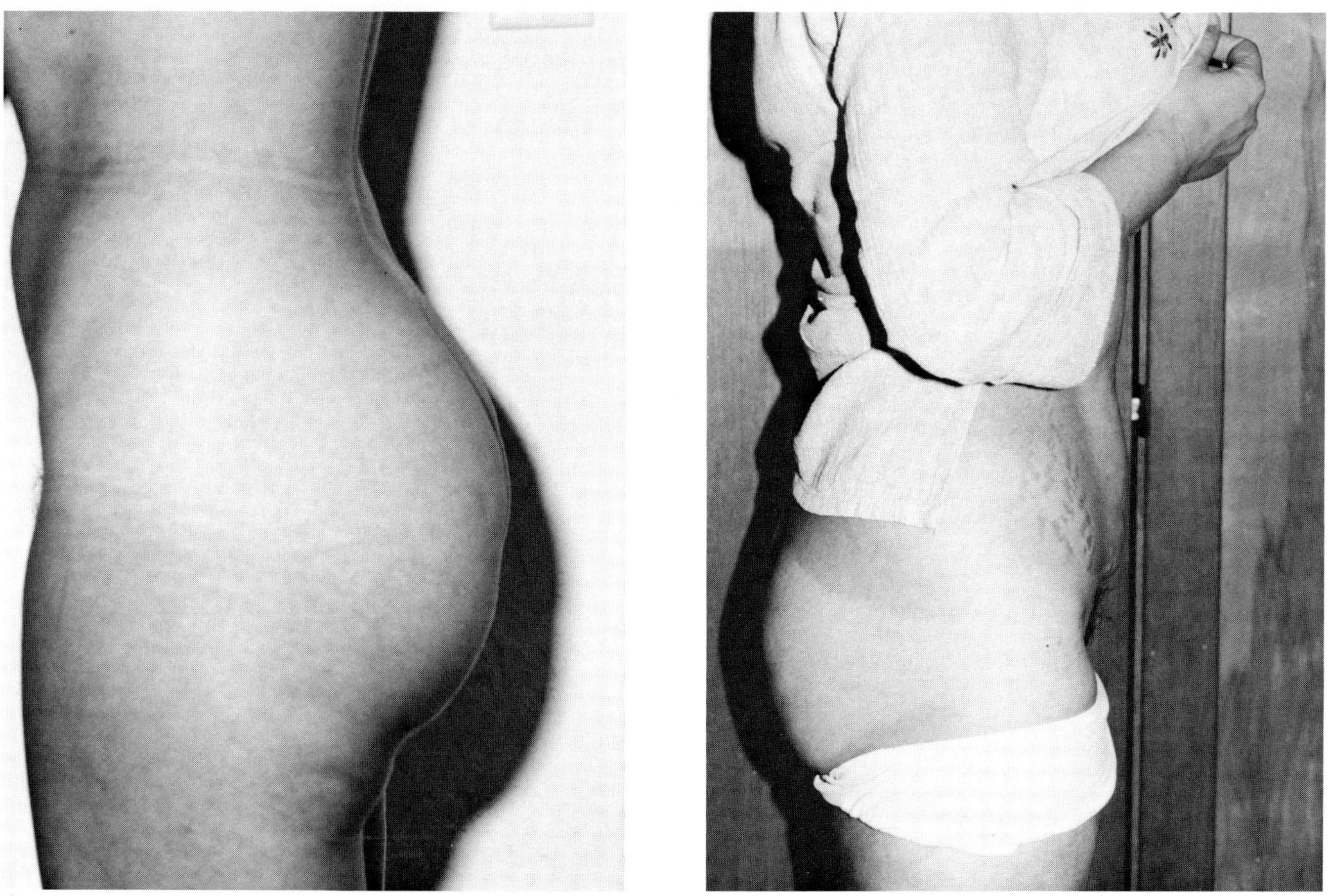

A B

Figure 5-20

A. Preoperative lateral photograph for buttock reduction showing slight rotation and shadowing due to flash position and proximity to the background.

B. Preoperative lateral abdominoplasty photograph. The abdomen is not in sharp focus, and the background is distracting. The arm positioning and presence of the clothes are distracting.

action. Unauthorized use of pictures of patients is one of the more frequent violations of a patient's right to privacy. It is immaterial that the pictures of the patient are taken and published in professional journals or medical books or used in the interest of medical education, knowledge, or research. The patient's consent should be in writing and should state specifically that to which the patient consents. Sample photographic consent forms are shown in the appendix to the book.

SUMMARY

The most sophisticated photographic equipment, when used improperly, can yield poor results. The method described herein has evolved from trial and error, and from consultation with professional and amateur photographers alike.

Eliminating variables helps to produce consistency in clinical photography. The use of automatic electronic flash, predetermined distance settings, viewfinder grid composition with anatomic landmarks, and standard poses and points of focus, as described, will enable the aesthetic plastic surgeon to make accurate and reproducible photographs.

REFERENCES

1. Chappel, J. G., and Stephenson, K. L. Photographic misrepresentation. *Plast. Reconstr. Surg.* 45:135, 1970.
2. Dickason, W. L., and Hanna, D. C. Pitfalls of comparative photography in plastic and reconstructive surgery. *Plast. Reconstr. Surg.* 58:166, 1976.
3. *Medicolegal Forms with Legal Analysis.* Chicago: American Medical Association, 1981.
4. Morello, D. C., and Bernard, R. W. Quality Clinical Photography. Presented at the American Society for Aesthetic Plastic Surgery meeting, Houston, 1981.
5. Morello, D. C., Converse, J. M., and Allen, D. Making uniform photographic records in plastic surgery. *Plast. Reconstr. Surg.* 59:366, 1977.
6. Reeder, R. C. *Sourcebook of Medical Communication.* St. Louis: Mosby, 1981.
7. Tebbetts, J. B. Personal communication. 1982.

II. Rhinoplasty

6. Septorhinoplasty

Paule Regnault
Rollin K. Daniel

Rhinoplasty remains the most challenging and intriguing of aesthetic procedures. Successful results require a well-defined set of aesthetics, a thorough understanding of nasal anatomy, and a broad repertoire of surgical techniques. Ultimately, the final result is determined by selection of surgical maneuvers that can only be guided by experience, especially an understanding of surgical cause and effect. This chapter emphasizes the essential triad of anatomy, aesthetics, and principles that the experienced surgeon can hopefully use to achieve a greater consistency of excellent results.

HISTORY

Although nasal reconstruction has been performed since antiquity, aesthetic nasal surgery began only in the 1880s. Detailed reviews of its evolution have been written by Rogers [129] and McDowell [89], as well as Fomon and Bell [47]. In 1891, John Roe [128] of Rochester, New York, published the first paper on reduction rhinoplasty. He showed remarkable results in photographic case reports and popularized endonasal incisions. Weir [158] introduced numerous external excisions for the exceptionally large nose. Reduction of the nasal hump was the principal step in the operation, as evidenced by Joseph's name for the operation, *Hockerabtragung* ("hump removal"). Refinement of the nasal tip was of limited importance, as is shown in the anatomic drawings and operative techniques of the period. Jacques Joseph [75–77] is considered the father of modern aesthetic rhinoplasty because of his systematic approach to the operation, development of specialized instruments, and publication of a monumental textbook on the subject, *Nasenplastik und sonstige Gesichtsplastik.* These accomplishments occurred over a 33-year period beginning with his first publication in 1898, a second dissertation in 1902 describing 10 patients operated on using a midline dorsal external incision, a subsequent report in 1904 detailing perfection of Roe's intranasal approach as performed on 100 patients, and culminating in his magnificent textbook in 1931.

In 1951 Brown and McDowell [17] published their classic text, *Plastic Surgery of the Nose,* which summarized both aesthetic and reconstructive nasal surgery. Although multiple operations were shown, their approach to the osseous cartilaginous hump was largely an extension of Joseph's basic technique. Tip refinements included descriptions of a "hockey stick" incision into the everted alar domes. As they had similarly affected cleft-lip surgery, Brown and McDowell brought a predictable rhinoplasty technique to the majority of plastic surgeons. Throughout the 1950s, otolaryngologists began to present their techniques with the contributions of Cottle [27, 28], Fomon [46–48], Goldman [53–56], and Anderson [2–5]. Emphasis was placed on nasal respiration and routine correction of septal deviations.

Starting in the 1960s, plastic surgeons began to take a more conservative approach, with preservation of tissues and an artistic flair designed to achieve maximum aesthetic improvement with minimum anatomic disruption. Millard [94–99] popularized the intracartilaginous incision, which reduced the number of incisions, as well as molding of the alar base and rim. Skoog [143, 144] presented his method of hump removal and reinsertion as a means of closing the "open roof" in large prominent noses. By 1978, McDowell [89] reported that all the major contributions to rhinoplasty surgery had been made and most new articles were simply "rehashes" of previous ones. As inevitably follows such statements, a virtual explosion of knowledge occurred. The work of Sheen [134–140], Rees [118–120], Peck [110–112], and Tardy [151–154] introduced a new level of finesse to replace the three-step rhinoplasty. This period has been characterized by conservative remodeling of tissues rather than radical resection, a refined tip crowning the nose rather than mere reduction to fit the nasal profile, and an endomucosal dissection preserving nasal physiology. Although surgical techniques may not have changed radically, the standard of excellence has risen dramatically.

PATHOPHYSIOLOGY AND CLASSIFICATION

If one excludes posttraumatic deformities, the pathology of aesthetic rhinoplasty is a disproportional anatomy of either hyperplasia or hypoplasia involving the entire nose or certain parts, as based on the patient's perception of the ideal. Since classification is merely an aid in deciding on the optimal operation, rhinoplasty requires, first and foremost, an *aesthetic* classification followed by a *proportional* three-dimensional analysis of the nasal parts, and then an *anatomic* evaluation of each structure.

The surgeon must have a definite method of assessing nasal aesthetics. A vague feeling of what is normal will not suffice for preoperative planning, nor will mere correction of abnormal parts serve as an operative technique. Rather, one must develop an aesthetic appreciation of the nose. On the basis of Sheen's observation [138], the five aesthetic components of the nose are evaluated (radix, dorsum, tip, columella-lip, and nasal base) as seen in the three views from which the nose is usually observed (frontal, lateral, and oblique). The nose must obviously be in relation to other facial components, especially the chin and forehead, as well as the patient's stature. As a three-dimensional structure, the nose has three planes: length, height, and width. The obvious classification is to determine the degree of deviation in each plane according to certain landmarks. Longitudinally, the nose should pass from a nasofrontal angle of about 30 degrees to a definite tip with a columella-lip angle of approximately 100 degrees. Vertically, the customary facial angle is 36 degrees, with a radix not less than 1.5 cm and a nasal tip rarely exceeding 2.5 cm in height. Nasal width should be along a divergent concave radix touching a line dropped from the inner canthus. This approach is of value only in dealing with the extremes of each dimension. However, when dimensional concepts are applied to each structural component, they begin to elucidate the problems. For example, failure to recognize short nasal bones or thin lateral crura can have catastrophic consequences.

Once the three-dimensional characteristics of each component are assessed, one is better able to select the optimal operative procedure to achieve the desired aesthetic result. For example, if the nasal tip is too wide, as determined aesthetically by a broad three-point light reflex, and has a bifid tip with separated domes composed of thick alar cartilages, remodeling can be effected by suturing the medial crus. However, this surgical approach must be based on a careful analysis of the three-dimensional aspects of the nasal tip: (1) length, short or plunging tip; (2) vertical, insufficient, or excessive projection; and (3) transverse, narrow or wide tip. Thus, the preceding example of suturing the medial crus to correct the bifid tip was a one-dimensional solution that assumed normal projection and adequate length as well as favorable characteristics of the cartilage and overlying skin. In assessing the problem, one must pass full circle from aesthetics to dimensional proportions to component parts.

CONSULTATION

A significant amount of time should be spent establishing the patient-doctor relationship [58]. In contrast to the rhytidectomy consultation, during which gentle preauricular tension demonstrates the potential result, or the breast augmentation consultation, during which insertion of prostheses into a brassiere can produce a facsimile, there is no method of truly indicating how the "new" nose will appear. Further complicating the visit is the explanation of inherent limitations caused by the patient's skin and osseocartilaginous configuration as well as the vagaries of healing, especially the delay of 6 to 12 months before the final result is visible. For these reasons, many surgeons favor two consultations—the first for evaluation and general assessment and the second several weeks later for detail discussion, often employing photographs of the patient.

Medical History

The history must determine specific requests, motivation, and psychologic stability. As noted by Peterson [113], numerous questions are asked to define the problem.

1. What is wrong with the nose? A deliberately vague question allows the patient to define the problem as being aesthetic, functional, or both.
2. What would you like changed? The patient will usually have a definite answer—either an aesthetic change or

breathing improvement. Once aware of the problem, one can take a more general nasal history.

3. Have you ever injured your nose? Do you have difficulty breathing or allergies? If previous trauma has occurred, one should document whether medical treatment was necessary and any sequelae. The question of breathing difficulty can unleash a limitless discussion. Additional inquiries concern medications, nasal sprays, nosebleeds, and medical consultation. How is the condition now: better or worse? Have you ever had surgery on the nose before? It is important to ask this question directly, as many patients will either omit any mention of prior surgery or forget significant procedures.
4. How is your general health? One can use this opportunity to inquire into the patient's general well-being, both physical and mental. A brief review of systems, medications, type of work, family status, and life satisfaction is obtained. One should ask about any nervous or psychiatric problems. Also, the patient's current condition is often revealed by the question, "How is life treating you these days?"
5. What specifically do you want changed? Can you show me in the mirror? Most patients will point to a definite hump or squeeze a bulbous tip. Further elaborations will point out that the nose is "too wide, too long, or too big." One must be careful of the patient who cannot specify the desired changes. By forcing patients to demonstrate the alteration on themselves the surgeon is reinforcing the concept that surgery merely alters their own existing tissues and does not miraculously substitute a new nose.
6. Why do you want the surgery now? What do your family and friends think? Most patients will have thought about surgery for several years but will not seek it until they reach the appropriate age or achieve adequate financial resources. Be wary of the patient who desires surgery as a means to an end, i.e., career advancement or improved relationships. A supportive or at least understanding family is desirable. If a parent or spouse is strongly opposed, a second consultation is planned and separate discussion held with each. Ultimately, one's obligation is to the patient, but several months' delay will often allow time for reconciliation.
7. Have you ever had any cosmetic surgery and were you satisfied with the result? Have you ever seen another physician regarding surgery on your nose? This direct question is helpful in determining the patient's motivation and ability to handle potential complications. Throughout the history-taking process one is attempting to gain rapport with the patient and to obtain an understanding of the patient's objectives.

Motivation

The specific objectives of most patients seeking an aesthetic rhinoplasty can be divided into four broad categories: (1) type changes, (2) specific changes, (3) proportional changes, and (4) refinement (Fig. 6-1). Patients requesting a type change frequently have a large aquiline, or "beak," nose and wish it altered to a straighter, shorter nose with a slightly elevated tip. Orientals and blacks occasionally request a more "Caucasian" nose [41, 149]. In a classic article, Flowers [44] described the polymorphic types of "oriental" noses and a cohesive approach to their modification. Another group desires change in a specific structure: a large hump or a bulbous tip. Other patients say that they like their nose but find it just too big and want the overall size reduced. Increasingly, patients are seeking refinement of nasal aesthetics to reach a finer balance of the parts, i.e., narrower in the middle third, lowering of the dorsum, and a more delicate tip. The surgeon must explore the patient's motivations, being certain that persons who want type changes will be truly satisfied and not psychologically stressed by loss of their heritage and that those who want proportional change realize that it is rarely achieved and they will look different.

With regard to patient population, one may arbitrarily define certain subgroups: (1) adolescent females, (2) males, (3) middle-aged females, (4) older individuals, (5) non-Caucasians, and (6) neurotics or psychotics. Adolescent females react well to major changes in their noses. Their acceptance and rapid integration of the new nose probably reflect continuation of the dramatic body changes that have occurred in the transition of puberty [52]. Chin implants and other alterations are readily accepted. Male patients can be divided into three subgroups: posttraumatic, homosexual, and aesthetic. Most posttraumatic patients want the nose straight, the breathing improved, and a humpless profile. The homosexual male is frequently demanding and perfectionistic but ultimately an agreeable and grateful patient. With the exception of those with large "beaks," the male seeking purely aesthetic improvement must be approached cautiously. The junior author routinely refers them to a psychiatrist for evaluation. Thus far, surgery has been deemed acceptable in half and cautionary in a quarter, and psychotherapy without surgery has been recommended in a quarter. If this precaution seems excessive, Hinderer's chilling account [70] of Dr. Anon's murder by a male rhinoplasty patient is testimony to the "nose-penis" relationship. Increasingly, middle-aged patients are requesting septorhinoplasty along with blepharoplasty or rhytidectomy. When asked, "Why have surgery now?" they usually answer, "I wanted to have my nose fixed as a teenager but my parents wouldn't let me," or "I didn't have the money until now." One should beware of patients who suddenly decide to change their nose as this action may be a substitute for dealing with a life crisis or other problem. One should avoid the patient who wants to have the operation done immediately. Gorney's admonitions on how to evaluate aesthetic patients is particularly valuable [65]. Individuals in their late fifties and sixties are now seeking rhinoplasty. Their most common complaints are drooping of the nasal tip and increased size, which are associated with old age [109]. In order to avoid loss of identity, dramatic changes should *not* be done and remodeling of the nasal tip is often sufficient, rather than a complete septorhinoplasty with fracturing of brittle nasal bones.

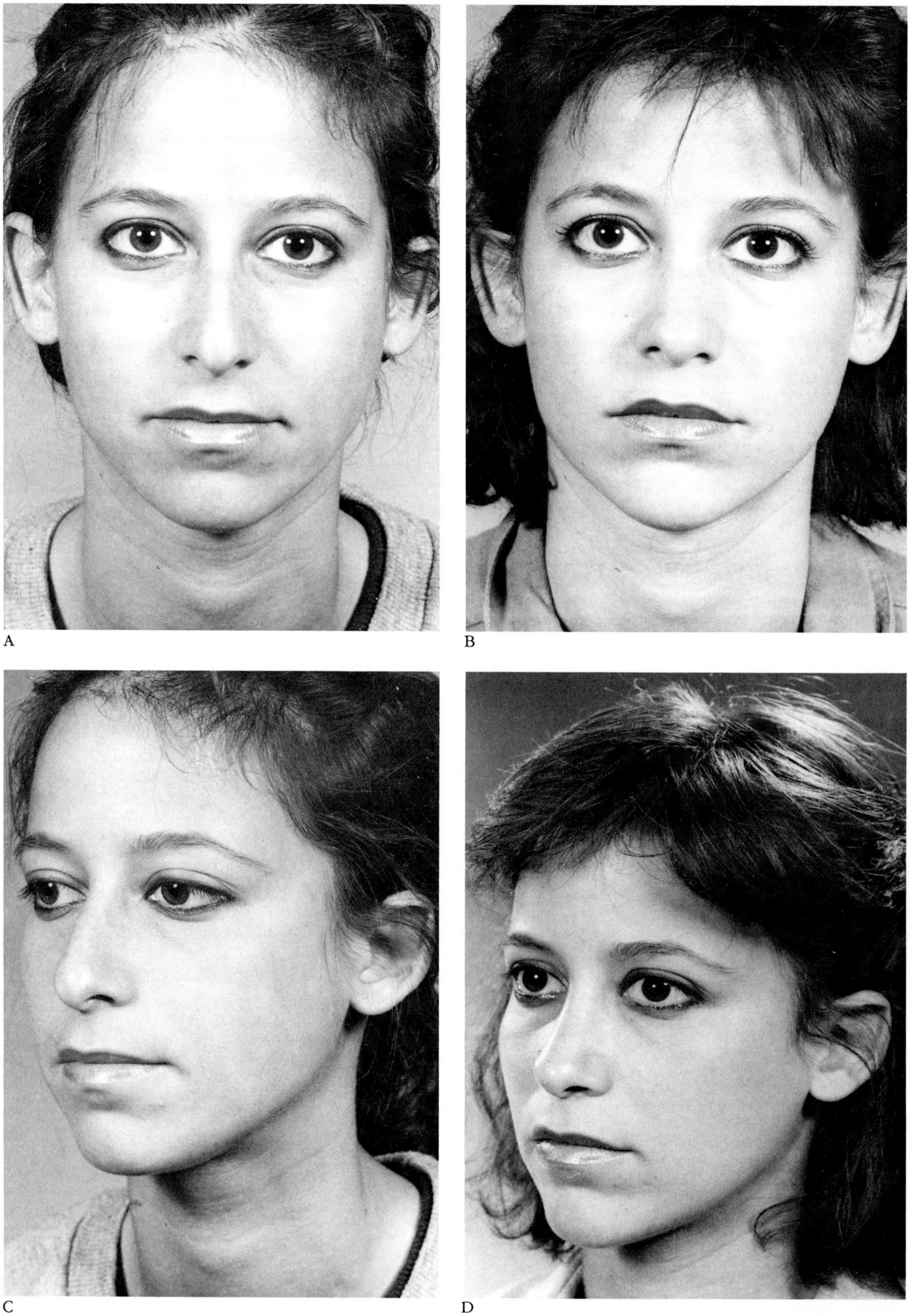

Figure 6-1. The different motivations for seeking rhinoplasty.
A–D. Patient requested a smaller, softer nose that would not dominate her face—a type change.

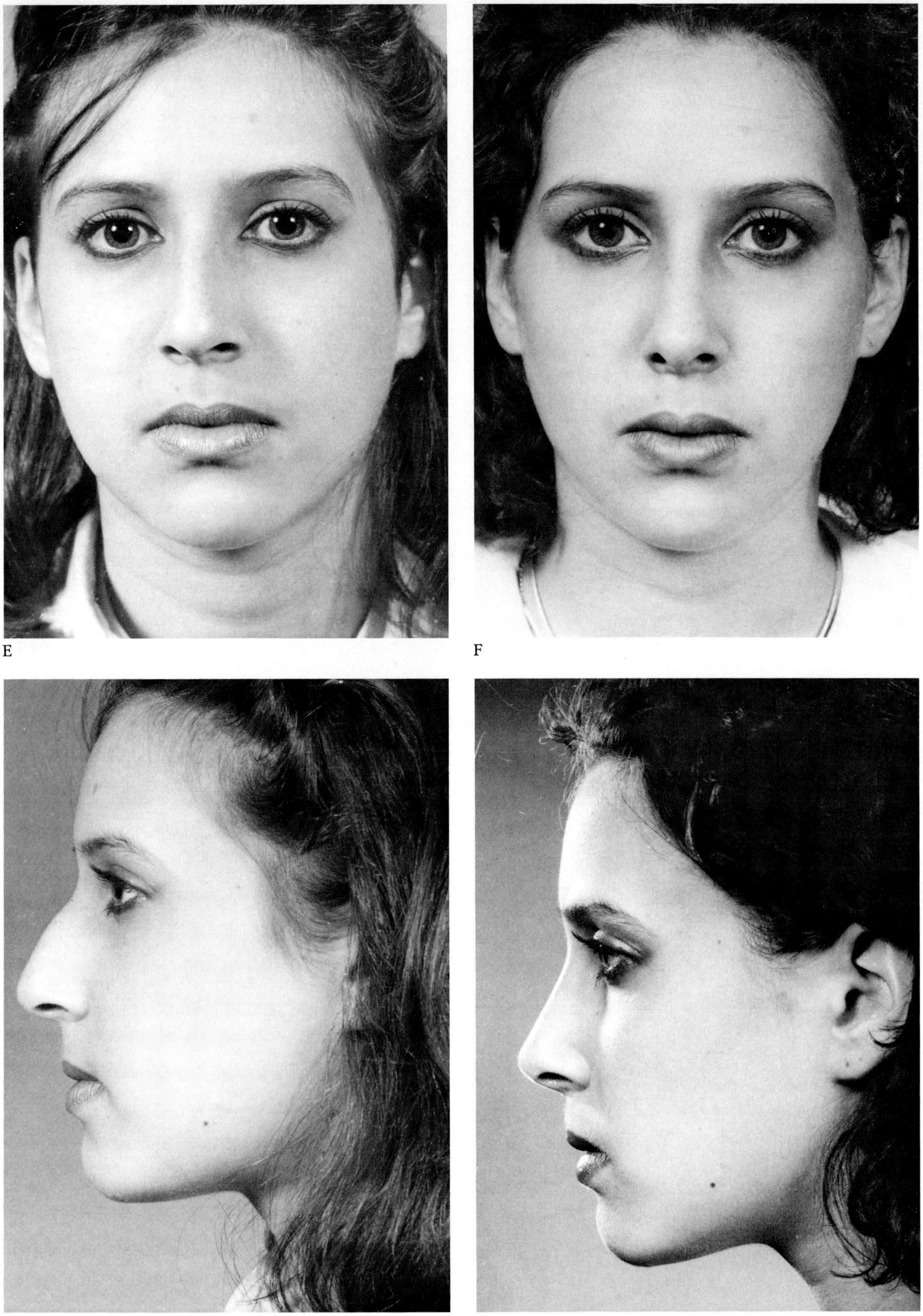

Figure 6-1 (continued)
E–H. A 17-year-old specifically sought elimination of the hump without any tip elevation—a specific change.

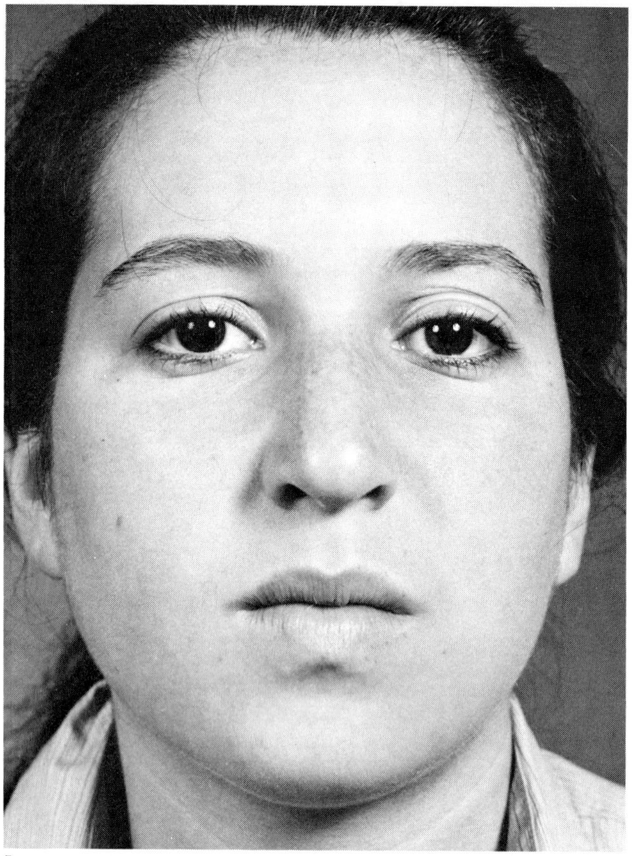

I

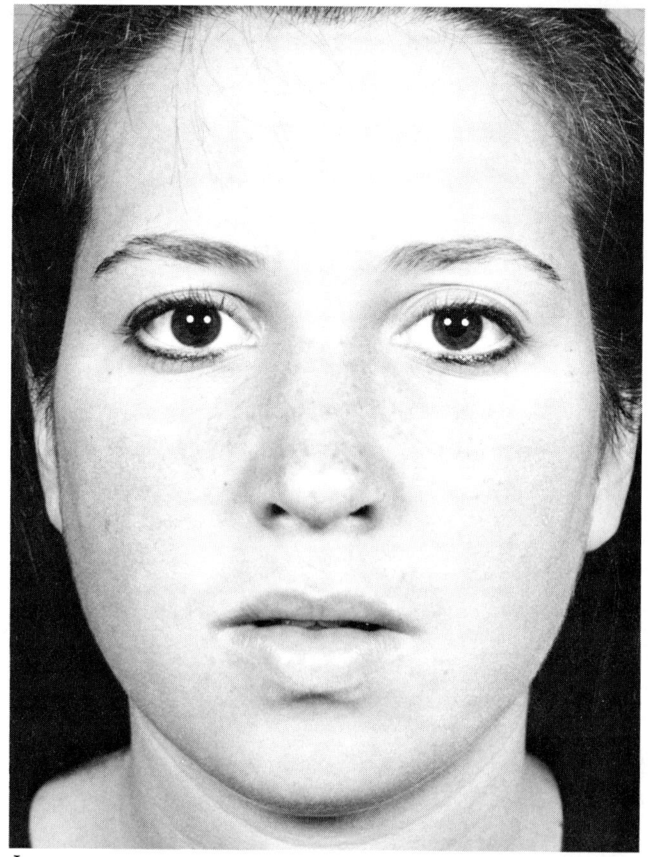

J

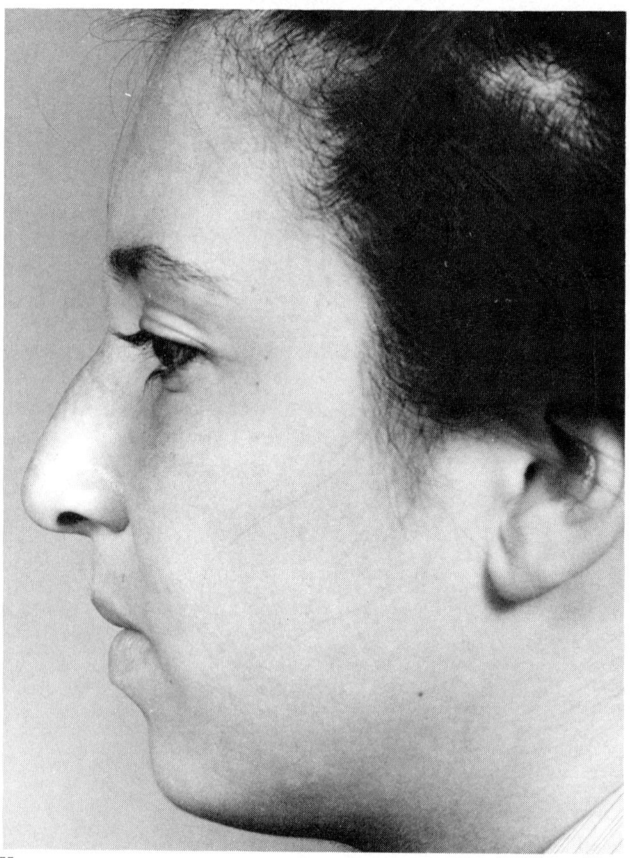

K

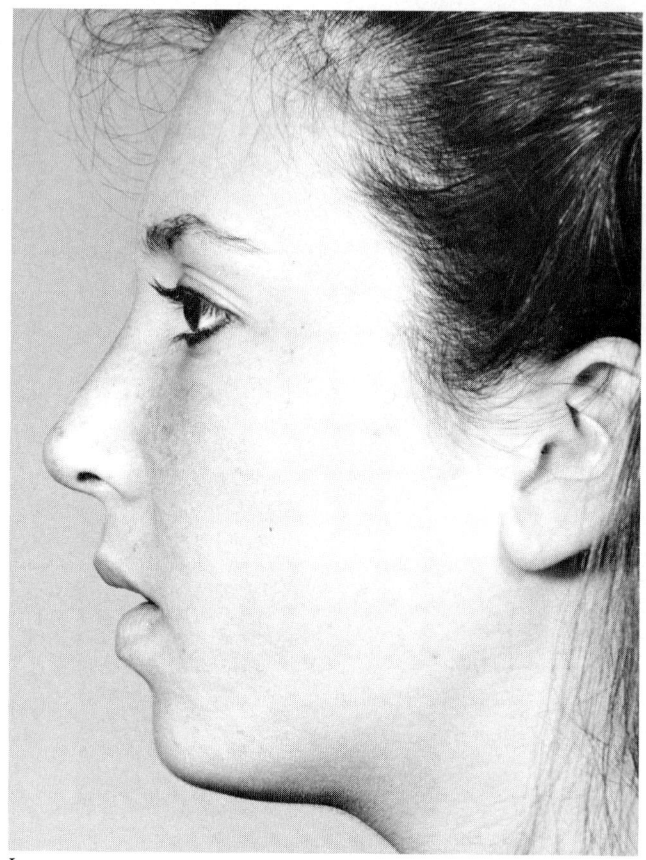

L

Figure 6-1 (continued)
I–L. A 16-year-old wanted her "own nose, only smaller and nicer"—a proportional change.

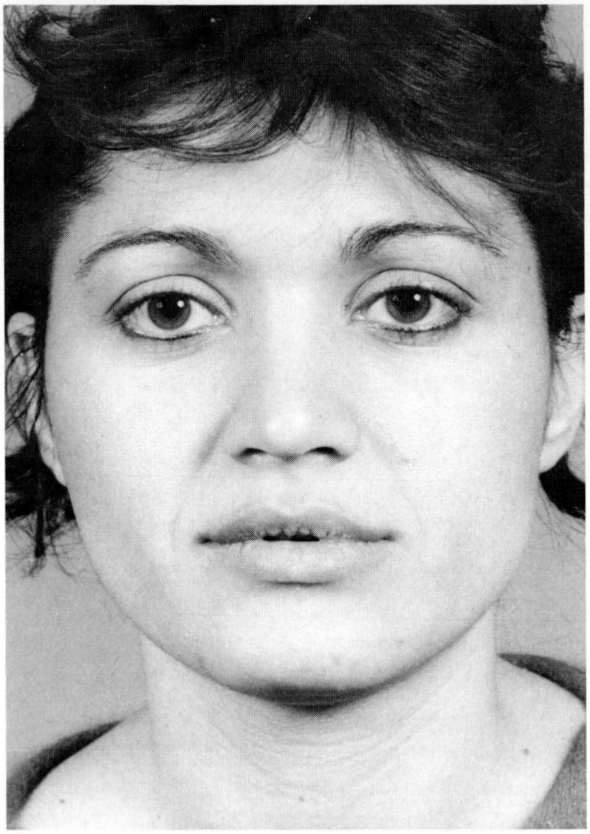

M

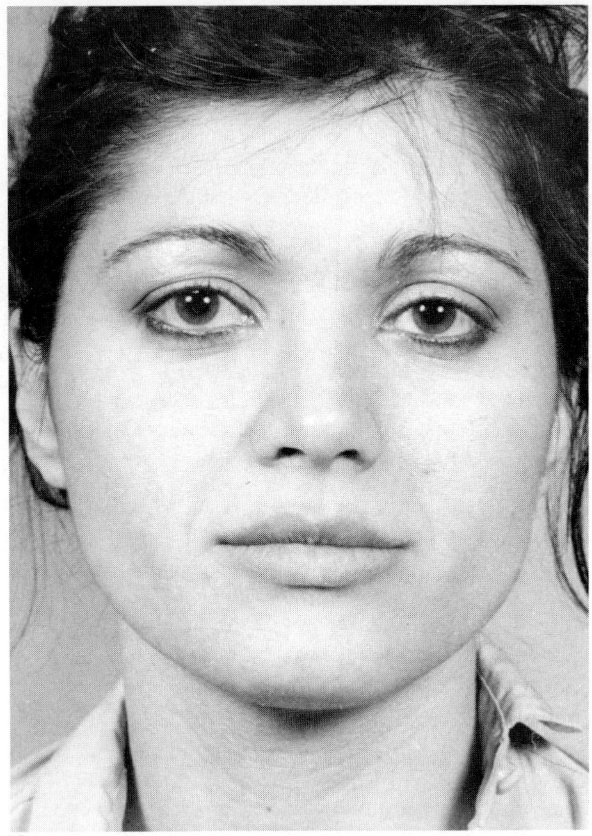

N

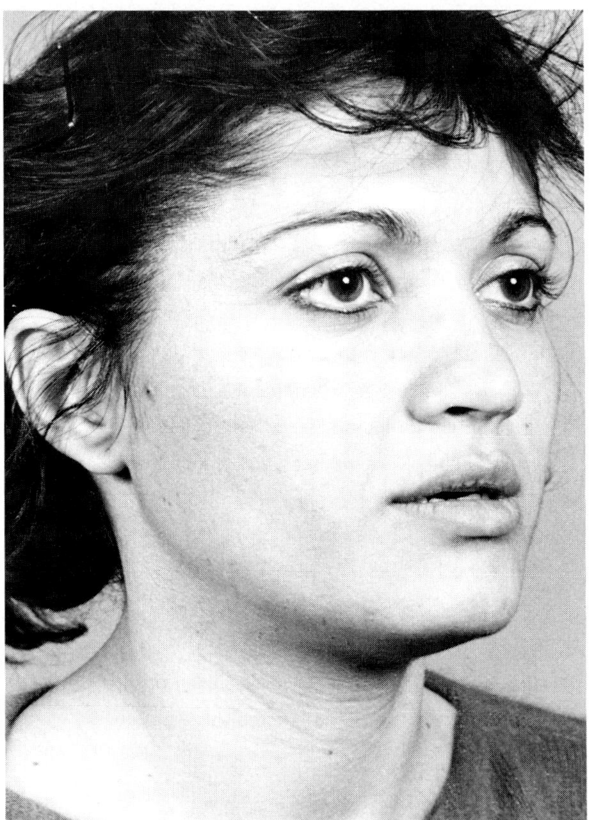

O

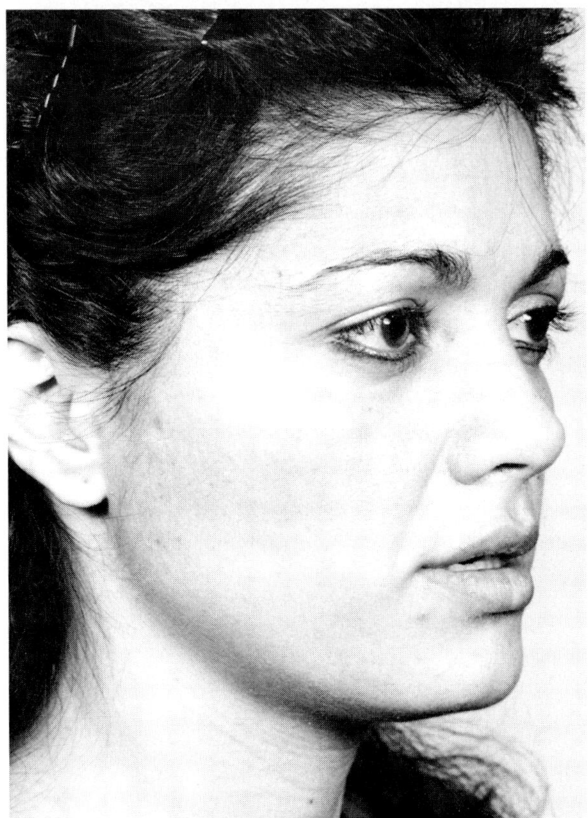

P

Figure 6-1 (continued)
M–P. A 23-year-old desired an aesthetically pleasing nose—a refinement.

Physical Examination

Examination must determine the characteristics of each component part, the potential for modification, and evolution of an operative plan. Throughout the consultation, the surgeon has the opportunity to assess the patient's general appearance, demeanor, and presentation. The relative relationship between face and nose is carefully defined. As stressed by Fomon [46] and Peterson [113], one should try to characterize the facial type (round, oval, rectangular, or triangular) as well as the relationship to forehead (convex, perpendicular, sloping, receding), lips, and upper and lower jaws (protruding, receding).

The *external nose* is carefully examined and palpated. The overall configuration of the nose is analyzed, its dimensions in all three planes are assessed and any prominent deformities are noted. The length is essentially the distance from the radix to the columella, with potential changes confined to the leading edge of septum and medial crura. The dorsal height is determined primarily in the profile view and tip projection on basal view. The width is evaluated at the radix, the bony base above the piriform aperture, and the alar base. Deviation of the nose is checked from above and confirmed by placing small dots 5 mm apart along the septum.

Critical skin factors are thickness, elasticity, composition, and condition. If the skin is thick and inelastic, with numerous sebaceous glands, it will drape poorly, and true "tip definition" will be difficult. Thin elastic skin allows better definition but must be elevated in a deep plane to avoid dermal damage and visible surgical sequelae. One should also note any scars from previous trauma or excisions, dermatologic conditions, and telangiectasia.

The configuration, size, and position of the nasal bones are determined by observation and palpation. The nasofrontal angle, the width of the nasal root, and the cephalic extension of the hump are measured. An estimate of the hump's bone-cartilage composition is made. The relationship of the upper lateral cartilages to the septum and alar cartilages is carefully examined, as is pinching on forced inspiration. The degree of overlying subcutaneous tissue is noted.

Each component of the lobule and its adjacent tissues must be carefully assessed: alar cartilages, columella, septum, and nostrils. Is the lobule itself excessively projected, retracted, pointed, or rounded? Where are the domes? What are the dimensions and thickness of the lateral alar cartilages? Are the lateral crura too long, with scroll formation at the upper laterals, or are they thin delicate strips with a sesamoid-filled gap? Are the lateral crura too wide, with arching of the nostril, or are they angulated superiorly, producing a parenthesis tip? Is there a significant asymmetry? Are the medial crura separated in the midline, splayed inferiorly, or pushed downward? Is the columella too high, too short, too wide, or very delicate? What is the nasolabial angle, what is the relative length of the upper lip, and what happens to the tip on forced smiling? The nasal spine and leading edge of the septum are palpated through the columella. The width of the nasal base is assessed on frontal view relative to the inner canthi and the columella-alae angle. With the head tilted back, the lobule-nostril ratio, nostril configuration, and any visible septal deviation are determined.

The *internal nose* is now examined. If an accurate internal exam is not done, one may encounter unsuspected high septal deviations, turbinate hypertrophy, and other deformities, which will either force additional surgery or preclude attainment of the desired result. A general guide as to airway patency is provided by compressing one nostril and determining with the back of a hand the amount of air on forced expirations. Gorney [64, 66] has detailed the optimal method of examining the internal nose as follows:

1. Examine the patient in a sitting position with a head rest.
2. Explain what is to be done and show the patient the speculum. Then look inside the nose, assessing the condition of the septum and turbinates.
3. With a bayonet forceps, insert a small wad of cotton soaked in 2% cocaine. Wait several minutes for mucosal vasoconstriction to occur, which results in dilatation.
4. Extract the cotton. Then, using a headlight (tightly focused fiberoptic or a headband mirror) and a narrow-bladed speculum, look into the nose.
5. Examine the septum. Look up to see high deviations, down to see septovomerine shelves. Is the cartilage fractured, overlapped, perforated, or displaced?
6. Check the turbinates. What is their color, size, condition?

Aesthetic Goals

Following a thorough exam, the patient's objectives are reviewed, the physical exam is summarized, and a realistic assessment of the expected result is presented. Statements that "The hump can be removed," "The tip can be elevated and narrowed" are often followed by the question, "But what will it look like?" Previously plaster casts were used to demonstrate potential changes, but tissue is not so easily sculptured or wound healing so certain. Utilization of preoperative and postoperative photographs of other patients is truly irrelevant and may imply a legal guarantee of equal results. The logical solution is to use photographs of the patient, either projected color slides with changes drawn in erasable ink on a screen, or prints that are reversed and placed on an x-ray view box with changes drawn in pencil. This technique implies a second consultation. Instant photographs represent an alternative, although high-quality photographs are essential prior to surgery.

Informed Consent

The patient must realize that every effort will be made to achieve the desired objectives. However, the inherent anatomic structures and the uncertainty of wound healing will influence the result. Final assessment is not possible before 1 year.

1. Bruising and ecchymosis vary with the individual but are usually minimal by 2 weeks. Rarely, conjunctival hemorrhage will occur and last for 6 to 8 weeks.
2. In contrast, swelling will persist for up to 1 year but will decrease over the radix by 1 month, the dorsum by 2 months, and the tip by 9 months.
3. Sensation is decreased over the dorsum and usually returns by 3 months.
4. Some degree of nasal obstruction is expected and may persist for 6 to 8 weeks.
5. The basic objective remains an aesthetically pleasing nose that complements the face. The "perfect nose" is impossible to achieve.

Patient Preparation

1. No aspirin or aspirin-containing medication should be taken for 2 weeks prior to surgery.
2. Photographs are an important part of the surgical record and serve as references during surgery.
3. Although the operation is relatively painless, all pain medications should be filled prior to surgery.

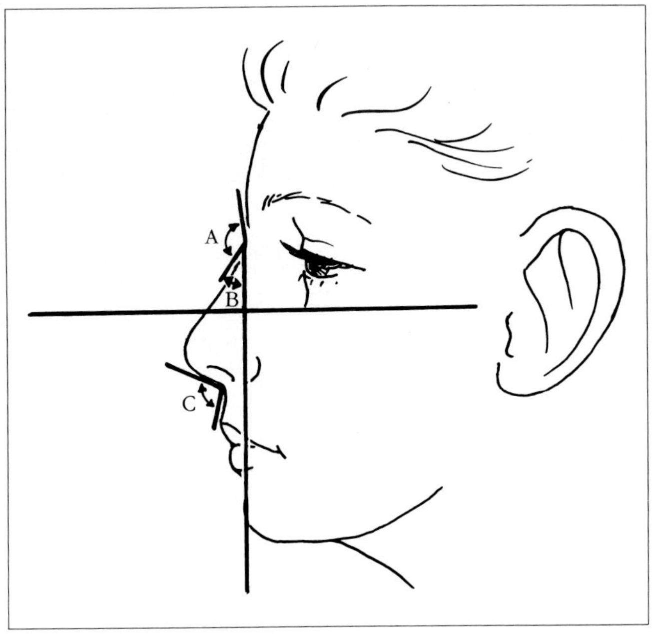

Figure 6-2. The three most useful facial angles for preoperative assessment.
A. The obtuse nasofrontal angle (average 125 degrees).
B. The acute angle of nasal projection (23–37 degrees).
C. The critical nasolabial angle (90–110 degrees).

SURGICAL ANATOMY

In contrast to breast or torso surgery, which deals with anatomy that is rarely complex, nasal anatomy is *a critical factor* in determining selection of operative technique and in limiting the attainable result. The surgeon must understand the anatomic basis of the visible nasal deformities ranging from the short nasal bone syndrome to the parenthesis tip [138]. Otherwise, application of a standard operation that gives good results in most cases will produce a disaster in certain anatomic variations.

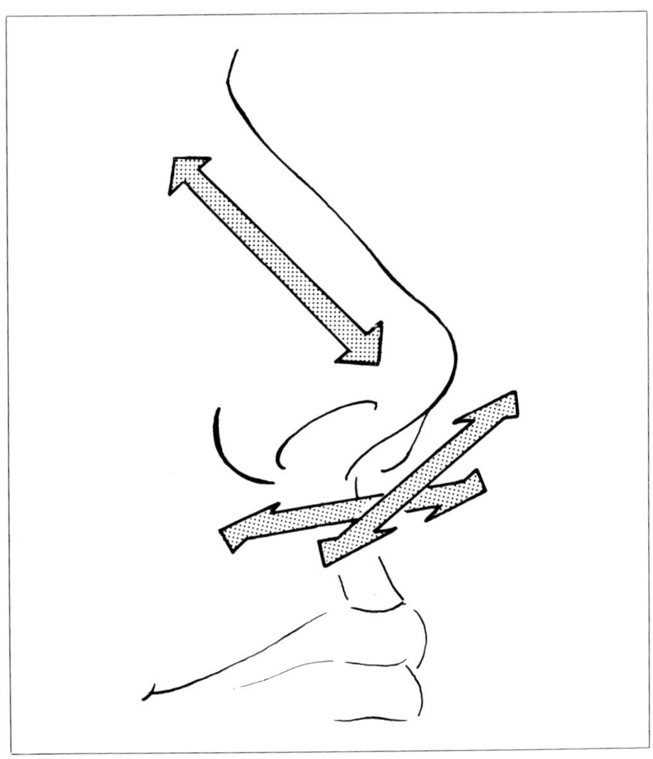

Figure 6-3. The three planes of the nose: sagittal, vertical, and transverse.

Topography

Since the nose is the central and most prominent facial feature, it must have both a harmonious relationship and an intrinsic beauty [17]. The most important facial planes are the Frankfort horizontal, a line passing between the infraorbital foramen and the highest part of the tragus, and the vertical facial plane, a line passing from nasion to menton going through the vermilion of the upper lip but anterior to the lower lip [47]. As shown in Figure 6-2, the facial angles include the following: (1) nasofrontal angle, between the forehead and bony dorsum, indicating forehead slope and nasal projection (obtuse, approximately 125 degrees), (2) angle of nasal projection, classically between the nasomenton line and the bony dorsum (approximately 23–37 degrees), and (3) nasolabial angle, between the base of the nose and upper lip with its apex at the subnasal point, indicating the relationship of the nose to the lip (in males, 90 degrees; in females, 110 degrees).

The nose is a three-dimensional entity with three planes: (1) sagittal (length), (2) vertical (height), and (3) transverse (width) (Fig. 6-3). Directional changes will be described as cephalic to caudal in the sagittal plane, poste-

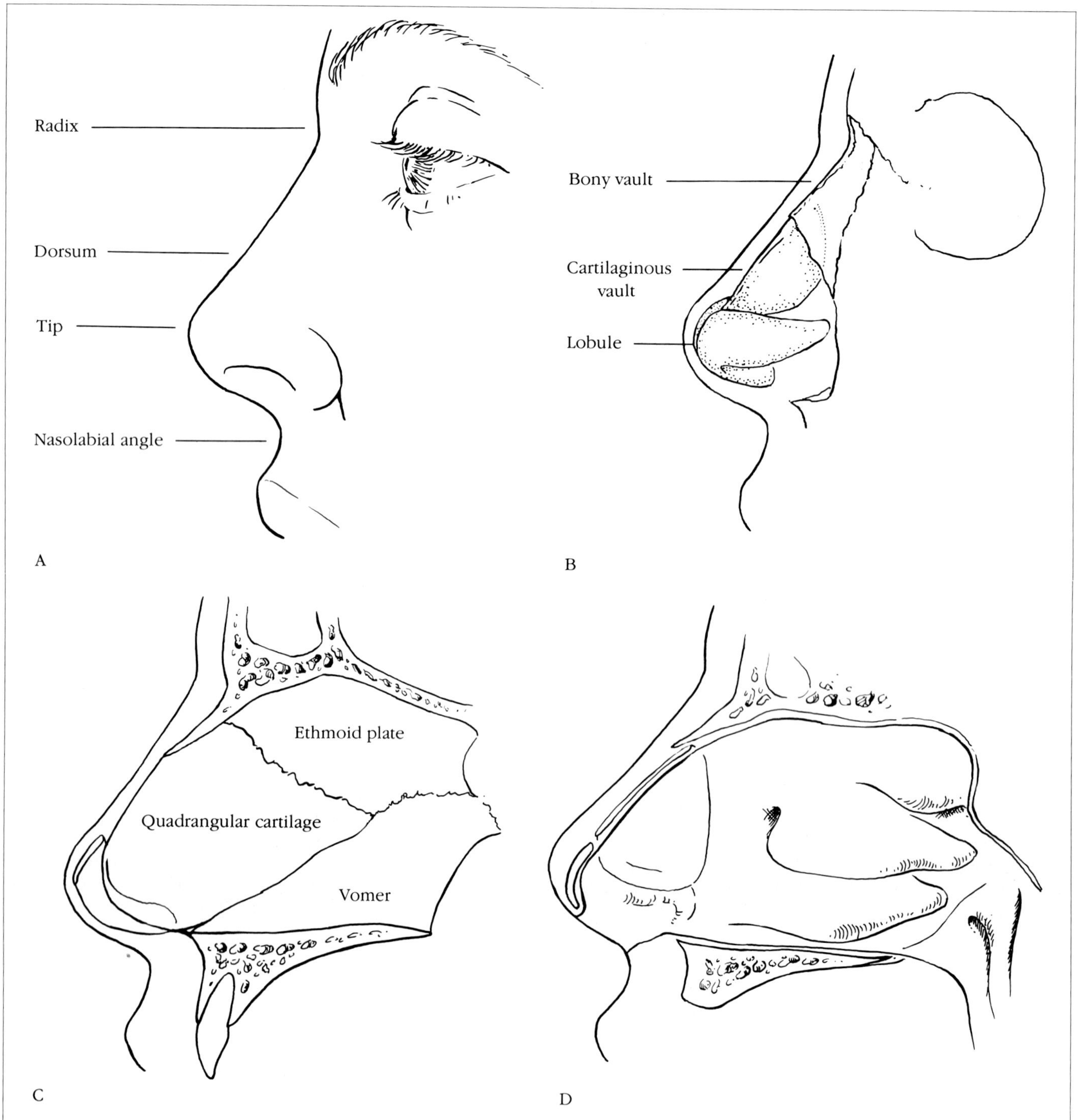

Figure 6-4. The nasal anatomy.
A. The nasal topography consists of radix, dorsum, tip, and nasolabial angle.
B. The basic components are the bony vault, cartilaginous vault, and lobule.
C. The midline septum is composed of cartilage (quadrangular cartilage) and bone (vomer, ethmoid plate).
D. The lateral walls are composed of three turbinates plus the lower lateral and alar cartilages.

rior to anterior in the vertical plane, and medial to lateral in the transverse plane. Significant deviation in any direction produces visible abnormalities. Terminology of the nasal components varies between anatomic and surgical perspective. The aesthetic units of the nose will be classified according to Sheen [138]: radix, dorsum, nasal tip, columellar-alar complex, and nasal base. Surgically, the nose will be divided into three components: bony vault, cartilaginous vault, and lobule [100]. The latter subdivision reflects both the proportional thirds of the nose and its anatomic components (Fig. 6-4).

Soft Tissue Coverage

The nasal skeleton is covered by skin, subcutaneous tissue, and muscles with their fascia. The skin is thinner and more mobile in the upper half, thicker and more adherent distally. Numerous sebaceous glands in the nasal tip can produce an oiliness and porosity that limit tip definition. The skin becomes thin again along the alar margins and columella. Variable amounts of subcutaneous tissue may be found between the alar cartilages and overlying the upper lateral cartilages. However, the skin-to-skin apposition of the nostril margin renders it vulnerable to notching and disfigurement from poorly executed rim incisions. Blood vessels and nerves pass within the subcutaneous tissue above the muscle fibers.

The nasal muscles consist of partially overlapping superficial and deep layers that function as either elevators or depressors (Fig. 6-5). The central procerus and the parallel levator labii superioris serve to shorten the nose by elevation of the tip and alae respectively. In contrast, the nasalis (alar part) and depressor septi nasi serve to lengthen the nose and dilate the nostrils. The nasalis consists of two distinct portions, both of which arise from the maxilla. The transverse part passes upward and medially to the bridge of the nose, becoming an aponeurosis that fuses with its opposite counterpart and the aponeurosis of the procerus. In contrast, the alar portion arises from the maxilla medially and deeper to the transverse portion before passing directly downward to the alae. The transverse part of the nasalis tends to compress and contract the nose, acting as an antagonist of the procerus. Surgically, one elevates the dorsal musculature to gain access and exposure, while occasionally transecting the procerus to deepen the nasion and to facilitate removal of the hump. The lower musculature—the depressor septi and the alar part of the nasalis—is often transected to prevent downward traction of the nasal tip on smiling, a maneuver that can temporarily reduce teeth exposure on maximum smiling.

Bony Vault

The bony vault encompasses the nasal bones, the nasal process of the maxilla, and the nasal part of the frontal bone. Each component can vary enormously in size and shape, thus altering the nasal contour. For example, Hovorka [73] found a diverse number of shapes, suture lines, and dimensions of the nasal bones with significant variations in width (7–24 mm) and length (8–33 mm). The paired nasal bones have the following borders: (1) superiorly, nasofrontal suture line; (2) medially, opposite nasal bone and perpendicular plate of ethmoid; (3) laterally, nasomaxillary suture line; and (4) inferiorly, overlap with the upper lateral cartilage. The quadrangular nasal bones are thicker superiorly and thinner inferiorly. The inferior juncture of the nasal bone and maxilla defines the pear-shaped piriform aperture. Each of the anatomic borders has a surgical significance.

Superiorly, the nasofrontal suture line is in the glabellar region at the level of the medial eyebrows. In contrast, the radix is at the medial canthal level, and it is at this point that transverse fractures are done to narrow the nose. This contrast between nasofrontal suture line and radix is poorly shown in most surgical texts. Virtually all transverse fractures are done at the radix and pass through the nasal bones rather than along natural suture lines. The surgical significance of the nasofrontal suture line occurs in cases in which maximum deepening of the glabellar is achieved by complete disarticulation of the nasal bones (Fig. 6-6). Medially, the nasal bones meet in the midline as a syndesmosis with the caudal half associated with the cartilaginous septum and the cephalic half articulated with the ethmoid plate. Laterally, the sidewalls of the bony vault are composed of the nasal frontal process of the maxilla and the nasal bones, which join at the nasomaxillary suture line. Lateral osteotomies pass totally within the maxillary bone. An exception is in order in the excessively wide nose, which may require "double-level" osteotomies—one at the higher nasomaxillary suture line and an inferior low-to-low lateral osteotomy [108]. The area of overlap between the nasal bone and upper lateral cartilage is referred to as the keystone area [101]. The close adherence of nasal bone to upper lateral cartilage is obvious in post-traumatic cases, in which the entire lateral wall is usually deflected. Occasionally, one sees avulsion of the upper lateral cartilage, producing a depression in the middle third; although usually traumatic, it may follow heavy-handed rasping of a dorsal hump.

Cartilaginous Vault

The wing-shaped triangular upper lateral cartilages serve as important regulators of airflow in the nasal passage. The borders of the upper lateral cartilages are the following: (1) superiorly, the nasal bones; (2) medially, the cartilaginous septum; (3) laterally, a *free border* abutting on dense fibrous connective tissue; and (4) inferiorly, the alar cartilages. From embryologic evidence and anatomic dissections, Straatsma and Straatsma [148] have clearly defined the structural relationships of the upper lateral cartilages to the nasal bone and septum (Fig. 6-7). The nasal bones overlap the upper lateral cartilage as a side-to-side apposition rather than an end-to-end approximation. The amount of upper lateral cartilage covered by the nasal bone ranges from 7 to 14 mm, with the intimate apposition separated only by a thin membrane consisting of fused periosteum

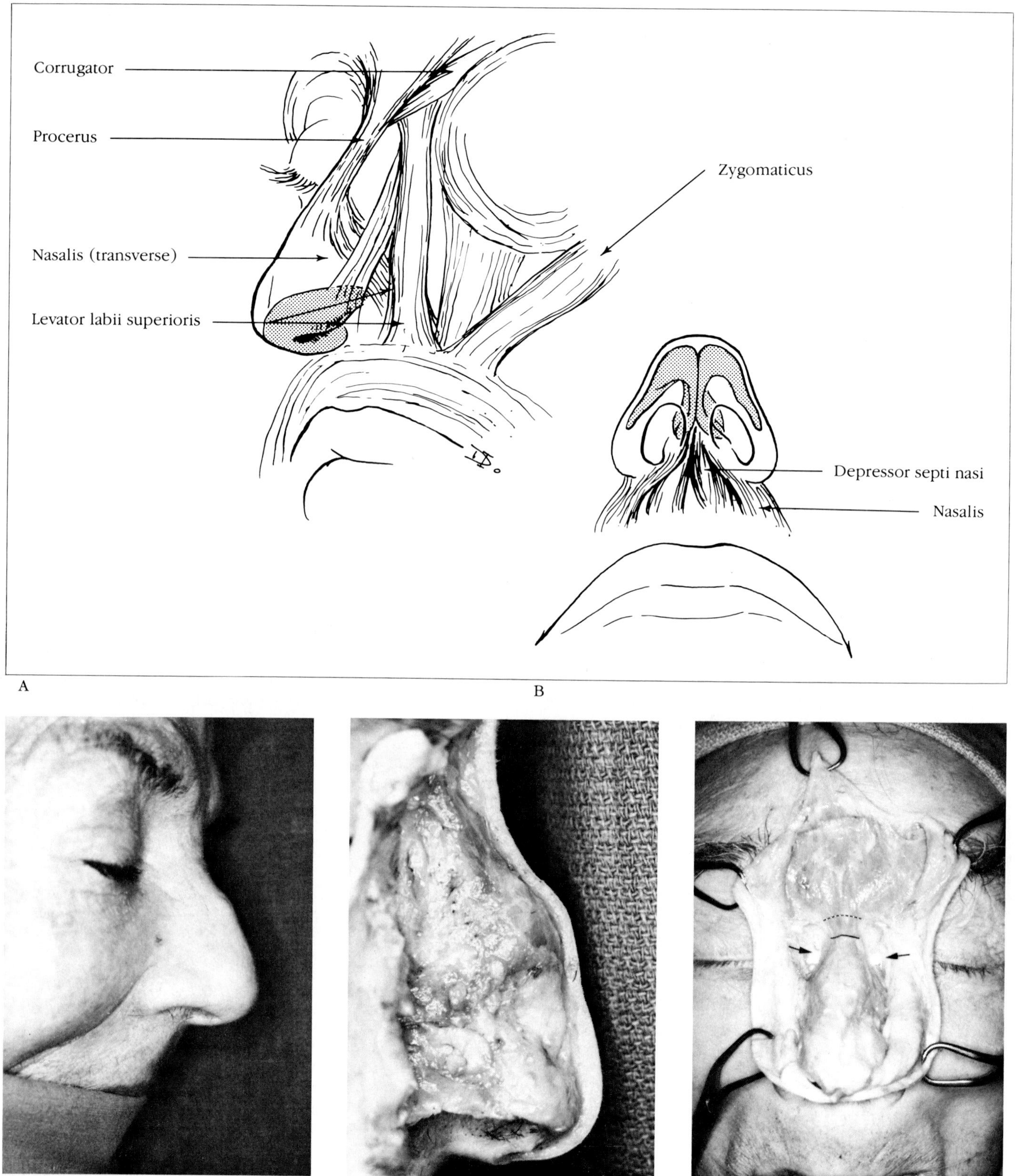

Figure 6-5. Muscles of the nose.

A. The superficial and deep nasal muscles function as constrictors and dilators of the nasal aperture.

B. The muscles of the nasal tip are the lateral nasalis and the more central depressor septi nasi, which may have to be divided to prevent tip descent on forced smiling.

C–E. Cadaver dissection demonstrating variation in soft tissue coverage and muscle distribution. Skin is thickest at the tip with obvious subcutaneous fat in the supratip area. The configuration of the nasion is determined primarily by the procerus and corrugator muscles. The arrows indicate the medial canthal ligaments, the solid bar denotes maximum cephalic continuation of the hump, and the dotted line indicates the nasofrontal suture line.

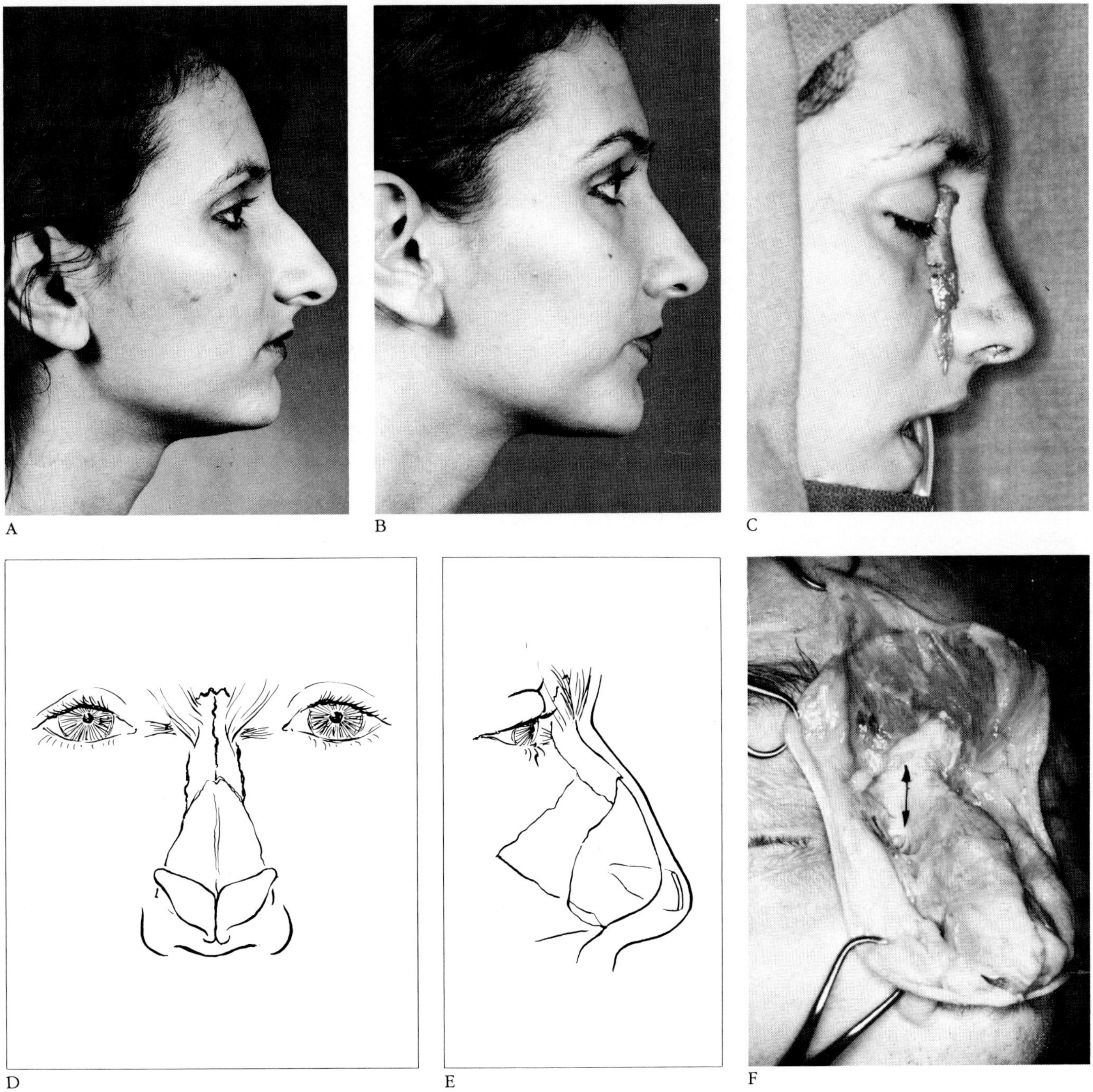

Figure 6-6. A patient with a high radix that required a disarticulation and reinsertion of a modified graft.

A. Since several of her friends had been given "little pixie noses with loss of ethnic identity," she requested a proportional reduction.

B. Result following a modified Skoog rhinoplasty, which satisfied the patient. The pupil-to-radix distance was shortened and a definite glabellar notch produced despite the sloping forehead.

C. Intraoperative photograph showing the disarticulated hump. Note the radix curvature *within* the resected dorsum, approximately 1 cm below the nasofrontal suture line.

D, E. The radix is at the level of the medial canthus while the nasofrontal suture lines approach the medial eyebrow.

F. As in this cadaver dissection, the distance from ligament to suture line is 12 mm.

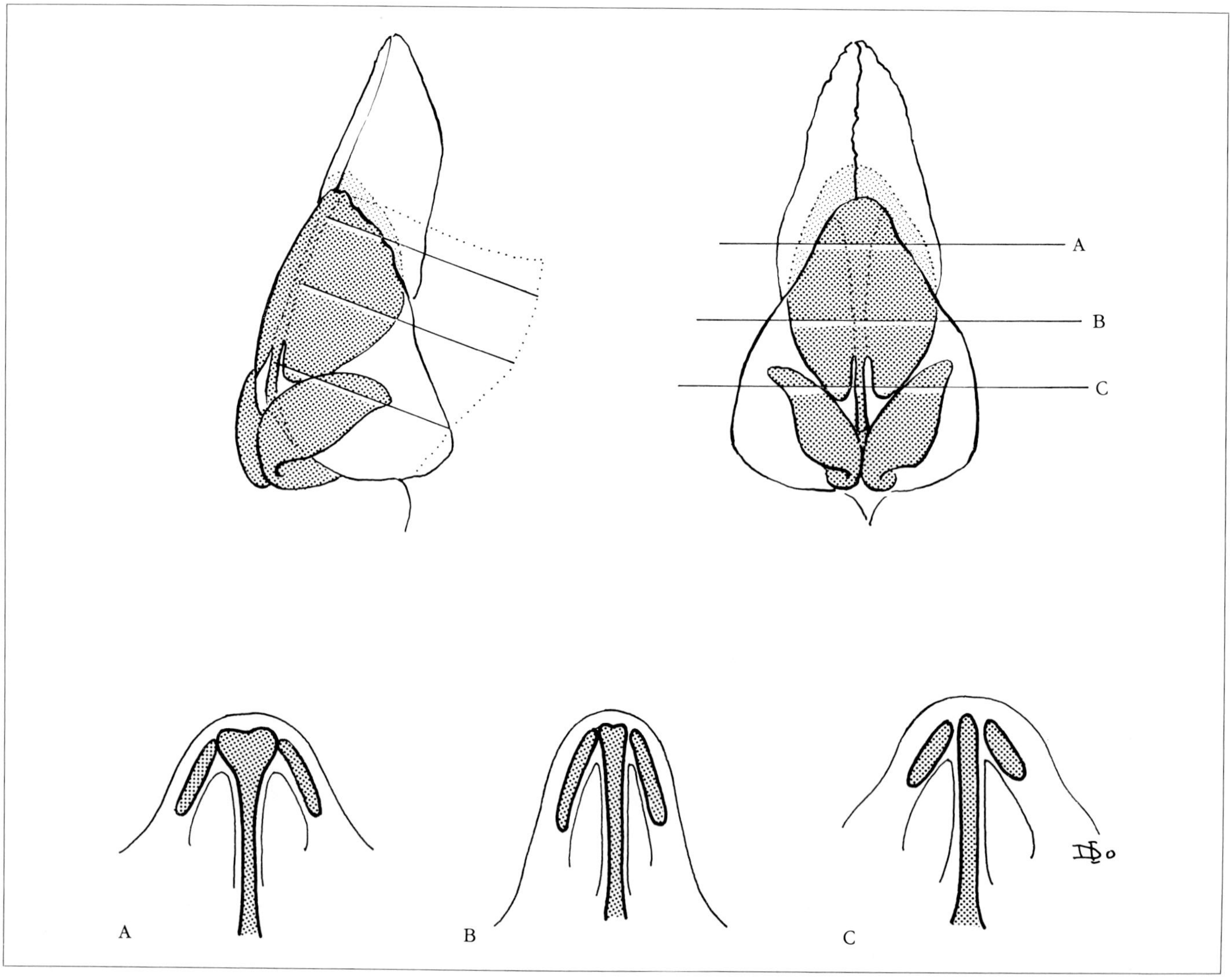

Figure 6-7. The relationship of the upper lateral cartilages to the septum (after Straatsma and Straatsma).
A. The Y-shaped septum dominates the dorsal profile and offers stability in the septal area.
B. The I-shaped septum and large width of the upper lateral cartilages constitute the middle third of the nose.
C. The straight septum and the separated upper lateral cartilages are quite mobile in the valve region.

and perichondrium. This overlap occurs embryologically as the membranous analog of the nasal bones lies superficial to the cartilaginous nasal capsule.

The upper lateral-septal relationship varies, depending on the anatomic level. As one moves toward the tip, the upper lateral cartilages gradually detach from the septum, creating the mobile inner valve, whereas the septum converts from a bifurcated Y shape with a supraseptal groove to a straight I beam. Throughout its passage, the cartilages meet in an end-to-end fashion separated by a narrow cleft of perichondrium, which widens caudally. Inferiorly, the juncture of upper lateral and alar cartilages constitutes an important anatomic landmark—externally the alar groove and internally the limen nasi (Fig. 6-8). The latter point marks the transition between vestibular skin and nasal mucosa as well as the site of intercartilaginous incisions. Usually, the alar cartilages overlap the upper lateral cartilage [36]. The extremes consist of a significant cartilage abutment producing a buckling "scroll" formation or separation by fibrous tissue interspersed with sesamoid cartilages [13]. Laterally, the upper lateral cartilages are separated from the piriform aperture of the maxilla by fibroareolar tissue that connects perichondrium to periosteum.

At surgery, the cartilaginous vault is seen to be composed of the upper lateral cartilages and the intervening cartilaginous septum. It comprises most of the "nasal hump" removed in a rhinoplasty, ranging from 50 percent in large humps to over 80 percent in smaller ones. As previously stated, the dorsal border is a broader Y at the nasal bones but a straight I shape by the septal angle. The central concavity is masked externally by the soft tissues. Unsuspected high septal deviations are occasionally revealed following hump removal and require immediate

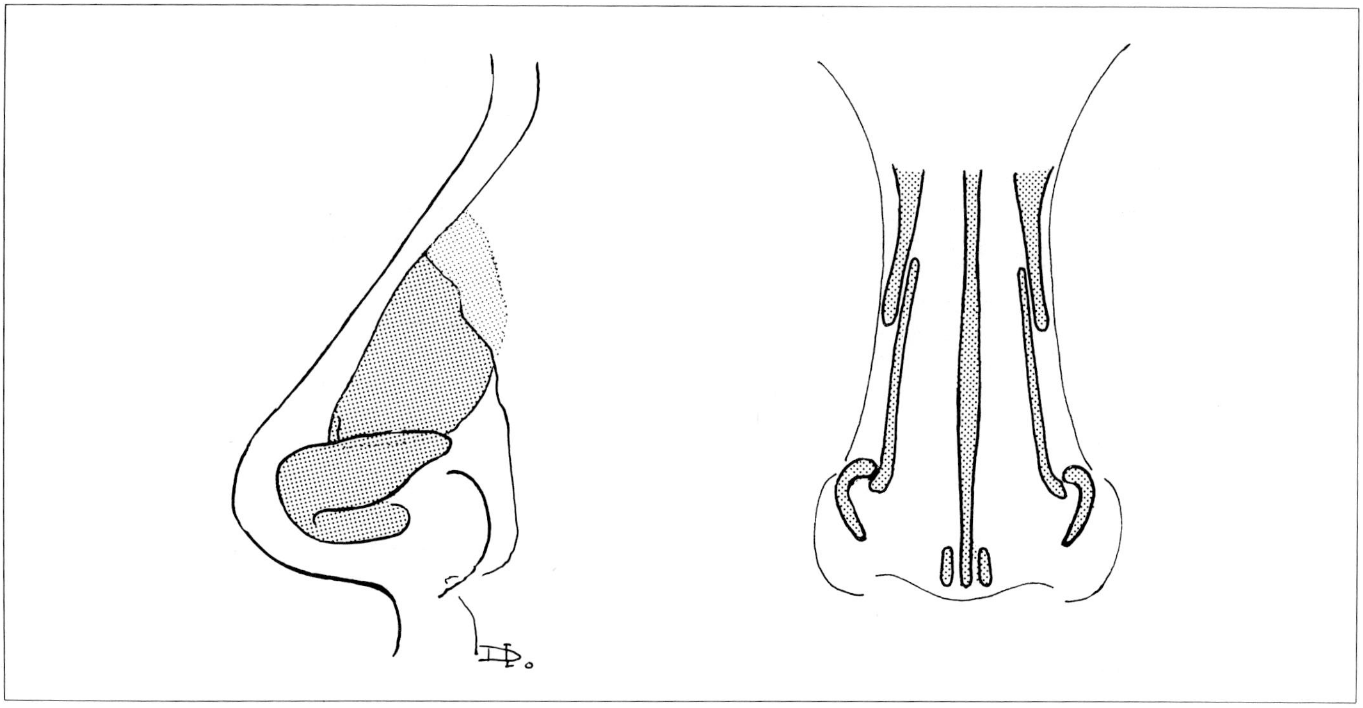

Figure 6-8. Superiorally, the upper lateral cartilages are overlapped by the nasal bones in a side-to-side fashion while inferiorally they form a scroll configuration with the alar cartilages in most cases. See also Figure 6-10.

correction. The upper laterals are "detached" from the septum in most rhinoplasties but remain structurally self-supporting because of their rigid bony adherence and unaltered lateral edge. In classic techniques, the caudal border of the upper laterals was routinely removed to allow shortening of the nose. However, numerous strictures in the valve area and external pinching have led to a more conservative preservation except in extremely long noses or where bulging is a problem.

Lobule

Anatomically, the lobule or lower nose is composed of the nasal tip, columella, and membranous septum, as well as their internal structures. It is highly mobile and without bony or cartilaginous continuity to the rest of the nose. In view of their impact on lobule shape, one may also include the nasal spine and the leading or caudal edge of the septum. The alar cartilages are paired arched structures that enclose the vestibule and are composed of medial and lateral crura. The borders of the alar cartilages are the following: (1) superiorly, overlap of or abutment to the caudal end of the upper lateral cartilages; (2) medially, apposition with its counterpart, ending in imbrication of the septum by the foot plates; (3) laterally, a free edge supported by the fibroareolar tissue of the alae; and (4) inferiorly, a free border covered by skin.

The nasal tip is composed of the skin, which is thicker and more glandular, subcutaneous tissue, and the alar cartilages. Bernstein [13–15] emphasizes that the term *dome* is used in at least three different contexts: anatomic, clinical, and surgical. Anatomically, the dome is the juncture of the medial and lateral crura, which may vary from a specified point to a broad curve (Fig. 6-9). As defined by Denecke and Meyer [32], the nasal tip curvature has two angles, medial and lateral, which are 2 to 3 mm apart. Others refer to a distinct dome that is the "point of union" of the lateral and medial crura. It is the authors' opinion that a diverse transition area, complete with buckling and even overlap, occurs, especially in thin cartilages, whereas a distinct dome is often present, especially in thicker cartilages. Surgically, one attempts to define a distinct dome, either preserving the one already present or creating a new one by judicious modification.

The shape of the tip is determined largely by its component parts whereas its "position" is determined by its abutting structures, i.e., cartilaginous septum, upper lateral cartilages, and nasal spine. Also important is the directional axis of the alar cartilages. Their normal axis is at a 45-degree angle from the dome through the lateral tail toward the pupil (Fig. 6-10). Deviations of this direction can produce significant deformities, such as the 90-degree axis of the parenthesis tip. The lateral crus varies greatly in its location and dimensions [67]. The lateral crus occupies only the medial half of the alae; the lateral half is composed of fibroareolar tissue. From 30 cadaver dissections, Natvig [101] found only one type of lateral crura configuration whereas Zelnik and Gingrass [162] reported five alar types based on intrinsic concavity and convexity. Marked asymmetries can occur when the lateral alae are of different types [79]. In addition, the external aesthetic expression of the lateral crura range from greatly convex in a bulbous tip to concave in the very sharp tip with collapsed nostrils. Also, the lateral crura may be quite narrow, with

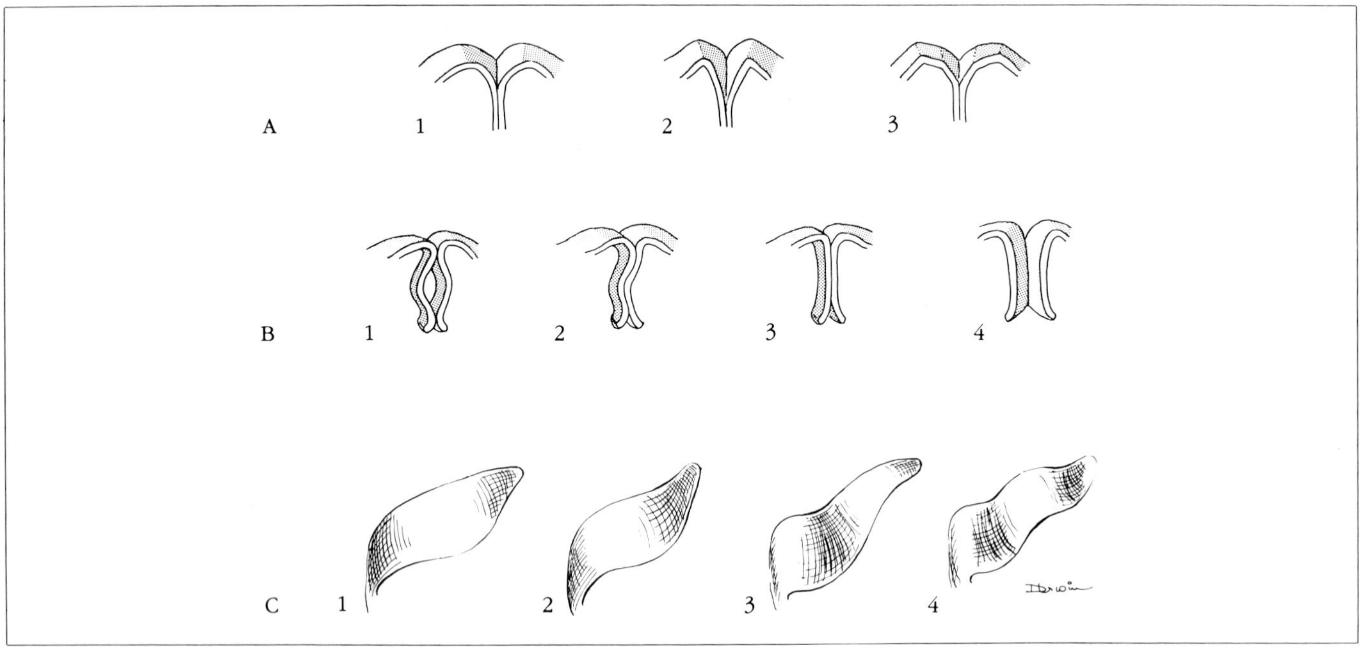

Figure 6-9. Anatomy of the alar cartilages.
A. The domes may present as (1) a broad curve, (2) a distinct point, or (3) a transition area with two definite angles.
B. The medial crura may have (1) opposite or (2) parallel curves or (3) a straight appearance, often with variable degrees of (4) bifidity.
C. The lateral crura can be described externally as having concavity and convexity. The more common types are (1) convex, (2) convex-concave, (3) concave-convex, and even (4) concave-convex-concave. One can see an example of these configurations in Figure 6-40.

multiply interspersed sesamoids in the delicate nose, or very wide, with scroll formation in the long nose. The lateral crura are easily separated from the overlying subcutaneous tissue but are more adherent to the underlying mucosa. Careful palpation will often reveal the dimensions and rigidity of the alar cartilages. Removal of subcutaneous tissue between and overlying the alar cartilages is often necessary in persons with thick skin. The inferior border of the alae is covered by a skin sandwich of external and vestibular lining that creates a "soft triangle" above the superomedial nostril aperture.

The columella consists of the medial crura and a variable amount of interposed subcutaneous tissue. The skin is quite thin, with direct attachment to the cartilage. Although Natvig [101] has discussed three types of medial crura configurations, we have found from clinical dissections that the medial crura are positioned like the covers of an upright open book, with often an asymmetric opening from the midline. Therefore, greater separation of the medial crura produces a bifid tip, which can be corrected by excision of the intervening soft tissue followed by suturing together of the medial crura or camouflaging with crushed cartilage grafts. The medial crura terminate in divergent foot plates that accommodate the caudal border of the septum and produce flaring of the columella base (Fig. 6-11). Excessive projection of the tip may be corrected by resection of a middle segment of the medial crura using a modified Lipsett technique [85, 120]. A wide columella infringing on the nostril is narrowed by removal of the foot plates. Deformities in the sagittal plane include the "hanging columella," which is often due to a protruding convex caudal septal border or wide medial crura. A greater challenge is complex spiral deformities with notching of the medial crura. The retracted columella may be congenital, traumatic, or surgical in origin but is due to deficient septal length rather than abnormalities of the medial crura. The position of the columella in the sagittal plane is dictated by the caudal septum. Therefore, the retracted columella can be corrected by either advancing it with a septal graft or camouflaging it with a columella graft.

The cartilaginous septum impinges on the tip anteriorly, is separated from the columella by the membranous septum, but is sandwiched by the medial crura posteriorly. The anterior septal angle represents the dorsal termination of the cartilaginous septum. It is a common misconception that the nasal septum provides support to the nasal lobule. Numerous anatomic and clinical dissections prove that in the majority of cases the leading edge of septum is many millimeters proximal to and below the domes, thus precluding any tip support [83] (Fig. 6-12). In addition, a triangular aponeurosis extends between the divergent lateral crura and covers the septal angle. Converse [23–25] referred to it as the "weak triangle" because of its fragile support for the dorsum (Fig. 6-13). On profile, it is the supratip area or point of tip differentiation. The caudal or leading edge of the septum is widely variable but generally has a convex bowing that forces the columella to hang 2 to 3 mm below the alar rim on profile view. In shortening the septum, one should maintain this convexity rather than producing a straight line. The membranous septum is

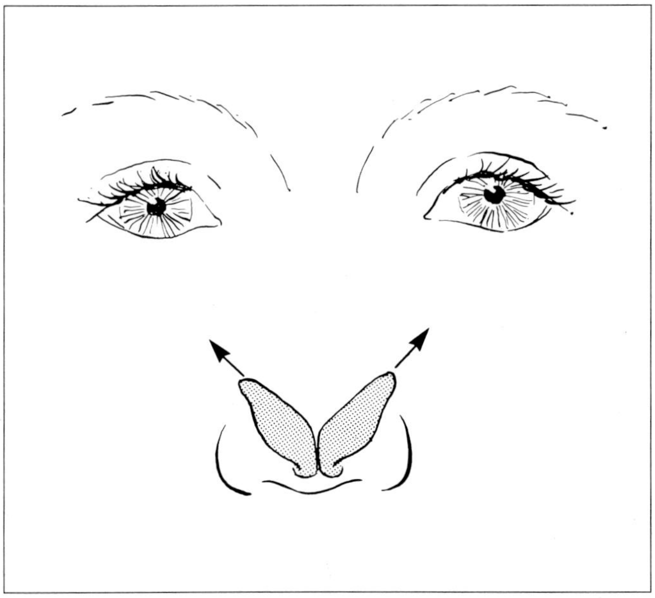

A

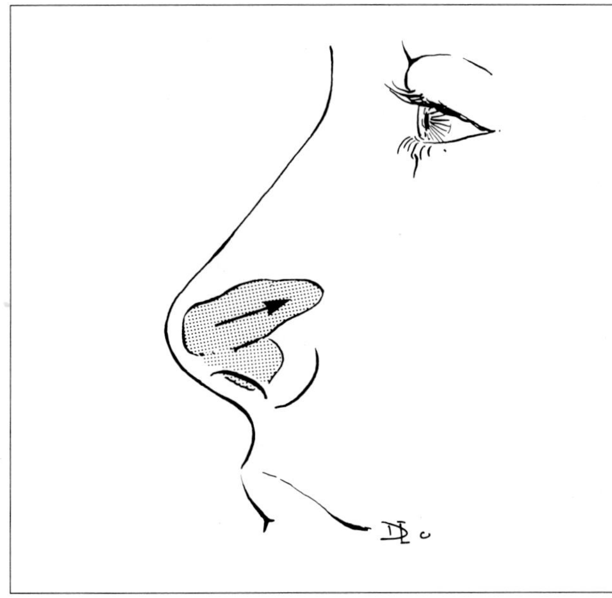

B

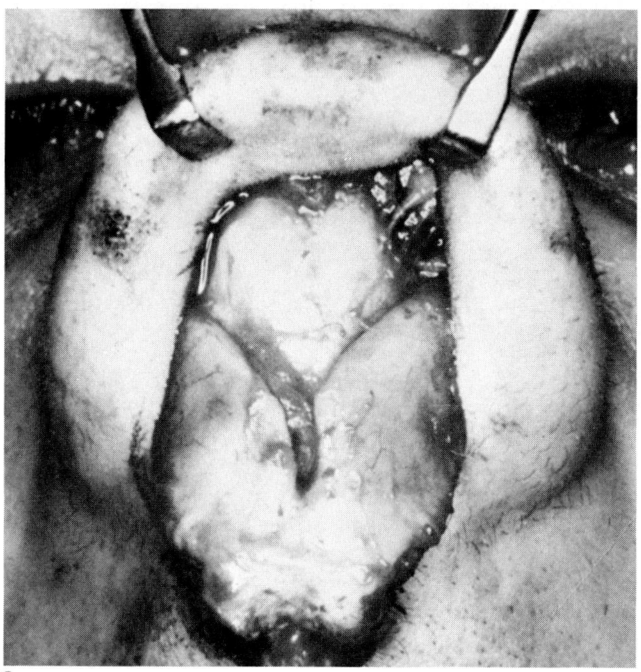

C

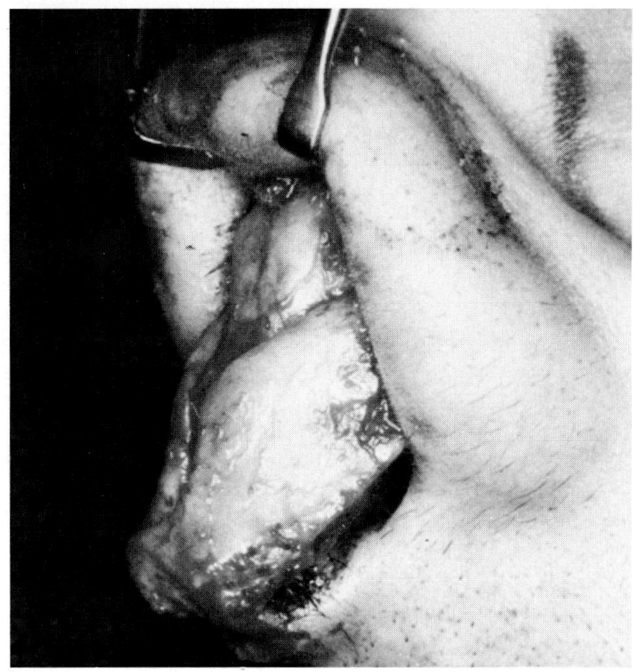

D

Figure 6-10
A, B. The axis of the alar cartilages is toward the pupil.
C. During an external rhinoplasty, the alar axis is readily apparent.
D. The convexity of the alar cartilages and their "scroll" formation with the upper lateral cartilages are evident as well as their projection above the septal angle.

composed of elastic tissue and allows movement of the columella. Posteriorly, the septum passes from the vomerine groove to the nasal spine. Since the foot plates of the medial crura overlap the septum above its base on the nasal spine, excessive width of the columella is not related to a bony prominence except in traumatic dislocation. Separation of the septum from the medial crura is present anteriorly but disappears posteriorly. Many surgeons limit their transfixion incision, thereby preserving tip support from this fixed basal point.

The relationship of the septum to the nasal spine and upper lip is both static and highly dynamic. Anatomically, the septum curves from the dorsum downward to rest on the nasal spine. The leading edge is usually slightly convex but may be greatly elongated, producing a plunging tip and an acute septolabial angle. Alternatively, the nasal spine may be elongated and projected, producing a similar clinical deformity. As pointed out by Aston and Guy [6], differentiation of the offending part can be determined by

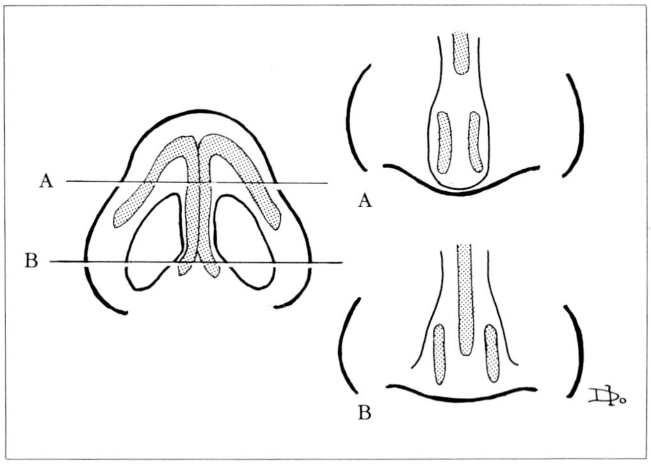

Figure 6-11. The relationship of the medial crura to the caudal edge of the septum.

A. On sagittal view in the upper portion of the columella, the medial crura are separated from the cartilaginous septum by the membranous septum.

B. In the lower third of the columella, the medial crura foot plates overlap the cartilaginous septum, thereby providing tip support.

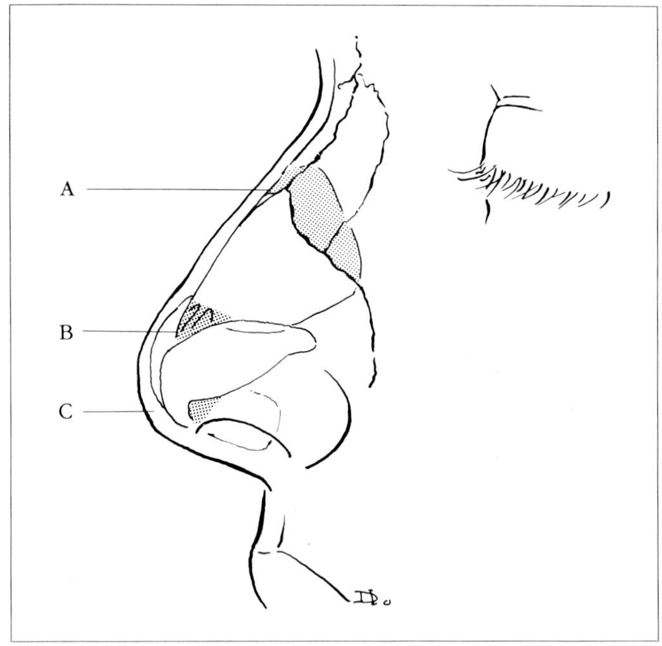

Figure 6-13. The three triangles of the nose.

A. The keystone area of nasal bones overlapping upper lateral cartilage.

B. The weak triangle of the supratip region, which may lack interposed cartilage framework.

C. The soft triangle below the alar cartilage where skin abuts skin.

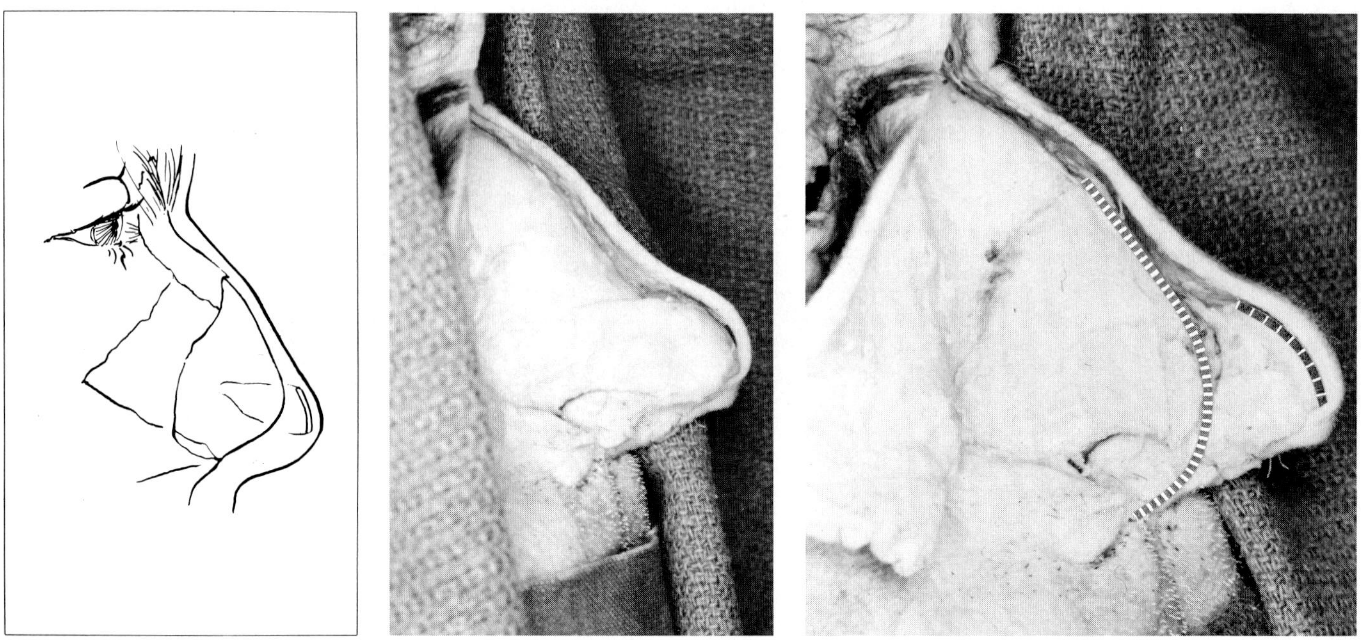

A B C

Figure 6-12. The relationship of the leading edge of the septum to the alar cartilages.

A. Schematically, on sagittal view, the leading edge of the septum is several millimeters proximal to and beneath the alar domes, thus precluding direct tip support.

B, C. In a cadaver dissection, removal of the alar cartilages *(dashed line)* reveals that the cartilaginous septum *(dotted line)* curves downward several millimeters proximal to the alar dome.

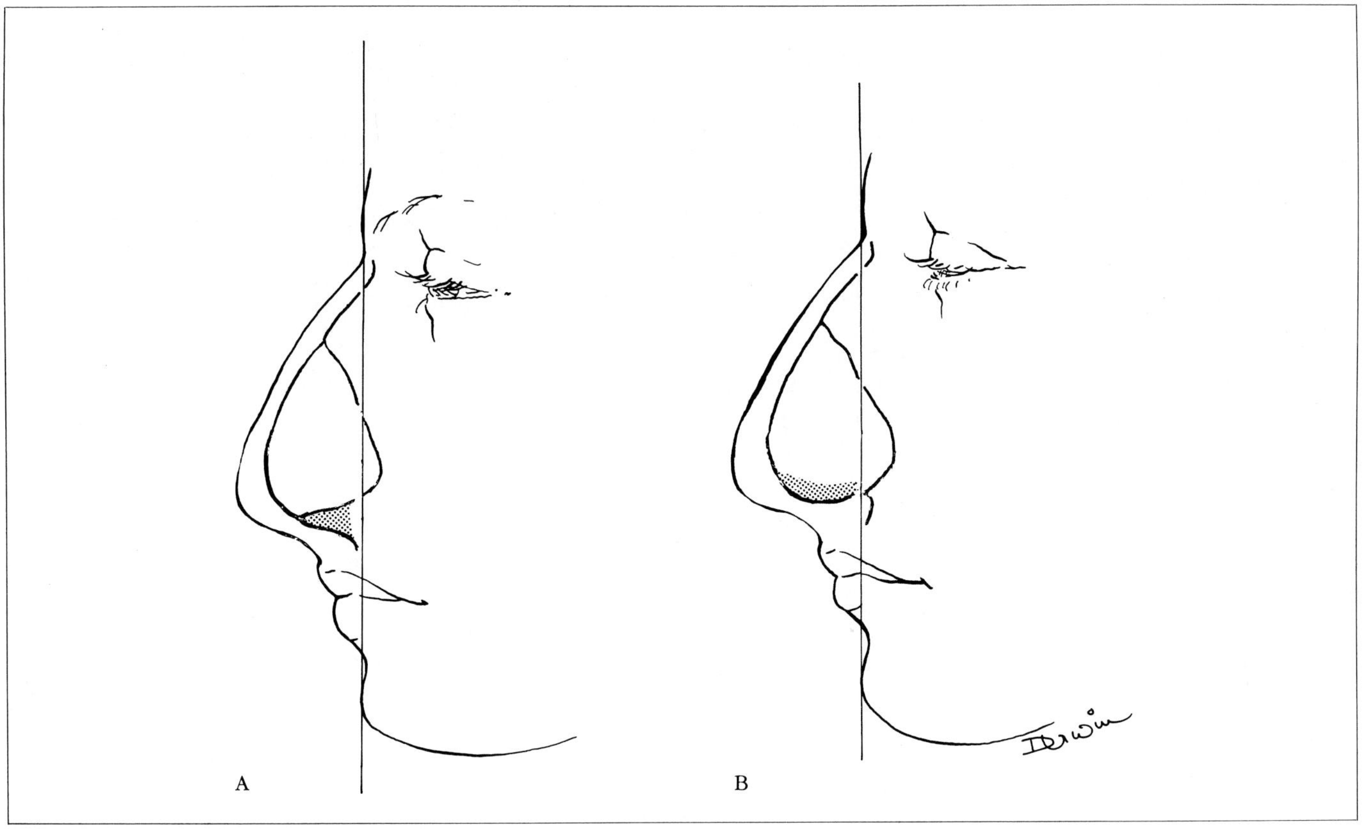

Figure 6-14. The crowded nasolabial angle can be caused by either the nasal spine or the cartilaginous septum.
A. The nasal spine projects beyond the facial plane.
B. The caudal edge of the septum is elongated while the nasal spine is proximal to the facial plane.

the relationship of the nasal spine to the facial plane. If the nasal spine is anteriorly projected, it is resected; when the problem is an elongated septum resting on a normal nasal spine, cartilage contouring is sufficient (Fig. 6-14). Relationship of the nose to the lips is critical in determining the nasolabial angles. Lips vary in their shape (square, tapering, ovoid) and dimensions (long, short). Of particular concern is the lip seal, whether easily achieved or forced. It is important to evaluate the nose-lip relationship both at rest and in animation. In many patients with a prominent dorsal hump and elongated septum, the lobule will move on talking and plunge on forced smiling. Action of the depressor septi nasi and nasalis muscle pulls the tip downward and is further compounded by the latter's interdigitation with the orbicularis oris, which retracts and shortens the upper lip. The depressor septi muscle passes from the maxilla through the columella and membranous septum to insert on the caudal septum. Transection of this muscle will eliminate significant rocking of the tip. The nasolabial angle is further influenced by projection of the alveolar process of the maxilla. In the aging patient, the nose is felt to elongate and become ptotic. However, Jost [78] analyzed 400 cases and found that the dorsal length is not altered but rather changes in the alveolar process, creating the illusion of a dropped tip in the older individual.

The paired nostrils are the external openings of the nose. The borders of the nostril are the following: (1) superiorly, the nostril rim with its "soft triangle"; (2) medially, the columella; (3) laterally, the alae; and (4) inferiorly, the nostril sill. They are composed of an aperture and its surrounding soft tissue. Sheen [138] states that the apertures should be elliptic to pear shaped and be 1 to 2 times the height of the lobule as viewed from below. This relationship has been defined as the nostril-lobule ratio and is between 1 : 1 and 2 : 1. The presence of small nostrils and a short columella signals a significant problem. The width of the apertures should be approximately half the nasal height at the midpoint on basal view. The nostril rim is composed of external nasal skin and vestibular skin separated by loose areolar tissue. As one passes from medial to lateral, the amount of intervening connective tissue increases, eventuating in the fibrocartilaginous alar tissue. The alae are composed of dense connective tissue without any cartilage. They are three-dimensional structures defined cephalically by the alar groove, laterally by the alar-facial groove, and medially by continuation into the nostril sill. The alar lobule varies in thickness and is often reduced in its transverse direction by alar wedge resections and occasionally narrowed vertically. The juncture of the alar lobule with the nostril sill is highly variable; the sill may be flat, the sill may be elevated, the columella base may be widely divergent, etc.

The nasal base has several important spatial relationships: (1) the columellar-alar angle, (2) the alar-basal angle, (3) the basal width, and (4) the nostril-lobule ratio. All these factors must be considered in determining preoperatively the indications for and type of alar modification.

Nasal Vestibule

The nasal vestibule is a skin cavity that denotes the beginning of the nasal passage. Its caudal border is the nostril, and its cephalic limitation is the limen vestibuli as defined by a cul-de-sac between the mucosal deflection of the upper lateral cartilage and the transition from skin to mucosal lining. The roof of the vestibule is apposed skin layers with vibrissae and then hairless skin applied to the concave undersurface of the lateral alae. The enclosed recess behind the nasal tip is called the atrium or ventricle. The juncture of the upper lateral cartilages with the septum and lateral alae constitutes the *nasal valve* and the upper border of the vestibule. The columella and membranous septum constitute the medial wall of the vestibule while the floor is composed of skin-covered alveolar process tissue back to the piriform aperture. Numerous physiologic processes begin within the vestibule, including particle filtration, resistance, and deflection of air currents. In addition, virtually all endonasal incisions are made within the vestibule, and distortion secondary to scarring can have serious repercussions.

Nasal Cavity

The nasal cavity is divided into two chambers by the septum, each of which has a roof, floor, lateral wall, and medial wall, the latter formed by the septum. The arching roof consists of nasal bone, nasal spine of the frontal bone, cribriform plate, and body of the sphenoid bone. The gently concave floor is formed anteriorly by the palatine process of the maxilla and posteriorly by the horizontal plates of the palatine bones. The irregular lateral wall is composed of the bony conchae or turbinates, whose physiologic importance will be discussed under Physiology. The medial wall is the osteocartilaginous nasal septum. The bony septum consists of two major components, the vomer and the perpendicular plate of the ethmoid, plus an inferior palatine base consisting of the crest of the palatine bone, the crest of the maxilla, and the nasal spine. The perpendicular plate of the ethmoid hangs downward, attaching to the vomer and the septal cartilage with numerous perforations for olfactory nerve fibers. The sloping rhomboid vomer extends from the body of the sphenoid anteriorly down to the bony palate. The crests of the bony palate serve as a supporting pedestal for the vomer. The nasal spine, projecting from the piriform crest above the concave floor of the vestibule, is most prominent in Caucasians.

The quadrilateral cartilaginous septum is derived from the body of the sphenoid and is the only unpaired structure in the nose (Fig. 6-15). Its borders are the following: (1) cephalically, the perpendicular plate of the ethmoid;

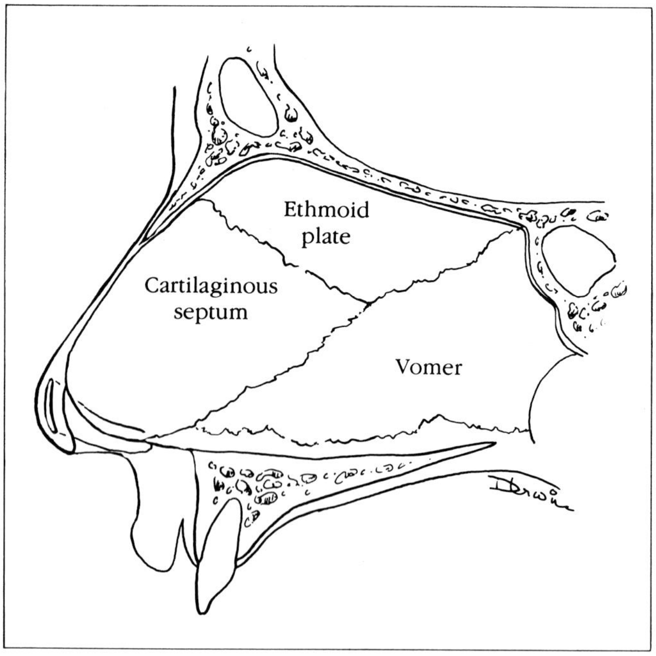

Figure 6-15. The nasal septum consisting predominantly of the quadrangular cartilage, the perpendicular plate of the ethmoid, and the vomer with the nasal spine projecting from the crest of the maxilla.

(2) anteriorly, the nasal bones proximally (it is free distally); (3) posteriorly, juncture with the vomerine groove and the nasal spine; and (4) caudally, a free border enclosed by the membranous septum. The relationship of cartilaginous septum to ethmoid is a somewhat fragile osseous cartilaginous suture line. Thus, fractures with deflection are quite common at this point, a fact confirmed in the attempt to harvest long septal grafts for dorsal reconstruction. Inferiorly, the juncture of the cartilage with the vomerine bone has been a subject of controversy, both as to its composition and as to its fibrous attachment. Many anatomists recognize a small vomeronasal cartilage, which is interposed between the two. Distinct separation of perichondrium and periosteum by a fibrous septum implies that elevation of the septum's mucosal coverage requires two dissection planes followed by severance of the intervening band. Deflection of septal cartilage out of the vomerine groove is a common problem in posttraumatic cases.

Blood Supply

The nose has a rich and variable vascular supply derived from the external and internal carotid arteries. The facial artery provides numerous branches; the superior labial artery has terminal septal and alar branches, and the lateral nasal artery ultimately communicates with the infraorbital branches. The nasal cavity is supplied predominantly by the anterior and posterior ethmoidal branches of the ophthalmic artery, by the sphenopalatine artery, and to a lesser degree by the greater palatine artery. Externally, the arteries are accompanied by paired venae comitantes; internally, cavernous plexus are present submucosally before forming distinct veins. The nasal lymphatics may form an anterior division, which passes superficially into the skin, terminating in the submandibular nodes, and a posterior division, which goes toward the retropharyngeal lymph nodes.

Nerve Supply

The external nose has both sensory and motor innervation, the latter arising from the facial (seventh) nerve. The nasal branches of the supraorbital nerve innervate the radix and upper lateral wall whereas the alar region is supplied by the nasal branches of the infraorbital nerve. The external branch of the anterior ethmoidal nerve innervates the dorsum of the nose, passing from beneath the nasal bones to lie on top of the upper lateral cartilages. The septum itself is innervated by the medial branches of the anterior ethmoidal nerve and the nasopalatine nerve. The lateral walls of the nasal cavity are supplied by multiple branches from the sphenopalatine ganglion and the anterior ethmoidal nerve.

Physiology

The five functions of the nose are respiration, filtration, humidification, heating, and protection. Filtration is basically accomplished by the vibrissae in the vestibule, and the mucus-cilia covering of the turbinates. Humidification and heating are related to the specialized vascular tissues regulated by parasympathetic and sympathetic fibers. The rich capillary system is augmented by venous sinuses whose sphincteric obstruction results in dramatic enlargement especially of the inferior turbinates. It is postulated that capillary perfusion controls temperature and humidity while sinus filling regulates mucosal thickness, thereby affecting airway resistance. Protection of the individual from bacteria and viruses is by both mechanical and chemical means; mechanical protection is due to the 20-minute transit time of the cilia for passage of the mucosal blanket into the nasopharynx. The nasal mucosa contains immunoglobulin A and muramidase.

The nose functions in respiration as a variable resistor to airflow. As noted by Proetz [116] and by Abramson and Harker [1], the small, horizontal nares direct inspired air upward and medially toward the turbinates rather than straight posteriorly along the nasal floor. The resulting parabolic curve ensures essential contact with the turbinates. Thus, the nares are the directors of airflow currents and if altered can cause dramatic changes; i.e., the plunging tip forces the air higher, producing eddies, while the retroussé tip directs the air along the nasal floor. The nostrils can be altered voluntarily: dilatation on expiration, contraction on inspiration.

As inspiration continues, a negative pressure develops and the nasal valve closes; inspiratory collapse occurs. The nose contributes approximately 30 percent of total airway resistance. Nasal resistance, as determined by the internal valve and turbinates, is essential for normal respiration and comfort. The internal valve is defined by the relationship of the upper lateral cartilages to the septum (Fig. 6-16). It measures approximately 10 to 15 degrees and is

Figure 6-16. The internal valve area.
A, B. Anatomically, the relationship of septum, upper lateral cartilage, and alar cartilages is critical in determining the normal configuration for ideal respiration.
C. On inspiration the valve is closed while on expiration it is opened. Any deviation of the septum can markedly affect respiration.

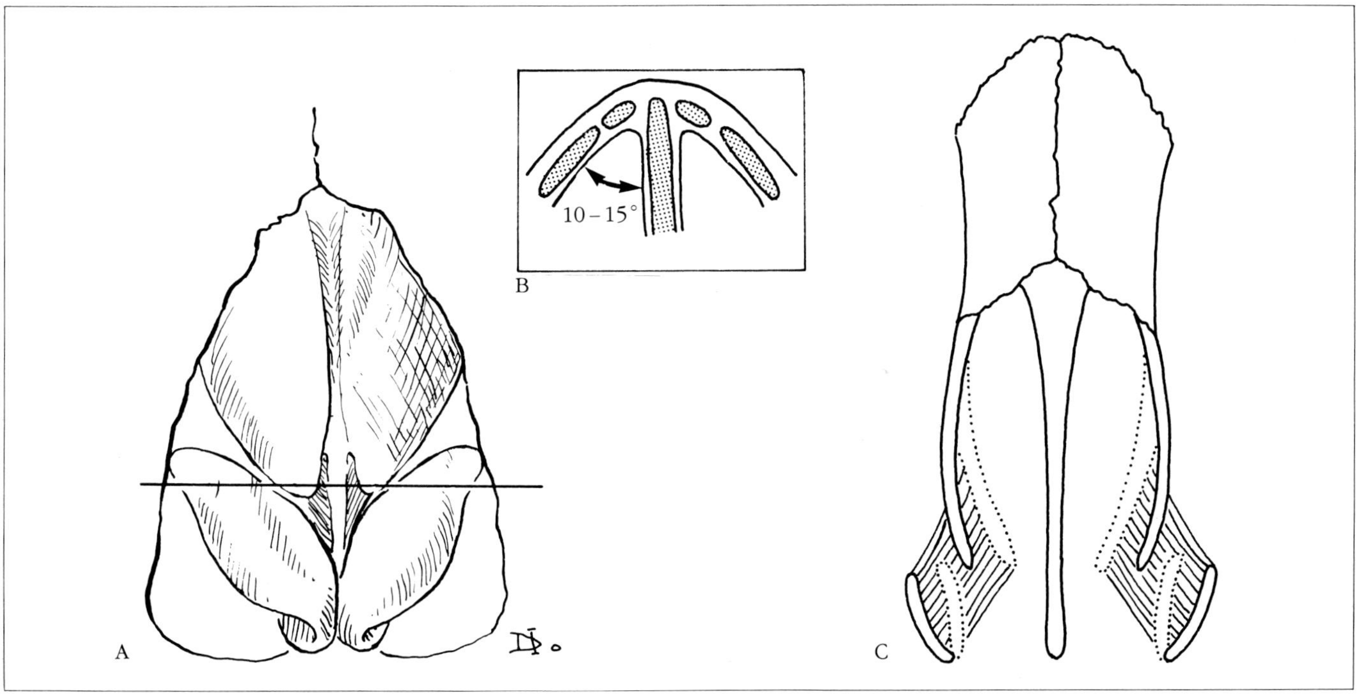

the narrowest part of the upper airway. This angle is influenced by both the condition of the septum and the aponeurotic connections of the upper lateral cartilage to the septum and the lateral crura. Deviation of the septum, excessive mucosal resection, synechia formation, and amputation of either the caudal end of the upper lateral or most of the lateral crura will result in narrowing of the angle, with respiratory obstruction. The importance of an open aperture and wide angle is demonstrated by the postrhinoplasty patient who shows improved respiration by lateral traction on the cheek, which opens the angle.

Additional resistance is provided by the turbinates, especially the inferior one with its venous plexus [22]. Although sensitive to noxious and emotional stimuli, a normal "nasal cycle" of congestion-decongestion exists with reciprocal changes on the two sides. Thus, total resistance is constant, but significant changes in the turbinates may occur every 3 hours [68]. In septal deflections, the turbinate on the concave side undergoes compensatory hypertrophy, thereby maintaining adequate resistance. With correction of the septal deviation, hypertrophic turbinates return to normal. Treatment of turbinate hypertrophy remains controversial; there are advocates for steroid injections [8], surgical resection [29, 30], cauterization, and sclerosing agents. Additional discussion of nasal physiology for rhinoplasty surgery is available elsewhere [9].

AESTHETIC CONCEPTS

Undoubtedly, the best discussion of nasal aesthetics is by Sheen in his text *Aesthetic Rhinoplasty* [138]. He divides the nose into five aesthetic units and discusses them from each view (frontal, oblique, and profile) (Fig. 6-17). This approach invites the reader to think, visualize, and grasp fundamental concepts that have been ignored too long in rhinoplasty surgery (Fig. 6-18). The following description is largely a distillate of Sheen's principles with additions from Joseph [77], Brown and McDowell [17], Fomon and Bell [47], and Rees [120].

Radix

The radix is the root of the nose and is part of the continuous uninterrupted line that passes from the medial orbital wall along the nasal bones and upper lateral cartilages to terminate at the domes. Common errors that are visible in the postoperative period include (1) nonparallel curves due to unequal mobilization of nasal bones, (2) breaks in the curve due to splintering of the nasal bone, (3) excessive narrowness due to overmobilization, and (4) excessive width following inadequate mobilization. In most cases, significant narrowing of the radix is *not* necessary, and one should avoid routine medial osteotomies and resection of bone in the radix.

Dorsum

Previously, improvement in the dorsum was demonstrated by lateral preoperative and postoperative photographs, but not on front view. Sheen has defined the dorsum as the structure that connects the radix with the lateral projection of the alar cartilages, producing "two divergent concave lines that are unbroken extensions of the superciliary ridges." The most common causes of breaks in the dorsal curves are septal deviations, low fractures of the nasal bones, and avulsion of an upper lateral cartilage. Fomon [46] has stressed that excessive reduction of the nasal hump can produce flatness in the middle third of the face, which gives the illusion of increased separation between the eyes. Brown and McDowell [17] stated that if one is to avoid a retruded face, "it is better to remove too little bony hump than too much." Following radical hump removal, one can often see the triangular outline of the bony vault into which the smaller cartilaginous vault descended. On lateral view, the dorsal line is relatively straight and ends at the tip, which on oblique view is the opposite dome of the alar cartilage and the highest point. Currently, the straight dorsum is in vogue and contrasts with the previous desire for a slightly "scooped" dorsum. In actuality, the scoop of the septal cartilage was designed to accentuate the differentiation of the tip from the dorsum. This desire reached its zenith in the Goldman tip, in which the domes were transected, the crura were sutured together, and the septum was cut in a cephalic direction and allowed to project 2 to 3 mm above the septum [55].

Tip

Four landmarks are defined on the nasal tip: (1) the point of tip differentiation from the dorsum, (2) the right dome, (3) the left dome, and (4) the columellar-lobular junction [138]. The critical line is the intracrural distance (ICD), and its apex should be the highest projection of the nose. These points are both palpable and visible especially the three-point light reflex of the nasal tip on front view. Any deviation from this equilateral triangle is readily visible. For example, (1) asymmetry of the domes from the midline can be seen, (2) a wide ICD produces a bulbous tip, and (3) a narrow ICD creates a single light reflex expressed as a small pinched tip. On lateral view the apogee of the ICD should be the highest point and be the definite end point of the profile. On oblique view the dome of the opposite ala should be the highest part of the nasal silhouette. Although evaluation of the dorsum is usually done on lateral view, the subtleties of tip analysis can best be observed on oblique view. The criteria of expertise in rhinoplasty surgery are no longer the dramatic cases of hump reduction but rather the subtle nuances of tip refinement that can be assessed only in oblique views.

Columellar-Alar Complex

On lateral view, the columella should be a visible structure, hanging 2 to 3 mm below the alar rims and parallel to them. The columella consists of two reverse curves joined at the columellar-lobular junction, with the upper part contributed by the tip and the lower part by the columella-lip angle. The caudal septum and nasal spine directly influence the shape of the columella curve. On front view,

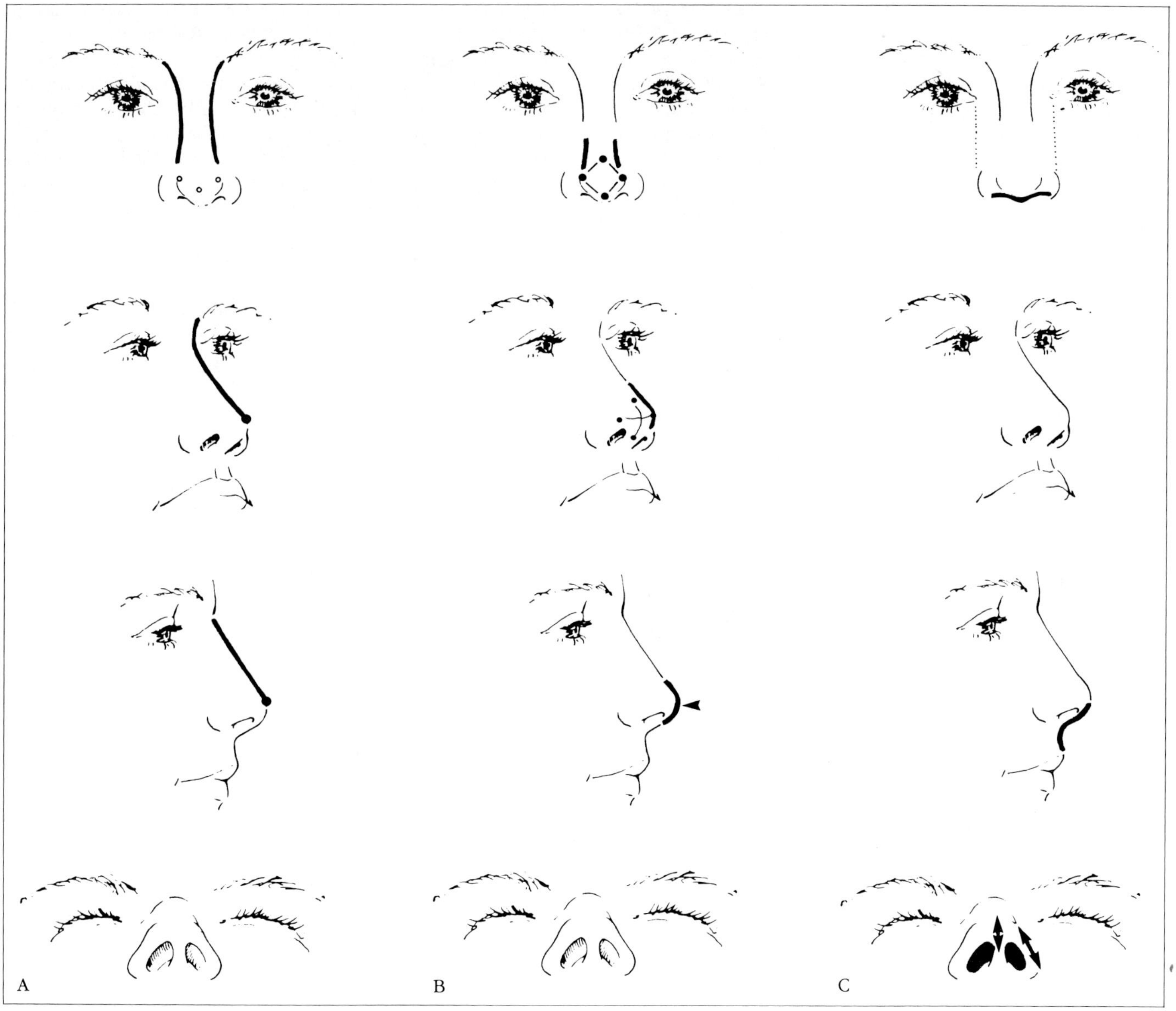

Figure 6-17. The nasal aesthetic "canons" of Sheen.

A. The radix, on frontal view, consists of parallel lines that converge from the supraorbital region at the root of the nose and then diverge slightly toward the three-point light reflex of the tip. On oblique and lateral view, the radix is the deepest point of the nasofrontal angle while the dorsum continues down to the nasal tip.

B. The nasal tip, on frontal view, consists of four points (point of tip differentiation, right dome, left dome, and columellar-lobular junction) and two interconnecting lines. On oblique view, the opposite dome should be the highest projecting part of the nose. On lateral view, the apogee of the intracrural distance should be the highest point and represent a definitive end point for the nose.

C. The nasal base, on frontal view, should have a slight seagull-in-flight appearance and fall within the intracanthal distance. On lateral view, the columella must have a definite break at the columellar-lobular juncture, an obtuse angle with the lip, and a "show" of 2 to 3 mm below the alae. On basal view, the nasal tip should be triangular, with almond-shaped nostrils approaching 60 percent of the height.

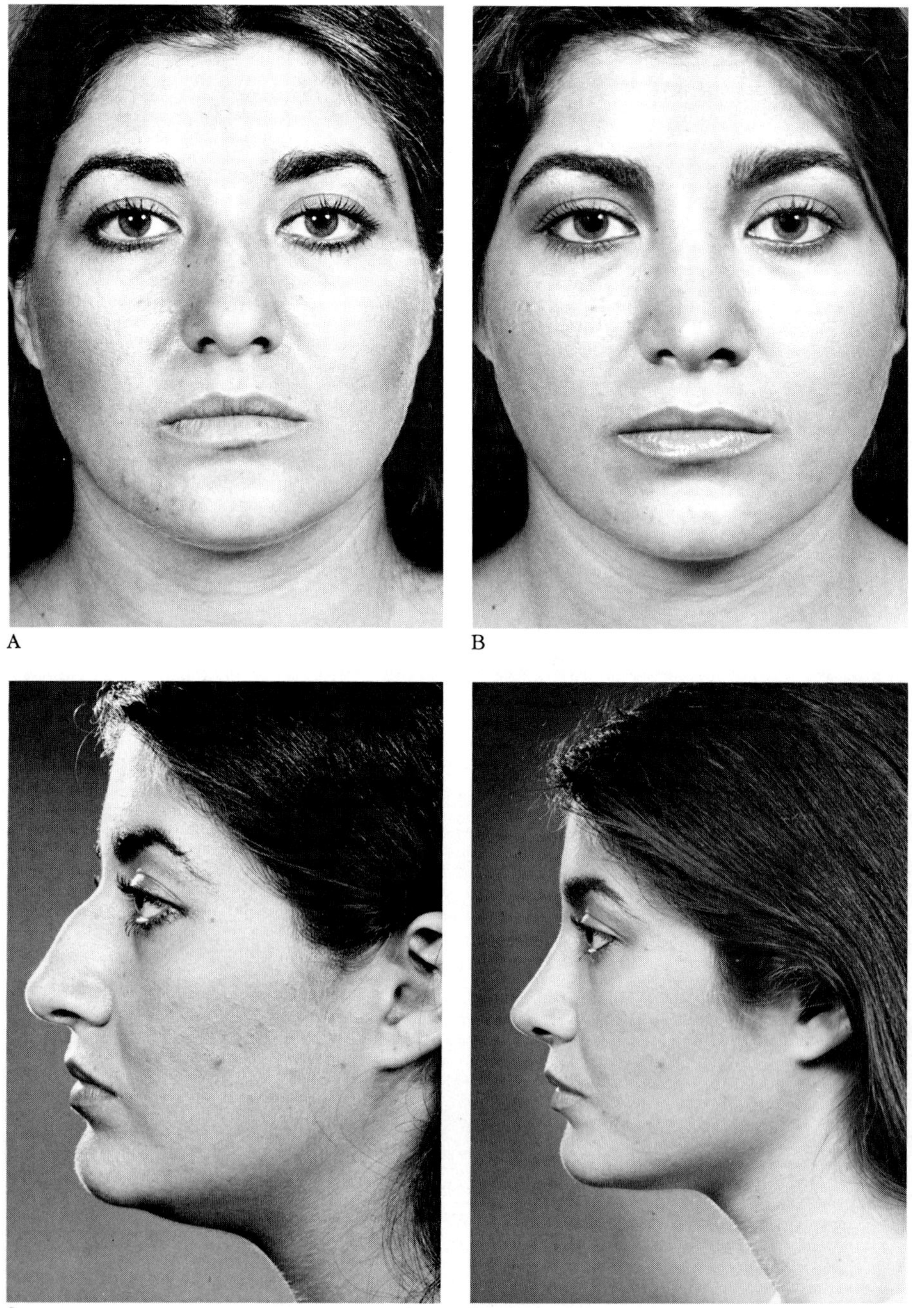

A B C D

Figure 6-18. The aesthetics of a rhinoplasty.

A. On frontal preoperative view, the radix is nicely curved, the domes are insufficiently defined, and the intracrural distance (ICD) is a bit wide.

B. Postoperatively, the concave parallel curves of the radix have been preserved while the light reflexes indicate a narrowing of the ICD, accomplished by suturing the medial crura.

C. On lateral preoperative view, the forehead slopes without adequate definition of the radix, the dorsal hump is approximately half bone and half cartilage, and the nasolabial angle is less than 100 degrees.

D. Postoperatively, the radix has been deepened, the dorsum is straight, and the nasolabial angle exceeds 100 degrees.

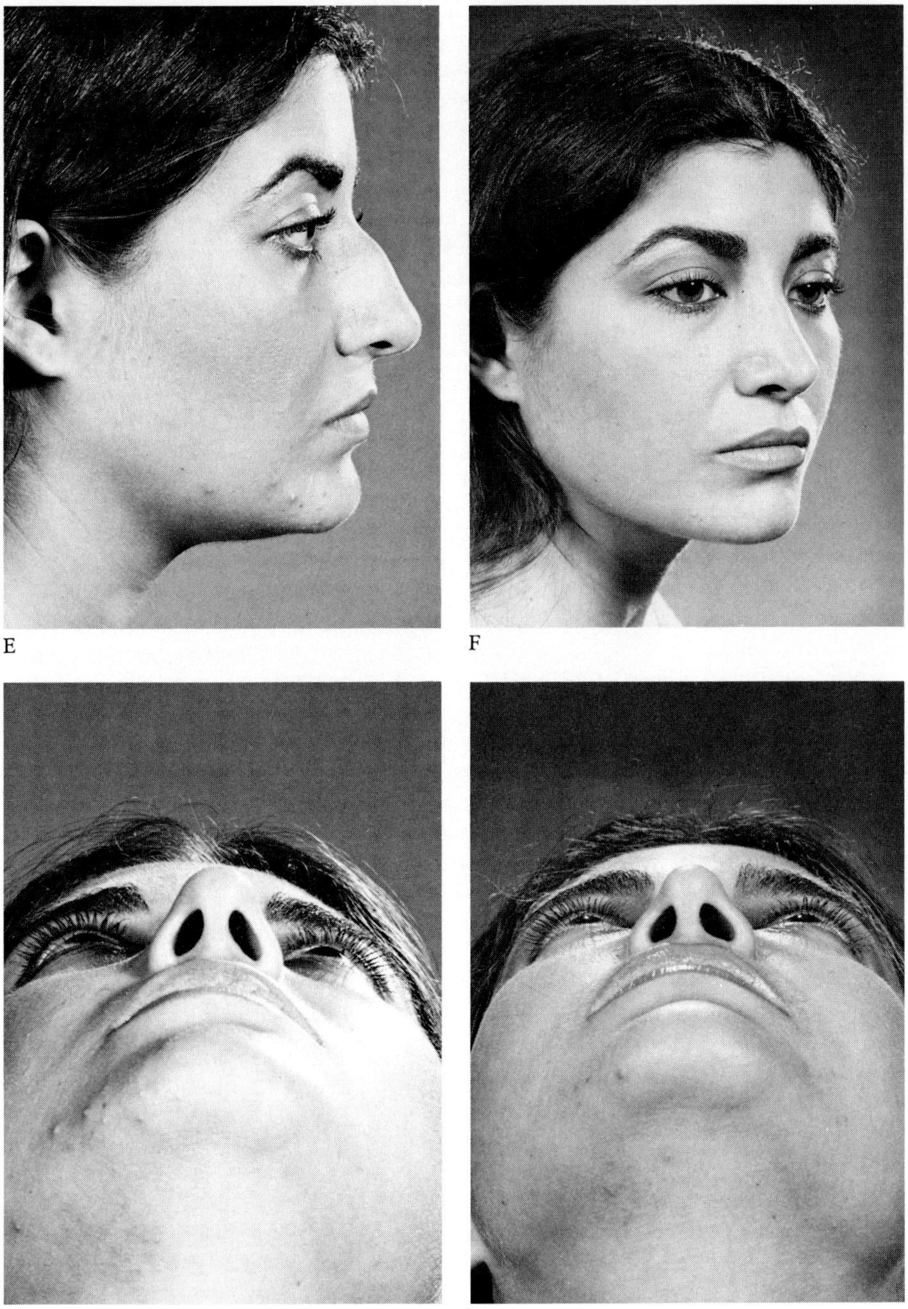

E F G H

Figure 6-18 (continued)

E, F. The importance of oblique views. Traditionally, the lateral view was used to demonstrate dramatic reduction of the hump. However, it is inadequate for meaningful analysis of the tip and the subtleties of nasal aesthetics, which are best shown on the oblique view.

G, H. On basal view, tip projection was preserved, but with slight broadening of the nostril base.

Sheen notes that the columellar-alar complex is like a "gull-in-flight," the columella being slightly lower than and parallel to the alar bases diverging from the midline of the columella. If this divergence is excessive, alar wedge resection is indicated, but if the alar plane is perpendicular to the nasal base, alar resection is rarely performed.

Nostrils

On basal view, the nostril-lobule complex has a triangular shape, the nostrils averaging 1 to 2 times the soft tissue portion of the lobule. The nostrils themselves should have an almond or elliptic shape with the greatest diameter at the nostril sill. Sheen stresses that the round nostril may reflect a lack of dorsal support, which can be corrected by augmenting the dorsum.

SURGICAL PRINCIPLES

Rhinoplasty is an operation that is constantly changing under the influence of technical refinements, functional necessities, and society's aesthetics [86]. For every surgical maneuver in a rhinoplasty, there is a fervent supporter and an adamant opponent. The domes of the alar cartilages that are currently so carefully preserved have previously been transected, crushed, or totally excised—all with good results as demonstrated photographically [115, 131]. Comparable diversity is found in hump removal, mucosal preservation, caudal septal resection, and alar wedges [87, 130, 159]. Ultimately, one must select a specific technique for the individual patient, and the following principles may serve as useful guidelines [130].

Preparations

If possible, the patient is seen the day before surgery to review the operative plan. For the busy practitioner, this final check reinforces an individualized approach and reduces the chances of performing a standardized "signature nose." Antibiotics are not given routinely and are used only if a silastic implant is inserted for chin augmentation. The patient is offered a choice of anesthesia, local infiltration with sedation or general anesthesia, and of surgical setting, inpatient or outpatient. The final choice is often determined by economic and age factors. We agree with Peck [110] that there is less bleeding with local anesthesia and one has total access to the face for determining structural relationships; besides, the patient can cooperate by smiling or opening the mouth. General anesthesia is essential for persons with labile personalities and those adamantly requesting it. The senior author uses local anesthesia in 65 percent and general anesthesia in 35 percent of cases, and all procedures are done in an office operating suite.

The patient is placed on a comfortable tiltable (30 degrees elevation) operating table with the head supported. The face is gently washed with Hibitane. Then the nose is again palpated and the internal nose examined with a nasal speculum. The following external reference marks are made: (1) the borders of the alar cartilages, including the domes, (2) the desired dorsal line from radix to dome, (3) the nasofacial line, and (4) alar wedges as planned. The surgical plan and preoperative photographs are placed adjacent to the surgical field. Two overhead lights are used, one placed inferiorly directed into the nasal cavity and the other transversely. The junior author routinely employs a fiberoptic headlight.

Local anesthesia consists of cocaine nasal packs and 6 to 10 ml of 1% Xylocaine with epinephrine 1 : 100,000. Approximately 4 ml of 4% cocaine is placed in a medicine glass and marked with a drop of methylene blue. Nasal packing is moistened with the solution, any excess is squeezed out, and then three strips are inserted—beneath the lower turbinate, adjacent to the middle turbinate, and high in the vault. Although controversy exists regarding cocaine toxicity, reports of significant morbidity and mortality from its use in rhinoplasty surgery have not been substantiated in the literature [42]. All cocaine-soaked gauzes are removed prior to commencement of the procedure. Using a 1½-in. No. 30 needle, 0.5 ml deposits of anesthesia are inserted in the glabellar region, beside the alar bases, and in the middle of the membranous septum (Fig. 6-19). Dingman [35] emphasizes that 6 to 10 ml of anesthesia is sufficient. From the glabellar point, it is possible to block both the supratrochlear and the infratrochlear nerve branches as well as the termination point of the lateral osteotomies. From the adjacent alar area, one can block the infraorbital nerves, the passage for the lateral osteotomies including the piriform aperture, and then transversely across the nasal base. From the membranous septum, one can place minute deposits along the planned incision lines and the leading edges of the septum, then high in the vault to facilitate the extramucosal approach, terminating underneath the nasal bones to constrict the external nasal branch of the anterior ethmoidal artery. If a septoplasty is required, direct infiltration of the mucosa is added. In general, a perimeter or field block is done to prevent distortion of the nasal architecture, especially the dorsum and tip. To be excepted are patients with very thin

Figure 6-19. Local anesthesia is instilled in minute quantities wherever incisions are planned and to block specific nerve branches.

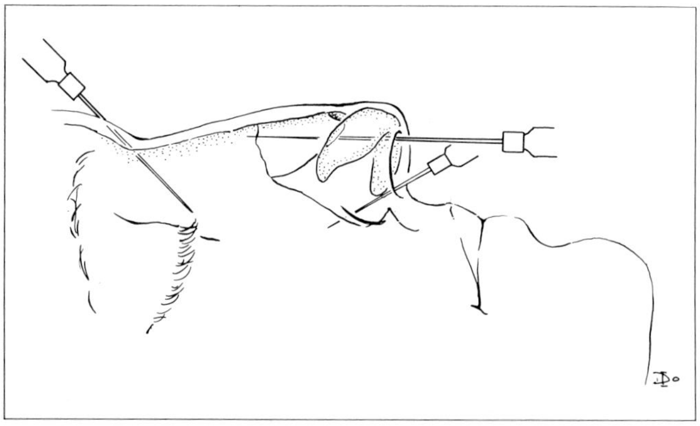

skin, those with large bony humps, and those having secondary rhinoplasties in whom hydrodissection is recommended. We do not routinely employ hyaluronidase or other enzymatic preparations to diminish postoperative edema. A similar sequence is used under general anesthesia to effect hemostasis. Several adjuncts are routinely employed with general anesthesia: (1) a Rey endotracheal tube whose natural curvature minimizes distortions, (2) a throat pack to allow suctioning of accumulated blood, thereby reducing the risk of postoperative aspiration, and (3) a positive pressure alarm device, which signals within 5 seconds any disconnection of the ventilation system that may occur beneath the drapes. At this point, the surgeon scrubs while the nurse preps, drapes the face, and cuts the vibrissae with Vaseline-covered scissors or a No. 15 blade, thus allowing 5 to 10 minutes for the anesthesia to work. Prior to commencement of surgery, the nose is packed inferoposteriorly with saline-soaked gauzes to prevent bleeding into the pharynx, which can alarm and agitate a sedated patient.

Operative Sequence

Establishment of the operative sequence is based in part on historical precedence, surgical concepts, patient factors, and the individual surgeon's preference (Table 6-1). As shown in Table 6-1, Joseph did his rhinoplasties in the following manner: (1) en-bloc removal of the osseocartilaginous hump, (2) lateral osteotomy with infractures, and (3) nasal tip plasty including transection of the alar cartilages. He used a saw with a knife at its base that allowed simultaneous cutting of the bony and cartilaginous portions. To avoid confusion, all modifications of the rhinoplasty operation will be discussed as departures from Joseph's classic technique. Subsequently, surgeons divided the hump into two parts, bony and cartilaginous, removing them separately with different instruments and in different sequence. Gradually, mastery of resecting the bony and cartilaginous vault was achieved, but problems remained with the nasal tip. The importance of tip surgery was clearly stated by Fomon [46]: "He who masters the tip, masters rhinoplasty." Since the nasal tip was the limiting factor, surgeons changed the operative sequence and began with the tip first. There is support for this concept: (1) Tip surgery is more delicate and should be done first while the surgeon is fresh, and before edema or bleeding obscures subtle nuances; (2) tip projection is often the controlling factor in a rhinoplasty, and it is easier to adjust the osseocartilaginous dorsum to the tip than the reverse; and (3) any difficulties in achieving the desired tip can be accommodated by modifications in the rest of the operative procedure. But exceptions exist: (1) Very large humps or plunging septums are removed first to allow the tip to assume a nondistorted position; (2) septal deviations, especially the lower leading portions, are straightened first to eliminate any influence on alar position; and (3) some patients have well-defined tips that do not require modification, while others require onlay grafts or aug-

Table 6-1. Operative sequence

Joseph	Rees	Sheen	Peck
Exposure	Exposure	Exposure	Exposure
Intercartilaginous incision	Intercartilaginous incision	Intercartilaginous incision	Intracartilaginous incision
Soft tissue elevation	Soft tissue elevation	Soft tissue elevation	Transfixion incision
Hump removal	Cartilaginous vault—knife	Cartilaginous vault—knife	Septal modification
En bloc-saw	Bony vault—elevator	Bony vault—elevator	Septal shortening
Osteotomies	Transfixion incision	Septal modification	Nasal spine resection
Lateral: low-to-low saw	Hump removal	Nasal spine resection	Nasal tip
Transverse: digital	Cartilage hump—scissors	Hump removal	Excess alar cartilages excised
Nasal tip	Bony hump—chisel	Bony hump—rasp	Tip refinement
Resection dome/mucosa	Osteotomies	Cartilage hump—No. 11 blade	Hump removal
Removal excess lateral alar cartilages	Lateral: low-to-low straight osteotome	Nasal tip	Bony hump—rasp
Septal modification	Transverse: digital	Delivery technique	Cartilage hump—No. 15 blade
Closure	Medial: optional	Direct excision lateral alar cartilages	Osteotomies
Upper lateral shortening	Nasal tip	Osteotomies	Lateral: low-to-high 4-mm chisel
Columellar suturing	Intracartilaginous incision	Lateral: low-to-high curved osteotome	Transverse: digital
Alar base shaping	Removal excess lateral alar cartilages	Transverse: digital pressure	Medial: unnecessary
	Closure	Medial: unnecessary	Closure
	Septal edge trim	Closure	Upper lateral shortening
	Upper lateral shortening	Septal edge trim	Columellar suturing
	Columellar suturing	Columellar suturing	Alar base shaping
	Alar base shaping	Upper lateral shortening	
		Alar base shaping	

Note: This sequence is the one commonly described. Obviously, these surgeons pick only the steps appropriate for the individual patient.

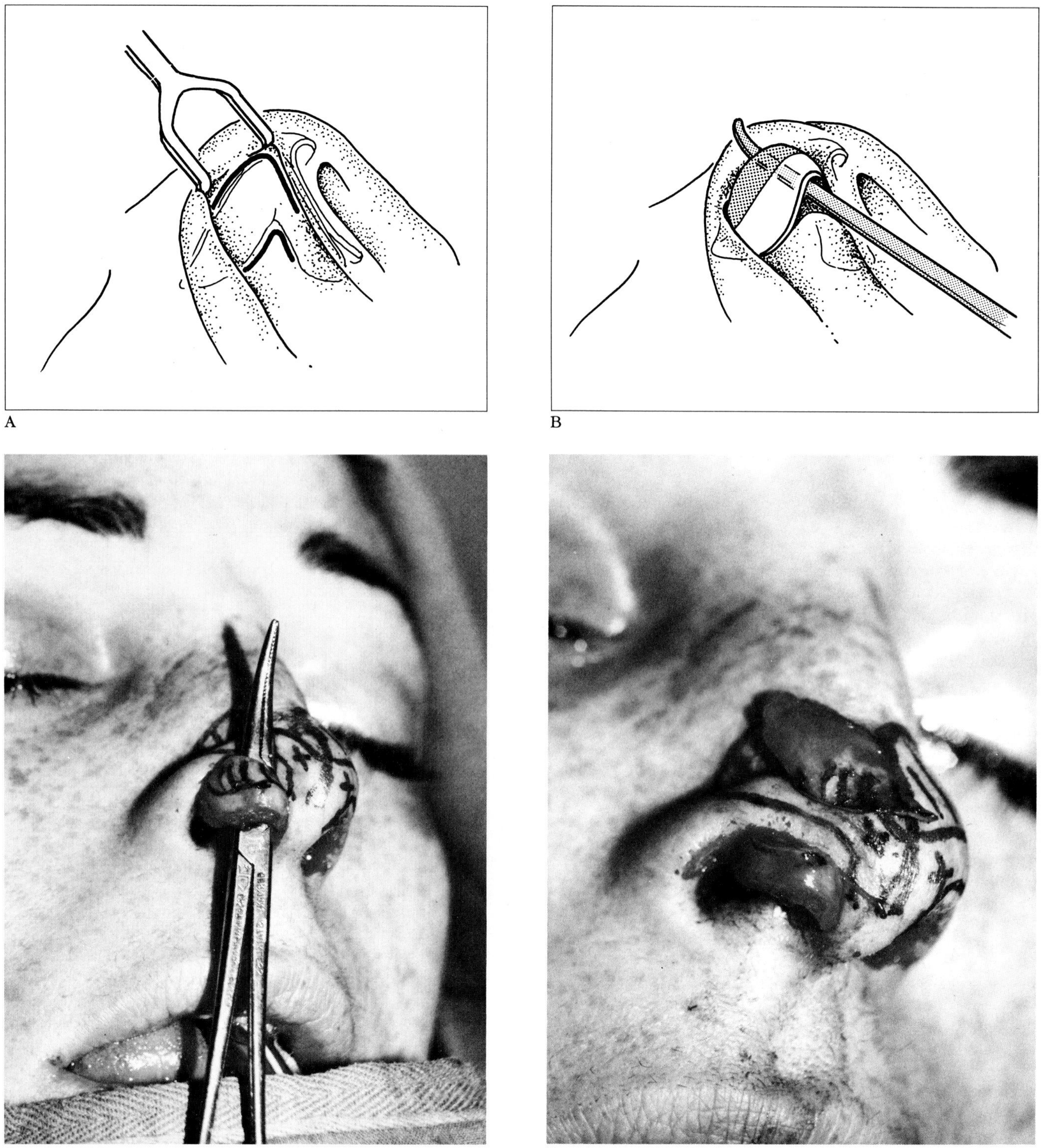

Figure 6-20

A, B. The delivery approach consists of intercartilaginous and infracartilaginous incisions, which allow the alar cartilage to be exteriorized.

C, D. Intraoperative photographs showing the delivered alar cartilage, of which a 4-mm strip will be preserved and the rest excised.

mentations. An additional factor to be considered is whether an operative step should be included or not. Obviously, only steps that are necessary to give the optimal result are incorporated into the final procedure. Broadbent and Woolf [16] have emphasized this principle: "Not all noses should have something done to everything."

Incisions and Exposure

As developed by Roe [128], endonasal incisions allow surgical access to structures without visible scars. If external incisions are reserved for special situations, the choice of incisions is largely dictated by the planned tip modification. The classic intercartilaginous incision is made at the visible limen vestibuli, representing the juncture of upper and lower lateral cartilages. From this point, the soft tissues over the upper lateral cartilages and the periosteum overlying the bony hump are elevated. From the intercartilaginous incision, one can gain access to the alar cartilages by adding an additional incision: (1) direct excision through the vestibular lining (Joseph), (2) hockey stick incision into the dome with eversion (Brown and McDowell), (3) a cartilage-splitting incision (Fomon), and (4) a marginal or infracartilaginous incision with delivery of the alar cartilages for direct modification (Anderson).

The "delivery approach" through combined intercartilaginous-infracartilaginous incisions allows direct visualization of the domes and excellent access to the subcutaneous tissues of the tip and facilitates suturing of the medial crus (Fig. 6-20). Thus, it is of value in difficult problem noses and for the surgeon with limited experience. As an alternative to the two-incision approach, one can use a single intracartilaginous or cartilage-splitting incision (Fig. 6-21). Its simplicity, speed, and minimal scarring are balanced by the need for greater precision of placement, limited access to the dome, and higher complication rate for the inexperienced. Friedman et al. [51] reviewed 673 rhinoplasties using various incisions and found that the delivery technique offered the greatest flexibility with the fewest complications. Ultimately, selection of incisions is dictated by the need for modification of the domes. If the tip is anatomically well defined with pleasing aesthetics, then an intracartilaginous incision is used, as it makes little sense to risk alar damage or obscure their definition with scarring. When significant changes in the domes are required, either in shape or dimensions, then a delivery technique is used.

The transfixion incision refers to separation of the columella from the septum with its length along the membranous septum a controversial point. Proponents argue that a complete transfixion incision facilitates exposure of the dorsum while providing access to the nasal spine and septum. Opponents stress that routine division of the membranous septum eliminates major tip support provided by the overlapping medial crural foot plates [88]. The additional criticism that straight-line scar contracture contributes to postoperative tip descent is poorly substantiated. A limited transfixion incision is done unless major modification of the lower septum and nasal spine is required.

Nasal Tip

The structures that contribute to the nasal tip are numerous: (1) medial and lateral crura plus their transitional dome, (2) upper lateral cartilages, (3) skin and subcutaneous tissue, (4) caudal margin of the septum–nasal spine, and (5) columella plus muscles crossing the membranous septum.

From a technical viewpoint, one must evaluate three characteristics of the tip: (1) projection, (2) position, and (3) size and shape. Aesthetically, the tip must be the highest point in the nasal profile and must be a definite

Figure 6-21
A, B. The intracartilaginous incision splits the alar cartilage into an inferior strip to be preserved and a superior portion to be removed.

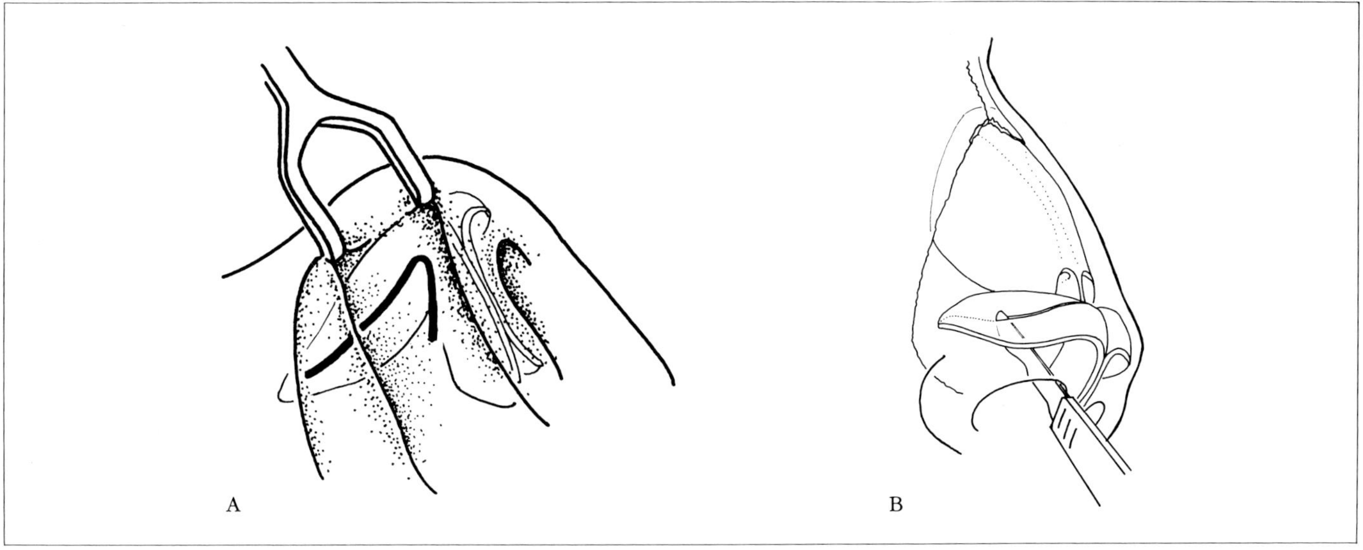

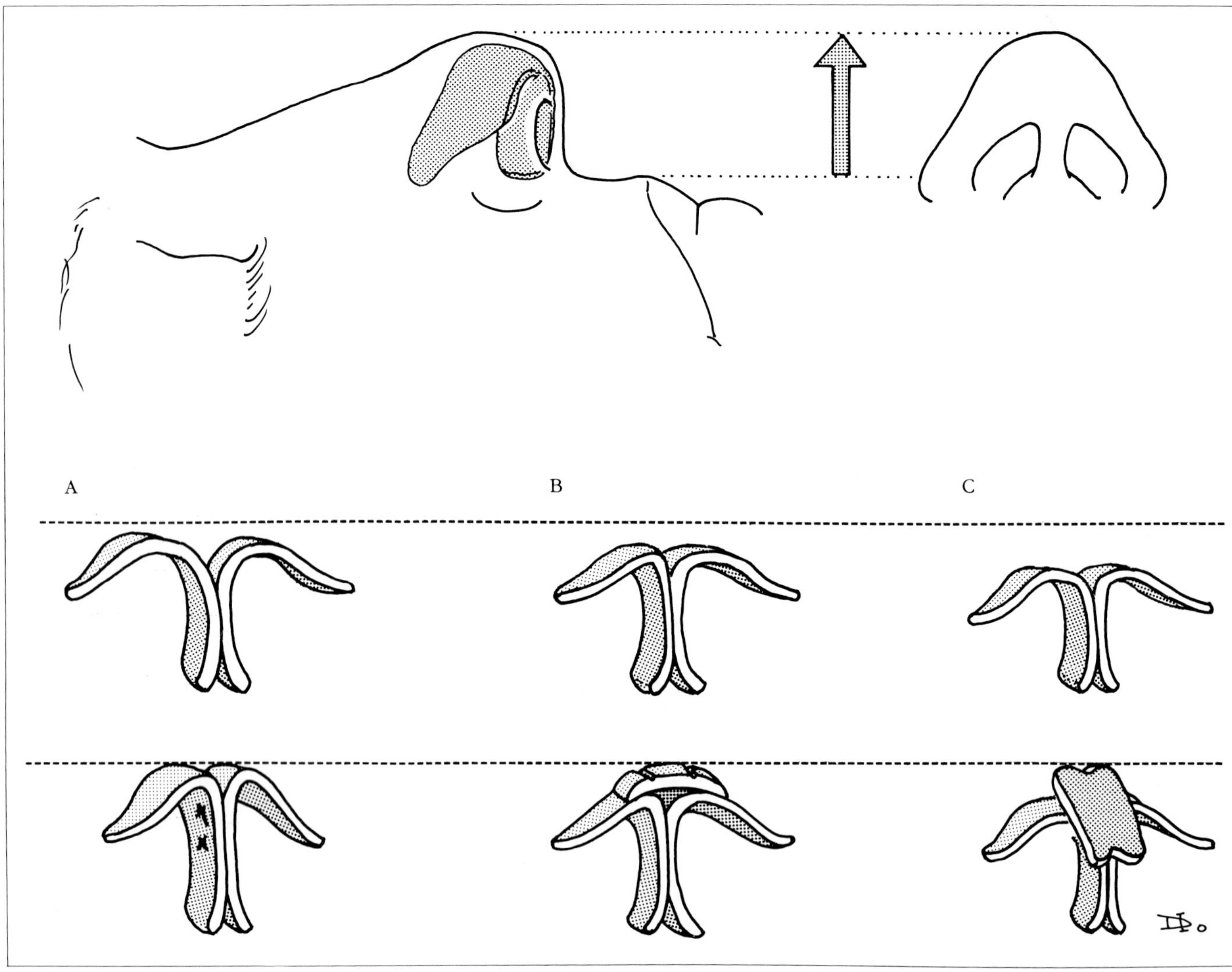

Figure 6-22. When existing tip projection is too low and increased height is desired, graded procedures are available.
A. For minor inadequacies, suturing of the medial crura will raise the domes.
B. For moderate deficiencies, a Peck onlay graft will augment the domes.
C. For extreme deformities, a Sheen tip graft will camouflage the normal domes while creating a new aesthetic tip.

entity that terminates nasal length. Tip projection is defined anatomically on basal view measuring from lip to nasal tip. Four possible conditions exist: (1) correct, (2) too high, (3) too low, and (4) noncorrectable, requiring either support from a strut or camouflage with a graft. Directly influencing the question of projection is the position of the tip or nasolabial angle, and whether tip rotation is necessary. If projection and position are correct, a high intracartilaginous incision is used with limited alar resection. By preserving the lateral accessory cartilage/aponeurotic complex, one maintains tip projection and avoids lateral collapse on deep inspiration. If the projection is *too low,* as shown in Figure 6-22, the degree of severity determines the method of treatment: (1) minor inadequacies require a high intracartilaginous incision, with preservation of the domes, resection of a prominent caudal septal margin or nasal spine, and release of any tethering of soft tissues; (2) moderate deficiencies call for not only the previous maneuvers but also a delivery technique, resection of any intracrural subcutaneous tissue, suturing of the medial crus and domes to obtain the desired projection, and then partial transection of the lateral crus to create new domes as well as consideration of a Peck onlay cartilage graft [112]; (3) extreme deformities often necessitate radical release of the soft tissues plus insertion of a Sheen tip graft [134] to create a more projected nasal tip. If the projection is *too high,* as shown in Figure 6-23, one must select the optimal technique based on the degree of severity: (1) minor diminution—a very low intracartilaginous incision with most of the cephalic lateral alar cartilage removed; (2) moderate reduction—a delivery technique with weakening of the medial crus and excision of the lateral end of the alar crus; and (3) maximum decrease—a modified Lipsett technique [85, 120] with resection of the middle portion of the medial crus.

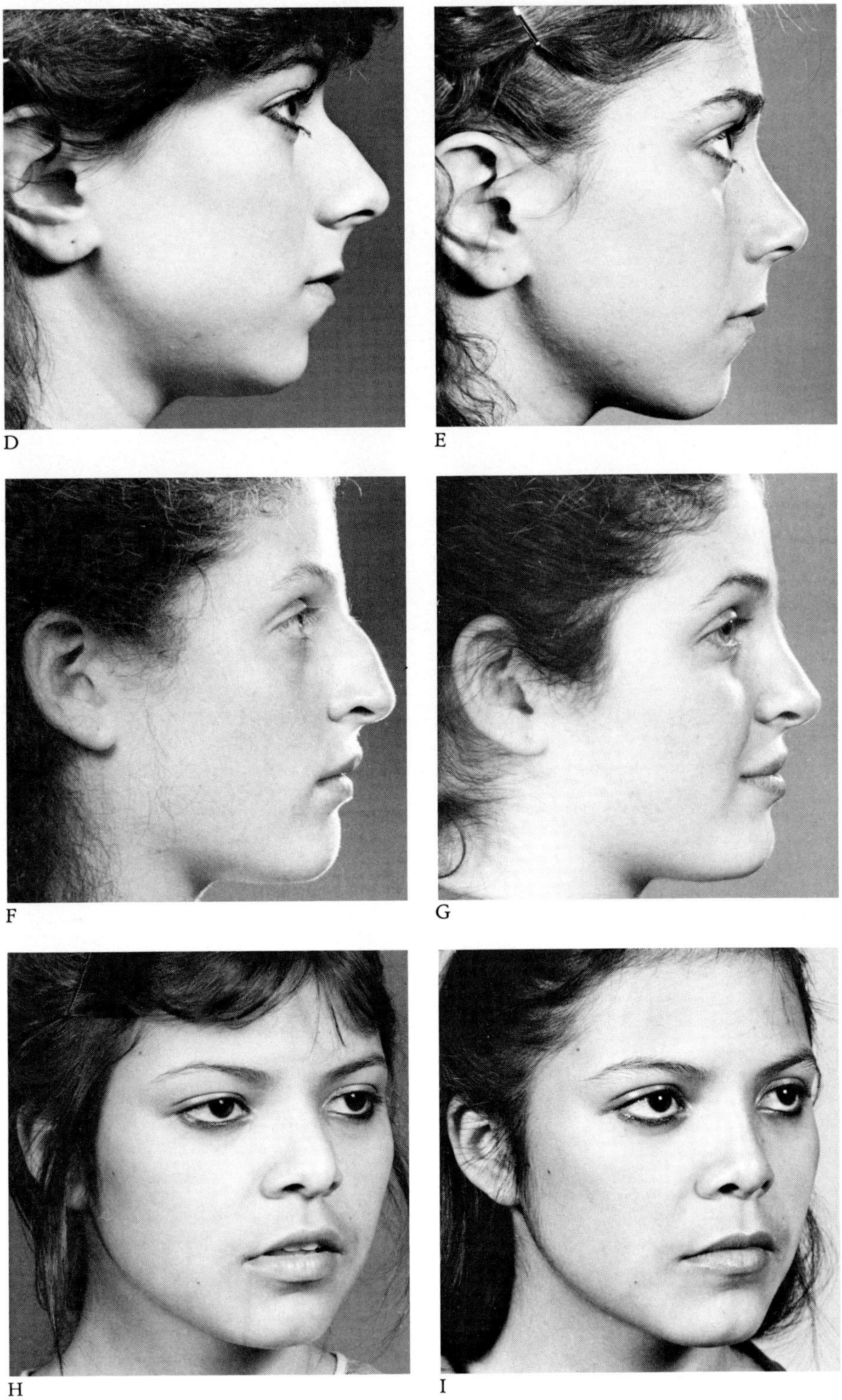

Figure 6-22 (continued)

D, E. Case of minor inadequacy of tip projection corrected by suturing of the medial crura. Patient refused chin augmentation.

F, G. Moderate inadequacy overcome by Peck onlay graft.

H, I. Severe tip flattening and lack of projection improved with Sheen TIP graft and Ortiz-Montesario graft to columella.

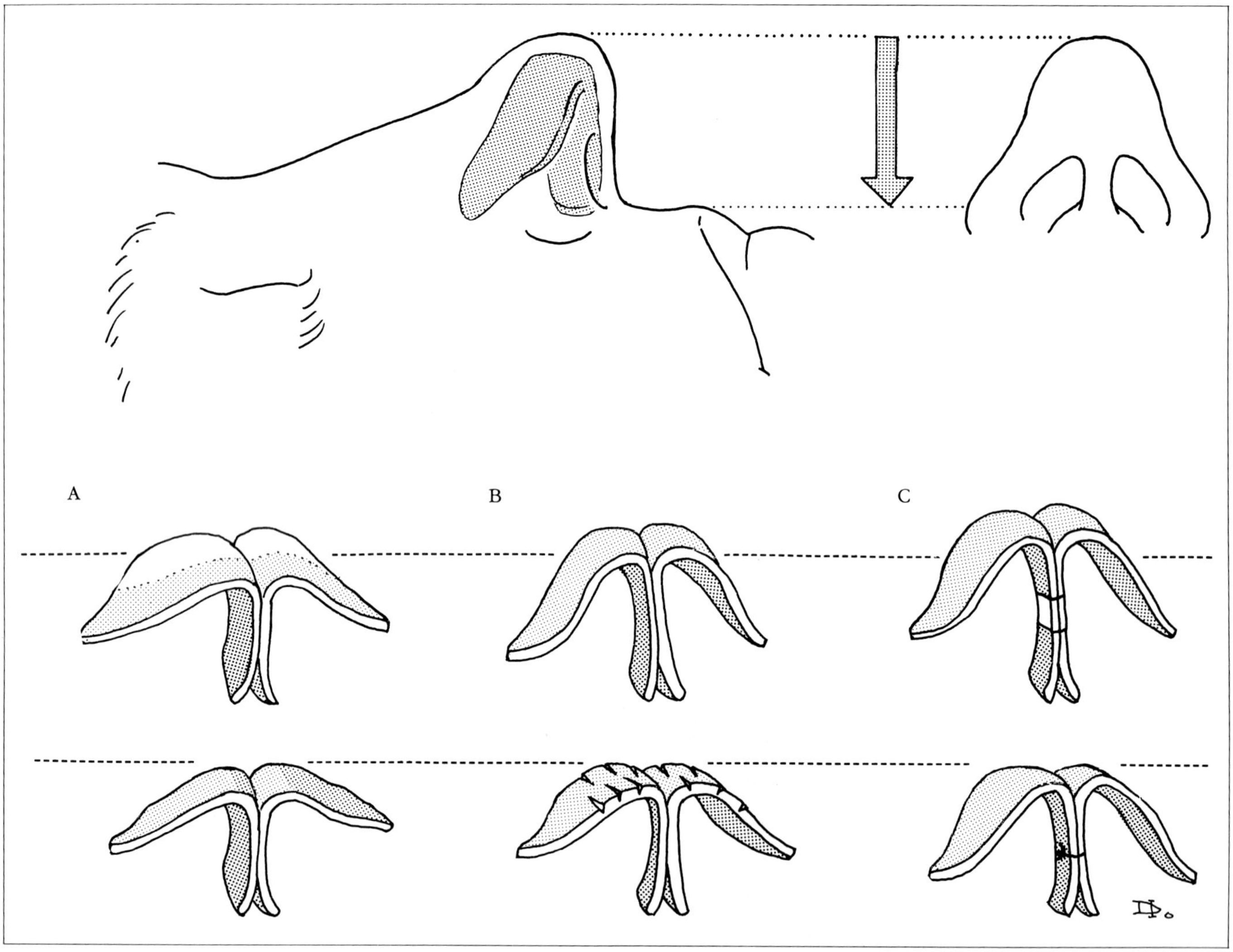

Figure 6-23. When existing tip projection is excessive and decreased height is essential, graded procedures are utilized.

A. For minor diminution, the upper portions of the alar cartilages are removed.
B. For moderate reduction, interdigitating partial-thickness cuts extending onto the medial crura are preferred.
C. For maximum decrease, a 2- to 4-mm segment of the medial crura with overlying skin is excised.
D, E. Minor excess projection improved by a low intracartilaginous resection.
F, G. Moderate projection decreased by weakening of the domes and excision of a lateral crural segment. Columella "show" achieved with an Ortiz-Montesario graft, while chin improved with a horizontal reduction genioplasty.
H, I. Severe projection with setback using a modified Lipsett technique.

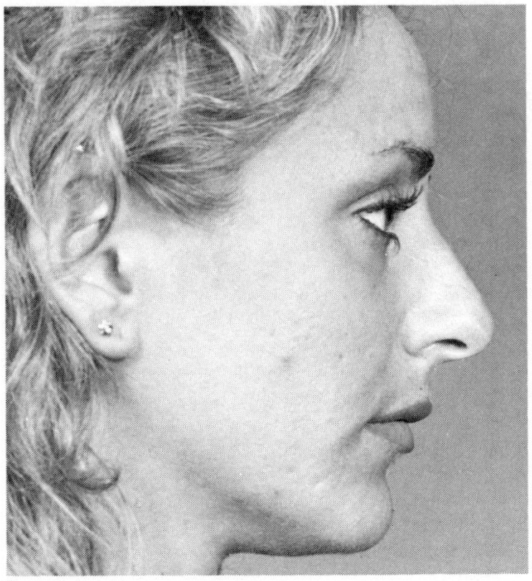
D

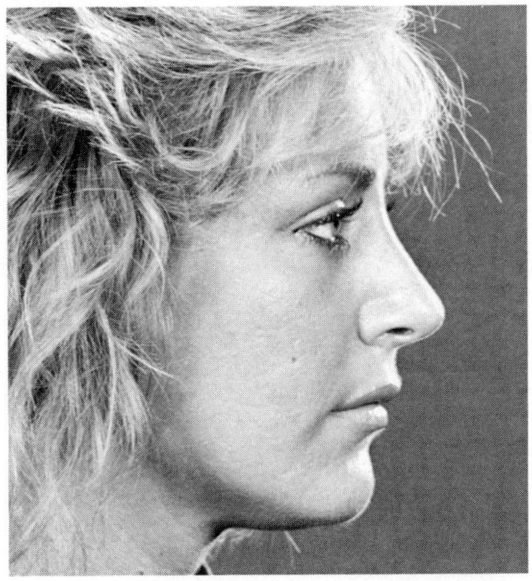
E

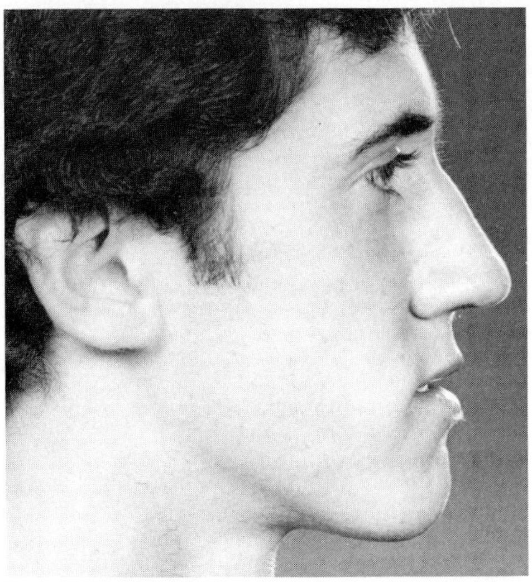
F

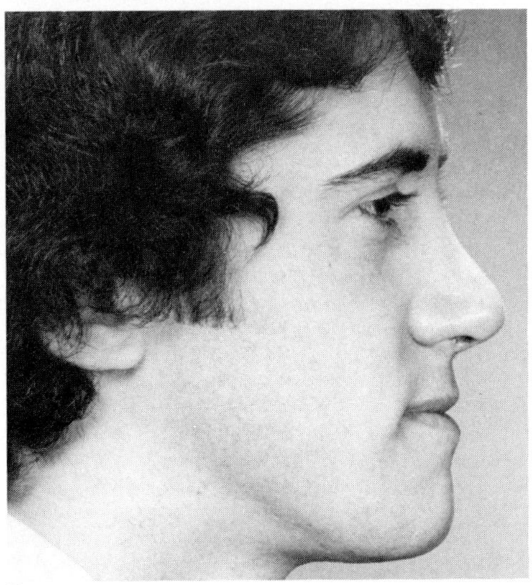
G

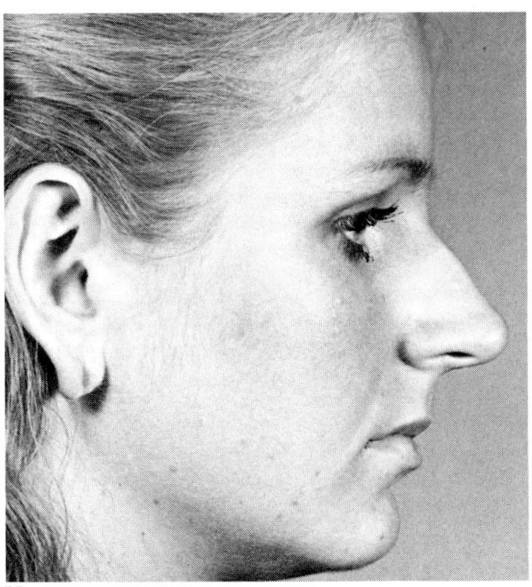
H

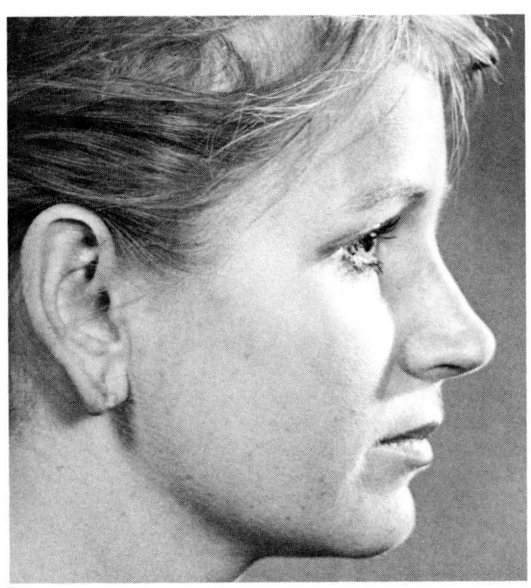
I

Figure 6-23 (continued)

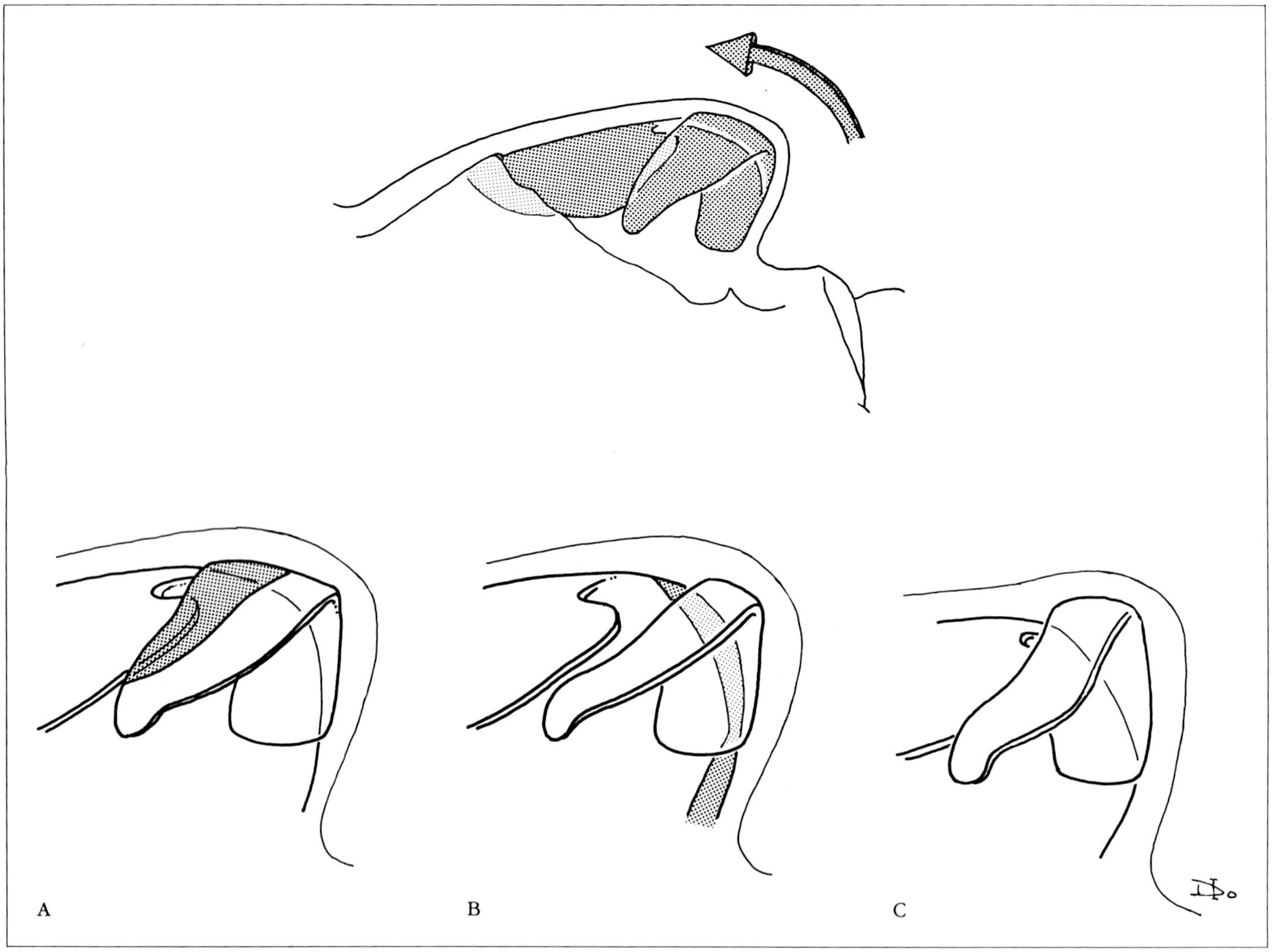

Figure 6-24. Achieving cephalic rotation of the nasal tip using a graded approach.
A. Excision of the upper portion of the alar cartilage.
B. Resection of a triangular portion of the septal cartilage.
C. The desired result.

Tip rotation in a cephalic direction is achieved routinely by two methods: (1) resection of the cephalic portion of the lateral crus, which breaks the downward projection caused by the abutment between upper and lower lateral cartilages, and (2) excision of a triangular segment of the caudal margin of the septum (Fig. 6-24). Frequently, it is necessary to excise the "scroll" of the upper lateral cartilage or to shorten its caudal projection. Webster [156, 157] has developed a third technique—a cartilaginous septal transfixion incision involving excision of a superiorly based triangle of septum with cephalic rotation of the entire nasal lobule.

Modification of the caudal margin of the septum is done as a progressive sequence to achieve three goals: (1) cephalic rotation of the tip, (2) shortening of nasal length, and (3) alterations in the nasolabial angle (Fig. 6-25). The line of excision on the septum should be convex in its anterior third to ensure normal projection of the columella below the alar rims on lateral views [110]. The superior portion of the excision achieves the cephalic rotation whereas the inferior portion shortens the nose and eliminates a hanging columella. Aston and Guy [6] differentiated two causes of an obtuse nasolabial angle; first, the more common caudal septum, and second, the prominent nasal spine as defined by its projection beyond the facial plane. The nasal spine is resected or rasped when encroachment into the lip occurs, as accentuated on smiling [147]. However, this maneuver should *not* be a routine part of every rhinoplasty and is probably necessary in less than 10 percent of patients. Rarely, patients will have a "hanging columella" that is due not to either of the above, but to an excessively wide medial crus. Randall [117] described a series of graded excisions of the medial crus including the overlying skin. Occasionally, one will encounter patients with a widely obtuse nasolabial angle and a hanging upper lip, often in consequence of surgery in which radical resection of the septum and nasal spine was done (Fig. 6-26). When it is not too severe or where previous surgery was not done, the angle can be partially closed by maxillary augmentation with a supramid mesh or a large cartilage graft, as described by Ortiz-Monasterio [104, 105].

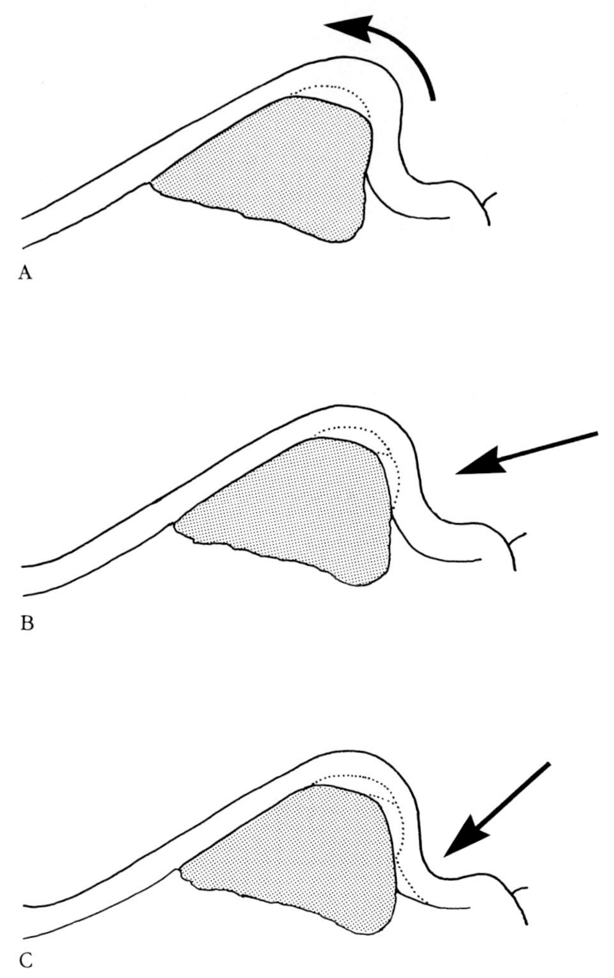

Figure 6-25. Modification of the caudal border of the septum.
A. The upper leading edge of the septum is excised to achieve tip rotation.
B. The caudal border is excised to shorten the length of the nose.
C. The nasal spine is reduced to deepen the nasolabial angle.

From evaluating long-term results, several guidelines have evolved: (1) The domes are *not* completely transected; (2) a 1- to 2-mm rim of alar crus is dangerous, whereas 3 to 4 mm offers security; (3) the upper outer "tail" of the lateral crus is not excised; (4) the medial crus is maintained; (5) thin cartilages require careful preservation, whereas thick cartilages can be maximally manipulated; (6) thin skin shows every deficiency while thick skin limits definition; and (7) the wide diversity of nasal tips requires maximum flexibility from the surgeon. The quality of the skin and underlying cartilages is a limiting factor, as to techniques employed and in terms of possible results. In the thin-skinned patient with delicate cartilages, the cartilages should be modified by scoring and sculpting rather than resecting the deformity; symmetry and preservation of structural integrity is critical. In the patient with heavy oily skin and thick cartilages, significant excision of both subcutaneous tissue and cartilage is essential, and occasionally darts placed at the domes. Further discussion of the nasal tip is found in Chapter 7.

Nasal Hump

In Joseph's classic rhinoplasty, the osseocartilaginous hump was removed en bloc, including the mucosal lining [77]. Subsequently, Brown and McDowell [17] utilized a single saw with diagonal orientation allowing the bony hump to be freed, and then the cartilaginous component was "sliced off" with a drawing knife. Irregularities were corrected with a rasp (bone) or excised with a knife (cartilage). Converse [26] removed the cartilaginous hump first, then altered the tip, then removed the bony hump. Rees [120] removes the cartilaginous hump first, then excises the bony hump with an osteotome. Peck [110] and Sheen [138] favor reduction of the bony hump with a rasp followed by sharp excision of the entire cartilaginous hump with a scalpel.

Currently, most surgeons prefer to remove the hump in two parts, except in very prominent noses, where sharp transection of the cartilaginous hump is followed by placement of a guarded osteotome with en bloc hump removal. Robin [125–127], Jost [78], and Anderson [2–5] extended Eitner's [39, 40] concept of an ***extramucosal approach*** so that the nasal mucosa along the septum and undersurface of the upper lateral cartilage–nasal bones is reflected downward prior to hump removal (Fig. 6-27). This approach reduces disruption of the internal valve, webbing of the vestibule, and postoperative bleeding. Although technically more difficult, the physiologic value of preserving the internal lining cannot be denied.

The basic objective of hump removal is to establish the new dorsal profile line in both the longitudinal and vertical planes. Since the profile is determined by both the osseocartilaginous hump and the skin-subcutaneous tissue covering, each factor must be considered. Wright [160] dissected 10 cadavers and performed hump removal, with these findings: (1) The skin was thickest (2–3 mm) over the root and lower lateral cartilage but thinnest (1 mm or less) over the hump area (rhinion); (2) a straight-line hump excision resulted in some degree of polybeak; (3) bony removal should generally be less and cartilaginous excision more; and (4) a final check should always be done to remove irregularities or debris. Anderson [2] routinely scooped the dorsum of the cartilaginous septum below that of the bony septum to accommodate the thicker soft tissue covering in the supratip area. As noted by Wright [161], reconstruction of a precise straight line following hump removal must accommodate the changes that occur in the nasal skin envelope: (1) The radix of the nose is rarely changed in most rhinoplasties and usually serves as a reference point; (2) since the average hump is mainly cartilaginous and not bony, the bone removal is less in a longitudinal dimension; (3) the stretched skin over the rhinion probably contracts to approach the thicker skin at either end; and (4) the thickness of the

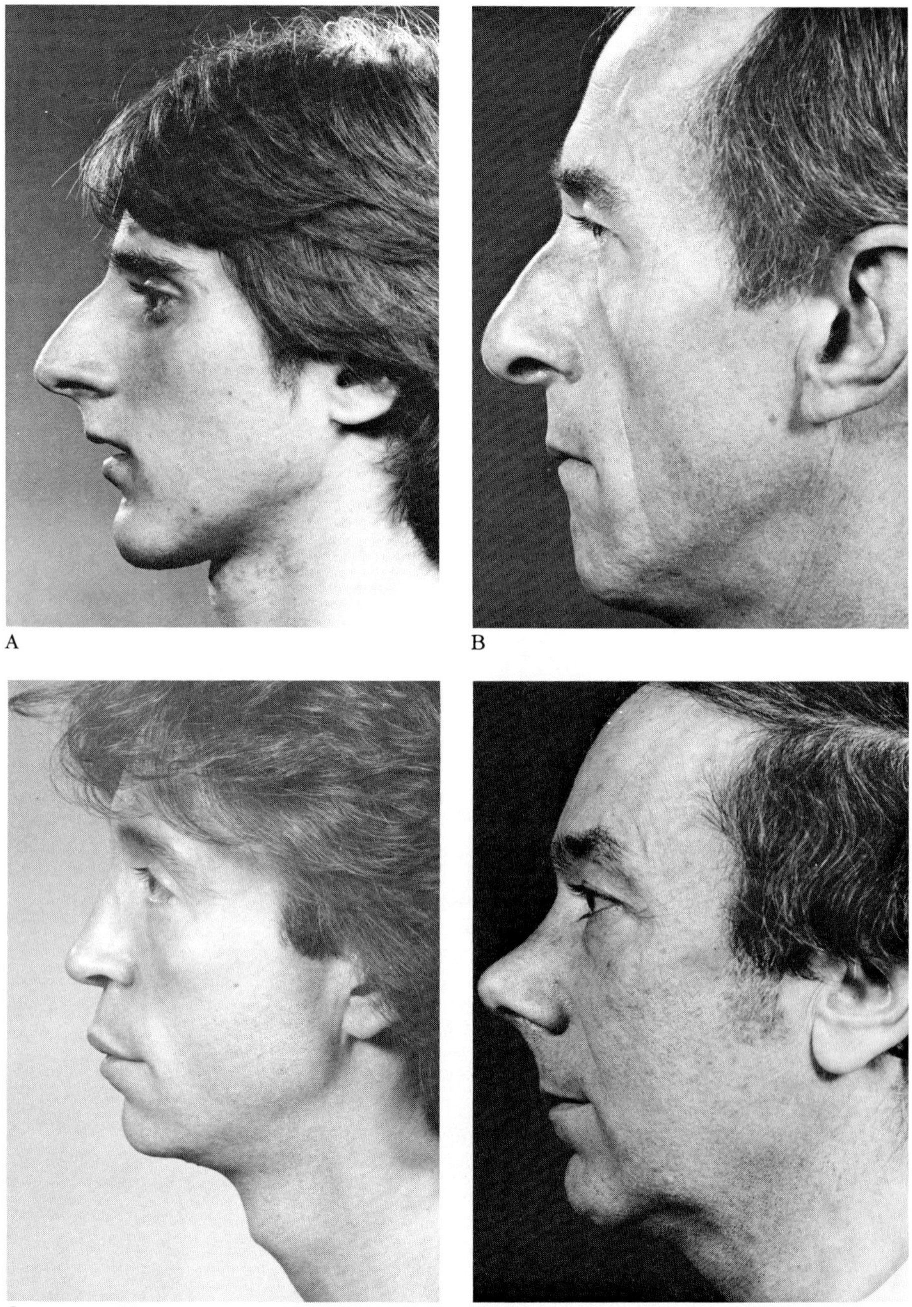

A B C D

Figure 6-26. Four problems related to the caudal border of the septum and nasal spine.

A. Patient with obvious projection of the nasal spine beyond the facial plane.

B. Patient with a hanging columella due to septal cartilage. Any resection of the nasal spine would accentuate a vertical hanging lip.

C. Secondary nasal deformity seen in consultation, with an acute nasolabial angle and hanging upper lip following excessive removal of the nasal spine.

D. Secondary nasal deformity seen in consultation, with an obtuse nasolabial angle following radical resection of the cartilaginous septum.

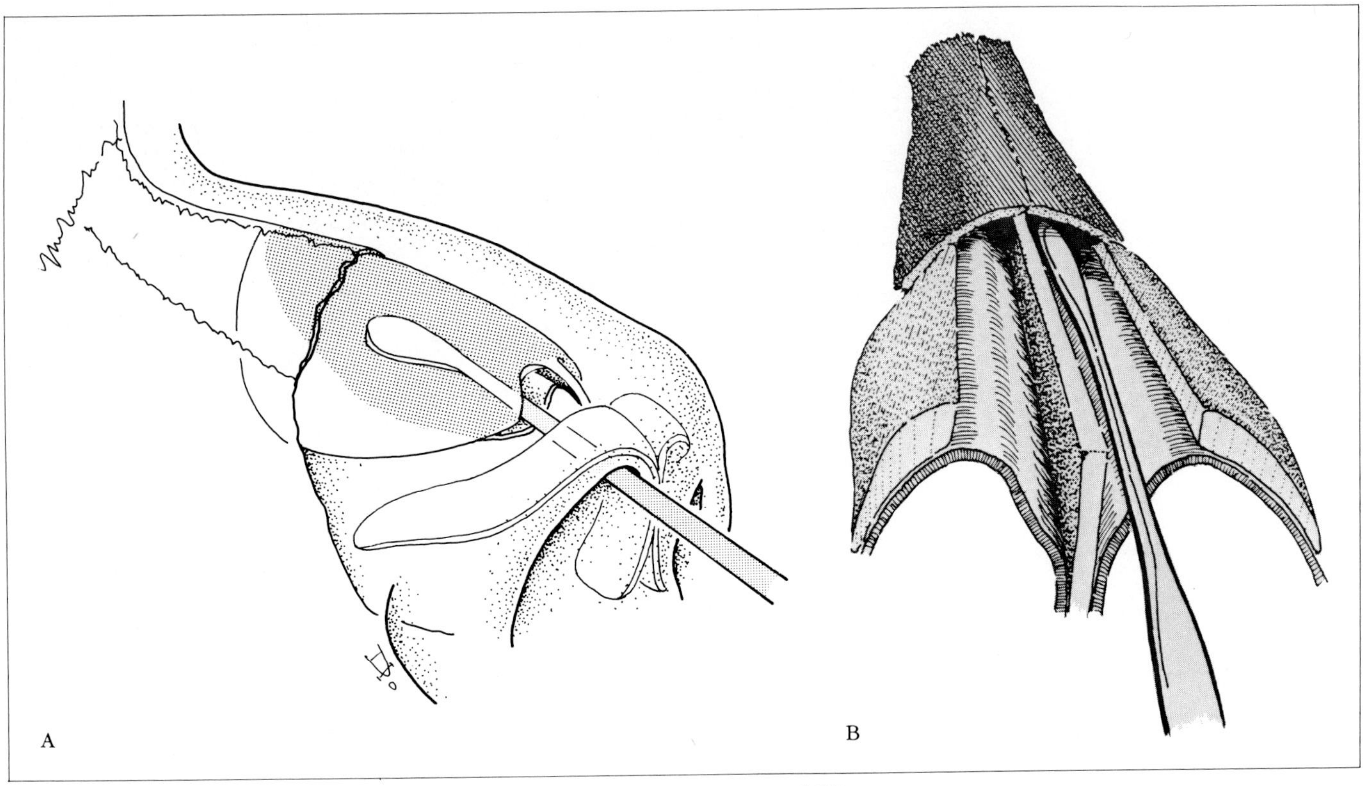

Figure 6-27
A, B. The extramucosal approach requires reflection of the mucosa downward from the dorsum. This mucosal preservation facilitates removal of the hump and minimizes trauma to the nasal valve area.

supratip skin is lessened directly by excision of subcutaneous tissue and indirectly by excision of the cephalic portion of the upper lateral cartilages. With fiberoptic lights, direct visualization of the septum is possible and a straight dorsal line can be achieved, but its projection above the nasofacial line is reduced and brought more nearly parallel.

In planning the dorsal hump removal, the following marks are made: (1) the desired nasofrontal angle at the radix, (2) the desired projection of the nasal domes, (3) an interconnecting line signifying the new dorsal profile, and (4) the juncture of nasal bones with upper lateral cartilages. Rather than grading humps on their projection, it is best to analyze them on their overall length and encroachment onto the nasofrontal angle (Fig. 6-28). In small and moderate humps that fall below or 2 mm above the intercanthal line, the bony portion is rasped down and the cartilaginous component excised with a sharp blade. For the large hump, an extramucosal approach is used and the individual components of the cartilaginous hump are transected with scissors. Then a sharp resection of the bony component is made with a Robin osteotome, thus achieving en bloc hump removal. One must avoid excessive hump removal as it can lead to flattening of the middle third of the face. However, certain large humps may require deepening of the nasofrontal angle and occasionally even complete disarticulation at the nasofrontal suture line. With large removals, an "open roof" deformity may exist that is virtually impossible to close by infracturing and often requires some method of covering with a graft. For this reason Skoog [143] developed the technique of reinserting the resected hump following its reduction and modification. The technique is particularly valuable in inadvertent asymmetric hump removals where the attached lateral nasal bone can be replaced along with the modified dorsum.

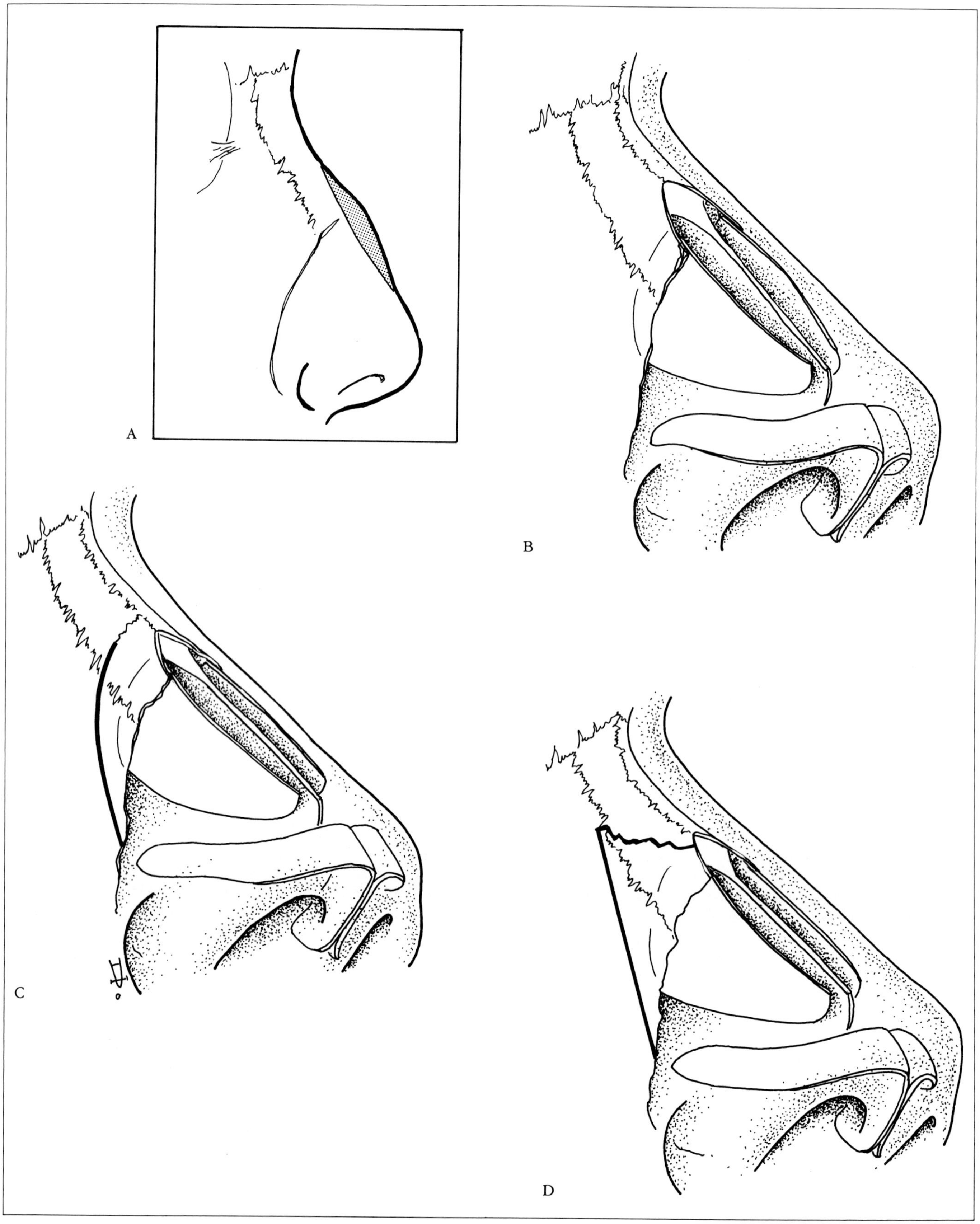

Figure 6-28. The interrelationship of hump removal and osteotomies required to close the open roof.

A, B. A *small hump* implies an aesthetically pleasing radix and an open roof that ends below the intercanthal line.

C. An angulated osteotomy is used for narrow noses. It incorporates both the lateral and transverse components.

D. A low-to-high osteotomy plus digital pressure will result in a transverse fracture line that passes beneath the intact bony pyramid.

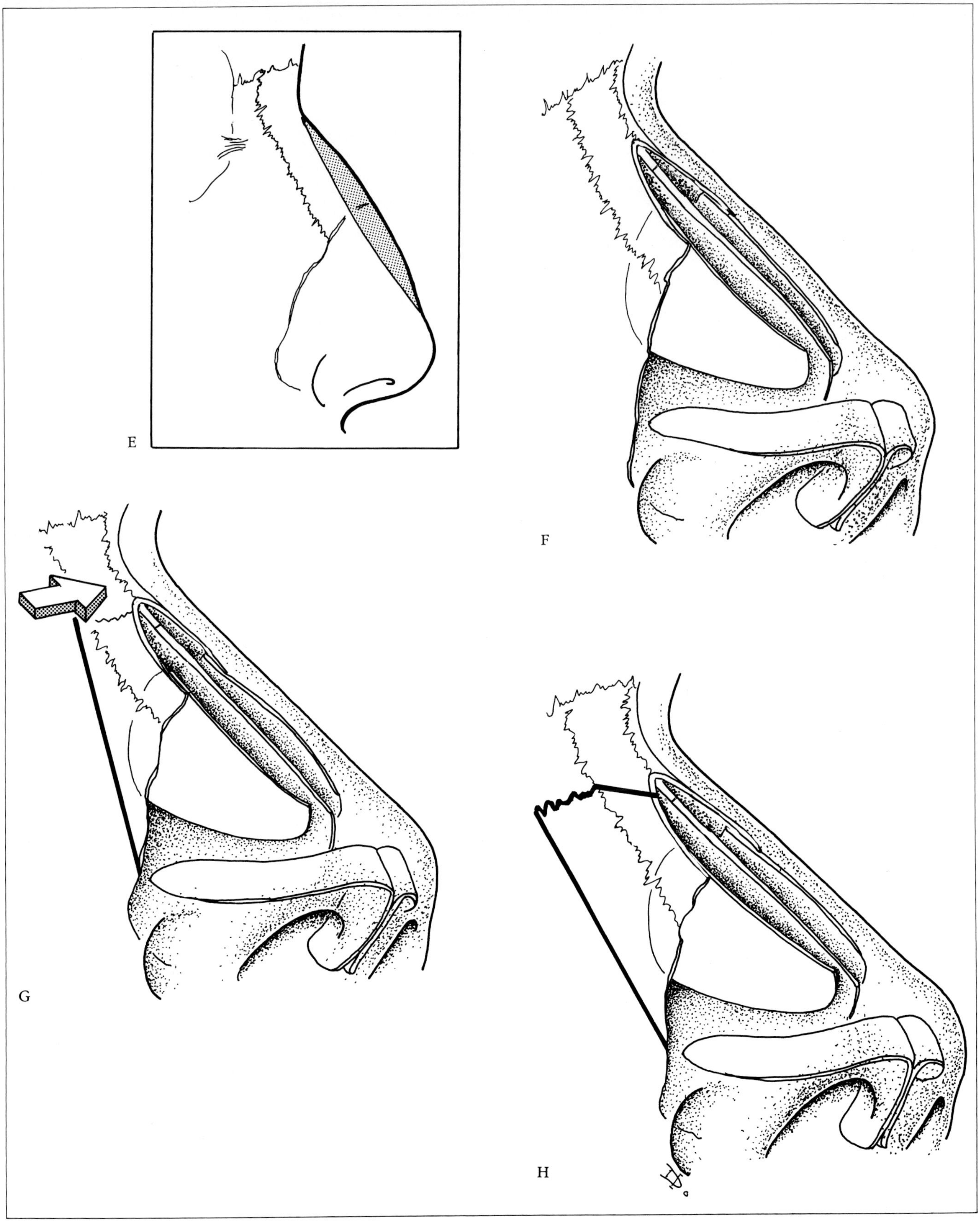

Figure 6-28 (continued)
E, F. A *moderate hump* extends to or slightly above the intercanthal line.
G. A low-to-high osteotomy plus digital pressure is effective in most cases.
H. In the wide nose with a moderate hump removal, a medial oblique osteotomy is done prior to a low-to-low osteotomy with medial movement accomplished by digital pressure.

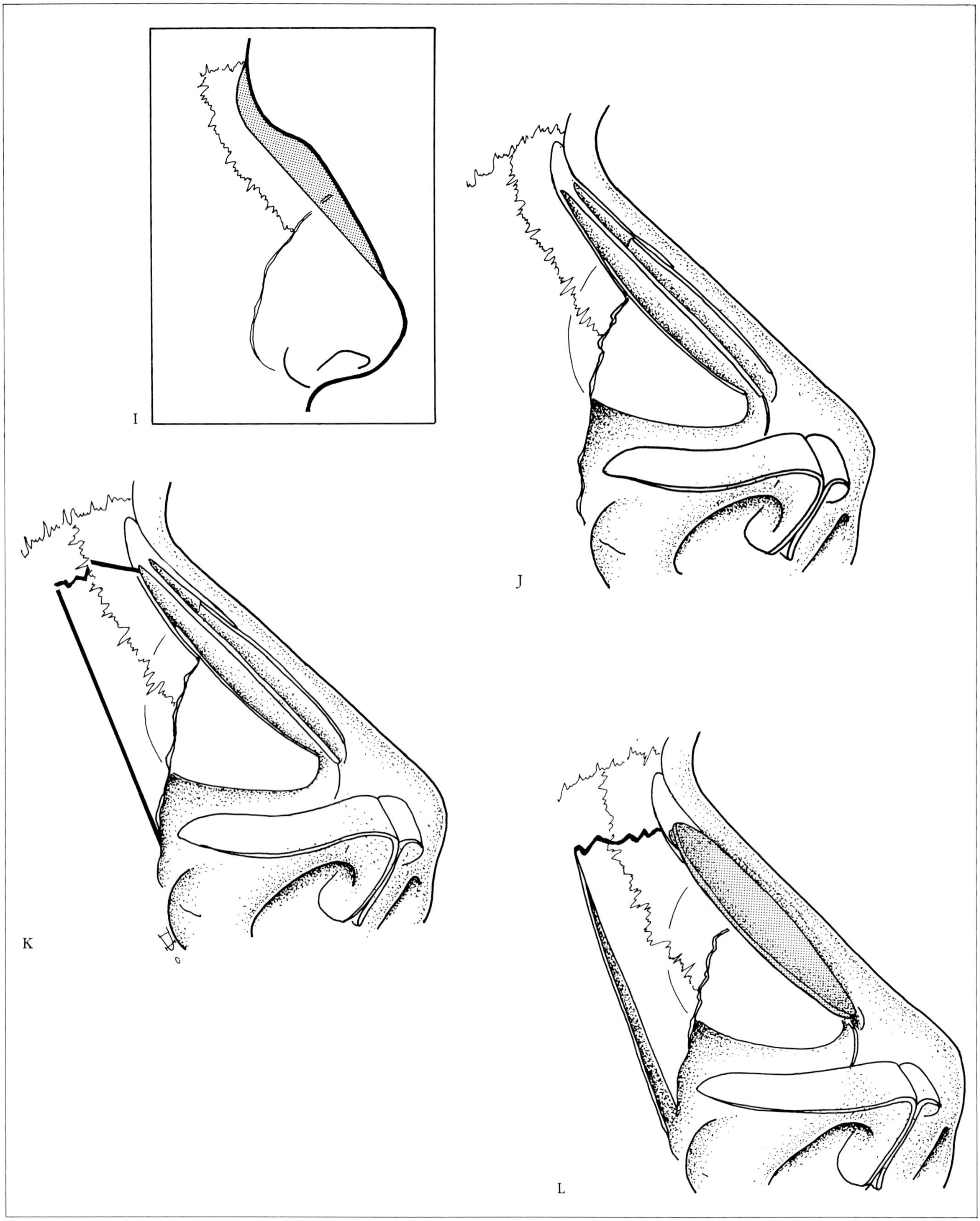

Figure 6-28 (continued)
I, J. A *large hump* extends to the nasofrontal suture line and deepens the nasofrontal groove.
K, L. A combined medial oblique and low-to-low osteotomy is done with optional insertion of a dorsal graft.

Osteotomies

Through a subperiosteal tunnel, Joseph [77] performed the lateral osteotomy with a saw and followed it by digital pressure to effect the transverse fracture, while the previous large hump removal obviated the need for medial osteotomies. Subsequently, Aufricht [7] began removing a bony web at the radix with a rongeur and then performing an "outfracture" with a medial osteotomy. Thick dorsal nasal bone was incorporated into the mobilized nasal bone, a "rocker effect" was produced that precluded medial movement [11]. Another concern was descent of the nasal bones into the nasal vault. Previously, lateral fractures were performed low in order to ensure body support for the lateral walls by the frontal process of the maxilla. However, radiographic studies have shown that bony contact is not maintained and that support of the lateral walls is by the overlying skin rather than a bony shelf. Therefore, widespread elevation of the skin overlying the bony dorsum is no longer done.

Narrowing of the bony nasal vault requires three fracture lines: (1) lateral—along the frontal process of the maxilla, (2) transverse—through the nasal bones, and (3) medial—parallel to the septum (Fig. 6-29). For discussion purposes, an *osteotomy* is a surgical procedure done with an osteotome or chisel that separates the bone into two parts, whereas a *fracture,* done with digital pressure, allows the bone to remain in approximate contact; the goal of both is to allow movement. The critical factor that must be determined is whether a single lateral osteotomy plus digital fractures is sufficient, or whether multiple osteotomies are required and in which sequence.

This decision is dictated in part by the extent of hump removal. Following removal of a large hump, the open roof extends above the intercanthal line, and the bony vault is easily narrowed by a lateral osteotomy plus a transverse fracture, which occurs close to the intercanthal line. In patients with small humps, the bony dorsum is left intact as the aesthetics are often excellent. As shown in cadavers, a low-to-high osteotomy plus digital pressure will narrow the bony vault but requires both transverse and medial fractures with the latter potentially disrupting the smooth dorsum. Since fractures caused by digital pressure are inherently uncontrollable, a controlled medial-oblique osteotomy is considered for selected cases. In contrast to the classic medial osteotomy, which was done as an outfracture following the lateral osteotomy, the medial oblique is done before the lateral osteotomy to preserve the dorsum. For moderate humps, an outwardly directed medial oblique fracture is used when the dorsal width is excessive and narrowing is required at a precise point. In small humps, a more parallel medial oblique fracture is done to preserve the smooth dorsum. Thus, planning the osteotomies for their aesthetic value is essential and one must not use a failure-determined sequence; i.e., if the lateral osteotomies plus digital pressure does not work, then keep adding osteotomies until total mobilization is achieved.

The location of the lateral osteotomies is highly variable with four common variations, each having inherent limitations: (1) a high-to-high osteotomy produces a visible steplike deformity along the lateral wall; (2) a low-to-low osteotomy passing within the frontal process of the maxilla; (3) a low-to-high osteotomy, which passes across the frontal process to end at the nasal bone-maxilla suture line; and (4) a sharply curved osteotomy preferred by Anderson and Peck, which combines the lateral and transverse components (Fig. 6-30). From our clinical experience, it has become apparent that the location of the lateral osteotomy should be dictated by a new concept—the need for narrowing the base width of the bony vault. The widest point on the base of the bony vault is marked with an X on the sitting patient. Once defined, an "angulated lateral osteotomy" is done beneath this maximum width. In effect, the angle ranges from straight (low-to-low) for maximum narrowing to gradual (low-to-high) to sharply curved (oblique), depending on the patient's deformity. Thus, closure of the open roof is the inherent objective, but placement of the lateral osteotomy is determined by the base width of the bony vault. In general, a straight osteotome is used for low-to-low lateral osteotomies (10%) and a curved osteotome for the more frequent low-to-high cases (90%). The guard is always placed submucosally, a maneuver whose adoption has led to a dramatic decrease in postoperative ecchymosis.

In standard textbooks, the transverse fracture line is often drawn at the level of the nasofrontal suture line and medial canthus. However, if one marks the radix on the skin, it closely corresponds with the medial canthal ligament and confirms that most transverse fractures pass through the body of nasal bones and not the nasofrontal suture line. If the transverse fracture cannot be accomplished by digital pressure, we use a 2-mm osteotome placed through a skin stab wound above the medial canthal ligament. Medial osteotomy, outfracturing, and removal of bony webs are reserved for those few patients requiring a narrowed radix or posttraumatic cases where mobilization of the nasal bones is often difficult.

Two important subgroups of patients require alternative techniques. The older individual frequently wants major changes in the nasal tip with minor hump excision. Thus, osteotomies are not required nor often desirable as comminution is inevitable. A second subgroup consists of individuals at the extremes of bony architecture—short nasal bones, the flattened dorsum, or massive humps. As emphasized by Sheen [138], fractures of short nasal bones and very narrow bony vaults can lead to visual separation of the bony cartilaginous vaults and cause respiratory obstruction. For these patients and those without humps, especially Orientals and blacks, dorsal augmentation is required. Following large hump removal, an "open-roof" deformity exists that must be closed by osteotomies and/or grafting. A modified hump is reinserted using the Skoog technique as described by Regnault and Alfaro [122].

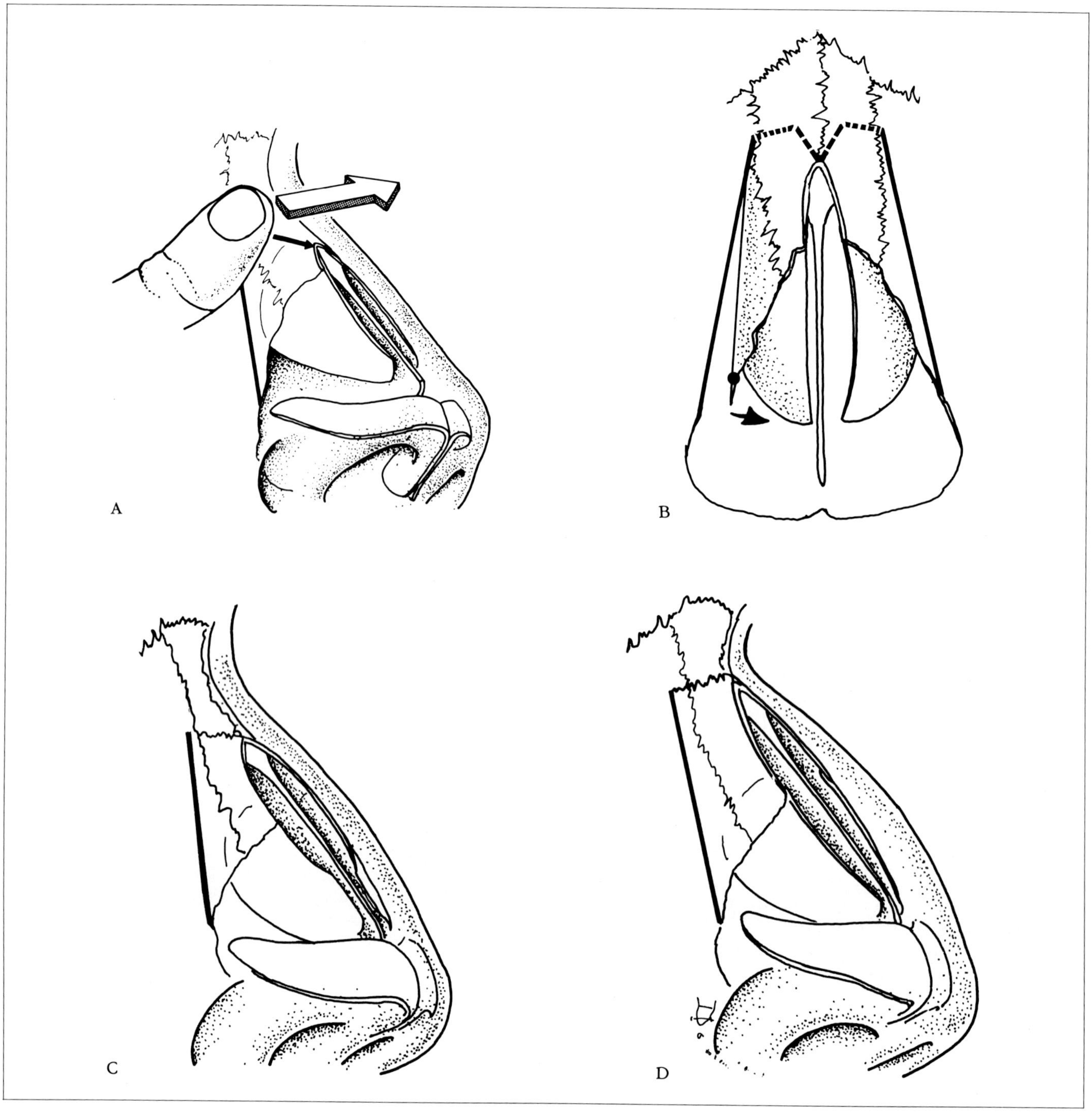

Figure 6-29. Medial movement of the nasal walls to close the open roof.

A. Digital pressure produces a fracture that passes along the plane of least resistance into the open roof.
B. The majority of medial movement occurs at the pyriform aperture, while the transverse fracture at the radix acts as a hinge.
C. In small humps, the transverse fracture line will be acutely angulated as it passes beneath the intact bony dorsum.
D. In moderate humps, the transverse fracture line will pass straight into the open roof.

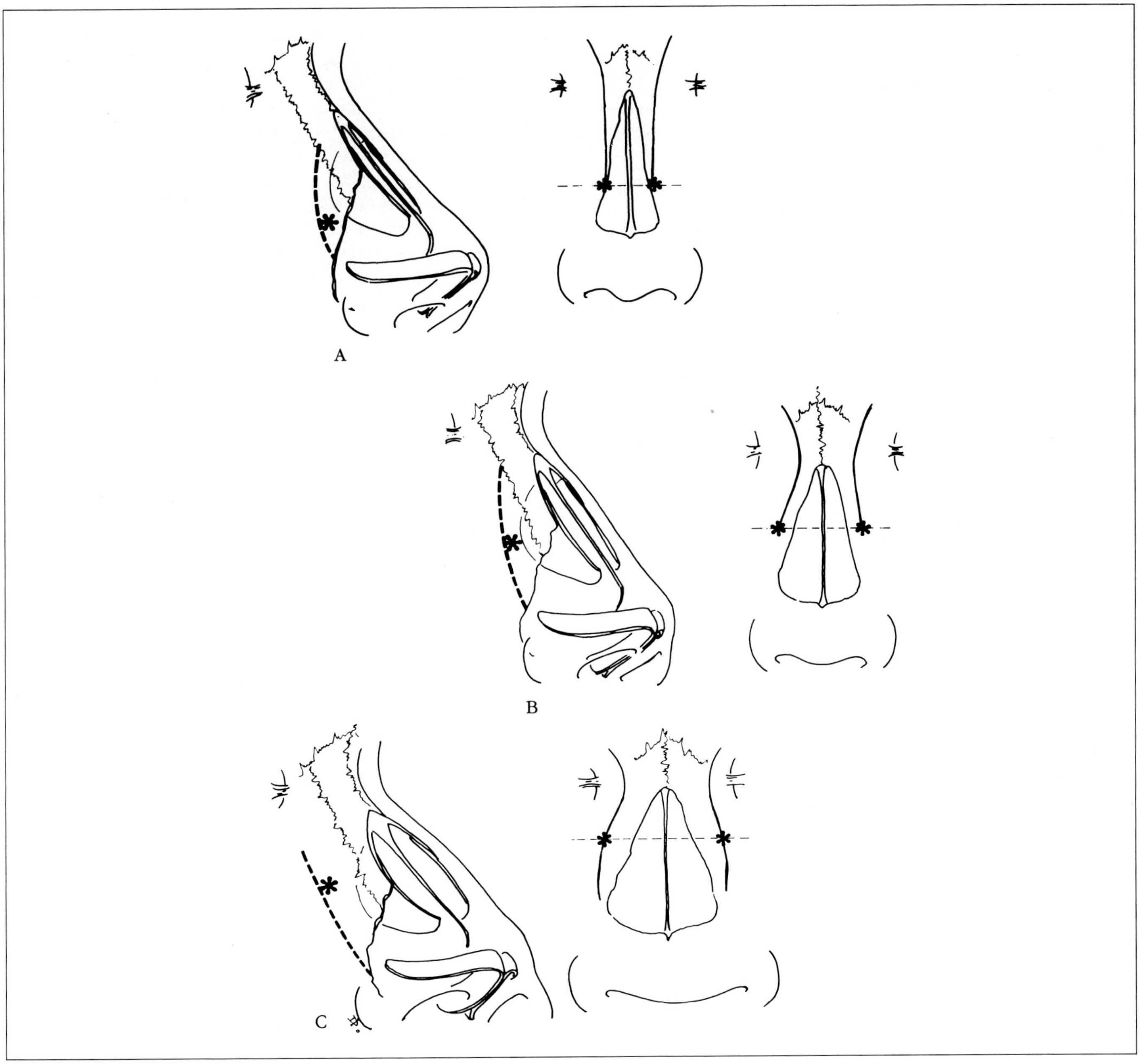

Figure 6-30. The X point for determining the type of lateral osteotomy.

A. In a narrow nose, the base bony width requires little movement and sharply angulated osteotomy is done.
B. In an average-width nose, a low-to-high osteotomy is used.
C. In a broad nose, a low-to-low osteotomy is used. The X point denotes the broadest point of the base width of the bony triangle as determined in the sitting patient.

Septum

Correction of septal deformities that cause respiratory obstruction and external deformities is an integral part of septorhinoplasty. The severity of the defects ranges from caudal deflections producing alar distortion and vestibular obstruction to serious osseocartilaginous displacement and total airway blockage. Since the subject is covered in great depth by Jost in Chapter 8, only a few principles will be presented here.

An accurate history and examination are essential in determining the etiology of airway obstruction, especially the significance of turbinate hypertrophy (allergic, compensatory, etc.) and septal deviation, which is the rule rather than the exception [8–10]. Whereas a submucous resection was performed in almost 100 percent of rhinoplasties by Aufricht [7], most surgeons now perform a limited septoplasty in about 10 to 25 percent of cases and treat the turbinates in 5 to 50 percent of patients complaining of respiratory obstruction. External deviations are readily visible and classifiable into bony (posterior or perpendicular plate of ethmoid), cartilaginous (caudal margin, midseptal), or combined. Internal deviations have been classified by locations, planes, and shapes (deflections, shelves, subluxation, overlaps). Careful preoperative examination, with a headlight, of normal and vasoconstricted mucosa is necessary, especially for detection of high and posterior septal deformities. Preoperatively, one must determine the location and type of septal deformity as well as the surgical procedure (septoplasty or resection). Internal obstructions are often correctable by limited procedures; external manifestations may require an endless combination of cross-hatchings, excisions, and eventually camouflage with dorsal grafts. The logical progression is correction of obstruction, deviation, and distortion.

With certain exceptions (severely displaced nasal deformities, friable mucosa, and chronic sinusitis), the septum is corrected as part of the aesthetic procedure [71]. Within the operative sequence, the senior author prefers to correct the septal deformity after removal of the dorsal hump and establishment of the new profile. As favored by Converse [26], this approach allows one to establish the definitive dorsum and then tailor the amount of septal excision, thereby maintaining adequate dorsal support and columellar projection. In contrast, the junior author corrects the septal problem before removing the dorsal hump. Gorney [64] prefers straightening the septum first as there is minimal bleeding and excellent visibility early. Also, modifications of the septum can cause significant changes in the dorsal line (elevation following correction of subluxation, depression following excision of caudal deflections). All resections are done through the transfixion incision, whereas isolated septoplasties are done through a classic Killian incision located 5 to 10 mm behind the caudal septal margin. Injection of the septum with isotonic saline or diluted local anesthetic performs hydrostatic dissection. Sharp dissection with either knife or scissors opens the subperichondrial plane and allows visualization of the bluish cartilage — "if it's not blue, it's not true." The extent of exposure is determined by the planned procedure: A submucous resection will require complete elevation on both sides; a septoplasty is confined to the concave surface of the deflection on one or both sides. Total exposure of the septum requires two planes of dissection — *subperiosteally* over the vomer and *subperichordially* over the quadrilateral septum with the intervening connective tissue sharply divided.

With current emphasis on conservation and the use of autogenous grafts for secondary surgery, extensive submucous resections are rarely performed. However, posterior bony deformities of vomer and ethmoid are excised with a double-action rongeur. Septal deflections associated with deviations of the anterior vomerine groove are corrected by fracturing the vomer and replacing it in the midline. Cartilaginous areas of overlap and shelf deformities are excised, with a 10-mm dorsal and caudal strut maintained. Most deflections in the midseptum are treated by scoring or cross-hatching the concave surface while preserving the attachment of the perichordium on the opposite side. Anterior deflections may be repositioned by being sutured to the nasal spine, directly excised if significant nasal shortening is required, or detached by means of a high septal transfixion incision with complete removal of the deformed portion followed by careful resuturing. After a radical submucous resection, many surgeons morselize the removed specimen and reinsert it between the mucosal flaps as support. Alternatively, the hump and alar cartilage remnants can be banked in occipital scalp for future use [138]. During the past 2 years, the approach described by Jost in Chapter 8 has been adopted with excellent results. Once the concepts are mastered, technical execution is far simpler than initially imagined.

Closure and Nasal Base

Prior to closing of the incision, a final check should be made of the entire nose. All debris and clots are removed by a curet or irrigation followed by suction. The nasal bones are palpated for any spicules, which are rasped down. The dorsal profile line can be checked visually and on palpation by pulling downward on the nasal tip. Resection of the caudal margin of the septum is checked by pushing the columella upward.

Closure of the nose is begun usually with a septocolumellar "transfixion suture." Joseph [77] attempted to elevate the tip with two superiorly angulated "orthopedic sutures" through the medial crus and septum. The effect was all too often a strangulated membranous septum, an obtuse nasolabial angle, and supratip swelling [31]. Currently, most surgeons feel that reliance on a transfixion suture to achieve tip elevation is futile. Rather, the goal is to bring the wound together with one or two transverse transfixion sutures of 4-0 catgut plus any additional septal sutures as required. The membranous septum is generally not excised, but the reflected mucosal lining may be partially removed following resection of a large protruding septal margin.

A check of the internal valve area is made. Any protruding portion of the upper lateral cartilage is trimmed con-

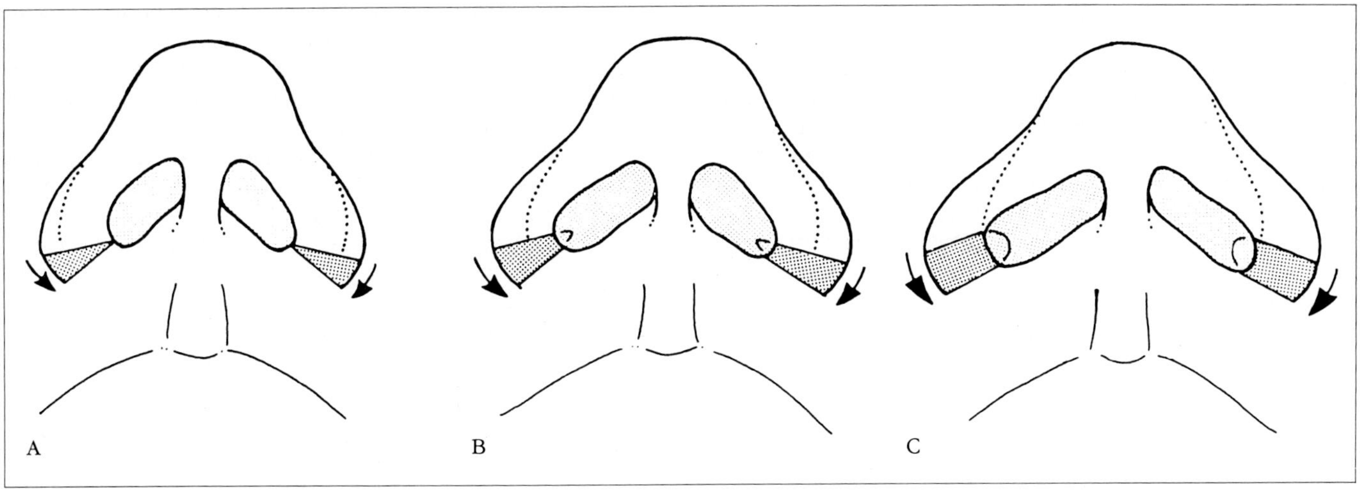

Figure 6-31. Sheen's two-surface approach for alar wedges.
A. Triangular excision for reducing the alae, but minimal effect on the nostril aperture.
B. A moderate decrease in the alae and minor diminution of the nostrils.
C. Maximum reduction of the alae and nostrils as well as significant narrowing of the alar base.

servatively and submucosally. Previously, Diamond [33] and others routinely excised the leading edge of the upper lateral cartilages to allow shortening of the nose—and did so early in the operation for better visualization. Next, all vestibular and rim incisions are closed with 5-0 plain catgut.

A decision is now made on whether modifying the nostril base is essential. Joseph frequently performed alar base reduction using a technique similar to Weir's, first, in a very large nose that required reduction in all dimensions, and second, if there was a dynamic flaring of the alar base secondary to lowering of the nasal tip. Millard added a third indication—artistic sculpting of the alar rims [94, 96]. Subsequently, alar wedges were performed with greater frequency, ranging from Lewis's 35 percent to Millard's 65 percent [84]. Unfortunately, significant complications began to occur: visible scars on the alar base, notching of the nostril sill, asymmetry, and excessive narrowing of the nostrils. In order to avoid these problems, one must have a clear understanding of the procedure's objectives and principles, as well as a careful surgical technique. Rees [120] uses alar base modification to narrow the nasal base and to shorten the nasal height. He excises a square segment of nostril floor to achieve narrowing but places the excision on the base of the alar lobule with a crescentic extension to achieve height reduction. Some vestibular skin is excised. Every effort is made to place the incisions in the natural groove. The procedures are considered an "adjunct" to enhance the results obtained with other procedures. Sheen [138] has different objectives based on a two-surface concept: first, modification of the alar lobule contour by excision of skin, and second, changes in the nostril perimeter by excision of vestibular skin. The mitigating factor is the relationship between the vertical plane of the alar lobule and the horizontal plane of the nasal base. Since an outward flare is normal, one should not rotate the alae when the alar-basal planes are perpendicular or inwardly displaced.

Additional patient variables that must be considered are (1) nostril width and configuration, (2) alar base–nostril floor juncture, which may be abrupt, blending, or a continuous curl, and (3) extent of flaring. When should the decision be made as to modifications of the alar bases? Preoperatively, certain patients can be diagnosed as requiring nasal base modification: (1) those who have a bulbous tip with alar bases extending beyond vertical lines dropped from the inner canthi, (2) those with a very projecting nose that will be lowered, and (3) those with abnormal axis of the nostrils, especially on more transverse orientation as seen on basilar view.

How should the alar base excision be done? As noted by Sheen [138], the "surgical look" is produced by notching of the nasal sill, which is avoided through maintaining a triangular medial flap, and by violation of the alar-facial groove, which is minimized by *always* placing the lower incision 1 to 2 mm above the groove. He alters the design of the alar base resection depending on the objective: (1) With excessive lobule and normal nostril, the wedge is placed entirely on the lobule (triangular); (2) with excessive lobule and redundant nostril, comparable amounts of lobule and vestibular skin (quadrangular) are used (Fig. 6-31). In contrast, Peck [110] does not excise vestibular skin whereas Stark [146] places the excision, not on the alar base, but more medially on the nostril floor. We prefer to sculpt the alar base and modify the nostrils as necessary using Sheen's principles.

Dressings

The dressing consists of intranasal pack, paper tape on the skin, and an overlying plaster cast. The purpose of the intranasal pack, which is done with a petrolatum-covered gauze, is to separate the raw surfaces, thereby preventing synechiae, and to promote coagulation from any oozing. Occasionally, a more generous packing will be necessary to compress septal flaps following submucous resection or severely comminuted "eggshell" nasal bones. The paper tape is designed to compress the dorsal skin gently and to help mold the nasal tip. The plaster cast serves to protect the nose, reduce edema, and reassure the patient. The nasal pack is removed on the second postoperative day unless extensive septal surgery has been performed, which delays its removal to the fourth or fifth day. Many surgeons have advocated no nasal packing and minimal dressings for short duration [150]. Prior to removal of the dressing on the seventh postoperative day, the patient is reminded that swelling will be present, that breathing will be partially obstructed for several weeks, and that occasional nonserious nosebleeds may occur [63].

SURGICAL TECHNIQUES

Technically, many surgeons conceive of a rhinoplasty as being three steps: tip modification, hump removal, and closure of the bony vault. With experience, execution becomes easier but improved results do not necessarily follow. Mastery of the rhinoplasty operation requires an understanding of "surgical cause and effect" as applied to an infinite variety of nasal anatomy. This understanding of the relationship between surgical technique and final appearance demands in-depth preoperative planning, detailed records of operative technique, frequent postoperative visits, and study of sequential photographs.

A Standard Technique

The senior author was taught to do rhinoplasties using the Joseph technique. However, selective acceptance and modification of new ideas have resulted in conversion from saws to osteotomes, from mucosal transection to mucosal preservation, from eversion of the alae to intracartilaginous incisions, and from subperiosteal to submucosal osteotomies. Numerous other innovations have been tried and either rejected or reserved for exceptional cases [121]. The following standard technique serves as a starting point and is modified to suit the individual patient (Fig. 6-32).

With the patient prepped and draped, the reference marks are made indicating the proposed changes in the alar cartilages, dorsum, and alar bases. Next, local anesthesia (0.50% Xylocaine with epinephrine 1:200,000) is injected both as a field block of the sensory nerves (infratrochlear, infraorbital, and anterior palatine) and to affect specific areas where dissection is planned (roof of nasal cavities, osteotomy sites, alar bases). In 90 percent of cases, an alar reduction is performed first via a crescentic excision just above the alar crease line. This maneuver reduces nasal flare, increases exposure, and provides access for the lateral osteotomies. Next, the intracartilaginous incisions are done, beginning in the dorsal area and passing laterally, with preservation of a 3- to 4-mm alar rim, and then medially as a transfixion incision through the membranous septum down to the nasal spine (Fig. 6-33). The alar cartilages are not removed until the dissection is complete. Elevation of the skin envelope is accomplished with small blunt scissors over the cartilaginous vault and with a periosteal elevator over the bony bridge. If a large hump is to be removed, as in a modified Skoog procedure, the undermining extends to the glabella, where the procerus and corrugator muscles are detached. The mucosa is separated from the upper alar cartilages, which are then removed leaving the lining intact. Certain modifications in the alae can be made, reducing the intact alar rim to 1 or 2 mm in width for thin-skinned patients with small tips, or excising cartilaginous triangles at the domes in thick-skinned patients with broad tips.

Next, an extramucosal dissection is done, beginning at the free border of the septum, with small sharp scissors. Previous injection of local anesthetic facilitates its separation. A submucosal elevator is passed along the cartilaginous septum and rolled outward to reflect the mucosa from the dorsal and upper lateral cartilages. Gentle dissection is continued up to the root of the nose. An en bloc hump removal is accomplished by dividing the cartilaginous components, the two upper lateral cartilages and septum, with straight scissors followed by separation of the bony component with a fine guarded osteotome (Robin type) (Fig. 6-34). Since the skin was elevated, the muscles were detached, and the mucosa was reflected downward, the hump is easily removed and preserved in one piece. The dorsum is inspected, any bone spicules are rasped smooth, and cartilaginous prominences are trimmed with scissors. The cartilaginous septal line is leveled accordingly and the lower edge modified as necessary for cephalic rotation, nasal shortening, or deepening of the nasolabial angle. The tip of the septal cartilage is rounded off, ensuring a tip differentiation. If septal abnormalities are present, they are corrected at this point but with preservation of an L-shaped remnant to prevent nasal collapse and columellar retraction.

Lateral osteotomies are performed to narrow the bone of the nasal pyramid and to close the open dorsal roof (Fig. 6-35). If alar wedges have been done, a narrow straight guarded osteotome is inserted through them; otherwise a small piriform stab wound is made. The guard is placed inside, thereby preserving the external periosteal and soft tissue attachments of the nasal walls [69]. This placement reduces the chances of nasal collapse and minimizes postoperative swelling. A low-to-low lateral osteotomy is done. A straight osteotome is then introduced in the midline, and the nasal bones are outfractured, completing the transverse fracture. Excess mucosa along the membranous septum is trimmed and the transfixion incision closed with two 4-0 Vicryl sutures; an effort is made to elevate the domes in relation to the septum. Each nostril is packed with petrolatum-covered gauze. The alar bases are closed first along the nostril base with an everting horizontal mattress suture followed by alar skin approximation with 6-0 silk. Micropore tape is applied to the skin and a preformed foam-backed aluminum splint taped on. The packing is removed 2 to 4 days postoperatively, the stitches in 5 to 6 days, and the splint at 1 week.

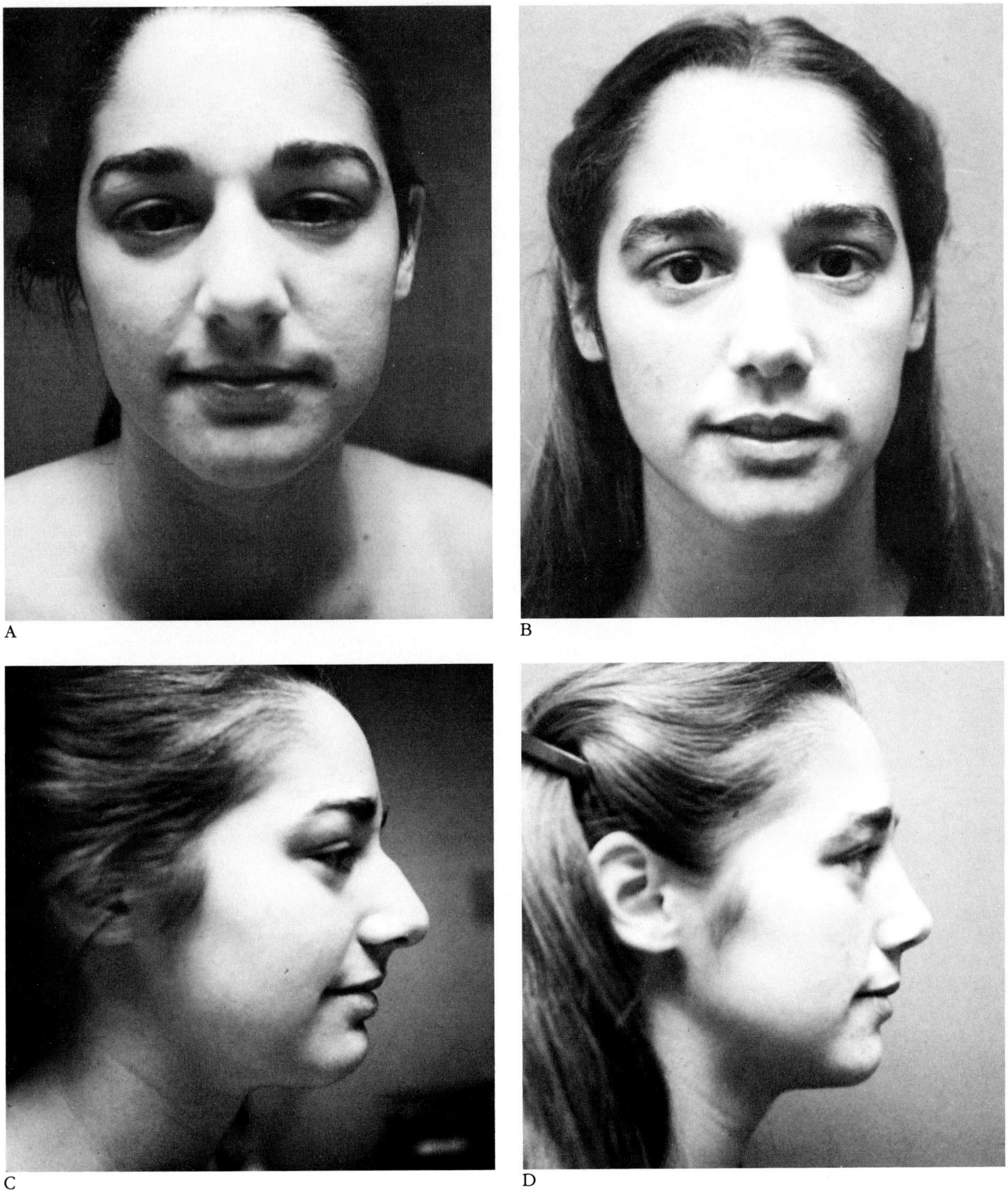

Figure 6-32
A, C. Patient with heavy thick skin, bulbous tip, dorsal hump, crowded nasolabial angle, and wide base.
B, D. Result following rhinoplasty with the atraumatic technique, demonstrating a more delicate tip, straight dorsum, open nasolabial angle, and narrower base.

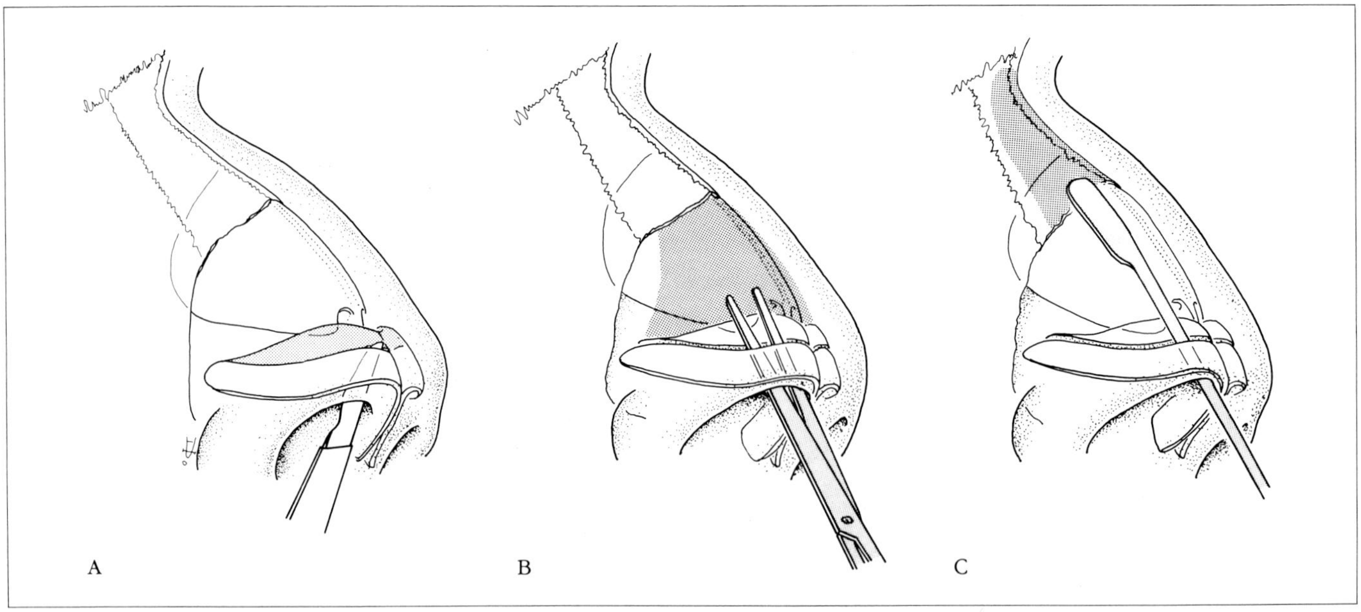

Figure 6-33
A. The intracartilaginous incision starts at the dome, leaves 3 to 4 mm of alar rim, and then reverses through the membranous septum to complete the transfixion incision.
B. The soft tissues overlying the cartilaginous vault are undermined with small blunt nose scissors.
C. A periosteal elevator is used to elevate the soft tissues over the bony vault.

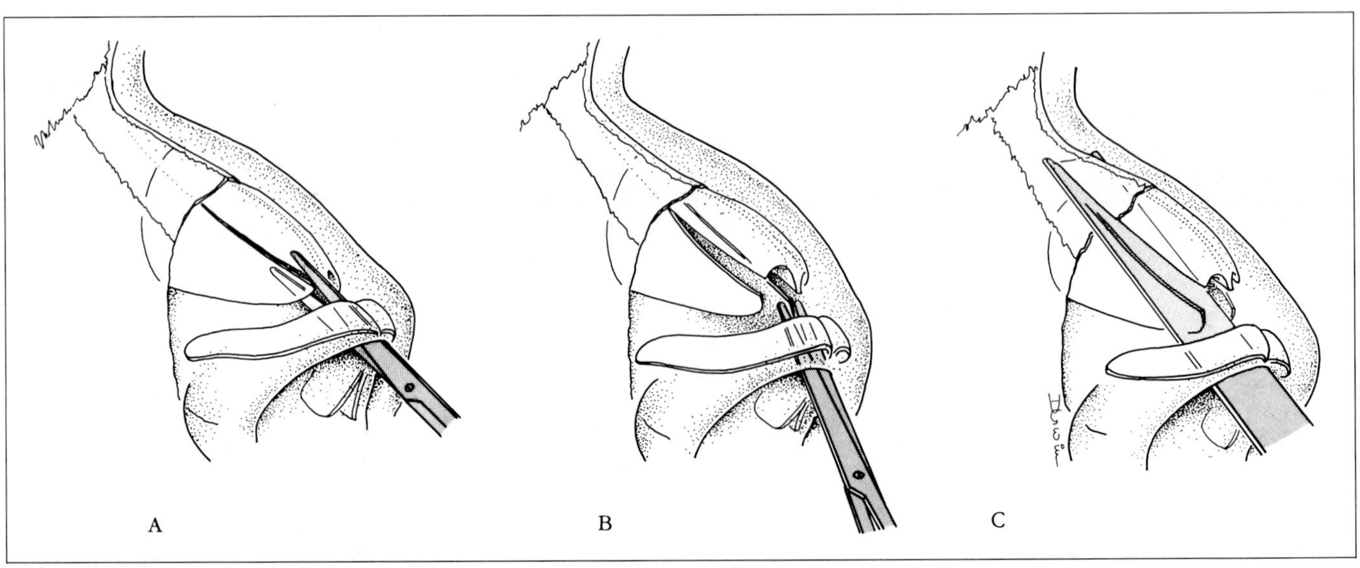

Figure 6-34. Following endomucosal dissection, the dorsal hump is removed in en bloc fashion.
A, B. The upper laterals and cartilaginous septum are divided, using straight scissors.
C. A fine guarded osteotome is inserted and the hump completely detached.

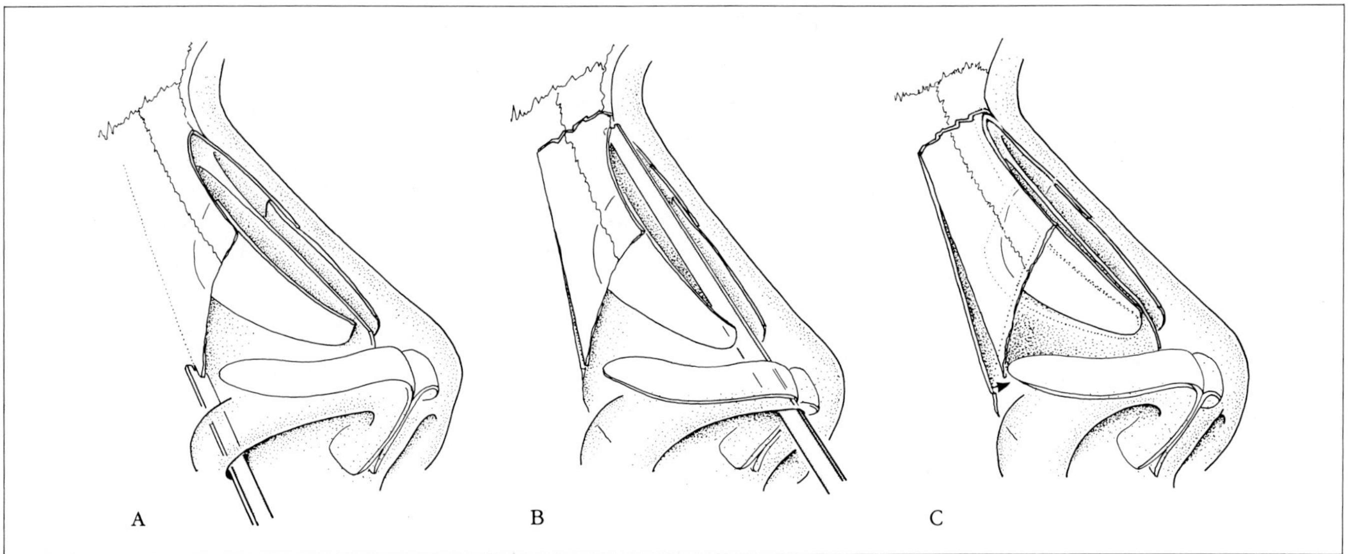

Figure 6-35. The osteotomies and fractures allow narrowing of the nose.
A. A low-to-low osteotomy is done with the guard on the mucosal side.
B. A straight osteotome is inserted medially and passed along the midline; then outfracturing is done.
C. Narrowing is accomplished by digital pressure, which completes the transverse fracture.

The advantages of this technique are the following: (1) It is minimally traumatic; (2) the incisions are few in number and limited in length; (3) the nasal valve and all mucosa are preserved; (4) it is economical in time and maneuvers; and (5) postoperative recovery is quick, as edema and ecchymosis are minimal. The principal disadvantages are that it requires precise preoperative planning, careful judgment of the cartilaginous excisions, and flawless execution of the osteotomies. Additional modifications and tip refinements may be difficult for the inexperienced.

The Controlled Rhinoplasty

Traditionally, rhinoplasty is a "blind operation" based on the surgeon's artistic concept and conducted by "feel" through a restricted exposure. Learning the procedure as a resident is difficult because direct observation is impossible, a second side is not available, and few surgeons are comfortable teaching it. In the early years of a practice, most surgeons will gratefully accept a majority of "good" results as pursuit of superb results often leads to excessive resection requiring complicated secondary procedures. Thus, a flexible controlled technique that maximizes visualization and minimizes downside risk has evolved, based on the contributions of Peck [110] and Sheen [138]. The junior author uses this operation in the majority of his cases (Fig. 6-36).

As with all rhinoplasties, careful preoperative evaluation and planning are essential. The five aesthetic components of the nose are assessed from the three planes of reference. Utilizing black-and-white photographs for additional information, a decision is made as to the need for a modification of each component part. Next, the structures are carefully palpated and the feasibility of potential surgical maneuvers is judged. Then, sketches are made of how to modify the cartilages, anterior septum, and dorsal hump as well as the anticipated fracture lines. The sequence of steps is usually tip-dorsum-septum-osteotomy-base.

The reference lines are marked, and the highest points of the two domes are dotted with needle and dye, much as otoplasty markings are made. Local infiltration is done in the standard fashion. Additional small amounts are instilled along the alar margin and tip, and high in the nasal vault, facilitating dissection and removal of subcutaneous tissue. The operation begins through infracartilaginous and intercartilaginous incisions, with the latter extended to the upper half of the membranous septum as a transfixion incision. With skin hook traction on the underside of the domes, the alar cartilages are separated from the overlying skin with blunt-tipped scissors. Once the two incisions are joined, the tip of a small hemostat is passed through the intercartilaginous incision and back out the nostril, thereby delivering the alar cartilages. Extension of the infracartilaginous incision medially to the upper one-third of the columella and the intercartilaginous incision laterally is often necessary. All overlying soft tissue is removed. The amount of alar rim to be preserved is measured—usually 3 to 4 mm; the excess upper alar cartilage is then excised. The lateral tail and underlying mucosa are kept intact. A decision is made as to the need for altering the shape or height of the crura; most often interdigitating cuts to narrow the width. It is essential that any modification of tip projection be made at this point to allow accommodation in subsequent dorsal changes. Scissors are used to undermine the nasal skin over the upper lateral cartilage. Beginning laterally, a subperiosteal tunnel is created over the nasal bones and a limited area elevated, using the Joseph elevator. With double hook traction, the leading edge of the cartilaginous septum is exposed and the subperichondral plane exposed. By means of a small elevator, a submucosa pocket is dissected longitudinally along the upper septum, beneath the hump medially and laterally under the upper lateral cartilages and nasal bones. Next, the bony hump is lowered with a rough rasp followed by a smoother one and then a fine rasp to smooth the edges, especially the upper caudal edge of the nasal bones. Free bony fragments are removed by irrigation with suction or a curet. Then, under direct vision afforded by a headlight and the Aufricht retractor, the cartilaginous hump is excised with straight scissors—first the upper laterals and then the cartilaginous septum. At this point the dorsal line is checked by downward traction on the tip. Any irregularities are shaved off under direct vision by a blunt-tipped No. 11 blade.

The anterior leading edge of the septum is modified submucosally as required, achieving the desired tip rotation, nasal shortening, and modification of the nasolabial angle. A convexity of the leading edge is maintained, and conservatism in nasal spine resection is practiced, the former achieved with straight scissors and the latter with small osteotomes. The lateral osteotomies are done through a small transverse incision in the piriform aperture with a 4-mm osteotome. A subperiosteal pocket is not dissected. Sequential linked cuts are made in a sloping direction from low to high, and the transverse fracture is initiated. The majority of transverse fractures are greenstick breaks resulting in sufficient movement at the piriform aperture to allow closing the "open roof" but without narrowing the radix. Final tip refinements are made as necessary, often suturing the crura or placing an onlay graft. Then the transfixion incision is closed with either a through-and-through mattress suture or individual interrupted sutures using 4-0 plain catgut. The length of the upper lateral cartilages is checked and any excess removed submucosally. The infracartilaginous incisions are closed with 5-0 plain catgut. The decision for alar base modification is usually made preoperatively, and this is performed as a final step, with a circumalar crescentic excision placed *above* the alar facial groove. If the nostrils

Figure 6-36. A controlled rhinoplasty performed on a 23-year-old art student who requested a more refined nose plus correction of the anterior septal deviation.
A, C, E. The cartilaginous vault is slightly curved to the left and the alar bases are at different levels. The tip is bulbous and plunging on anterior view despite an open nasolabial angle.
B, D, F. Postoperatively, the nose is straight, the tip light reflex narrower, the lobule triangular on basal view, and the caudal septum returned to the nasal spine.

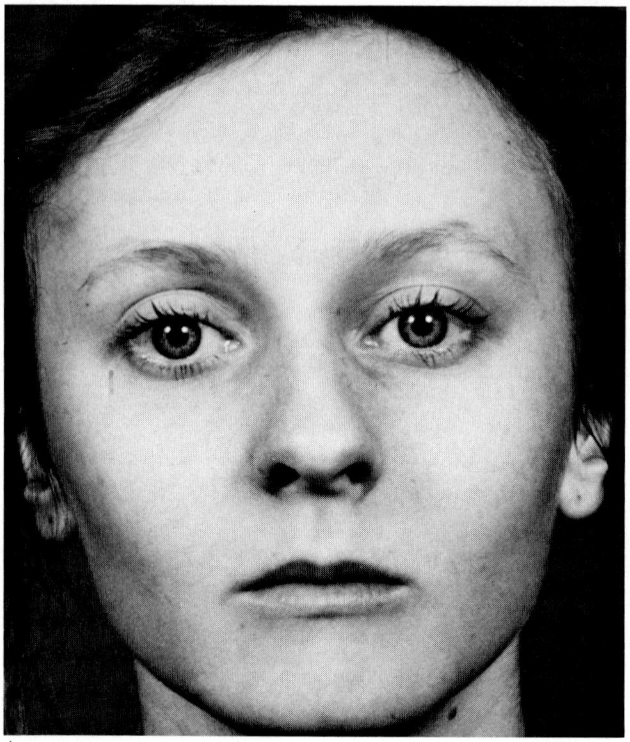
A

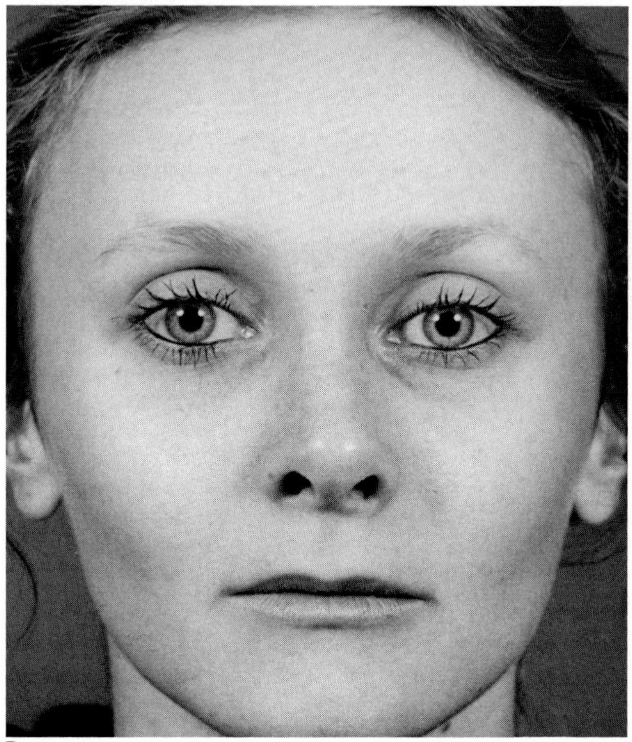
B

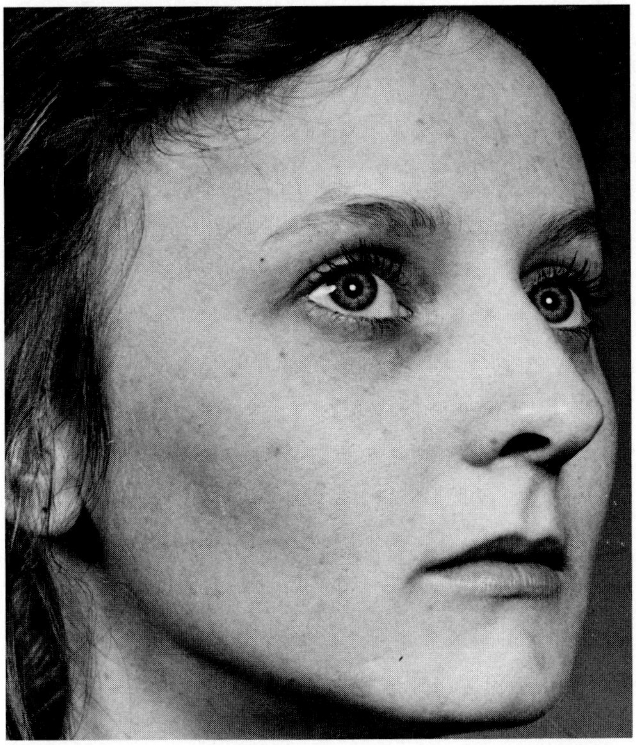

C

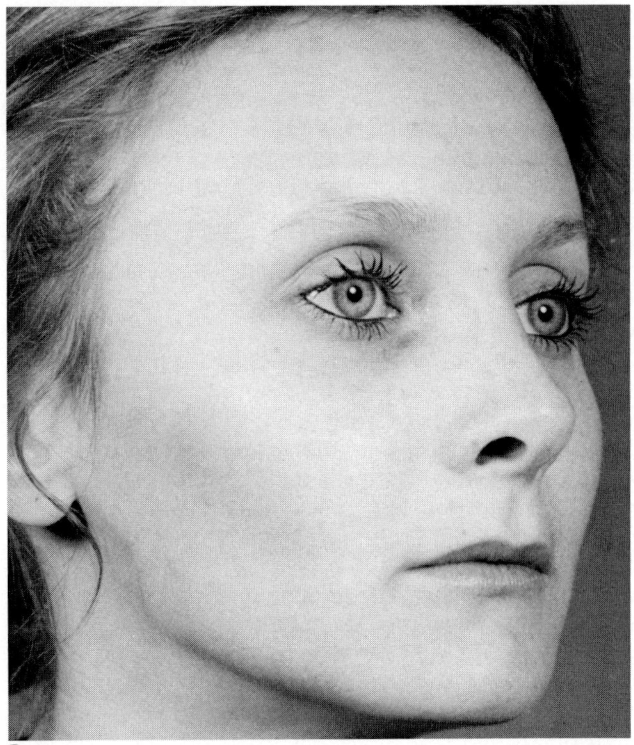

D

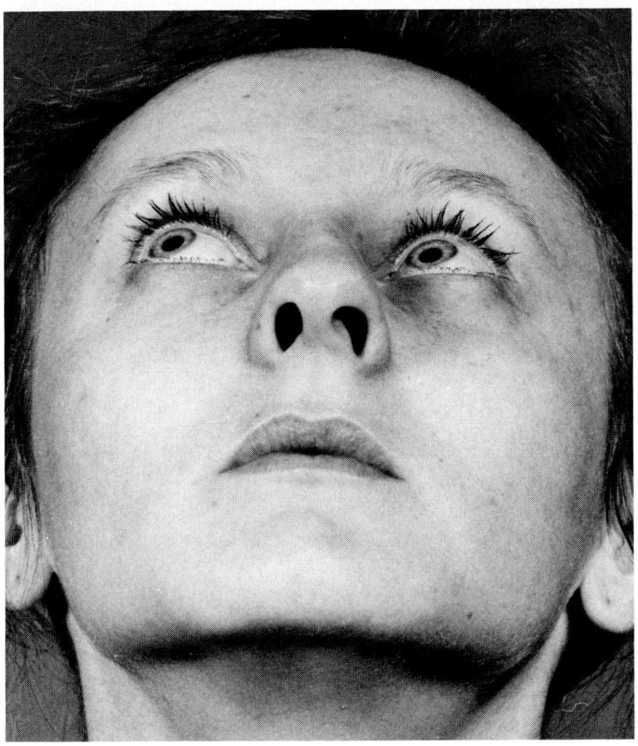

E

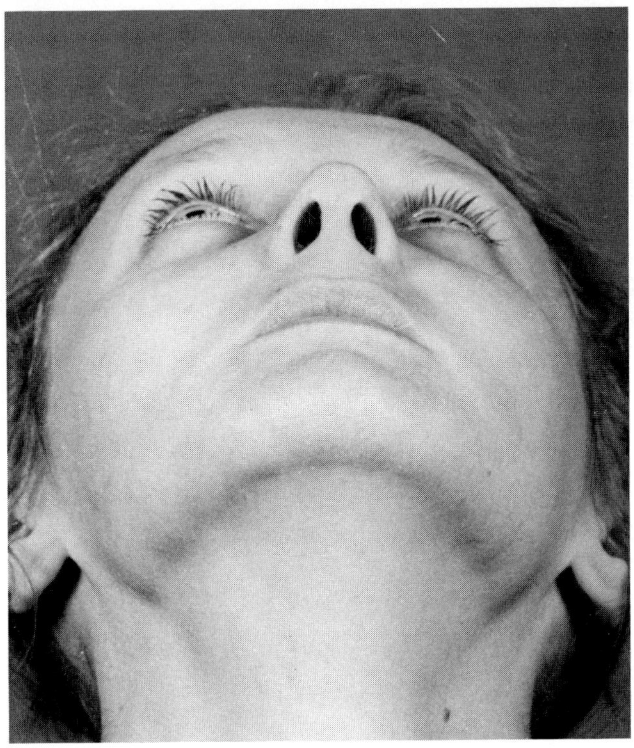

F

appear to flare following nasal tip modification, their width is reduced by a wedge excision in the nostril floor. A limited nasal pack is inserted to minimize synechiae. Then overlapping half-inch micropore tape is applied to the nose. A divided Telfa pad is placed slick side down to facilitate subsequent cast removal and cotton side up to ensure cast adherence. A plaster of paris cast is applied over the bony and cartilaginous vaults followed by a covering of half-inch adhesive tape.

The advantages of the controlled rhinoplasty are as follows: (1) Major tip modifications are done under direct vision, ensuring accuracy, symmetry, and conservatism; (2) all mucosa is preserved; (3) bony hump removal is rarely excessive because the rasp is used; (4) cartilaginous hump removal is incremental; (5) the osteotomies are exact without requiring continuation of initial alignment; (6) tip support is maximized; and (7) its inherent conservatism permits simple secondary revision rather than reconstruction.

Several disadvantages also exist: (1) Two separate incisions are required; (2) dissection is greater over the alar cartilages; (3) there is more fiddling with the osseocartilaginous dorsum; (4) more traumatic osteotomies produce greater postoperative ecchymosis; and (5) operating time is longer. However, the junior author considers the controlled rhinoplasty a safe, teachable method with minimal downside risk.

The External Rhinoplasty

Numerous external incisions have been used for performing rhinoplasty including the midline dorsal incision of Dieffenbach [34], the glabellar–lateral incision of Peterson [114], and the columellar incision of Rethi [123, 124]. A modification of the latter was utilized routinely by Sercer [132, 133] and Padovan [106, 107] in more than a thousand cases and was found to offer excellent exposure with minimal scarring (Fig. 6-37). The junior author uses the external technique, as described by Goodman [60–62] and colleagues, in approximately 7 percent of cases (33 out of 472) and finds it particularly valuable for certain aesthetic indications: (1) significant tip asymmetries, (2) complicated secondary cases, and (3) twisted noses with osseocartilaginous deviations (Fig. 6-38).

Following the instillation of local anesthesia and patient preparation, an inverted-V incision is drawn at the midcolumellar level. The skin on either side of the incision is dotted with dye at three points to ensure an accurate closure. Bilateral infracartilaginous incisions are completed first and the alar cartilages separated from the overlying soft tissue. Next, the midcolumellar incision is made with a No. 15 blade beginning at the notch and extending laterally with great care to avoid damaging the border of the medial crura. With blunt-tipped scissors the central columella is undermined up to the tip, and then the lateral skin edges are freed from the underlying me-

Figure 6-37. The external rhinoplasty.
A. A superiorly darted midcolumellar incision is made over the middle third of the medial crura; dots facilitate realignment on suturing.
B. It is combined with an infracartilaginous incision, which will allow an unparalleled exposure of the nasal anatomy.

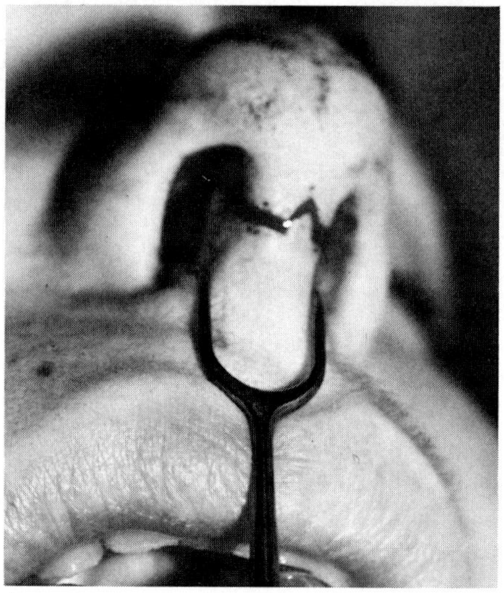
A

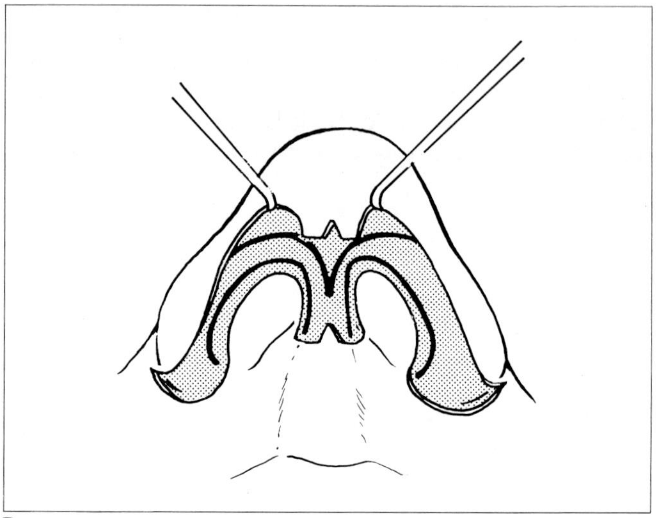
B

dial crura. With skin hook traction on the domes, the dissection is completed over the tip and beyond the weak triangle onto the upper lateral cartilages. Transmuscular dissection should be avoided by passing directly onto the cartilaginous dorsum. The subperiosteal plane is entered with the Joseph knife and the hump completely exposed.

Following skin elevation, the alar cartilages are modified according to size, shape, and projection. Abundant soft tissue can be removed from the tip area especially overlying and between the alar cartilages. Correction of bifidity and alar asymmetries and insertion of grafts are facilitated. Access to the anterior septum is gained by reflection of the mucosal lining in the weak triangle area, which can be continued to the anterior septal area. As in the extramucosal method, longitudinal tunnels are created beneath the dorsum. Total exposure of the septum is achieved by division of the upper lateral cartilages at their septal juncture and medial osteotomies of the nasal bone as required. With outward traction on the upper lateral cartilages and downward traction on the domes, unrivaled exposure of the septum is gained, permitting correction of the most twisted nose, a high septal deviation, or even perforations. The dorsal profile is lowered by means of heavy scissors—first the septal component and then the lateral walls [53]. The lateral osteotomies are performed through piriform aperture stab incisions with a guarded osteotome passed submucosally. Following the fractures, the degree of dorsal reapproximation is checked and the contour assessed. If medial movement was prevented by bony triangles in the radix, direct removal is possible, thus avoiding a "rocker" phenomenon. The upper laterals are sutured together with the septum using 4-0 Vicryl suture. Morselized cartilage grafts are inserted under direct vision to correct any depressions or asymmetries. The columella incisions are approximated with a midline subcutaneous 5-0 catgut suture and the skin edges closed with 6-0 silk. The infracartilaginous incision is sutured meticulously with 5-0 plain catgut. A standard dressing is applied. The patient is instructed to keep the columella incision line free of crusts using dilute hydrogen peroxide. The silk sutures are removed on day 4 or 5.

The advantages of the external approach are many: (1) One has total exposure of and free access to all structures; (2) tip modification is easier, especially suturing; (3) septal deviations can be totally corrected; (4) there is flexibility for dealing with difficult tips (bifid, bulbous, parenthesis, plunging) and diversity of cartilaginous vaults; (5) it is possible to evaluate and correct difficult secondary deformities; (6) teaching residents is facilitated because all structures and maneuvers are visible; and (7) studies of nasal anatomy and pathology are possible.

The disadvantages are few but formidable: (1) Any external scar may be unacceptable to the patient, no matter how fine; (2) the surgeon must adapt basic concepts and practiced techniques for a radically different exposure; (3) elevation of the skin envelope makes sequential assessment of the final results more difficult; and (4) resolution of tip swelling is undoubtedly slower. In contrast to Goodman, who employs the external approach for most of his rhinoplasties, we continue to follow Padovan's original indications with emphasis on asymmetries, twisted noses, congenital deformities, and difficult secondaries [106]. Within this context the results have been excellent and are clearly superior to those achieved with other types of external incisions [38].

Autogenous Grafts

The results of secondary rhinoplasty improved dramatically once the etiology was understood to be a deficiency rather than an excess of tissue in most cases. The void is best filled with autogenous tissue [93]. Subsequently, the value of cartilage grafts in primary rhinoplasty also became evident. Currently, the authors use autogenous grafts in more than 20 percent of primary rhinoplasties either to improve the profile line or as fillers to correct asymmetries. Our conviction is that it is better to utilize grafts of available tissue at the primary operation than to fabricate them from distant sources at a second procedure.

PRINCIPLES

Permanence of the grafts has often been questioned. However, Sheen [134], Lamont [82], and others have unequivocally demonstrated survival of the grafts for 10 to 20 years. Retention of the perichondrium is not necessary for survival, and it is usually removed. Many donor sites are available, including excised material (dorsal hump, alar cartilages, septum) or other sources harvested especially for the purpose (septum, vomer, ethmoid plate, concha) [37]. When grafts are employed as structural components, careful shaping is essential, especially beveling of the edges, whereas morselization is mandatory when the tissue is used as filler. Gentle crushing in a Cottle morselizer fragments the cartilage, eliminates its structural memory, and allows it to conform within the skin envelope. In contrast to secondary rhinoplasties, in which tight pockets ensure fixation, most structural grafts in primary cases should be positioned with guide sutures (5-0 plain catgut) passing through the graft and overlying skin. These sutures are merely taped to the skin and cut flush with the surface on removal of the dressing. Although applications are numerous, the three most common indications will be discussed: dorsal augmentation, tip projection, and asymmetries.

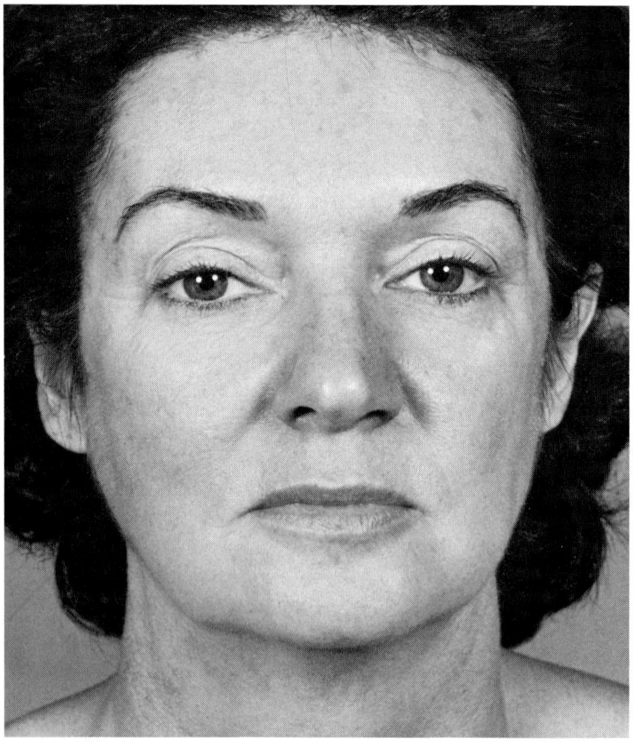

A

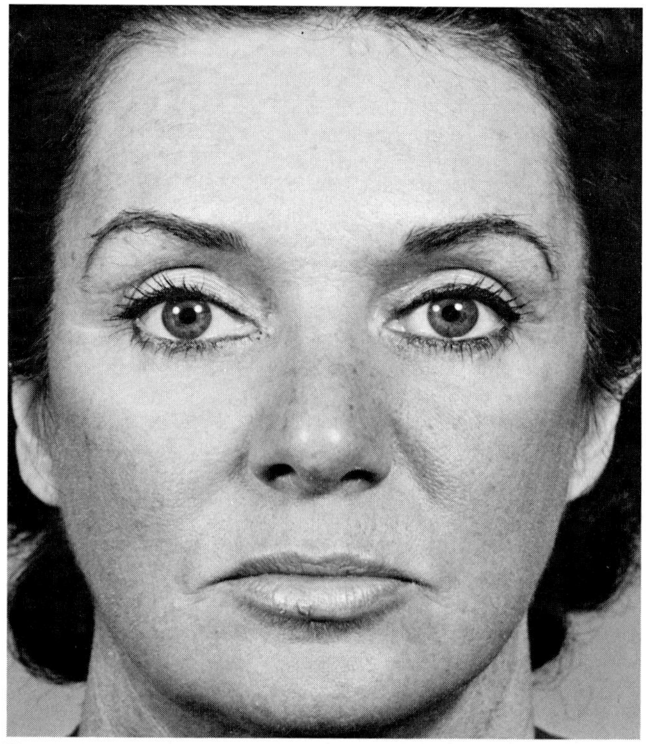

B

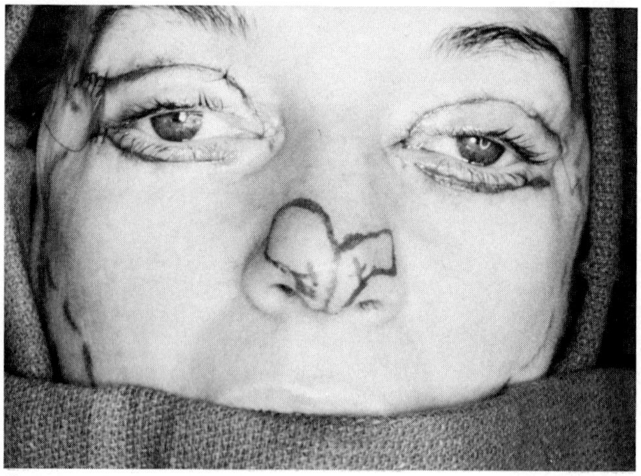

C

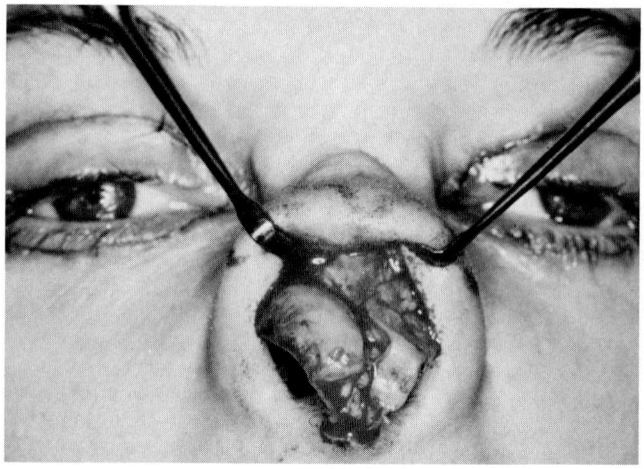

D

Figure 6-38

A, E. A 50-year-old patient sought facial rejuvenation including cervicofacial rhytidectomy, four-eyelid blepharoplasty, and septorhinoplasty.

B, F. Result following suturing of the domes, interdigitating cuts on the right alar cartilage, and onlay grafts of the left alar cartilage. Note subtle change in the tip light reflex.

C. On preoperative examination, a marked asymmetry of the alar cartilages was detected, which influenced domal locations and lateral configurations.

D. Because of the marked asymmetries, an external approach was used. Following elevation of the nasal skin, the right lateral alar cartilage is seen to be convex while the left is concave-convex-concave. Also, the domes are divergent in all three planes.

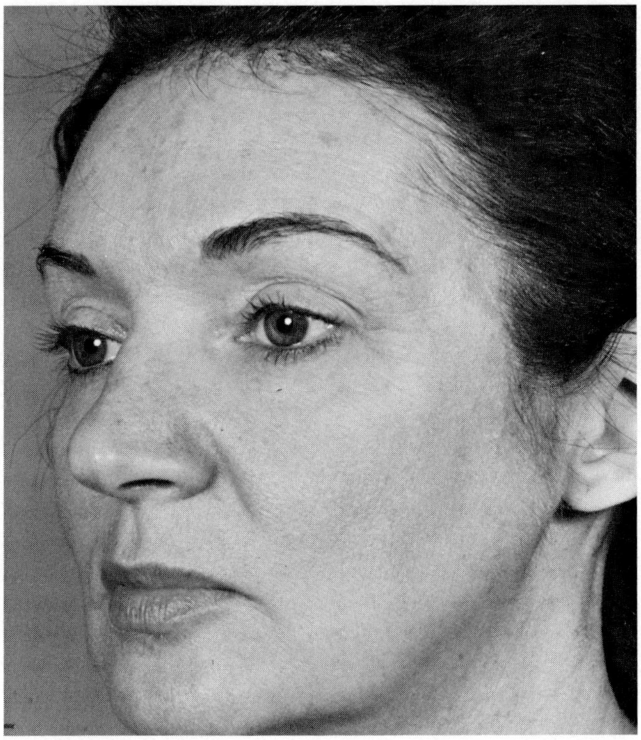

E

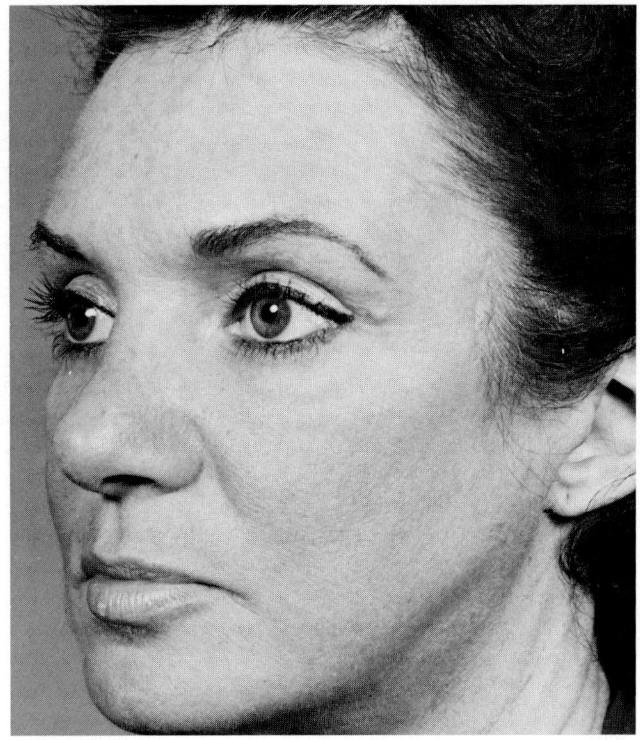

F

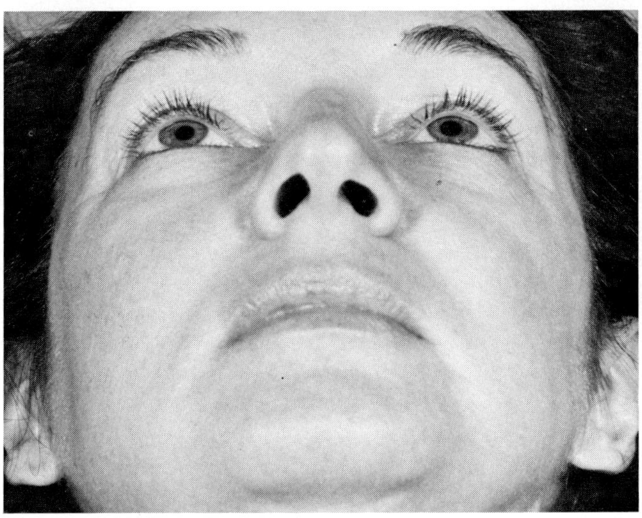

G

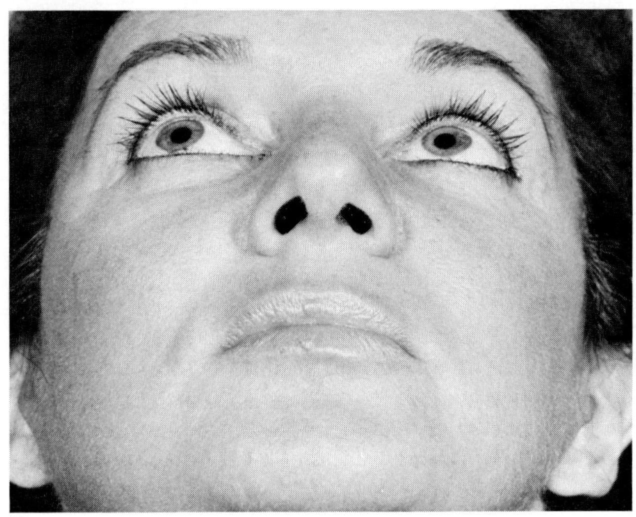

H

Figure 6-38 (continued)
G. Preoperative basal view. Note arching of right nostril and relative collapse of left nostril due to lateral crus asymmetry.
H. Postoperative basal view without visibility of scar.

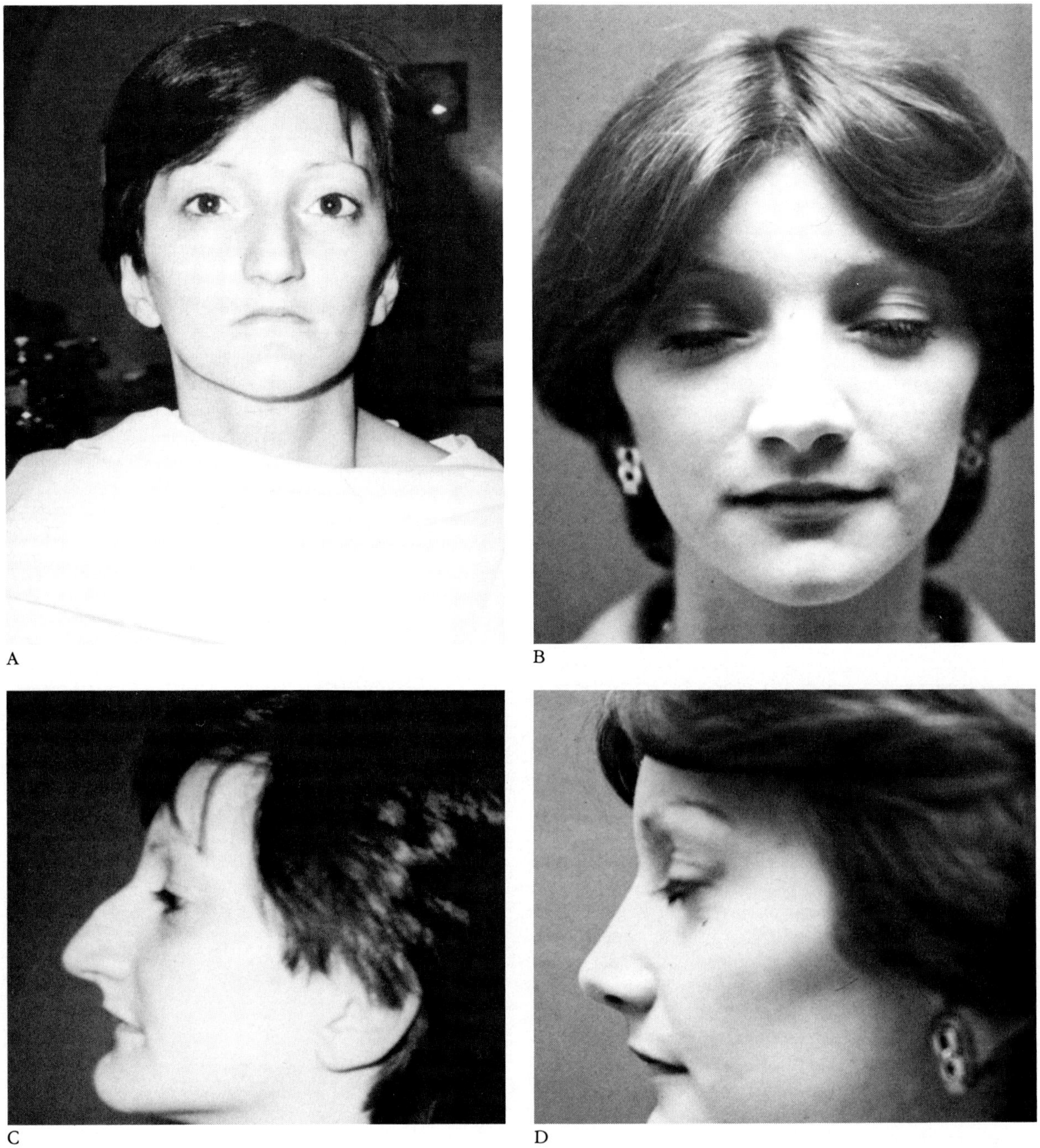

Figure 6-39
A, C. Patient with a massive "beak" and sloping forehead.
B, D. Result following a modified Skoog rhinoplasty with reinsertion of a modified hump.

DORSAL AUGMENTATION

Placement of dorsal grafts is either preplanned or an unfortunate necessity. A preoperative decision to use a dorsal graft includes the Skoog [143] procedure for management of the large dorsal hump, the short nasal bone syndrome, and concealment of curvatures not amenable to more radical surgery. The principle of autografting the nasal dorsum was first published by Cottle [27] and refined by Skoog [144]. Reinsertion of the resected hump is indicated for patients seeking nasal reduction without a change in shape and those with very large noses, especially if deepening of the glabellar area is planned. Our technique differs from Skoog's primarily in using extramucosal dissection and a razor-sharp thin double-guarded osteotome, which ensure en bloc resection (Fig. 6-39). Once the hump is removed, it is shaped and cleaned of septal remnants [122]. The external lining is left intact as it smooths the graft. It is reinserted and modified until the desired shape is achieved. With the graft in place, the bony and cartilaginous components match the osseocartilaginous framework and rarely require suture fixation to the septum. From experience with more than 200 cases, the senior author has found several advantages of hump reinsertion: (1) It serves as an internal splint, which avoids numerous secondary deformities in the large nose, especially middle-third retraction; (2) it provides a natural appearance without surgical stigmata; and (3) revisions, where necessary, are easily done by rasping or graft removal. The disadvantage is the technically demanding step of removing an en bloc hump and then judging the amount to be reinserted. Although not used routinely, this modified Skoog technique is ideal for the patient with a large nose, especially one requiring a deeper nasolabial angle.

In contrast, certain patients will present with short nasal bones or with a dorsal curvature in which concealment is preferred to a complete septorhinoplasty and submucous resection. As defined by Sheen [138], short nasal bones exist when the bony pyramid is less than one-third the distance from radix to septal angle and is characterized by a narrow upper vault and bilateral concavities in the cartilaginous vault. Nasal fractures in patients with this defect narrow the nose further and may impede respiration. Osteotomies are therefore contraindicated. A portion of the removed cartilaginous hump is reinserted as a dorsal graft to close the open roof and to support the middle vault. Concealment of deviated nasal components, as opposed to a deviation of the entire nose, can be achieved with judicious use of autogenous grafts. Where no hump removal is done, a long septal graft of cartilage and perpendicular plate of ethmoid can be harvested (Fig. 6-40). Heavy scissors are used to trim the graft, thereby avoiding separation into two components, and then the cartilage is carefully beveled. The primary error is too wide a graft, which can be avoided by assessing its width on lateral downward traction of the skin. Additional height can be achieved by stacking the grafts, placing smaller portions underneath rather than on top, which merely creates a new hump. For small dorsal irregularities, cartilaginous remnants are morselized and inserted as filler.

TIP GRAFTS

Insertion of cartilaginous grafts into the nasal tip is used in a spectrum from minor deformities requiring concealment (asymmetry, bifidity), which can be achieved with morselized cartilage, to moderate deficiencies corrected by dorsal augmentation using Peck's technique, to the most severe inadequacies requiring concealment plus creation of a new tip [112]. Sheen characterizes the tip with inadequate projection (TIP) as being a downward inclination toward the nasal spine, caused by a combination of a short columella and inadequate arch of the lower lateral cartilages [138]. The solution is to augment the inadequacy of tissue and to conceal the uncorrectable structures by creating an illusion of a new tip (Fig. 6-41). The tip grafts recommended by Sheen have the following attributes: (1) They are composed of septal cartilage; (2) they are quite large (20 mm long, 5–8 mm wide) and taper downward from a rounded or bidorsal top to an inferior notch; (3) insertion is through a rim incision with a 35-degree cephalic tilt; and (4) the base is at the columellar-lobular junction. With this approach, one can achieve significant tip projection creating the illusion of lengthening the nose and avoiding a rounded "snipped-off" appearance.

Chin

Since the nose-chin relationship is a critical determinant of facial balance, chin modification is required in approximately 10 percent of patients seeking improved appearance. If normal dental occlusion is present, correction is possible concurrent with septorhinoplasty and produces dramatic improvement. Conversely, failure to alleviate the imbalance can lead to persistent patient dissatisfaction focused on the nose rather than the primary chin deformity. Careful analysis of photographs using the intersecting Frankfort and facial planes can demonstrate the required adjustment to the patient and allow an objective decision [20].

AUGMENTATION MENTOPLASTY

Historically, chin augmentation was done by inserting the resected dorsum devoid of its lining through an external incision. Although undeniably effective, the dorsal hump is rarely large enough to correct the deficiency adequately. Therefore, silastic implants were developed and can be inserted through an intraoral incision placed 1 cm above the lower labial sulcus (Fig. 6-42). The pocket is developed by sharp dissection above the periosteum and extending laterally with preservation of the mental nerves. With implants having a marked midline, it is possible to center the prosthesis exactly and achieve the desired projection. The critical factors are making the lateral pocket sufficiently long to avoid bending, and placing the prosthesis over the bone, thereby avoiding downward droop or upward fullness. A double-layer closure of 4-0 Vicryl is used, and drains are not necessary. The implant is carefully held in place, ensuring sufficient downward pressure. Prophylactic antibiotics are used for 1 week.

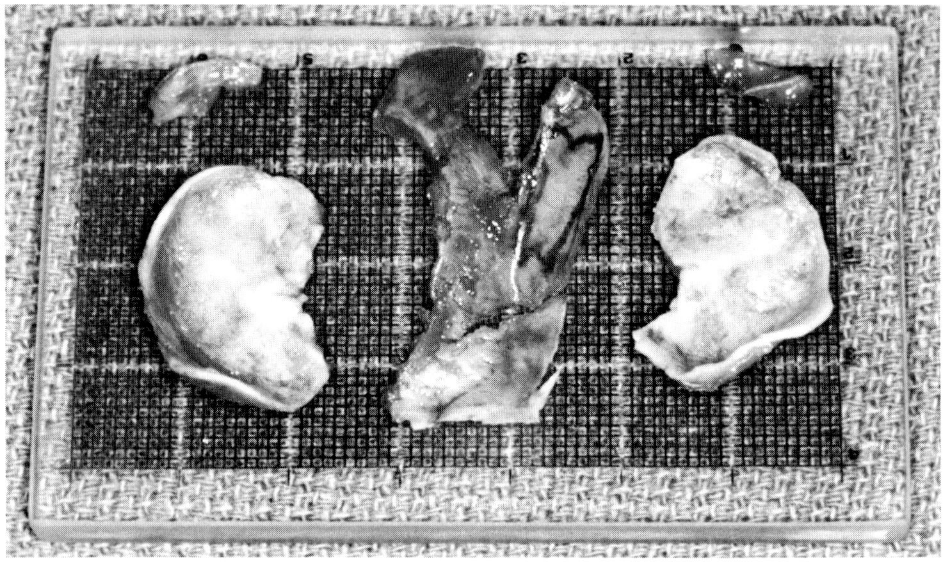

A

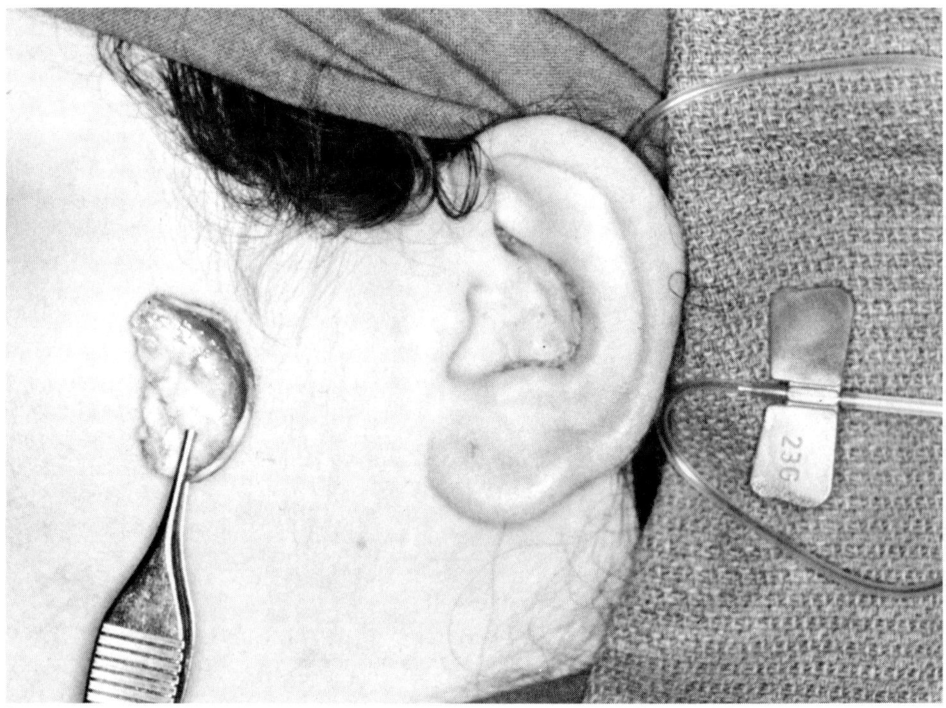

B

Figure 6-40

A. Autogenous graft materials include the resected alar cartilages, both conchae, and a large portion of the cartilaginous septum–perpendicular plate of ethmoid.

B. The conchal graft is harvested through an anterior incision.

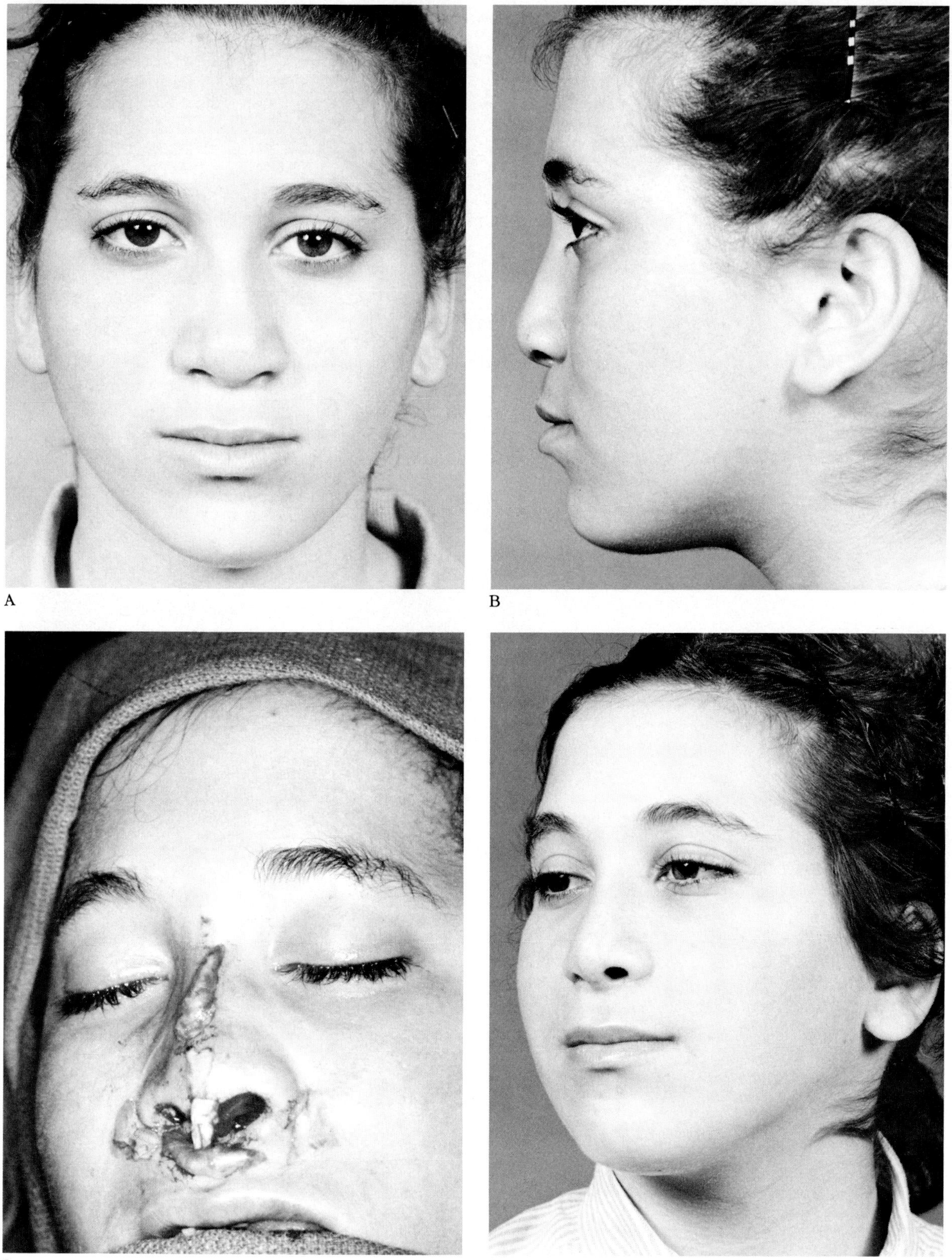

A B C D

Figure 6-41

A, B. A 15-year-old with marked nasal flattening, septal deviation, maxillary hypoplasia, and an acute nasolabial angle. Previous evaluation did not reveal any evidence of facial clefts.

C. Since the patient is a severe juvenile diabetic, allografts were considered contraindicated. Virtually every source of autogenous grafts was used to augment the nose and maxillary foundation.

D. Result showing marked improvement in appearance.

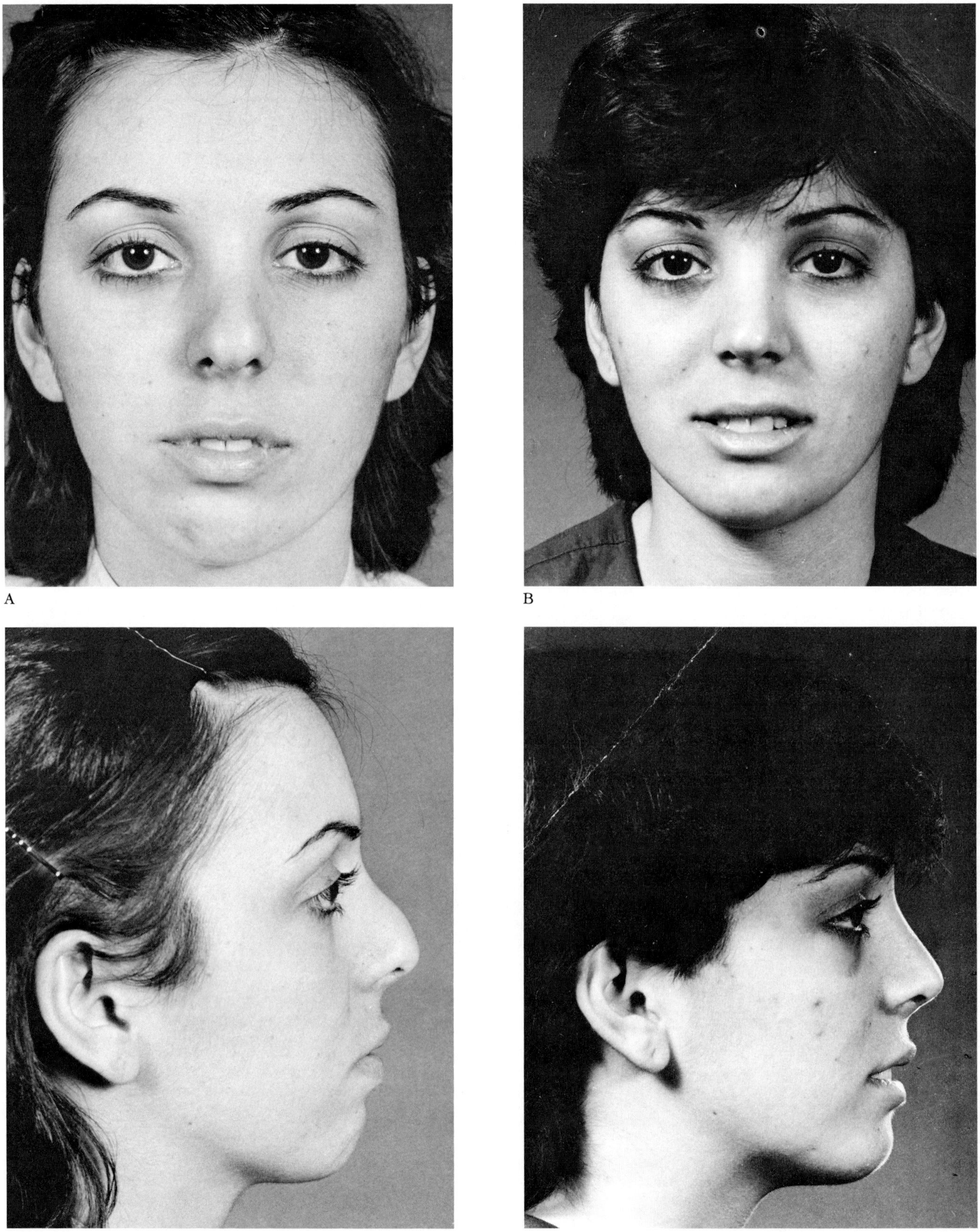

A B C D

Figure 6-42

A, C. A 19-year-old who requested septorhinoplasty. After consultation, the patient accepted the suggestion of a silastic chin implant.

B, D. A small implant was inserted through an intraoral incision producing a more aesthetic profile.

REDUCTION MENTOPLASTY
In an average plastic surgery practice, 1 to 2 percent of patients seeking septorhinoplasty will request reduction of a prominent chin. Approximately half will have an occlusal problem requiring an osteotomy while the rest can be treated by a local reduction mentoplasty [142]. The alternative procedures are a simple reduction of the mental prominence using a high-speed bur, as described by McKinney and Rosen [91], and a horizontal osteotomy with wedge excision, as discussed by Wolfe in Chapter 10. According to Kawamoto [80], reduction mentoplasty with a bur provides an unpredictable result, as evidenced by submental fullness, ptosis of the soft tissue pad of the chin on animation, or squared-off appearance. For reductions less than 8 mm, we routinely bur the prominence down, but for projections greater than 8 mm we do a horizontal osteotomy. Hybrid deformities of normal occlusion but abnormal mandibles are occasionally seen following previous orthodontia.

COMPLICATIONS

Despite the frequency of rhinoplasty and reported series of several thousand cases, statistical analysis of the incidence and types of complications has not been presented [18, 33]. Rather, retrospective analysis of randomly collected cases or small series are offered [81, 90] (Table 6-2). Comparison of the data would indicate that the type and occurrence of complications have not changed significantly during the last 20 years (1960–1980 [21]). However, experienced rhinoplasty surgeons feel that the more conservative procedures being practiced currently lead to fewer catastrophic complications, especially crucified noses.

Table 6-2. Complications

Complication	Klabunde/Falces (n = 300)	McKinney/Cook (n = 200)
Early		
Hemorrhage		
Intraoperative	1	0
Postoperative	6 (2%)	4 (2%)
Infection	5 (1.6%)	0%
Septal perforation	2	2 (1%)
Skin slough	0	0
Late		
Edema	18	
Ecchymosis	1	
Scar tissue	10	
Vestibular webbing	10	
Total	18.3% (5.5/30)	
Dissatisfaction		
Patient	14%	13%
Surgeon	32%	17%
Reoperation	29 (10%)	24 (12%)
Overall satisfaction	95%	90%

Intraoperative Complications

The primary problems of airway and patient compliance are related to anesthesia and to bleeding. A functioning airway is of paramount concern in rhinoplasty surgery. Local anesthesia preserves the gag reflex and allows cooperative deep breathing. However, anaphylactic reactions and cardiopulmonary collapse can occur, requiring the surgeon to be proficient in cardiac resuscitation and tracheostomy. General anesthesia provides a controlled airway but risks undetected disruption of the airway. This danger can be lessened by use of a positive pressure sensor that signals any interruption. Although satisfactory for a cooperative patient, local anesthesia is not ideal for certain individuals, including the psychologically immature, the very anxious, and those with cardiac problems. The problem of an increasingly hysterical patient and a frustrated surgeon who has yet to perform the osteotomies is familiar to all. These situations are best avoided by offering the patient a choice of anesthesia regimens. Intraoperative hemorrhage sufficient to interrupt the operative procedure is rare. Persistent bleeding that makes surgery more difficult does occur and may be attributed to prior ingestion of salicylate-containing drugs, bleeding disorders, or concurrent menses. Minimization is achieved by a detailed history of previous bleeding episodes (teeth extractions, minor trauma, nosebleeds), recommendation to avoid all aspirin-containing medicines for 2 weeks prior to surgery, and scheduling of patients in the middle of their menstrual cycle. Digital compression and intranasal packing should stop diffuse oozing whereas cauterization of a persistent bleeding vessel may be necessary.

Early Complications

During the first 6 to 8 weeks postoperatively the primary complaints are bruising, swelling, nasal obstruction, and a diffuse dissatisfaction that the nose does not look smaller or more refined. Reassurance and reinforcement of the expected resolution as discussed preoperatively are necessary.

HEMORRHAGE
Bleeding may occur immediately postoperatively or secondarily at 7 to 14 days. Early bleeding is most often associated with major osteocartilaginous septal resections. If it is copious or does not respond to head elevation with gentle compression, evaluation under direct vision is required. The procedure should be done in a well-equipped examining room complete with suction, cautery, illumination, and nursing assistance. Anterior bleeding may be controlled by cauterization whereas posterior bleeding requires nasopharyngeal packs. Severe hemorrhage mandates packing over inflated catheters, hospitalization, and sedation, with ligation of the internal maxillary artery as a desperate last resort. The more common event is epistaxis in the second postoperative week due to sloughing of

eschars and nasal cleansing by the patient. This occurrence can be lessened by meticulous closure of the incision lines plus warning the patient to avoid picking, blowing, or cleansing the nose. In cases not responding to elevation with gentle compression, cauterization of the bleeding point is followed by packing with Gelfoam or Oxycel.

HEMATOMA

Accumulation of blood beneath the dorsal skin, overlying the osteotomies, or within the septum may be generalized or localized. Diffuse enlargement of the nose may follow hemorrhage and require evacuation. Broadbent and Woolf [16] recommend primary insertion of a small intercath drain for persistent septal oozing. Bleeding is best avoided by preoperative preparations (limitation of salicylates, detailed history), limited dissections, and a conforming splint.

ECCHYMOSIS AND EDEMA

Bruising and swelling are normal occurrences following a rhinoplasty. Many surgeons try to minimize them by restricting periosteal elevation, delaying the osteotomies to the end of the procedure, and applying cold compresses or ice packs to the area as soon as possible. Although the authors favor the former combination, a number of surgeons rely on pharmacologic agents including diuretics and enzymes (hyaluronidase). If the patient has been properly prepared, acceptance of the edema requires reassurance that the expected regression will occur: dorsum (1 month), middle third (2 months), and tip (6–12 months). Occasionally patients will have scleral hemorrhage persisting for 3 to 6 weeks, or prolonged infraorbital ecchymosis due to breakdown of hemoglobin pigments.

INFECTION

As noted by McKinney and Cook [90], infections following rhinoplasty have decreased markedly to less than 1 percent despite the absence of prophylactic antibiotic coverage. Prevention is achieved by not operating on patients with active acne or pustules and by careful removal of all tissue fragments and blood clots that could provide a nucleus for infection. If a localized abscess occurs, it is best treated by incision and drainage, warm compresses, and broad-spectrum antibiotics that are adjusted for bacterial cultures—usually a penicillin-resistant *Staphylococcus aureus.* Although bacteremia is rare, associated complications can include staphylococcal endocarditis and meningitis [145]. A more chronic infection producing swelling and erythema can occur along the fracture lines (periostitis) or around small foreign-body fragments (paraffinomas).

SKIN

Skin problems can be divided into minor (pustules, allergic reaction, telangiectasia) and major (wrinkling, necrosis). Skin maceration and allergic reactions tend to occur in oily skin covered with adhesive compounds or tape, as they do in warm humid weather. Their occurrence can be minimized through drying of the skin, direct application of paper tapes, and early removal (4–5 days) in the summer months. Treatment should consist in expressing the pustules followed by a desquamating soap and application of topical steroid creams for allergic reactions. Telangiectasias may increase in patients with this propensity or develop de novo from a too superficial dissection. Fair-skinned patients with preexisting telangiectasia must be warned of a potential increase and told that it can be ameliorated by electrocautery or perhaps the Argon laser [103]. In thin-skinned patients, especially those undergoing secondary rhinoplasty, injection of the dorsal skin with very dilute local anesthetic performs a hydrodissection that will ensure a deep dissection. Also, use of a sharp-knife dissection over the oseocartilaginous vaults is recommended in these patients.

Wrinkling of the dorsal skin is a potential occurrence following large hump resections, especially in older individuals. It can be lessened by wider undermining of the dorsal skin over the upper lateral cartilages plus meticulous application of the initial paper tape dressing. Skin necrosis occurs rarely and is attributed to a combination of excessive pressure from the dressing, injection of local anesthetic, and idiosyncratic reaction. Prevention is best achieved by taping of the nasal tip rather than plaster and minute injections of local anesthetic into the nasal tip. Treatment must be conservative, with eschar separation followed by secondary healing or skin grafting.

LACRIMAL SYSTEM

Damage to the lacrimal apparatus with resulting epiphora and dacryocystitis is a theoretic complication as these have not been reported. From the studies of Flowers and Anderson [45], it is obvious that damage of the unprotected lacrimal sac is a common occurrence, but rarely is the nasolacrimal duct injured. Osteotomies performed on cadavers demonstrated a 33 percent (12 out of 37) incidence of lacrimal sac penetration whereas no permanent sequelae were found on 1000 clinical rhinoplasties.

SEPTAL PERFORATIONS

Perforation of the septum now occurs in 1 to 2 percent of septorhinoplasties. Many authors attribute this decrease to less radical resections, antibiotics, and early drainage of septal hematomas. Prevention is best ensured by conservative single mucosal flap elevation and cartilage scoring for septal deviation rather than radical resection. If the condition is symptomatic, treatment requires mucosal flaps from the nose or mouth. Although perforations were previously attributed to technical errors including damaged mucosa, the popularity of cocaine sniffing may be an etiologic factor.

Late Complications

Late complications are relatively rare except for nasal obstruction and patient dissatisfaction. Of all the problems associated with rhinoplasty, managing the patient with an unfavorable result is the most difficult. The demand for immediate revision must be rejected and the patient reassured that surgery probably will not be necessary [50].

OLFACTORY PROBLEMS

Alterations in the sense of smell for several months must be anticipated. Goldwyn and Shore [59] found that 80 percent of patients had normal olfaction at 2 weeks and all were normal by 2 months, thus negating the finding of Champion [19], who had reported subjective impairment of longer duration (6–18 months).

SCARS

Despite every effort at concealment, visible scars do occur after rhinoplasty. They may be located at the alar bases following wedge resection or along the membranous septum. Visible scars along the alar-facial groove are usually due to poor placement or excessive primary excision. Revision should be cautiously contemplated, and localized dermabrasion is preferred. Alar notching is produced by excessive vestibular resection and straight excisions rather than preservation of a medially based flap, as recommended by Sheen [138]. Visualization of a scar in the membranous septum most frequently occurs with retracted alae and a downwardly displaced columella. Secondary surgery is required.

VESTIBULAR NARROWING

Decrease in the vestibular aperture along the internal valve can be considered a cicatricial progression from adhesions to webbing to stenosis. Small adhesions that develop between the granulating septum and the opposite turbinate can be sharply transected and recurrence prevented by nasal packing for 2 weeks. The more complex webbing, which occurs high in the vestibule, may progress to circular scarring with stenosis. The former is secondary to loss of mucosa and aggressive shortening of the caudal end of the upper lateral cartilages while the latter is due to circular incisions (membranous septum, intercartilaginous plus piriform), and excessive mucosal resection and poor wound closure. Sheen [138] defines four grades of vestibular atresia: I (0–15%), no treatment necessary; II (15–40%), impedance of respiration, treatment beneficial; III (40–75%), partial impedance, aggravated by exertion, surgery required; and IV (more than 75%), virtual respiratory cripple, surgery mandatory. For grades I and II, local flaps or Z-plasty may be sufficient, but as severity increases, resection of the scar tissue is essential followed by full-thickness retroauricular skin grafts.

NASAL OBSTRUCTION

Postrhinoplasty rhinitis is manifested by partial nasal obstruction and occurs in virtually all patients [9]. It is due to transient mucosal edema and crusting along suture lines. Although it is not avoidable, patients should be told preoperatively that some "stuffiness" and sense of obstruction is common but should resolve spontaneously within 2 to 3 weeks. In contrast to this acute episode, there are certain patients who develop a persistent obstruction [141]. Beekhuis [12] reviewed 1000 consecutive rhinoplasties and found that 10 percent had some nasal obstruction, usually due to enlargement of the inferior turbinates and correctable by *intra*mucosal steroid injections. On inspection, the turbinates are seen to be exceedingly large, press against the septum, and have a normal color. Beekhuis also discussed evaluation of nasal obstruction in consulting patients seeking secondary rhinoplasty after primary surgery elsewhere. The etiologic factors were divided into (1) persistence of the preoperative condition (high septal deflections, caudal dislocation of the septum, turbinate hypertrophy), (2) obstructive rhinitis, (3) intranasal obstructions (adhesions, webs), and (4) inadequate support for the lobule (alar collapse) [155].

Results

SHORT-TERM RESULTS

Despite the infinite complexity and challenges of rhinoplasties, the vast majority of patients are satisfied with their result. A recent retrospective review by McKinney and Cook [90] of 200 patients indicates a satisfaction rate of 87 percent, which rose to 91 percent following revisions in 12 percent of patients. With regard to the 24 revisions, 11 nasal tips were considered too bulbous, necessitating reduction of the alar rim from 5 mm down to 2.5 to 4.0 mm; five required modification of the nasal bones, either rasping of spurs or adjusting infractures; and two patients each had prominences of the cartilage dorsum and leading edge of septum, while one patient had a prominent nasal spine. These figures reveal the small revisions that are characteristic of a conservative primary rhinoplasty. The absence of numerous grafts and extended procedures indicates a finesse type of rhinoplasty.

Undoubtedly, the early postoperative period is most tranquil for the surgeon who carefully selects and informs his patients. The patient must accept the fact that final tip definition may require 6 to 12 months and that revision is not possible or indicated before 1 year.

LONG-TERM RESULTS

Unlike other facial aesthetic procedures, in which aging and life crises can have catastrophic consequences, rhinoplasty tends to offer a primary and permanent change. As noted by Goldwyn [57], the true culprit in rhinoplasty is not time but faulty surgical technique. Broadbent and Woolf [16] found that good results remain good while poor results do not get any better. Thus, the commitment to detailed records, frequent follow-up, and critical self-analysis is an essential part of rhinoplasty surgery. For readers interested in surgical techniques and their long-term consequences, the work of Webster and Smith [157] is particularly valuable.

REFERENCES

1. Abramson, M., and Harker, L. A. Physiology of the nose. *Otolaryngol. Clin. North Am.* 6:623, 1973.
2. Anderson, J. R. A new approach to rhinoplasty. *Trans. Am. Acad. Ophthalmol. Otolaryngol.* 70:183, 1966.
3. Anderson, J. R. New approach to rhinoplasty: A five-year appraisal. *Arch. Otolaryngol.* 93:284, 1971.
4. Anderson, J. R. A personal technique of rhinoplasty. *Otolaryngol. Clin. North Am.* 8:559, 1975.

5. Anderson, J. R., and Rubin, W. Retrograde intramucosal hump removal rhinoplasty. *Arch. Otolaryngol.* 60:346, 1958.
6. Aston, S. J., and Guy, C. L. The nasal spine. *Clin. Plast. Surg.* 4:153, 1977.
7. Aufricht, G. Joseph's rhinoplasty with some modifications. *Surg. Clin. North Am.* 51:299, 1971.
8. Baker, D. C. Treatment of obstructing inferior turbinates with intranasal corticosteroids. *Ann. Plast. Surg.* 3:253, 1979.
9. Baker, D. C. Rhinoplasty: Physiology. In T. D. Rees (ed.), *Aesthetic Plastic Surgery.* Philadelphia: Saunders, 1980. P. 66.
10. Baker, D. C., and Strauss, R. B. The physiologic treatment of nasal obstruction. *Clin. Plast. Surg.* 4:121, 1977.
11. Becker, O. J. Plastic Surgery of the Nose. In O. J. Becker, *Principles of Otolaryngologic Plastic Surgery.* Rochester, Minn.: American Academy of Ophthalmology and Otolaryngology, 1952.
12. Beekhuis, G. J. Nasal obstruction after rhinoplasty: Etiology and techniques for correction. *Laryngoscope* 86:540, 1976.
13. Bernstein, L. Applied anatomy in corrective rhinoplasty. *Arch. Otolaryngol.* 99:67, 1974.
14. Bernstein, L. A basic technique for surgery of the nasal lobule. *Otolaryngol. Clin. North Am.* 8:599, 1975.
15. Bernstein, L. Surgical anatomy in rhinoplasty. *Otolaryngol. Clin. North Am.* 8:549, 1975.
16. Broadbent, T. R., and Woolf, R. M. Rhinoplasty. In E. H. Courtiss (ed.), *Aesthetic Surgery: Trouble, How to Avoid It and How to Treat It.* St. Louis: Mosby, 1978. Pp. 75–96.
17. Brown, J. B., and McDowell, F. *Plastic Surgery of the Nose* (rev. ed.). Springfield, Ill.: Thomas, 1965.
18. Bruck, H. G. Corrective rhinoplasty: A study of 5,000 personal cases. *Arch. Otolaryngol.* 97:441, 1973.
19. Champion, R. Anosmia associated with corrective rhinoplasty. *Br. J. Plast. Surg.* 19:182, 1966.
20. Coburn, R. J., Rees, T. D., and Horowitz, S. Mentoplasty. In T. D. Rees (ed.), *Aesthetic Plastic Surgery.* Philadelphia: Saunders, 1980. P. 770.
21. Cohen, S. Complications following rhinoplasty. *Plast. Reconstr. Surg.* 18:213, 1956.
22. Cole, P. Nasal turbinate function. *Can. J. Otolaryngol.* 2:259, 1973.
23. Converse, J. M. Corrective surgery of nasal deviations. *Arch. Otolaryngol.* 52:671, 1950.
24. Converse, J. M. The cartilaginous structures of the nose. *Ann. Otol. Rhinol. Laryngol.* 64:220, 1955.
25. Converse, J. M. Corrective surgery of the nasal tip. *Laryngoscope* 67:16, 1957.
26. Converse, J. M. Corrective Rhinoplasty. In J. M. Converse (ed.), *Reconstructive Plastic Surgery* (2nd ed.). Philadelphia: Saunders, 1977. P. 1040.
27. Cottle, M. H. Nasal roof repair and hump removal. *Arch. Otolaryngol.* 60:408, 1954.
28. Cottle, M. H., and Loring, R. M. Corrective surgery of the external pyramid and the nasal septum for restoration of normal physiology. *IMJ* 90:119, 1946.
29. Courtiss, E. H. Resection of obstructing inferior nasal turbinates. Reply. (Letter to the Editor.) *Plast. Reconstr. Surg.* 63:719, 1979.
30. Courtiss, E. H., Goldwyn, R. M., and O'Brien, J. O. Resection of obstructing inferior nasal turbinates. *Plast. Reconstr. Surg.* 62:249, 1978.
31. Daniel, R. K., and Lessard, M. L. Rhinoplasty: A graded aesthetic anatomical approach. *Ann. Plast. Surg.* In press.
32. Denecke, H. J., and Meyer, R. *Plastic Surgery on Head and Neck.* New York: Springer-Verlag, 1967.
33. Diamond, H. Rhinoplasty techniques. *Surg. Clin. North Am.* 51:317, 1971.
34. Dieffenbach, J. *Die operative Chirurgie.* Leipzig: Brockhaus, 1845.
35. Dingman, R. O. Local anesthesia for rhinoplasty and the nasal septum in rhinoplastic surgery. *Plast. Reconstr. Surg.* 28:251, 1961.
36. Drumheller, G. W. Topology of the lateral nasal cartilages: The anatomical relationship of the lateral nasal to the greater alar cartilage, lateral crus. *Anat. Rec.* 176:321, 1973.
37. Dupont, C., Cloutier, G. E., and Prevost, Y. Autogenous vomer bone graft for permanent correction of the cartilaginous septal deviations. *Plast. Reconstr. Surg.* 38:243, 1966.
38. Ecker, H. A. A direct approach to the more severely deformed cleft lip nose. *Plast. Reconstr. Surg.* 67:369, 1981.
39. Eitner, E. *Kosmetische Operationen.* Berlin: Springer-Verlag, 1932.
40. Eitner, E. Verletzungen der Nase und ihre kosmetische Behandlungen. *Wien. Med. Wochenschr.* 84:307, 1934.
41. Falces, E., Wesser, D., and Gorney, M. Cosmetic surgery of the non-Caucasian nose. *Plast. Reconstr. Surg.* 45:317, 1970.
42. Feehan, H. F., and Mancusi-Ungaro, A. The use of cocaine as a topical anesthetic in nasal surgery: A survey report. *Plast. Reconstr. Surg.* 57:62, 1976.
43. Fenton, R. S. Surgery of the nasal dorsum. *Can. J. Otolaryngol.* 7:24, 1978.
44. Flowers, R. S. The surgical correction of the non-caucasian nose. *Clin. Plast. Surg.* 4:69, 1977.
45. Flowers, R. S., and Anderson, R. Injury to the lacrimal apparatus during rhinoplasty. *Plast. Reconstr. Surg.* 42:577, 1968.
46. Fomon, S. *Cosmetic Surgery: Principles and Practice.* Philadelphia: Lippincott, 1960.
47. Fomon, S., and Bell, J. W. *Rhinoplasty—New Concepts: Evaluation and Application.* Springfield, Ill.: Thomas, 1970.
48. Fomon, S., and Syracuse, V. R. Routine technic of a typical rhinoplasty. *IMJ* 94:242, 1948.
49. Fred, G. B. Role of depressor septi nasi muscle in rhinoplasty. *Arch. Otolaryngol.* 62:37, 1955.
50. Fred, G. B. Postoperative drooping of the nasal tip after rhinoplasty. *Arch. Otolaryngol.* 67:177, 1958.
51. Friedman, W. H., Oliver, M., and Biller, H. F. Evaluation of nasal tip surgery. *Laryngoscope* 85:1539, 1975.
52. Goin, M. K., and Goin, J. M. *Changing the Body.* Baltimore: Williams & Wilkins, 1981.
53. Goldman, I. B. Rhinoplasty: Its surgical complications and how to avoid them. *J. Int. Coll. Surg.* 13:285, 1950.
54. Goldman, I. B. Surgical tips on the nasal tip. *Eye Ear Nose Throat Monthly* 33:583, 1954.
55. Goldman, I. B. The importance of the medical crura in nasal-tip reconstruction. *Arch. Otolaryngol.* 65:143, 1957.
56. Goldman, I. B. Rhinoplastic sequelae causing nasal obstruction. *Arch. Otolaryngol.* 83:151, 1966.
57. Goldwyn, R. M. *The Unfavorable Result in Plastic Surgery.* Boston: Little, Brown, 1972.
58. Goldwyn, R. M. *The Patient and the Plastic Surgeon.* Boston: Little, Brown, 1981.
59. Goldwyn, R. M., and Shore, S. The effects of submucous resection and rhinoplasty on the sense of smell. *Plast. Reconstr. Surg.* 41:427, 1968.
60. Goodman, W. S. External approach to rhinoplasty. *Can. J. Otolaryngol.* 2:207, 1973.
61. Goodman, W. S., and Charbonneau, P. A. External approach to rhinoplasty. *Laryngoscope* 84:2195, 1974.
62. Goodman, W. S., and Charles, D. A. Technique of external rhinoplasty. *Can. J. Otolaryngol.* 7:13, 1978.
63. Gordon, H. L., and Baker, T. J. Primary cosmetic rhinoplasty.

Clin. Plast. Surg. 4:9, 1977.
64. Gorney, M. The Septum in Rhinoplasty: Form and Function. In D. R. Millard (ed.), *Symposium on Corrective Rhinoplasty.* St. Louis: Mosby, 1976. P. 180.
65. Gorney, M. Malpractice. In E. H. Courtiss (ed.), *Aesthetic Surgery: Trouble, How to Avoid It and How to Treat It.* St. Louis: Mosby, 1978. P. 180.
66. Gorney, M. Personal communication. December 17, 1981.
67. Gunter, J. P. Anatomical observations of the lower lateral cartilages. *Arch. Otolaryngol.* 89:61, 1969.
68. Hasegawa, M., and Kern, E. B. The human nasal cycle. *Mayo Clin. Proc.* 52:28, 1977.
69. Hilger, J. A. The internal lateral osteotomy in rhinoplasty. *Arch. Otolaryngol.* 88:119, 1968.
70. Hinderer, U. T. Dr. Vazquez Anon's last lesson. *Aesthetic Plast. Surg.* 2:375, 1977.
71. Horton, C. E. Combined Septoplasty and Rhinoplasty. In F. W. Masters and J. R. Lewis (eds.), *Symposium on Aesthetic Surgery of the Nose, Ears, and Chin.* St. Louis: Mosby, 1973.
72. House, H. P. Submucous resection of the inferior turbinal bone. *Laryngoscope* 61:637, 1951.
73. Hovorka, O. *Die aussere Nase.* Wein: Holder, 1893.
74. Janeke, J. B., and Wright, W. K. Studies on the support of the nasal tip. *Arch. Otolaryngol.* 93:458, 1971.
75. Joseph, J. Ueber die operative Verkleinerung einer Nase (Rhinomiosis). *Berl. Klin. Wochenschr.* 40:882, 1898; also in *Plast. Reconstr. Surg.* 46:178, 1970.
76. Joseph, J. Intranasale Nasenhockeragtragung. *Berl. Klin. Wochenschr.* 42:650, 1904.
77. Joseph, J. *Nasenplastik und sonstige Gesichtsplastik Nebst einem Anhang ueber Mammaplastik.* Leipzig: Kabitzsch, 1931.
78. Jost, G. *Atlas de Chirurgie Esthétique Plastique.* Paris: Masson, 1975.
79. Jost, G., Vergnon, L., and Hadjean, E. Les asymétries nasales postopératoires. *Ann. Chir. Plast.* 20:173, 1973.
80. Kawamoto, H. K., Jr. Discussion of "Reduction mentoplasty" by P. McKinney and P. B. Rosen. *Plast. Reconstr. Surg.* 70:151, 1981.
81. Klabunde, E. H., and Falces, E. Incidence of complications in cosmetic rhinoplasties. *Plast. Reconstr. Surg.* 34:192, 1964.
82. Lamont, E. On nasal tip projection. (Letter to the Editor.) *Plast. Reconstr. Surg.* 57:228, 1976.
83. Lessard, L., and Daniel, R. K. Surgical anatomy of the nose. *Arch. Otolaryngol.* In press.
84. Lewis, J. R., Jr. *Atlas of Aesthetic Plastic Surgery.* Boston: Little, Brown, 1973.
85. Lipsett, E. M. A new approach to surgery of the lower cartilaginous vault. *Arch. Otolaryngol.* 70:42, 1959.
86. Masters, F. W., and Lewis, J. R., Jr. *Symposium on Aesthetic Surgery of the Face, Eyelid, and Breast.* St. Louis: Mosby, 1972.
87. Masters, F. W., and Lewis, J. R., Jr. *Symposium on Aesthetic Surgery of the Nose, Ears, and Chin.* St. Louis: Mosby, 1973.
88. McCurdy, J. A., Jr. Surgery of the nasal tip: Current concepts. *Ear Nose Throat J.* 56:238, 1977.
89. McDowell, F. History of rhinoplasty. *Aesthetic Plast. Surg.* 1:321, 1978.
90. McKinney, P., and Cook, J. Q. A critical evaluation of 200 rhinoplasties. *Ann. Plast. Surg.* 7:357, 1981.
91. McKinney, P., and Rosen, P. B. Reduction mentoplasty. *Plast. Reconstr. Surg.* 70:147, 1981.
92. Meyer, R., and Kesselring, U. K. Sculpturing and reconstructive procedures in aesthetic and functional rhinoplasty. *Clin. Plast. Surg.* 4:15, 1977.
93. Meyer, R., and Kesselring, U. K. Surgical correction of the unusually short nose. *Aesthetic Plast. Surg.* 1:271, 1977.
94. Millard, D. R. External excisions in rhinoplasty. *Br. J. Plast. Surg.* 12:340, 1960.
95. Millard, D. R. Adjuncts in augmentation mentoplasty and corrective rhinoplasty. *Plast. Reconstr. Surg.* 36:48, 1965.
96. Millard, D. R. Alar margin sculpturing. *Plast. Reconstr. Surg.* 40:337, 1967.
97. Millard, D. R. Rhinoplasty. *N. Engl. J. Med.* 281:485, 1969.
98. Millard, D. R. Secondary corrective rhinoplasty. *Plast. Reconstr. Surg.* 44:545, 1969.
99. Millard, D. R. (ed.). *Symposium on Corrective Rhinoplasty.* St. Louis: Mosby, 1976.
100. Natvig, P. Anatomy of the Nose. In D. R. Millard (ed.), *Symposium on Corrective Rhinoplasty.* St. Louis: Mosby, 1976. P. 40.
101. Natvig, P., et al. Anatomical details of the osseous-cartilaginous framework of the nose. *Plast. Reconstr. Surg.* 48:528, 1971.
102. Neivert, H. Reduction of nasofrontal angle in rhinoplasty. *Arch. Otolaryngol.* 53:196, 1951.
103. Noe, J. M., et al. Postrhinoplasty "red nose": Differential diagnosis and treatment by laser. *Plast. Reconstr. Surg.* 65:661, 1981.
104. Ortiz-Monasterio, F., and Olmedo, A. Rhinoplasty on the mestizo nose. *Clin. Plast. Surg.* 4:89, 1977.
105. Ortiz-Monasterio, F., Olmedo, A., and Oscoy, L. O. The use of cartilage grafts in primary aesthetic rhinoplasty. *Plast. Reconstr. Surg.* 67:597, 1981.
106. Padovan, I. F. External approach in rhinoplasty. *Surg. ORL Lug.* 3–4:354, 1966.
107. Padovan, I. F. Combination of extranasal and intranasal approach in surgery of the nasal pyramid and nasal septum. *Can. J. Otolaryngol.* 4:522, 1975.
108. Parkes, M. L., Kamer, F., and Morgan, W. R. Double lateral osteotomy in rhinoplasty. *Arch. Otolaryngol.* 103:344, 1977.
109. Patterson, C. N. The aging nose: Characteristics and corrections. *Otolaryngol. Clin. North Am.* 13:275, 1980.
110. Peck, G. C. Aesthetic Rhinoplasty. In W. C. Grabb and J. W. Smith (eds.), *Plastic Surgery* (3rd ed.). Boston: Little, Brown, 1979. P. 424.
111. Peck, G. C. Aesthetic Rhinoplasty II. In J. N. Barron and M. N. Saad (eds.), *Operative Plastic and Reconstructive Surgery.* Edinburgh: Churchill Livingstone, 1980. Pp. 747–758.
112. Peck, G. C. The onlay graft for nasal tip projection. *Plast. Reconstr. Surg.* 71:27, 1983.
113. Peterson, R. A. Preoperative Evaluation for Rhinoplasty. In D. R. Millard (ed.), *Symposium on Corrective Rhinoplasty.* St. Louis: Mosby, 1976. P. 56.
114. Peterson, R. A. Open-Flap Rhinoplasty. In D. R. Millard (ed.), *Symposium on Corrective Rhinoplasty.* St. Louis: Mosby, 1976. P. 83.
115. Pollet, J., and Weikel, A. M. Some technical considerations in primary rhinoplasty. *Aesthetic Plast. Surg.* 1:25, 1976.
116. Proetz, A. W. Physiology of the nose from the standpoint of the plastic surgeon. *Arch. Otolaryngol.* 39:514, 1944.
117. Randall, P. The direct approach to the "hanging columella." *Plast. Reconstr. Surg.* 53:544, 1974.
118. Rees, T. D. Current concepts of rhinoplasty. *Clin. Plast. Surg.* 4:131, 1977.
119. Rees, T. D. Rhinoplasty in the older adult. *Ann. Plast. Surg.* 1:27, 1978.
120. Rees, T. D. *Aesthetic Plastic Surgery.* Philadelphia: Saunders, 1980.
121. Regnault, P., and Alfaro, A. Aesthetic Rhinoplasty I. In J. N.

Barron and M. N. Saad (eds.), *Operative Plastic and Reconstructive Surgery.* Edinburgh: Churchill Livingstone, 1980. Pp. 729–745.
122. Regnault, P., and Alfaro, A. The Skoog rhinoplasty: A modified technique. *Plast. Reconstr. Surg.* 66:578, 1980.
123. Rethi, A. Raccourcissement du nez trop long. *Rev. Chir. Plast.* 4:85, 1934.
124. Rethi, A. Right and wrong in rhinoplastic operations. *Plast. Reconstr. Surg.* 3:361, 1948.
125. Robin, J. L. Rhinoplastie extra-muqueuse côntrolée avec mesure pré-opératoire de la modification du profil. *Ann. Chir. Plast.* 18:119, 1973.
126. Robin, J. L. Extramucosal method in rhinoplasty. *Aesthetic Plast. Surg.* 3:171, 1979.
127. Robin, J. L. The preplanned rhinoplasty. *Aesthetic Plast. Surg.* 3:179, 1979.
128. Roe, J. O. The correction of angular deformities of the nose by subcutaneous operation. *Med. Rec. N.Y.* 40:57, 1891.
129. Rogers, B. O. Early Historical Developments of Corrective Rhinoplasty. In D. R. Millard (ed.), *Symposium on Corrective Rhinoplasty.* St. Louis: Mosby, 1976. P. 18.
130. Rogers, B. O. Symposium on rhinoplasty. *Clin. Plast. Surg.* 4:1, 1977.
131. Rubin, F. F. Permanent change in shape of cartilage by morselization. *Arch. Otolaryngol.* 89:64, 1969.
132. Sercer, A. Dekortikation der Nase. *Chir. Maxillofac. Plast.* 1:149, 1958.
133. Sercer, A., and Mundnich, K. *Plasticke Operationen an der Ohrmuschel.* Stuttgart: Thieme, 1962.
134. Sheen, J. H. Achieving more nasal tip projection by use of small autogenous vomer or septal cartilage grafts. *Plast. Reconstr. Surg.* 56:35, 1975. (Discussion by C. E. Horton, *Plast. Reconstr. Surg.* 56:211, 1975.)
135. Sheen, J. H. Secondary rhinoplasty. *Plast. Reconstr. Surg.* 56:137, 1975.
136. Sheen, J. H. Finesse in Rhinoplasty. In D. R. Millard (ed.), *Symposium on Corrective Rhinoplasty.* St. Louis: Mosby, 1976. P. 263.
137. Sheen, J. H. Secondary Rhinoplasty Surgery. In D. R. Millard (ed.), *Symposium on Corrective Rhinoplasty.* St. Louis: Mosby, 1976. P. 133.
138. Sheen, J. H. *Aesthetic Rhinoplasty.* St. Louis: Mosby, 1978.
139. Sheen, J. H. Colloquium: Rhinoplasty. *Ann. Plast. Surg.* 1:601, 1978.
140. Sheen, J. H. A new look at supratip deformity. *Ann. Plast. Surg.* 3:498, 1979.
141. Sherman, A. H. A study of nasal airway function in the postoperative period of nasal surgery. *Laryngoscope* 87:299, 1977.
142. Simons, R. L., and Lawson, W. Chin reduction in profileplasty. *Arch. Otolaryngol.* 101:207, 1975.
143. Skoog, T. A method of hump reduction in rhinoplasty. *Arch. Otolaryngol.* 83:283, 1966.
144. Skoog, T. *Plastic Surgery.* Philadelphia: Saunders, 1975.
145. Slavin, S. A., et al. An investigation of bacteremia during rhinoplasty. *Plast. Reconstr. Surg.* 71:196, 1983.
146. Stark, R. B. *Aesthetic Plastic Surgery.* Boston: Little, Brown, 1982.
147. Stoksted, P., and Gutierrez, C. Obtaining a gentle contour to the columella by modifying the maxillary spine. *Plast. Reconstr. Surg.* 68:689, 1981.
148. Straatsma, B. R., and Straatsma, C. R. The anatomical relationship of the lateral nasal cartilage to the nasal bone and the cartilaginous nasal septum. *Plast. Reconstr. Surg.* 8:443, 1951.
149. Stucker, F. J. Non-caucasian rhinoplasty. *Trans. Am. Acad. Ophthalmol. Otolaryngol.* 82:417, 1971.
150. Stucker, F. J., and Ansel, D. G. A case against nasal packing. *Laryngoscope* 88:1314, 1978.
151. Tardy, M. E. Rhinoplasty tip ptosis: Etiology and prevention. *Laryngoscope* 83:923, 1973.
152. Tardy, M. E., and Becker, O. J. Surgical Correction of Facial Deformities. In J. J. Ballenger (ed.), *Diseases of the Nose, Throat and Ear.* Philadelphia: Lea & Febiger, 1977. P. 23.
153. Tardy, M. E. Rhinoplasty in midlife. *Otolaryngol. Clin. North Am.* 13:289, 1980.
154. Tardy, M. E. *Rhinoplasty.* Baltimore: Williams & Wilkins, 1984.
155. Thomas, J. N. S.M.R.: A two year follow-up survey. *J. Laryngol. Otol.* 92:661, 1978.
156. Webster, R. C. Advances in surgery of the tip: Intact rim cartilage techniques and the tip-columella-lip esthetic complex. *Otolaryngol. Clin. North Am.* 8:615, 1975.
157. Webster, R. C., and Smith, R. C. Rhinoplasty. In R. M. Goldwyn (ed.), *Long-Term Results in Plastic and Reconstructive Surgery.* Boston: Little, Brown, 1980. P. 576.
158. Weir, R. F. On restoring sunken noses without scarring the face. *N.Y. Med. J.* 56:449, 1892.
159. Wright, W. K. Lateral osteotomy in rhinoplasty. *Arch. Otolaryngol.* 78:70, 1963.
160. Wright, W. K. Study on hump removal in rhinoplasty. *Laryngoscope* 77:508, 1967.
161. Wright, W. K. Surgery of the bony and cartilaginous dorsum. *Otolaryngol. Clin. North Am.* 8:575, 1975.
162. Zelnik, J., and Gingrass, R. P. Anatomy of the alar cartilage. *Plast. Reconstr. Surg.* 64:650, 1979.

BIBLIOGRAPHY

Aiach, E., and Gomulinski, L. Resection controlee de la busse nasale osseuse au niveau de l'angle naso-frontal. *Ann. Chir. Plast.* 27:226, 1982.

Anderson, J. R. Twenty-five helpful hints in rhinoplasty. *Trans. Pac. Coast Otoophthalmol. Soc.* 51:113, 1970.

Anderson, J. R. Straightening the crooked nose. *Trans. Am. Acad. Ophthalmol. Otolaryngol.* 76:945, 1972.

Anderson, J. R. Colloquium: Rhinoplasty. *Ann. Plast. Surg.* 1:598, 1978.

Anderson, J. R., and Rubin, W. Management of combined external nasal and septal deformities. *J. La. State Med. Soc.* 108:258, 1956.

Armstrong, D. P. Aggressive management of the hanging columella. *Plast. Reconstr. Surg.* 65:513, 1980.

Arons, M. S. Dr. Frank McDowell on grafts to the nose. Correspondence. *Plast. Reconstr. Surg.* 70:118, 1982.

Aufricht, G. Combined nasal plastic and chin plastic: Correction of microgenia by an osteocartilaginous transplant from a large hump nose. *Am. J. Surg.* 25:292, 1934.

Aufricht, G. A few hints and surgical details in rhinoplasty. *Laryngoscope* 53:317, 1943.

Aufricht, G. Surgery of the radix and bony nose: Preliminary report of a new type of nasal clamp. *Plast. Reconstr. Surg.* 22:315, 1958.

Aufricht, G. Rhinoplasty and the face. *Plast. Reconstr. Surg.* 43:219, 1969.

Baarsma, E. A. External septorhinoplasty. *Arch. Otorhinolaryngol.* 224:169, 1979.

Baum, S. J. Nasal projection. *Arch. Otolaryngol.* 103:262, 1977.

Becker, O. J. Problems of the septum in rhinoplastic surgery. *Trans. Am. Acad. Ophthalmol. Otolaryngol.* 55:244, 1951.

Beekhuis, G. J. Nasal tip projection. *Eye Ear Nose Throat Monthly* 51:30, 1972.

Beekhuis, G. J. Saddle nose deformity: Etiology, prevention, and treatment; augmentation rhinoplasty with polyamide. *Laryngoscope* 84 : 2, 1974.

Beekhuis, G. J. Surgical correction of saddle nose deformity. *Trans. Am. Acad. Ophthalmol. Otolaryngol.* 80 : 596, 1975.

Berman, W. E. Surgery of the nasal tip. *Otolaryngol. Clin. North Am.* 8 : 563, 1975.

Berman, W. E. Secondary rhinoplasties and composite grafts. *Trans. Am. Acad. Ophthalmol. Otolaryngol.* 84 : 952, 1977.

Bernstein, D. Oblique osteotomies in septorhinoplasty. *Int. Surg.* 52 : 250, 1969.

Bernstein, D. Homologous nasal hump implant. *Arch. Otolaryngol.* 98 : 385, 1973.

Bernstein, L. Symposium on corrective rhinoplasty. *Otolaryngol. Clin. North Am.* 8 : 547, 1975.

Berson, M. I. Prevention of deformities in corrective rhinoplasty. *Laryngoscope* 53 : 276, 1943.

Birrell, J. F. Nasal polypi and the deviated nasal septum. *Practitioner* 205 : 762, 1970.

Bloom, S. M. The problem of implants in rhinoplasty. *Arch. Otolaryngol.* 71 : 778, 1960.

Blue, J. A. Rhinitis medicamentosa. *Ann. Allergy* 26 : 425, 1968.

Boo-Chai, K. Augmentation rhinoplasty in the Oriental. *Plast. Reconstr. Surg.* 34 : 81, 1964.

Brennan, H. G., and Parkes, M. L. Septal surgery: The high septal transfixion. *Int. Surg.* 58 : 732, 1973.

Briant, T. D. R., Paradisgarten, A., and Jansen, V. Surgery of the nasal tip. *Can. J. Otolaryngol.* 2 : 217, 1973.

Bridger, P. Physiology of the nasal valve. *Arch. Otolaryngol.* 92 : 543, 1970.

Buttler, J. Work of breathing through the nose. *Clin. Sci.* 19 : 55, 1960.

Caronni, E. P. A new method to correct the nasolabial angle in rhinoplasty. *Plast. Reconstr. Surg.* 50 : 338, 1972.

Cinelli, J. A. Correction of the combined elongated nose and recessed naso-labial angle. *Plast. Reconstr. Surg.* 21 : 139, 1958.

Cinelli, J. A. Lengthening of the nose by a septal flap. *Plast. Reconstr. Surg.* 43 : 99, 1969.

Cinelli, J. A. Physiologic Rhinoplastic Principles. In W. H. Maloney (ed.), *Otolaryngology.* New York: Harper & Row, 1971.

Clayman, L. Z. Resection of obstructing inferior nasal turbinates. (Letter to the Editor.) *Plast. Reconstr. Surg.* 63 : 718, 1979.

Cottle, M. H. Modified nasal septum operations. *Eye Ear Nose Throat Monthly* 29 : 480, 1950.

Cottle, M. H. The structure and function of the nasal vestibule. *Arch. Otolaryngol.* 62 : 173, 1955.

Cottle, M. H. Concepts of nasal physiology as related to corrective nasal surgery. *Arch. Otolaryngol.* 72 : 11, 1960.

Coursey, D. L. Staphylococcal endocarditis following septorhinoplasty. *Arch. Otolaryngol.* 99 : 454, 1974.

Courtiss, E. H. Septorhinoplasty of the traumatically deformed nose. *Ann. Plast. Surg.* 1 : 434, 1978.

Crikelair, G. F. Reduction rhinoplasty. *Plast. Reconstr. Surg.* 26 : 626, 1960.

Crysdale, W. S. Septorhinoplasty surgery in children. *Can. J. Otolaryngol.* 2 : 211, 1973.

Cucin, R. L. An aid to tailoring the alar cartilages in tip rhinoplasty. *Plast. Reconstr. Surg.* 65 : 828, 1980.

Daley, J. Retaining a correct septolabial angle in rhinoplasty. *Arch. Otolaryngol.* 39 : 348, 1944.

Daley, J. Introduction of an artistic point of view in regard to rhinoplastic diagnosis. *Arch. Otolaryngol.* 42 : 33, 1945.

Daley, J. Role of columellar and septocolumellar sutures in rhinoplasty. *Arch. Otolaryngol.* 45 : 178, 1947.

Davis, P. K. B. The complications of silastic implants: Experience with 137 consecutive cases. *Br. J. Plast. Surg.* 24 : 405, 1971.

de Avelar, J. M. Personal contribution for the surgical treatment of the Negroid nose. *Aesthetic Plast. Surg.* 1 : 81, 1976.

De Lara Galindo, S., Cuspinera, De G., E., and Ramirez, C. Anatomical and functional account on the lateral nasal cartilages. *Acta Anat.* (Basel) 97 : 393, 1977.

Deutsch, H. J. Septoplasty in nasal surgery. *J. Med. Soc. N.J.* 65 : 647, 1968.

Diamond, H. P., and Pitman, G. H. Rhinoplasty. *Ann. Plast. Surg.* 1 : 582, 1978.

Dingman, R. O., and Walter, C. Use of composite ear grafts in correction of the short nose. *Plast. Reconstr. Surg.* 43 : 117, 1969.

Drumheller, G. H. Septal reconstruction in the deficient nose. *Rhinology* 14 : 189, 1976.

Dufourmentel, C., and Mouly, R. *Chirurgie Plastique.* Paris: Flammarian, 1959.

Edwards, N. Septoplasty: Rational surgery of the nasal septum. *J. Laryngol. Otol.* 89 : 875, 1974.

Ellis, M. S. Suture technique for caudal septal deviations. *Laryngoscope* 90 : 1510, 1980.

Falces, E., and Gorney, M. Use of ear cartilage grafts for nasal tip reconstruction. *Plast. Reconstr. Surg.* 50 : 147, 1972.

Feit, L. J. Undermining and redraping in rhinoplasty. *Trans. Am. Acad. Ophthalmol. Otolaryngol.* 80 : 540, 1975.

Fine, I. J. Goldman technique in nasal septal surgery. *Arch. Otolaryngol.* 59 : 141, 1954.

Flemming, I., and Jazbi, B. Rhinoplasty in children. *Otolaryngol. Clin. North Am.* 10 : 33, 1977.

Flowers, R. S. Augmentation rhinoplasty by the intra-oral route. *Plast. Reconstr. Surg.* 54 : 570, 1974.

Fomon, S., and Bell, J. W. Rhinoplasty: A fine art. *Arch. Otolaryngol.* 85 : 685, 1967.

Fomon, S., et al. Physiologic surgery of the nares. *Arch. Otolaryngol.* 47 : 608, 1948.

Fomon, S., et al. Plastic repair of the obstructing nasal septum. *Arch. Otolaryngol.* 47 : 7, 1948.

Fomon, S., et al. New approach to ventral deflections of the nasal septum. *Arch. Otolaryngol.* 54 : 356, 1951.

Fomon, S., et al. Physiological principles in rhinoplasty. *Arch. Otolaryngol.* 53 : 256, 1951.

Fomon, S., et al. Postoperative elongation of nose. *Arch. Otolaryngol.* 64 : 456, 1956.

Fomon, S., et al. The nasal hump problem. *Arch. Otolaryngol.* 79 : 164, 1964.

Francesconi, G. Treatment of deflection of the anterocaudal portion of the nasal septum. *Plast. Reconstr. Surg.* 51 : 342, 1973.

Fredericks, S. Tripod resection for "Pinocchio" nose deformity. *Plast. Reconstr. Surg.* 53 : 531, 1972.

Freer, O. T. The correction of deflections of the nasal septum with a minimum of traumatism. *J.A.M.A.* 38 : 636, 1902.

Freer, O. T. Deflections of the nasal septum: A critical review of the methods of their correction by the window resection, with a report of 116 operations. *Ann. Otol. Rhinol. Laryngol.* 14 : 213, 1905.

Fries, R., Platz, H., and Haidenthaler, A. Surgical correction of cartilaginous nasal septum deformities. *J. Maxillofac. Surg.* 6 : 163, 1978.

Fry, H. J. H. Modified septal reconstruction for deflected nasal septum. Correspondence. *Med. J. Aust.* 1 : 188, 1967.

Fry, H. J. H. Nasal skeletal trauma and the interlocked stresses of the nasal septal cartilage. *Br. J. Plast. Surg.* 20 : 146, 1967.

Fry, H. J. H. Nasal trauma: 1. Recent advances in the understanding of fresh nasal trauma. *Med. J. Aust.* 1 : 1059, 1967.

Fry, H. J. H. The distorted residual cartilage strut after submucous resection of the nasal septum. *Br. J. Plast. Surg.* 21 : 170, 1968.

Fry, H. J. H. The pathology and treatment of haematoma of the nasal septum. *Br. J. Plast. Surg.* 22 : 331, 1969.

Fry, H. J. H. Judicious turbinectomy for nasal obstruction. *Aust. N.Z. J. Surg.* 42 : 291, 1973.

Gibson, T., and Davis, W. B. The distortion of autogenous cartilage grafts: Its causes and prevention. *Br. J. Plast. Surg.* 10:257, 1958.

Gilbert, J. G., and Feit, L. J. The nasal aponeurosis and its role in rhinoplasty. *Arch. Otolaryngol.* 61:433, 1955.

Gilchrist, A. G. Surgery of the nasal septum and pyramid. *J. Laryngol. Otol.* 88:759, 1974.

Gill, J. A. Management of the difficult septum. *Arch. Otolaryngol.* 78:42, 1963.

Gipson, M., and Connolly, F. H. The incidence of schizophrenia and severe psychological disorders in patients 10 years after cosmetic rhinoplasty. *Br. J. Plast. Surg.* 28:155, 1975.

Gnudi, M. T., and Webster, J. P. *The Life and Times of Gaspare Tagliacozzi, Surgeon of Bologna (1545–1599).* New York: Reichner, 1950.

Goldman, I. B. New technique in surgery of the deviated nasal septum. *Arch. Otolaryngol.* 64:183, 1956.

Goldman, I. B. Removal of the nasal hump. *Arch. Otolaryngol.* 74:51, 1961.

Goldman, I. B. Principles in rhinoplasty. *Minn. Med.* 50:833, 1967.

Goldwyn, R. M. *Long-Term Results in Plastic and Reconstructive Surgery.* Boston: Little, Brown, 1980.

Gonzalez-Ulloa, M. Quantitative principles in cosmetic surgery of the face (profileplasty). *Plast. Reconstr. Surg.* 29:186, 1962.

Gonzalez-Ulloa, M., and Stevens, E. The role of chin correction in profileplasty. *Plast. Reconstr. Surg.* 41:477, 1968.

Goode, R. L., and Ross, J. Columellar advancement for nasal tip elevation. *Laryngoscope* 83:1123, 1973.

Gottschalk, G. H. An improved septoplasty: The microsurgical suture technique. *Ann. Plast. Surg.* 1:30, 1978.

Gray, L. The deviated nasal septum: I. Aetiology. *J. Laryngol. Otol.* 79:567, 1965.

Gray, L. The deviated nasal septum: II. Prevention and treatment. *J. Laryngol. Otol.* 81:806, 1967.

Gray, L. The deviated nasal septum: III. Its influence on the physiology and disease of the nose and ear. *J. Laryngol. Otol.* 81:953, 1967.

Griesman, B. L. Muscles and cartilages of the nose from the standpoint of a typical rhinoplasty. *Arch. Otolaryngol.* 34:431, 1944.

Griesman, B. L. Base of the nose: Anatomy and plastic repair. *Arch. Otolaryngol.* 51:541, 1950.

Guerrero-Santos, J. Cosmetic repair of the acute columellar-lip angle. *Plast. Reconstr. Surg.* 52:246, 1973.

Hage, J. Collapsed alae strengthened by conchal cartilage: The butterfly cartilage graft. *Br. J. Plast. Surg.* 18:92, 1964.

Hay, G. G. Psychiatric aspects of cosmetic nasal operations. *Br. J. Psychiatry* 116:85, 1970.

Hay, G. G., and Heather, B. B. Changes in psychometric test results following cosmetic nasal operations. *Br. J. Psychiatry* 122:89, 1973.

Heetderks, D. R. Observations on the reaction of normal nasal mucous membrane. *Am. J. Med. Sci.* 174:231, 1927.

Hinderer, K. H. Diagnosis of anatomic obstruction of the airways. *Arch. Otolaryngol.* 78:660, 1963.

Hinderer, K. H. *Fundamentals of Anatomy and Surgery of the Nose.* Birmingham: Aesculapius Publishing Co., 1971.

Horton, C. E. Achieving more nasal tip projection by the use of a small autogenous vomer or septal cartilage graft. Commentary. *Plast. Reconstr. Surg.* 56:211, 1975.

Huffman, W. C., and Lierle, D. M. Transoral lateral osteotomy of the nose. *Plast. Reconstr. Surg.* 25:45, 1960.

Huizing, E. H. Septum surgery in children: Indications, surgical technique and long-term results. *Rhinology* 17:91, 1979.

Ionescu, R., and Todea, B Subperichondromucous resection of the nasal septum without postoperative tamponade of the nasal mucosa, followed up in 1,000 cases over a 10 year period. *Otorinolaringol.* 10:69, 1965.

Janeke, J. B., and Wright, W. K. A study of nasal fracture healing. *Arch. Otolaryngol.* 97:253, 1973.

Jeppesen, F., and Windfeld, I. Dislocation of the nasal septal cartilage in the newborn. *Acta Obstet. Gynecol. Scand.* 51:5, 1972.

Johnson, C. M., and Anderson, J. R. The deviated nose: Its correction. *Laryngoscope* 87:1680, 1977.

Johnson, N. E. Secondary surgery of the septum. *Otolaryngol. Clin. North Am.* 7:75, 1974.

Joseph, G. Preliminary discussion of the thick septum problem. *Rev. Laryngol. Otol. Rhinol.* (Bord.) 5:111, 1967.

Jost, G., Meresse, F., and Torossian, F. Etude de la jonction entre les cartilages lateraux du nex. *Ann. Chir. Plast.* 18:175, 1973.

Jost, G., Vergnon, L., and Hadjean, E. Les asymétries nasales postopératoires. *Ann. Chir. Plast.* 20:173, 1973.

Juri, J., Juri, C., and Elias, J. C. Ear cartilage grafts to the nose. *Plast. Reconstr. Surg.* 63:377, 1979.

Kean, H. One stage repair of the twisted nose. *Eye Ear Nose Throat Monthly* 53:502, 1974.

Kern, E. B. Rhinomanometry. *Otolaryngol. Clin. North Am.* 6:863, 1973.

Kern, E. B. Surgery of the Nasal Valve. In G. A. Sisson and M. E. Tardy (eds.), *Plastic and Reconstructive Surgery.* Stuttgart: Theime, 1975.

Kerth, J. D., and Bytell, D. E. Revision in unsuccessful rhinoplasty. *Otolaryngol. Clin. North Am.* 7:65, 1974.

Knorr, N. J. Feminine loss of identity in rhinoplasty. *Arch. Otolaryngol.* 96:11, 1972.

Kosoy, J. Nasal surgery and airway resistance. *Laryngoscope* 89:1655, 1979.

Krmpotic-Nemanic, J., et al. Morphological and histological changes responsible for the droop of the nasal tip in advanced age. *Acta Otolaryngol.* (Stockh.) 71:278, 1971.

Lacy, G. M., and Conway, H. Recovery after meningitis with convulsions and paralysis following rhinoplasty: Cause for pause. Report of a case. *Plast. Reconstr. Surg.* 36:254, 1965.

Lamont, E. Rhinoplasty: Securing the graft. *Ann. Plast. Surg.* 4:84, 1980.

Lawson, V. G. Management of the twisted nose. *J. Otolaryngol.* 7:56, 1978.

Le Pesteur, J., and Firman, F. Reflexions sur L'auvent cartilagineux nasal. *Ann. Chir. Plast.* 22:1, 1977.

Lewis, M. L. Prevention and correction of cicatricial intranasal adhesions in rhinoplastic surgery. *Arch. Otolaryngol.* 60:215, 1954.

Lichtenstein, L. M., and Norman, P. S. Pathogensis of Allergic Rhinitis. In M. Samter (ed.), *Immunological Diseases.* Boston: Little, Brown, 1971.

Little, S. W. Management of enlarged turbinates. *Va. Med. Monthly* 90:484, 1963.

Maliniac, J. W. Prevention and treatment of sequelae in corrective rhinoplasty. *Am. J. Surg.* 50:84, 1940.

Mannheim, U. L. Surgery of the turbinate bones and the piriform crest. *Rhinology* 14:65, 1976.

Maran, A. G. The role of septoplasty and the submucous resection. *Clin. Otolaryngol.* 4:307, 1979.

Martin, H. Surgery of the crooked nose. *Arch. Otolaryngol.* 92:583, 1970.

Matthews, D. The nose tip. *Br. J. Plast. Surg.* 21:153, 1968.

May, M., and West, J. W. The "stuffy" nose. *Otolaryngol. Clin. North Am.* 6:655, 1973.

McCabe, B. F. The problem of the collapsing upper lateral cartilage. *Ann. Otol. Rhinol. Laryngol.* 88:524, 1979.

McCurdy, J. A., Jr. Reduction of excessive nasal tip projection with a modified Lipsett technique. *Ann. Plast. Surg.* 1:478, 1978.

McGrew, R. N. Sudden blindness secondary to injections of common drugs in the head and neck: I. Clinical experiences. *Trans. Am. Acad. Ophthalmol. Otolaryngol.* 86:152, 1978.

McGrew, R. N. Sudden blindness secondary to injections of common drugs in the head and neck: II. Animal studies. *Trans. Am. Acad. Ophthalmol. Otolaryngol.* 86:152, 1978.

McIndoe, A., and McLaughlin, C. R. Advances in plastic surgery. *Practitioner* 169:427, 1952.

McKinney, P., and Miller, W. Nasal xeroradiography. *Br. J. Plast. Surg.* 27:352, 1974.

McKinney, P., and Shively, R. Straightening the twisted nose. *Plast. Reconstr. Surg.* 64:176, 1978.

Millard, D. R. The triad of columella deformities. *Plast. Reconstr. Surg.* 31:370, 1963.

Millard, D. R. Corrective rhinoplasty. *Mod. Trends Plast. Surg.* 2:300, 1966.

Millard, D. R. Congenital nasal tip retrusion and three little composite ear grafts. *Plast. Reconstr. Surg.* 48:501, 1971.

Millard, D. R. The versatility of a chondromucosal flap in the nasal vestibule. *Plast. Reconstr. Surg.* 50:580, 1972.

Millard, D. R. Three very short noses and how they were lengthened. *Plast. Reconstr. Surg.* 65:10, 1979.

Millard, D. R. The alar cinch in the flat, flaring nose. *Plast. Reconstr. Surg.* 65:669, 1980.

Mink, P. J. *Physiologie der Obern Luftwege.* Leipzig: Vogel, 1920.

Natvig, P. Some aspects of the character and personality of Jacques Joseph. *Plast. Reconstr. Surg.* 47:452, 1971.

Natvig, P. *Jacques Joseph: Surgical Sculptor.* Philadelphia: Saunders, 1982.

Naumann, H. H. On the Physiology of the Nasal Cavity. In J. Conley and J. T. Dickinson (eds.), *Plastic and Reconstructive Surgery of the Head and Neck.* Stuttgart: Thieme, 1972.

Negus, V. E. *The Comparative Anatomy and Physiology of the Nose and Paranasal Sinuses.* London: Livingstone, 1958.

Neivert, H. Principles and mechanics of surgery of the bony nasal vault. *Arch. Otolaryngol.* 61:585, 1954.

Neuner, O. A simple procedure for correction of the hump nose. *Br. J. Plast. Surg.* 24:375, 1971.

Norman, P. S. Allergic rhinitis and sinusitis. *Postgrad. Med.* 54:94, 1973.

O'Brien, M. A. Current concepts of nasal septal surgery. *J. Laryngol. Otol.* 82:987, 1968.

O'Connor, G. B., and McGregor, M. W. Secondary rhinoplasties: Their cause and prevention. *Plast. Reconstr. Surg.* 15:404, 1955.

O'Connor, G. B., et al. The bulbous nose. *Plast. Reconstr. Surg.* 39:278, 1967.

Ogura, J. H., et al. Nasal obstruction and the mechanics of breathing: Physiologic relationship and the effects of nasal surgery. *Arch. Otolaryngol.* 83:135, 1966.

Ogura, J. H., Unno, T., and Nelson, J. R. Nasal surgery: Physiologic considerations of nasal obstruction. *Arch. Otolaryngol.* 88:288, 1968.

Ortiz-Monasterio, F., Lopez-Mas, J., and Araico, J. Rhinoplasty in the thick-skined nose. *Br. J. Plast. Surg.* 27:19, 1974.

Ortiz-Monasterio, F., and Olmedo, A. Corrective rhinoplasty before puberty: A long-term follow-up. *Plast. Reconstr. Surg.* 68:381, 1981.

Papangelou, L. Correction of the nasal septum deviation: A new conservative technique. *J. Laryngol. Otol.* 86:83, 1972.

Papangelou, L. Surgery of the nasal septum. *J. Laryngol. Otol.* 92:653, 1978.

Parisier, S. C. Correction of deviated nose: Interim septal surgery vs combined approach. *Arch. Otolaryngol.* 92:60, 1970.

Parkes, M. L., and Brennan, H. G. High septal transfixion to shorten the nose. *Plast. Reconstr. Surg.* 45:487, 1970.

Patterson, C. N. Reconstructive septonasoplasty. *Arch. Otolaryngol.* 84:121, 1966.

Patterson, C. N. Symposium: The supra-tip in rhinoplasty: A dilemma: I. Theories and causes of supra-tip convexities. *Laryngoscope* 86:45, 1975.

Patterson, C. N., and Powell, D. G. Facial analysis in patient evaluation for physiologic and cosmetic surgery. *Laryngoscope* 84:1004, 1974.

Pearson, B. W., and Goodman, W. S. S.M.R., septoplasty, and the surgical relief of nasal obstruction. *Can. J. Otolaryngol.* 2:238, 1973.

Peck, G. C. Rhinoplasty Surgery. In D. R. Millard (ed.), *Symposium on Corrective Rhinoplasty.* St. Louis: Mosby, 1976. P. 8.

Peck, G. C. The difficult nasal tip. *Clin. Plast. Surg.* 4:103, 1977.

Peer, L. A. An operation to repair lateral displacement of the lower border of the septal cartilage. *Arch. Otolaryngol.* 25:475, 1937.

Pers, M. An operation for the correction of snub-nose deformity. *Scand. J. Plast. Reconstr. Surg.* 7:64, 1973.

Pitanguy, I. Surgical importance of a dermacartilaginous ligament in bulbous noses. *Plast. Reconstr. Surg.* 36:247, 1965.

Pitanguy, I. *Aesthetic Plastic Surgery of Head and Body.* Berlin: Springer-Verlag, 1981.

Planas, H. The twisted nose. *Clin. Plast. Surg.* 4:55, 1977.

Pollet, J. Three autogenous struts for nasal tip support. *Plast. Reconstr. Surg.* 49:527, 1972.

Pollet, J., and Baudelot, S. Séquelles de la chirurgie esthétique de la base du nez. *Ann. Chir. Plast.* 12:185, 1967.

Pollet, J., and Weikel, A. M. Revision rhinoplasty. *Clin. Plast. Surg.* 4:47. 1977.

Proetz, A. W. Respiratory air currents and their clinical aspects. *J. Laryngol.* 67:1, 1953.

Reed, G. F. Nasal obstruction: Causes and treatment. *Postgrad. Med.* 54:464, 1963.

Rees, T. D. Nasal plastic surgery in the Negro. *Plast. Reconstr. Surg.* 43:13, 1969.

Rees, T. D. An aid in the treatment of supratip swelling after rhinoplasty. *Laryngoscope* 81:308, 1971.

Rees, T. D. Colloquium: Rhinoplasty. *Ann. Plast. Surg.* 1:597, 1978.

Rees, T. D., Krupp, S., and Wood-Smith, D. Secondary rhinoplasty. *Plast. Reconstr. Surg.* 46:322, 1970.

Reich, J. Post-traumatic deformity of the nasal skeleton. *Med. J. Aust.* 1:821, 1966.

Reidy, J. P. The nasal septum. *Ann. R. Coll. Surg. Engl.* 43:141, 1968.

Richardson, J. R. Turbinate treatment in vasomotor rhinitis. *Laryngoscope* 58:834, 1048.

Ritter, F. N. The vasculature of the nose. *Ann. Otol. Rhinol. Laryngol.* 79:468, 1970.

Roe, J. O. The deformity termed "pug nose" and its correction by a simple operation. *Med. Rec.* 31:621, 1887.

Rogers, B. O. Secondary and Tertiary Rhinoplasty. In *Transactions of the 4th International Congress of Plastic and Reconstructive Surgery.* Amsterdam: Excerpta Medica, 1969. Pp. 1065–1071.

Rogers, B. O. Rhinoplasty. In R. M. Goldwyn (ed.), *The Unfavorable Result in Plastic Surgery.* Boston: Little, Brown, 1972.

Rogers, B. O. The role of physical anthropology in plastic surgery today. *Clin. Plast. Surg.* 1:439, 1974.

Rogers, B. O. Secondary and Tertiary Correction of Postrhinoplastic Deformities: Some Dos and Don'ts. In D. R. Millard (ed.), *Symposium on Corrective Rhinoplasty.* St. Louis: Mosby, 1976. P. 23.

Roydhouse, N. A new look at the crooked nasal septum or septoplasty in children. *N.Z. Med. J.* 65:686, 1966.

Rudolph, R. *Pseudomonas* infection in the postoperative nasal septum. *Plast. Reconstr. Surg.* 70:87, 1982.

Safian, J. *Corrective Rhinoplastic Surgery.* New York: Hoeber, 1935.

Safian, J. A critical review of recent literature on rhinoplasty. *Plast. Reconstr. Surg.* 2:463, 1947.

Safian, J. Deceptive concepts of rhinoplasty. *Plast. Reconstr. Surg.* 18:127, 1956.

Safian, J. Fact and fallacy in rhinoplastic surgery. *Br. J. Plast. Surg.* 11:45, 1958.

Safian, J. The split-cartilage tip technique of rhinoplasty. *Plast. Reconstr. Surg.* 45:217, 1970.

Safian, J. Personal recollections of Professor Jacques Joseph. *Plast. Reconstr. Surg.* 46:175, 1970.

Sanders, S. H. Allergic rhinitis and sinusitis. *Otolaryngol. Clin. North Am.* 4:565, 1971.

Saunders, W. H. Septal dermoplasty: Ten years experience. *Trans. Am. Acad. Ophthalmol. Otolaryngol.* 72:153, 1968.

Seeley, R. D. Reconstruction of the nasal tip: A new technique. *Plast. Reconstr. Surg.* 3:594, 1948.

Seltzer, A. P. The nasal septum: Plastic repair of the deviated septum associated with a deflected tip. *Arch. Otolaryngol.* 40:433, 1944.

Seltzer, A. P. The surgically induced saddle nose. *Eye Ear Nose Throat Monthly* 30:350, 1951.

Seltzer, A. P. Cautions in rhinoplastic surgery. *Eye Ear Nose Throat Monthly* 32:85 1953.

Seltzer, A. P. Submucous resection: Prevention of septal perforation. *J. Natl. Med. Assoc.* 62:342, 1970.

Sheen, J. H. Absorption of small bone graft in nasal tip. (Letter to the Editor.) *Plast. Reconstr. Surg.* 56:332, 1975.

Sheen, J. H. The Small Dorsal Hump. In *Transactions of the 6th International Congress of Plastic and Reconstructive Surgery.* Paris: Masson, 1975. P. 479.

Shehadi, S. I. Reducing the eyelid edema and ecchymosis that occur after corrective rhinoplasty. *Plast. Reconstr. Surg.* 49:508, 1972.

Ship, A. G. Alar base resection for wide flaring nostrils. *Br. J. Plast. Surg.* 28:77, 1975.

Siegel, M. I. The role of the cartilaginous nasal septum in midfacial growth. Correspondence. *Plast. Reconstr. Surg.* 65:93, 1980.

Siegler, J. The place of septal replacement operation in treatment of nasal obstruction. *J. Laryngol. Otol.* 87:153, 1973.

Silver, A. G. Pitfalls in rhinoplasty. *Eye Ear Nose Throat Monthly* 31:556, 1952.

Simons, R. L. Adjunctive measures in rhinoplasty. *Otolaryngol. Clin. North Am.* 8:717, 1975.

Smith, H. W. Nasal hump implant. (Letter to the Editor.) *Arch. Otolaryngol.* 98:435, 1973.

Smith, H. W. Saddle nose. (Letter to the Editor.) *Arch. Otolaryngol.* 98:435, 1973.

Smith, T. W. As clay in the potter's hand: A review of 221 rhinoplasties. *Ohio Med. J.* 63:1055, 1967.

Smith, T. W. Osteotomy and infraction in rhinoplasty. *Arch. Otolaryngol.* 100:266, 1974.

Smithdeal, C. D. The significance of correction of the anterior septum in rhinoplasty. *South. Med. J.* 61:931, 1968.

Smithdeal, C. D. The sequential septo-rhinoplasty. *Laryngoscope* 85:1216, 1975.

Snell, G. E. D. A history of rhinoplasty. *Can. J. Otolaryngol.* 2:224, 1973.

Snyder, G. B. Rhinoplasty in the Negro. *Plast. Reconstr. Surg.* 47:572, 1971.

Snyder, G. B., et al. A new chin implant for microgenia. *Plast. Reconstr. Surg.* 61:854, 1978.

Soss, T. L. The allergic patient and rhinoplasty procedures. *Otolaryngol. Clin. North Am.* 7:845, 1974.

Spector, M. Indications for a submucous resection. *Arch. Otolaryngol.* 70:334, 1959.

Spina, V., Kamakura, L., and Psillakis, J. A new method for correction of the prominent nasal tip. *Plast. Reconstr. Surg.* 51:416, 1973.

Stallings, J. O., and Sessions, D. G. Airway obstruction due to prolapse of the lower lateral cartilages in saddle deformity. *Laryngoscope* 82:515, 1972.

Stark, R. B., and Frileck, P. F. Conchal cartilage grafts in augmentation rhinoplasty and orbital floor fracture. *Plast. Reconstr. Surg.* 43:591, 1969.

Steiss, C. F. Errors in rhinoplasty and their prevention. *Plast. Reconstr. Surg.* 28:276, 1961.

Stevens, M. H. General anesthesia in nasal septal surgery. *Ear Nose Throat J.* 56:22, 1977.

Stranc, M. F., and Robertson, G. A. A classification of the nasal skeleton. *Ann. Plast. Surg.* 2:468, 1979.

Stucker, F. J. Non-Caucasian rhinoplasty. *Trans. Am. Acad. Ophthalmol. Otolaryngol.* 82:417, 1971.

Stucker, F. J., and Smith, T. E. The nasal bony dorsum and cartilaginous vault. *Arch. Otolaryngol.* 102:695, 1976.

Takemiya, S., et al. Bilateral rhinomanometry using pneumotachometer. *Jpn. J. Otolaryngol.* (Tokyo) 66:985, 1963.

Tamerin, J. A. Subtotal removal of the upper and lower lateral cartilages and overlying adipose tissue in rhinoplasty. *Plast. Reconstr. Surg.* 40:40, 1967.

Tamerin, J. A. Five most important points in a reduction rhinoplasty. *Plast. Reconstr. Surg.* 48:214, 1971.

Taylor, M. The origin and functions of nasal mucus. *Laryngoscope* 84:612, 1974.

Thompson, H. S. Preoperative selection and counseling of patients for rhinoplasty. Editorial. *Plast. Reconstr. Surg.* 50:174, 1972.

Togawa, K., and Konno, A. Aerodynamic studies on the effect of nasal septal plasty. *Rhinology* 15:173, 1977.

Toranto, I. R. Mentoplasty: A new approach. *Plast. Reconstr. Surg.* 65:875, 1982.

Trop, J. L., and Golden, J. S. Rhinoplasty in transsexuals. *Plast. Reconstr. Surg.* 55:593, 1975.

Vetter, U., Pirsig, W., and Heinze, E. Growth activity in human septal cartilage: Age-dependent incorporation of labelled sulfate in different anatomic locations. *Plast. Reconstr. Surg.* 71:167, 1983.

Walter, C. Composite grafts in nasal surgery. *Arch. Otolaryngol.* 90:622, 1969.

Walter, C. The Nasal Septum. In M. M. Paparella and D. A. Shumrick (eds.), *Otolaryngology* (vol. 3). Philadelphia: Saunders, 1973.

Walter, C. D. Secondary nasal revision after rhinoplasties. *Trans. Am. Acad. Ophthalmol. Otolaryngol.* 80:519, 1975.

Webster, G. V. Skin excision in reduction rhinoplasty. *Plast. Reconstr. Surg.* 51:289, 1973.

Webster, R. C., Davidson, T. M., and Smith, R. C. Curved lateral osteotomy for airway protection in rhinoplasty. *Arch. Otolaryngol.* 103:454, 1977.

Webster, R. C., Davidson, T. M., and Smith, R. C. Browplasty as an adjunct to rhinoplasty. *Head Neck Surg.* 1:112, 1978.

Webster, R. C., et al. Columella-splitting incisions in rhinoplasty. *J. Otolaryngol.* 8:417, 1979.

Weimert, T. A., and Yoder, M. G. Antibiotics and nasal surgery. *Laryngoscope* 90:667, 1980.

Wexler, M. Post-rhinoplastic complications. *Eye Ear Nose Throat Monthly* 31:553, 1969.

Wexler, M. R. Nasal septum: Experimental and clinical correlation of surgery and injury. *Laryngoscope* 81:1409, 1971.

Wexler, M. R. Surgical repair of the caudal end of the septum. *Laryngoscope* 87:304, 1977.

Willemot, J. Correction of old nasal deviations. *Plast. Reconstr. Surg.* 43:430, 1969.

Willemot, J. The crooked or twisted nose. *Eye Ear Nose Throat Monthly* 49:42, 1970.

Williams, J. E. The pinched nasal tip. *Clin. Plast. Surg.* 4:41, 1977.

Williams, R. I. Functions of the nasal septum as related to septal reconstructive surgery. *Laryngoscope* 63:212, 1953.

Williams, R. I. Physiology of the nose in reconstructive surgery. *Rocky Mt. Med. J.* 51:352, 1954.

Williams, R. I. The nasal index: anthropological and clinical. *Ann. Otol. Rhinol. Laryngol.* 67:171, 1956.

Williams, R. I. Hemitransfixion approach to problems of the nasal septum. *Laryngoscope* 77:1116, 1967.

Williams, R. I. Nasal Physiology. In M. M. Paparella and D. A. Shumrick (eds.), *Otolaryngology* (vol. 1). Philadelphia: Saunders, 1973.

Wright, W. K. Symposium: The supra-tip in rhinoplasty: A dilemma: II. Influence of surrounding structure and prevention. *Laryngoscope* 86:50, 1975.

Wright, M. R., and Wright, W. K. A psychological study of patients undergoing cosmetic surgery. *Arch. Otolaryngol.* 101:145, 1975.

7. *Aesthetic Rhinoplasty of the Nasal Tip*

George C. Peck

Nasal tip surgery is one of the most challenging areas of plastic surgery, for every case presents a new and dynamic problem. The surgeon is constantly faced with the realization that any mistake will show up in the final result. The nasal tip will constantly be there for the patient and the world to see. In order to avoid mistakes and perform predictable, reproducible, and, most important, pleasing results, the surgeon must thoroughly understand the dynamic aesthetic anatomy and the surgical techniques directly related to a given problem. This chapter offers insights from my 25 years of experience dealing with rhinoplastic problems.

PLANNING

Successful surgery always requires careful planning. In my practice I use the following format:

1. Examination of the patient
2. Analysis of the problem
3. Establishment of a surgical plan
4. Review of preoperative photographs

The patient's consultation begins with a thorough understanding of the problem as stated and described by the patient. I must know what the patient hopes to gain from the surgery and I must decide whether the goals are realistic. As I talk to the patient, I begin my evaluation. I usually examine the nasal tip and its relationship to the entire face for balance and symmetry. I examine its relationship to the bridge, glabella, forehead, upper lip, chin, and neck, discreetly making notes of my findings.

Once the visual examination of the nasal tip is completed, the physical examination begins. This involves a close inspection and palpation of the nasal tip and all related structures. The examination will tell me certain basic facts that are essential for good planning. Most important is the nasal tip projection. I want to know whether it is too high, too low, or about right. The tip is examined and the extent of width and bulbousness determined. These findings will directly affect the surgical planning.

In the profile view, I observe the nasolabial angle and the entire lip-columella-lobule complex. I then look at the relationship of the nasal tip to the nasal bridge. Palpation gives me a clue to the rigidity, thickness, and support of the lower laterals. I palpate the nasal spine and the caudal end of the septum. Palpation also helps to determine the skin condition. Is it thick or thin? How will it drape over our osseocartilaginous framework? Is it laden with sebaceous glands? The examination continues with the intranasal inspection. Are there septal deflections, either low or high? Low deflections will almost always produce a crooked tip; high deflections may affect nasal physiology.

When all problems have been ascertained and written up on a chart, I always asterisk the most important defects and concentrate my efforts on devising a plan that will correct them. For example, in a patient with a hanging columella, this problem must be satisfactorily corrected if the patient is to be happy with the result. A generally good result from the surgeon's point of view is meaningless unless the patient is satisfied.

The final step in planning a rhinoplasty is photographing the patient. The photographs must be standardized (I prefer a 5- × 7-in. size) and should include serious and smiling profiles, serious and smiling front views, a worm's-eye view, and an oblique view. These are best taken in black and white with a high-quality camera in order to give good detail while preventing distortion. The light must show all shadow lines (I prefer fixed lights rather than flash). The photographs are then studied in detail, and the information they supply, together with that gained in the course of the physical examination, will enable me to develop a definitive surgical plan.

During surgery, the photographs should be displayed on the x-ray viewer and constantly used as a reference. This is essential, for when the patient lies on the operating table the surgeon's perspective of lines and angles of the nose will change. The same thing applies to the total facial appearance and balance; position can make a long nose appear normal.

AESTHETIC SURGICAL ANATOMY

Lower Lateral Cartilages

These paired fibroelastic cartilaginous structures produce the skeletal support for the nasal tip pyramid. They have three surgically important components—the lateral crus, the dome, and the medial crus (Fig. 7-1).

LATERAL CRUS
This structure provides the skeletal support for the lateral wall of the nasal tip pyramid and also supplies bulk for the nasal tip. Modification (sculpturing) of the lateral crus will create the necessary aesthetic lines. The bilateral sculptured lines will impart a gull-wing design to the nasal tip, which is the desired and preferred aesthetic effect (Fig. 7-2). Cephalad to the sculptured line (intracartilaginous incision) a section of lower lateral cartilage will be removed together with contiguous fibrofatty tissue, producing a "level discrepancy" at the sculptured line. Cephalad to this line nothing remains between the external skin and the internal vestibular lining. Below the line is a full thickness of external skin, fibrofat, lower lateral cartilage, and internal vestibular skin. As light strikes the level discrepancy it will cast a shadow, and it is this shadow that will create the good aesthetic lines of the nasal tip. In essence, this is the same as a scar that has a level discrepancy between its two sides. Even in the thick-skinned nose there will be some degree of level discrepancy.

DOME
This structure provides height for the nasal tip projection. An important surgical anatomic consideration is the structure or structures that provide nasal tip elevation and support, but first we must understand the functional anatomy of the nasal tip pyramid.

It is the septal cartilage and medial crura that provide the tent-post support for the nasal tip pyramid. However, this support does not give the nasal tip (lobule) the necessary projection. This essential aesthetic detail is afforded by the domes of the lower lateral cartilage. Nasal tip projection is therefore comprised of these two important components. Surgical reconstruction may involve one or both, depending on the problem.

MEDIAL CRUS
This structure provides tent-post support in the columella for the nasal tip pyramid. Together with the septal cartilage, it lends support to the pyramid; however, the septum

Figure 7-1

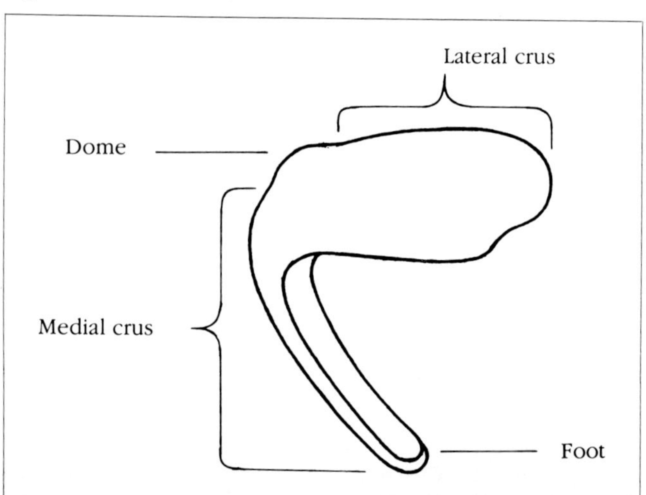

Figure 7-2

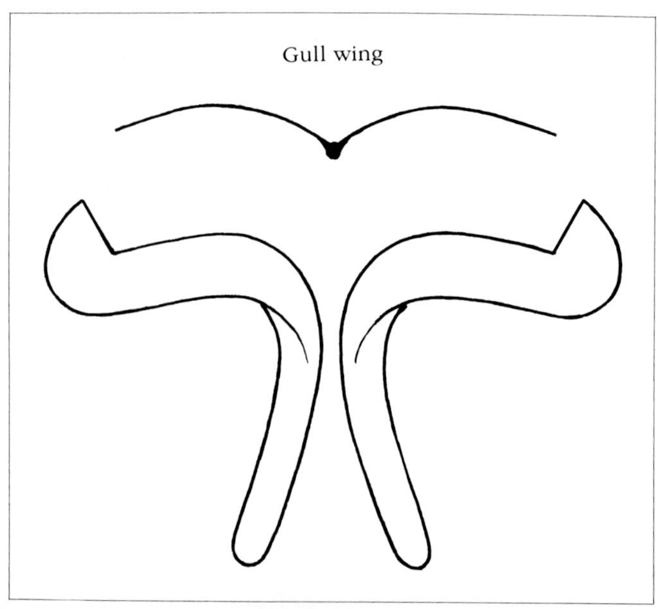

provides the bulk of this support. Its intimate attachment to the skin of the columella makes separation difficult. In some conditions the feet of the medial crura, together with dense fibrous tissue, create too much bulk at the base of the columella.

Septum

This hyaline, cartilaginous structure in the nasal tip area separates the anterior right and left nasal passageways. The caudal end lends the most support to the nasal tip pyramid. In addition to its function as upright support, the downward projection of the caudal border gives the aesthetic lines to the columella. It is the primary producer of the lip-columella-lobule complex, which is so important to the profile.

As mentioned earlier, the septum is the primary support for the nasal pyramid. If the nose had no lower laterals, the septal tent-post effect would produce a sharp, pointed, unaesthetic tip. The dome areas of the lower laterals lie over the tent post, providing the softness for the nasal tip. This subtle nasal tip projection gives the nasal tip a pleasing aesthetic effect.

Figure 7-3 shows the entire lip-columella-lobule complex and lines. In a female, the nasolabial angle should be greater than 90 degrees whereas in the male 90 degrees is satisfactory. The columella profile line should create an obtuse angle, as shown in the drawing. Contributing to this line is the nasal spine prominence or lack of prominence. If the nasolabial angle is less than 90 degrees, it will give the appearance of a recessed maxilla. In the crowded-lip deformity, either the nasal spine or the septal cartilage may be too prominent and extend caudad too far into the upper lip.

The caudal edges of the medial crura may contribute to columellar defects such as irregularity, asymmetry, or hanging. However, surgery in this area is rare, as these are not usually the primary anatomic problems.

Figure 7-3

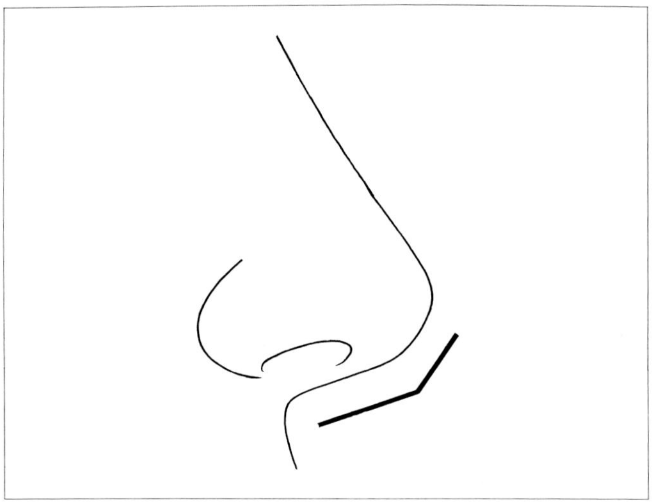

Figure 7-4

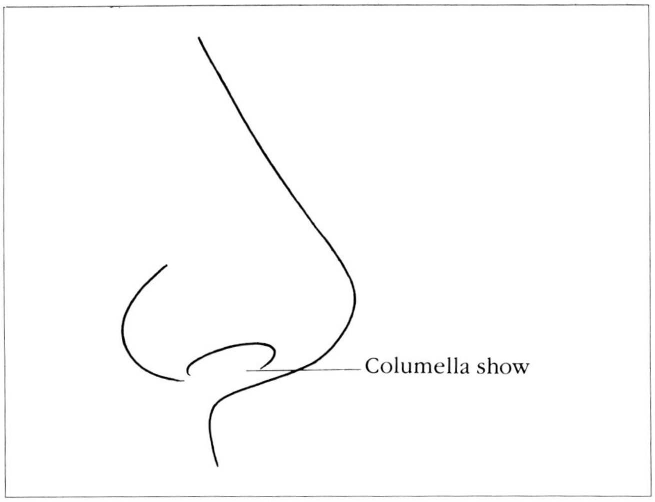

Alar Rims

The external nasal opening is formed by the alar rim laterally and the columella medially. Good profile aesthetics will have an arching alar rim with the columella showing below the rim in the profile view (Fig. 7-4). An alar rim that hides the columella in the profile view makes the nasal tip appear bulky and the nose overlong. Conversely, too much arch allows too much septum to show. The worm's-eye view tells us about flaring. It is important to remember that a reduction rhinoplasty essentially reduces nasal tip projection. It lowers the tent post; consequently, the sides become baggy and lateral alar rim flaring is caused.

ANATOMIC DEFORMITIES CLASSIFIED

Anatomic deformities are classified as follows:

- I. Nasal tip projection
  - A. Primary support
    - 1. Short septum
      - a. Congenital
      - b. Traumatic
      - c. Postsurgical
    - 2. Abnormally high septum
  - B. Lower lateral projection
    - 1. Flat or blunted
    - 2. Too high
- II. Bulbous tip
  - A. Lateral crus of lower lateral
    - 1. Too large
    - 2. Too thick
  - B. Thick skin
- III. Wide tip
  - A. Slightly
  - B. Moderately
  - C. Extremely

IV. Profile
  A. Long nose—glabella to tip of lobule
  B. Columella
    1. Recessed (snubbed)
    2. Hanging
  C. Nasolabial angle
    1. Acute
    2. Wide
  D. Drooping lobule
V. Alar rims
  A. Flaring
  B. High arch
  C. Veiling

SURGICAL TECHNIQUES

First, the basic conservative rhinoplasty is performed in almost all cases (Fig. 7-5). If used correctly, this technique burns no bridges. After completing the basic operation, I can evaluate the nasal tip and do whatever else is necessary. The following ancillary techniques are used for the more important problems.

Nasal Tip Projection

The loss of projection following rhinoplasty has always been an unsolved problem. The surgeon must understand that the removal of portions of the lower laterals reduces volume in the nasal tip pyramid, causing a collapse of the nasal tip pyramid in all planes. Therefore, it is easy to understand what happens to a nose with good normal projection prior to surgery. The modification of the lower laterals will produce a loss of the subtle tip projection that is desired for good aesthetics. It is for this reason that we vary the position of the intracartilaginous incision.

LACK OF PRIMARY SUPPORT

Short Septum. SEPTAL STRUT. If the septum is present, a submucous resection is done, and a septal cartilage graft is taken for the strut.

EAR CONCHAL CARTILAGE GRAFT. Where the septum has had previous surgery or trauma, septal cartilage will not be available. I then use the autogenous ear cartilage. An incision is made in the skin behind the ear, and the cartilage strut is taken from the straightest area of the concha. Straightening can be done with the Rubin morselizer, although this will have little bearing on the final result (as will become obvious later).

TECHNIQUE. The graft is to be inserted between the medial crura of the columella (Fig. 7-6). An infracartilaginous incision is made high in the columella. A pocket is dissected between the medial crura down to the nasal spine and up into the lobule. The strut is placed in the pocket and the length trimmed as necessary so that it extends from the spine to the lobule tip. The strut should not lie in the columella below the edges of the medial crura or it will distort the columella and flatten the important obtuse angle. The graft is held in position by through-and-through sutures.

One can now understand why the slight curves or thinness of the concha will have no bearing on the end result. The graft is sandwiched between the medial crura, and as they heal, the columella gains its support from the combination of all three structures.

LACK OF LOWER LATERAL DOME PROJECTION

Even in the patient with good primary support in the columella there may still be a flat or blunted nasal tip.

Technique. A graft of cartilage, approximately 4 × 9 mm, is taken from the ear conchal cartilage (Fig. 7-7). The graft should be taken so that its convex curve will simulate the curvature and fullness of the nasal tip. An infracartilaginous incision is made at the medial crural side of the dome of the lower lateral cartilage. With sharp dissecting scissors, a pocket is developed horizontally across the domes at the position at which augmentation of the tip projection is desired. The onlay cartilage graft is inserted into the pocket. We try to make the pocket only large enough to accommodate the graft. (If necessary, additional layers of graft can be added.) In a short nasal tip projection, the tent post of the cartilage graft will provide the necessary support and elevation. However, it is almost always necessary to combine this technique with a subtle augmentation of the lobule projection (Fig. 7-8). This is done with an onlay graft positioned over the existing domes and over the projecting end of the strut graft. The onlay softens the point of the strut and provides a more anatomically aesthetic nasal tip.

EXCESSIVE LOWER LATERAL DOME PROJECTION

Excessive projection is common in the Pinocchio nasal tip. This is an extremely rare condition, and most noses that appear to have the problem will reduce satisfactorily with the basic technique. In any event, it is better to have a larger nose with good anatomic lines.

Technique. Lateral rotation of the lateral crus and dome (Fig. 7-9) is employed.

Bulbous Tip

In the bulbous tip the first step, as always, is the basic technique. This should always reduce the fullness as related to the lower lateral cartilages. If it does not, the problem may be too much remaining lateral crus in the alar rim. I would then check the remaining width using a retrograde dissection, and if it were greater than 3 mm (in this type of case), I would reduce it to 3 mm.

Many bulbous tip cases are related to thick skin. We must *never* overreduce the size of a nose with thick, heavy skin. The skin will not redrape adequately, and there will be a subsequent fullness remaining, especially in the supratip area.

The preferred technique for thick-skin problems is very conservative reduction in size, the goal being to create good lines rather than small size. Many tips will also be enhanced by the addition of an onlay nasal tip graft, which forces the tip to have a better projection to the lobule.

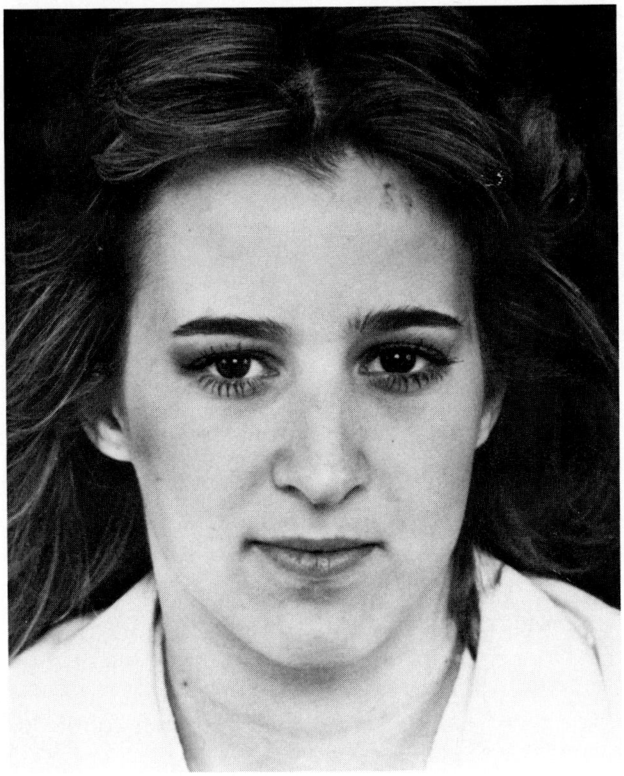

A

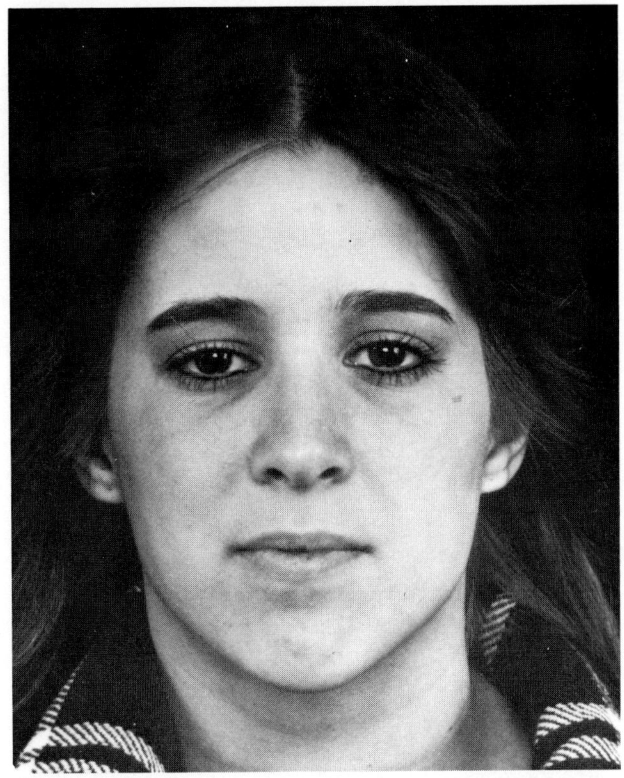

B

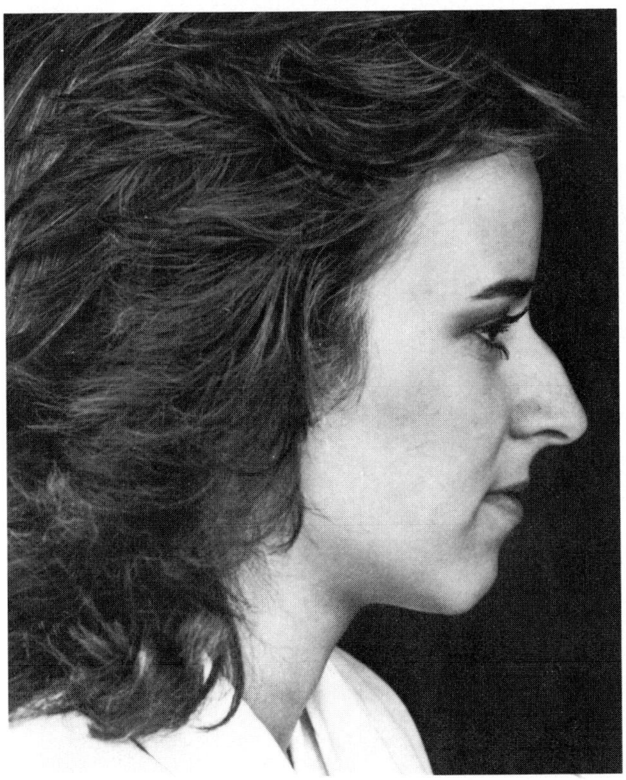

C

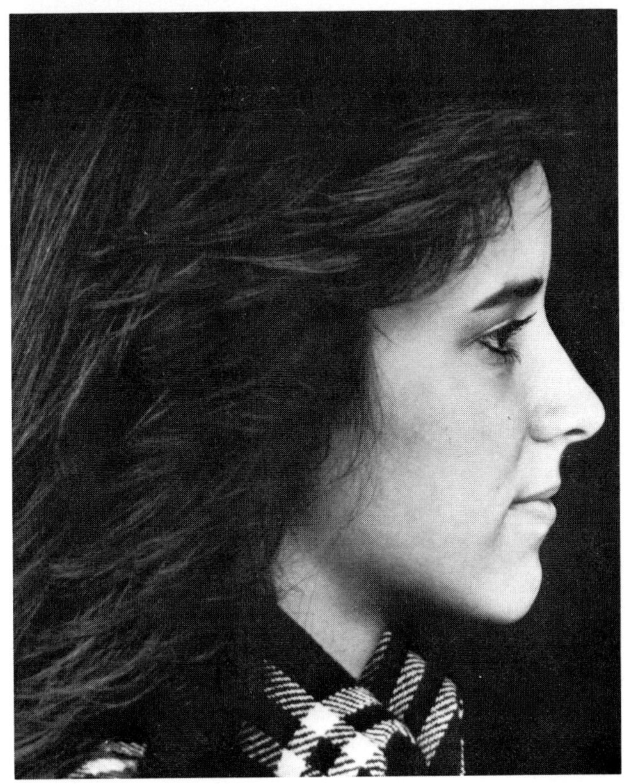

D

Figure 7-5
A–D. Primary rhinoplasty of a 20-year-old patient, with postoperative photographs 1 year later.

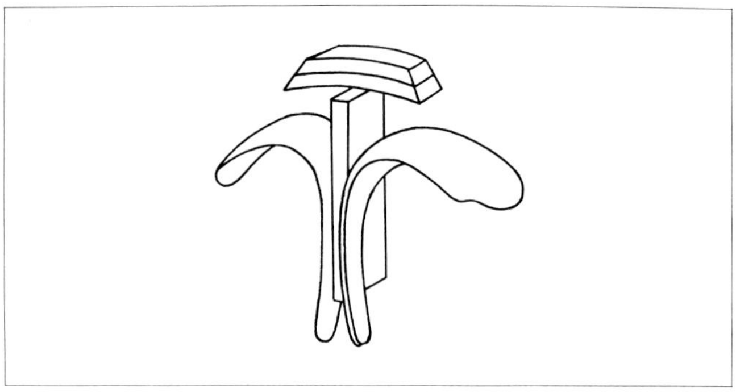

Figure 7-6

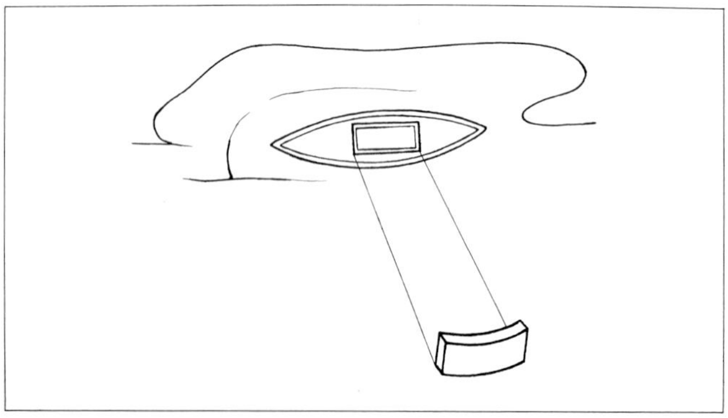

Figure 7-7

Wide Tip

SLIGHTLY TOO WIDE AFTER BASIC RHINOPLASTY
The rationale is to weaken the dome by cross-cutting so as to create a sharper dome angle (Fig. 7-10).

WIDE
The rationale is to decrease the lineal length of the lateral crus that is producing the wide nasal tip. Cross-cutting is done at the height of the nasal tip (Fig. 7-11), and the lateral crus is shortened by excision of a section laterally.

Profile

LONG NOSE
The rationale is to shorten the overall length of the nose from the glabella to the tip of the nasal lobule. The entire caudal end of the septum is elevated as it projects downward into the columella. After the septal cartilage is shortened, concern is with the correct lines at the nasolabial angle and at the obtuse angle.

COLUMELLA
Recessed (Snubbed) Columella. The rationale is to lengthen the columella's downward projection. If there is sufficient looseness to the columella skin, the following maneuver is undertaken.

TECHNIQUE. Through an infracartilaginous incision in the columella, a pocket is developed caudal to the medial

Figure 7-8
A, B. Primary rhinoplasty with augmentation of nasal tip projection utilizing hump cartilage for onlay graft. Postoperative photograph is 2 years later.

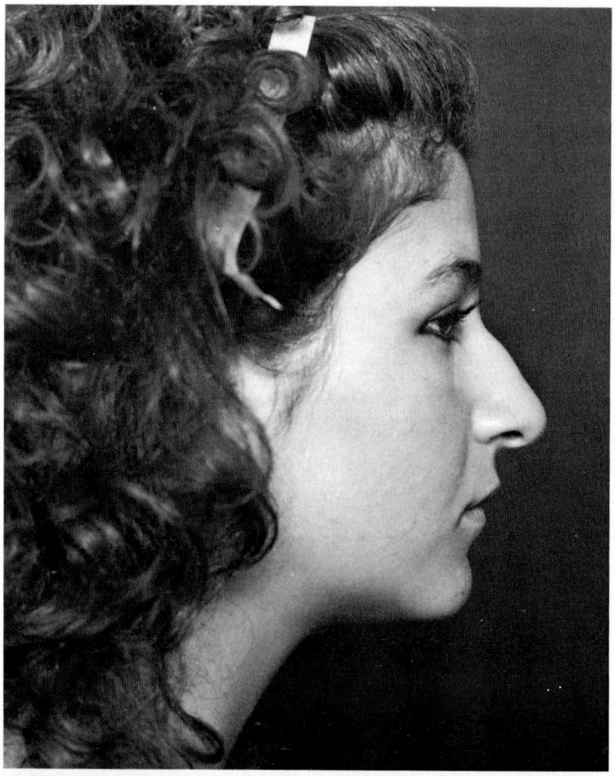

A

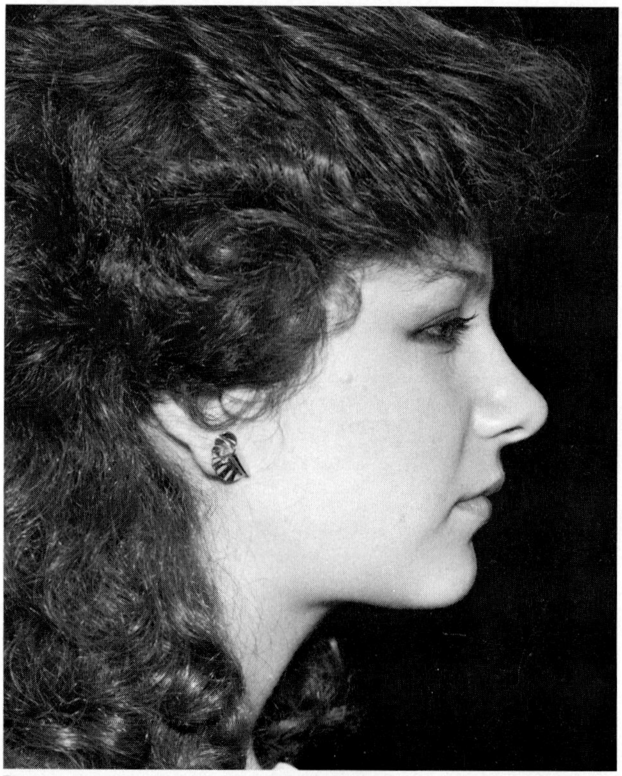

B

crura. An autogenous conchal cartilage graft is inserted. In some cases, better pocket dissection may be obtained by an intraoral approach, beginning at the nasal spine. After insertion of the graft, the obtuse angle *must always* be inspected. Placing a larger graft in the columella and a smaller piece at the angle creates an obtuse angle effect. From the front view, the piece creating the angle should have a triangular configuration to simulate the front view of this area. The triangular graft is only a filler graft and should not put tension on the lobule skin. If greater projection of the nasal tip is required, an additional *onlay* graft should be inserted into a separate pocket overlying the domes of the lower lateral cartilage.

If the columella is so short as not to be amenable to this technique, it will be necessary at some point to rotate flaps of internal nasal lining to augment the columella. At a later point, the cartilage grafts can be inserted.

Figure 7-9. A–C

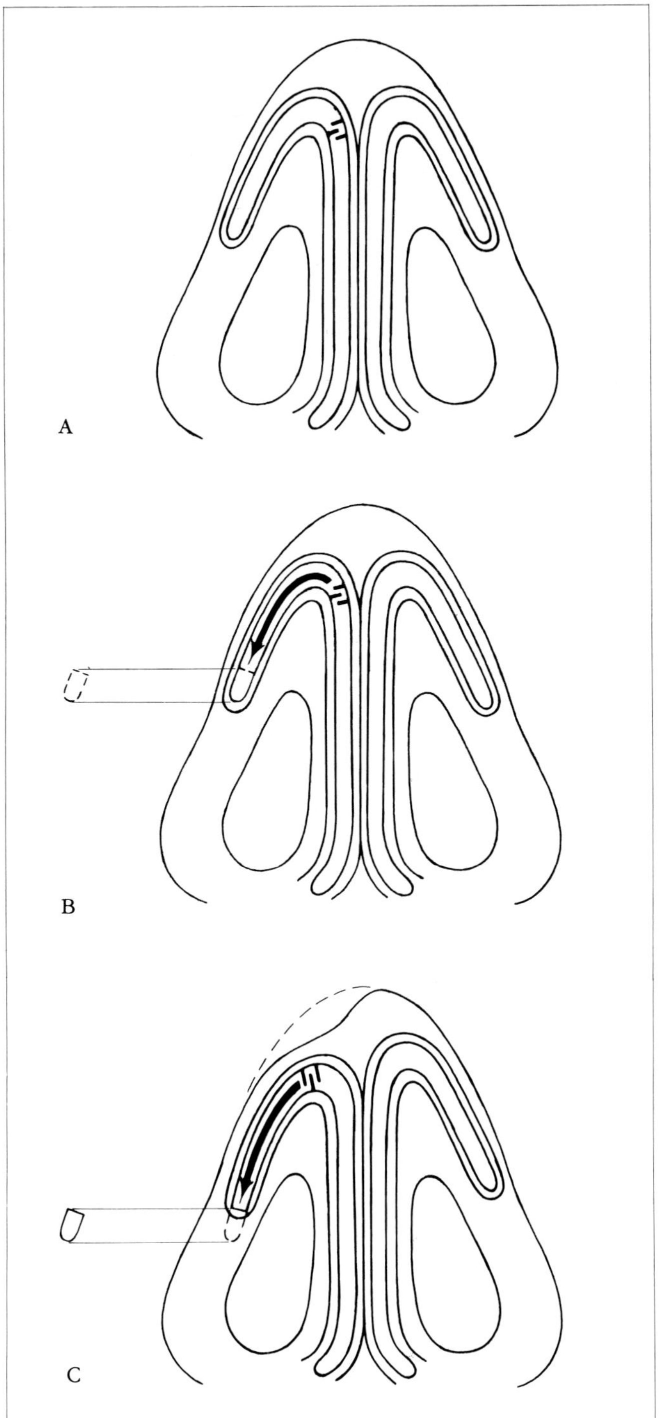

Hanging Columella. TECHNIQUE. The first step is always to shorten the caudal end of the septum. It is rarely necessary to trim the membranous columella or the medial crura. (Many of the older textbooks showed the problem to be the membranous columella, but I rarely find that this is the case.)

NASOLABIAL ANGLE

This angle should never be less than 90 degrees. In a male it should be 90 degrees, and in a female it should be greater than 90 degrees.

Technique for Acute Angle. An incision is made intranasally at the foot of the medial crus. A pocket is developed at the junction of the columella and lip, and ear conchal cartilage or septum grafts are inserted. It will usually take multiple layers and much more than anticipated. The horizontal dimension of the graft should usually be less than 1 cm. I have stopped using alloplastic materials in this area since they inevitably produce problems, such as erosion into the anterior buccal sulcus.

Technique for Wide Angle. The correct angle is created by trimming the caudal end of the septum.

Nasal Spine and Crowded Lip. On occasion, the nasal spine may be prominent, creating an undesirable fullness

Figure 7-10

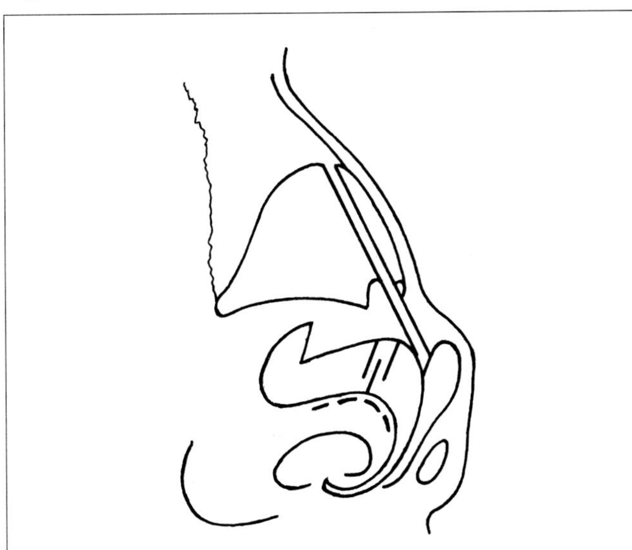

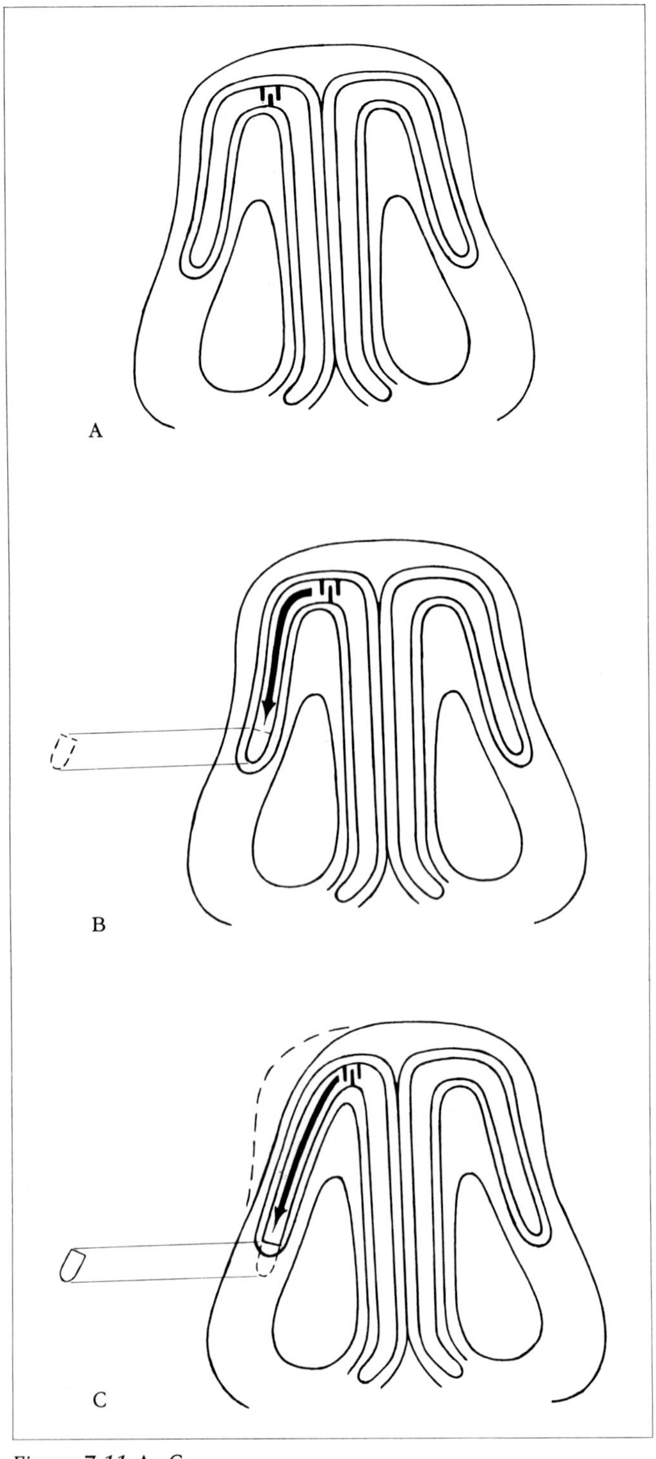

Figure 7-11. A–C

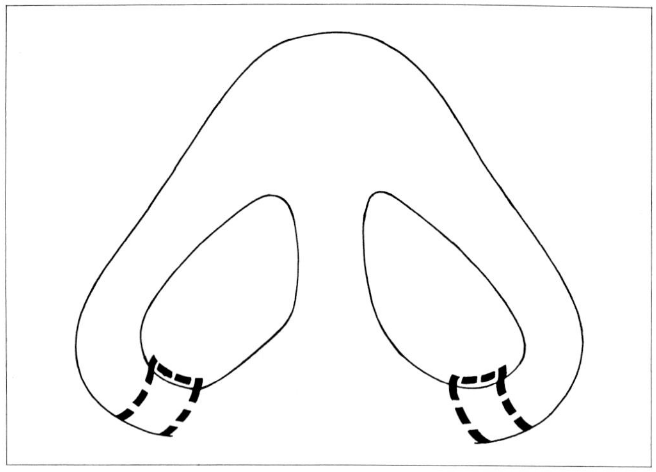

Figure 7-12

at the nasolabial angle. In many patients it is almost as if the caudal end of the nose grew into the upper lip. Through a transfixion incision, the nasal spine is exposed and a *portion* removed with a small bone rongeur. *Never* remove all of the nasal spine.

DROOPING LOBULE

A drooping lobule is a difficult problem that may require multiple solutions. We are concerned with the lobule that does not rotate upward after the obtuse angle has been created in the caudal septal cartilage.

This problem is usually a result of lack of tip lobule projection, and an onlay graft may be sufficient to solve it. Or an onlay nasal tip cartilage graft combined with a filler triangular graft may be the solution.

Alar Rims

FLARING

Use a modified Weir technique (Fig. 7-12).

COLLAPSE

HIGH ARCH

The rationale is to add a shaped ear cartilage graft. An incision is made intranasally in the alar rim lateral to the site of the graft. The graft is taken from the ear concha so as to simulate the shape and convexity of the rim. The pocket in the rim is developed from the incision. Blowing up the site with infiltration of anesthetic aids the dissection of the pocket, and the graft is inserted.

VEILING

The rationale is to trim the alar rim to the desired curvature. Outline the desired curvature (arch) on the alar rim and trim accordingly. The excision must always be pie-shaped so that the resulting incision line lies at the caudal alar margin. Since the incision line represents a curve, healing will tend to straighten the curve, and our result is always less curvature then we had expected.

Supratip Fullness

In order to solve this problem one must understand all of the possible causes.

THICK SKIN

As already mentioned, the overreduction of a thick-skinned nose can prevent draping, with subsequent supratip fullness. The correction is to make the nose larger. Start with one or more onlay nasal tip grafts. In some cases a complete reconstruction of nasal size will be necessary, utilizing a strut and dorsal onlay graft.

FIBROFATTY TISSUE
The inadequate removal of this tissue can produce a fullness in the supratip area. Such tissue will not only fill out the supratip area but mask the level discrepancy created at the sculptured lines. Surgical correction is removal of the fibrofatty tissue.

SUPRATIP SEPTUM
The inadequate lowering of the supratip septum is a very common cause of supratip swelling and produces the parrot-beak deformity. Surgical correction is simply to shave the septal cartilage in the supratip area.

GULL-WING INCISION
The gull-wing incision produces a V-shaped level discrepancy in the supratip area. If the sculpturing incisions leave too much dome cartilage in the supratip area, there will be excessive fullness.

UPPER LATERALS
The upper laterals may project down into area in which we are attempting to obtain the level discrepancy. This is almost never the case if we do not shorten the nose.

COMPLICATIONS

Complications in rhinoplastic surgery are extremely rare. The following are several that I have encountered.

Infection

In the past 25 years, I have seen one true nasal infection, which responded to the specific antibiotic. I routinely use prophylactic antibiotic for 3 days postoperatively if the nasal passageways are packed. I have always used tetracycline, 250 mg qid.

Bleeding

I have been called back to the hospital on account of postoperative bleeding no more than three times. If the packing is loose, the addition of more packing may suffice. In one case in which bleeding persisted, I completely removed the packing and put in new packing, and the bleeding subsequently stopped. I always do screening bleeding tests and always include these in my preadmission testing.

Persistent Ecchymosis

In a few patients the ecchymosis persisted for a number of months, but I never had a case in which ecchymosis did not ultimately clear.

Marked Swelling

The swelling and ecchymosis in my present patients is far less than it was 15 or more years ago. I am sure this decline is directly related to the conservative techniques, fewer incisions, less undermining, careful lateral osteotomy, no periosteal elevation, etc.

I have not found enzymes helpful, but I routinely use an antihistamine. (Orinade spansules are given bid.) *Crushed* ice in surgical gloves covers the eyes for a good part of the first 2 postoperative days.

Vestibular Scar Contractures

Vestibular skin must *never* be excised. Incisions should be minimal, as described in basic technique. The elimination of the intercartilaginous incision preserves the internal nasal valve and prevents scarring. The intracartilaginous and transfixion incisions are separated by vestibular lining so that there are two separate incisions. Thus, an extended curved incision, which tends to straighten with healing and produces a vestibular contracture, is prevented.

8. Posttraumatic Nasal Deformities

Guy Jost

CORRECTION OF THE POSTTRAUMATIC NOSE

The first question to be asked about correction of the posttraumatic nose is: Can septoplasty and rhinoplasty be performed simultaneously? The answer is simple: The two operations should be done at the same stage because it is impossible to obtain a straight dorsum without performing a septoplasty, while rhinoplasty affords better visualization of the dorsal septal deformity.

The second question is: Should one correct the septum first and then the nose or vice versa? In my experience, it is safer to begin with correction of the nasal tip, then do the subperiosteal and subperichondrial undermining, and finally perform the rhinoplasty (resection of the hump, lateral and paramedial osteotomies as required) [1]. It is only at the end of the operation that the septoplasty is done, in order to avoid complete separation of the septum from the rest of the nose.

Septoplasty is done, not septal resection. Small resections are often required by the pathologic deformity, and we must avoid the temptation to perform large systematic resections. Our goal is to recreate the normal plane and complete the anatomy of the septum, avoiding catastrophic septal perforations or a progressive saddlenose deformity. Thus, we have to follow two apparently contradictory rules:

1. Do not interrupt the continuity of the septal cartilage. Particularly, try to avoid removal of pieces of cartilage.
2. Try to obtain maximal weakening of the septal cartilage. In other words, break all the springs that stop the cartilage from finding its normal shape and position.

PATHOPHYSIOLOGY AND CLASSIFICATION

Septal deformities can be divided into four categories.

Transnostril Foreign Body

This deformity is frequently associated with a shortening of the nose or with a retracted columella. One nostril is obstructed by the caudal border of the septum while the other nostril is obstructed by the crest created by the folding of the septum. This crest is acute, and more or less parallel to the caudal border. The dorsum is deviated toward the crest. In its depth, the nasal fossa is obstructed by the subluxation of the septal vomerine border behind the crest (Fig. 8-1).

Vertical Crest

This is the same deformity as the transnostril foreign body, but the crest is vertical and the anterior slope larger. One

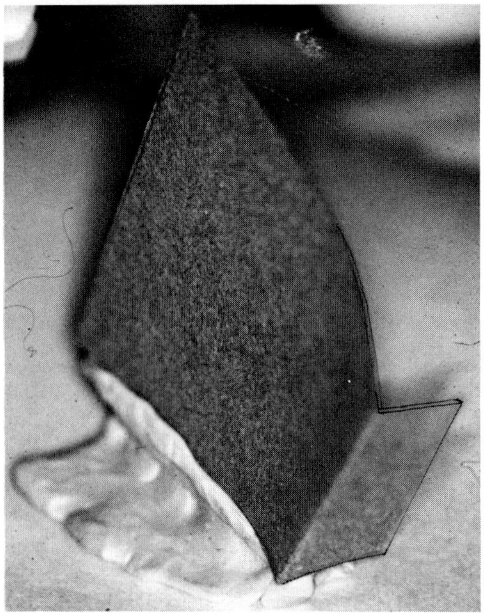

A

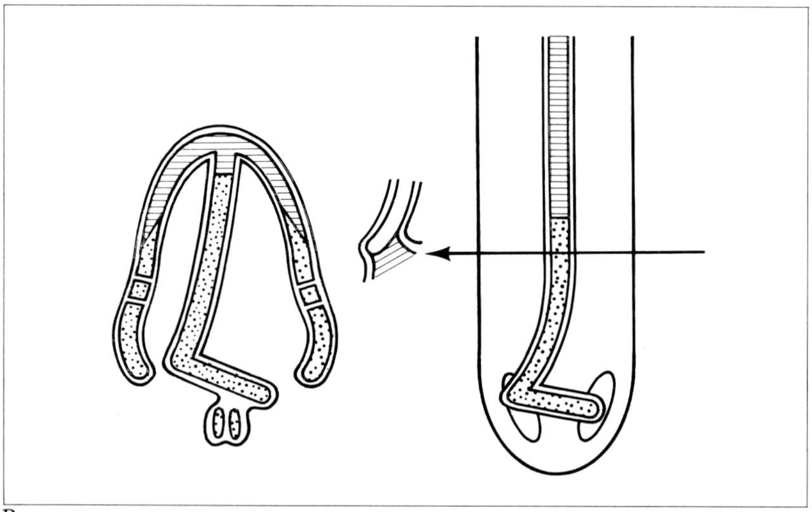

B

Figure 8-1
A, B. Transnostril foreign body. The right nostril is obstructed by the crest. The left nostril is obstructed by the displaced caudal border of the septum. In its depth, the right nasal fossa is obstructed by displacement of the septal cartilage along the border of the vomerine bone.

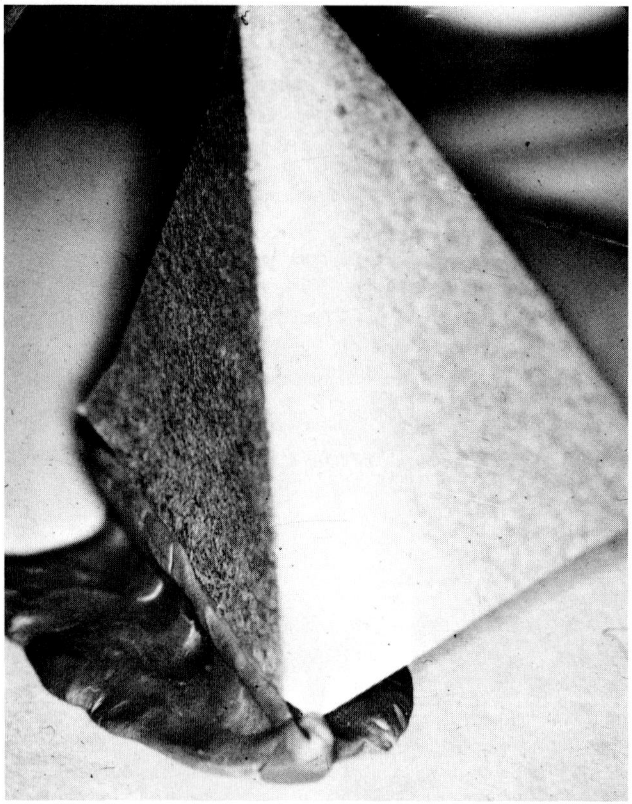

A

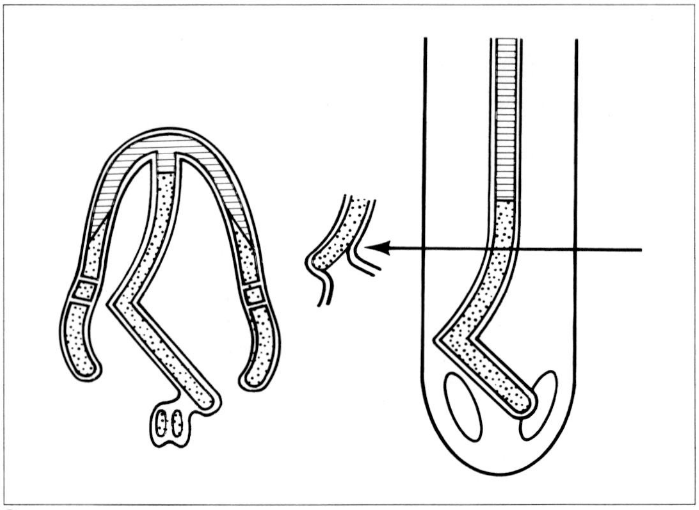

B

Figure 8-2
A, B. Vertical crest. The right nasal fossa is obstructed by the crest and, in its depth, by displacement of the vomerine border of the cartilage. The left nostril is obstructed by displacement of the leading edge of the cartilaginous septum.

nostril is obstructed by the septal caudal border. In its depth, the opposite nasal fossa is obstructed by the vertical crest and behind it by the subluxation of the septal vomerine border (Fig. 8-2).

Curved Deformity

Nostril and nasal fossa are obstructed on the same side. The nostril is obstructed by the septal caudal border while the nasal fossa is obstructed by the subluxation of the septal vomerine border from its vomerine groove (Fig. 8-3).

So-Called Overlappings

Other deformities are relatively rare and difficult to describe, particularly following significant trauma. However, the overlapping of two pieces of cartilage is very exceptional. More frequently, overlapping between the ethmoidal lamina perpendicularis and the cartilaginous septum occurs. When we dissect a so-called cartilaginous overlapping, we find it is in reality an accordionlike deformity, which is nothing other than a transnostril foreign body, or a vertical crest, extremely folded, thereby creating two folds rather than a true overlap.

Figure 8-3
A, B. Curved deformity. The left side is completely obstructed. The left nostril is blocked by displacement of the leading edge of the septum and the left nasal fossa by displacement of the vomerine border.

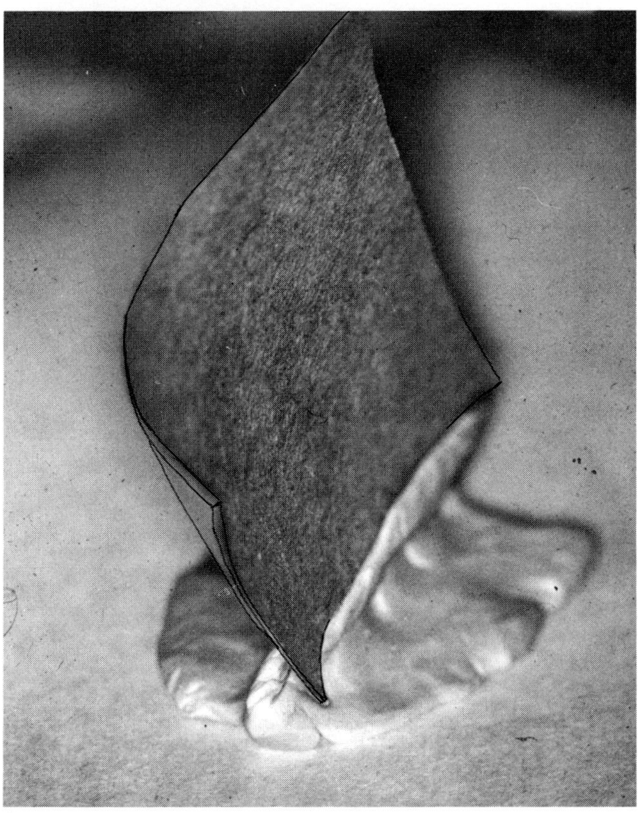

A

SURGICAL TECHNIQUES

In all cases, a bilateral subperichondrial dissection is done. This maneuver is the only way to expose the deformity.

Transnostril Foreign Body

The transnostril foreign body is the only deformity that warrants systematic resection followed by reinsertion of a piece of cartilage. First, the anterior slope of the folded cartilage is removed. This piece is usually straight and without irregularities. Second, the posterior slope, which is usually irregular and curved, is resected and thus the posterior septal edge becomes straight. Third, the anterior slope, which has been reshaped "on the table," is inserted and sutured with two stitches—one on the nasal spine and the other forward on the free edge of the septum (Figs. 8-4 and 8-5).

Vertical Crest

The vertical crest is slightly more difficult to correct. The anterior slope of folded cartilage is much larger than the anterior slope of the foreign body deformity. Thus, it would be dangerous to remove it completely and reinsert it. It is safer not to separate completely the two slopes and so leave a superior "pedicle." Therefore, the nasal hump is resected first, because hump resection following septoplasty would risk interference with the cartilaginous "pedicle" and lead to a completely free anterior slope. Surgical correction of the vertical crest involves initial separation of the anterior slope from the posterior by incising along the crest (Fig. 8-6). However, this incision does not reach the dorsal border of the septum, and a pedicle is left in place. Next, the anterior slope is put in the right sagittal place, but the nasal fossa is still obstructed by the posterior slope. At this point, two solutions are possible. First, we can merely resect the posterior slope, but in doing so, we fail to respect the rule of septal continuity.and risk creating a

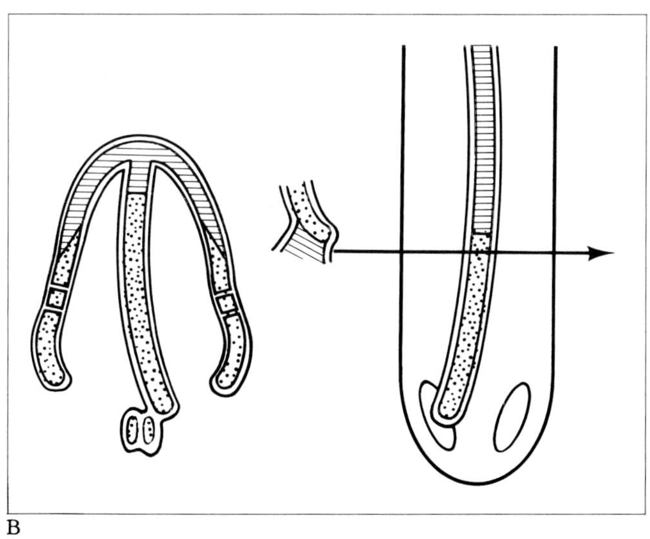

B

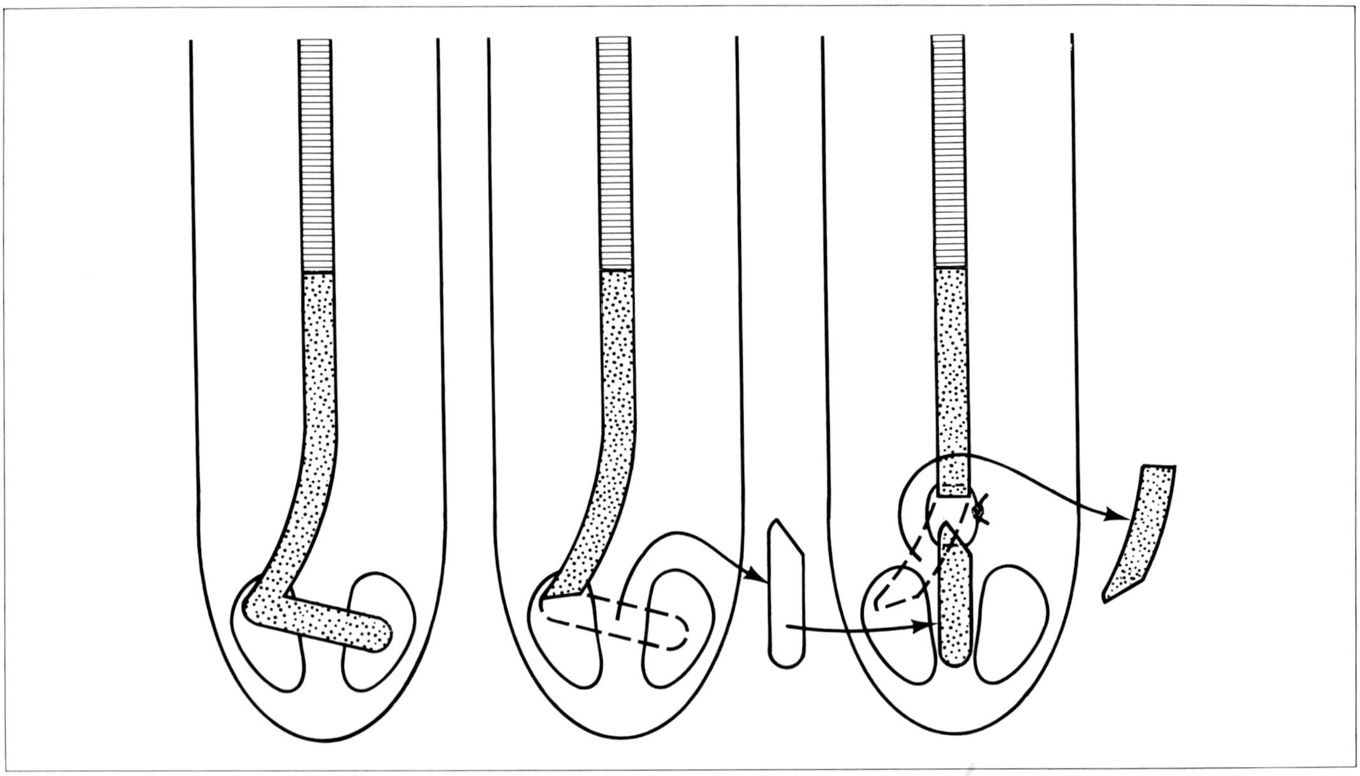

Figure 8-4. Correction of transnostril foreign body deformity. The anterior slope is removed. Then the posterior slope is removed. The anterior slope, which is usually straight, is reinserted and fixed in place. The curved posterior slope is used as graft material or discarded.

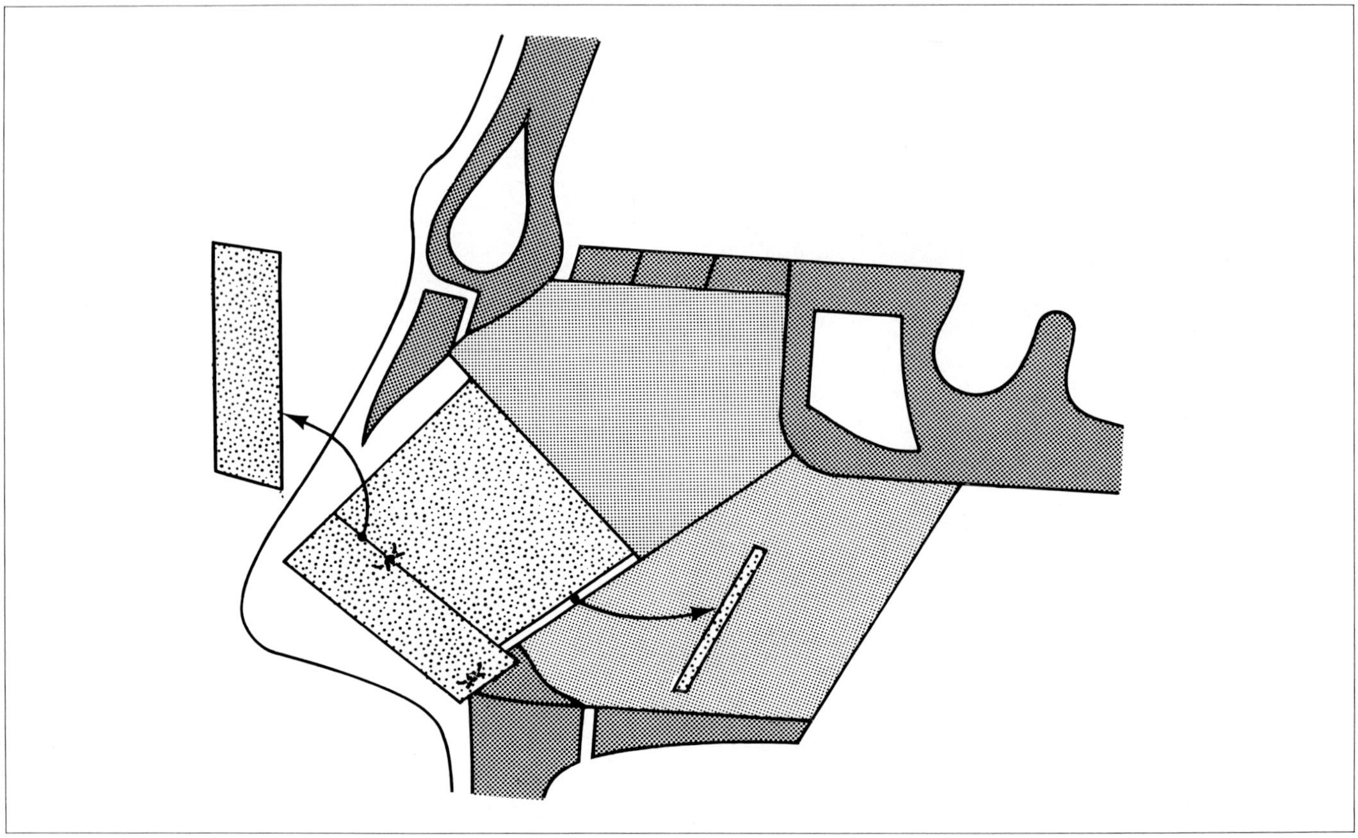

Figure 8-5. Correction of transnostril foreign body.

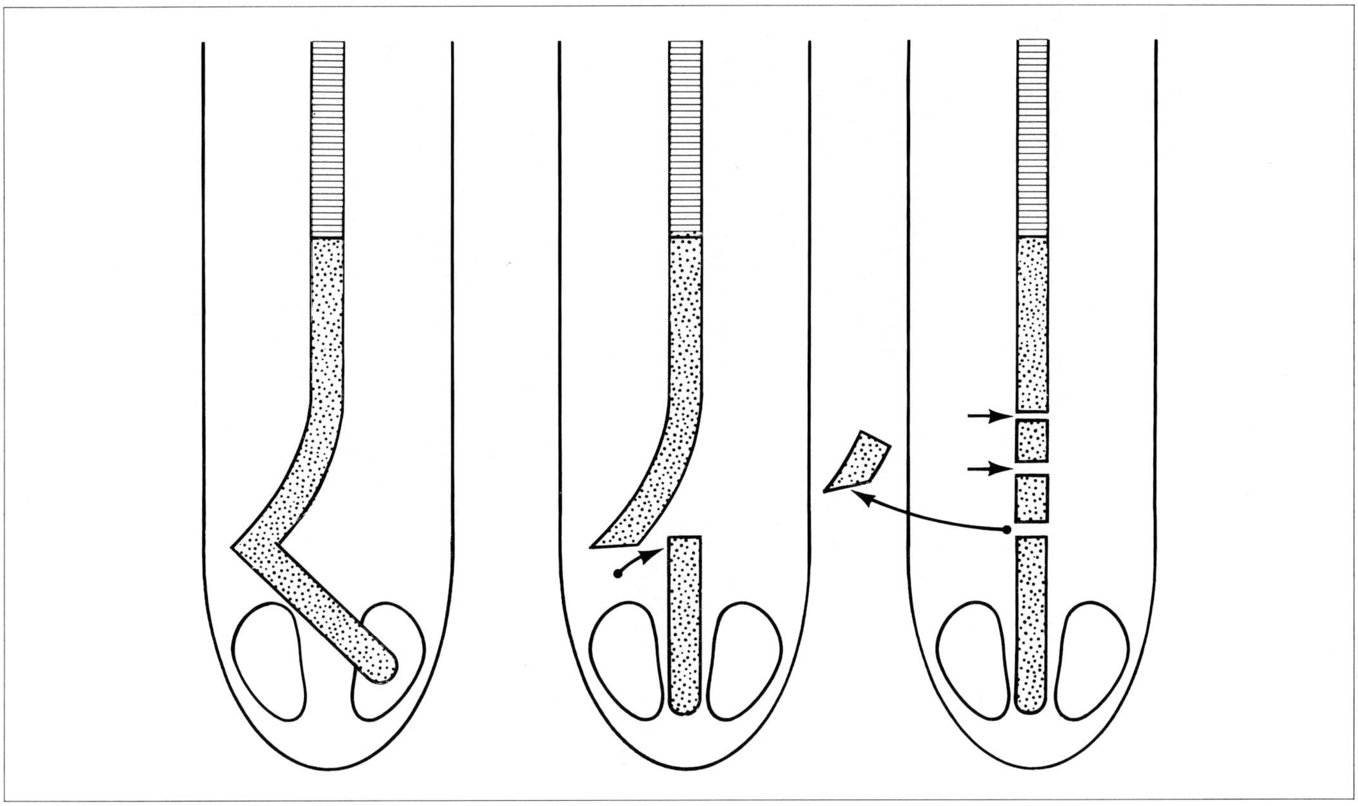

Figure 8-6. Correction of vertical crest deformity. The anterior slope is freed, leaving a continuity along the dorsum. Then, if possible, the posterior slope is weakened and left in place. It is resected only if necessary.

perforation (Fig. 8-7A). Thus, resection is done only if we are absolutely certain that the mucous membrane was elevated without damage. Alternatively, we can weaken the posterior slope and allow it to assume a normal position (Fig. 8-7B).

Curved Deformity

Correction of a curved deformity appears easy but in reality is the most complicated. The reasons are that the "spring effect" of the cartilage is a dominant force and that there is no real excess of cartilage. Any resection would potentiate septal collapse. Therefore, one must correct the distortion and relieve the internal stresses while preserving all tissue. To accomplish these goals a procedure is used that gives maximal weakening of the cartilage without disturbing septal continuity (Fig. 8-8). It consists of a "spiral incision," called the "Chinese serpentine" because of its similarity to those found in the Far East (Fig. 8-9). It is best to begin the spiral incision behind the nasal spine and to pass counterclockwise. It is possible to start anywhere depending on the type of deviation and the location of the spring. At the end of the incision in the center of the cartilage, it is necessary to resect a small piece of cartilage to allow the septum to settle.

Posterior Overlappings

At the level of the ethmoid plate, the work is easier because bone does not have the same spring effect as cartilage and can be fractured without interrupting its continuity (Fig. 8-10). In addition, the resection is safer because the mucous membrane is thicker and a lower level resection will not weaken the nasal pyramid. At the level of the vomer, the vomerine cartilaginous border must be resected if it is subluxated along the side of the bone. If the vomer is thin and oblique, it is separated from the palate and put in a normal vertical position by being fractured between the open blades of a Killian speculum. If the vomer is thick and constitutes a larger bony obstruction it must be resected. In the two preceding situations, the Joseph saw is useful. The mucous membrane is carefully separated from cartilage and bone and protected with an Aufricht retractor.

In summary, these deformities can be corrected by separation from the vomer, incision, weakening, and, rarely, resection. However, maintaining the result in good alignment is critical. One of two methods is used: either a U stitch or a fan dressing. The goal is to overcorrect a little the reduction of the cartilage on the columellar border. With the U stitch a nylon suture is passed through the strong periosteum of the nasal spine (Fig. 8-11). Then the suture goes through the inferior angle of the septum from the deviated side to the opposite side and back the other way, ending on the deviated side. When the suture is

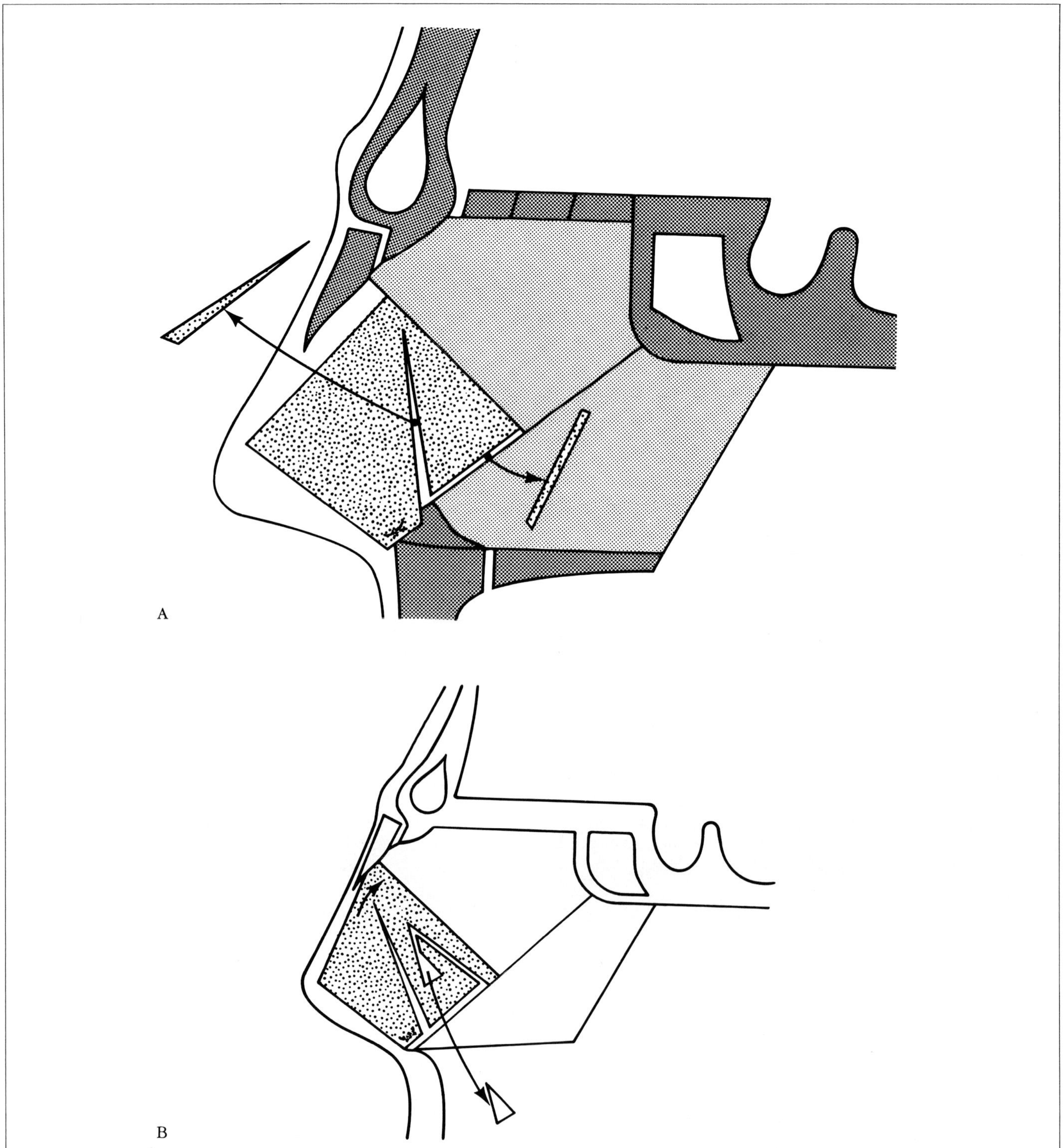

A

B

Figure 8-7. Correction of a vertical crest may require simple repositioning of the posterior slope (A) or a serpentine modification (B).

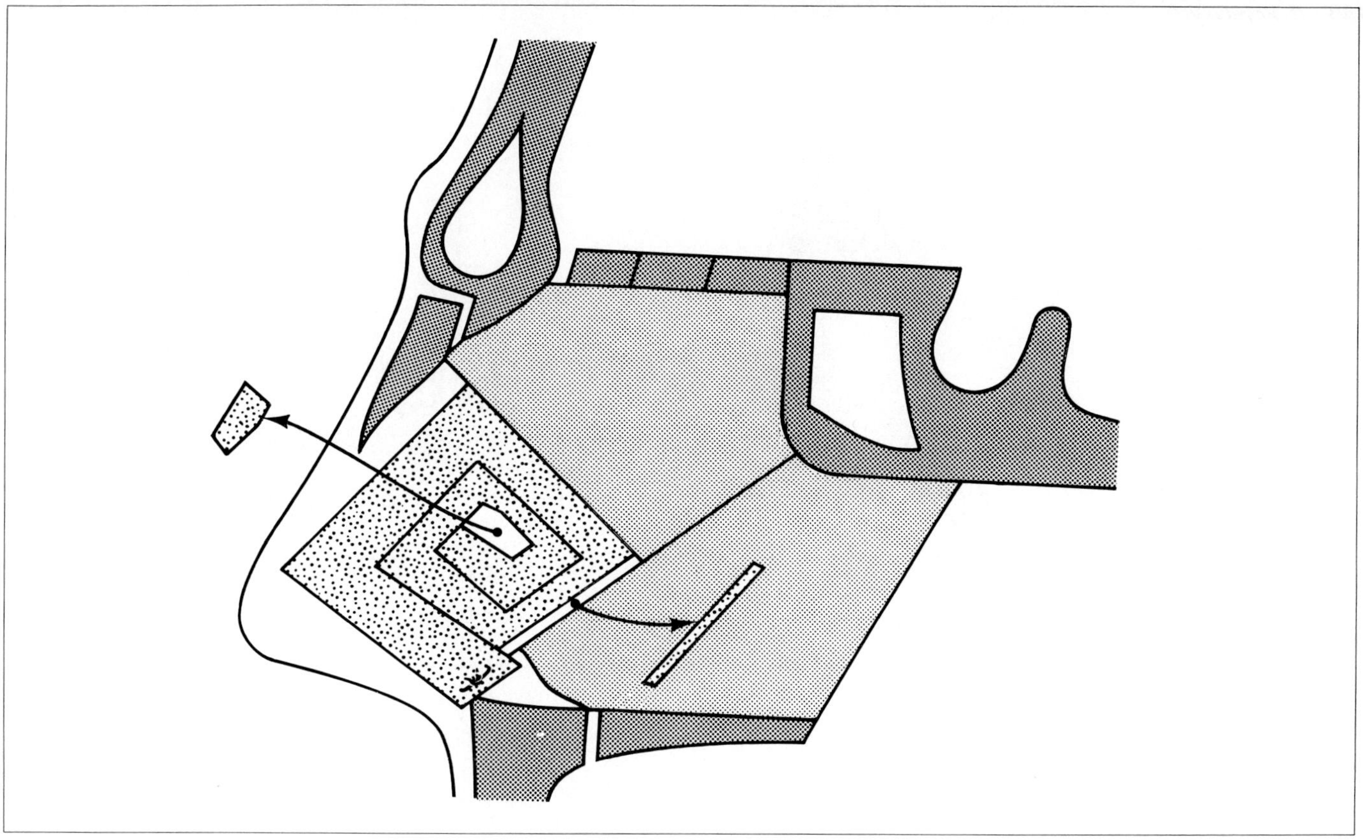

Figure 8-8. Weakening of a curved deformity by a spiral incision. Note excision of deviated portion along the vomerine groove and excision of central portion to allow displacement of parts.

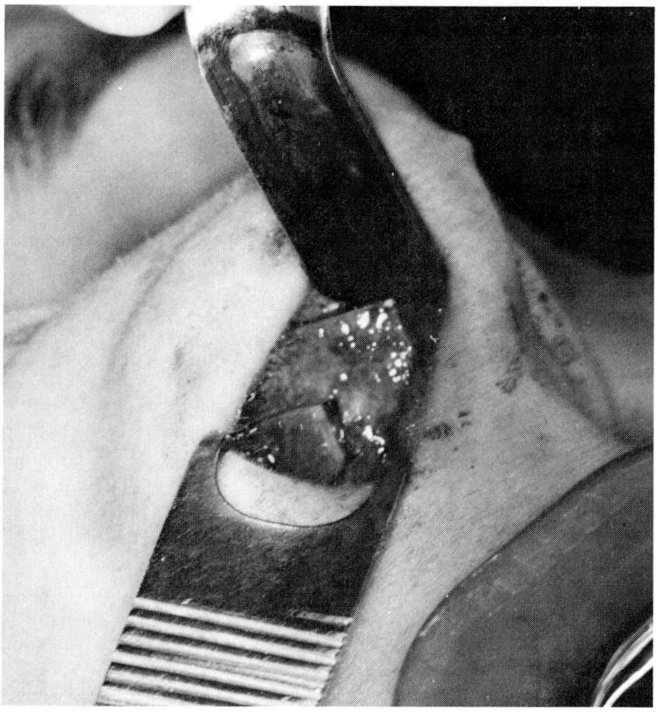

A

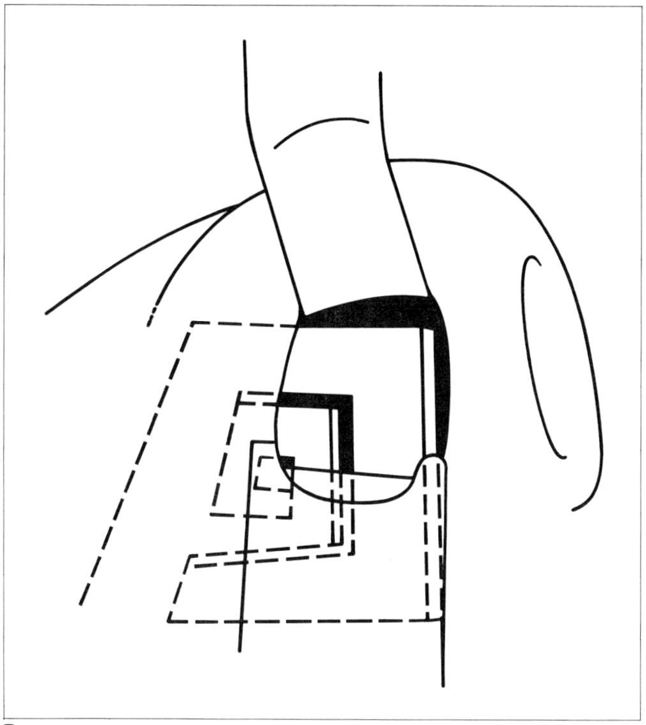

B

Figure 8-9
A, B. "Chinese serpentine," with portion visible through the nostril and extent of incision on schematic diagram.

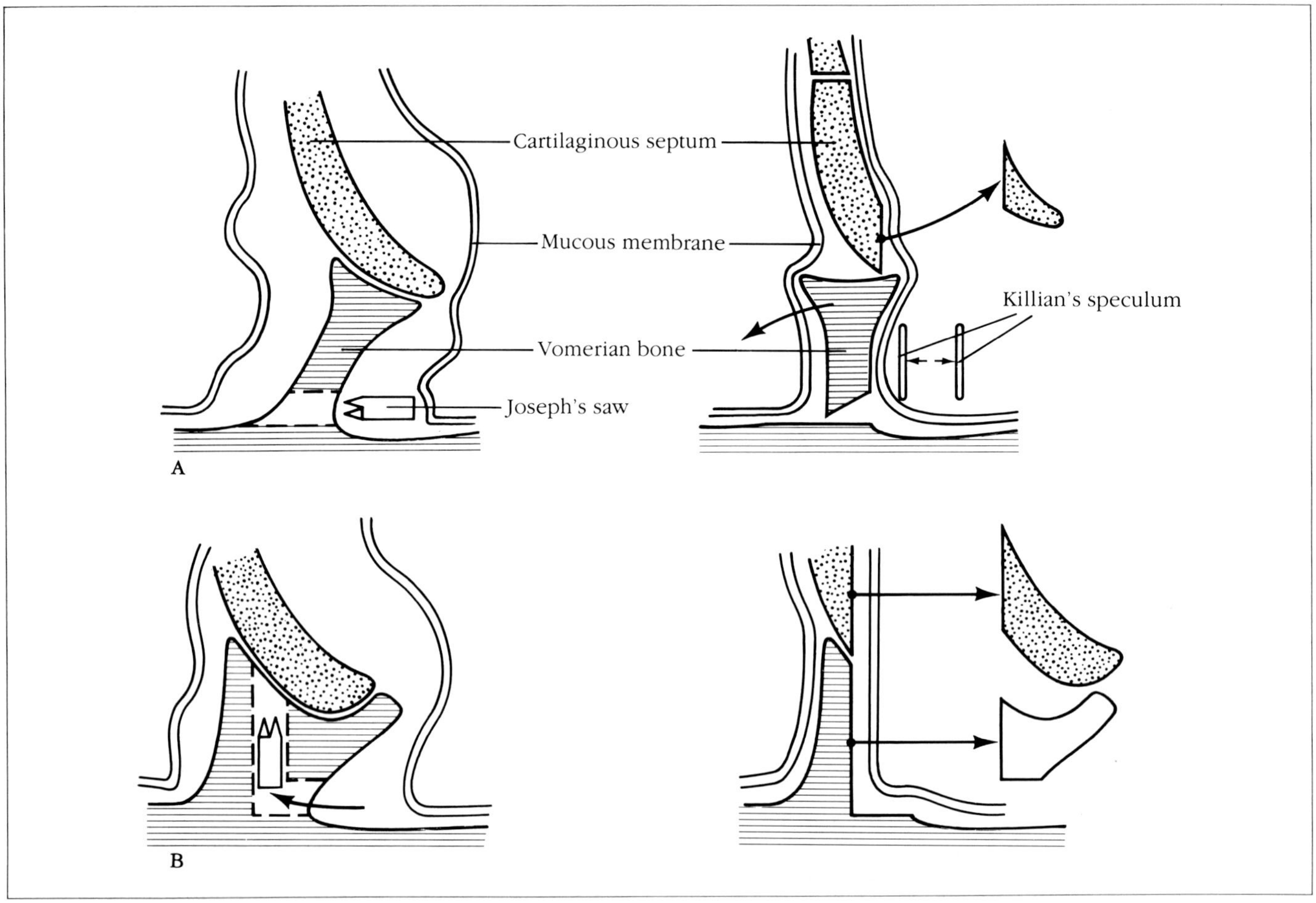

Figure 8-10
A. Resection of a deviated vomerine crest. Following elevation of the mucosa, the cartilaginous deviation is resected; then the vomer is weakened with the saw and fractured with the Killian's speculum.
B. Resection of a massive vomerine crest. This is done using the Joseph saw, with the mucosa protected by an Aufricht retractor.

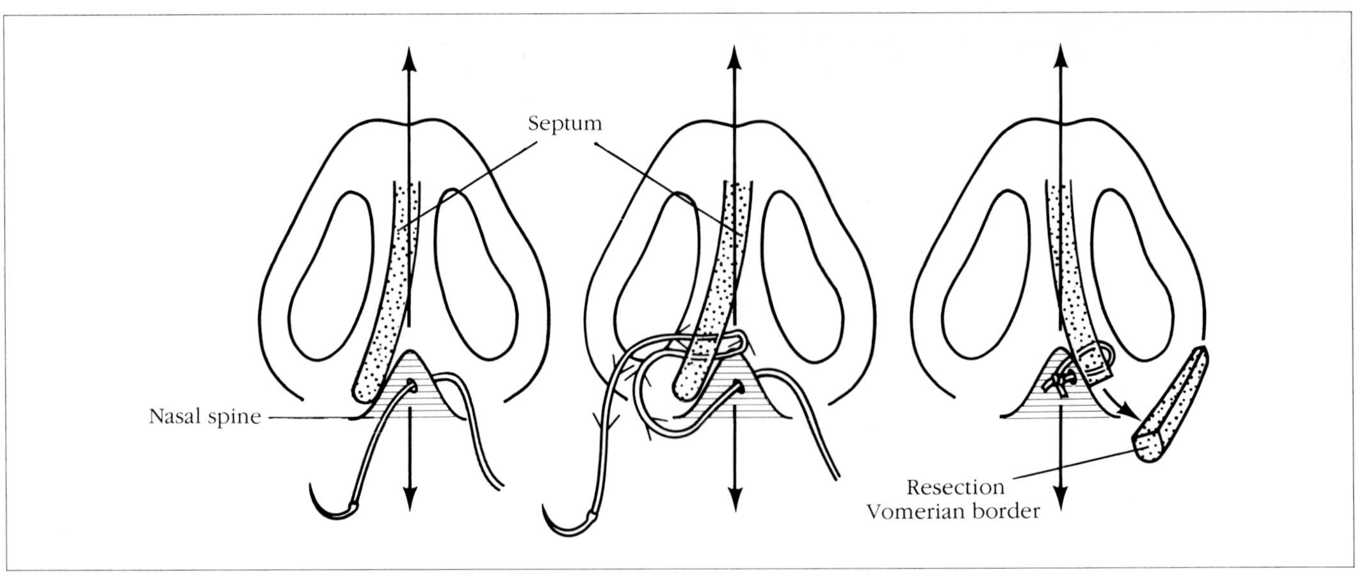

Figure 8-11. Lateral U stitch producing a slight overcorrection of the deviation of the leading edge of the septum.

tightened, the inferior angle crosses over the nasal spine and is held on the side opposite the deviation. A definite overcorrection is created and strongly fixed by an unabsorbable suture. Alternatively, the medial crura can be separated to receive the inferior angle of the septum, which will be buried in good position after the mucosal sutures.

It is my conviction that nasal packings are uncomfortable and even dangerous. They create a risk of infection. Often they do not work exactly where we want them to. They have a tendency to take a spherical shape that produces too little compression in some places and too much in others while completely blocking nasal breathing. Therefore, I use splints held in place by a transverse U stitch. In order to cover the maximum surface, four splints are inserted. They are cut from x-ray film (Fig. 8-12). Two splints, which will be inserted in one nostril, are put together and perforated at two points, anterior and posterior. The anterior perforations are done at the same point. However, the posterior perforations are done at different levels—close to the *superior* border for the external splint and close to the *inferior* border for the internal splint. Thus, when the nylon suture is tightened, the external splint extends upward to the dorsum while the internal splint extends downward to the nasal floor. The two splints on each side are diverging like an open fan. The splints are easy to introduce as their width is smaller than the width of the nostrils. When the knot is tightened, the posterior splint diverges so that it covers a maximum of surface without completely obstructing the nose (Fig. 8-13). The maneuver is similar to creating a ship in a bottle. The ship is inserted with the masts lying on the deck, and once it is in position they are raised by being pulled on a thread. The actual steps are as follows:

1. The suture is passed through the two anterior perforations of the right splints.
2. Passing through the mucosa and cartilaginous septum anteriorly, the suture is brought out the nostril and the left splint is prepared.
3. The suture is passed through the anterior perforation of the left splint, then the posterior perforation of the left splints (close to the inferior border for the external, close to the superior border for the internal).
4. The needle is then brought back into the nose and passed through the mucosa and cartilaginous septum posteriorly.
5. The left fan is introduced through the nostril in a collapsed form.
6. The suture is tightened to open the left fan. The degree of opening is controlled by pushing up the external splint with the tip of a dissecting forceps.
7. With the needle outside the nostril, it is passed through the posterior perforation of the right splint—again through the superior border of the internal splint and the inferior border of the external splint.
8. The right splint is introduced through the right nostril.
9. The right fan is opened by pulling on the suture. We can verify that the fan is opened by pushing the external splint upward.
10. The suture is knotted and the tails are left a bit long to facilitate their removal at 7 or 10 days—sometimes longer in complex cases.

Although cumbersome to describe, the splints can be made up ahead of time and autoclaved, allowing insertion in 1 or 2 minutes.

TECHNIQUE OF RHINOPLASTY

When the nose is both deviated and hypertrophied, it is necessary to resect more on one side than on the other. Personally, I think it is better to perform this resection at the level of the dorsum than at the level of the lateral osteotomy, as suggested by other surgeons. Also, it is often necessary to reinsert systematically tissue that has been excised. Thus, at the end of the operation we often have a gap between the two lateral walls (one gap if the septal dorsal border is lower than the lateral walls, two gaps if the dorsal border is slightly higher).

The best way to obtain a well-designed dorsum is to reinsert tissue to fill the gap. *In all rhinoplasties for correction of humped noses,* I practice *systematic reinsertion,* but in a very different manner from Skoog's. In my opinion, Skoog did a systematic hyperresection, creating a too curved nose, which he corrected by introducing the main portion of the resected hump. I do not use this procedure. I do not make a hyperresection. The nasal profile, rather than being changed by insertion of the graft, remains the same. It is not the objective of the graft to establish the new profile line; instead it has the following characteristics:

1. It is very thin and can be considered not as a real graft but as an "inducer of good scarring" that helps the dorsum to acquire a nicely rounded shape (Fig. 8-14).
2. The reinsertion is not an onlay graft like Skoog's but an inlay graft. Thus, we have to take care that the dorsal border of the septum will be half a millimeter lower than the dorsal edges of the lateral walls.
3. Last but not least, the grafting must be performed in association with the systematic use of the extramucosal method, which implies *preservation of the continuity between septal and lateral mucous membrane.*

Thus, we create two "mucosal domes," which constitute the floor of a pocket beneath the dorsal skin (Fig. 8-15). This mucosal floor protects the reinserted graft and keeps it from falling into the nasal fossa. In the posttraumatic nose, the reinserted graft is particularly useful: The free piece lying along the dorsum conforms to the plaster and corrects the asymmetry. In the saddlenose, this piece restores a normal dorsum.

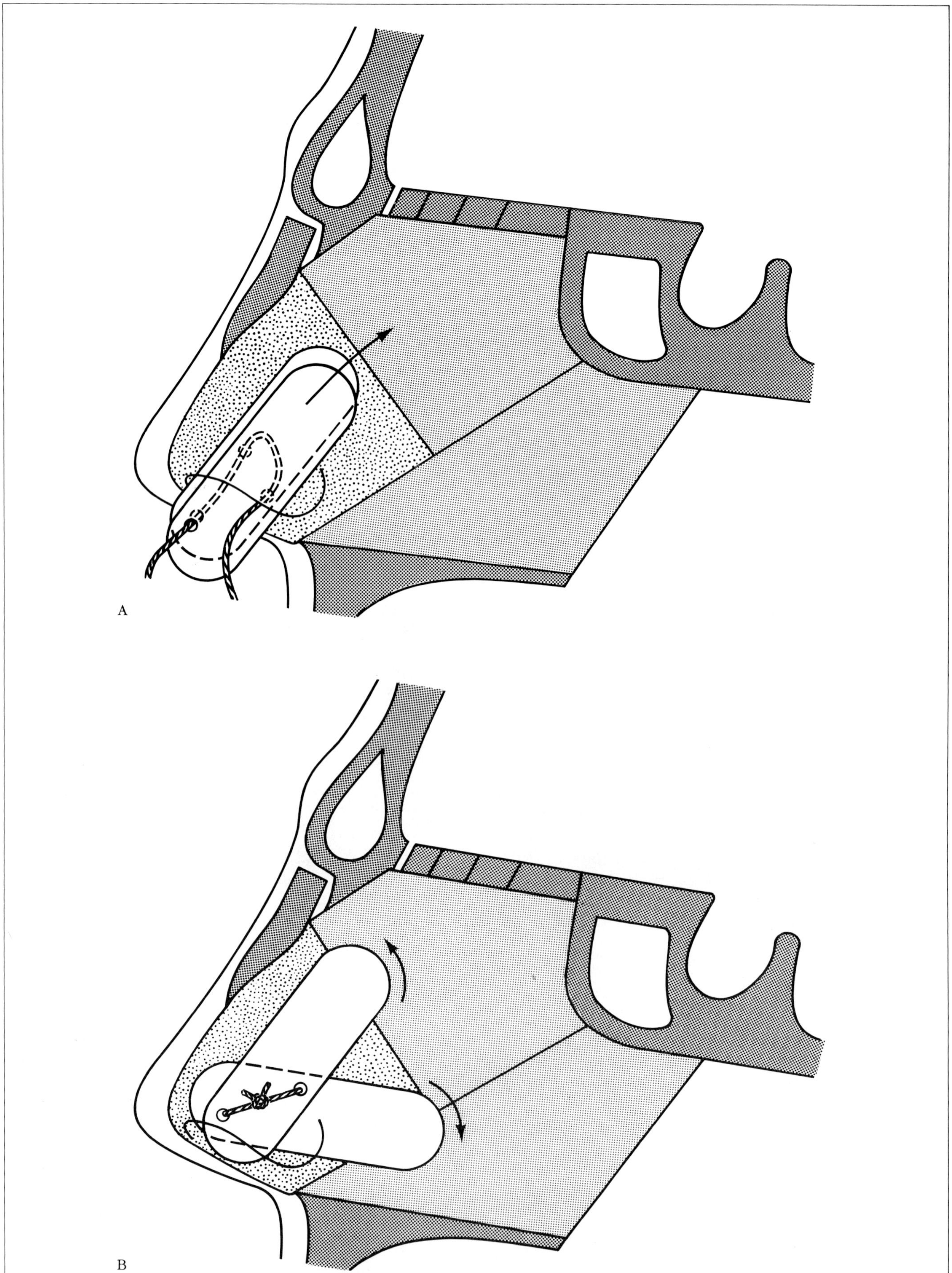
A
B

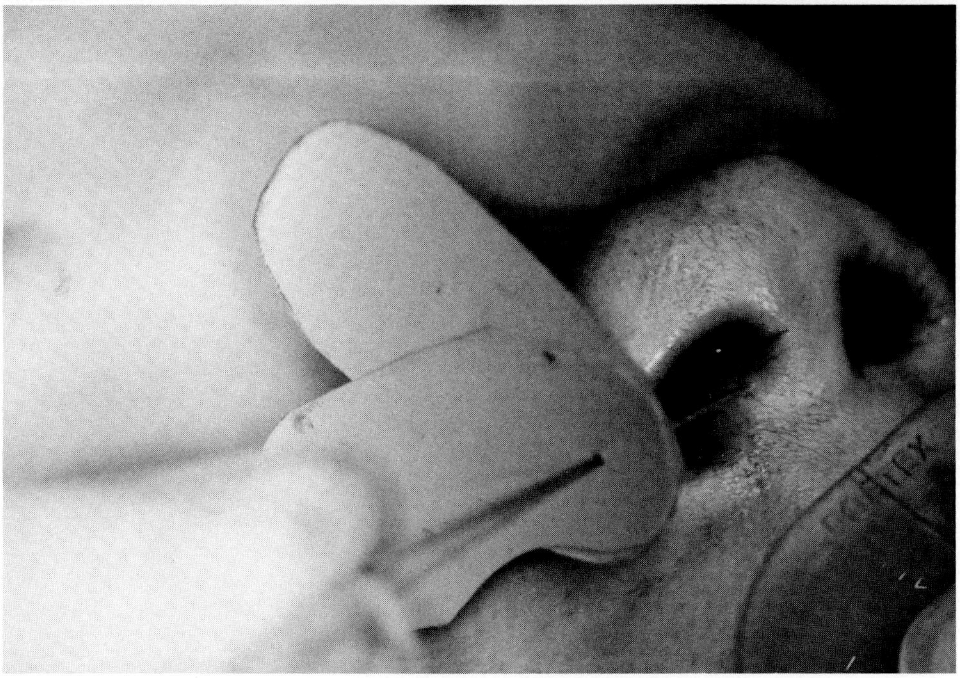

Figure 8-13. The two anterior perforations have been made, and the needle is about to pass through the septum.

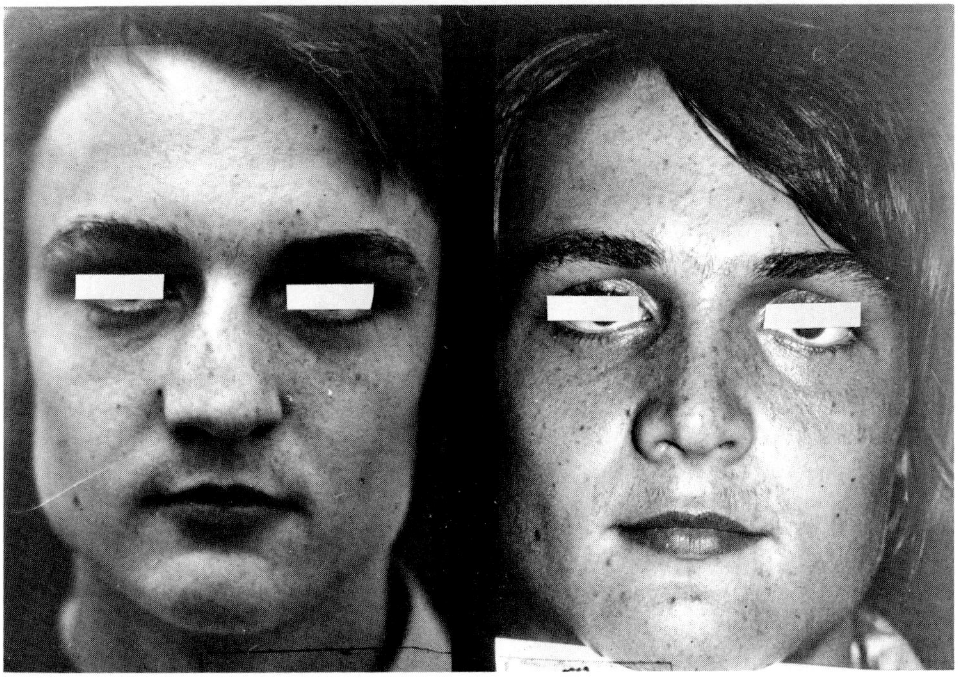

Figure 8-14. Patient with marked nasal deviation and the result following septorhinoplasty with reinsertion of a thin portion of the hump to serve as an "inducer."

Figure 8-12
A. The "shut fan" nasal splint is introduced through the nostril.
B. The "fan" is opened by pulling the suture.

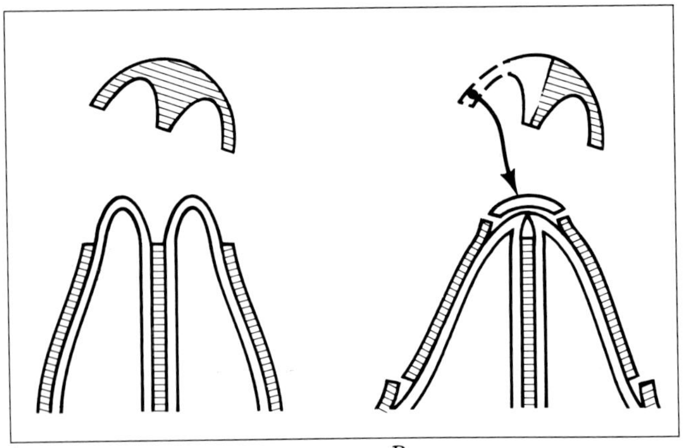

A B

Figure 8-15. Extramucosal method.
A. The two mucosal domes are dissected and preserved.
B. A portion of the hump is placed over the mucosal domes to recreate a nice round dorsum.

There are three ways to shape the reinserted graft:

1. The ideal way is to have a piece that is partly osseous and partly cartilaginous recreating the normal anatomy of the dorsum. Unfortunately, this is rarely possible because the bone is often too thick or too curved. The ideal is achieved only if the resected hump is composed of a very straight thin bone, as thin as a nail. In that case, we can shape a fine graft that is one-quarter osseous and three-quarters cartilaginous (Fig. 8-16).
2. More frequently, we use the two pieces of upper lateral cartilage resected with the hump. The two pieces are elevated from the bone, care being taken to dissect the thin bevel that is articulated with the inner part of the bone. These two pieces are turned head to tail and pressed together by being crushed between the teeth of a forceps (Fig. 8-17).
3. Sometimes the hump is inadequate for creating a dorsal graft. I try not to use the alar cartilages because of their longitudinal curve and straight width. Despite excision and morselization, the alars have a tendency to curl badly when in place. Septal cartilage can be used, but it is very thick and its borders risk creating abnormal palpable edges (Fig. 8-18). Hence it is necessary to crush them strongly with a screw crusher. This crusher has a plane surface on one side and straight parallel incisures on the other. Thus, the crushed cartilage curls slightly on its width, contributing to formation of a nice rounded shape for the dorsum (Fig. 8-19).

Figure 8-16. Systematic reinsertion of a portion of the nasal hump.
A. The reinsertion is partly osseous and partly cartilaginous. The desired portion is traced on the resected hump.
B. Only a quarter of the reinsertion graft is osseous.
C. The reinsertion graft is shown in place over the skin. The bony part must be straight and thin as a nail.

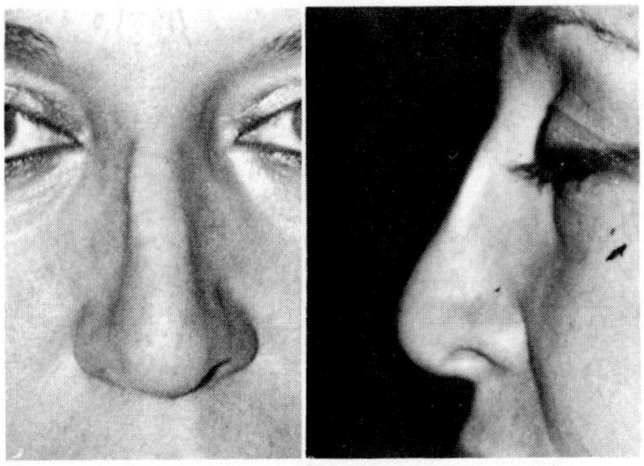

A B

Figure 8-18

A, B. If the septal cartilage is not morselized, its borders will be visible and will literally incise the skin from the inside. This septal cartilage graft is readily visible at 1½ years following insertion.

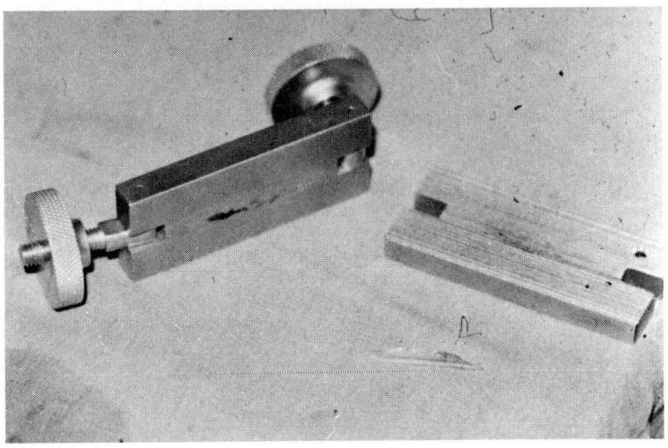

A

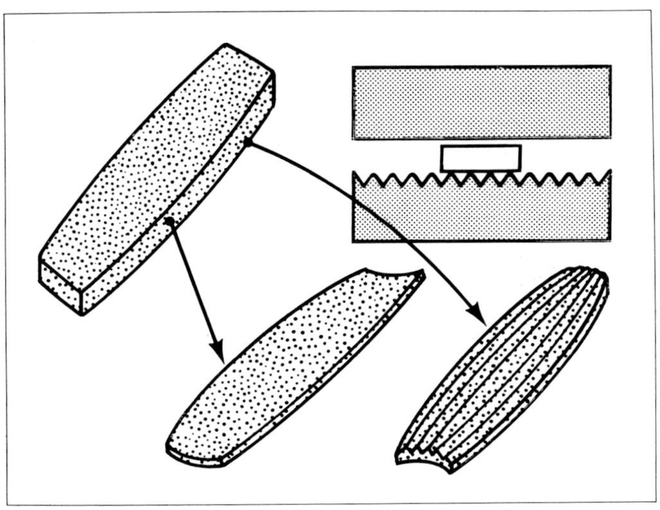

B

Figure 8-19

A, B. Screw crusher with one flat surface and the other surface with longitudinal incisures, allowing the graft to curl on its width.

CORRECTION OF POSTOPERATIVE SADDLENOSES

Saddlenose deformity is seen following too extensive resection of the septum and must be corrected. Also, some patients will have a subluxation of the columellar border into one nostril following trauma of congenital etiology. As previously noted, this subluxation can be associated with several different septal deformities that are more posterior. Unfortunately, most patients with postsurgical saddlenose deformities did not have a mere resection of the subluxated septum but total removal. Consequently, normal support between the nasal spine and the dorsum is absent. A saddlenose resulting from lack of support is due to three mechanisms: (1) trauma, (2) retraction of mucous membrane, and (3) catastrophic constriction of an anterior septal perforation that contracts the dorsum and columella.

Iliac or cartilaginous grafts can be used for the correction of these deformities. However, two simpler methods are available.

1. Utilization of an autogenous graft from the hump. Very frequently the patients have, before the accident, a hyper-

Figure 8-20. A part of the hump is used to reconstruct the septum. The bony part is fixed to the nasal spine. The cartilaginous part is fixed to the edge of the remaining septum or to one of the upper lateral cartilages.

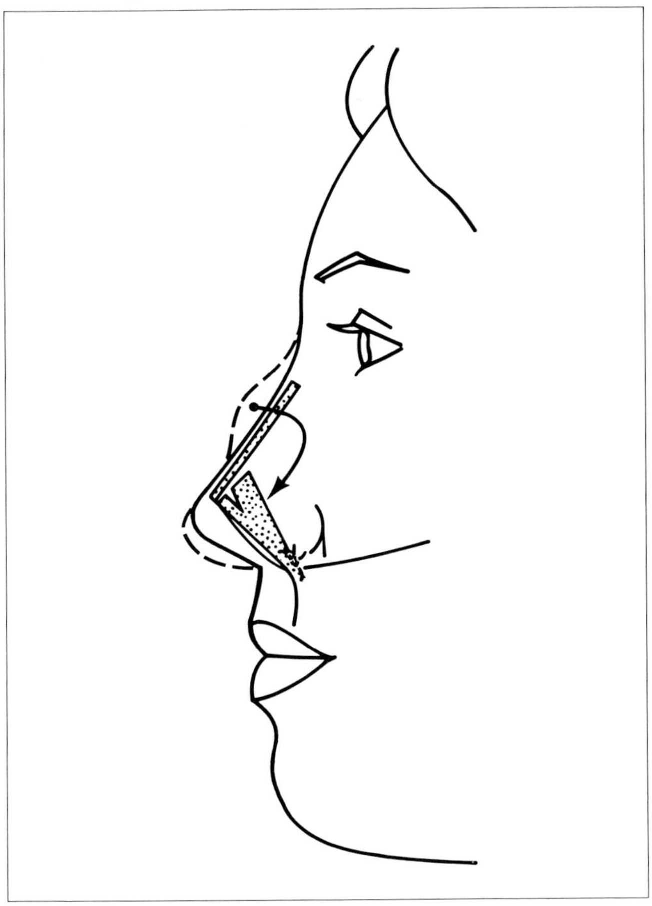

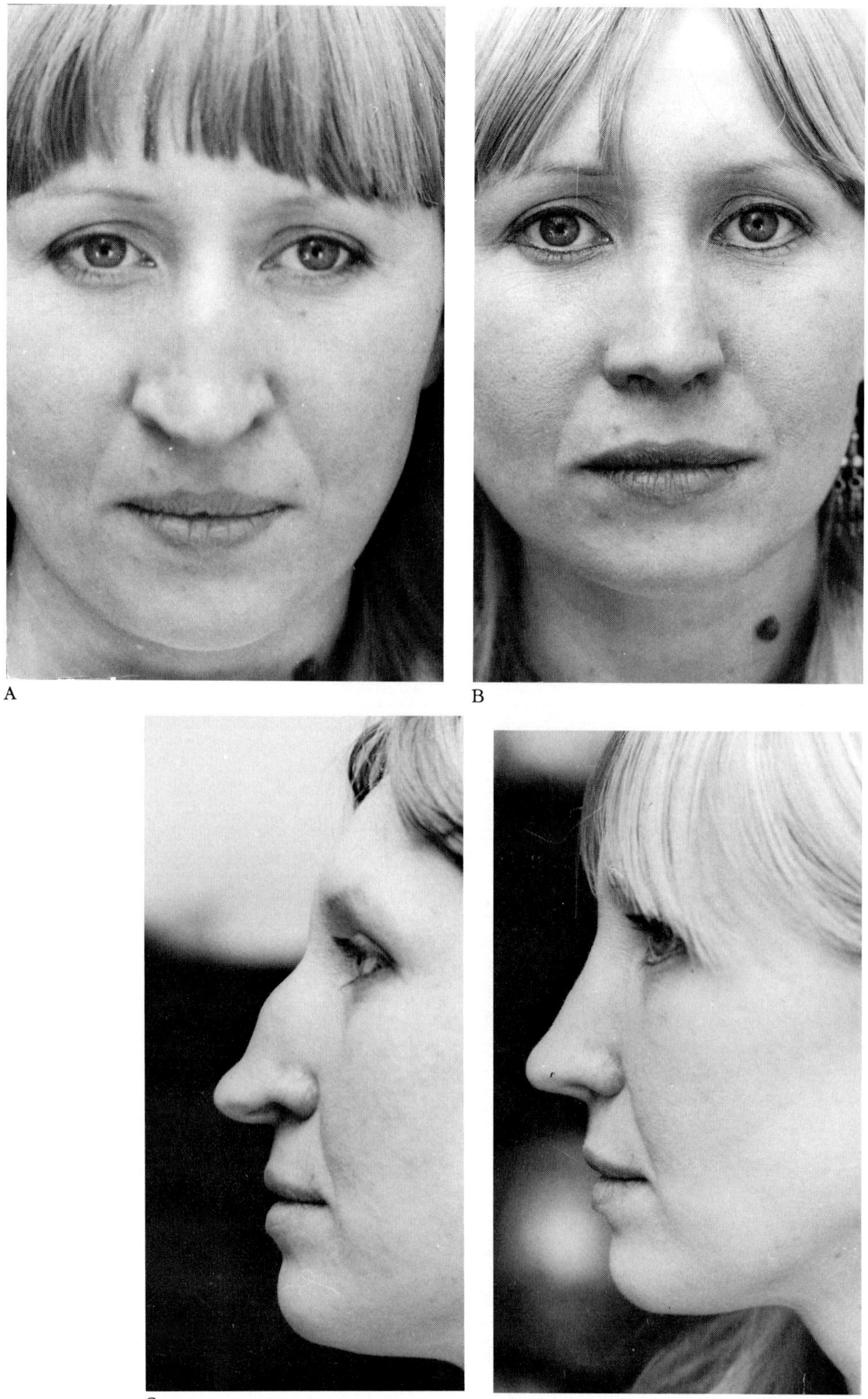

A B C D

Figure 8-21

A–F. Patient with postsurgical saddlenose deformity corrected by reconstruction with osseocartilaginous hump components: bone for tip support, cartilage for dorsal support.

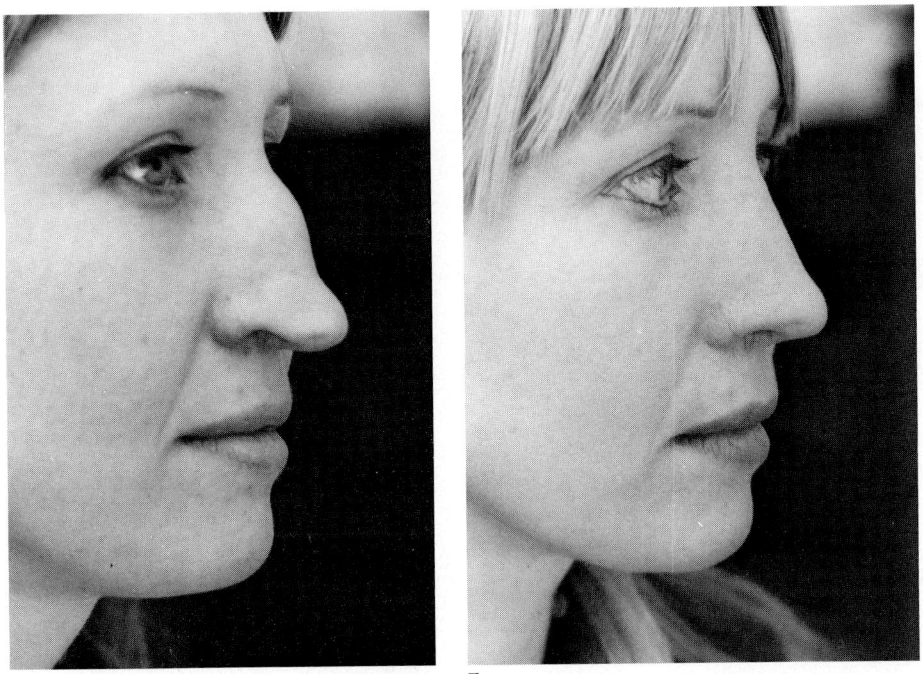

E F

Figure 8-21 (continued)

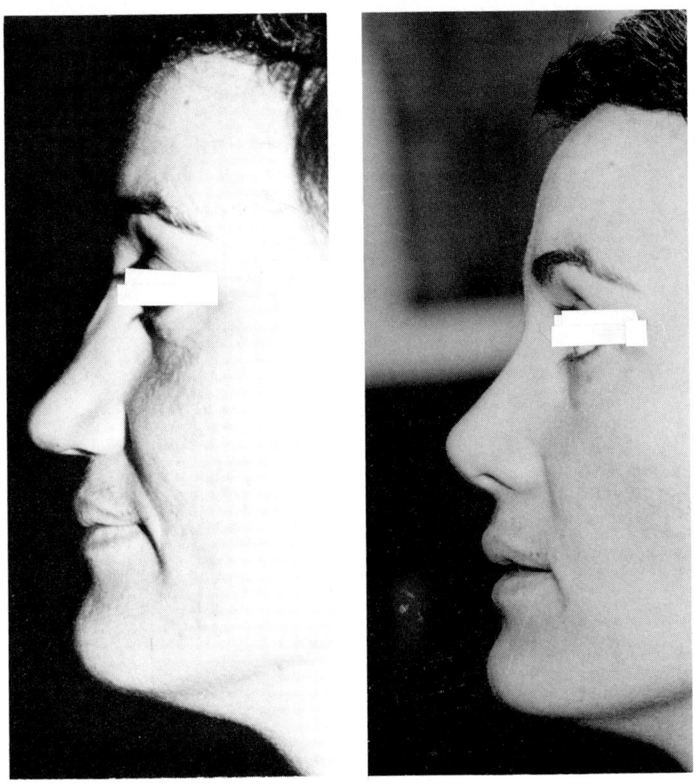

A B

Figure 8-22

A, B. Nasal deformity corrected by Millard composite alar flaps and cartilaginous graft to dorsum.

trophic or even humped nose. After drooping of the nasal tip, the hump is exaggerated and a "false" hump appears in consequence of the septal retraction. If a graft is done, the hump is resected first. The resected hump is used to build a new septum provided a straight strong piece is available. The bony part of the hump is fixed on the nasal spine while the cartilaginous portion is fixed to a lower lateral cartilage or to the edge of the remaining septum (Fig. 8-20). A reinsertion graft is placed along the dorsum. Thus, the hump can be used to produce an "economic" L-shaped graft. Since the graft is composed of local tissues, it takes without any difficulty and gives a permanent result (Fig. 8-21).

2. Millard's composite flaps. If we do not have a hump available and there is inward contraction of the columella, Millard's composite alar flaps are used. These flaps are taken from the enlarged alar cartilages. They have an anterior pedicle at the level of the domes. They are composite; the two cartilaginous strips (from one-third to two-thirds of the lateral crus) are still lined with mucosa. The two flaps are rotated downward and inward, filling the gap that appears after caudal traction on the columella. The cartilaginous surfaces are compressed together, while the mucosal surfaces are sutured to the septal mucosa and the columella. These flaps are particularly valuable for correcting the "pig nose" or retroussé tip by lowering the columella and slightly elevating the alar cartilages. Also, they provide strong septal support by elevating the tip and correcting the saddlenose. Here, too, insertion of a slight dorsal cartilaginous graft is useful (Fig. 8-22).

REFERENCE

1. Jost, G. *Atlas de Chirurgie Esthétique Plastique.* Paris: Masson, 1975.

9. Secondary Rhinoplasty

Rodolphe Meyer
Ulrich K. Kesselring

Even in expert hands a certain number of rhinoplasties are less than ideal, proving unsatisfactory for the patient and occasionally only for the surgeon. These cases require a secondary operation, which should, if possible, always be performed by the original surgeon.

The following structures are often modified in a primary rhinoplasty: (1) bony pyramid, (2) cartilaginous pyramid, (3) nasolabial angle, (4) tip, alae, and columella, (5) septum, (6) vestibule, (7) nasal cavity, and (8) skin. Any or several of these structures can subsequently be deficient or redundant, asymmetric, or irregular, thereby producing an unaesthetic deformity.

We distinguish the following indications for a secondary rhinoplasty: (1) insufficient removal of the hump, (2) supratip deformity, (3) excessive removal of the hump, (4) saddlenose, (5) deformities of the cartilaginous framework, (6) too short a nose and columella deformities, (7) secondary bone deformities, (8) septal perforation, and (9) stenosis of the nares.

INSUFFICIENT REMOVAL OF THE HUMP

In the standard rhinoplasty, hump removal includes resection of the cartilaginous and bony components of a prominent hump (Fig. 9-1A). In the extramucosal technique these structures are severed with no cutting of the nasal mucosa, which had been pushed down after having been dissected from the septum and after the upper lateral cartilages have been severed from the septum (Fig. 9-1B).

The most frequent cause for insufficient hump removal is inadequate resection of the dorsal portion of the cartilaginous septum at its cranial end, the part that usually lies between the nasal bones and is sometimes difficult to remove (Fig. 9-2). The treatment in such a case is a simple secondary resection of the septal excess.

Another cause for a persistent hump is an incomplete or insufficient trimming of the upper lateral cartilages after they have been severed from the septal cartilage (Fig. 9-3). The corrective intervention is quite simple here also and consists in trimming down the excess upper lateral cartilage.

SUPRATIP DEFORMITY

This very common complication takes the form of a hard or soft hump just above the tip in the region of the weak triangle. It can be the result of inadequate technique but also represents an unpredictable pitfall in the path of the most experienced surgeon. It seems that there are two types of supratip elevations: the polly beak of the novice,

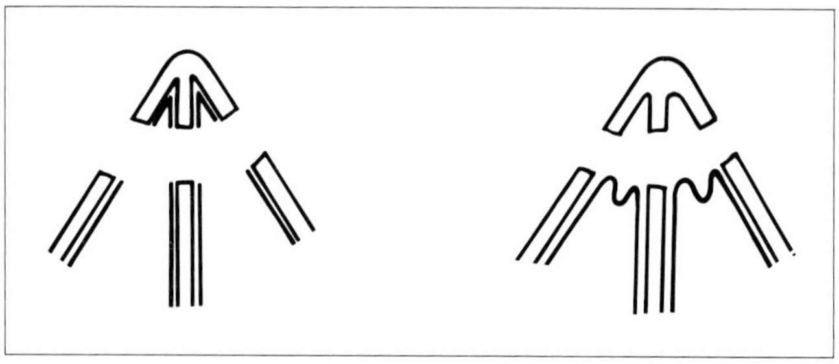

Figure 9-1
A. The classic hump resection severs the nasal lining.
B. The hump resection using the extramucosal approach leaves the mucosa of the nasal vault intact.

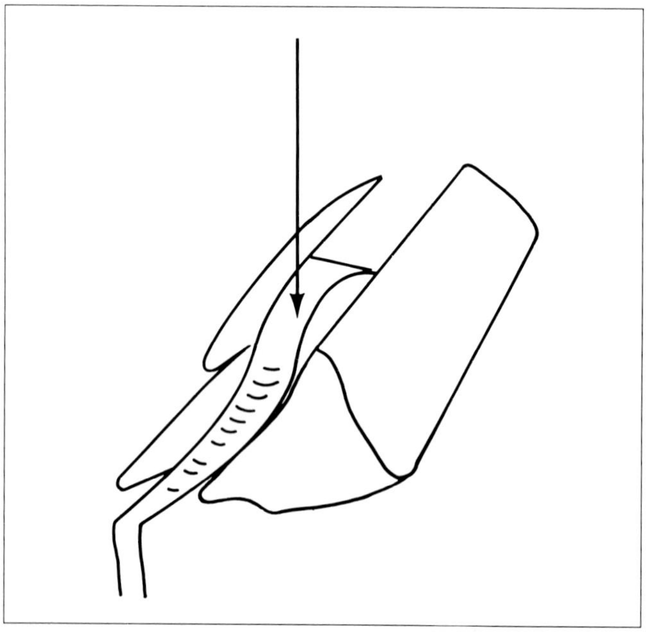

Figure 9-2. Insufficient removal of the dorsal cephalic portion of the cartilaginous septum causes a residual hump deformity.

resulting from inadequate resection, and the polly beak of the experienced plastic surgeon, resulting from excessive surgery. The causes are many and for this reason a precise diagnosis must be made before one proceeds to a secondary operation. Usually one can observe (1) insufficient lowering or trimming of the dorsal border of the septum, (2) insufficient trimming of the dorsal borders of the upper lateral cartilages, (3) insufficient trimming of septal mucosa, (4) excessive resection of intranasal lining, (5) excessive resection of alar cartilage domes, (6) uncompensated short columella, (7) inherent thickness of the skin and subcutaneous tissue, and (8) misplaced or misshapen grafts or implants.

If the septal dorsum is not sufficiently lowered, a postoperative convexity of the supratip area results. To prevent this after removal of a nasal hump, one removes a strip from the septal cartilage just above the lower anterior

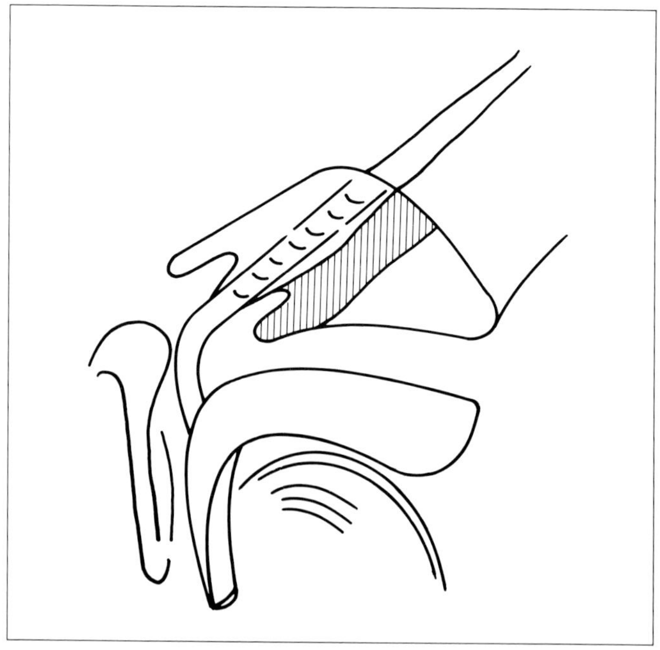

Figure 9-3. Another cause for a persistent hump but at a lower position is insufficient trimming of the upper lateral cartilages.

angle. The surplus subcutaneous tissue can sink into this recess. Lipsett even recommended cutting a small depression in the cartilage at this point (Fig. 9-4). At the end of a primary rhinoplasty there must be a slight concavity just above the nasal tip; in secondary procedures the depression must be even deeper.

If at the end of the operation one leaves a straight dorsum just above the tip, a hump is unavoidably formed with fibrous tissue because of the lateral compression of the dressing. It is important to create a slight supratip depression by means of tight horizontally placed adhesive tape strips (Fig. 9-5). Careful application of the dressing tape is important as it precludes a dead space in the region of the weak triangle. In patients with a thick skin even more caution is required as the skin adapts itself poorly to the underlying tissue. In patients with a primary hooked nose and relatively short columella the risk of a secondary supratip deformity is increased.

Insufficient trimming of the dorsal border of the upper septal cartilage has already been discussed under Insufficient Removal of the Hump.

If in the primary rhinoplasty the hump is resected without use of the extramucosal technique, the septal mucoperichondrium must be trimmed lower than the dorsal border of the septum. Otherwise, it may grow across the dorsum to unite with the opposite mucoperichondrium, becoming interposed between the skin and the septal cartilage (Fig. 9-6). This is one reason why the extramucosal technique is advantageous since there is no cutting of the mucoperichondral vault under the cartilaginous arch of the upper laterals—at least not in the caudal part of that vault. It is, however, obvious that in using the extramucosal method we have to be careful to push the preserved

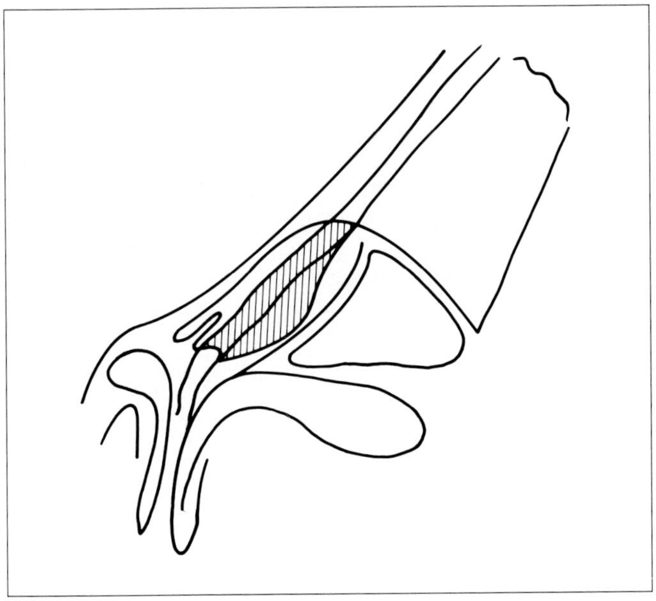

Figure 9-4. A small depression cut into the septal cartilage can help minimize a supratip deformity.

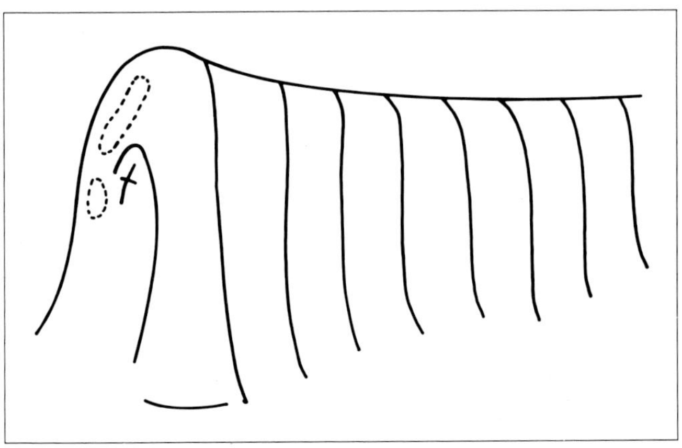

Figure 9-5. It is important to emphasize the supratip depression by means of a tight dressing.

mucoperichondral vault toward the lumen in order to avoid its interposition at the roof.

On the other hand, in the posterior or cephalic part of the nasal cavity, resection of the mucoperiosteal vault is of no importance because in that region a perfect alignment of the bones must be achieved in order to avoid an open roof.

Excessive Resection of Intranasal Lining

This error during primary surgery leads to scar retraction in the vestibules and compensatory scar hypertrophy in the soft tissue between the upper and lower lateral cartilages. Correction is done by careful removal of scar tissue or in extreme cases by increasing the vestibular lining with skin grafts or small composite grafts taken in the inner aspect of the crus helicis of the ear.

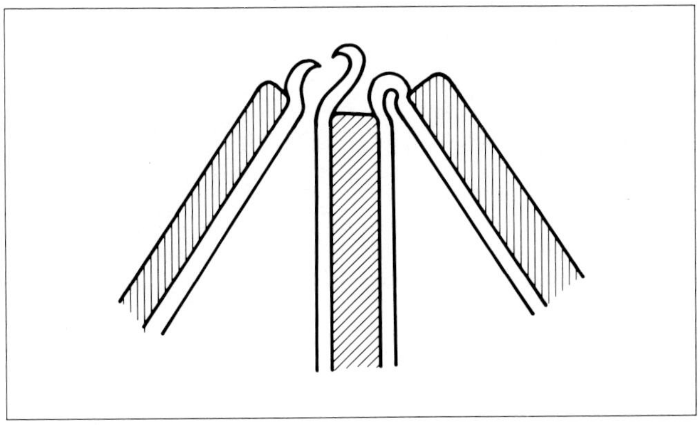

Figure 9-6. Insufficient trimming of the septal mucoperichondrium in primary classic rhinoplasty can lead to union of the two leaves across the dorsum.

Excessive Resection of Alar Cartilage

There are cases in which the dorsal profile cannot be lowered as much as desired for lack of development of the nasal tip. One has to rebuild the tip by sculpturing the lower lateral cartilages, which in those cases of parrot's beak deformity are altered and often excessively reduced. There is a lack of prominence of the alar cartilages, which has been insufficiently proportioned in relation to the profile. For preventing this failure, Wright [20] and others advise shaping the nasal tip before reducing the dorsum in patients with thick skin. The lack of tip projection caused by excessive resection of the alar cartilages at the domes must be compensated for with struts and support mechanisms such as mattress sutures at the remaining stumps of the lower lateral cartilages (Fig. 9-7). The concomitant advancement of the columella after rearrangement of the alar cartilages is provided by inserting a batten of cartilage, as will be explained later.

Uncompensated Short Columella

Failure to elongate the columella and advance the tip of the nose produces a supratip thickening with a hooked tip. In secondary surgery, corrections must be made utilizing all technical possibilities in the same way as in excessive resection of alar cartilage.

Inherent Thickness of the Skin and Subcutaneous Tissue

In this case the supratip swelling is accentuated by fibrous tissue formation in the dead space between the dorsal skin and the septal border. The thicker the skin of the tip and the dorsum, the more obvious the deformity will be. This is the deformity we can consider unpredictable up to a certain degree. It is the soft tissue "polly beak" that can occur after a rhinoplasty accomplished by the best specialist.

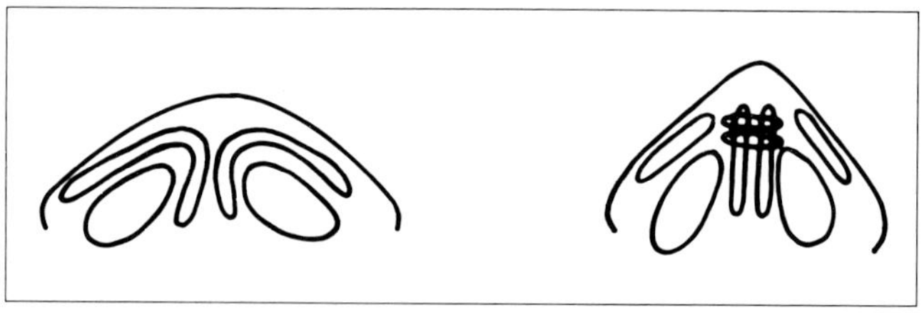

Figure 9-7. Cartilage struts and support mechanisms such as mattress sutures can provide tip projection.

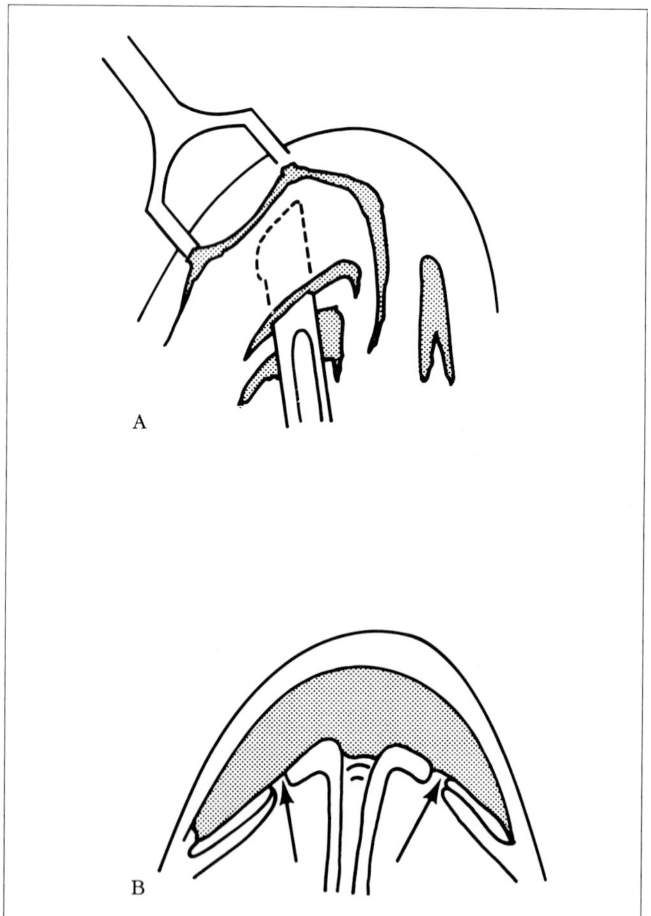

Figure 9-8
A. Retrograde beveled incision through the fibrous tissue.
B. Section showing the dissection planes in a supratip deformity.

Sometimes one can correct the parrot's beak 6 to 12 months after primary surgery by removing fibrous tissue from the weak triangle through a bilateral intercartilaginous incision. From there, one proceeds in a retrograde manner using an eversion technique for the alar cartilages. Beginning on the right side, the incision is enlarged with the scalpel cutting through the fibrous tissue in a beveled way toward the border of the nostril, meticulously preserving the skin lining of the lateral vestibular wall (Fig. 9-8). The external surface of the remaining alar cartilage is dissected from the thickened skin with small blunt scissors, and this detachment is extended, medially joining the fibrous tissue situated in front of the anterosuperior angle of the septal cartilage. Anteriorly, the intercartilaginous incision is carried through fibrous tissue into the membranous septum, reaching the posterior edge of the medial crura of the alar cartilage. Still preserving the vestibular skin at the dome of the lower lateral cartilages, the incision and dissection are continued onto the anterior dorsal border of the quadrangular cartilage, where a depression is created according to Lipsett [9]. At this point a strip of cartilage is often dissected and removed together with the scar tissue. The sharp dissection is then carried across the upper lateral cartilage until the line of the dorsum begins to look normal and does not need to be lowered. The extension of scar tissue removal in the membranous septum and columella was defined at the beginning of the procedure. Behind the lobule there is rarely fibrous tissue requiring removal. This delicate and meticulous maneuver is repeated on the opposite side until the undersurface of the whole fibrocartilaginous complex is completely freed from the new underlying skeleton of the stable part of the nose (Fig. 9-9).

Next, the most dangerous and delicate part of the correction is done: the undermining of the skin in the tip and supratip area, which must be in the right layer not too far from and not too close to the dermis. Again we use fine blunt scissors and begin just behind the tip. It is that point in primary surgery where the suspensory ligament (fascia superficialis) that supports the tip is cut through in order to give a certain degree of independence to the tip-columella complex. This is important in primary as well as in secondary procedures because it allows an upward shift of the cartilaginous and soft structures of the lobule. Once the skin of the whole supratip area is completely freed from the fibrous subcutaneous layer, the scar tissue complex can be removed en bloc together with the detached strip of cartilage. This small piece of cartilage will be useful as graft for supporting the tip. Projection of the tip is not achieved after excision of the supratip area. For this purpose, the strip of cartilage is shaped to a triangular or oval graft and introduced into a superficial pocket at the very tip of the nose, created through a small marginal incision at the anterior border of the columella. The pocket in the tip and lobule should not communicate with the now empty supratip pocket. The anterior one with its cartilaginous strut can now be shifted forward, accentuating tip protrusion (Fig. 9-9C,D, and Figs. 9-10 and 9-11).

At this point the dorsal profile, tip, and columella are checked and eventually perfected by reimplanting a small strip of cartilage longitudinally in the supratip area.

EXCESSIVE REMOVAL OF THE HUMP

This secondary deformity is a very serious complication and difficult to repair. The lack of sufficient dorsum creates a flat middle third of the face, and often an open vault or open roof configuration completes the complication. But besides the unaesthetic appearance it is also

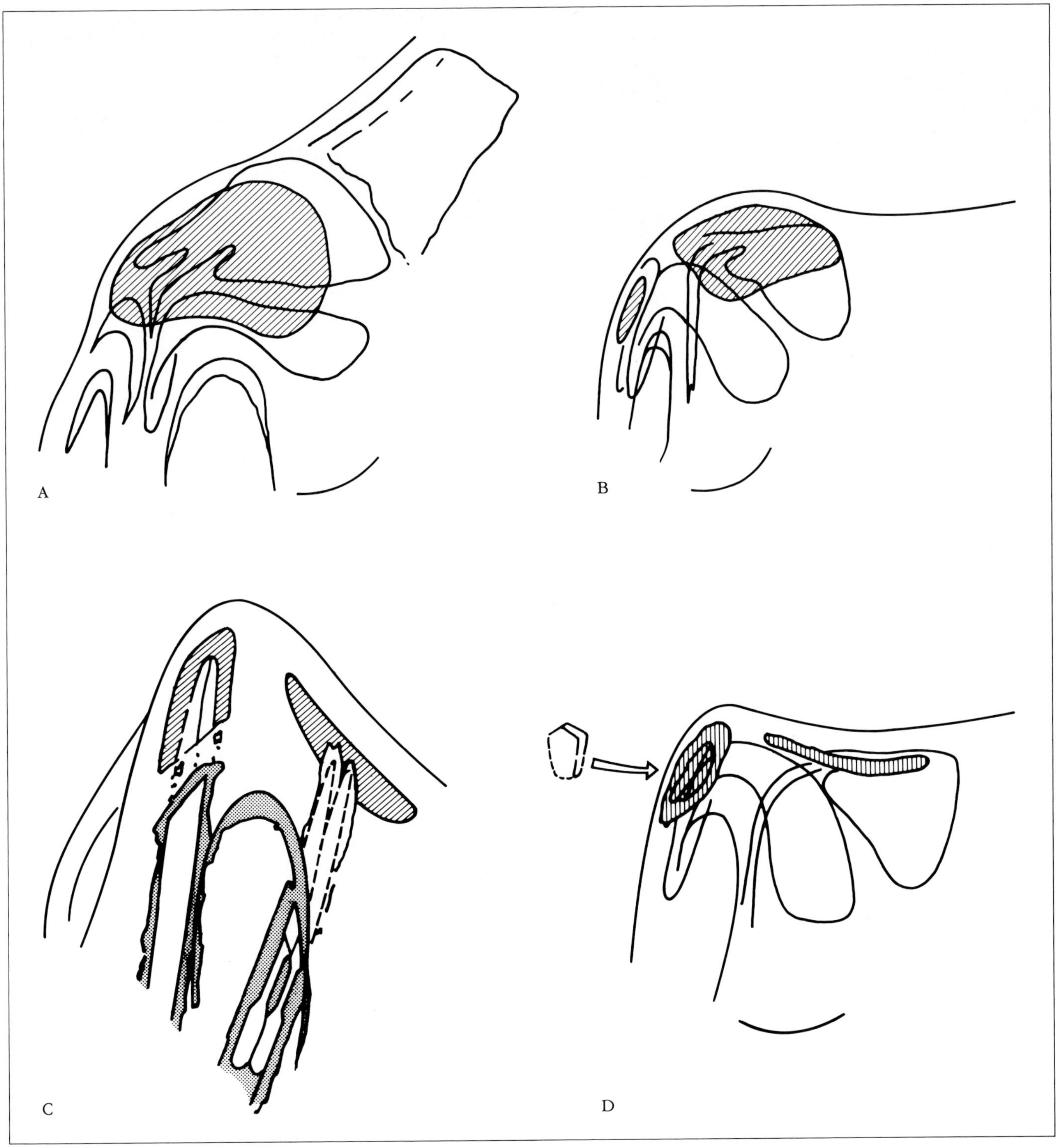

Figure 9-9
A, B. The fibrocartilaginous complex has to be dissected and scar removed carefully from the adjacent tissues.
C, D. The tip protrusion is accentuated by the cartilage grafts placed in a separate pocket in the lobule. The supratip pocket is left empty.

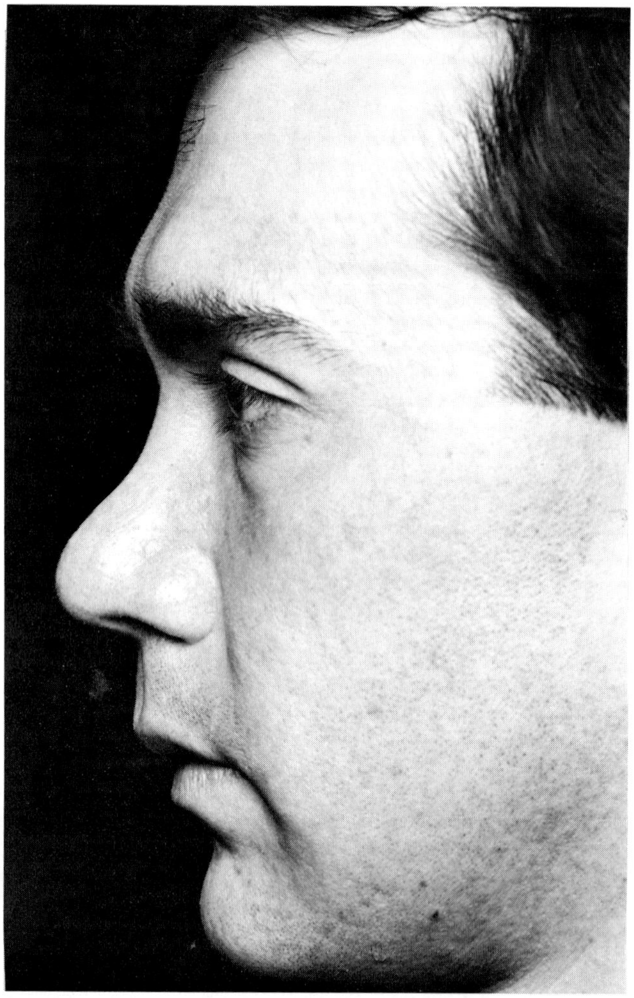

A

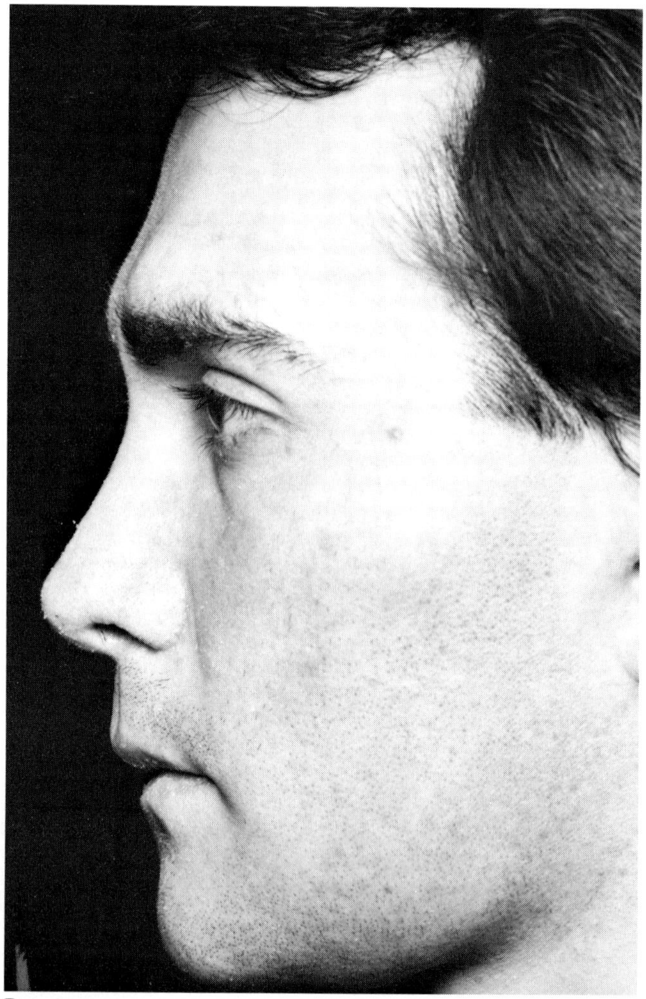

B

Figure 9-10
A, B. Polly beak corrected by utilizing the techniques of scar excision and cartilage grafts to the tip.

frequently the augmented sensibility and tenderness of the nasal dorsum that make the patient complain. The latter symptom is probably caused by the unprotected nasal mucosa that lies directly beneath the external nasal skin.

Treatment for this complication is median displacement of both nasal bones and both frontal processes of the maxilla, the infracturing being performed in such a way that the bones cannot separate again. If these maneuvers alone do not lead to a satisfactory configuration, one has to introduce grafts (dermal grafts or fascia, cartilage, or bone) or synthetic implants such as silicone or Proplast.

Since the nasal bones heal by fibrous union and not by callus in secondary rhinoplasty, the excessive fibrous tissue encountered at the osteotomy lines has to be reduced by excision. Mobilization of the bones must be complete and clean. As in revision procedures, the mobilization and displacement of the nasal bones in order to bring the dorsal edge into contact with the septum are not as easy as in primary surgery. More often we have to use a Walsham or Ash forceps to outfracture or infracture the bones. Because a saddlenose can be produced by too much infracturing, which allows the nasal bones to drop into the piriform aperture, Rees [16] and others preserve the periosteum along the lateral osteotomy, hoping that this attachment will keep the fractured bone from descending (Fig. 9-12).

SADDLENOSE

One of the more common nasal deformities is the saddlenose. It can be congenital or acquired; in the latter case the cause can be syphilitic, traumatic, or iatrogenic. The most common cause for a postoperative saddlenose is a badly executed septal resection. Extensive removal of the cartilaginous septum leads to subsequent collapse of the remaining bridge. Too radical infracturing of the nasal bones during an aesthetic rhinoplasty can also lead to a saddlenose when the bone fragments drop into the piriform aperture.

Many patients with saddlenose complain about obstructed nasal breathing. As a rule, it can be observed that

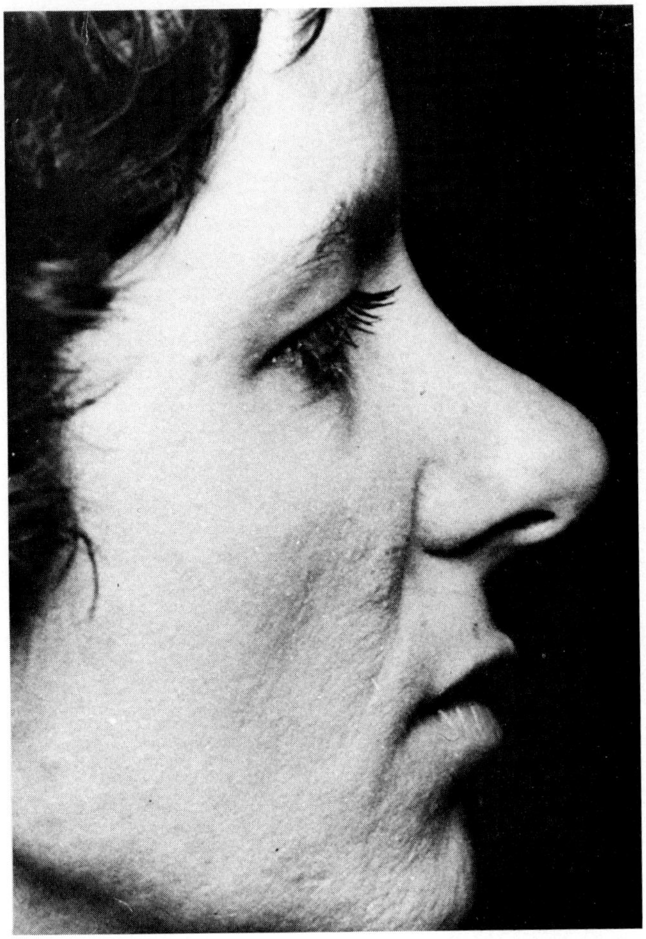

A

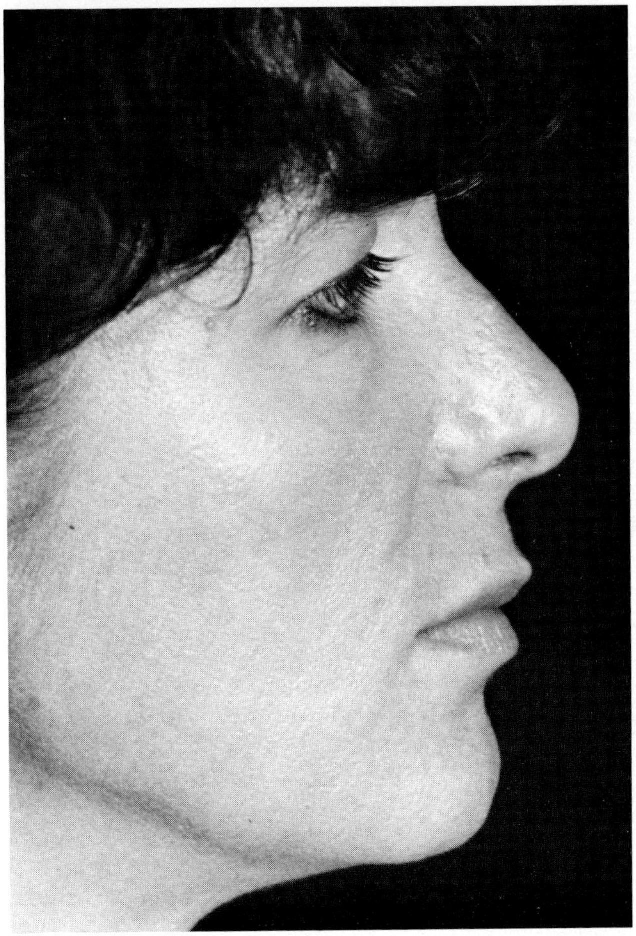

B

Figure 9-11
A, B. Fibrous thickening in the tip and supratip area before and after reduction and remodeling.

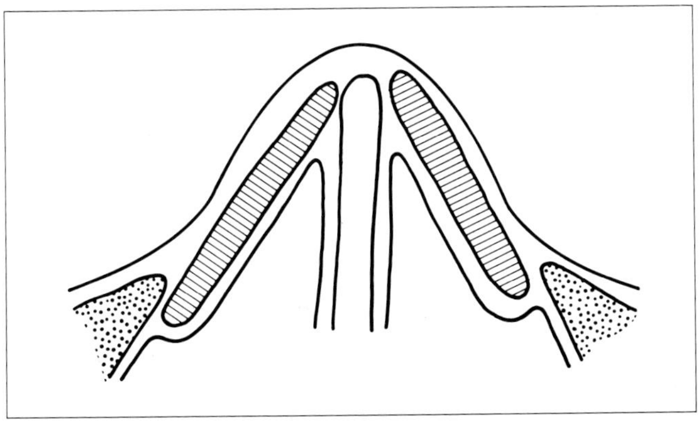

Figure 9-12. Preservation of the periosteum can keep the fractured bones from descending and falling into the piriform aperture.

the nasal cavity is sufficiently free and wide enough, but both vestibules are narrowed. The normally oval or slit-shaped valve area at the transition from vestibule to nasal cavity is flattened from above. The lumen is either a round or flat oval. This deformity directs the airflow downward toward the inferior meatus, thus changing the normal physiologic conditions that direct the airflow upward to the middle meatus and olfactory organ. This abnormal pattern can be relieved by correction of the saddlenose, which presents both a functional and a cosmetic indication.

A pseudosaddlenose, at times referred to as an "apparent" saddle, is usually the result of excessive projection of the nasal tip in contrast to a fairly normal dorsal profile. There are also combinations of true and pseudosaddlenose in which the bony and cartilaginous dorsum is lowered too much and the tip is extremely projected.

While the pseudosaddlenose is usually corrected by lowering the tip and performing new osteotomies, the true saddlenose can be corrected in many different ways. The choice of procedure depends on the degree of saddling and on what grafting material is available. We have always preferred autogenous grafts to allografts. A slight saddlenose can ordinarily be corrected with grafts taken from septal, lower lateral, upper lateral, or ear cartilage.

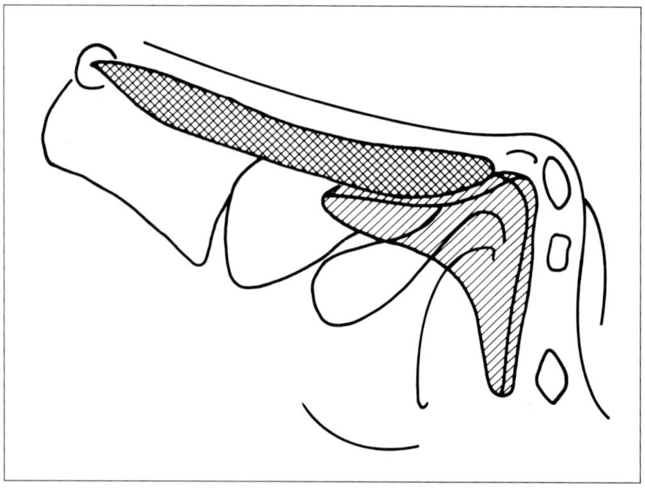

Figure 9-13. A bone graft from the iliac crest can be used in combination with a septocolumellar pillar harvested in the posterior part of the septum.

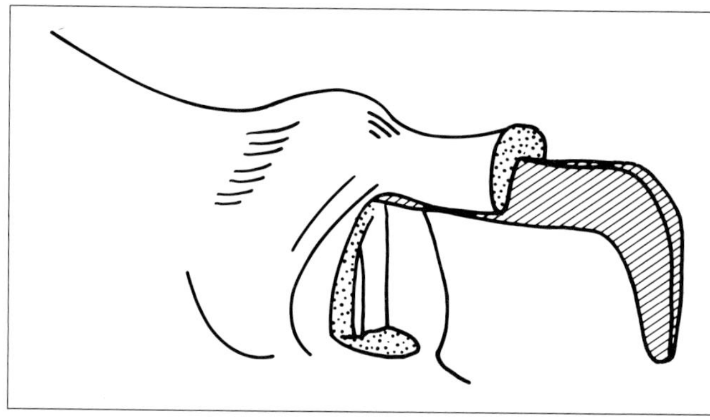

Figure 9-14. The best access for the insertion of a large cartilage graft is gained by transection of the columella.

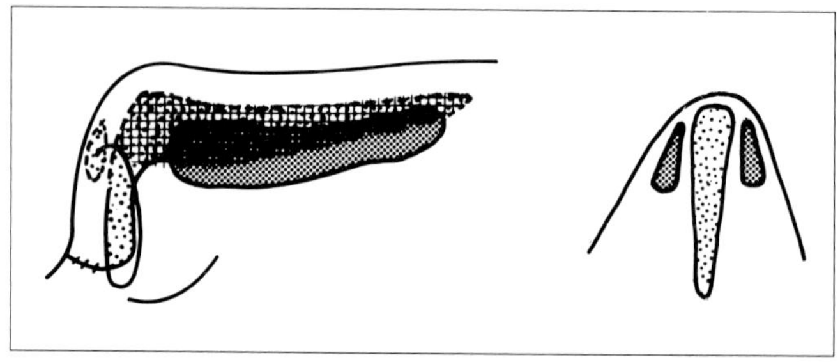

Figure 9-15. One has to be aware of the inherent tensions in cartilage grafts and counteract them by means of relieving incisions and two additional grafts.

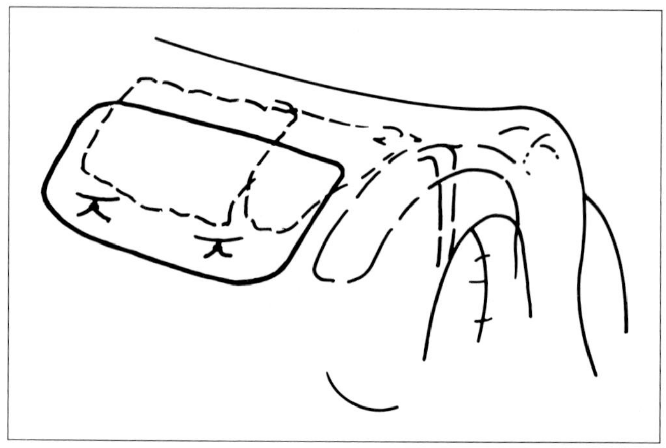

Figure 9-16. Transnasal mattress sutures guarantee initial immobilization in the correct position.

The bony and cartilaginous vault is usually narrowed after mobilization by osteotomies. For smaller depressions, especially in the middle third of the dorsum, the cartilage grafts are cut into little struts, which are placed at the side of the depressions. If the hole that has to be filled is rather large, we like to fix the grafts by external transnasal mattress sutures.

For the very large saddlenose, significant cartilage or bone grafts are necessary; if they are not available, alloplastic implants can be used. One must decide whether a straight or an L-shaped graft is called for, depending on whether tip support is required. If an L-shaped graft is needed, it is usually taken from the eighth, ninth, or tenth rib. A bone graft from the iliac crest can also be used together with a septocolumellar pillar from the posterior part of the septum (Fig. 9-13; see also Fig. 9-24). If this is not available, cartilage from the ear concha can be employed. The incision of choice is gained by an open roof procedure with section of the columellar base. The incision is carried through the membranous septum and extended into the vestibular intracartilaginous incision (Fig. 9-14). As stated, the alar cartilage can be reached in the usual way by the eversion technique. The bed for the graft at the dorsum and in the columella can be prepared under direct vision. Depending on the deformity, the dorsal graft can be short, resting on the bony vault, or long, ending at the glabella. A hole drilled into the frontal bone serves as anchorage.

If costal cartilage is used, we have to compensate for the inherent tensions described by Davis and Gibson [2], which may distort the sculptured graft. For this purpose, we make several relieving incisions and add on either side a narrow parallel graft having a counteracting force (Fig. 9-15).

In most cases, complete osteotomies are inevitable in order to push the bony structures forward, increasing protrusion of the dorsum in addition to the grafting. The narrowed bones and the graft are held in place by transcutaneous, transmucosal, and transseptal mattress sutures, which pass through the osteotomy lines and if necessary through the upper lateral cartilages (Fig. 9-16). The contact of the dorsal graft with the bony dorsum has to be firm. Fibrine adhesive can be used to increase the consolidation. Tape dressing and plaster splinting are left for 10 days. The results can be rather dramatic (Fig. 9-17).

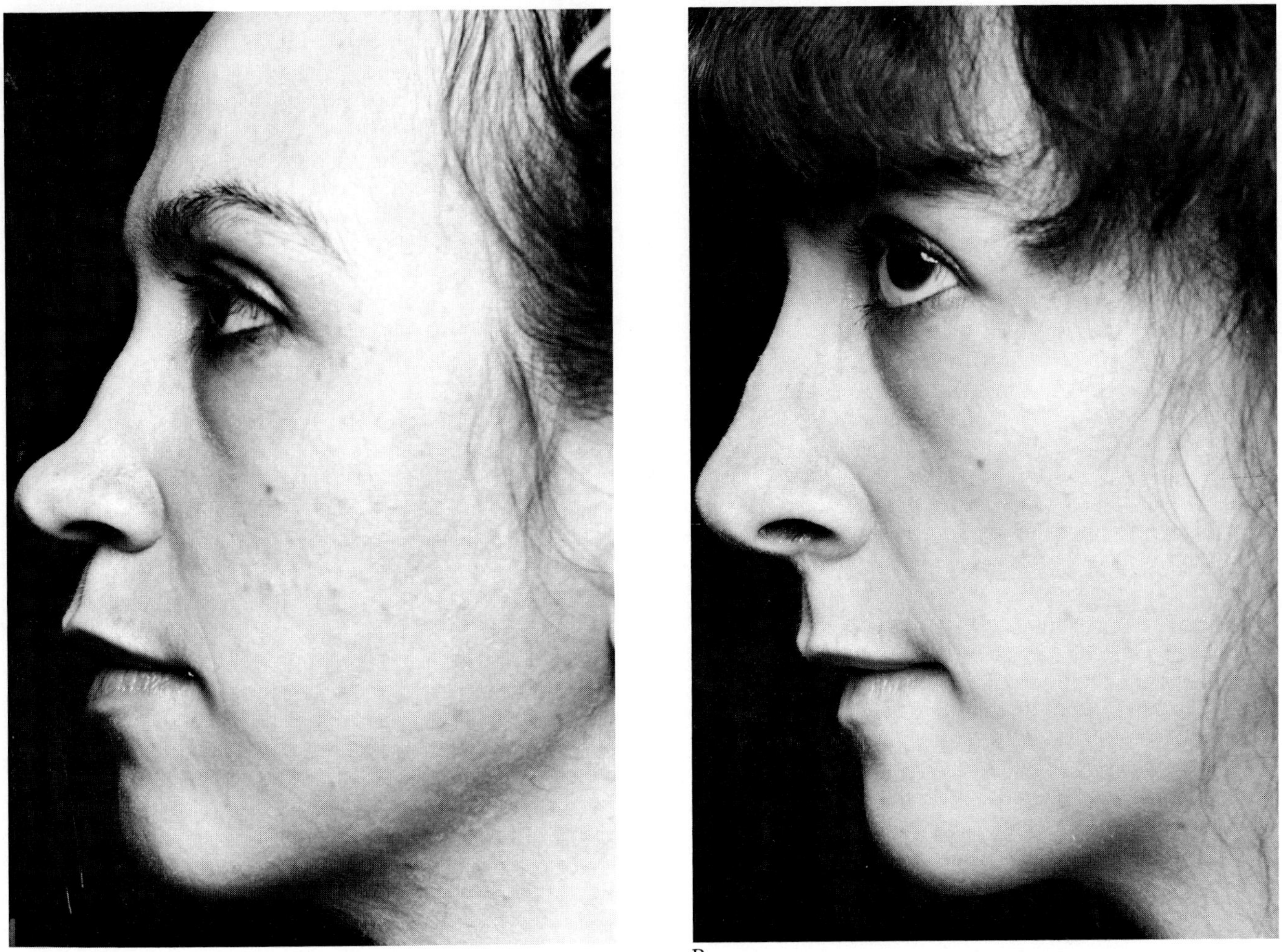

A B

Figure 9-17
A, B. Saddlenose corrected by L-shaped rib cartilage graft (preoperative and postoperative view).

DEFORMITIES OF THE CARTILAGINOUS FRAMEWORK AND TIP

The nasal tip and the nostrils are shaped essentially by the lower lateral cartilages, which enclose the anterior part of the two vestibules like the claws of a lobster. For correction and reshaping of the tip, the lower lateral cartilages must be modified. Access can be obtained in different ways: (1) a marginal incision for the delivery technique, (2) an intracartilaginous, transcartilaginous, or cartilage-splitting incision (the same incision but with different names), (3) an intercartilaginous incision for eversion or retrograde technique, (4) the transcolumellar incision for the decortication method of Rethi [17] and Erich [5], and (5) the columella circumcising incision of Gillies [7] and Potter [15].

In about 80 percent of revisions we choose the delivery technique through an infracartilaginous incision. This approach gives us the best view of the whole cartilaginous arch and easy access for the remodeling of the dome.

The intracartilaginous approach is indicated in cases in which the alar borders are retracted and fibrous thickening is present on the vestibular surface. It permits lowering of the alar rim by cartilage grafting if necessary (see below). It also permits important marginal resections that otherwise would interfere with a delivery technique.

The retrograde eversion is done through the intercartilaginous incision and has already been mentioned in conjunction with supratip deformity. It is also utilized if at the same time a Rethi [17] or a Potter [15] type of incision is chosen—for example, insertion of an L-graft. In all these cases, a bipedicled flap or delivery technique would be hazardous.

In secondary rhinoplasty every millimeter of cutaneous vestibular lining has to be preserved, and the triangular skin resection often performed in primary rhinoplasties is absolutely contraindicated for correction of supratip subcutaneous thickening.

The decortication method of Rethi [17] consists of bilateral marginal incisions extended to the lateral side of the columella and meeting in a transection between its anterior and middle third. We use this access mainly for the correction of cleft lip noses or in selected cases of columellar deformities such as retractions. The Erich [5] approach follows the same concept, but the incision line is curved instead of angulated.

Transsection of the columella at its base as proposed by Gillies [7] and Potter [15] gives maximal freedom for the access to the lower lateral cartilages. We have extended this incision into the membranous septum for the purpose of graft introduction under direct vision (see Saddlenose) [12].

In revisional tip surgery we encounter several typical secondary deformations: (1) the bifid or cleft tip, (2) the pinched nose, (3) the collapsing ala, (4) the depressed upper alar border, (5) various asymmetries and irregularities of the tip, and (6) the collapsed tip.

Bifid or Cleft Tip

This deformity is caused by a too generous resection of the cartilaginous arch in the medial crura, creating a dead space between the residual stumps into which the overlying skin of the tip can sink. The deformity is corrected by suturing the remnants of the dome as well as the crura together after having excised the intervening scar tissue. Sometimes it is necessary to interpose a small cartilage graft between the remaining stump and the skin to obliterate the depression.

Pinched Nose

Excessive removal of vestibular skin accompanied by segmental resection of alar cartilage too far laterally is the cause of the pinched nose. It can produce an anterior vestibular stenosis. A delivery or intracartilaginous incision can be used. The segmental loss of cartilage has to be compensated for by cartilage grafts, procured either from the upper border of the lateral crus, from the septum, which is often too thick and has to be thinned, or from the auricle.

These tiny grafts are fixed with a transalar 5-0 nonabsorbable mattress suture tied over a sheet of plastic material (Fig. 9-18). If inner lining has to be replaced or added, we have found that the best results are obtained with composite grafts from the ear concha or the inner side of the crus helicis.

Collapsing Ala

This is a similar deformity that has the same etiology and often the same secondary treatment (Fig. 9-19A). When ala collapse is due to inherent weakness or flaccidity, it is sufficient to perform an extramucosal dissection with section of the upper lateral cartilage at its insertion to the septum and fixation of this mobilized triangular cartilage by transalar mattress sutures.

Depressions at the Upper Border of the Ala

These depressions are also a secondary cartilage deficiency problem. They have to be corrected by means of small cartilage inlays fixed with mattress sutures (Fig. 9-19B).

Tip Deformities

Tip deformities range from slight asymmetries to gross deformities, torsions, skin irregularities, and furrows, which must be corrected at different levels. First of all, the alar cartilages have to be revised and trimmed symmetrically. Missing or notched cartilages have to be replaced or bridged with cartilage grafts (Fig. 9-19C). Minor skin irregularities can be corrected by collagen injections. Major irregularities and *furrows* mandate meticulous undermining and sometimes have to be underlaid with grafts of meshed cartilage, dermis, or fascia. Of utmost importance is precise fixation with mattress sutures, tied once again over transparent plastic sheets that allow inspection of the skin (Fig. 9-20).

Figure 9-18
A. Pinched nose produced by too much removal of the lateral alar cartilage segment.
B. Correction by bilateral insertion of a cartilage graft into the weak ala and fixation by transalar mattress sutures.

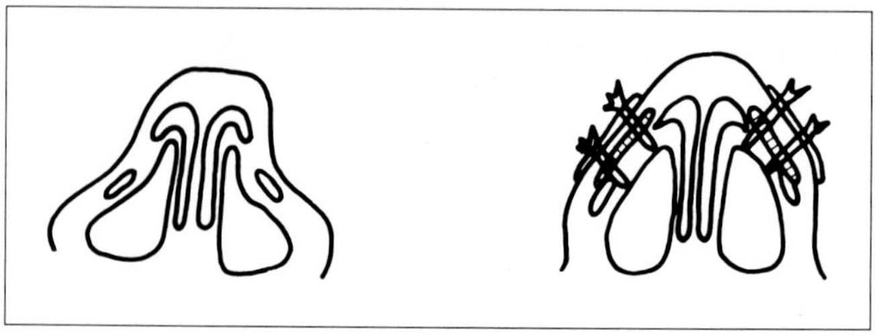

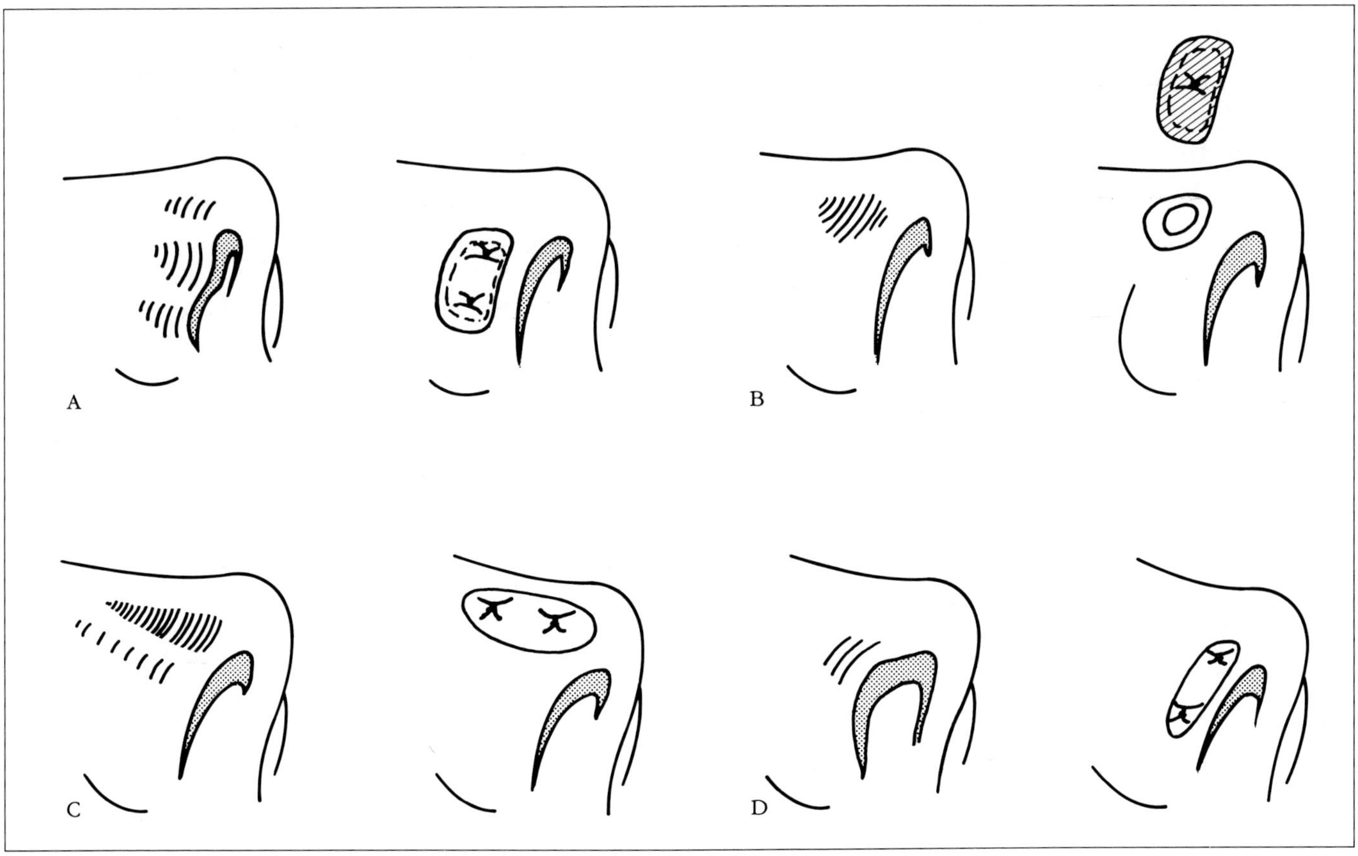

Figure 9-19
A, B. Transalar mattress suture tied over a transparent plastic sheet in correction of pinched nose or collapsed ala.
C. Similar correction of furrows of the tip.
D. Marginal mattress suture in correction of retracted alar rim.

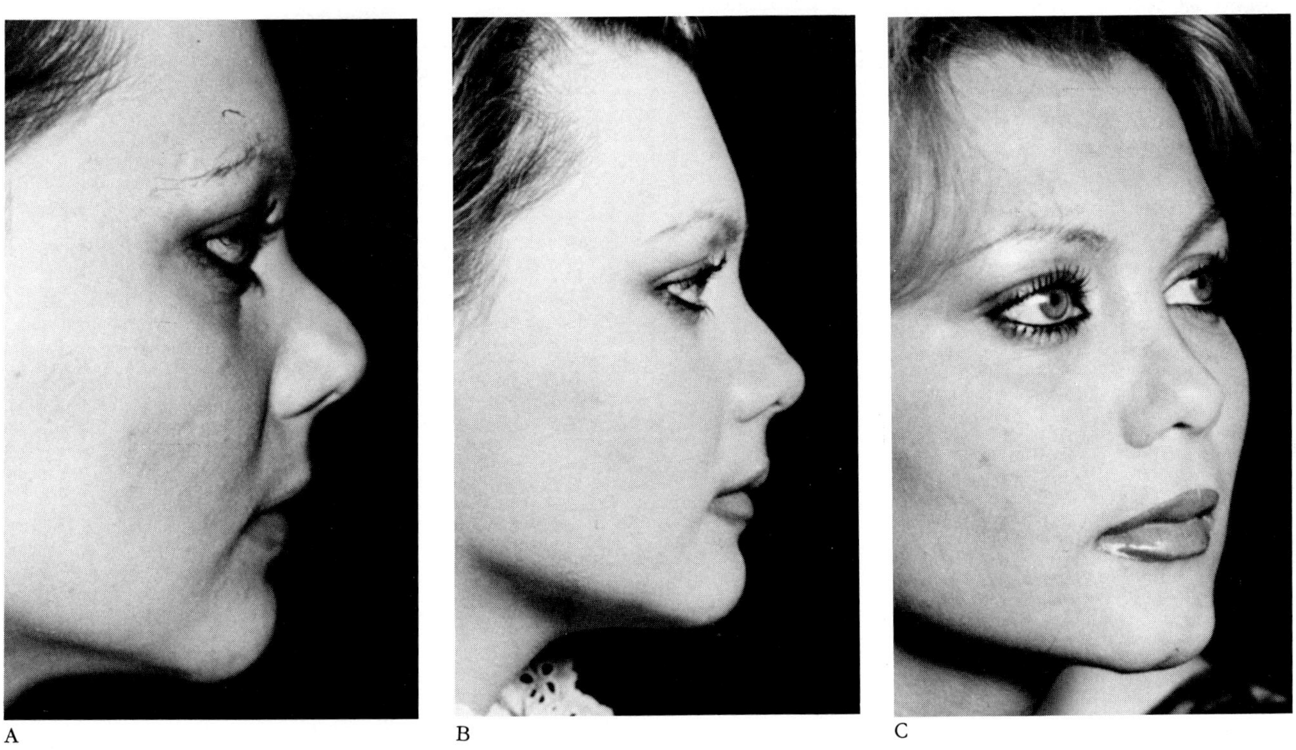

Figure 9-20
A–C. Furrows before and after correction.

Collapsed Tip

This rare iatrogenic deformity represents a summation of all the previously described deformities together in one patient. It is caused by a subtotal resection of the lateral crura of the alar cartilage as well as too generous resection at the medial crura (Fig. 9-21). Deprived of its support, the skin of the nostrils becomes flabby and is collapsed most of the time and especially during inspiration. The lobule-tip complex can also be distorted and weak. The repair is done by cartilage grafting at the tip. Either we place a convex alar cartilage graft in the whole tip or a small cartilage strut is sufficient. The graft is introduced in the way we have been doing it routinely in about 80 percent of our primary and secondary rhinoplasties for the last 20 years [3] (Fig. 9-22A). This technical detail has also been emphasized by Sheen [19] (Fig. 9-22B,C). Fixation with mattress sutures and extremely careful splinting are essential.

THE SHORT NOSE AND COLUMELLA DEFORMITIES

In this section three deformities are discussed: too high an alar rim, the hidden columella, and the retroussé or pig snout nose.

The *alar rim that is too high* has to be corrected by a simple equalizing border resection fore and aft of the alar arch. It is a problem of missing skin and missing cartilage. To repair this deformity, we choose the infracartilaginous incision of the delivery technique for access and dissect the vestibular skin bluntly down to the alar rim (Fig. 9-23). A strip of the upper part of the alar cartilage is then inserted in this marginal pocket, pushed downward in order to outfold the former vestibular skin, and fixed by two mattress sutures in its new position. The mattress sutures are as always tied on a plastic sheet in order to avoid marks on the nasal skin. Overcorrecting is necessary to obtain a good late result (Fig. 9-24).

The *hidden columella* is due either to a too generous resection of the caudal part of the septal cartilage or to a skin resection in that region, or even sometimes to a combination of these two errors. It can be corrected in three different ways depending on the degree of deformity.

Basically, we try to obtain an augmentation in length by inserting cartilage from the septum, ala, or ear in three possible places at the caudal end of the nose. One is a pocket formed by blunt dissection between the medial crura of the alar cartilage through a transfixion incision (Fig. 9-25). Another is the anterior superficial pocket in the columella created by blunt dissection, again subcutaneously. The third is the space between membranous septum and columella tissue, which we fill with cartilage once the mucosal layer of the transfixion is sutured on one side. In cases in which we use the Rethi [17] or a similar incision we can put a vertical cartilage strut in the columellar stump and then pull the sectioned columella at the end of the operation over this vertical cartilage (Figs. 9-26 and 9-27).

Inconsiderate resection of septal cartilage and nasal lining can lead to a too short nose culminating in the grotesque deformity of a so-called pig snout nose. Usually, the nasal skin can be stretched, but the nasal lining, especially the mucosa, is too restricted. For this reason, the mucosa has to be pulled down as an entity in continuity with the perichondrium and the periosteum of the septum as well as the mucosal lining of the upper lateral cartilages. The latter have not been severed previously at their insertion to the anterosuperior ridge of the septum. To allow caudal displacement of this "sleeve," the mucoperios-

Figure 9-21. Usual segmental resection at the medial crura for tip reduction. Depending on the amount of resection, collapsed tip can result.

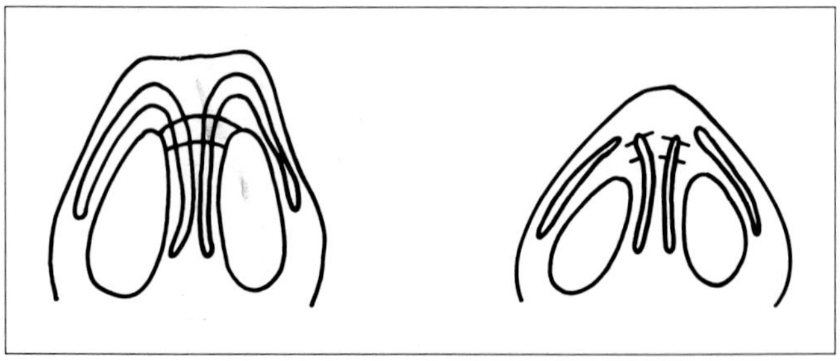

Figure 9-22

A. A small cartilage tip graft is used routinely in about 80 percent of our primary and secondary rhinoplasties. The design corresponds to that published by Denecke and Meyer in 1967.

B. The Meyer-Sheen lobular onlay. An oval rectangular or trapezoid graft from the septal cartilage is inserted in a bluntly dissected superficial pocket in the tip-lobule area.

C. For accentuating the double angle in the tip-columella profile, we put another smaller piece into the base of the lobule.

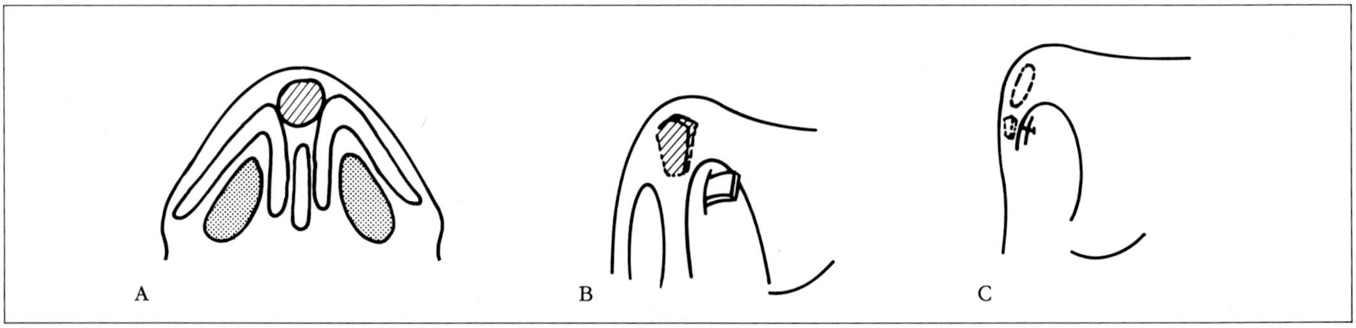

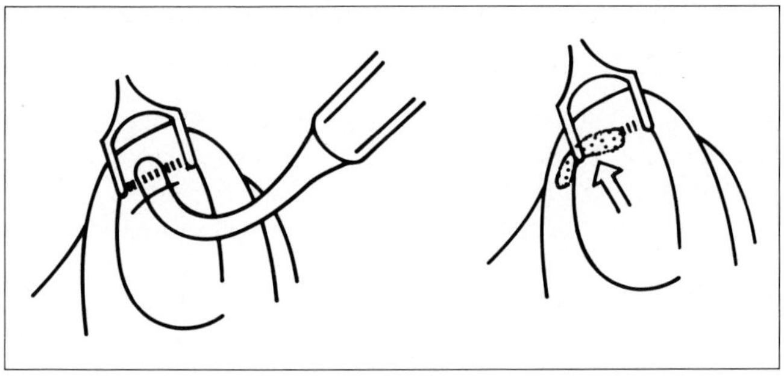

Figure 9-23. The too high alar rim brought down by an outfolding procedure including a caudal cartilage graft fixed with two mattress sutures.

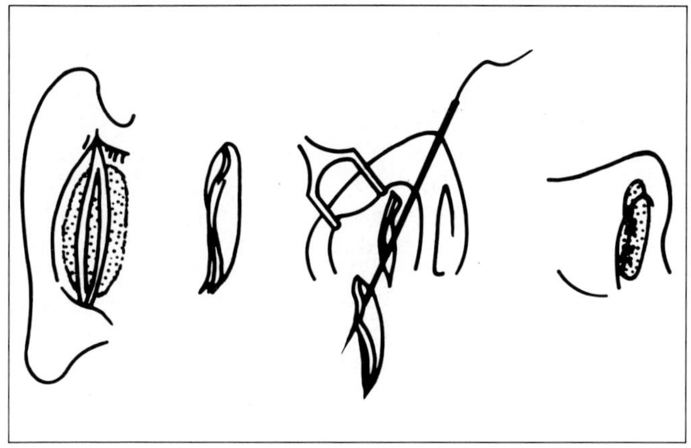

Figure 9-25. For correction of a hidden columella several kinds of cartilage grafts can be used. Here a composite strut of ear cartilage is introduced through a transfixion incision for correction of a hidden columella.

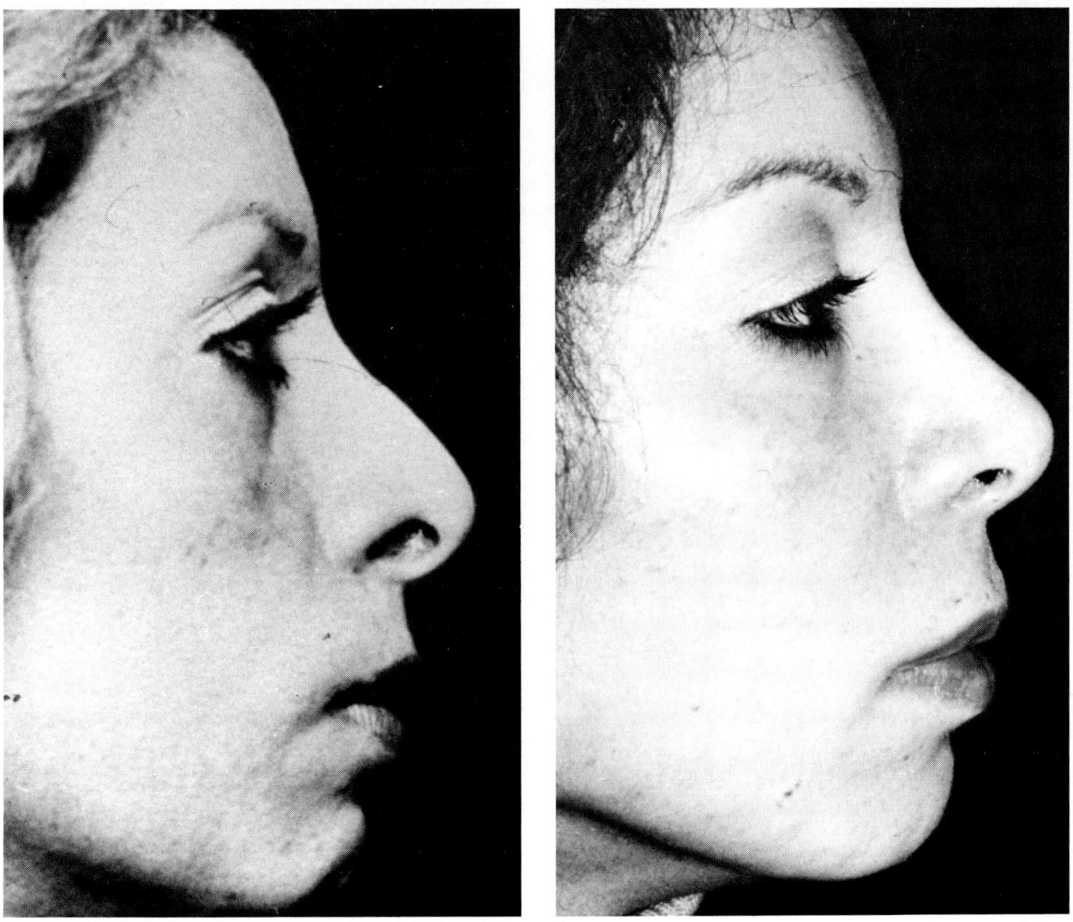

A B

Figure 9-24
A, B. Too high alar rim before and after surgical lowering.

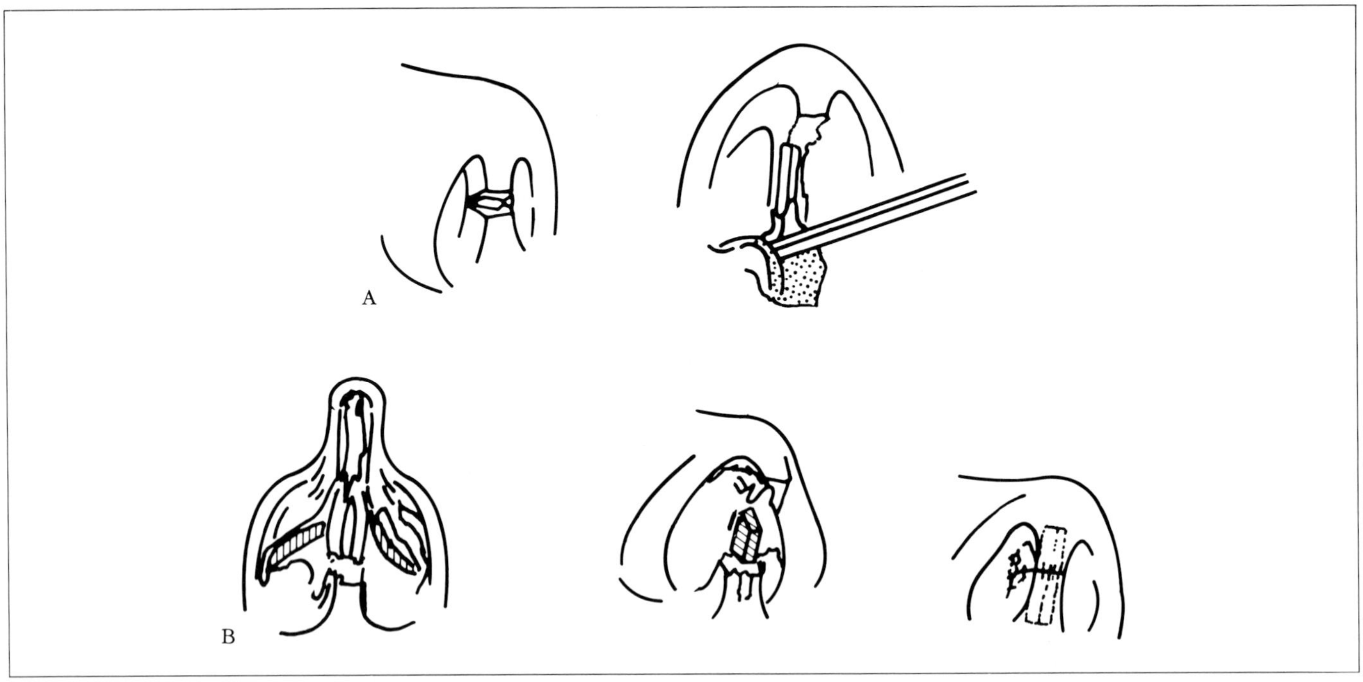

Figure 9-26
A, B. Using transcolumellar incisions we can place a vertical cartilage strut in the columellar stump and then pull the sectioned columella over this vertical cartilage.

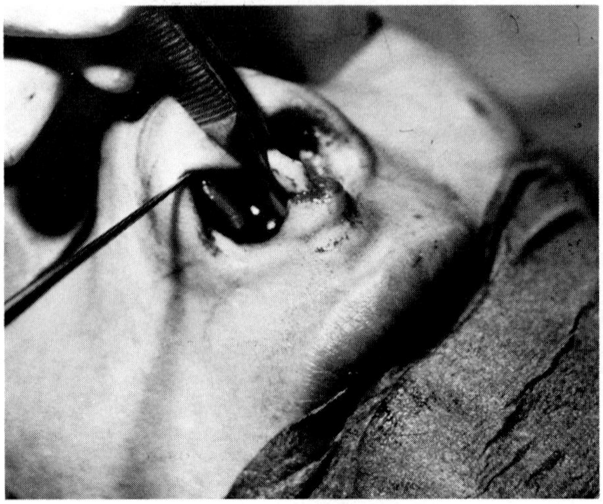

Figure 9-27. Cartilage strut introduced into the columellar.

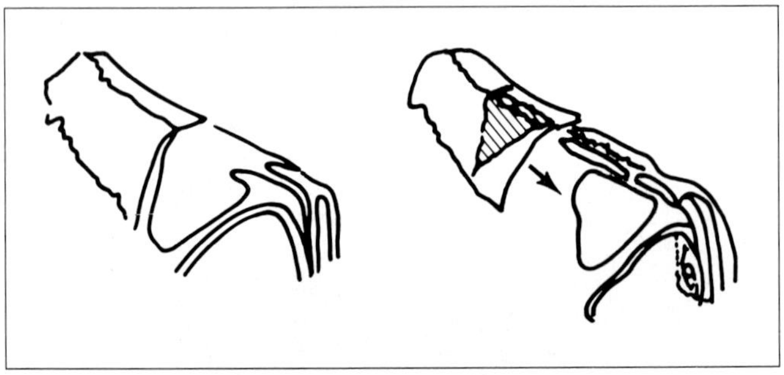

Figure 9-28. In a lengthening procedure that involves skin and nasal lining the mucosa has to be pulled down as a single entity including (1) the mucoperichondrium and mucoperiosteum of the septum and (2) the upper laterals with their mucosa. A relaxing vertical incision at the anterosuperior border of the septum facilitates this downward movement.

teum must be incised at its cranial end (Fig. 9-28). Obviously, in order to preserve the mucoperichondrium vault an extramucosal procedure must be done. Although often identified with its French advocates [8, 14, 18], it was described for the first time by Eitner [4] in 1932 and later by Fomon [6] and Denecke and Meyer [3]. Once the downward movement is achieved, a "spacer" has to be put at the caudal end of the too short septum where it will be covered by both leaves of the mucoperichondrium (Fig. 9-29). Transfixing mattress sutures are used. In extreme cases in which the height of the septum has been reduced too much, we employ, as in the saddlenose, an L-shaped costal cartilage graft for the augmentative-lengthening procedure (Fig. 9-30).

SECONDARY BONE DEFORMITIES

After precise approximation of the dorsal edges of the nasal bones, it becomes obvious whether the transverse

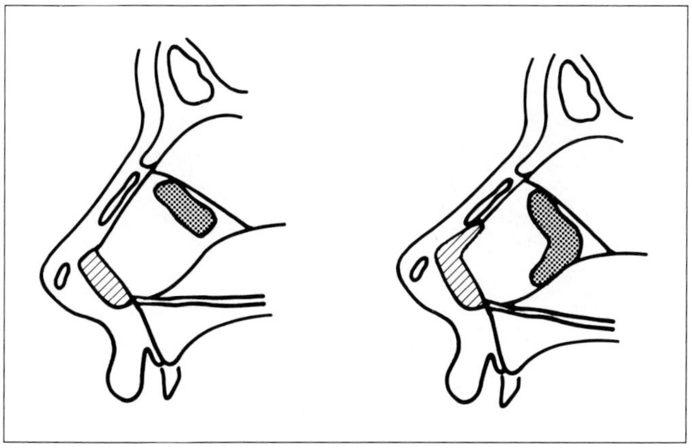

Figure 9-29. Additional length is provided by introducing a spacer at the caudal end of the septum. This cartilage can be harvested in the septum itself and may have either a rectangular or a boomerang shape.

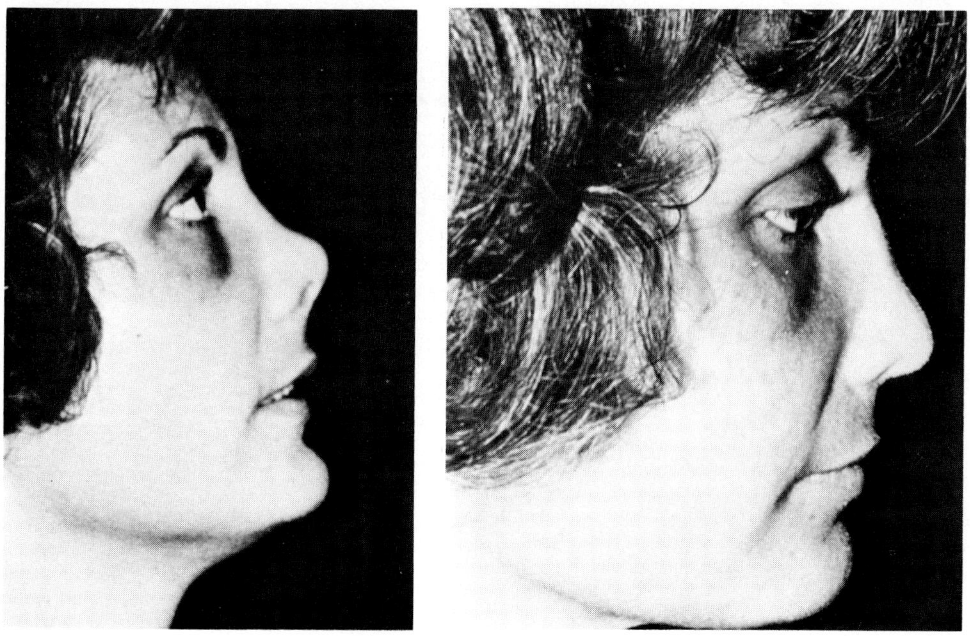

Figure 9-30. This extreme case of a pig snout nose was corrected in the described manner.

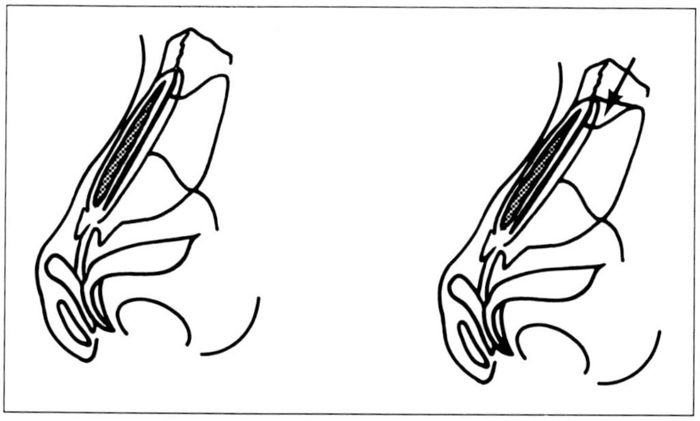

Figure 9-31. Remaining spurs caused by incorrect osteotomies have to be refractured or removed with a biting forceps.

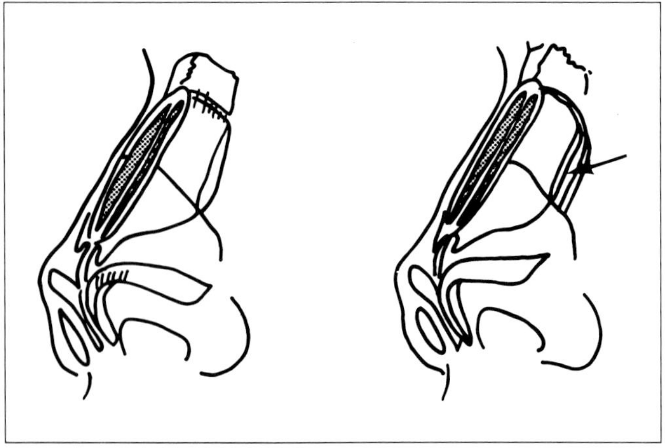

Figure 9-32. Imprecise lateral osteotomies can lead to a pathognomonic step deformity. This has to be corrected by a secondary, more lateral osteotomy.

osteotomy is truly horizontal or is angulated with medial spur formation. This defect occurs most often in noses with thick bones. If such a spur is present, it must be mobilized with the curved chisel and removed with the Luer or Levignac biting forceps (Fig. 9-31). The narrowed nose with its raised dorsum must be held in place for at least 10 days in a slightly exaggerated narrow position by transnasal mattress sutures and splinted with plaster of Paris. The suture material is 4-0 nylon on a straight needle going through the nasal cavity, the septum, and the other nasal cavity using the osteotomy bone gap to pass. Imprecise lateral osteotomies have to be recut, thus eliminating the step deformity (Fig. 9-32).

SEPTAL PERFORATIONS

The closure of septal perforations is in itself a subject that could fill an entire chapter of a book [11]. Anterior perforations up to a diameter of 30 mm can be closed in one stage by a procedure similar to that described for lengthening the nose: extramucosal dissection, mobilization of the whole mucoperichondrium and mucoperiosteum at the roof of the nose, the four-fifths of the septum, and the anterior floor of vestibule and cavity [13]. The detached lateral cartilages are severed from the septum and follow the advancement of the mucoperichondral flap. The perforation in the middle of the two flaps can usually be closed by approximation of the borders. The hole in the cartilage can be filled with cartilage from the basal or posterior aspect of the septum or with fascia or by the pushdown procedure of Cottle [1] (Fig. 9-33).

If the diameter of the perforation exceeds 30 mm, surgical closure is not very promising even with this method. Alternatively, a more complicated technique can be used [11]. It is a three-step method in which a spoon-shaped distant flap from the oral vestibule with a piece of cartilage attached is first inserted into the perforation and then severed from its pedicle after the cartilage fragment, which is covered with mucous membrane on both sides, has grown into the septum.

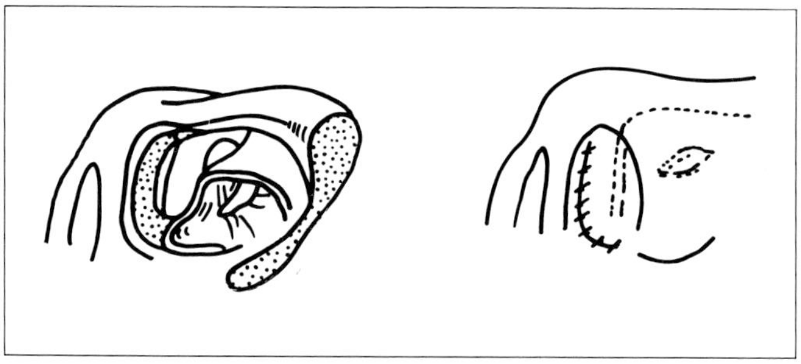

Figure 9-33. The same principles employed in a lengthening procedure can be used for closure of a septum perforation: By extramucosal access the whole mucoperichondrium and mucoperiosteum is mobilized.

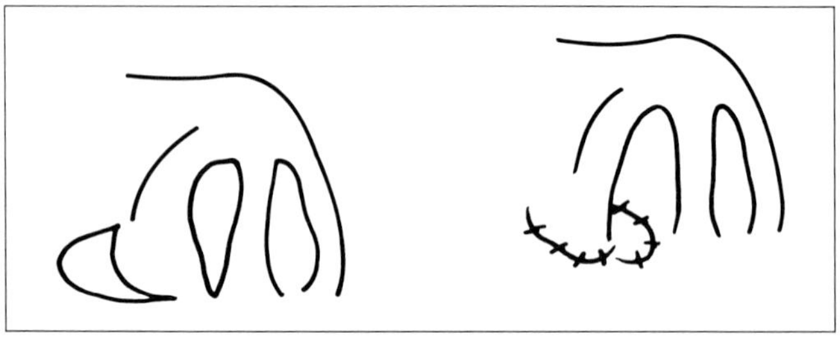

Figure 9-34. A sickle-shaped island flap from the nasolabial angle can be transferred to the floor of the vestibule in order to correct vestibular stenosis.

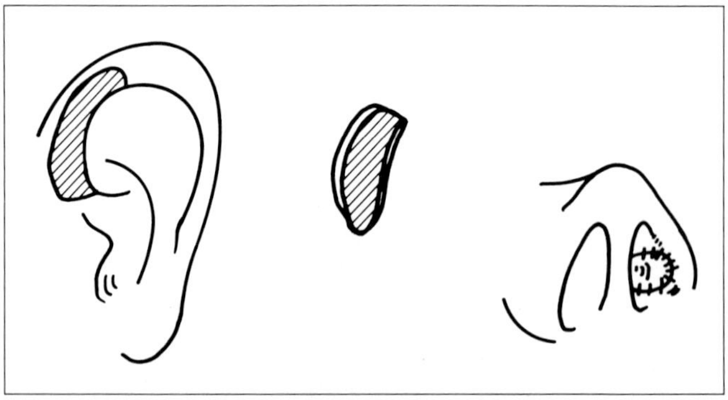

Figure 9-35. For widening the vestibule and the anterior part of the nasal cavity in more severe stenoses, a gutter-shaped composite graft is taken from the anterior crus helicis to fill the defect after excision of scar tissue.

STENOSES OF THE NARES

The correction of postoperative vestibular stenosis is sometimes rather difficult. Recurrence is frequent after inadequate surgery. The procedure we utilize most frequently makes use of a perialar half-moon–shaped island flap transferred to the floor of the vestibule and an auricular composite graft for widening the lateral vestibular lining [12]. Thus, the alar base is completely detached in order to be sutured to the original place once the island flap is pulled medially into the vestibular defect. The donor defect at the alar base is closed by approximation, thus spreading the nostril (Fig. 9-34). The composite graft, which we usually take from the minor aspect of the crus helicis, where the skin is extremely adherent to the cartilage, serves as lining for the alar defect after the excision of scarred tissue on the lateral wall of the vestibule. Such gutter-shaped composite grafts are suitable for widening of the vestibule, even reaching past the valve into the anterior part of the nasal cavity (Fig. 9-35). Additional methods for correcting stenosis of the nares are discussed elsewhere [12].

REFERENCES

1. Cottle, M. H. Nasal atrophy, atrophic rhinitis, ozenia. *Int. Coll. Surg.* 29:472, 1958.
2. Davis, W. B., and Gibson, T. Absorption of autogenous cartilage grafts in man. *Br. J. Plast. Surg.* 9:177, 1956.
3. Denecke, H. J., and Meyer, R. *Corrective and Reconstructive Rhinoplasty. Plastic Surgery on Head and Neck* (vol. 1). New York: Springer-Verlag, 1967.
4. Eitner, E. *Kosmetische Operationen, ein kurzer Leitfaden fur den Praktiker.* Wien: Springer, 1932.
5. Erich, J. B. A technic for correcting a flat nostril in cases of repaired harelip. *Plast. Reconstr. Surg.* 12:320, 1953.
6. Fomon, S. *Cosmetic Surgery: Principles and Practice.* Philadelphia: Lippincott, 1960. Pp. 329–332.
7. Gillies, H. D. *Operative Surgery,* Vol. 1. London: Grey-Turner, 1931.
8. Jost, G. Défaut de projection de la pointe du nez. *Ann. Chir. Plast.* 17:245, 1972.
9. Lipsett, E. M. A new approach to the surgery of the lower cartilaginous vault. *Arch. Otolaryngol.* 70:42, 1959.
10. Meyer, R. Correction of Rhinoplasty Complications. In *Transactions of the 8th International Congress of Plastic and Reconstructive Surgery.* Melbourne: Butterworths, 1971.
11. Meyer, R. Nasal-septal Perforation and Nostril Stenosis. In R. M. Goldwyn (ed.), *The Unfavorable Result in Plastic Surgery.* Boston: Little, Brown, 1972.
12. Meyer, R., and Kesselring, U. K. Sculpturing and reconstructive procedures in aesthetic and functional rhinoplasty. *Clin. Plast. Surg.* 17:90, 1972.
13. Meyer, R., and Kesselring, U. K. Surgical correction of the unusually short nose. *Aesthetic Plast. Surg.* 1:271, 1977.
14. Pollet, J. Rhinoseptoplastie. *Ann. Chir. Plast.* 17:90, 1972.
15. Potter, J. Some nasal tip deformities due to alar cartilage abnormalities. *Plast. Reconstr. Surg.* 15:202, 1955.
16. Rees, T. D., and Wood-Smith, D. *Cosmetic Facial Surgery.* Philadelphia: Saunders, 1974.
17. Rethi, A. Right and wrong in rhinoplastic operations. *Plast. Reconstr. Surg.* 3:361, 1948.
18. Robin, J. L. Rhinoplastie extramuqueuse controlée avec mesure préopératoire de la modification du profil. *Ann. Chir. Plast.* 18:119, 1971.
19. Sheen, J. H. *Aesthetic Rhinoplasty.* St. Louis: Mosby, 1978.
20. Wright, W. K. General principles of lateral osteotomy and hump removal. *Trans. Am. Acad. Ophthalmol. Otolaryngol.* 65:854, 1961.

III. Facial Procedures

10. Aesthetic Procedures on the Chin

S. Anthony Wolfe

This chapter presents one individual's approach to chin deformities, and it may, at first reading, seem unnecessarily complex or difficult to many surgeons performing primarily aesthetic surgery.

Craniofacial surgery is having its effect on other areas of plastic surgery, and aesthetic surgery is certainly no exception. One does not have to be a craniofacial surgeon, however, to use the direct osteoplastic procedures described here. The procedures are quite simple and will allow the aesthetic surgeon to deal with a much greater range of deformities than is possible with alloplastic implants alone. This approach is based on fundamental principles of reconstructive plastic surgery: Return displaced or misplaced structures to their proper position and keep them there, and replace what is missing with like tissue [8].

There is nothing original in this chapter, and I express my gratitude and debt to my teachers for all of the techniques that were used. Millard [13] brought the combination of submental and submandibular lipectomy to its current state. Obwegeser [14], Converse [2, 3], and Tessier [18] have been responsible for development of most of the techniques currently used in plastic surgery of the facial skeleton. I believe that the combination of these soft tissue and hard tissue techniques will allow the surgeon to obtain results that by other methods would be elusive. I have chosen to let the cases themselves carry most of the discussion, since I think plastic surgeons are more likely to believe documented results than words.

HISTORY

Horizontal osteotomy of the mandibular symphysis with advancement was first described in the German literature in World War II by Hofer [10], and subsequently by Trauner and Obwegeser [19] and Converse and Wood-Smith [5]. Because of the subsequent development of alloplastic substances for chin implantation [17], procedures that directly alter the bone of the chin have been used more often in major maxillofacial reconstruction and have not found a frequent use in aesthetic surgery.

ANATOMY

That portion of the face we know as the chin can be defined in terms of both overlying soft tissue and underlying osseous structures. With regard to the *soft tissue,* the chin extends superiorly to the labiomental fold (generally at the level of the lower labial sulcus) and inferiorly to the submental-cervical crease. Laterally, it blends into the skin of the cheek at a point below the oral commissure, along a line where jowl formation takes place because of the more

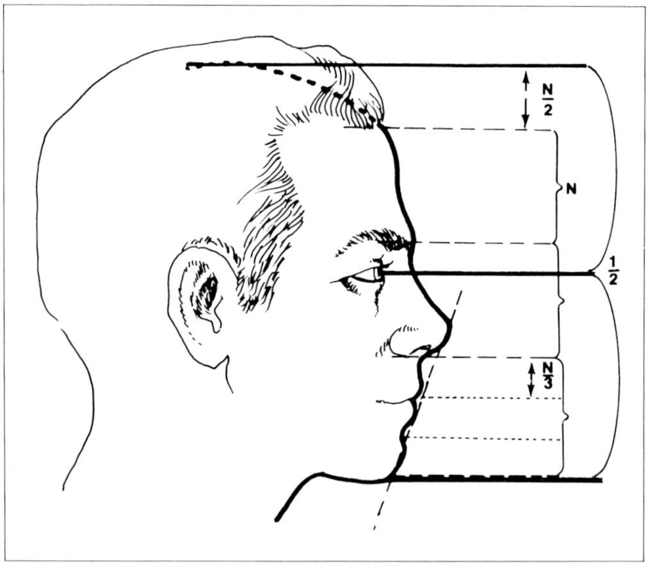

Figure 10-1. Schematic representation of the anatomic relationship of the chin.

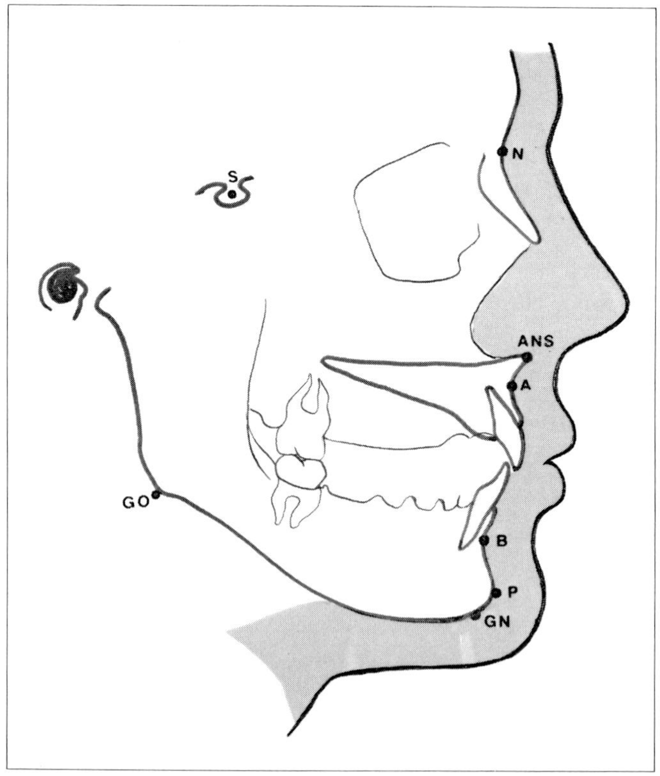

Figure 10-2. Hard tissues of the facial skeleton. S = sella; N = nasion; ANS = anterior nasal spine; P = pogonion; GN = gnathion; GO = gonion.

rapid drooping of the cheek skin, which is unattached to underlying bone.

Since the time of da Vinci and Dürer, artists have appreciated a number of harmonious and pleasing relationships of the chin to other portions of the face. These relationships derive from the study of Caucasian faces and do not necessarily hold true for blacks or Orientals. As noted in Figure 10-1, one-third of the vertical dimension of the face is occupied by the area from the base of the columella to the bottom of the chin. The upper lip occupies one-third of this area, and the lower lip and chin, two-thirds. On lateral profile with the head in the Frankfort horizontal, the convexity of the chin is found at about the same anteroposterior projection as the convexity of the glabella, and the chin point should touch or extend beyond the projection on a line drawn from the tip of the nose to the lower lip [15].

Muscles of the chin include the transverse fibers of the orbicularis oris superiorly, the vertically oriented mentalis, quadratus labii inferioris, and triangularis, as well as some fibers from the platysma that extend up over the symphysis. All of these are innervated by branches of the facial nerve.

Sensory nerve supply comes through the continuation of the inferior alveolar nerve exiting through the mental foramen and becoming the mental nerve. The mental foramen is located at the base of the second bicuspid or between the second bicuspid and the first molar. The foramen may vary in its position and in some cases may be double. In patients with severe developmental abnormalities of the mandible, such as lateral facial microsomia with absent temporomandibular joint, the mental foramen may not be present.

Hard tissue points on or near the chin used by orthodontists in facial skeletal cephalometric analysis include those shown in Figure 10-2:

B, the deepest point on the outer portion of the mandibular alveolar process beneath the central incisor

Pogonion, the most anterior part of the convexity of the mandibular symphysis

Gnathion, the most inferior point on the contour of the chin

Gonion, the most anterior point on the convexity of the mandibular angle

PATHOPHYSIOLOGY AND CLASSIFICATION

Deviations from the ideal normal can occur in the (1) sagittal plane (excessive or inadequate anteroposterior projection), (2) vertical plane (excessive or inadequate height), and (3) transverse plane (deviation of the chin point to one side).

In patients with significant malocclusion due to mandibular retrognathia, adequate chin projection cannot be adequately obtained without mandibular advancement, and in patients with class III malocclusion and mandibular prognathism, adequate reduction of the chin cannot be properly performed unless the entire body of the mandible is moved back into a proper skeletal relationship with the maxilla. It is not the purpose of this chapter to describe in detail procedures that alter occlusion; the reader is referred to existing textbooks on maxillofacial surgery [1, 2].

CONSULTATION

Although some patients will cite their chin as the chief complaint, others who do not look at themselves in profile may not be aware of a deficient chin. This is certainly the case for patients requesting rhinoplasty, and to a lesser extent for patients asking about a face-lift.

This is one of the few areas in plastic surgery where one may ethically suggest something to patients that they have not brought up themselves. The chin and nose are inextricably related, as are the chin and neck. I have never had a patient become offended by having the chin brought into the discussion.

I explain to the patient what I would propose for the chin and, if it is to be an adjunct to another procedure, why it could be expected to give a better overall result. I explain the pros and cons of implant versus osteotomy, mentioning the lack of a foreign body and greater resistance to infection, as well as the need for general anesthesia. It is worthwhile to mention that intermaxillary fixation is not required and the dental occlusion is not changed, since some patients may confuse a genioplasty with an osteotomy of the mandible to correct malocclusion.

I have not yet had a patient choose an implant over a genioplasty, but this fact may be misleading because I do not use chin implants and also because a number of patients may have chosen to go elsewhere for surgery (with a chin implant) after their initial consultation with me.

SURGICAL TECHNIQUES

Alternatives

For lesser degrees of retrogenia, either alloplastic chin implants or a chin advancement can be used. Both methods have their advantages and disadvantages. The term *chin advancement* seems the simplest way to describe the horizontal osteotomy of the mandibular symphysis with sliding advancement of the lower fragment. *Genioplasty* is a nondescript term that does not describe what plastic procedure is being done to the chin.

Chin Augmentation with Alloplastic Substances

The principal advantage of a silastic implant is that it can be placed under local anesthesia. The significant disadvantages are that it must be placed above the periosteal layer and therefore in the muscle, and it may shift position or cause a crinkling distortion of the chin on smiling (Fig. 10-3). Sometimes the edges of the implant can be seen. If the implant is placed beneath the periosteum, erosion into the underlying mandible may occur [7, 16] and may threaten the roots of the underlying teeth (Fig. 10-4). There is a higher rate of infection, which can occur years after the implant has been placed if there is adjacent dental or other type of infection, or minor trauma [11].

Figure 10-3
A, B. On smiling, a distortion of the chin is evident, caused by a violation of the muscle layer of the chin.

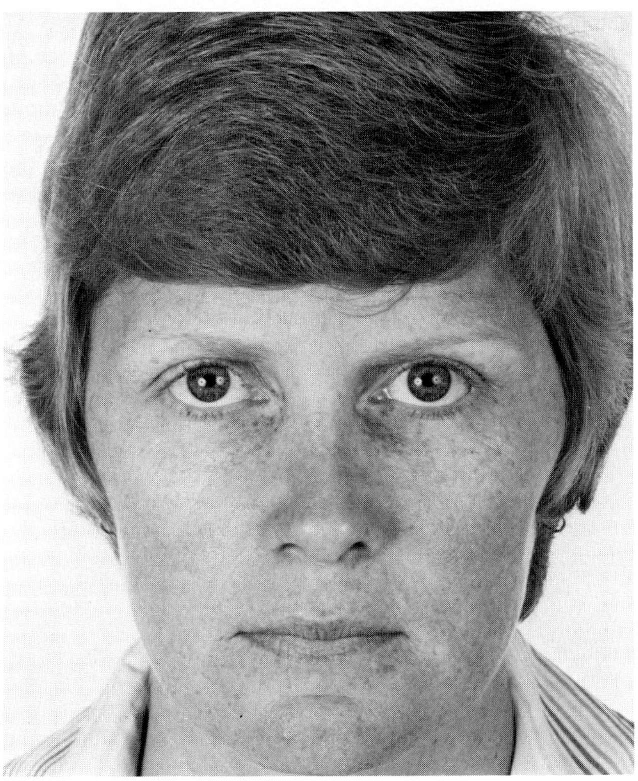

A

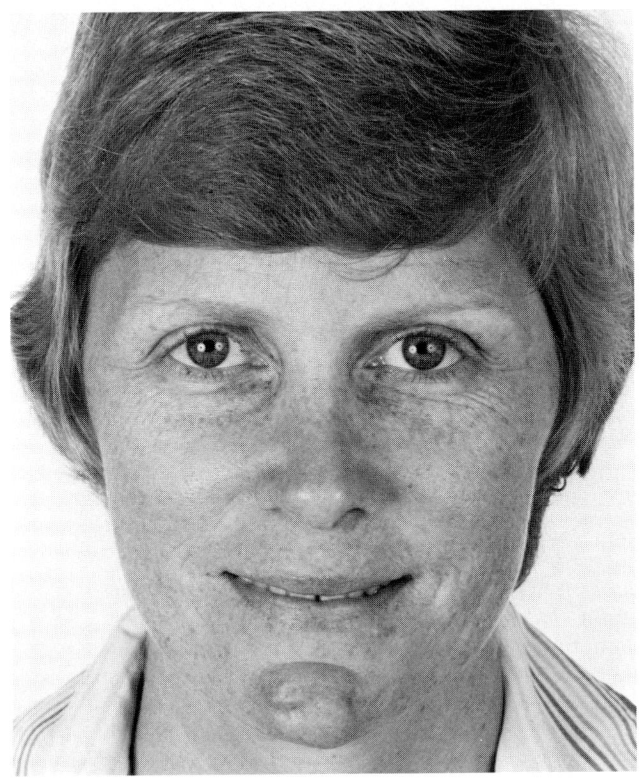

B

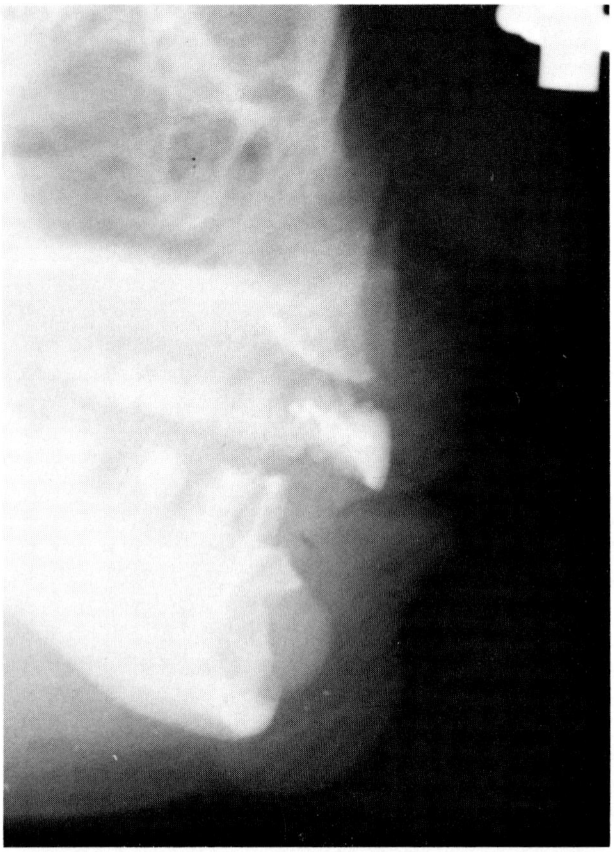

Figure 10-4. Erosion of a silastic chin implant 8 mm into the mandibular symphysis, with a threat to the underlying canine roots.

Chin Advancement

The advantage is that since no foreign body is used, resistance to infection is greater than with alloplastic substances, particularly when the blood supply of the lower symphysial fragment is maintained. In all of the procedures that will be described, care is taken to maintain at least a portion of the attachment of the genioglossus, geniohyoid, and anterior bellies of the digastric muscle that attach to the inferior border of the lower fragment. Besides providing blood supply and making this a bone-muscle "flap" rather than a free bone graft, such management ensures that an anterior pull on the lower fragment will be transmitted to these muscles, which seems to help in the correction of the slack neck in the same way as does the posterior pull on the platysma and superficial fascia (SMAS). The effect of chin advancement on the neck is shown in Figures 10-5, 10-6, and 10-7.

The procedure is performed in the subperiosteal plane; therefore there should be no disturbance of the overlying musculature. A solid osteosynthesis, once healed, will not shift. Certain patients, because of the configuration of their mandible, will not get a good result from a chin implant (Fig. 10-8).

The primary disadvantage is that general anesthesia is required in most cases. The procedure can be performed with adequate control of pain with bilateral inferior alveolar nerve blocks and blocks of the mental nerves, but the difficulty here may be more in controlling the airway than in controlling pain (Fig. 10-9). Power equipment is required and a hospital setting. The question of resorption of the advanced fragment will be discussed later.

In one category of patients, those with a mild degree of retrogenia, either a chin implant or a chin advancement if properly performed will give equally good results. Both procedures, improperly performed, will give a bad result, and a bad result from badly performed chin advancement will be more difficult to correct than a bad result from a poorly performed chin implant.

More pronounced degrees of retrogenia or macrogenia, and all deformities in the vertical or transverse plane, are correctable only by osteotomies of the chin.

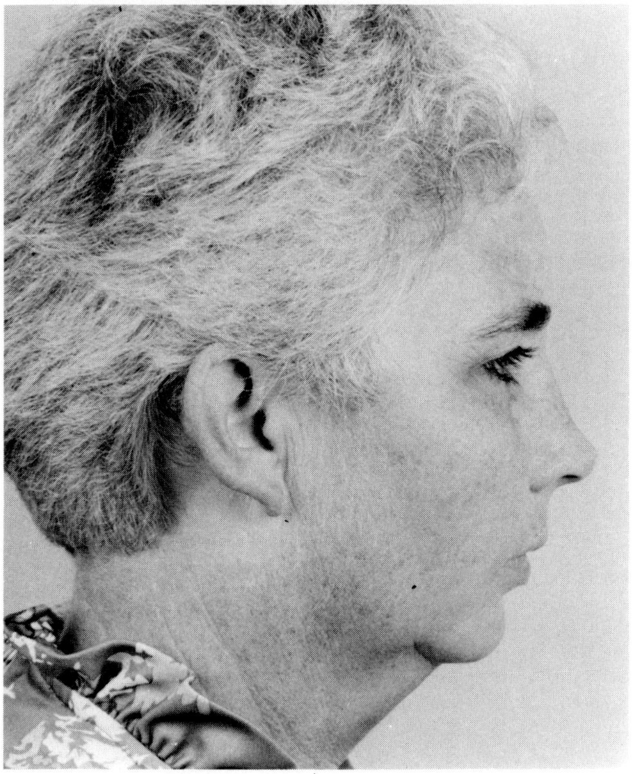

A

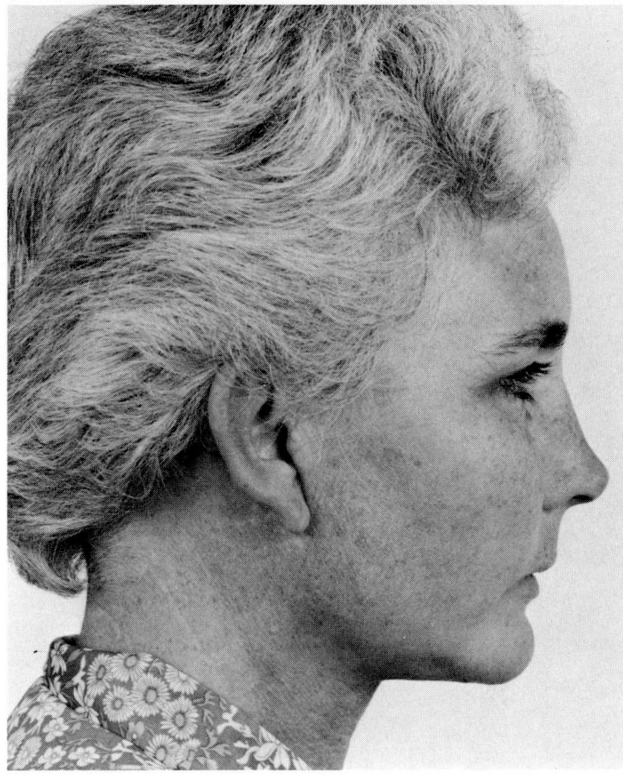

B

Figure 10-5

A–C. Before and after meloplasty, submental lipectomy, and chin advancement (performed at same sitting). No weight loss on the part of the patient. The improvement in the neck line is due to removal of fat and skin, posterior pull on the SMAS, and anterior pull on the muscles attached to the lower symphysial fragment. (From S. A. Wolfe, Chin advancement as an aid in correction of deformities of the mental and submental regions. *Plast. Reconstr. Surg.* 67:624, 1981.)

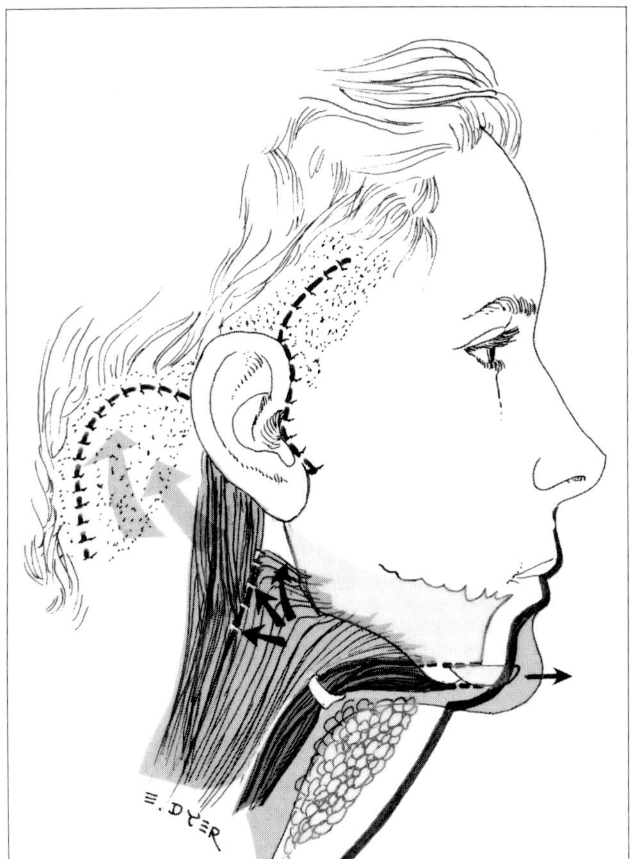

C

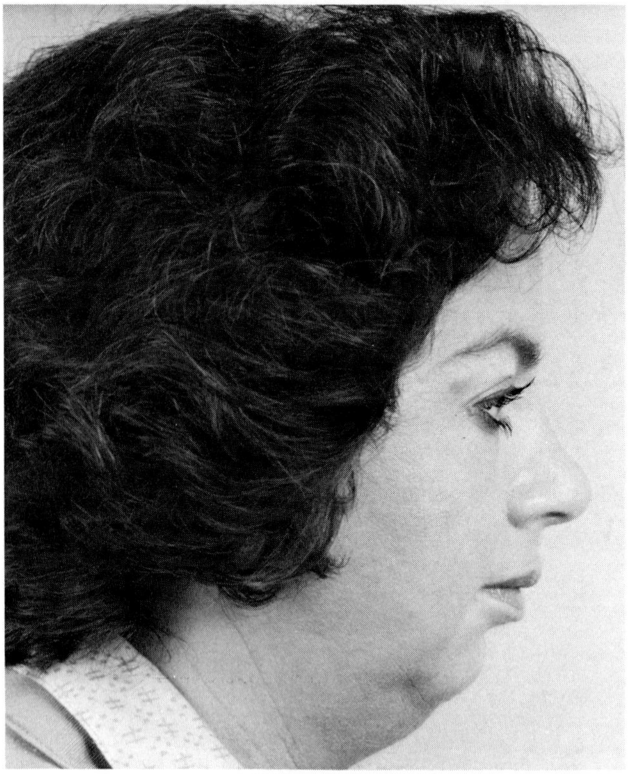

A

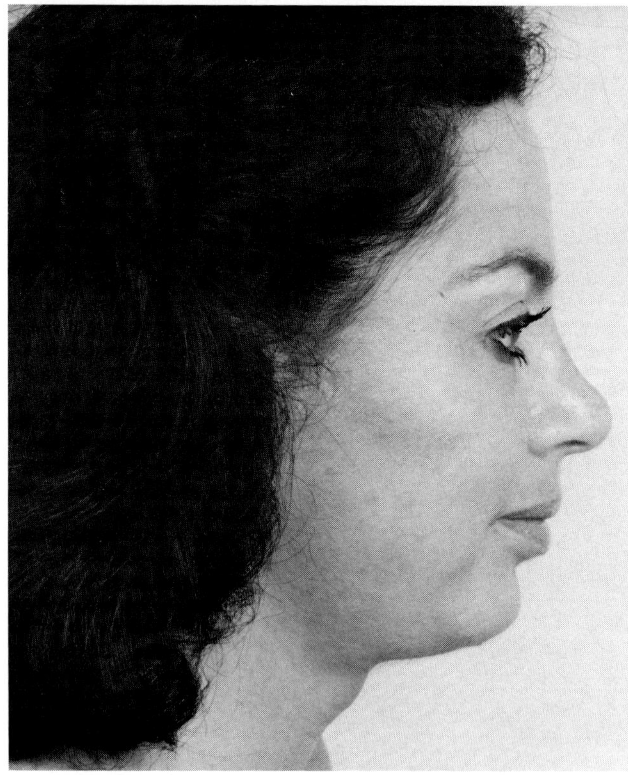

B

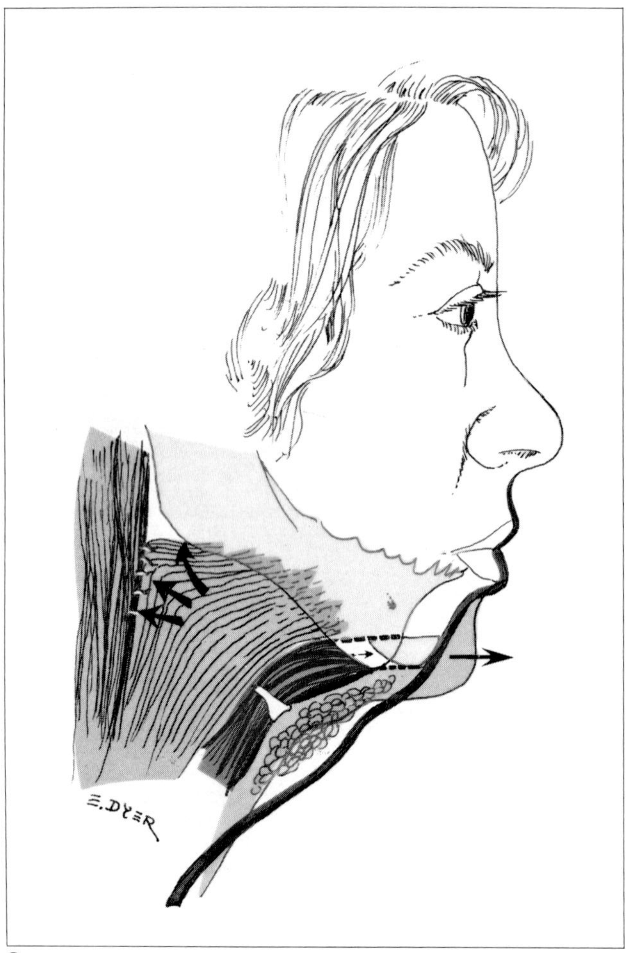

C

Figure 10-6
A–C. This patient had an identical procedure to that of the patient in Figure 10-5 and is of similar weight and age. The result differs because of the more anterior and inferior position of the hyoid, which is the limiting factor.

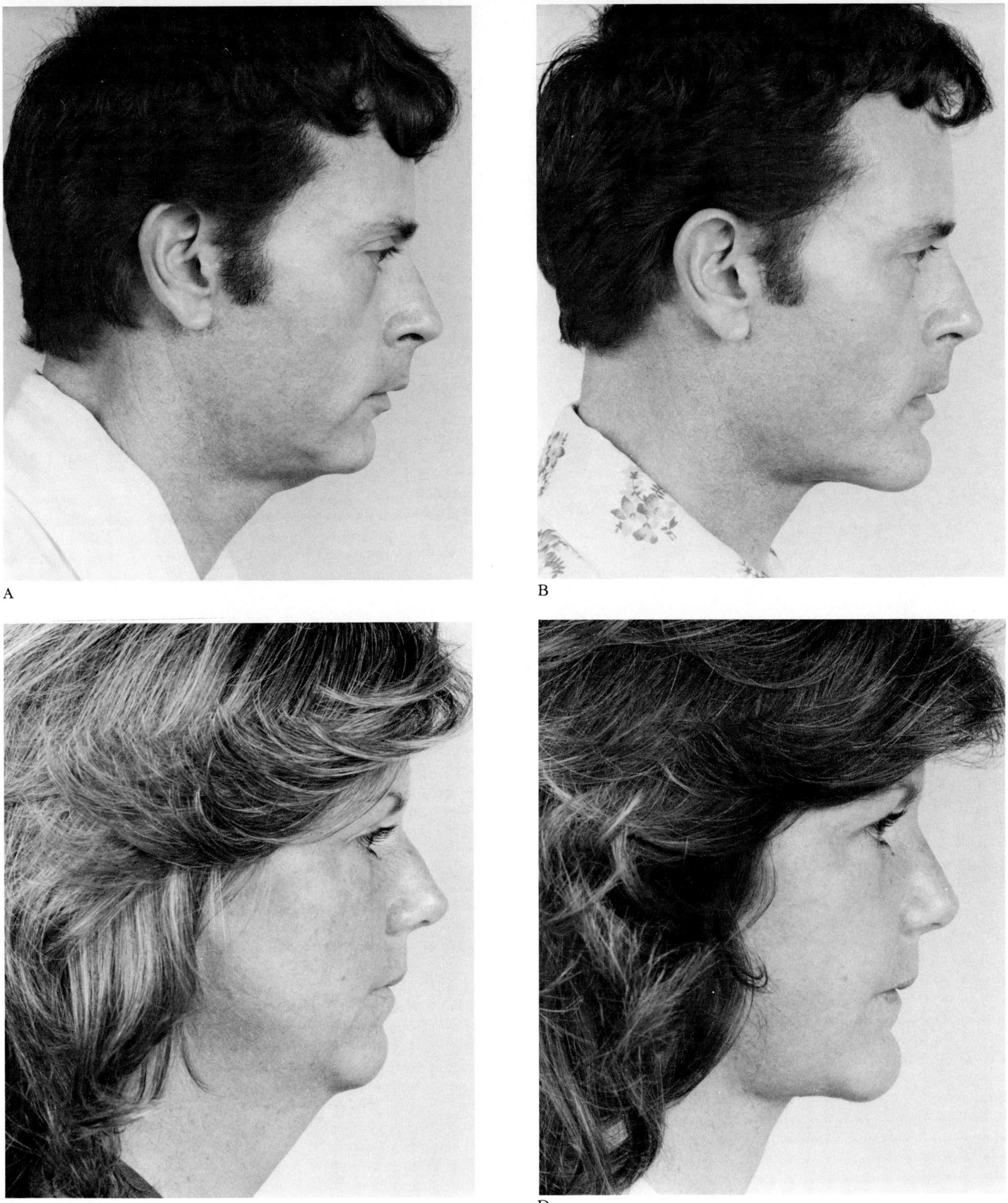

A B C D

Figure 10-7. The range of application for chin advancement.

A, B. This patient has only a chin advancement without any further intervention in the submental region, showing the very definite effect of the anterior pull on the lower symphysial fragment with attached musculature.

C, D. This 24-year-old patient was of normal weight and was unhappy about her "flabby" neck. Chin advancement, meloplasty, and submental lipectomy gave an improved neck line and a slightly heavy chin.

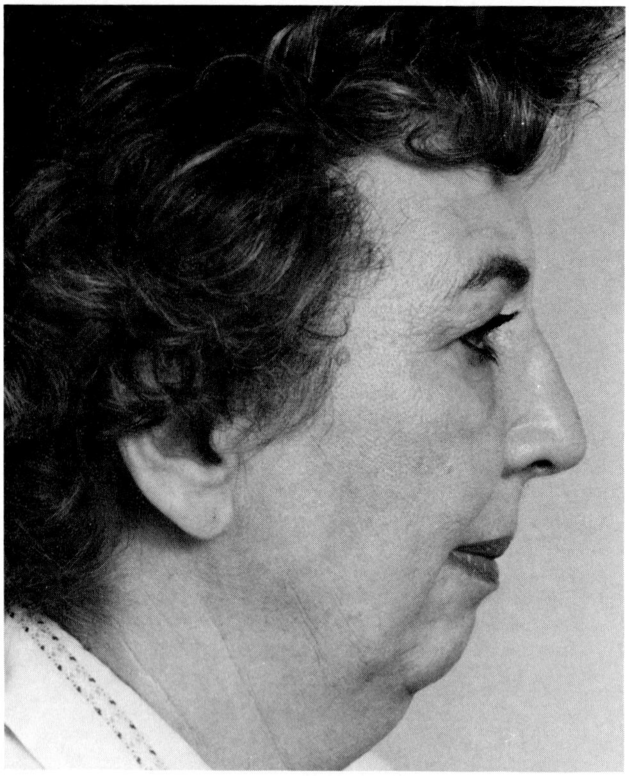

E

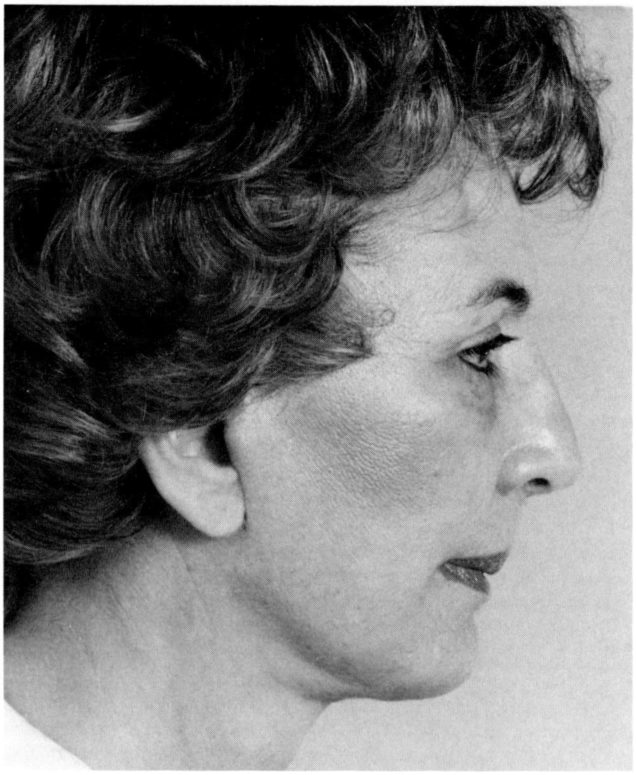

F

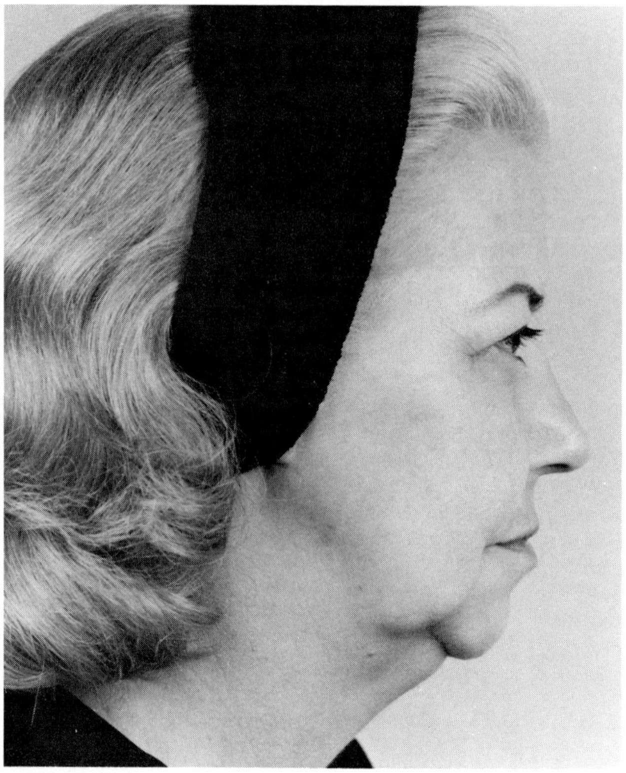

G

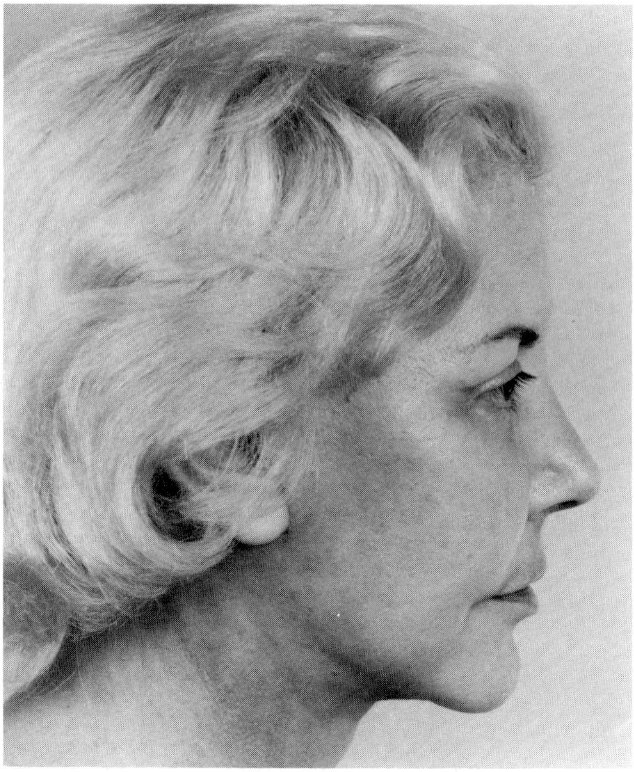

H

Figure 10-7 (continued)

E, F. After a chin advancement, meloplasty, and submental lipectomy this patient had a considerable improvement in her neck line, but postoperatively the submandibular glands were noticeable. These glands when prominent can be removed through the meloplasty incision, although it is not an easy procedure.

G, H. The combination of meloplasty, submental lipectomy, and chin advancement give a good result even in the patient with an edentulous mandible. Although a mandible without teeth loses much of its vertical height, there is less loss in the anteroposterior dimension and ample bone remains for the advancement.

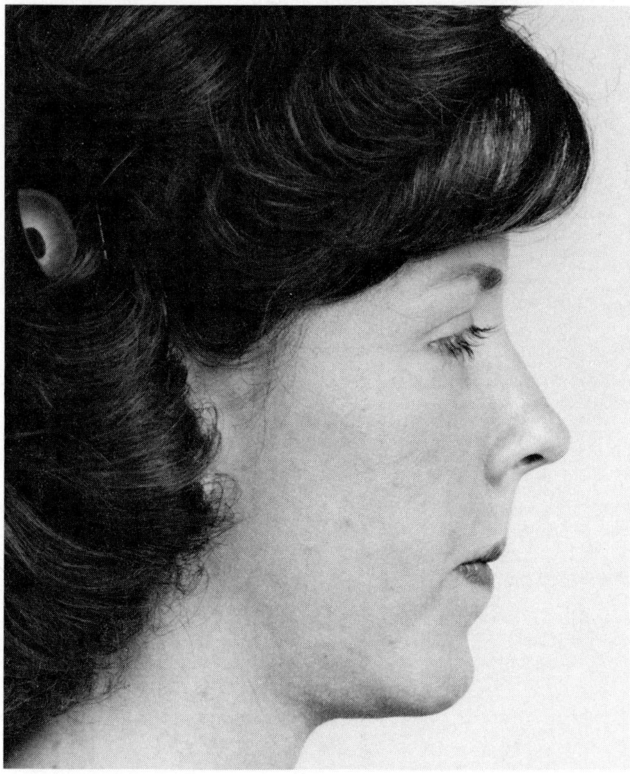

A

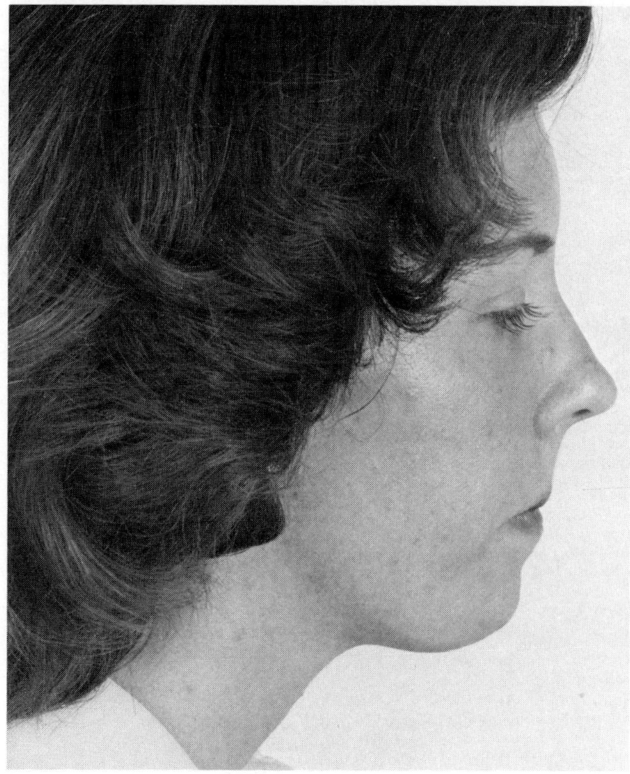

B

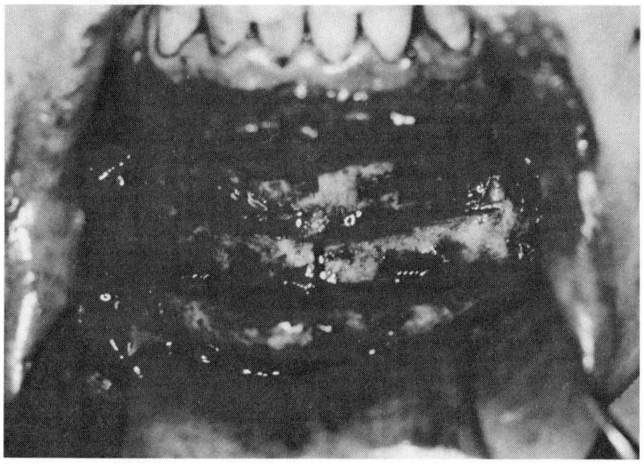

C

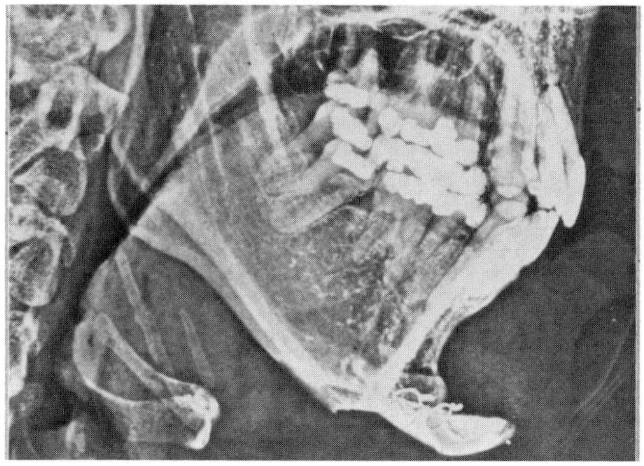

D

Figure 10-8

A. This patient is shown preoperatively with her third chin implant, of Proplast, which did not please her. The two previous attempts used silastic. The basic problem was not in the material used but in the configuration of her mandible, which did not permit an implant to be placed over the lower border of the symphysis.

B. Result that finally pleased the patient.

C. The Proplast was removed (the operative photo shows 5 to 6 mm of resorption beneath the position of the Proplast just above the advancement fragment; the right mental nerve is evident) and the lower border of the symphysis advanced.

D. X-ray film shows the degree of advancement—about 10 mm.

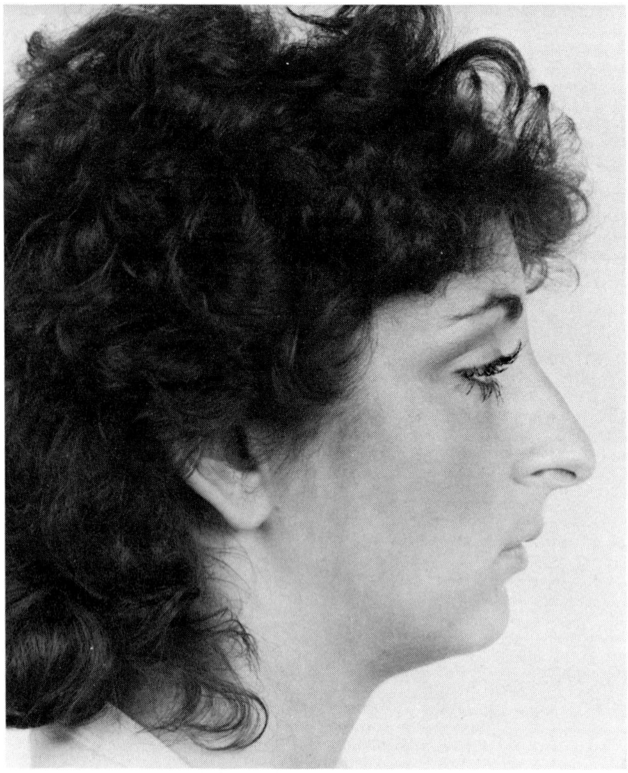

A

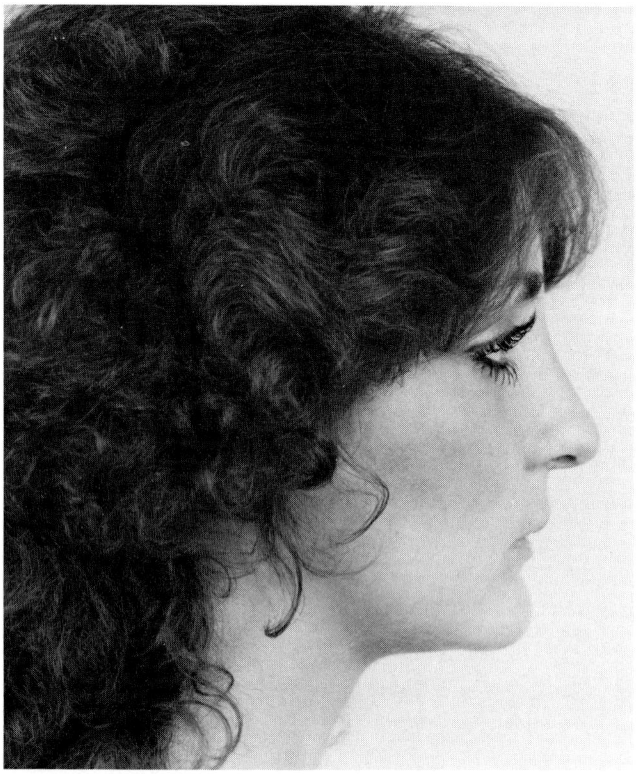

B

Figure 10-9

A, B. This patient underwent rhinoplasty and chin advancement under local anesthesia, but general anesthesia is preferred for reasons mentioned in the text. (From S. A. Wolfe, Chin advancement as an aid in correction of deformities of the mental and submental regions. *Plast. Reconstr. Surg.* 67:624, 1981.)

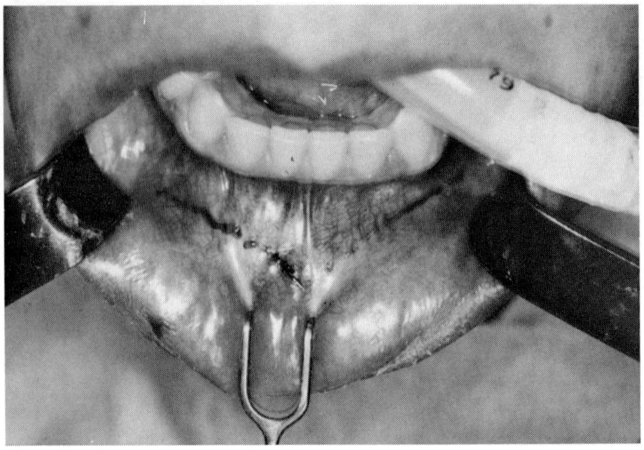

A

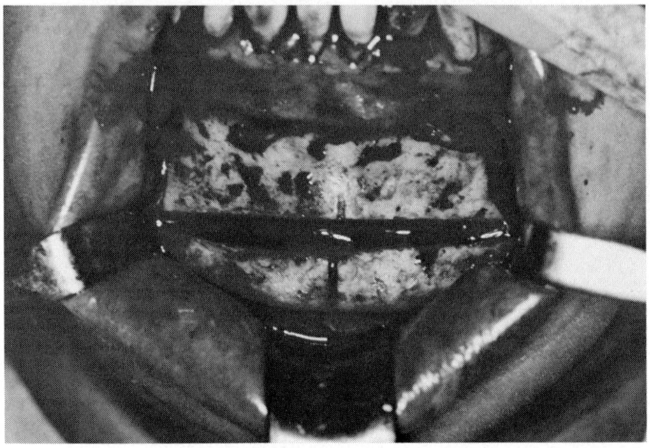

B

Figure 10-10

A. The incision is made well on the labial side of the lower labial sulcus, sparing the frenulum.

B, C. The midline is scored, and the osteotomy is made entirely with the oscillating and reciprocating saws.

D. Muscles attached to the posterior border of the advancement fragment. Bleeding can still be seen from the bone of the advancement fragment.

E, F. Passage of the four osteosynthesis wires.

G, H. After tightening of the wires and a rigid osteosynthesis.

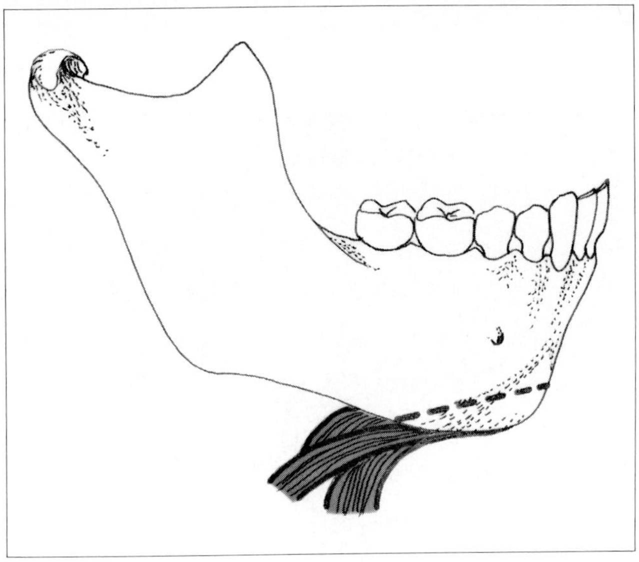
C

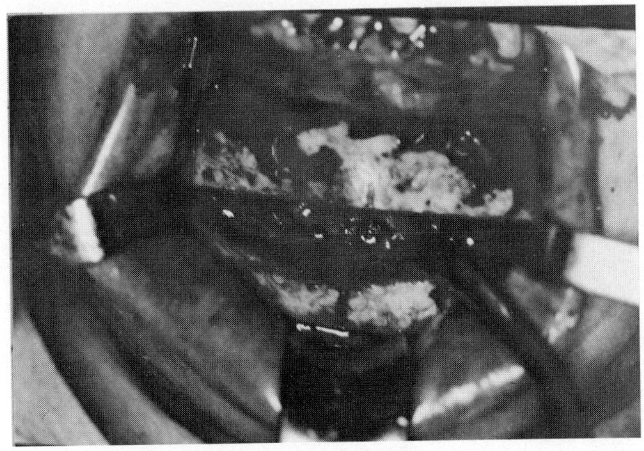
D

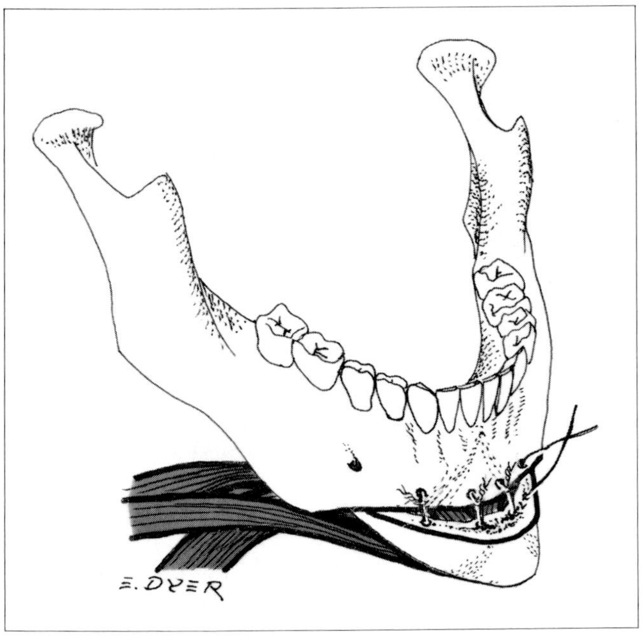

E

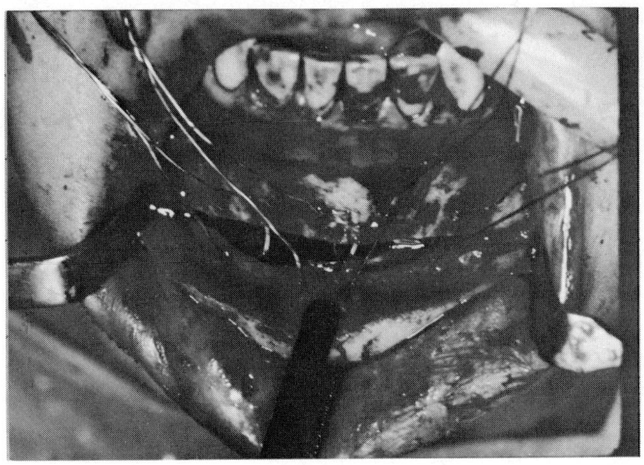
F

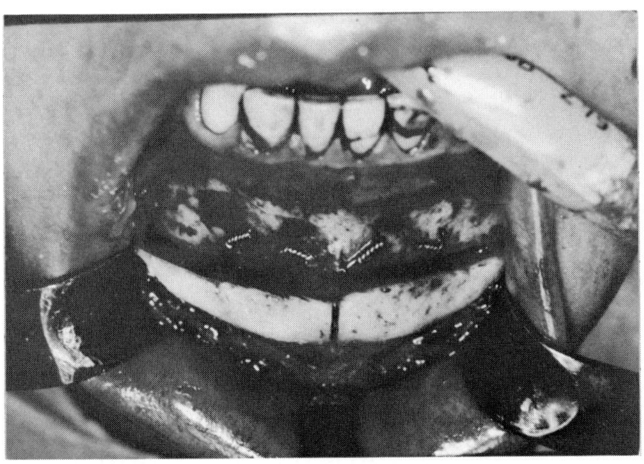
G

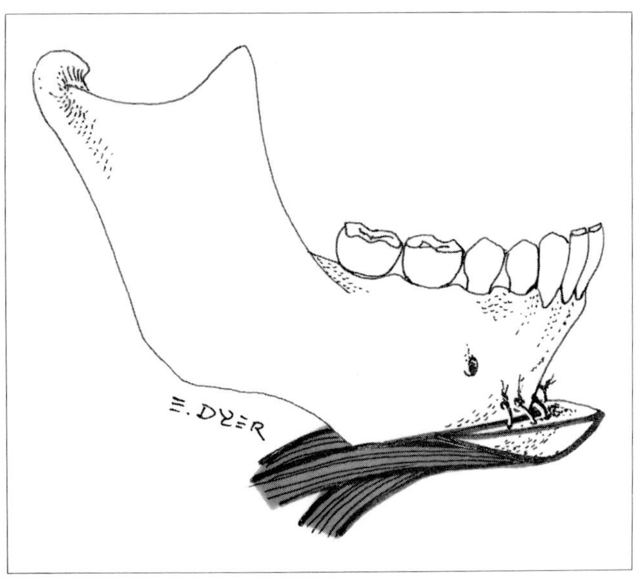

H

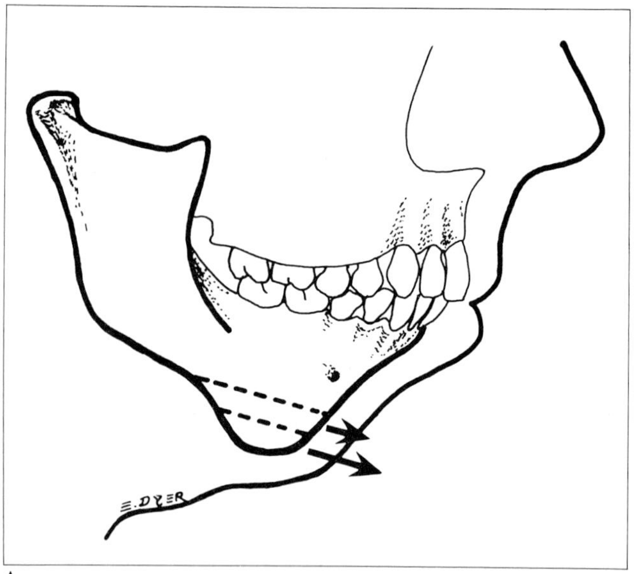

A

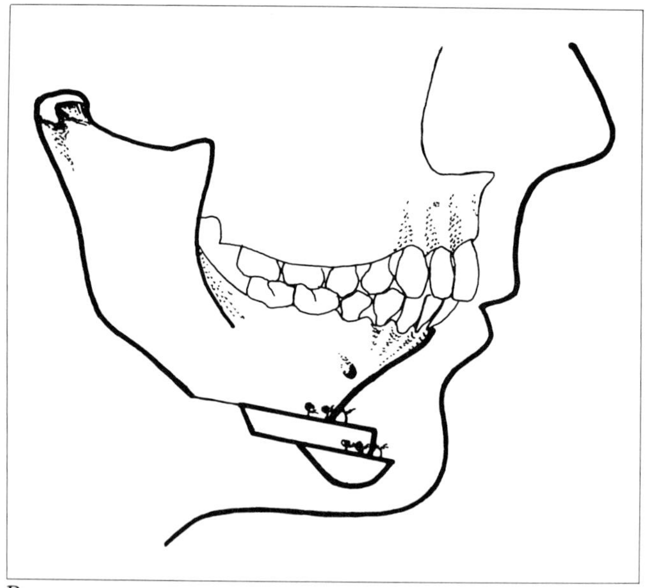

B

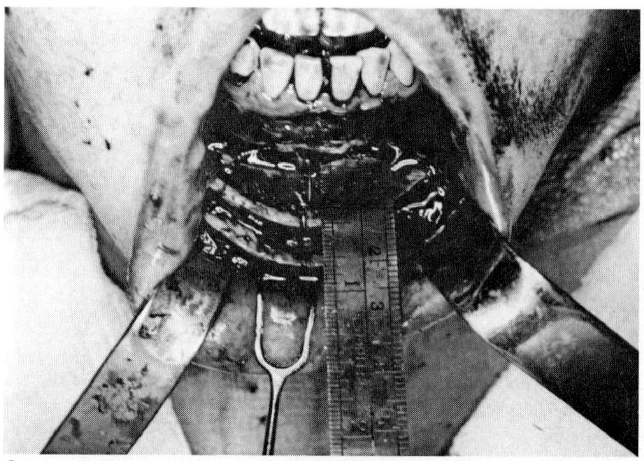

C

Figure 10-11
A–C. A two-tiered advancement, properly designed, can provide an increase in both the anteroposterior and vertical dimensions of the chin.

SAGITTAL ADVANCEMENT (MINOR)

Either oral or nasal intubation can be used. The procedure can be performed in conjunction with a rhinoplasty or meloplasty, or other procedure. A detailed description will be given of the chin advancement since this is the most commonly used procedure and the other procedures represent only minor variations on it.

Antibiotics (penicillin being the drug of choice) are given intraoperatively and for several days following the procedure. Infiltration of the lower labial sulcus is done with a 1:500,000 epinephrine-saline solution. The incision is made on the labial side of the lower labial sulcus, sparing the frenulum (Fig. 10-10A). Dissection is immediately taken to the subperiosteal plane, and a degloving of the mandibular symphysis is carried out, with visualization and preservation of the mental nerves. A vertical line is scored on the symphysis from the interincisive space downward to the lower border of the symphysis, and perpendicular to this the line for the transverse osteotomy is scored on the symphysis (Fig. 10-10B, C). Great care must be taken to establish that the latter is an *absolutely* horizontal line. The osteotomy is performed with either an oscillating or a reciprocating power saw (my preference is Aesculap). The cut should be even, straight, and carried completely through both cortical layers of the symphysis. The lateral portion of the osteotomy, beneath the mental foramen, is usually the hardest to perform; it is best to use a reciprocating saw, and the saw cut should be carried completely through the posterior border. If one attempts to do this portion of the osteotomy with an osteotome, the posterior border will generally fracture in such a way that advancement of the inferior fragment is impeded and the offending bone will need to be burred down. The lower fragment, when completely freed, is grasped with a bone-holding clamp and pulled forward against the still-attached muscles (Fig. 10-10D) until the desired degree of advancement is obtained—usually between 8 and 12 mm. Four interosseous wires (0.040 mm) are passed through the posterior cortex of the inferior fragment and the anterior cortex of the superior fragment (Fig. 10-10E, F). As the wires are tightened, a very rigid osteosynthesis should be obtained and no wiggling of the lower fragment should be possible (Fig. 10-10G, H). The advanced fragment can then be tailored as required with an acrylic bur. The incision is closed in two layers with chromic catgut. Drainage is generally not necessary; a lightly compressive dressing of ¼-in. paper tape is placed across the chin to keep the lip and chin in contact with the underlying bone. With properly functioning equipment, the procedure generally takes about 15 minutes.

SAGITTAL ADVANCEMENT (MODERATE)

If more advancement is required, a two-tiered advancement can be performed and more than 20 mm of advancement obtained (Figs. 10-11 and 10-12). If possible, muscular attachments should be maintained to both of the

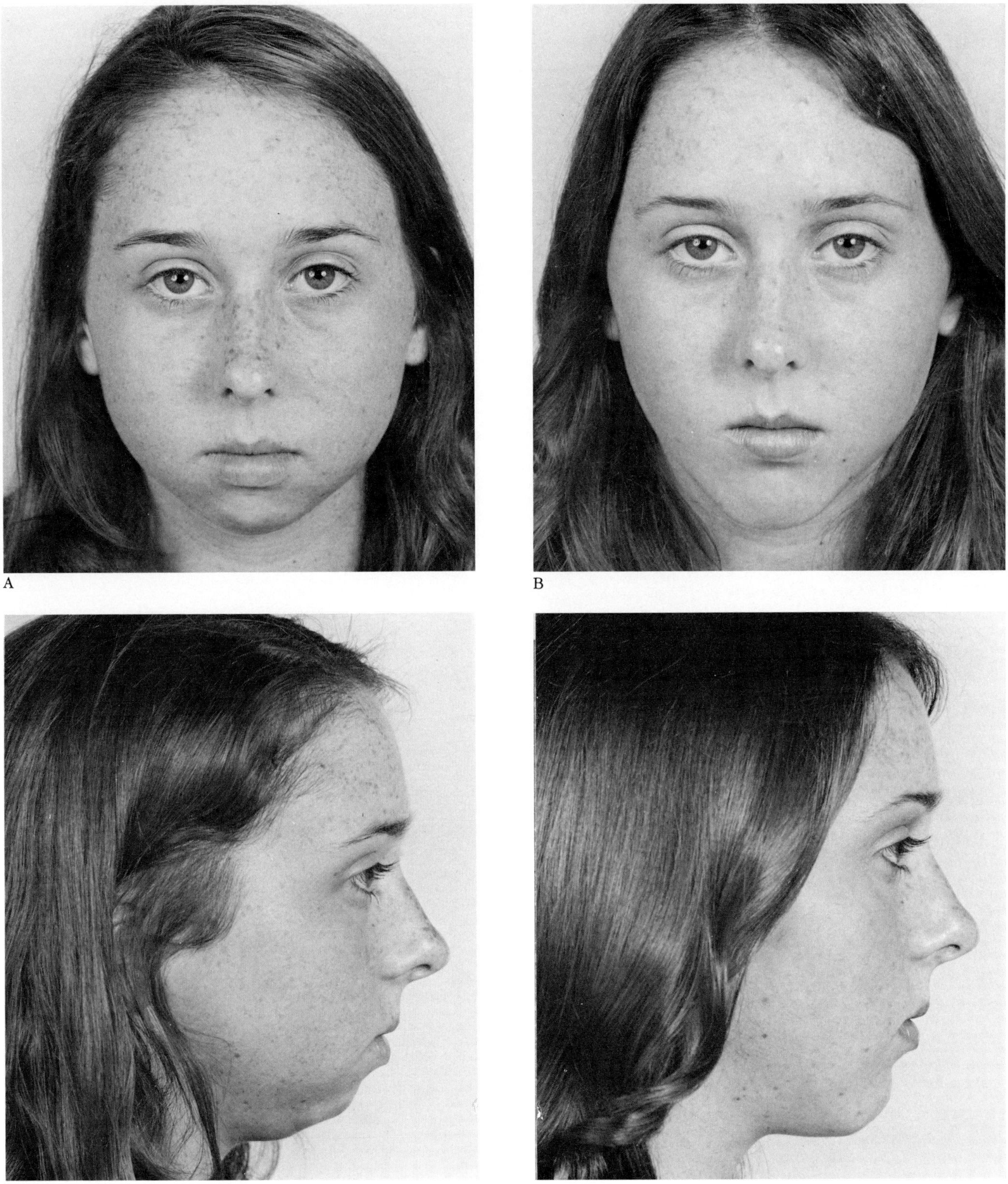

Figure 10-12
A–D. This patient had muscle attachments maintained to both fragments. She is shown 1½ years postoperatively. There had been about 50 percent resorption of the lower fragment and negligible change in the upper fragment. The overall result is nevertheless much more than could have been obtained with a chin implant.

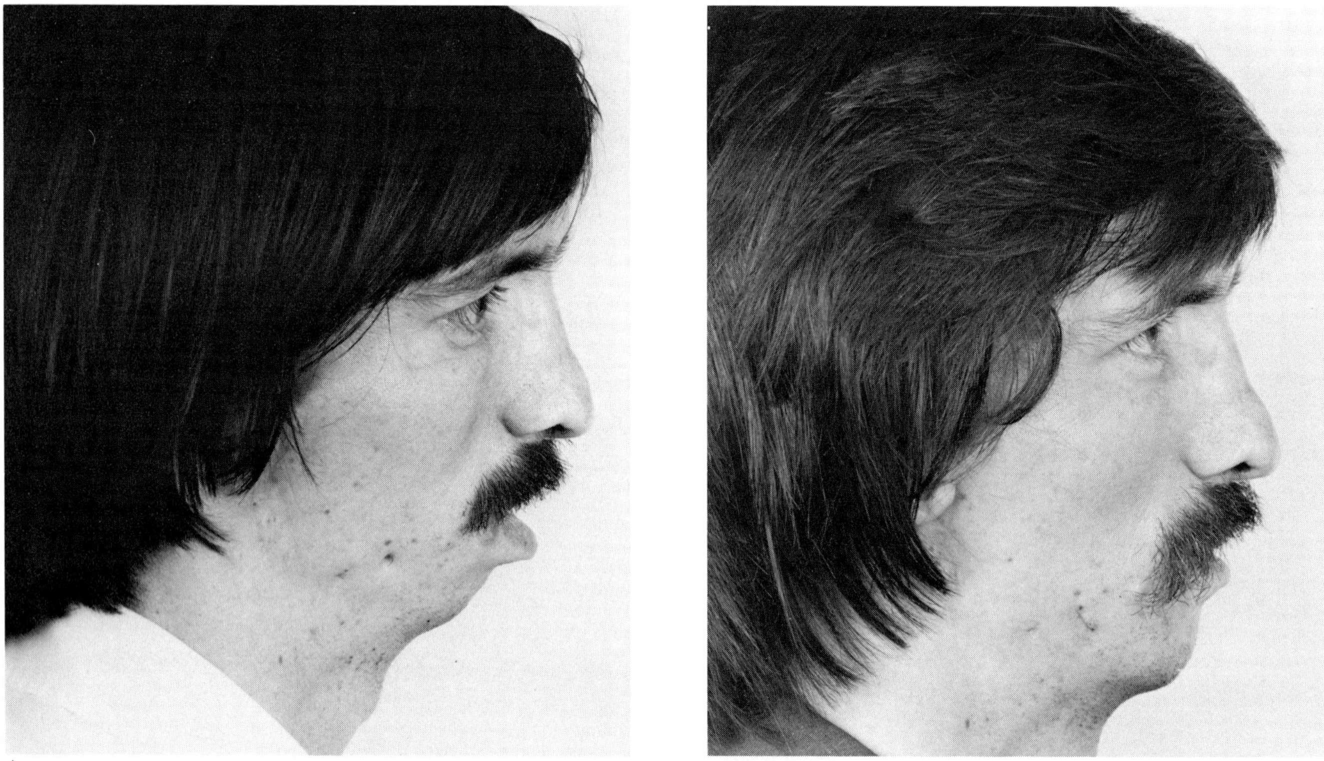

A B

advanced segments. A three-tiered osteotomy is possible in some cases, but I have not done this.

SAGITTAL ADVANCEMENT (MAXIMUM)
If a chin advancement has already been performed and more projection is still required, my preference is to use an autogenous costal cartilage graft on top of the previous chin advancement. Two pieces of cartilage are wired together for up to 15 to 20 mm of further projection. The pieces are tailored, and this cartilage sandwich is wired into place on top of the lower border of the symphysis (Fig. 10-13). Such a procedure is preferable in this scarred area to an alloplastic implant because of the greater resistance to infection, and free cartilage grafts to the chin seem to hold up well with time in contrast to free bone grafts.

Sagittal Reduction

Generally, sagittal reduction requires correction of an underlying mandibular prognathism and is thus beyond the scope of this chapter.

Vertical Shortening

If there is excessive vertical height of the chin but adequate projection, it is better to remove bone from above the lower osteotomy line and preserve the lower border with its attached musculature (Figs. 10-14 and 10-15). Removing excessive bone with a bur alone is likely to give a flat chin without an adequate labiomental crease, and a pouch of redundant skin may hang down underneath the chin in the submental area.

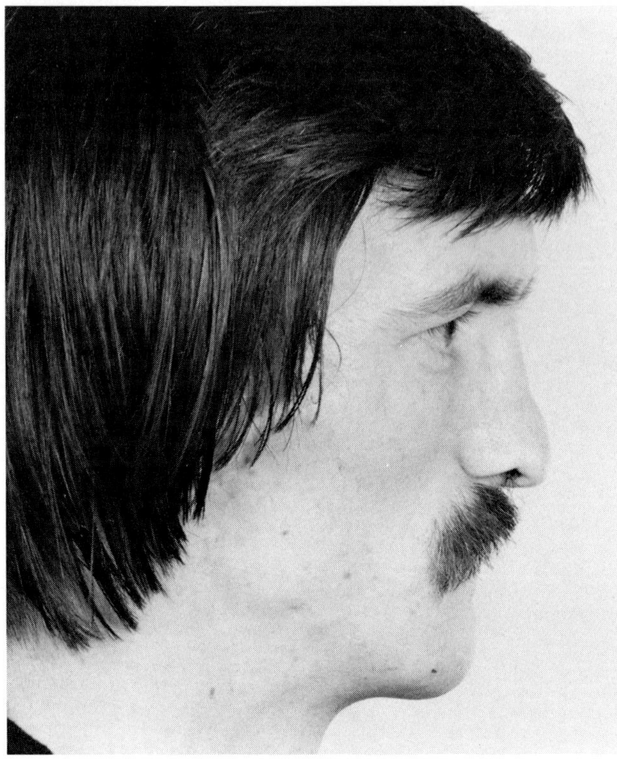

C

Figure 10-13
A–C. Patient with Treacher Collins–Franceschetti syndrome shown before and after a "jumping" chin advancement, which has both shortened and advanced the chin. The scars on the cheeks resulted from extrusion of silastic implants performed elsewhere.

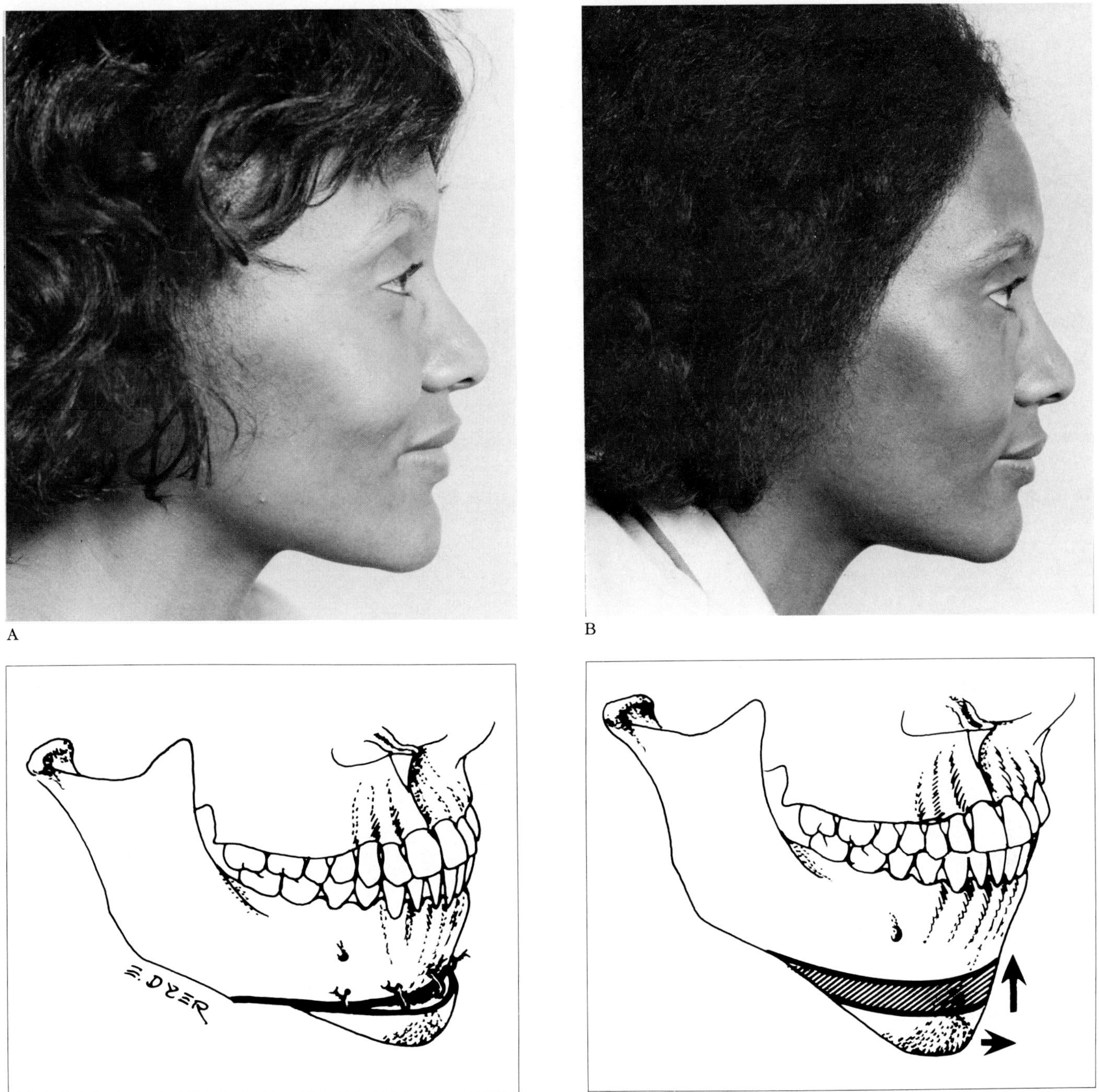

A B C D

Figure 10-14
A–D. Shortening of the vertical dimension of the chin is best performed by preserving the muscular attachments to the lower fragment and removing an appropriate strip of bone above this.

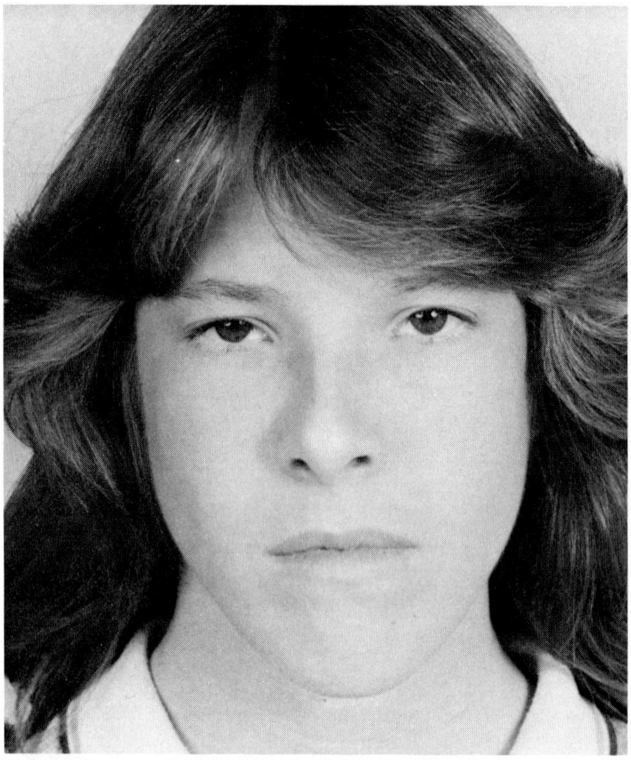
A

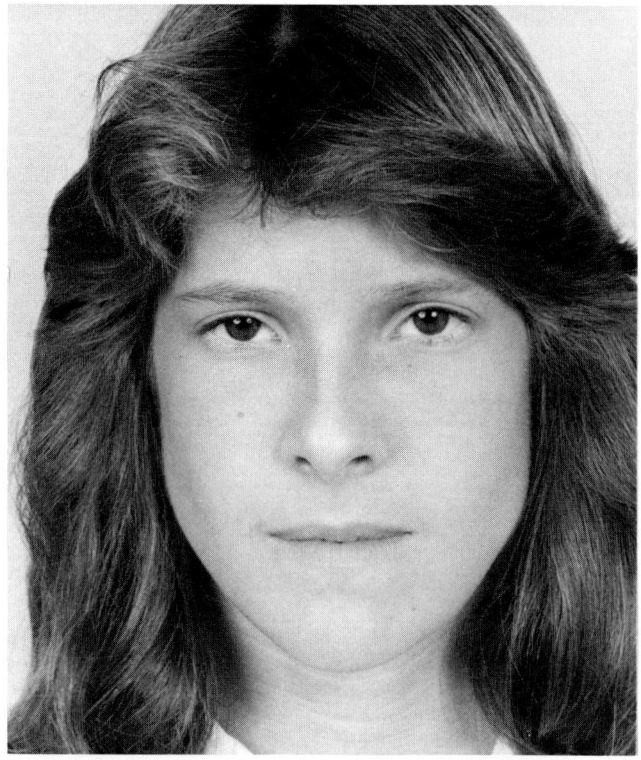
B

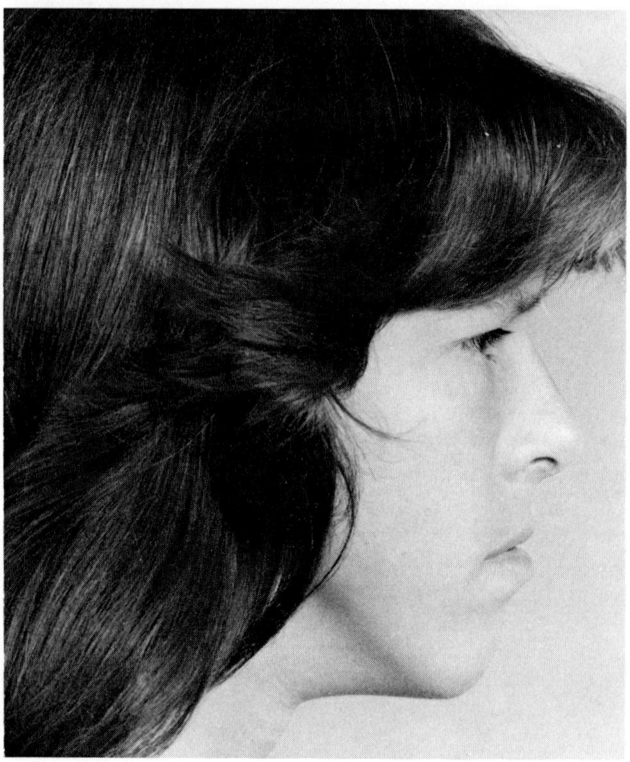
C

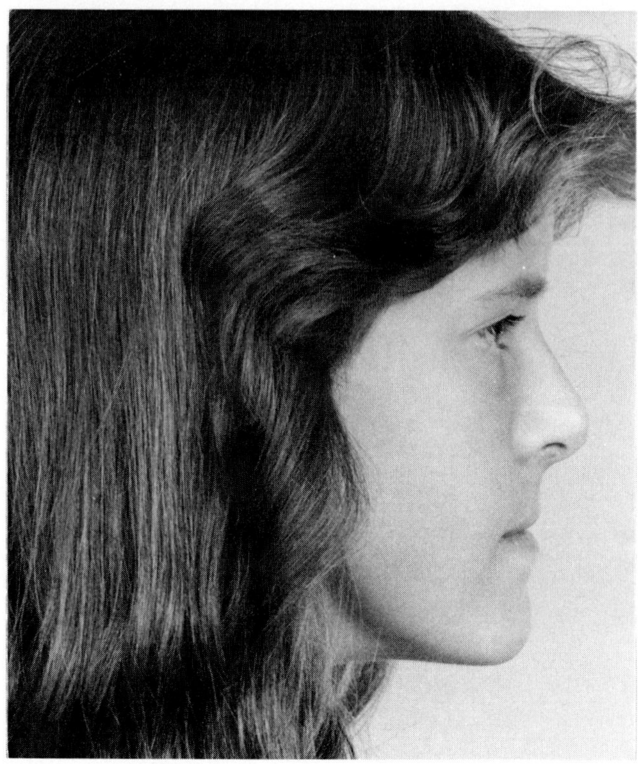
D

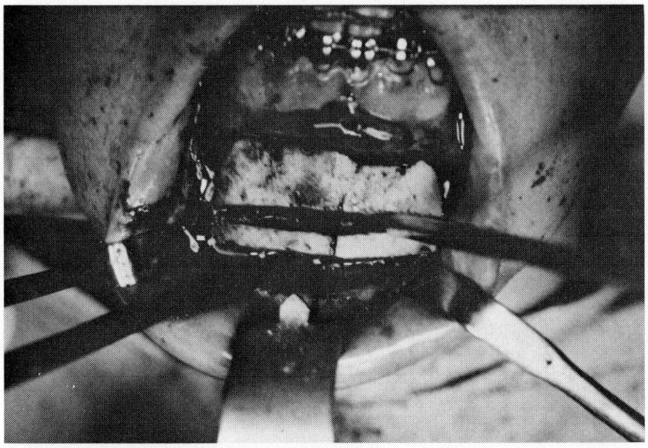

E

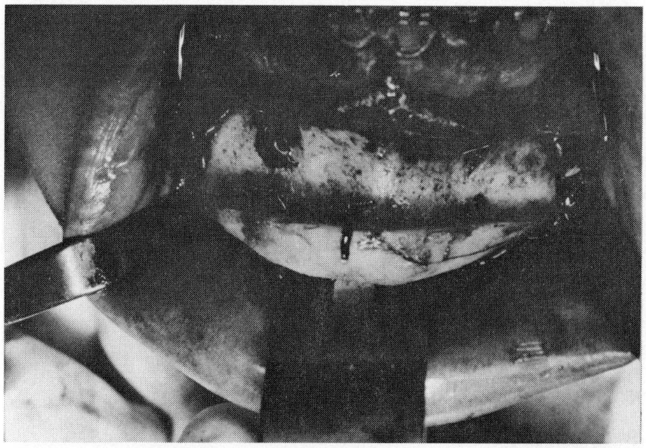

F

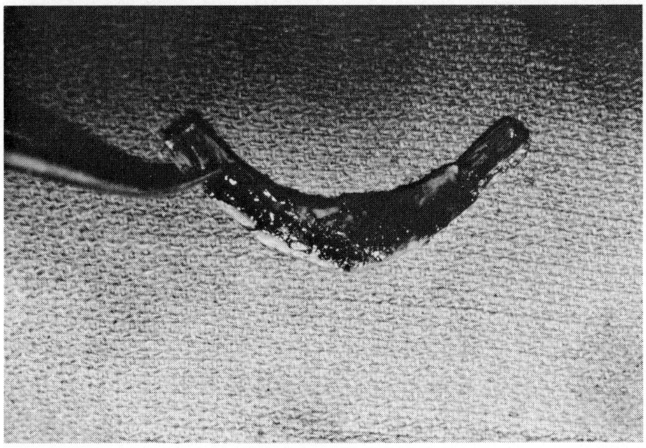

G

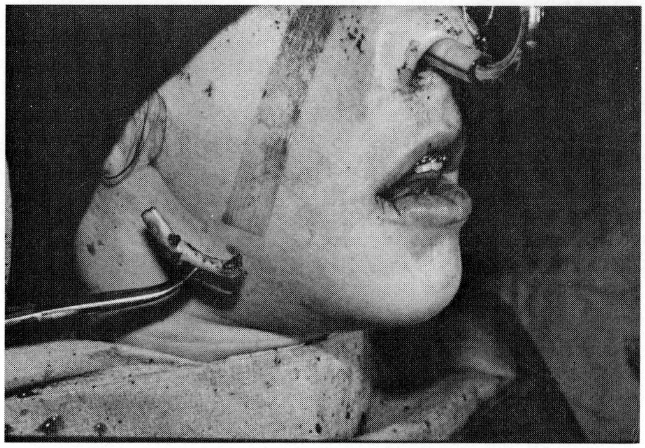

H

Figure 10-15
A–H. In this patient the chin was shortened vertically, the lower border fragment advanced and moved to the patient's right, and the strip of bone that was removed cut into two pieces and used as onlay bone grafts to help camouflage an obtuse gonial angle. This type of result would be impossible to obtain without a direct intervention on the bone.

Vertical Increase

A short chin can be lengthened with an interpositional bone graft by performing the same procedure in reverse (Fig. 10-16). An interpositional bone graft will hold up, whereas an onlay bone graft, in my experience, will not (Fig. 10-17).

Asymmetric Deformities

If asymmetry of the chin is present, a triangular portion of bone can be removed on one side and used as a bone graft on the other side, the central point of the chin being shifted to the desired position.

Combined Procedures

If one wishes to shorten the chin and at the same time provide more forward projection, the lower fragment is "jumped" up on top of the upper segment of the mandible and kept in place with wires, which are tightened from beneath. With this maneuver the chin is shortened by 8 to 10 mm and generally advanced 12 to 14 mm (Fig. 10-18).

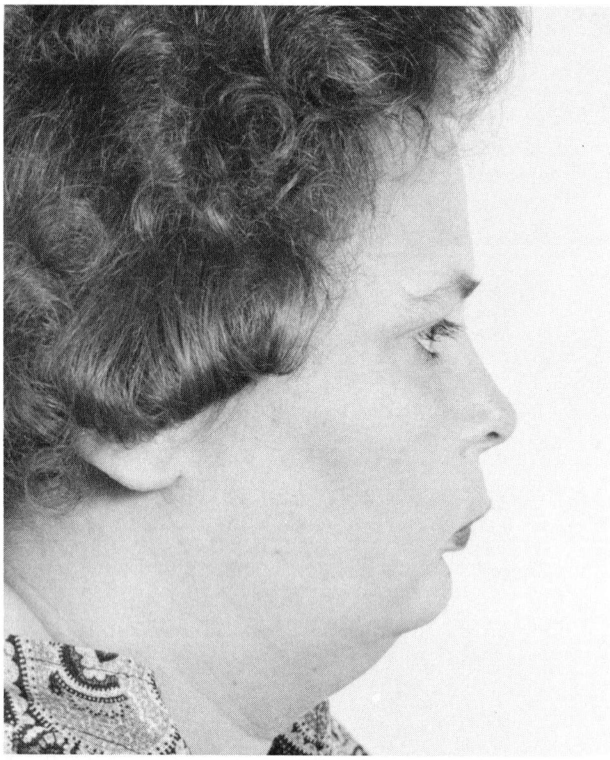

A

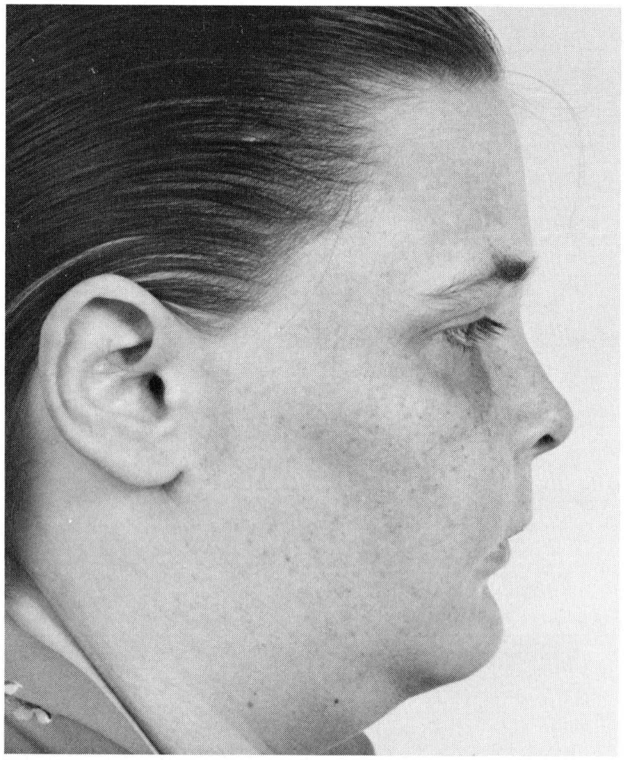

B

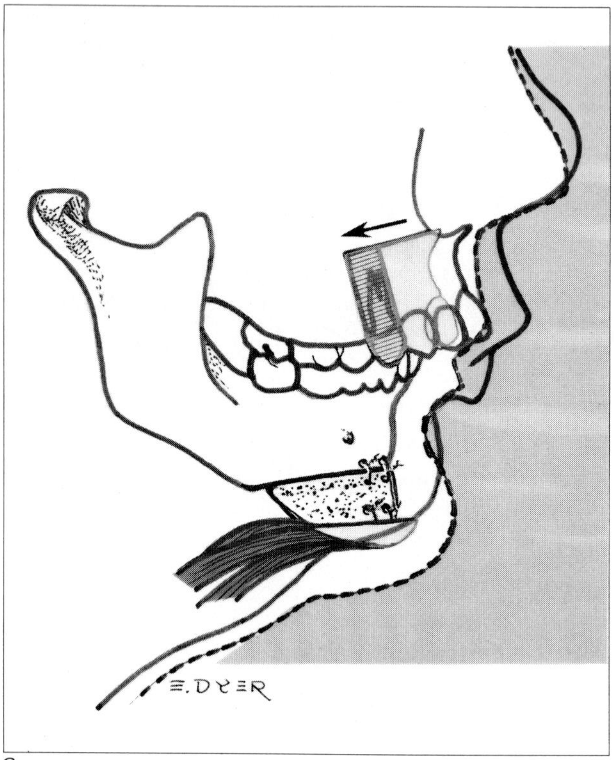

C

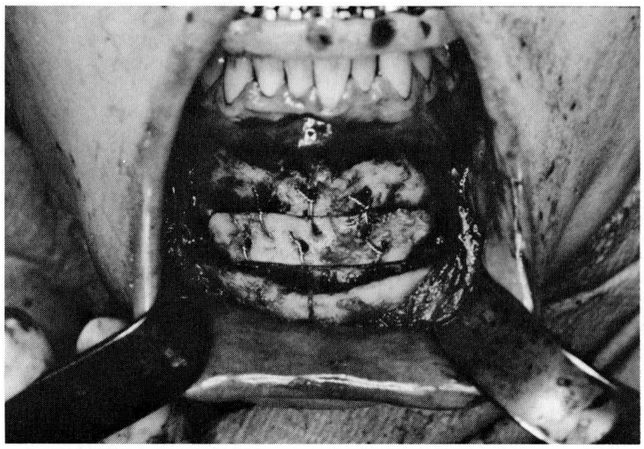

D

Figure 10-16

A–D. Before and after multiple maxillary osteotomies and extraction of three bicuspids performed in the downfractured position after Le Fort I osteotomy, as well as a downward and forward movement of the advancement fragment with an interpositional iliac bone graft. After adequate weight loss, the soft tissue deformity of the neck will be corrected.

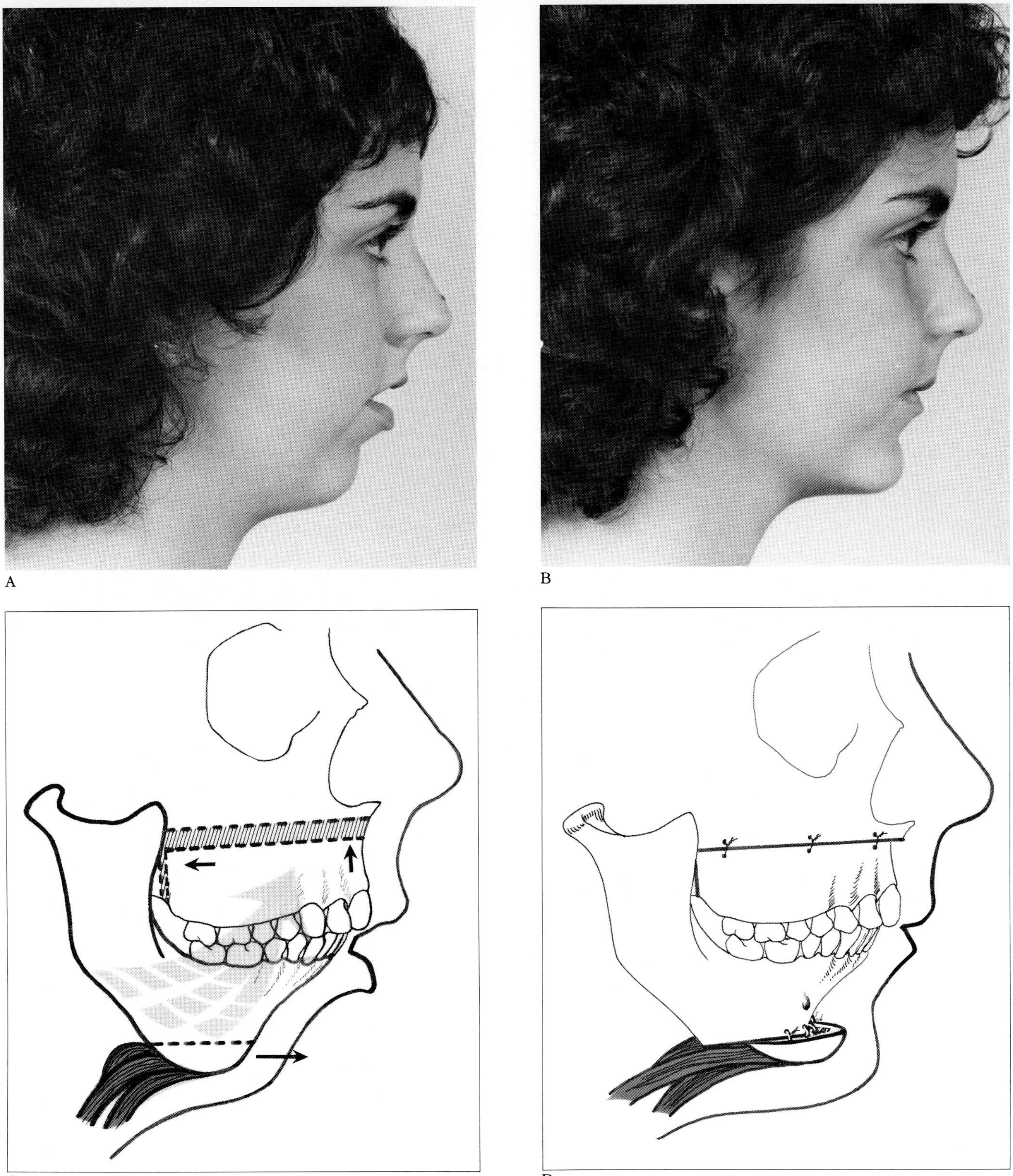

A B C D

Figure 10-17

A–D. In the long-face syndrome due to vertical maxillary excess, the upward movement of the maxilla permits autorotation of the mandible, which in itself brings the chinpoint forward. Chin advancement is generally performed as well, as in this patient, in whom occlusion (the relationship between the maxillary and mandibular teeth) was not changed, but the occlusal plane was raised relative to the cranial base.

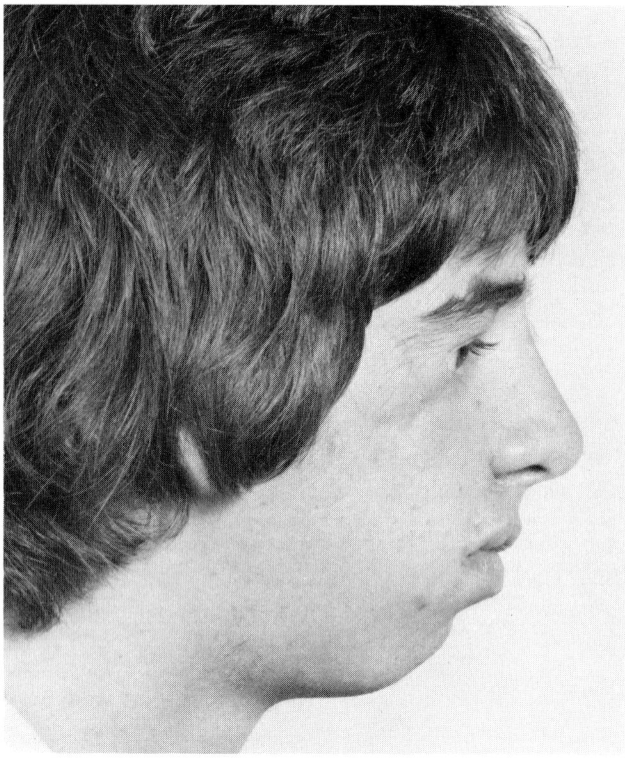

A

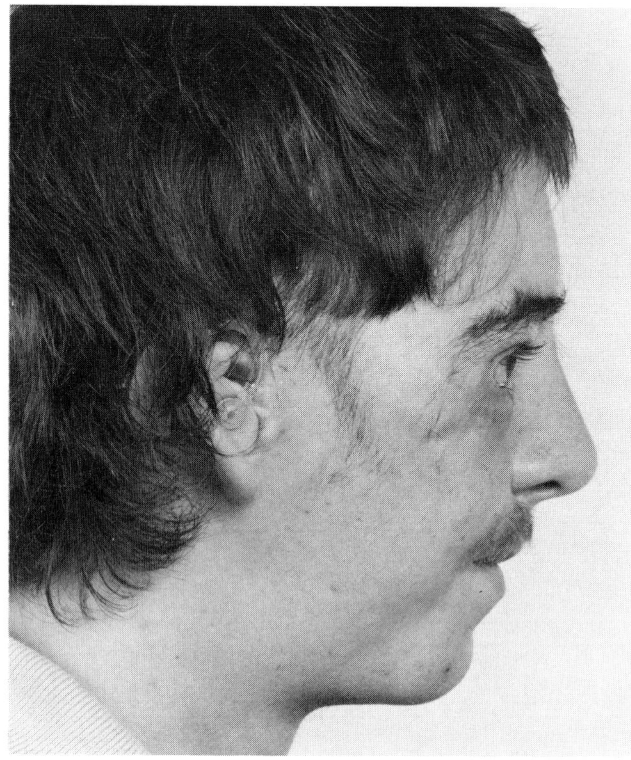

B

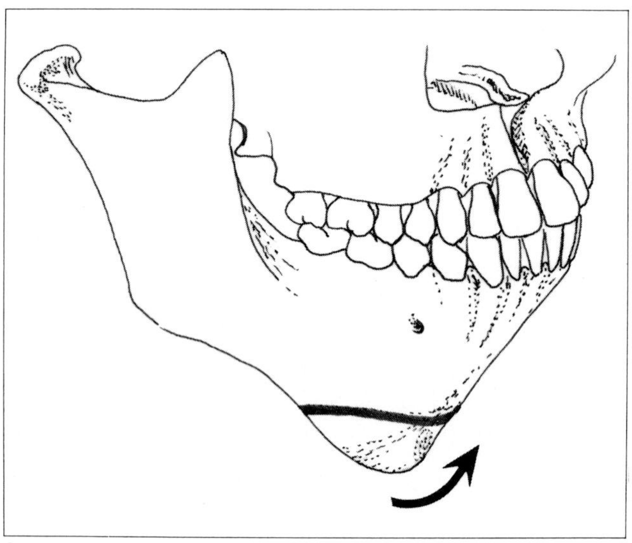

C

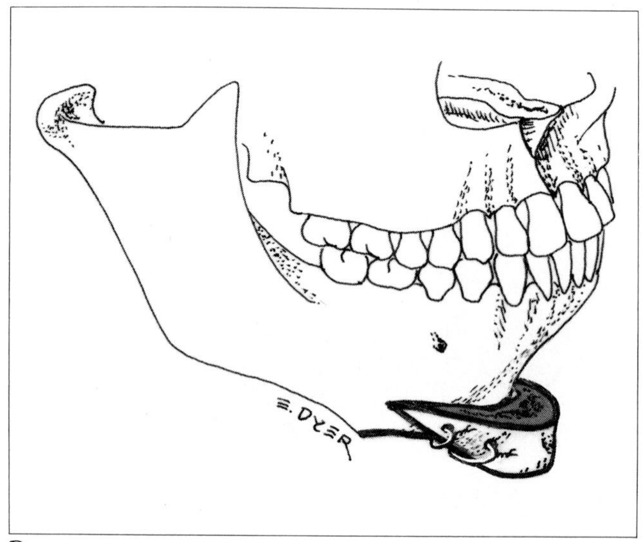

D

Figure 10-18
A–D. Patient with bilateral facial microsomia shown before and after chin advancement and finally after a costal cartilage graft performed over the chin advancement.

COMPLICATIONS

Chin Advancement

In 234 varied osteotomies of the chin, the following complications have been encountered [20].

1. Displacement of the lower-border of fragment requiring rewiring (one case) (long-face syndrome plus jumping genioplasty)
2. Suture line bleed on second postoperative day requiring a suture and compression as in the patient shown in Figure 10-8.
3. Excessive projection of chin requiring removal of a portion of the advanced fragment with a bur (Fig. 10-19)
4. Persistent pain after 1 year in central portion of chin (one case) (improved considerably after removal of all wires)

There have been no infections when only an osteotomy has been performed. One patient, who had an interpositional bone graft, developed a postoperative wound abscess, which cleared with antibiotics and drainage and eventual removal of wires without alteration of the shape of the chin.

There has been no permanent numbness of the lip, although most patients experience transient numbness and paresthesias in the lip for the first month or two.

Complications that have not been encountered but that are possible are the following:

1. Hematoma, requiring drainage
2. Fracture of the mandible if one attempts to perform a significant portion of the procedure with an osteotome
3. Avulsion of the mental nerve with permanent numbness of the lip
4. Damage to the roots of the teeth if the osteotomy is performed above the level of the mental foramina, or if the secondary dentition has not completely erupted

Resorption represents perhaps the greatest theoretic objection to chin advancement. As mentioned above, my limited experience with free iliac bone grafts to augment the chin has shown significant resorption in time ranging from 75 to 100 percent. For this reason, if a free graft is required, I prefer costal cartilage, which seems to hold up much better.

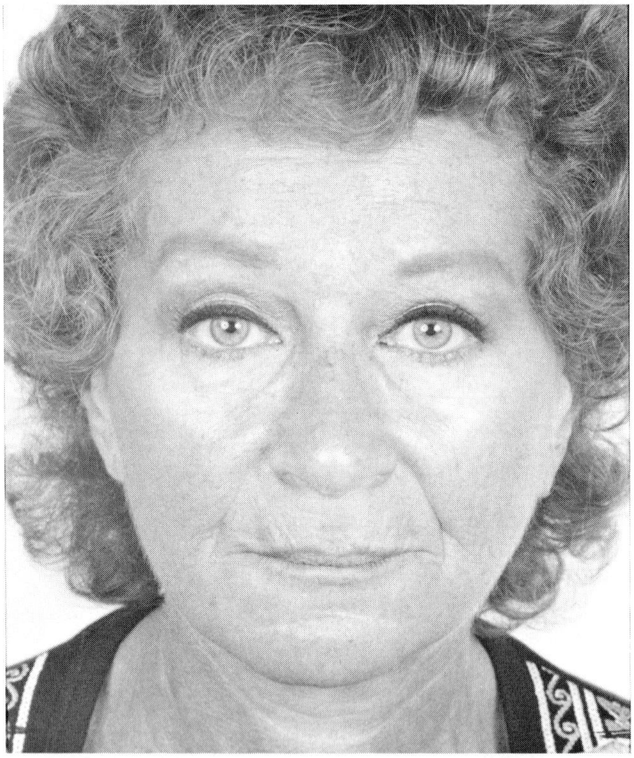

A

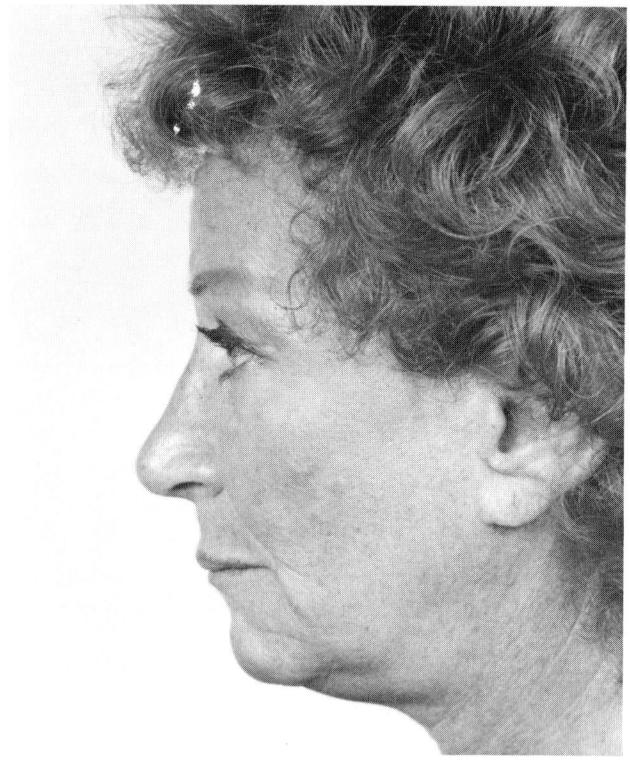

B

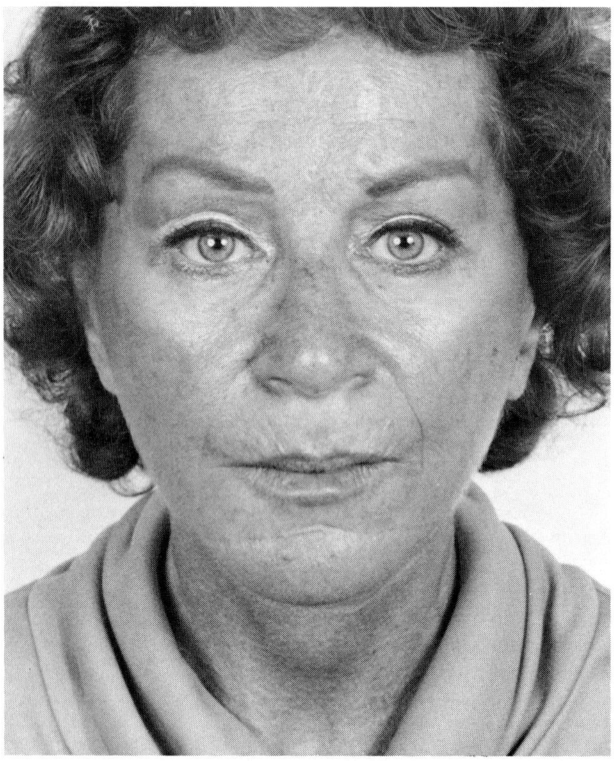

C

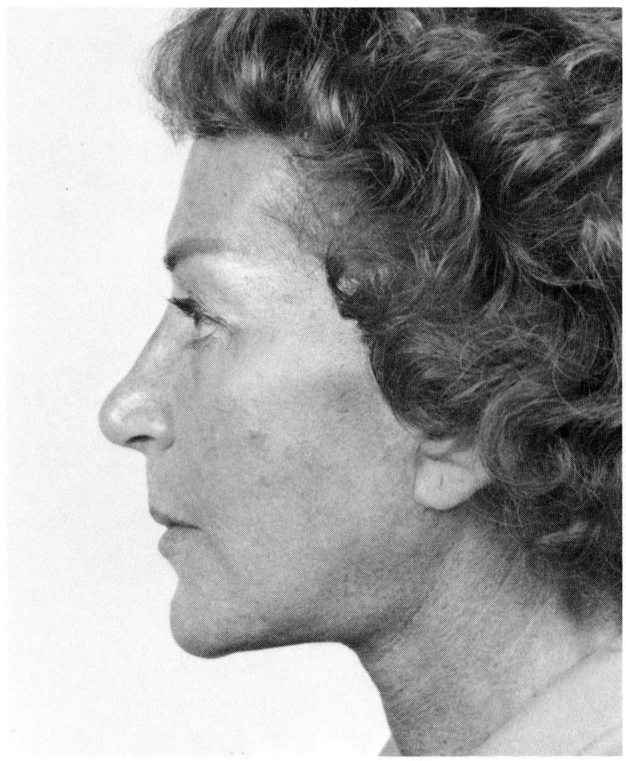

D

Figure 10-19. Secondary correction.

A, B. A 55-year-old woman shown preoperatively. She has had a face-lift and chin implant in the past.

C, D. Two months postoperatively. In addition to the bone work, she also had a forehead-lift, lower lid blepharoplasty, secondary face-lift, and submental lipectomy.

E. X-ray films show significant erosion of the chin implant into the symphysis, threatening the roots of her remaining teeth.

F. Adequate denture fit cannot be obtained because of obliteration of the lower labial sulcus. A vestibuloplasty cannot be performed over the underlying chin implant.

G. The chin implant at operation, showing area of erosion, greater than 1 cm superiorly into bone.

H, I, J. Horizontal osteotomy of symphysis with downward and forward movement of inferior fragment and an interpositional iliac bone graft. Further cancellous bone placed in erosion cavity from the chin implant.

K. Following vestibuloplasty with a split-thickness skin graft.

L. Dentures can now be comfortably worn.

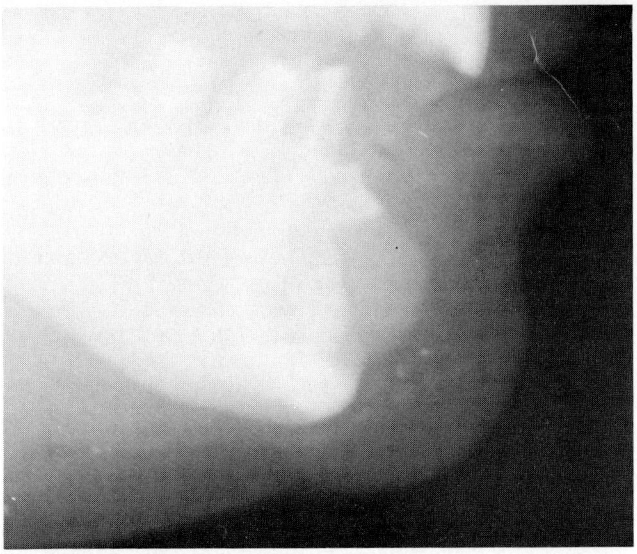
E

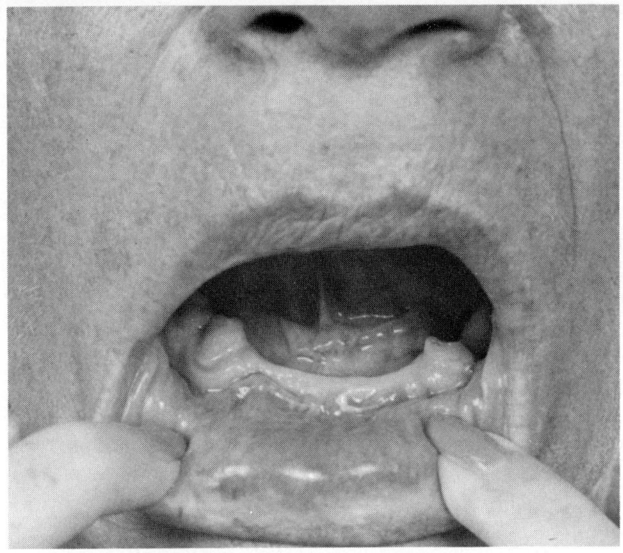
F

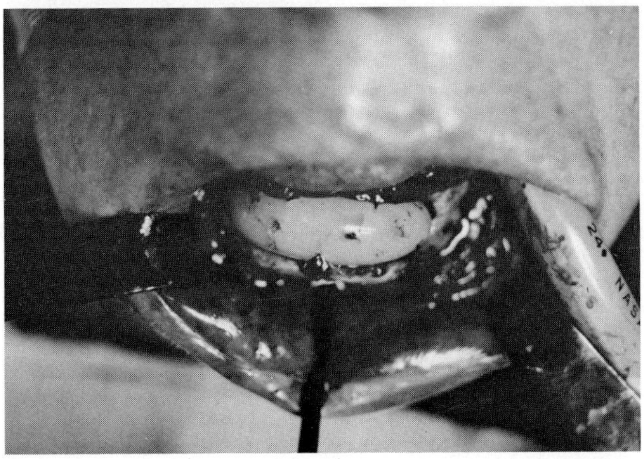
G

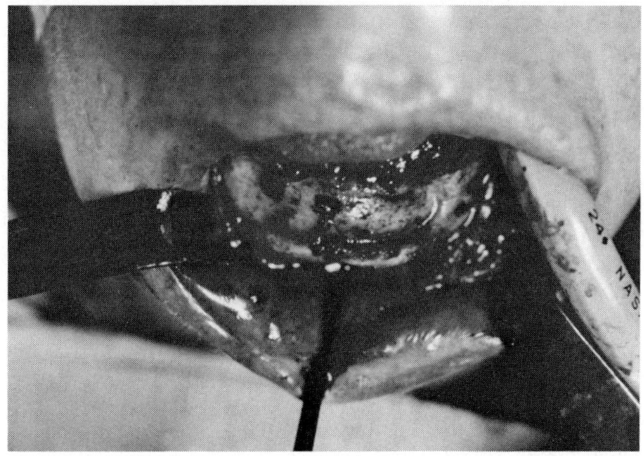
H

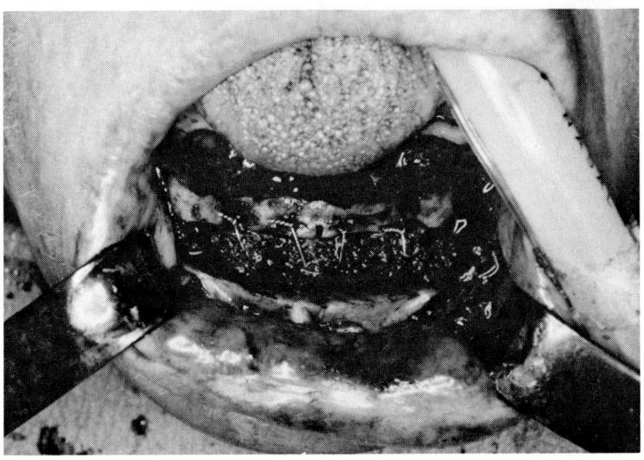
I

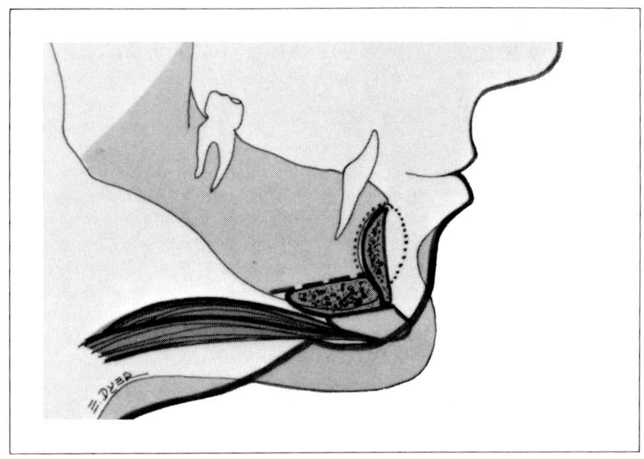
J

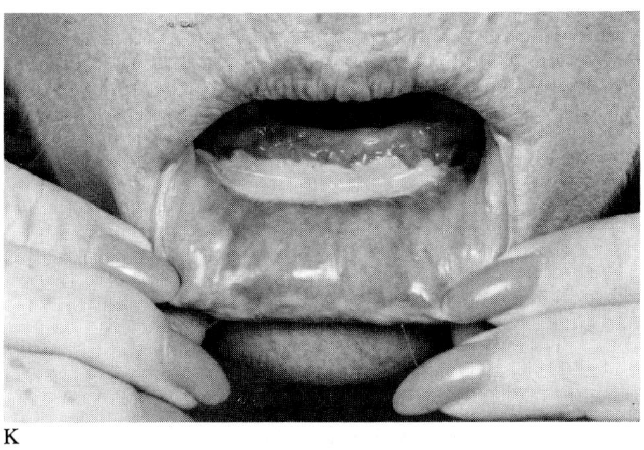
K

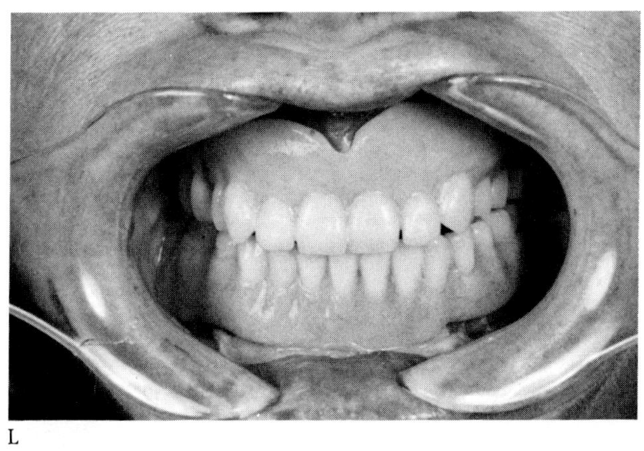
L

If the lower symphysial fragment is completely stripped of its muscular periosteal attachments, it becomes in essence a free graft. Converse [2] reported on 40 cases followed cephalometrically and found some smoothing of the upper border of the advanced fragment with only minimal changes in the degree of projection. In most of these patients the lower fragment had been completely stripped of soft tissue attachments, indicating a different biologic behavior of iliac and mandibular symphysial bone [4].

Other cephalometric studies [6, 9] of cases in which muscular attachments were maintained have confirmed this observation, showing bone apposition beneath the lateral border of the advanced fragment as well as rounding of the sharp upper border [12]. Our experience has been similar in most patients undergoing chin advancement for cosmetic purposes. Of course, in patients with major congenital anomalies and a significant deficiency of soft tissue, the tightness of the skin and muscle drape over the advanced fragment will cause a greater eventual degree of resorption.

Secondary Surgery

If secondary surgery is required in a patient who has a chin implant, the implant is removed and the problem dealt with by a direct osteoplastic approach, depending on the problem.

CONCLUSION

Osteotomies of the chin that do not alter occlusion will considerably broaden the scope of deformities the aesthetic surgeon can treat. Certain deformities of the chin—mainly symmetric retrogenia—can be successfully treated by either an alloplastic chin implant or chin advancement; deformities in all other planes will require a direct intervention on the bone.

REFERENCES

1. Bell, W. H., Proffit, W. R., and White, R. P. *Surgical Correction of Dentofacial Deformities.* Philadelphia: Saunders, 1980.
2. Converse, J. M. *Surgical Treatment of Facial Injuries* (vol. 2). Baltimore: Williams & Wilkins, 1974. P. 1081.
3. Converse, J. M. *Reconstructive Plastic Surgery.* Philadelphia: Saunders, 1977.
4. Converse, J. M. Personal communication, 1979.
5. Converse, J. M., and Wood-Smith, D. Horizontal osteotomy of the mandible. *Plast. Reconstr. Surg.* 34:464, 1964.
6. Fitzpatrick, B. N. Genioplasty with references to resorption and the hinge sliding genioplasty. *Int. J. Oral Surg.* 3:247, 1974.
7. Friedland, J. A., Loccaro, P. J., and Converse, J. M. Retrospective cephalometric analysis of mandibular bone absorption under silicone rubber chin implants. *Plast. Reconstr. Surg.* 57:144, 1976.
8. Gillies, H., and Millard, D. R. *The Principles and Art of Plastic Surgery.* Boston: Little, Brown, 1959.
9. Hinds, E. C., and Kent, J. N. Genioplasty: The versatility of horizontal osteotomy. *J. Oral Surg.* 27:690, 1969.
10. Hofer, O. Die osteoplastiche Verlangerung des Unterkiefers nach von Eiselsberg bei Mikrogenia. *Dtsch. Zahn. Mund. Kieferheilk.* 27:81, 1957.
11. Hoffman, S. Loss of a silastic chin implant following a dental infection. *Ann. Plast. Surg.* 7:484, 1981.
12. McDonnell, J. P., McNeill, R. W., and West, R. A. Advancement genioplasty: A retrospective cephalometric analysis of osseous and soft tissue changes. *J. Oral Surg.* 35:640, 1977.
13. Millard, D. R., Jr., Garst, W. P., and Beck, R. L. Submental and submandibular lipectomy in conjunction with a facelift in the male or female. *Plast. Reconstr. Surg.* 49:385, 1972.
14. Obwegeser, H. L. The indications for the correction of the mandibular deformity of the sagittal splitting technique. *Br. J. Oral Surg.* 1:157, 1964.
15. Ricketts, R. Keystone triad: I. Anatomy, physiogenetics and clinical references. *Am. J. Orthod.* 50:244, 1964.
16. Robinson, M., and Shuken, R. Bone resorption under plastic chin implants. *J. Oral Surg.* 27:116, 1969.
17. Safian, S. Progress in nasal and chin augmentation. *Plast. Reconstr. Surg.* 37:446, 1966.
18. Tessier, P. Definitive plastic surgical treatment of the severe facial deformities of craniofacial dysostoses: Crouzon's and Apert's diseases. *Plast. Reconstr. Surg.* 48:419, 1971.
19. Trauner, R., and Obwegeser, H. Surgical correction of mandibular prognathism and retrogenia with consideration of genioplasty. *Oral Surg.* 10:677, 1957.
20. Wolfe, S. A. Chin advancement as an aid in correction of deformities of the mental and submental regions. *Plast. Reconstr. Surg.* 67:624, 1981.

11. Otoplasty

Ray A. Elliott

Correction of congenital prominence of the ears has been a popular topic in the surgical literature for more than a century. Most historians identify Dieffenbach's report in 1845 [4] as the earliest contribution, and Luckett's report in 1910 [13] as the first recognition of a failure of folding of the anthelix. Following these early reports, a myriad of surgical techniques and technical refinements appeared, the majority of which directed attention to the anthelix roll. More recently, aesthetic surgeons have shown an appropriate concern for dealing with problems of the concha and the lobule as well. The quality of result has been vastly improved by a better understanding of the contribution of these various components, and attention to their individual correction.

PATIENT SELECTION

Candidates for any elective aesthetic surgery must be carefully selected; otoplasty for the correction of ear prominence is no exception. Poorly motivated patients and emotionally unstable patients will be difficult, if not impossible, to please and pose a risk that requires a mature, objective evaluation. The experienced aesthetic surgeon has learned to identify and deal with these problems. The primary goal of aesthetic surgery must be patient satisfaction (Fig. 11-1), and this begins with astute patient selection.

Indications

The strongest indication for the surgical treatment of prominent ears is well-motivated patient desire. Family and friends are usually aware of the deformity and may provide a stimulation for correction, but a patient of any age must express a personal interest in treatment.

The very young patient may well be conscious of an unusual prominence of his or her ears, but name-calling by uninhibited peers, particularly outside of the protection of the home, will often provide cruel evidence of an awareness of others. Unusually prominent ears may provoke an unrelenting barrage of verbal or even physical abuse that will challenge the emotional security of all but the strongest youngster. Social withdrawal and aggression are extremes of behavior that may result. A reasonable goal of early treatment of significant deformities is the prevention, correction, or modification of these problems.

The motivation of adults, particularly male patients, may be more difficult to evaluate. Latent hostility toward parents and society is not uncommon. When the surgical result is good and yet the patient is not satisfied, the surgeon must be critical of his preoperative evaluation and patient selection. Although there is a recognized incidence of fleeting depression following elective aesthetic

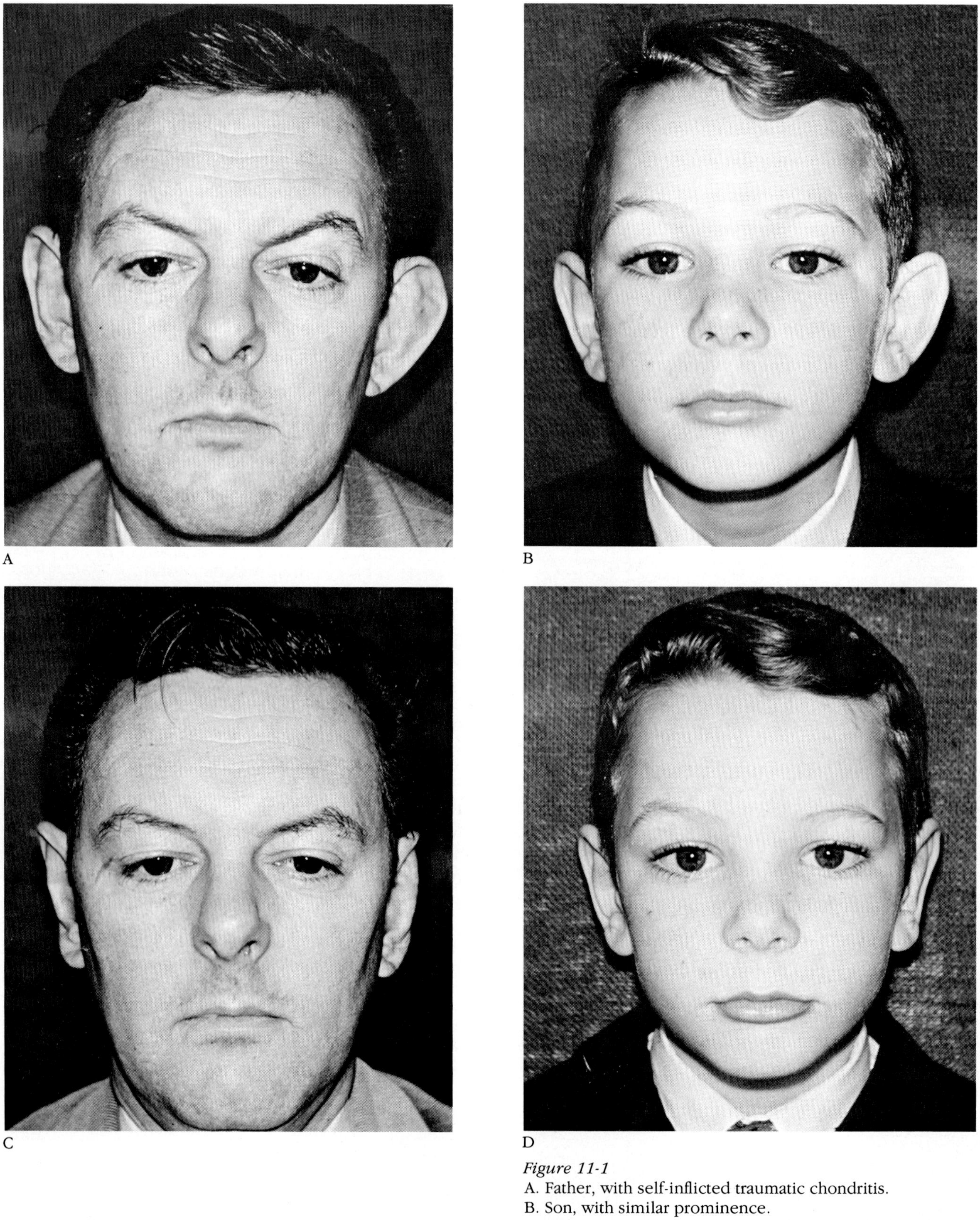

A B C D

Figure 11-1
A. Father, with self-inflicted traumatic chondritis.
B. Son, with similar prominence.
C. Father wanted his ears "back as far as possible" and was pleased with hidden helix (created before conchal repositioning was known).
D. Son's ears were positioned with more aesthetic relationship of helix and anthelix.

surgery in the adult population, more lasting dissatisfaction despite a good result is more often traced to unrealistic expectations, inadequate preoperative counseling, or deep-seated emotional problems.

Contraindications

Obviously, one major concern in the selection of patients for elective surgery is medical risk. The significance of the deformity must be weighed against the potential risks to the patient. Only patients with a near-zero risk should be considered for office surgery.

Although many patients can be treated under local anesthesia, general anesthesia may be a better choice for very young, apprehensive, or uncooperative patients. Strong motivation is a factor in the choice of anesthesia and setting. The desire of the patient to have a general anesthetic or a hospital setting will not necessarily contraindicate treatment, but the surgeon should be on guard with respect to motivation when patients over 10 years of age insist on a general anesthetic after the surgeon counsels a preference for local anesthesia.

The experienced aesthetic surgeon will usually be able to identify patients with unrealistic expectations or severe emotional problems. If good improvement can be anticipated, operation is seldom withheld if the deformity is significant and the patient is reasonably stable, but tactful referral for preoperative psychiatric evaluation is advised for borderline emotional risk patients if there is uncertainty.

Figure 11-2
A. Prominence of ears in 11-month-old patient.
B. Same patient at age 10 years

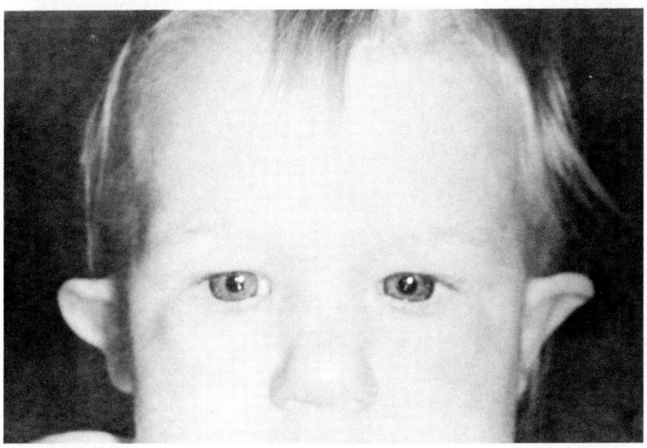

A

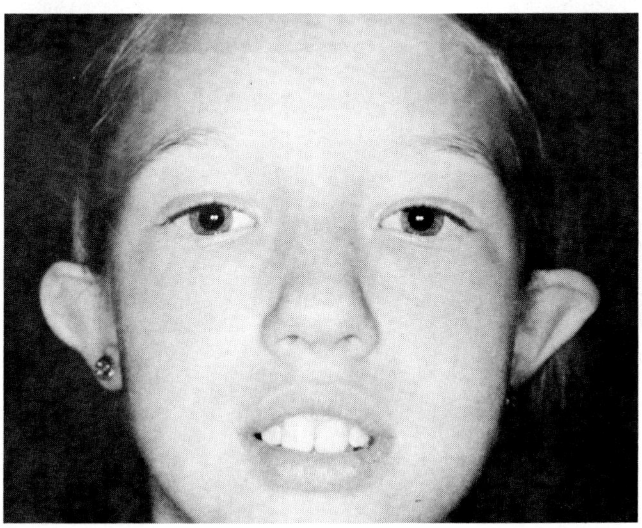

B

Patient Age

The deformity is usually apparent at birth, and parental concern may prompt early consultation (Fig. 11-2). The size and position of the ear continue to change for a number of years. One study [1] has indicated that 85 percent of ear development occurs by the third year, with width and position changing very little after age 10. Although vertical length of the ear continues to increase slightly for many years, this measurement causes scant concern in the treatment of the prominent ear.

In view of the above information concerning emotional problems and ear development, 4 or 5 years of age may be the ideal age for surgery. I routinely recommend the correction of significant deformities before school age to avoid the major source of psychic trauma. Minor deformities and those effectively hidden by hairstyling are delayed until at least 10 years of age, when patient motivation becomes more evident and correction with local anesthesia is frequently feasible.

Not all patients are seen this early. In our private practice, the median age for the initial consultation is 11 years, with the vast majority seen between the ages of 8 and 13 years. The oldest patient in our series of more than 200 cases is 43 years of age.

EVALUATION OF DEFORMITY

The measured distance from the lateral plane of the helix to the postauricular scalp tends to be less than 2 cm in the aesthetic ear. A more prominent ear will usually have a failure of anthelix folding, a deep concha, malposition of the concha, or a combination of these (Fig. 11-3). Isolated prominence of the lobule, Darwin's tubercle, and a variety of other less common problems will also be encountered. Asymmetry is common; hence, the ears should be evaluated separately.

Anthelix

When normal folding of the anthelix fails to occur, the conchal-scaphoid angle exceeds the 90-degree norm and a varying degree of prominence of the ear results. A defi-

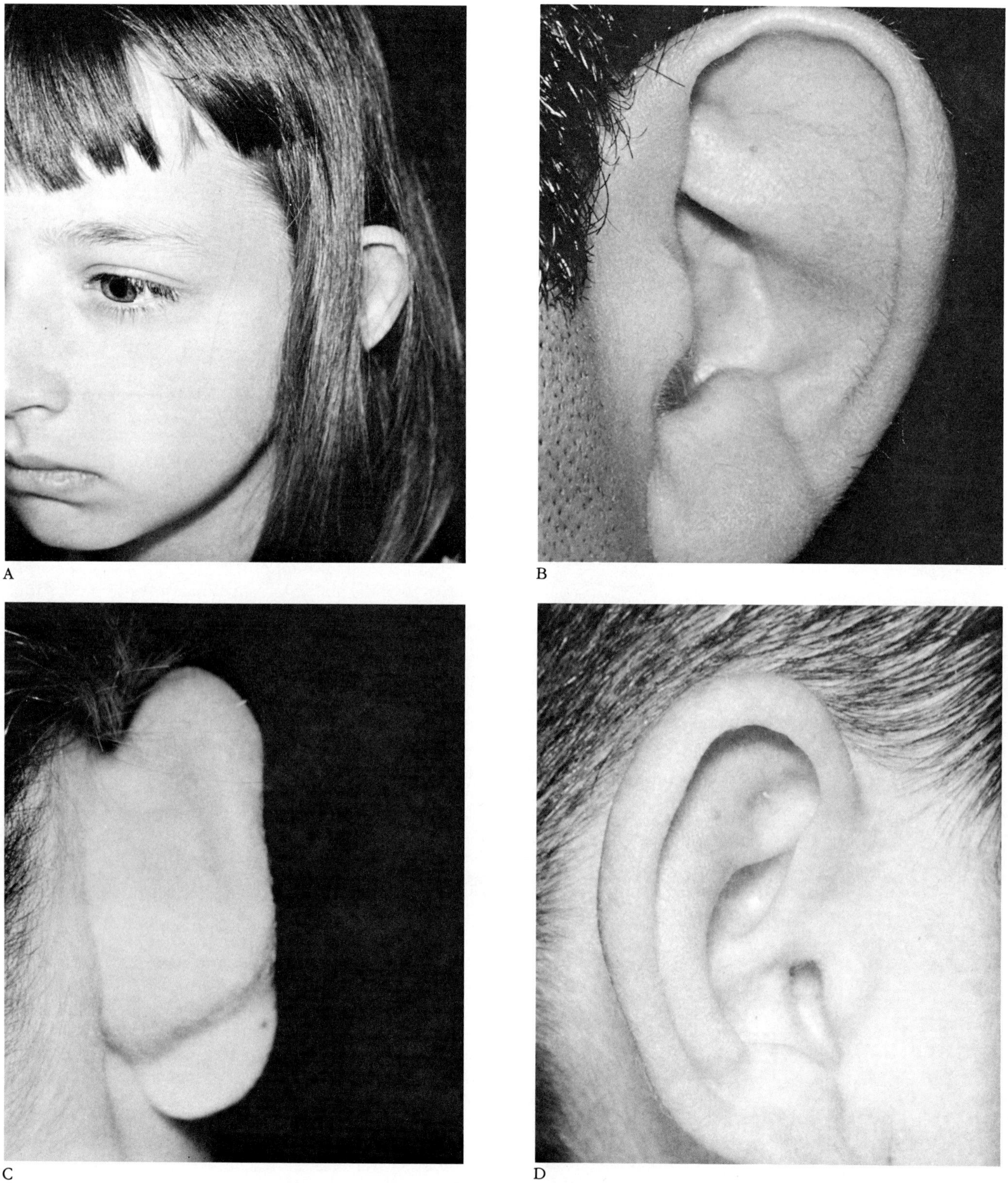

Figure 11-3. Evaluation of the deformity.
A. Prominence is difficult to hide.
B. Failure of anthelix folding.
C. Hypertrophic concha, most noticeable on posterior view.
D. Malposition of concha, obscures part of scapha on lateral view.

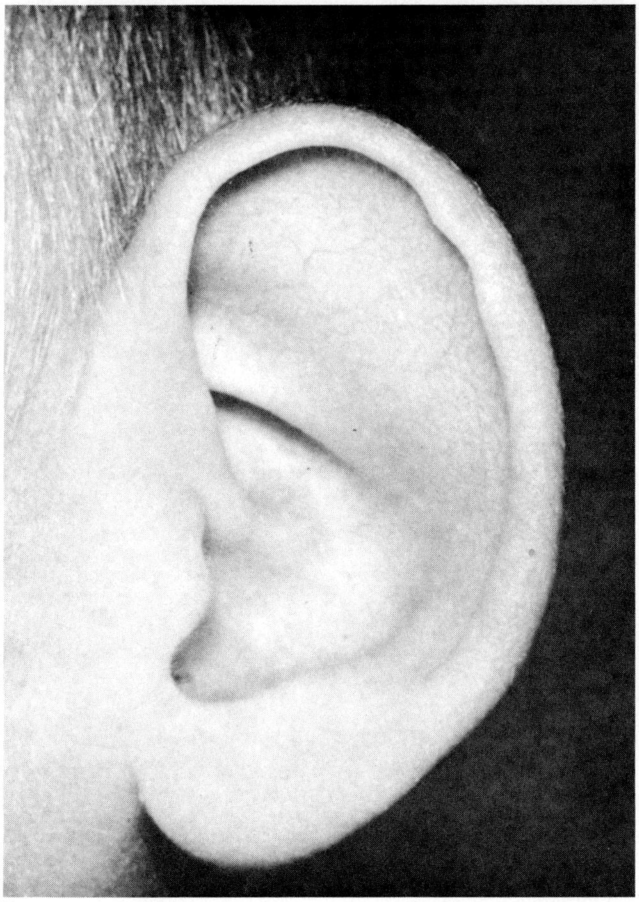

E

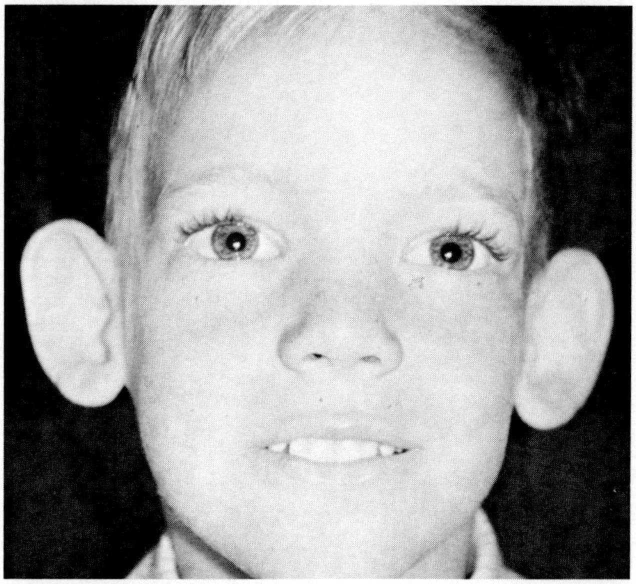

F

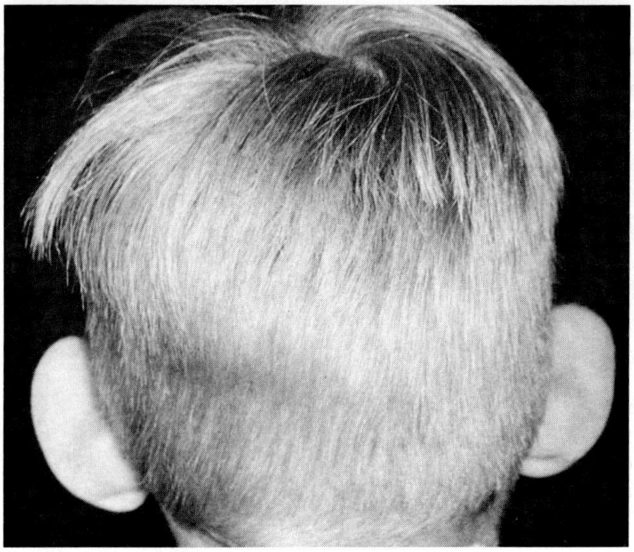

G

Figure 11-3 (continued)
E, F, G. A combined deformity evident in all views.

ciency of folding is frequently limited to the upper one-half or one-third of the ear but may involve the entire anthelix. An isolated flattening of the lower portion, with normal folding of the upper pole of the ear, has not been observed except as a complication of treatment, the latter being referred to us as a reverse telephone deformity (see Results and Complications).

Failure of anthelix folding is noticeable in all views. A winglike prominence of the ears is seen in the frontal and rear views, and the lateral view reveals projection of the helix toward the viewer, obscuring some or all of the scapha.

Concha

Prominence of the concha as a cause of ear protrusion may result either from an abnormally large and deep concha or from malposition of the concha. It is important to distinguish between these etiologic factors, as the proper plan of treatment for each is different.

HYPERTROPHY

The abnormally large and deep concha with lateral displacement of a normal anthelix is not readily detected on the lateral view. The size and depth of the enlarged concha is fully appreciated on the frontal, frontal-oblique, and rear views. The conchal-scaphoid angle is normal in the pure deformity.

MALPOSITION

Lateral displacement of the otherwise normal concha, associated with a normal anthelix roll and conchal-scaphoid angle, will, by contrast, be evident on the lateral view because the forward tilt of the ear obscures some or all of the scapha. An unusual visualization of the normal anthelix will be seen on the frontal view, while increased exposure of the concha dominates the rear view.

Combinations

Any of the described problems of the anthelix and concha can be seen in combination. Hypertrophy and malposition of the concha are commonly associated. Either conchal deformity can be seen in combination with a failure of anthelix folding, and when all three of these deformities are present to a significant degree, the ear prominence is likely to be most severe, and evident in all views.

Other Deformities

A variety of less common deformities may occur in isolation and in association with the described anthelix and conchal deformities. Darwin's tubercle, prominent anthelix, enlarged scapha, diminutive helix, gross enlargement of the ear, and enlarged or malpositioned lobule will all be encountered. Cup-ear, shell-ear, and satyr-ear are challenging deformities that are not traditionally included in a discussion of prominent ears.

AESTHETIC GOALS

Correct identification of the cause of ear prominence is the single most important step toward selection of the proper treatment plan. However, one must also predetermine the aesthetic goals of surgical treatment. This step is logically accomplished by a sound familiarity with the anatomy of the normal ear and a resolute effort to create a duplicate. Although patient satisfaction is the prime goal, the conscientious surgeon will strive for a perfection that will satisfy even the most discerning and critical eye. Well-motivated patients are often very grateful for a gross improvement and may be unaware of the potential for a better result, but the surgeon is not relieved of the responsibility to analyze the results, both short- and long-term, in search of refinements in contour and position. The reconstructed ear should not be readily identified as such.

Protrusion

Although there is a remarkable range of difference in the appearance of normally acceptable ears in the general population, as a reasonable goal the plane of the reconstructed ear should be singular from the upper pole through the lobule. Even a slight residual protrusion of the upper pole will detract from the result, while an isolated slight protrusion of the lobule may be less distressing. A significant relative prominence of both the upper and lower poles, nicknamed the telephone deformity, is totally unacceptable, as is the reverse deformity—a marked relative protrusion of the middle third of the ear.

The lateral plane of the reconstructed ear, as measured at the midpoint of the concha, should lie 1.8 cm (±0.2 cm) from the skin of the mastoid prominence. The retroauricular curvatures of the skull will result in a lesser distance at the upper pole and a greater distance to the skin surface behind the lobule. Overcorrection, like undercorrection, can easily exceed the range for acceptable appearance.

Anthelix

The vast majority of prominent ears will require some correction of an anthelix component. The normal anthelix, tightly constructed inferiorly, widens into a gentle roll as it curves upward and forward to divide into a small, sharp-edged inferior crus and a broader, rounded superior crus. Preservation or reconstruction of the curvature, normal width, and smooth roll of the anthelix, including the important superior crus, is essential to an aesthetic ear. Congenital abnormalities of the inferior crus are rare.

Sharp ridges, vertical post, irregular contours, too wide or too narrow a roll, or a malpositioned roll can be created by the surgeon. These will be discussed under Results and Complications.

Helix

The normal helix originates on the anterior floor of the concha, but at times the root extends well into the concha. The occasional prominent extension across the conchal floor is known as a transverse bar (see Fig. 11-12D). The helix overhangs the ear in a 180-degree fold along its course around the upper pole and becomes more tubelike in its descent before blending with the lobule inferiorly.

An increase in the width and prominence of the helix at the outer border of the upper pole is referred to as Darwin's tubercle (see Fig. 11-18A). Much like the transverse bar and prominence of the tail of the helix, this curious variation requires attention only if unduly prominent. An abnormal prominence of the tail of the helix has been described by many authors, along with a recommendation for amputation or reduction. A word of caution! Positioning of the tail of the helix is frequently the key to control of the lobule. In more than 200 otoplasties I have yet to see an indication for trimming this structure.

Distortion of the helix must be avoided and its smooth arc preserved. Ideally, the entire vertical course of the helix should be visible beyond the anthelix on the frontal view. The abnormal appearance of the ear with a hidden helix is well known to surgeons who elect to reduce a hypertrophic concha by increasing the anthelix roll.

Lobule

The soft fibrofatty appendage at the lower pole of the aesthetically pleasing ear will vary considerably in its size and attachment to the adjacent cheek. The lobule size should bear some reasonable relationship to the size of the ear; reduction by wedge excision is much more feasible than enlargement.

Protrusion of the lobule is a more frequent problem, the correction of which has generated ongoing interest and reams of misinformation concerning the role of medial skin excision. Skin excision is rarely needed if the tail of the helix with its attachment to the lobule is preserved and repositioned. This important concept will be discussed further.

Sulcus

The postauricular sulcus is important to the aesthetic appearance of the ear, particularly from the posterior view. Obliteration of the sulcus should no longer be seen after cosmetic otoplasty for congenital prominence. With proper treatment of the underlying problems already discussed, the excision of skin can be limited to the removal of the excess. Although advocated by early authors as a definitive treatment for prominence, tightening the skin is now fairly well established as being unnecessary with modern techniques. A few authors still describe obliteration of the sulcus behind the lobule to control its protrusion, but this is not recommended. Control of the tail of the helix is the key to control of the attached lobule. Surgeons who resect the tail will probably need to resort to skin excision and potential obliteration of the lower sulcus, but this is unfortunate.

Symmetry

It may be difficult or impossible to achieve absolute symmetry, particularly with asymmetric deformities, but this should be a constant goal. With the reversible techniques available to the aesthetic surgeon, differences of less than 1 or 2 mm of measured prominence can be achieved routinely, even when differences in contour persist. Fortunately, the two ears are rarely viewed together, and variations are not uncommon in the general population. Hence absolute symmetry, although a goal, is not necessarily essential for patient satisfaction. Peers may be more critical, and the conscientious surgeon will see even the most subtle differences.

SURGICAL PRINCIPLES

The procedure(s) selected for the treatment of prominent ears should be simple, reproducible, and reversible, giving the maximum aesthetic result with the lowest possible risk of recurrence and a near-zero risk of compounding the problem. The already sensitized patient undergoing elective cosmetic surgery has a low tolerance for complications and untoward results.

General Precautions

Gentle tissue handling, careful hemostasis, and sterile technique are essential. The excellent blood supply of the ear decreases the hazard of infection, but poor technique and hematoma can reverse this fortune.

Cartilage

Cartilage may require thinning, release of spring, excision, or relocation. Although common with earlier techniques, thinning of anthelix cartilage is seldom used today. Thinning has always been somewhat unpredictable, resulting too frequently in a sharp ridge rather than a soft roll. Disrupting the perichondrium and the surface of the cartilage on the front of the ear by scratching or scoring will release the cartilage spring and permit a more gentle folding.

Excess cartilage, particularly of the concha, can be excised, but sharp edges and distortions must be avoided. Reduction of the concha can be accomplished with an anterior or a posterior approach, but judgment of position and contour is easier with the anterior approach, and the scar is seldom noticeable. Incisions through the cartilage for other than excision should be avoided if possible. Techniques that require such incision(s) will have an incidence of sharp edges, and a miscalculation may not be reversible.

Skin

Increasing tension on the skin closure is neither a desirable nor a reliable method for controlling cartilage spring or for positioning the ear. Skin excision is usually limited to removal of any excess in the posterior sulcus. With modest undermining the extra anterior skin associated with a conchal reduction redrapes without bunching. Lobule reduction may be indicated occasionally, but control of the lobule position seldom requires posterior skin excision if the tail of the helix is preserved and used for this purpose.

Sutures

Although occasionally rejected with a localized infection, nonabsorbable sutures cause less tissue reaction than absorbable sutures and do not lose their strength. Since dark sutures may be visable beneath the thin ear cover, clear or white material is best for buried sutures.

Absorbable sutures are feasible for posterior skin closure in the absence of tension, and removal is not usually needed if plain catgut is chosen. Thus, retraction of the ear is obviated in the early postoperative course, and the advantage in the treatment of young children is evident. The delayed absorption of chromic catgut and polyglass sutures is a disadvantage; suture tracts may form before the sutures are absorbed. If nonabsorbable sutures are used for skin closure, they should be removed in 4 or 5 days to avoid these epithelial tracks.

Splinting

The position of the reconstructed ear should be maintained during healing and protected until stable. A soft compression dressing that follows the contours and holds the desired position affords comfort and decreases edema and ecchymosis (see Fig. 11-19). However, a dressing is not a substitute for good hemostasis and will not prevent a hematoma. Persistent pain deserves prompt attention for a possible complication. The ear should be protected from unintentional stress until healing is complete and the position has been stabilized by normal fibrous fixation.

SURGICAL TECHNIQUE

Selection of the proper treatment plan depends on an accurate analysis of the deformity. The selected technique(s) must then be directed at the specific problem(s).

History

The history of ear surgery has been detailed in Chapter 1, but some further discussion is warranted to develop the origin of the recommended techniques.

ANTHELIX

Until the late 1960s most authors ignored the concha in their enthusiasm to produce a more natural anthelix. A variety of procedures advocated thinning or through-and-through incisions to define the anthelix. Most of these were combined with either subcutaneous or buried sutures to hold the new position. Both anterior and posterior approaches were described.

Perhaps the most important contributions were those of Mustardé [14], who proposed a reversible suture technique without incisions, and Stenstrom [17], who scratched the anterior surface of the cartilage to break the spring. When these two techniques were in essence later used in combination, the incidence of recurrence seen with each alone was virtually eliminated. Mustardé's suture technique was modified and refined by use of a greater number of smaller mattress sutures to create a more gently curved anthelix and superior crus. Stenstrom's observation that cartilage springs toward the intact surface led to prompt acceptance of anterior scoring of the cartilage, but suture fixation of the cartilage fold was clearly preferred to the skin excision Stenstrom had proposed.

CONCHA

A review of the history of otoplasty for prominent ears published in the early 1970s [11] mentioned the concha in a single sentence. Most earlier reviews ignored the concha entirely.

Reduction. In 1952 the author, then a rotating intern on the plastic surgery service, recognized the hypertrophic concha and devised a procedure for its reduction via an anterior approach. This procedure gained limited attention in 1965 [5] and was published in 1972 [8], after it had been used in more than 100 cases. A posterior approach for conchal reduction was proposed in 1973 by Courtiss et al. [3].

Repositioning. In 1965 Owens and Delgado [15] published their experience with a conchal-mastoid suture technique for correcting malposition of the concha. Furnas [9] popularized this technique with his paper in 1968, and the author [6, 7] suggested the development of a definite pocket for the concha as a modification.

LOBULE

The recent otoplasty literature has routinely included consideration of prominence of the lobule. Most of the basic techniques used for lobule control today were introduced a decade or more ago, but many surgeons remain confused about the choice.

Skin Excision and Fixation. Much has been written about skin excision for control of the lobule, but, as previously mentioned, perhaps the value of this technique has been overstated. In 1969 Spira et al. [16] advocated suturing the dermis of the lobule to scalp periosteum, and in 1978 Furnas [10] recommended a modification in which he fixed the fibrofatty tissue of the lobule to the insertion of the sternocleidomastoid muscle.

Tail of the Helix. In 1959 I watched Webster control the lobule by repositioning the tail of the helix. His valuable contribution, subsequently published in 1969 [18], was cited by Beernick et al. [2] 10 years later in a report of 131 corrections using this technique.

Author's Preference

After review of the options and influenced by 30 years of fascination with otoplasty for the correction of prominent ears, during which time many worthwhile techniques and refinements have been presented, I found certain preferences evolving. Although most authors can report satisfaction with their own technique(s), the procedures I have selected are based primarily on the work of others, with the addition of a few original thoughts and several refinements. All of these techniques can be used individually or in combination to correct the specific deformity or deformities identified in an analysis of the defect.

ANTHELIX RECONSTRUCTION

Some deformities can probably be successfully managed by mattress sutures alone if the cartilage is thin, and perhaps by anterior scoring alone if a large posterior skin ellipse is removed, but recurrences will be seen. I routinely combine anterior scoring and mattress sutures to ensure more dependable results. Removal of an ellipse of posterior skin affords the usual exposure and is judged to eliminate the bunching of excess skin.

CONCHAL REDUCTION

Today I reserve reduction for the very deep concha and usually combine this technique with a repositioning. Mild and moderate hypertrophy is treated by repositioning alone. The anterior approach is preferred for conchal reduction because of the ease with which the ear position can be judged and distortions prevented. Fortunately, the scar is seldom noticeable.

CONCHAL POSITIONING

As emphasized by Furnas [9, 10], conchal-mastoid sutures can be used to reduce the posterior conchal wall contribution to a prominent ear. I believe, however, that a definite pocket should be created for the concha. Sacrifice of the posterior auricular muscle and the fibrofatty tissue overlying the mastoid process is of no consequence; routine excision prevents these structures from acting as a fulcrum to cause protrusion of the anterior wall and tragus, or from limiting the setback.

LOBULE CONTROL

The tail of the helix is the key to the control of the lobule in most cases.The lobule is left adherent to the tail of the helix, and the latter is repositioned on the posterior surface of the concha. Occasionally, a small posterior skin excision is added for additional setback, but a sulcus is always preserved. Reduction of a large earlobe is accomplished easily with a full-thickness wedge excision. The lobule attachment to the cheek can be increased by partial cleft excision, but this is an unusual cause of prominence.

MISCELLANEOUS PROCEDURES

I do not hesitate to wedge-excise a Darwin's tubercle or perform a crescent-shaped excision on a broad scapha if these deformities are prominent. Transverse wedge reduction of a grossly enlarged ear often requires a triangular excision of scapha above and below the wedge to obviate distortion. The correction may be especially gratifying when the deformity is unilateral.

Procedure

The preparation for surgery, operative techniques, and postoperative care presented here reflect the author's preference. They are distilled from a personal experience with many of the techniques described in the surgical literature and refined by a critical ongoing analysis of the results obtained.

PREPARATION

The hair is washed the evening before surgery and again just before surgery. The surgical permission and consent forms, laboratory data, and photographs are checked. Young children are prepared for general anesthesia; either ketamine or oral-tracheal intubation with another agent is used at the discretion of the anesthetist. Adults and older children are treated as outpatients with premedication and local anesthesia.

Draping. After cleansing of the face, neck, ears, and scalp, the entire head is exposed in the operative field. Stockinet or adherent plastic drapes can be used to isolate the ears, but to little advantage (Fig. 11-4). The more open exposure has been used safely for rhytidectomy for many years, and patients seem to be more comfortable.

Marking. The ear is folded manually, and the centerline of the anthelix and its superior crus are marked on the skin to outline the area for anterior undermining. With experience, perforation of the cartilage with needles dipped in dye is not required for suture techniques, as the placement and result of each suture are readily visualized. Incisions for conchal reduction and postauricular excision are marked.

Anesthesia. A solution of 2% lidocaine with 1 : 100,000 epinephrine is injected into the posterior sulcus and beneath the skin of the anterior and posterior surfaces of the ear. Besides providing anesthesia, this technique facilitates dissection and aids hemostasis. Patients under general anesthesia are injected in the same way.

OPERATION

Where the deformity is bilateral, the more prominent ear is corrected first and used as a pattern for the second ear. An attempt at symmetry is routine, but patients and family are cautioned that an exact match is not always obtainable. The head can be turned for intraoperative comparison of the ears as required, but the face is turned away from the operating surgeon to give full exposure of the ear during the procedure.

Approach. Exposure of the anthelix and concha is begun posteriorly with excision of an ellipse of skin and subcutaneous tissue. The excision extends from the upper pole of the ear to the inferior limit of the concha. The upper extension is needed for exposure of the superior crus and is not usually required when only a conchal repositioning is planned. The width of the skin excision is estimated conservatively to match the anticipated excess.

When only a conchal repositioning is required, the excision is centered on the posterior sulcus. Anytime an anthelix reconstruction is planned, the ellipse is moved onto the posterior surface of the concha to facilitate the exposure (Fig. 11-5).

Conchal reduction is achieved through a separate anterior incision several millimeters within the concha. This curved incision follows the entire length of the concha to permit the necessary exposure of the cartilage. Anterior scoring of the cartilage can be accomplished via the posterior approach, but I prefer a small vertical anterior incision above the tail of the helix.

Anthelix, Superior Crus, and Lobule. These three parts of the ear are considered together in many reconstructions (Figs. 11-6 and 11-7). After elevation of the posterior flap to expose the bare surface of the scapha and superior crus and the tail of the helix, I undermine the anterior surface of the ear in the intended position of the anthelix and superior crus and score the cartilage with the Dingman otoabrader (Fig. 11-8).

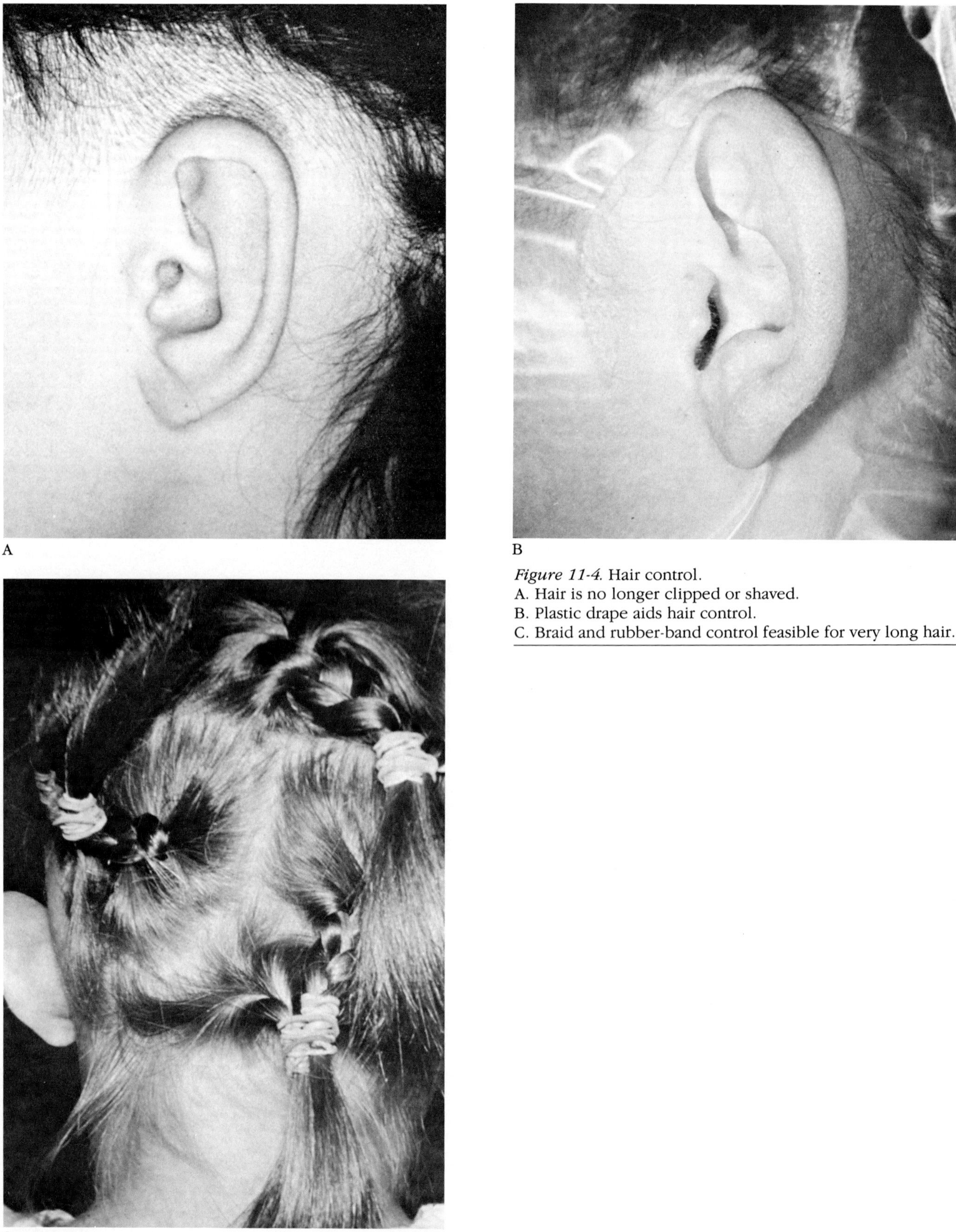

A

B

C

Figure 11-4. Hair control.
A. Hair is no longer clipped or shaved.
B. Plastic drape aids hair control.
C. Braid and rubber-band control feasible for very long hair.

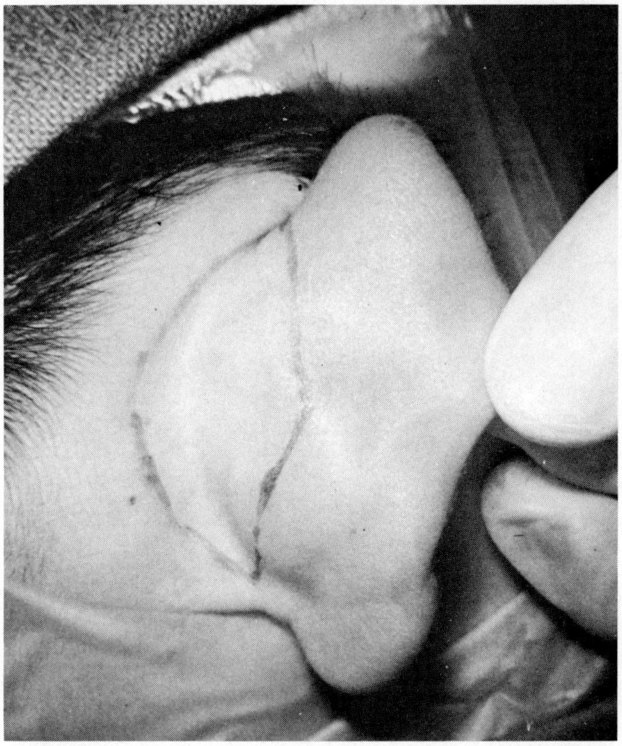

A

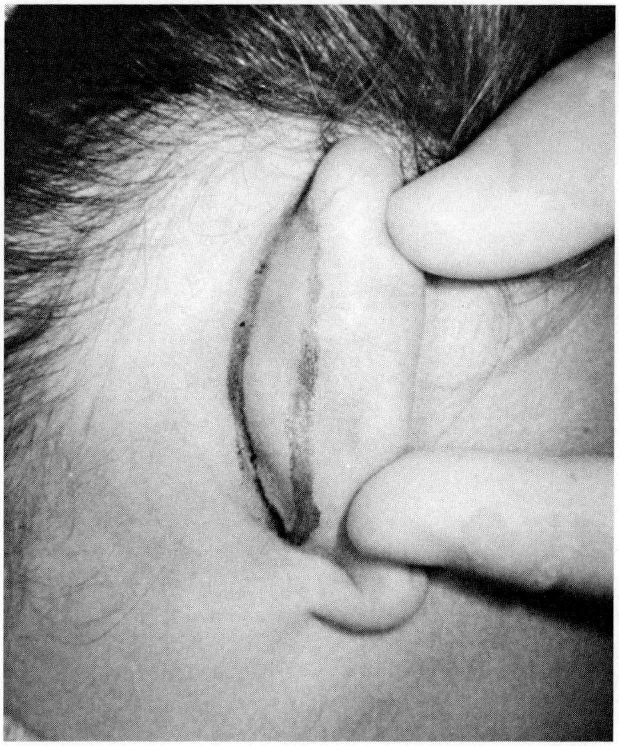

B

Figure 11-5. Posterior approach with excision of skin excess.
A. Excision centered on sulcus for conchal repositioning.
B. Excision on concha for combined deformities.

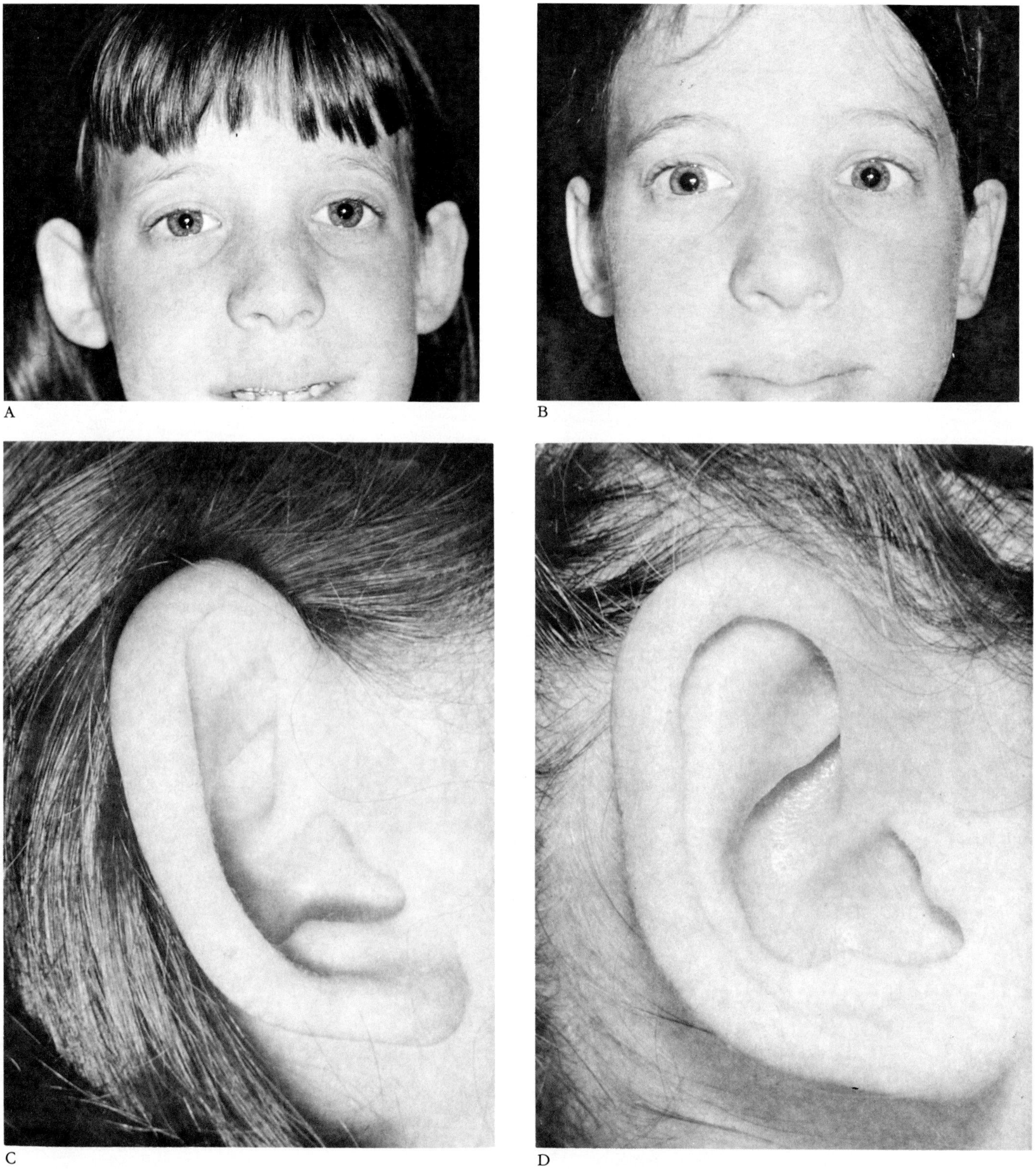

Figure 11-6. Anthelix reconstruction.
A. Preoperative front view.
B. Postoperative front view.
C. Preoperative lateral view.
D. Postoperative lateral view.

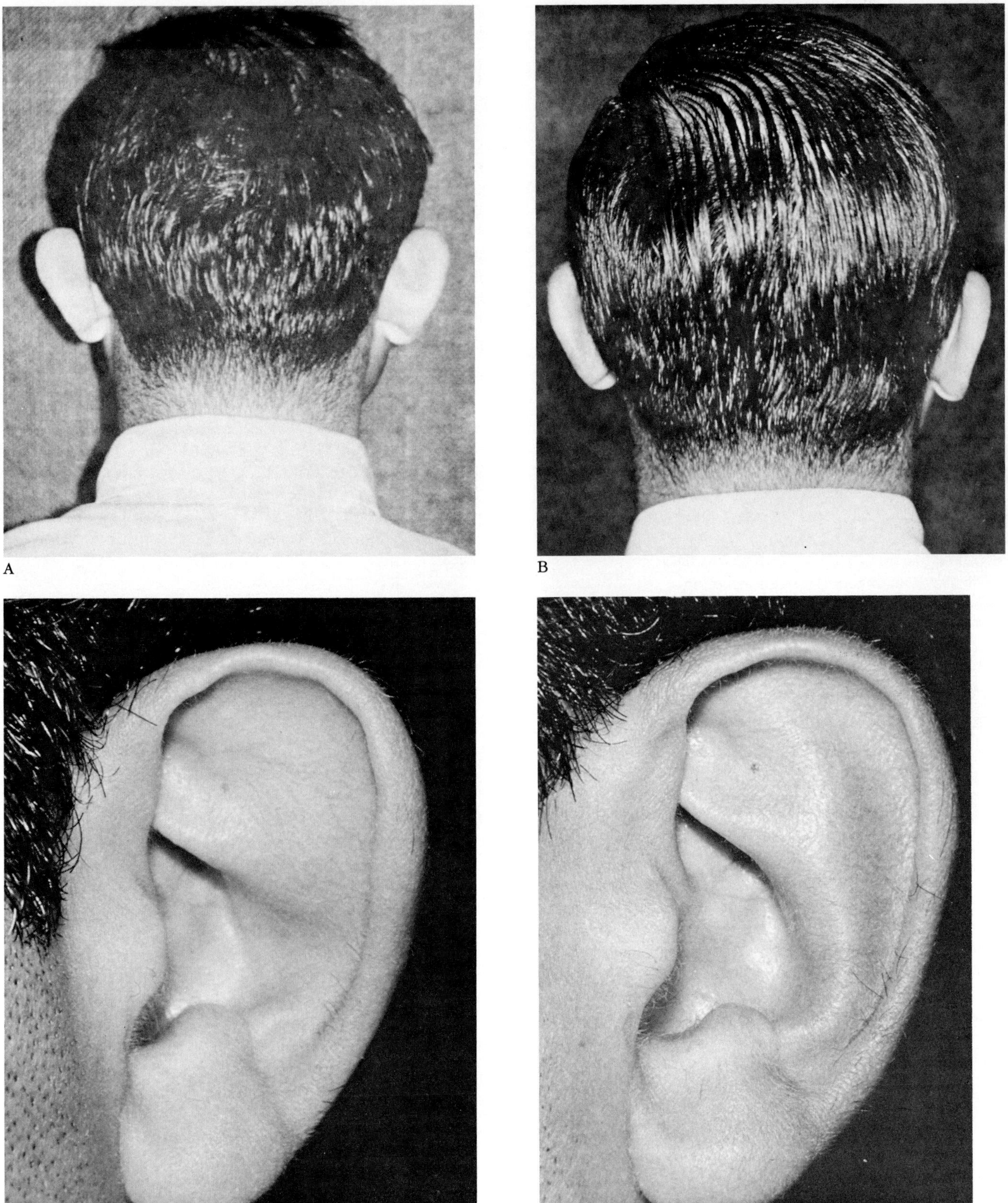

A B C D

Figure 11-7. Anthelix reconstruction.
A. Preoperative posterior view.
B. Postoperative posterior view.
C. Preoperative frontal-oblique view.
D. Postoperative frontal-oblique view.

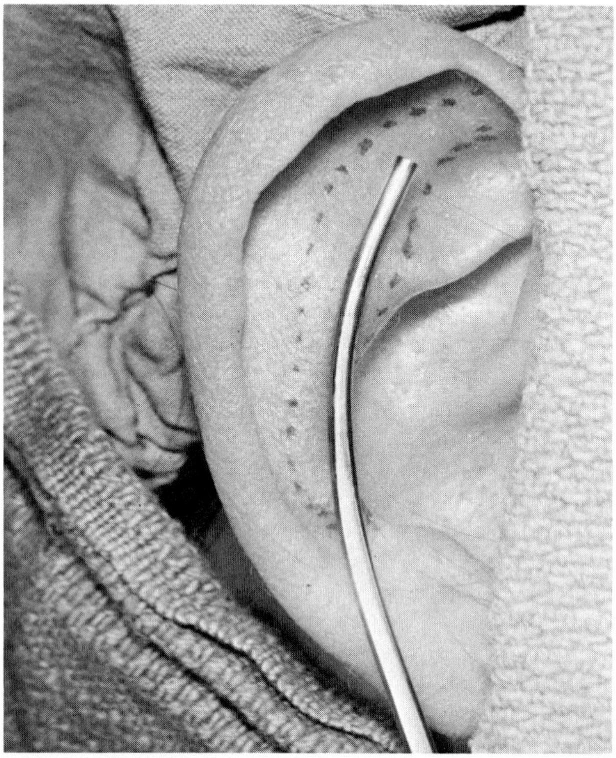

Figure 11-8. Otoabrader for anterior scoring.

The tail of the helix is exposed only on its posterior surface and is not dissected. The first suture is placed to draw the tail of the helix onto the posterior surface of the concha until the adherent lobule is in proper position. The exact effect is clearly visible, and this nonabsorbable suture is replaced until accurate. Such control of the lobule will afford a complete correction in most instances. Occasionally, a small posterior skin excision or reduction of the lobule will be needed but is best delayed until final skin closure.

Another four or five mattress sutures are placed posteriorly in radial fashion from inferior to superior to form a gently curved anthelix fold and superior crus of desired width (Fig. 11-9). Each suture, including the one through the tail of the helix, is tested as placed and then tied in order from inferior to superior, being tightened only enough to give the desired effect at that level. Any distortion is easily detected and promptly corrected by replacement of the offending suture(s) or use of additional sutures.

The correction is limited to the portion of the ear that contributes to the specific deformity. The flexibility of this technique and its complete evaluation and reversibility during the procedure clearly make it an attractive choice.

Conchal Reduction. As previously noted, the approach for reduction of the concha is through an anterior incision that follows the curve of the concha (Figs. 11-10 and 11-11). The incision, several millimeters from the rim of the concha, follows the length of the concha and is carried through the cartilage. Both surfaces of the cartilage are undermined, allowing the ear to be recessed into the desired position; then the overlapping excess of concha is excised. The length of the incision is planned to avoid distortion as the defect is closed by edge-to-edge approximation of cartilage with two nonabsorbable sutures. The knots are tied on the posterior surface.

This is a simple, accurate technique that permits evaluation of the exact effect before resection, and direct vision obviates gaps and overlapping. Anterior skin is seldom excised as liberal undermining prevents wrinkling in most cases, and the anterior scar has not presented a problem in more than 100 cases.

Conchal Repositioning. The conchal-mastoid suture technique has been modified to prepare a definite pocket for the concha (Figs. 11-12 and 11-13). Furnas [9] stressed the importance of preserving the posterior auricular muscle and left much of the fibrofatty tissue as protection for the sensory nerve, but in our experience this occasionally resulted in a fulcrum that created prominence of the tragus. Others have reported an incidence of recurrence with conchal-mastoid sutures alone [2].

Excision of the posterior auricular muscle and all of the fibrofatty tissue overlying the mastoid fascia creates a pocket for the concha. Usually two tacking sutures are used to fix the concha to the mastoid fascia. The placement of the sutures is judged to give the desired residual exposure of the posterior wall of the concha. Distortion of the external auditory meatus must also be considered and avoided. Recurrence of the deformity has not been seen with this technique.

Combined Deformities. The described procedures can be used in any combination, some requiring a minor revision to improve their compatibility (Figs. 11-14 and 11-15). When a flat anthelix, hypertrophic concha, and malposition of the concha all contribute to the deformity, the usual sequence of correction is anthelix reconstruction, conchal reduction, and then conchal repositioning. However, in this combination, a mild hypertrophy of the concha may be corrected by the anthelix folding, and moderate hypertrophy may require only the addition of conchal repositioning. Conchal reduction by cartilage excision is reserved for selected cases; the need can usually be judged in advance (Figs. 11-16 and 11-17). In borderline cases, conchal repositioning should be tested before committing to conchal reduction, and always after reconstruction of the anthelix. Whenever conchal reduction is combined with folding sutures, the anterior incision through the conchal cartilage is placed just far enough below the rim to avoid those sutures.

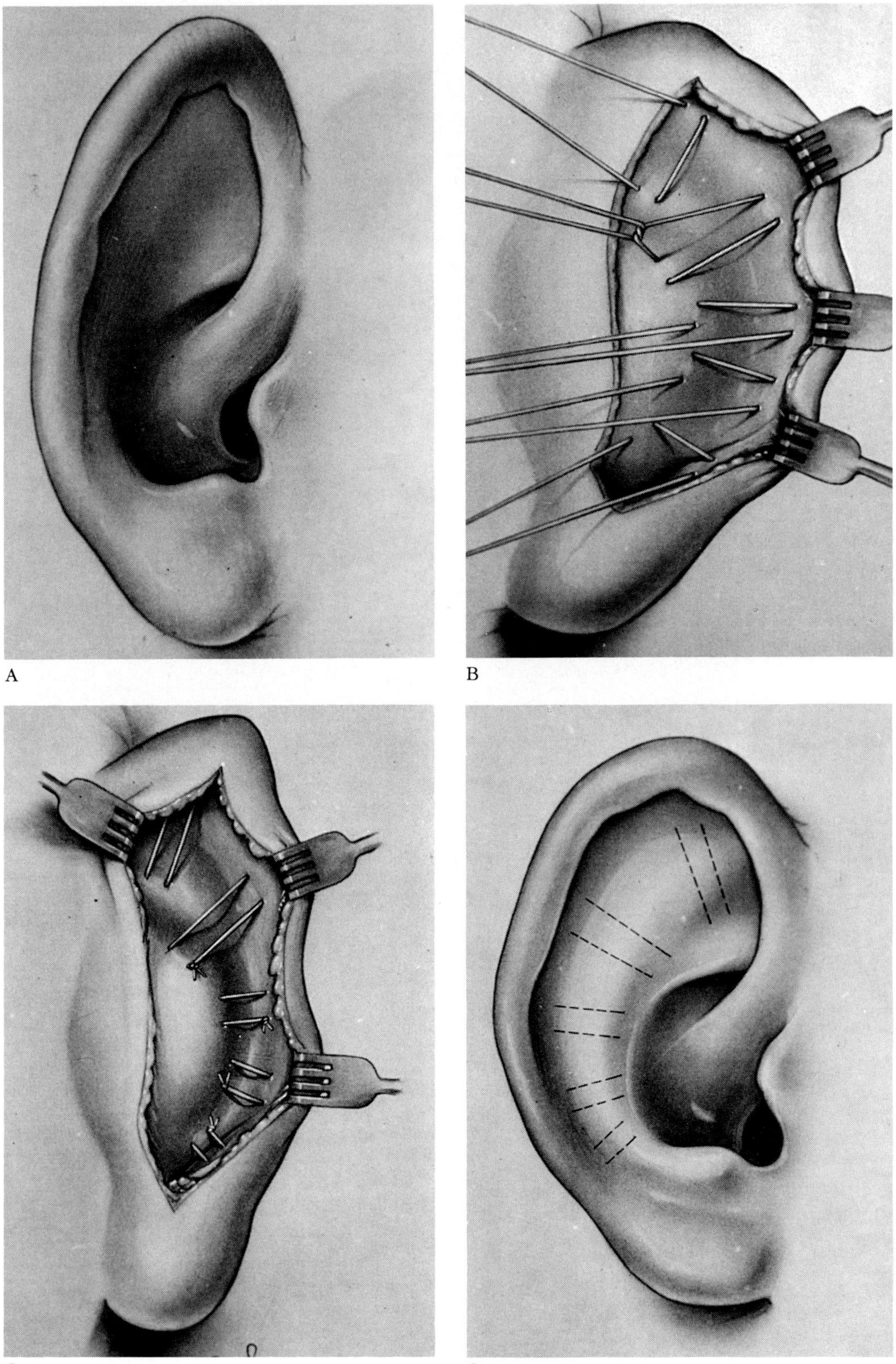

Figure 11-9. Suture technique for anthelix, superior crus, and lobule control.

A. Failure of anthelix fold.
B. Mattress sutures for anthelix and superior crus folding. Suturing tail of helix to concha controls lobule position.
C. Each suture tightened only enough to give desired effect at that level.
D. Radial placement produces curved roll.

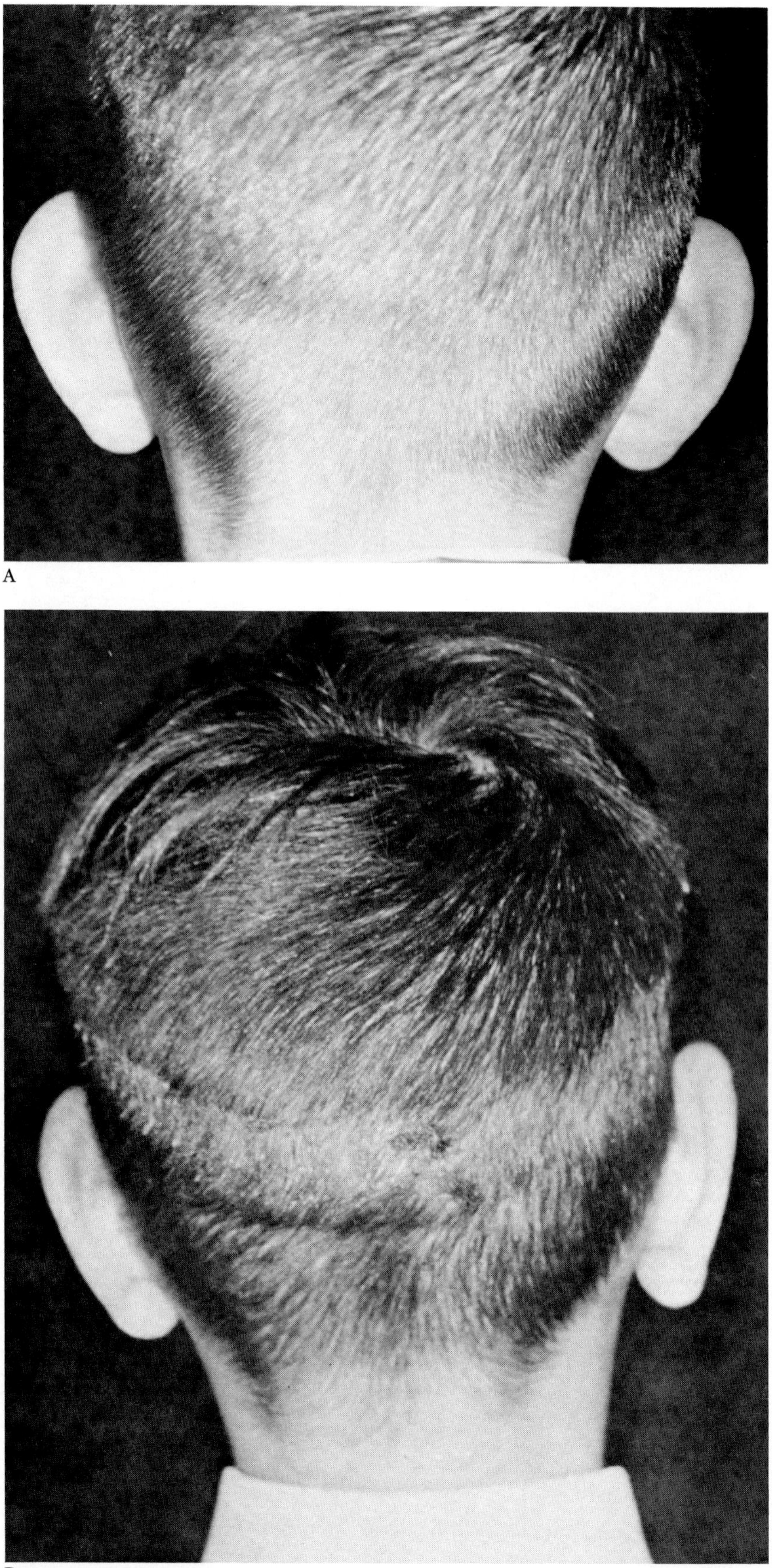

A

B

Figure 11-10. Conchal reduction.
A. Preoperative posterior view.
B. Postoperative posterior view.

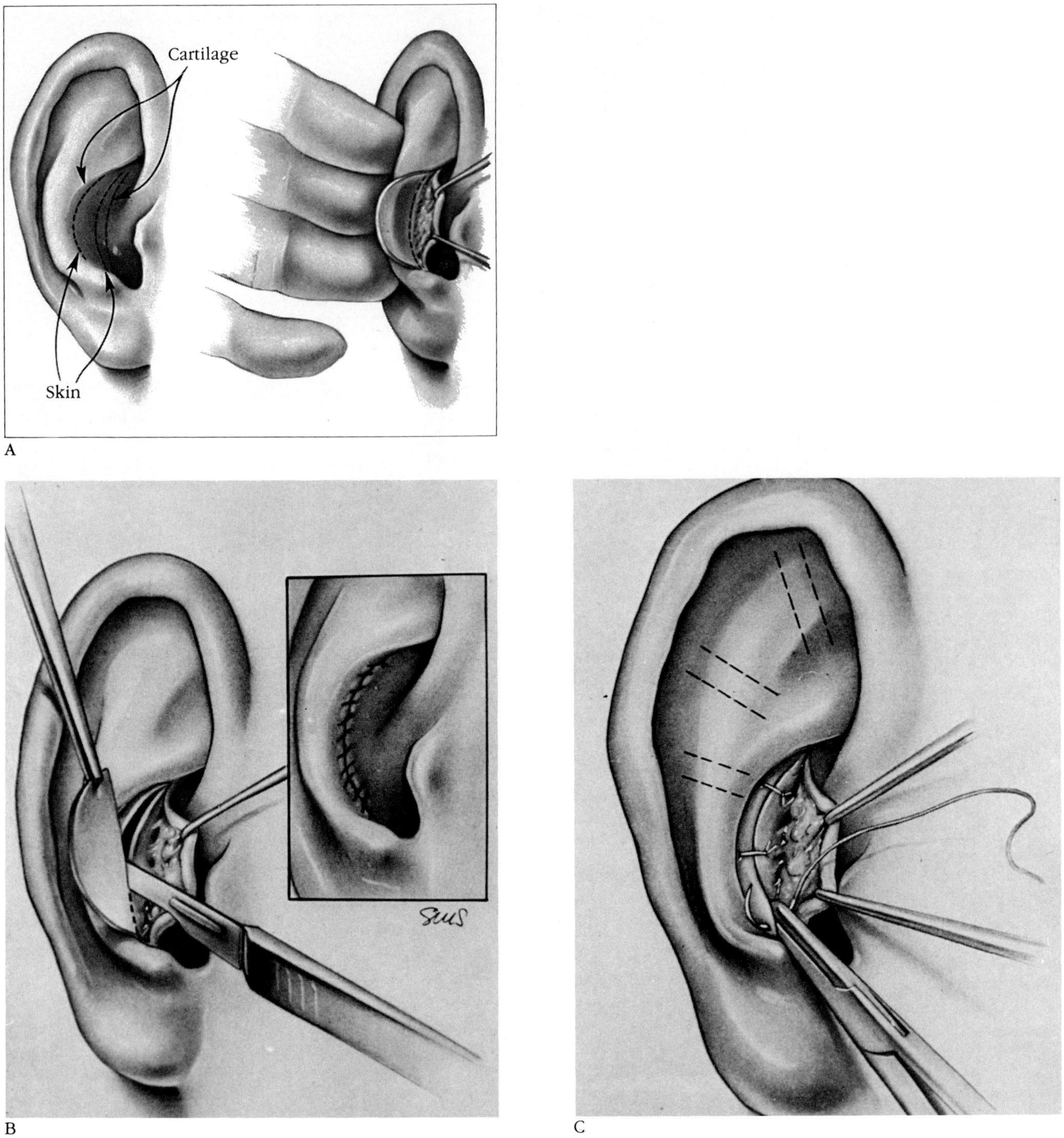

Figure 11-11. Anterior approach for conchal reduction.
A. Skin excision high on conchal wall. Excess cartilage easily judged by overlap. Skin seldom excised.
B. Skin excision obviated by undermining.
C. Cartilage defect sutured. Technique is compatible with anthelix reconstruction and conchal repositioning.

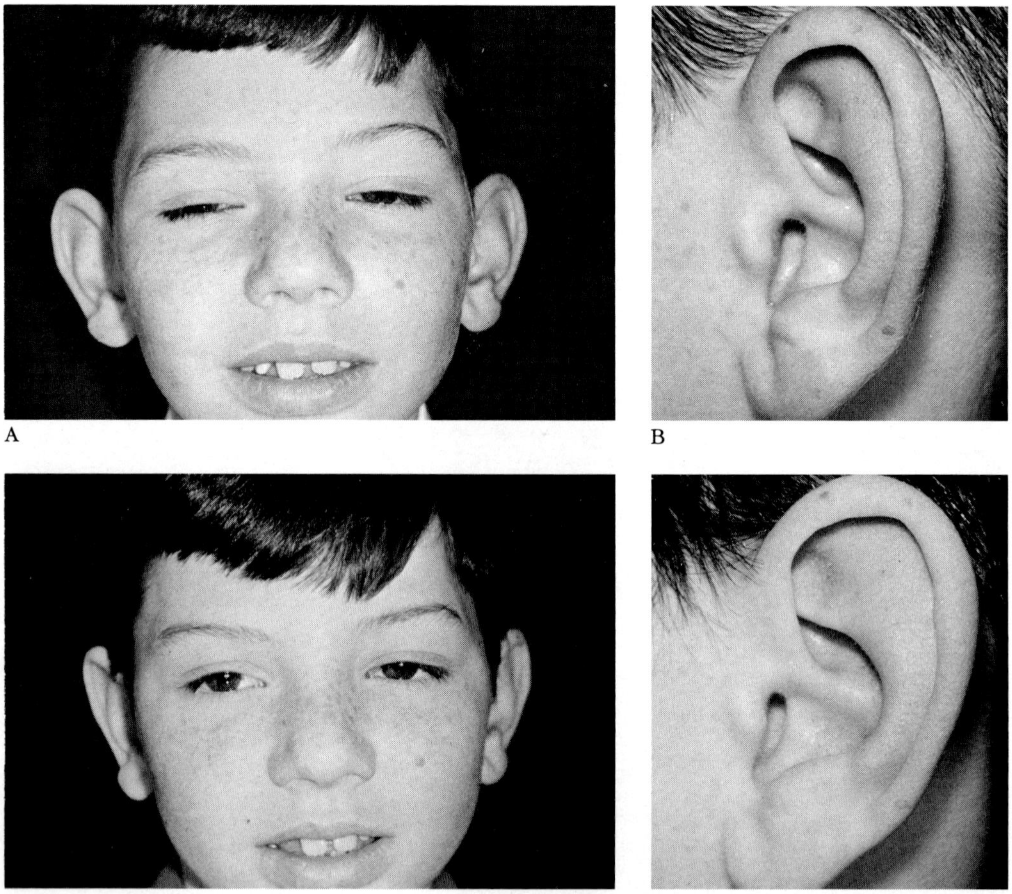

A B C D

Figure 11-12. Conchal repositioning.
A. Preoperative front view.
B. Preoperative lateral view, partially obscured anthelix.
C. Postoperative front view.
D. Postoperative lateral view. Note mild transverse bar.

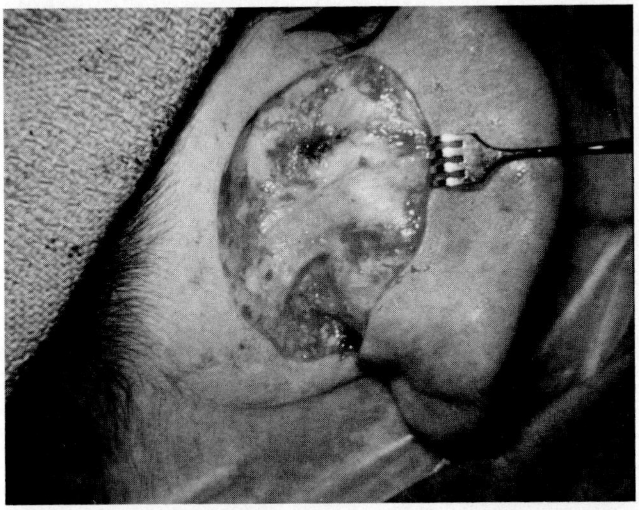

A

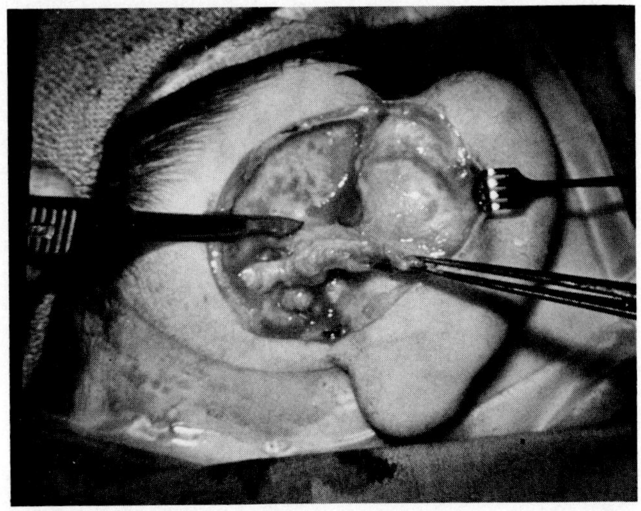

B

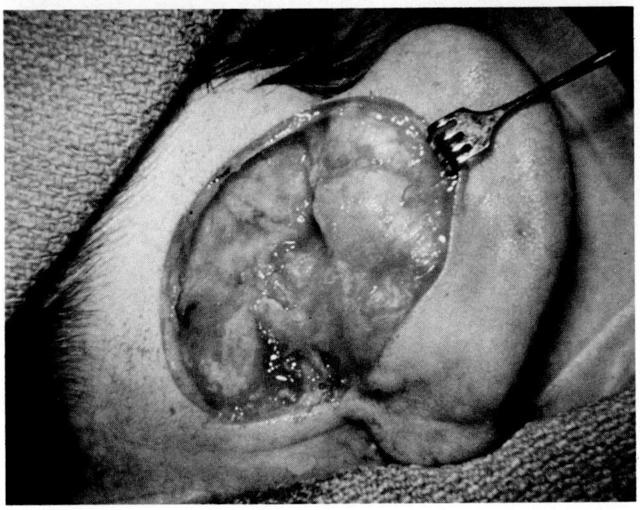

C

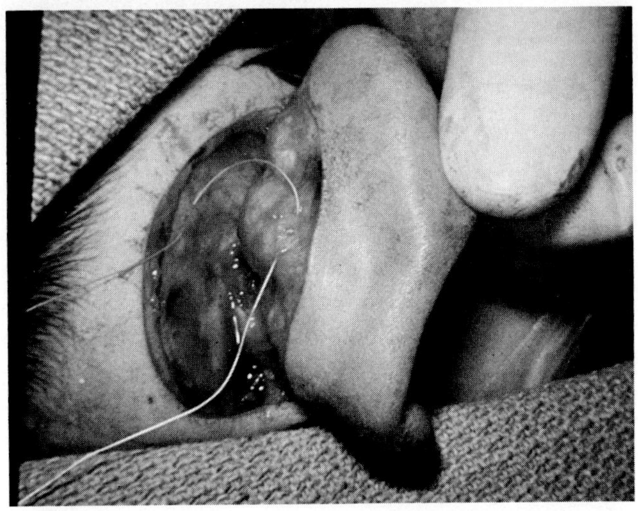

D

Figure 11-13. Conchal repositioning.

A. Postauricular muscle and fibrofatty tissue may create a fulcrum.
B. Excision of postauricular muscle and fibrofatty tissue is an important modification of the technique used by Owens and Delgado, as well as Furnas.
C. Liberal pocket on mastoid fascia.
D. One or two sutures will position concha in pocket.
E. Technique compatible with anthelix suture reconstruction.

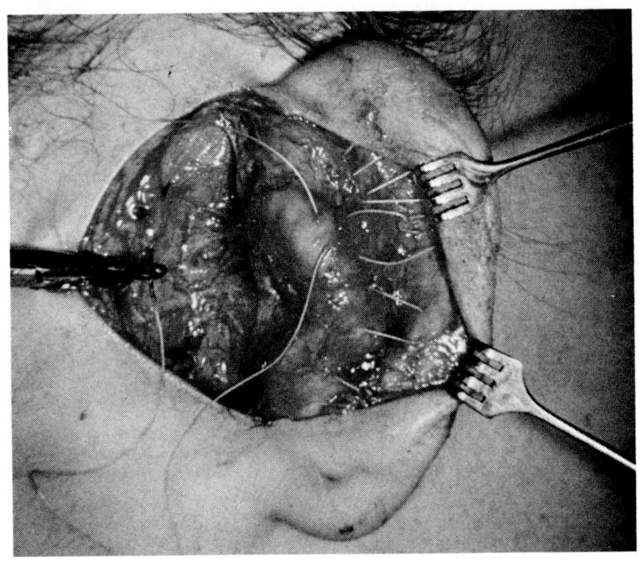

E

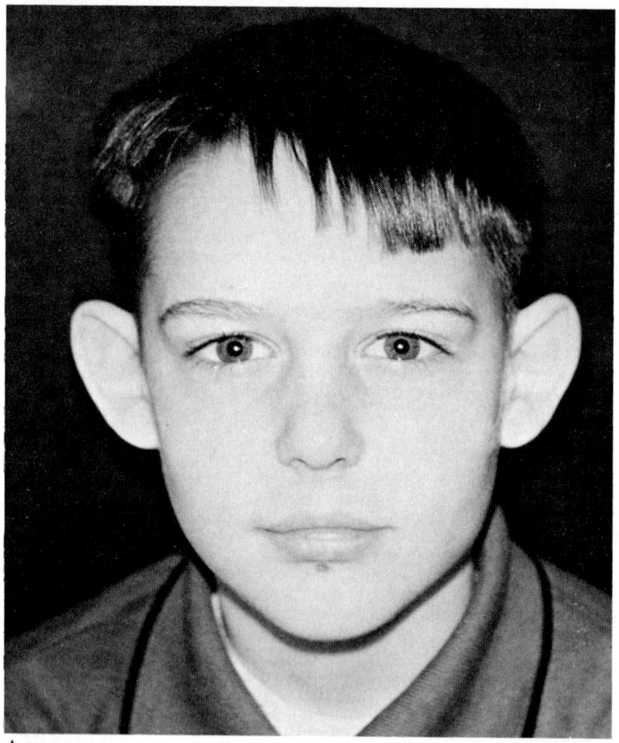

A

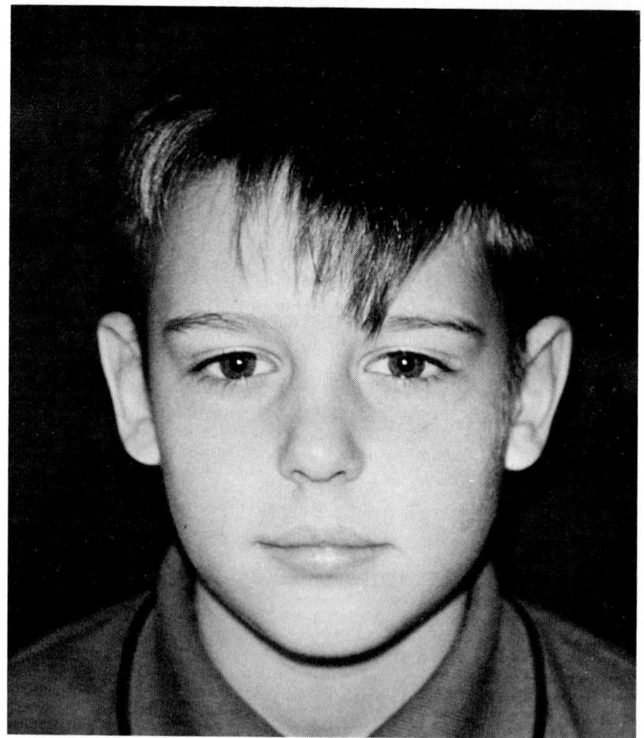

B

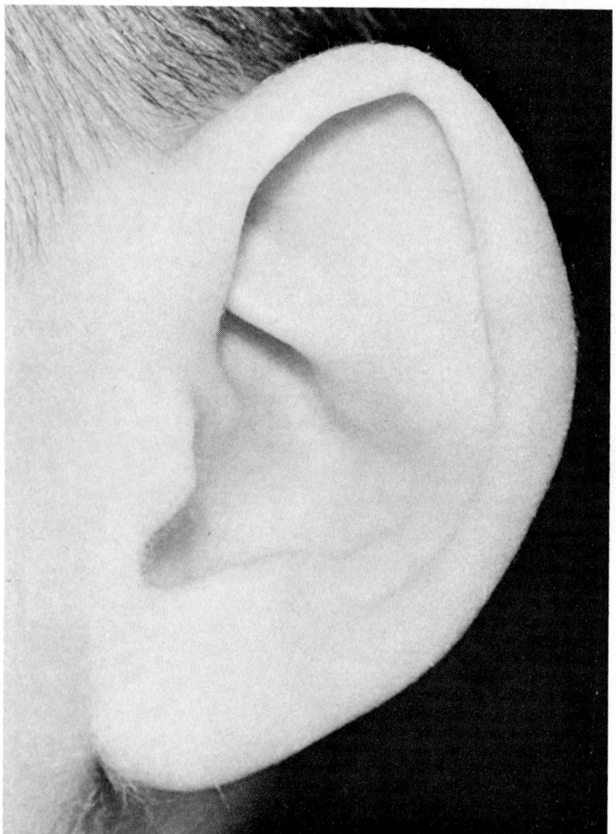

C

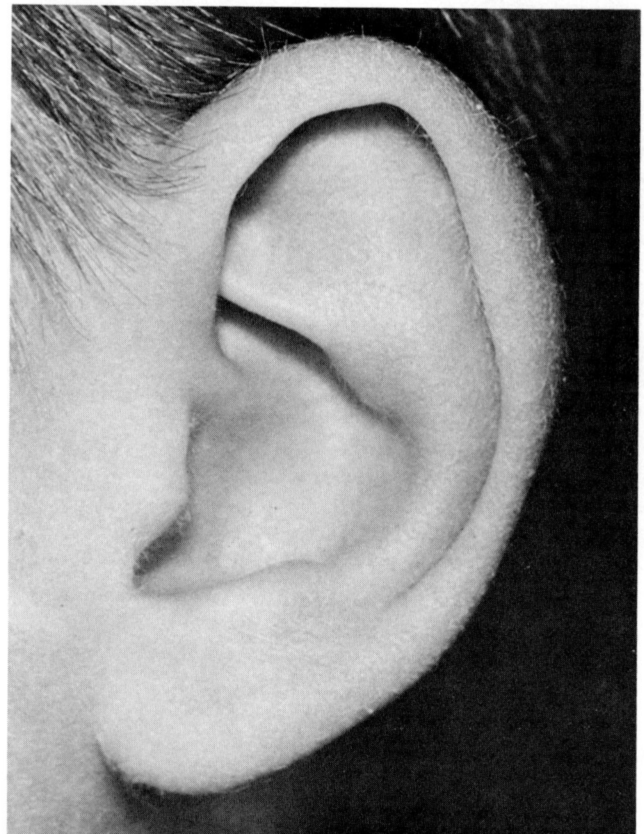

D

Figure 11-14. Combined anthelix reconstruction and conchal repositioning.
A. Preoperative front view.
B. Postoperative front view.
C. Preoperative frontal-oblique view.
D. Postoperative frontal-oblique view.

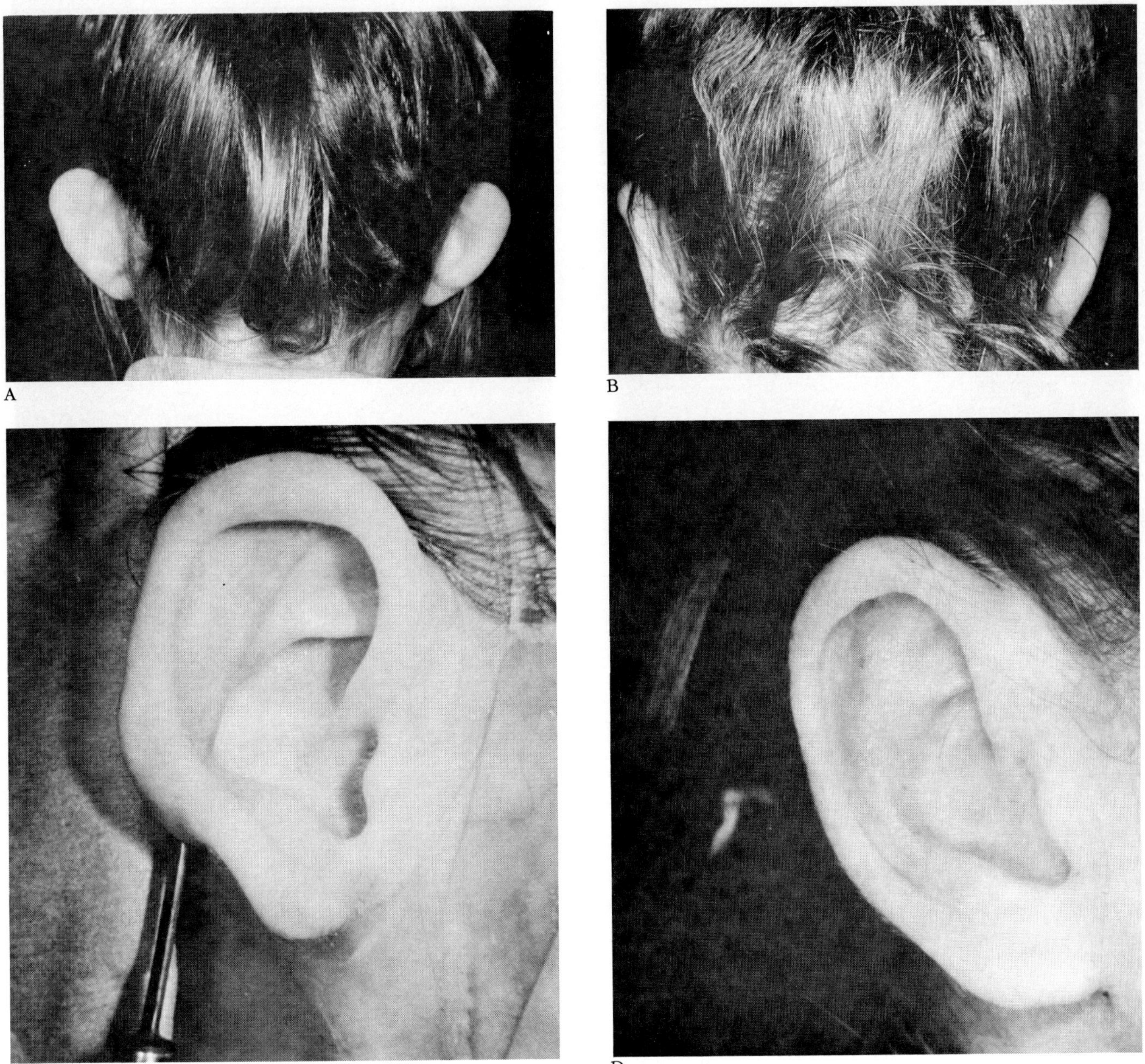

A

B

C

D

Figure 11-15. Combined anthelix reconstruction and conchal repositioning.
A. Preoperative posterior view.
B. Postoperative posterior view.
C. Operative view of anterior scoring.
D. Reconstructed anthelix fold and superior crus.

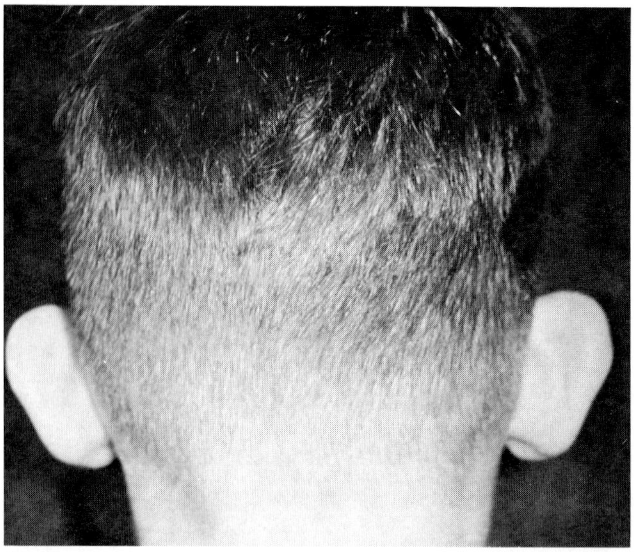

A

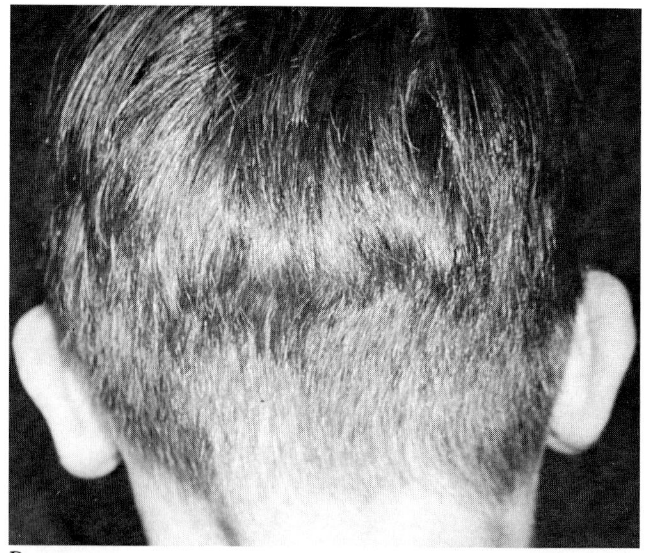

B

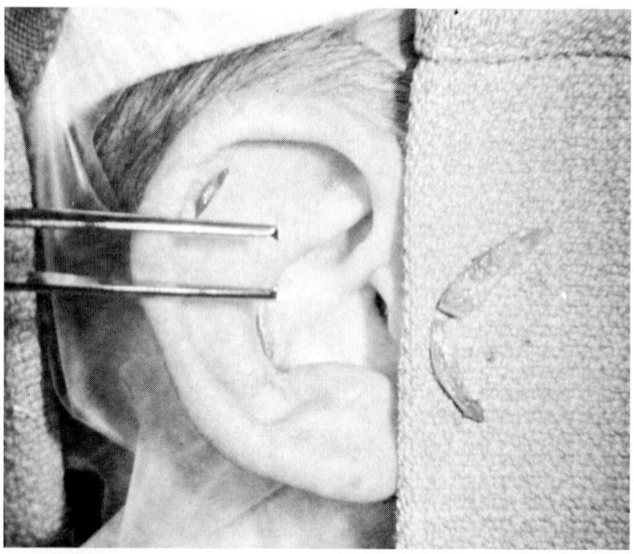

C

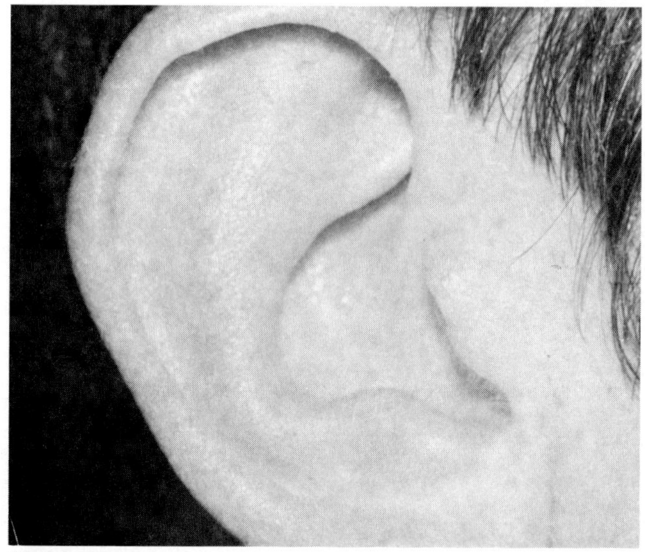

D

Figure 11-16. Combined superior crus reconstruction and conchal reduction.

A. Preoperative posterior view.

B. Posterior view 7 months postoperatively.

C. Operative view of incision for scoring, and specimen from concha.

D. Result 7 years postoperatively.

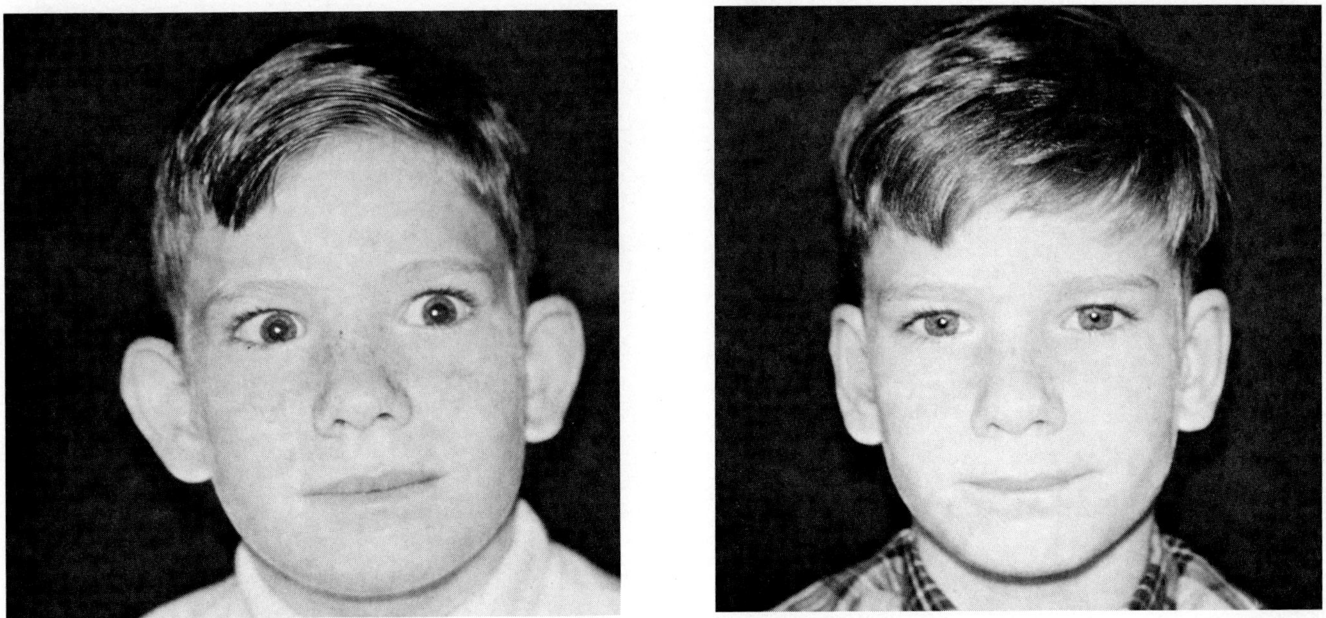

A

B

Figure 11-17. Combined anthelix reconstruction, conchal reduction, and conchal repositioning.
A. Preoperative front view.
B. Postoperative front view.

If flattening of the anthelix is limited to the upper part of the ear, including the superior crus, the approach will vary with the type of conchal deformity. If a setback of the concha is required, the standard posterior exposure is chosen for placing the folding sutures. If conchal reduction is planned and excessive posterior sulcus skin excision or conchal-mastoid sutures are not required, exposure for the folding sutures can be gained through an incision or excision directly behind the affected part, but scars are hidden better in the sulcus. For convenience, the incision for scoring the anterior surface is made higher on the scapha at the lowest part of the deformity.

After the ear prominence has been corrected, additional deformities such as a prominent Darwin's tubercle or a very broad residual scapha can be evaluated and treated, as previously described (Fig. 11-18). Any residual prominence of the lobule should also be corrected at this time. The surgeon should not complete the operation without the sincere feeling that he has reconstructed the very best possible contour, position, and symmetry. Adjustments will become less frequent with experience, but there will be an occasional need. Secondary procedures should be rare.

Skin Closure and Dressing. Posterior wounds are closed in a single layer with a continuous 5-0 plain catgut suture supplemented by interrupted sutures as required to maintain eversion of the edges. Anterior incisions are closed with either nonabsorbable or absorbable 6-0 everting sutures.

The incisions are covered with medicated gauze. Several thicknesses of gauze, trimmed to accommodate the concha, are placed behind the ear, and the anterior recesses are packed with fluffed gauze (Fig. 11-19). The fluff dressing is held lightly in place with a single strip of tape extending from neck to forehead, and mild compression is provided by a soft gauze roll and an Ace bandage, further secured with tape.

POSTOPERATIVE CARE

Most patients, even those requiring general anesthesia, are treated as outpatients. Hospitalized patients are frequently discharged on the day of surgery. Instructions for back elevation, limited activity, and avoidance of sweating are routine. Pain, especially after the first 12 hours, is not a common complaint and may herald a complication.

Normally the compression dressing is maintained for a week after an anthelix reconstruction or conchal reduction. Three or four days is sufficient after simple conchal repositioning except in the very young or uncooperative patient. The dressing is usually quite comfortable, affords good protection from early injury, and may reduce swelling and bruising, but it is not a substitute for good hemostasis and will not prevent a hematoma.

Patients are instructed to avoid traction on the ears for at least a month. Some protection with a stocking cap or other device is recommended for night wear during this period. Cleansing is important, especially in the posterior sulcus, and patients are instructed to accomplish this without displacing the ear. The first postoperative photographs are taken after 4 months and repeated after at least 1 year.

Results and Complications

The described procedures have provided the flexibility needed to correct the majority of prominent ear deformities. They have given a natural appearance to the corrected ear and a predictable degree of retroposition in almost

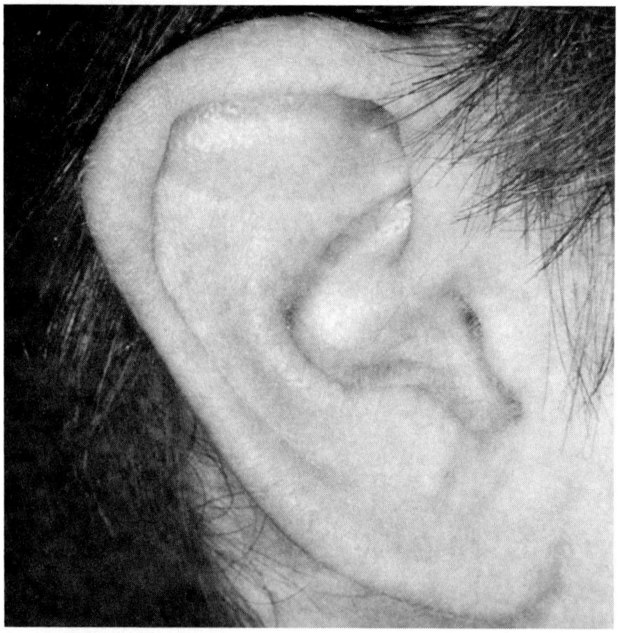

A

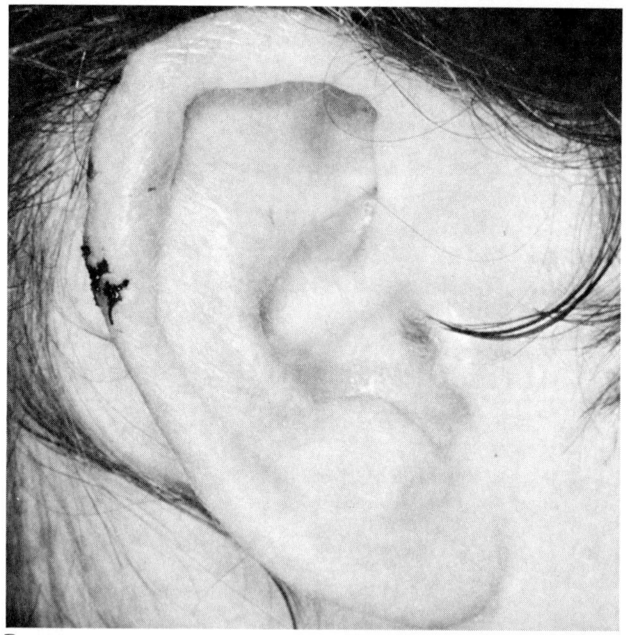

B

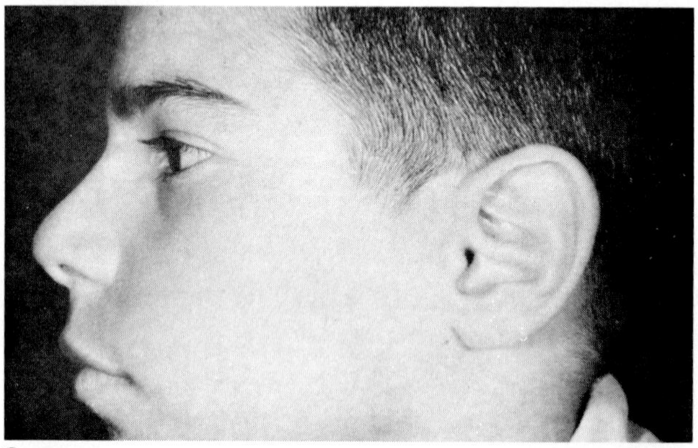

C

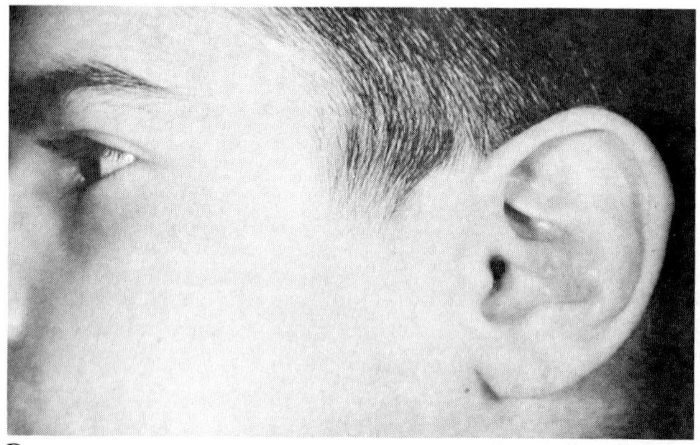

D

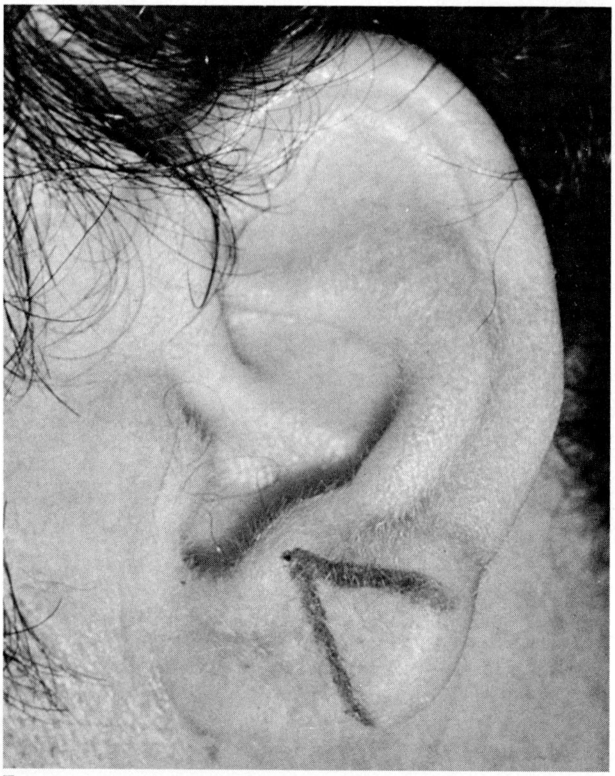

E

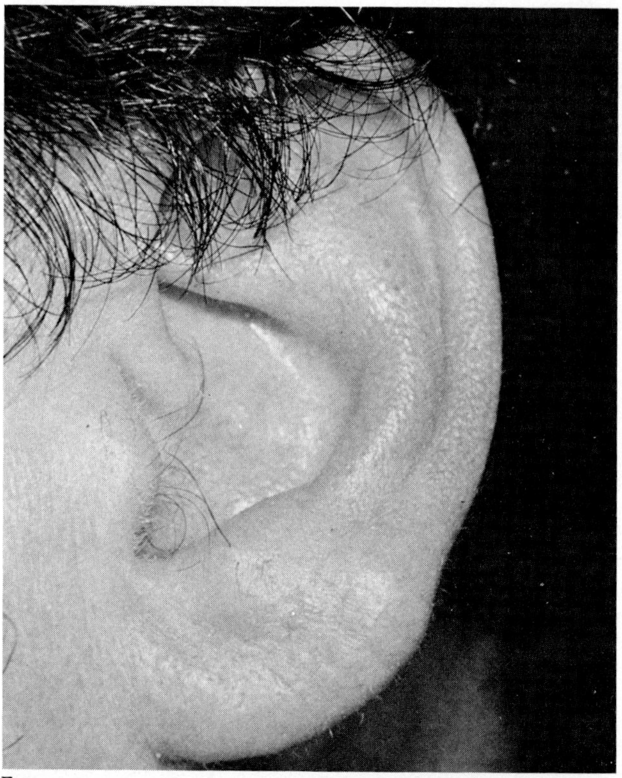

F

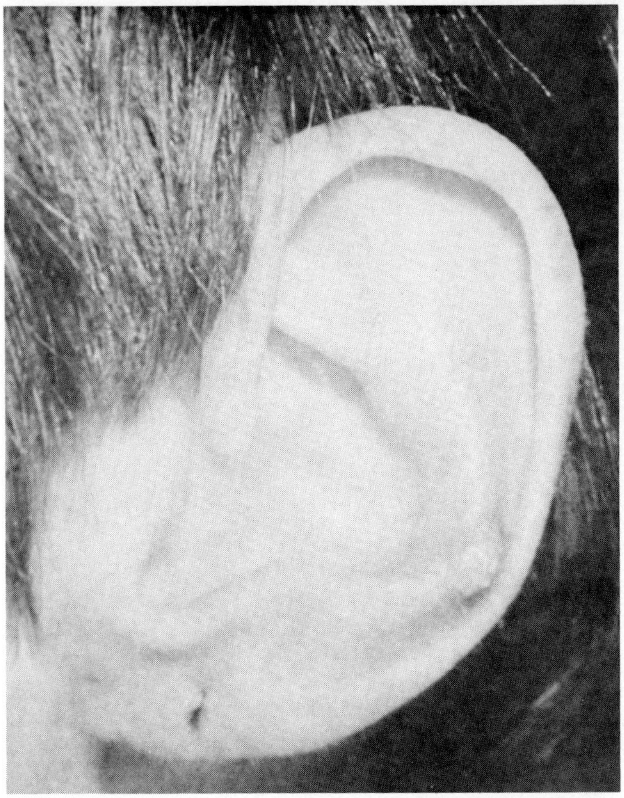

G

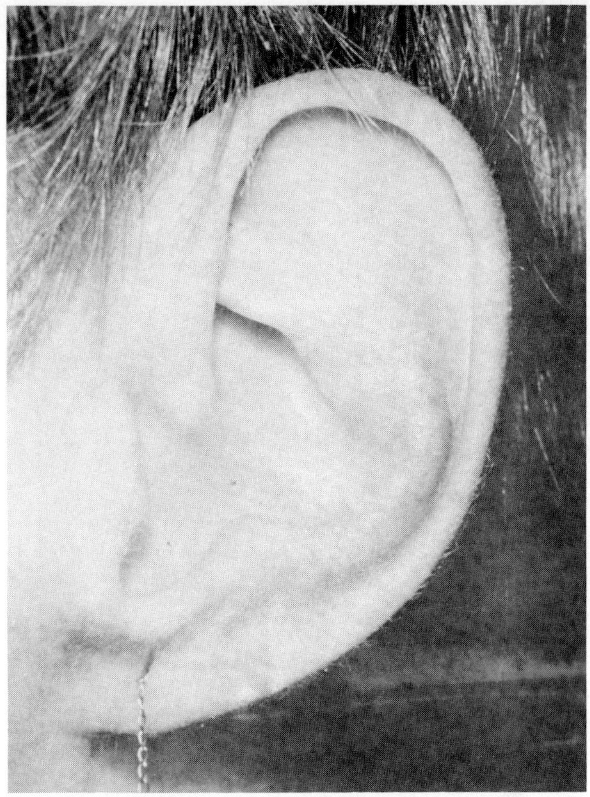

H

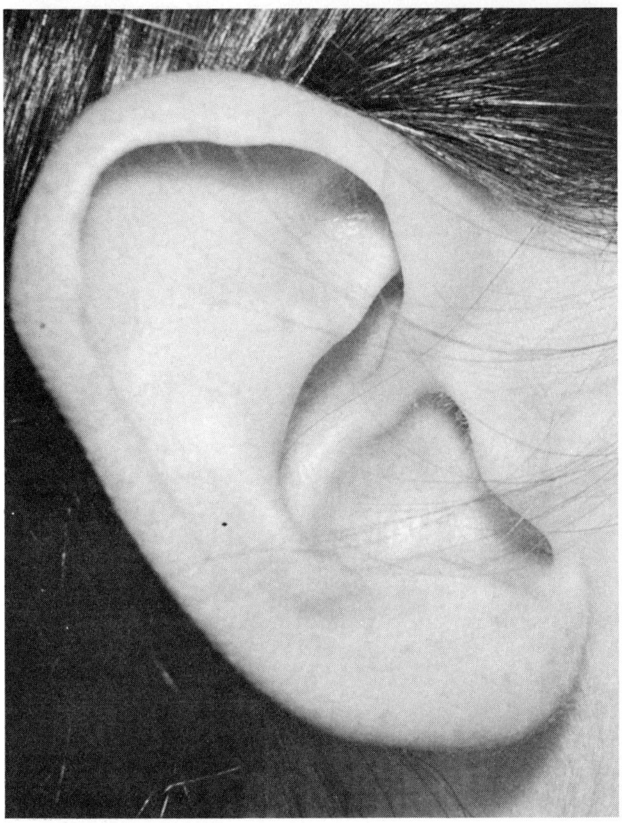

I

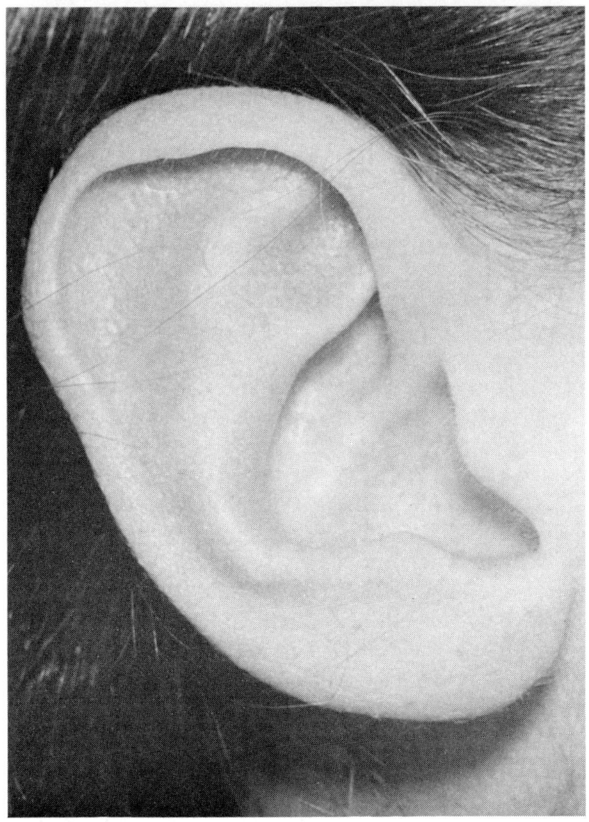

J

Figure 11-18. Miscellaneous deformities, preoperative and postoperative.

A, B. Darwin's tubercle, excised. (Courtesy of J. Hoehn.)
C, D. Transverse bar, excised.
E, F. Large earlobe, wedge reduction.
G, H. Prominent anthelix with chronic infection, cartilage trimmed.
I, J. Borderline enlarged scapha, helped by roll reconstruction (same patient as in Fig. 11-3A).

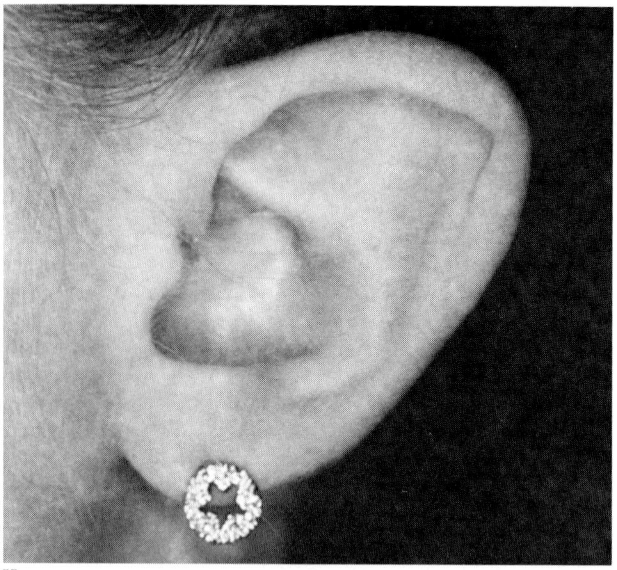

K

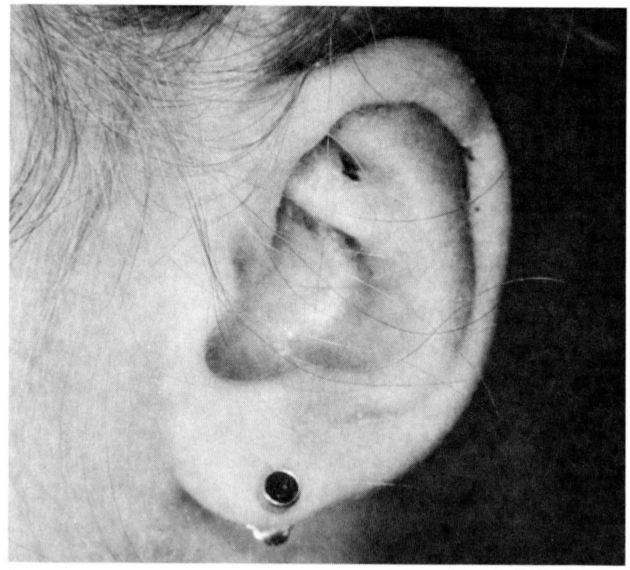

L

Figure 11-18 (continued)
K, L. Large scapha, wedge reduction with relocation of superior crus (same patient as in Fig. 11-2).

every case. The usual operative measurement of 1.8 cm from the anterior surface of the helix to the scalp has rarely exceeded 2 cm in the long-term follow-up.

Combining specific correction of the concha with anthelix reconstruction has obviated the problems of hidden helix and excessively wide anthelix seen with procedures limited to the anthelix. The latter techniques could not routinely match the natural appearance obtained with the composite approach and have been abandoned. Likewise, procedures that require through-and-through incisions to form the anthelix can seldom match the soft anthelix roll achieved with the combined scoring and suture technique. Acute folds and sharp edges are virtually impossible to correct.

Overcorrections and undercorrections still occur occasionally because of human inconsistency on the part of the surgeon, but recurrence of the deformity of the anthelix has not been seen since anterior scoring was added to the suture technique, and there have been no failures of the modified conchal-mastoid suture procedure. The conchal reduction technique has also been totally reliable.

The subcutaneous nodules on the anterior surface of the ear that occurred with Kaye's [12] technique were unfortunate, for this simple procedure gave equally fine contours and control of anthelix folding. It did not provide, however, for the important control of the tail of the helix. Interestingly, there have been no visible nodules associated with the anterior approach to conchal reduction, probably because the knots are buried on the posterior surface. The occasional late extrusion of a permanent suture as a foreign body has been of no significance except for the annoyance for the patient and surgeon. Fibrous fixation has held the correction without exception. This normal fixation accounts for much of the difficulty encountered in secondary procedures.

Secondary Procedures

Recurrence of the deformity may result from early postoperative trauma or a failure of the procedure. Reoperation carries a good prognosis if the cause of the failure is discovered and corrected.

The variety of deformities that can be produced by an inexperienced surgeon or by improper treatment selection is legend (Fig. 11-20). A number of these problems arise with alarming frequency. Most can be prevented, but not all can be corrected. A complete discussion of the specific deformities is beyond the scope of this chapter. They have been detailed elsewhere by the author [6, 7] and are recommended for careful study. Suffice it to say that contour irregularities, overcorrection, undercorrection, and malposition of the reconstructed part are seen most commonly. Fixed irregularities and malposition of the anthelix roll are difficult if not impossible to correct. Undercorrections of almost any type can usually be improved by secondary surgery. Some overcorrections can be revised by release of the fibrous fixation and graft replacement of missing tissues, but the result is seldom completely satisfactory.

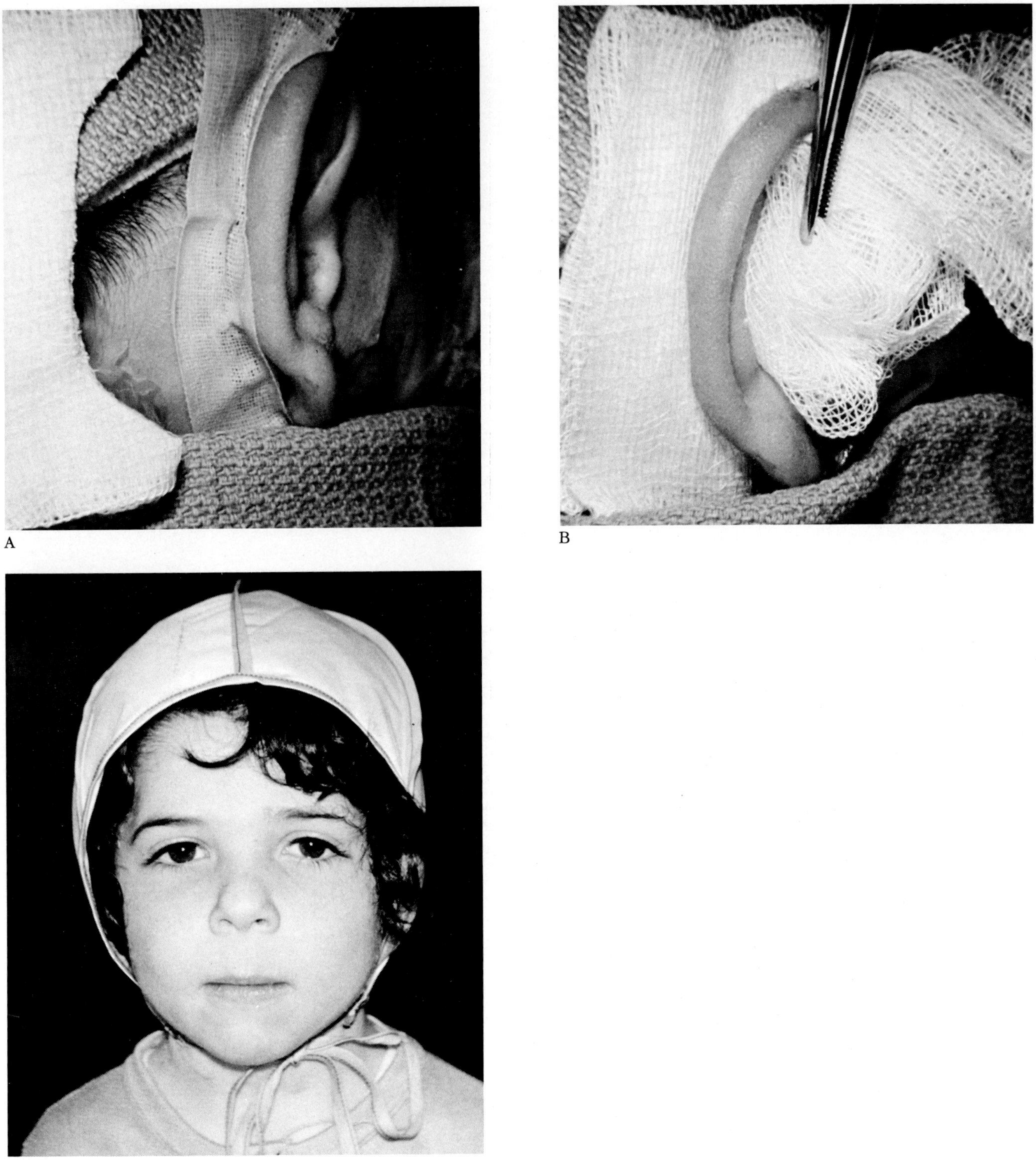

A B C

Figure 11-19. Postoperative protection.
A. Position splinted for safety.
B. Mild compression on all surfaces adds comfort.
C. Night protection advised for 1 month after surgery.

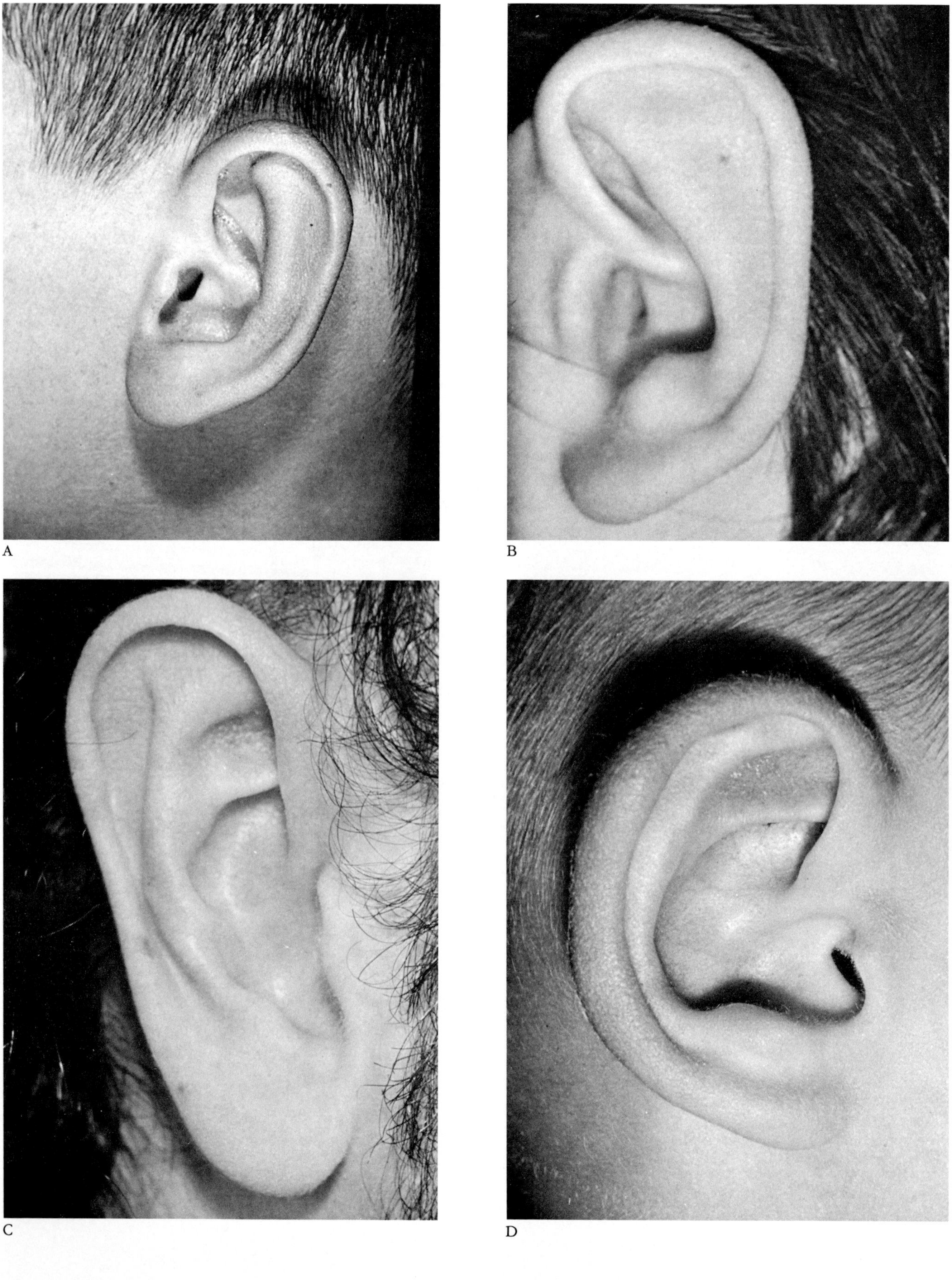

A B C D

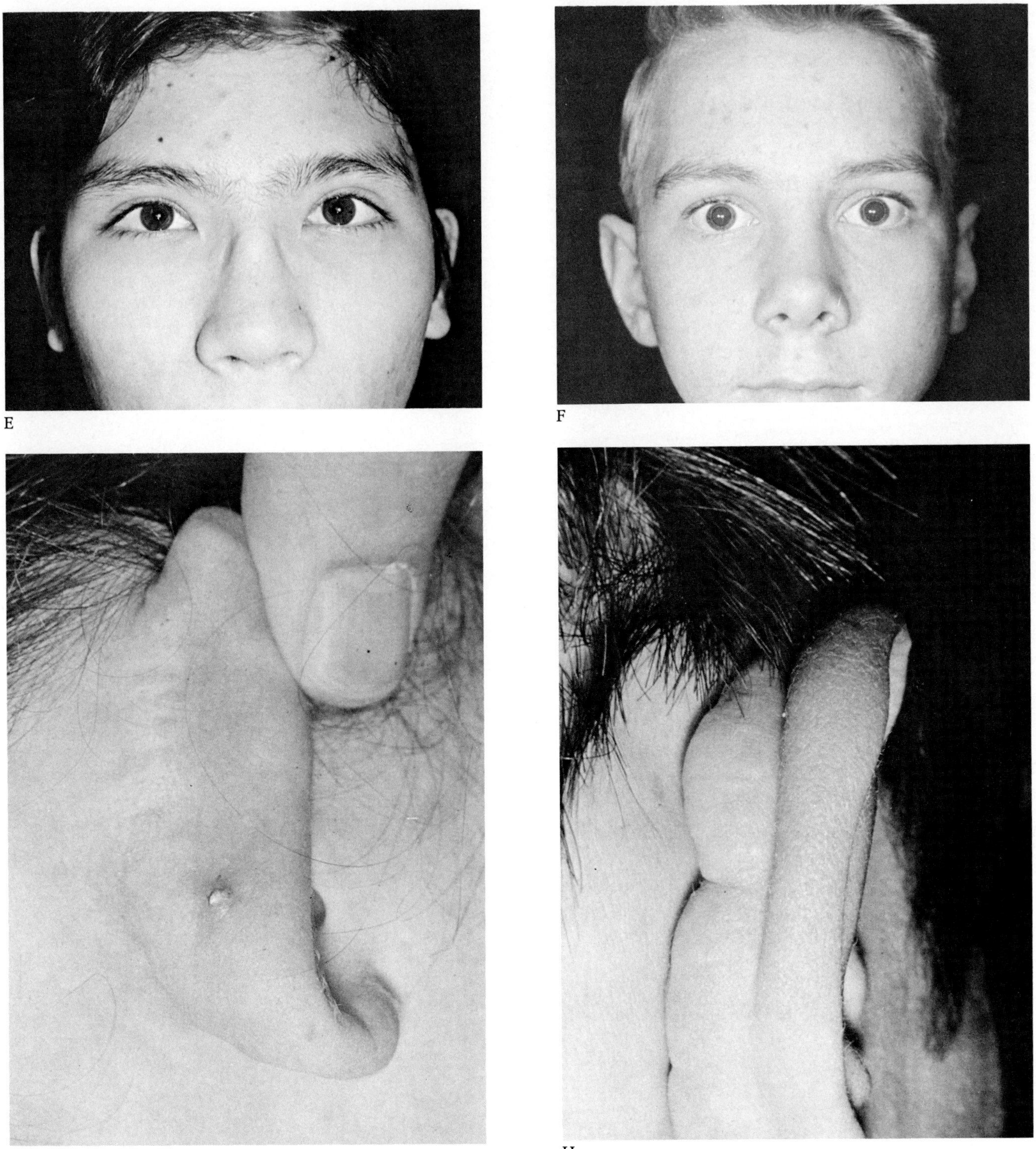

E F G H

Figure 11-20. Complications, iatrogenic.
A. Vertical post, may deform helix rim.
B. Malposition of anthelix.
C. Irregular anthelix.
D. Sharp anthelix.
E. Telephone deformity, relative conchal deficiency.
F. Reverse telephone deformity, relative conchal excess.
G. Suture granuloma and shallow sulcus.
H. Keloid scar, seen only postauricularly or on lobule.

CONCLUSION

Otoplasty for the correction of prominent ears is a complex procedure requiring a careful analysis of the deformity and selection of a treatment plan directed at the specific cause(s).

The patient with this problem usually comes for treatment because of name-calling or social rejection, either real or imagined. Early operation is urged to prevent further or permanent psychic trauma.

Congenital prominence of the ear is commonly due to a failure of the anthelix folding, overgrowth of the concha, malposition of the concha, or a combination of these deformities. The procedures detailed in this chapter have proved to be the most reliable for reconstruction of an ear in the range of normal appearance and have most consistently met the most important challenge: *patient satisfaction.*

REFERENCES

1. Adamson, J. E., Horton, C. E., and Crawford, H. H. The growth pattern of the external ear. *Plast. Reconstr. Surg.* 36:466, 1965.
2. Beernick, J. H., Blocksma, R., and Moore, W. D. The role of the helical tail in cosmetic otoplasty. *Plast. Reconstr. Surg.* 64:115, 1979.
3. Courtiss, E. H., Webster, R. C., and White, M. F. Otoplasty: Direct Surgical Approach. In F. W. Masters and J. R. Lewis, Jr. (eds.), *Symposium on Aesthetic Surgery of the Nose, Ears, and Chin.* St. Louis: Mosby, 1973.
4. Dieffenbach, J. F. *Die operative Chirurgia.* Leipzig: Brockhaus, 1845.
5. Elliott, R. A. Otoplasty for prominent ears. *Surg. World News* June, 1965.
6. Elliott, R. A. Complications in the treatment of prominent ears. *Clin. Plast. Surg.* 5:479, 1978.
7. Elliott, R. A. Otoplasty. In E. H. Courtiss (ed.), *Aesthetic Plastic Surgery: Trouble—How to Avoid It and How to Treat It.* St. Louis: Mosby, 1978.
8. Elliott, R. A., and Hoehn, J. G. Otoplasty. *Int. Micr. J. Aesthetic Plast. Surg.* 1972A.
9. Furnas, D. W. Correction of prominent ears by concha-mastoid sutures. *Plast. Reconstr. Surg.* 42:189, 1968.
10. Furnas, D. W. Correction of prominent ears with multiple sutures. *Clin. Plast. Surg.* 5:491, 1978.
11. Georgiade, N. G., and Still, J. History of Otoplasty for Correction of Prominent Ears. In F. W. Masters and J. R. Lewis, Jr. (eds.), *Symposium on Aesthetic Surgery of the Nose, Ears, and Chin.* St. Louis: Mosby, 1973.
12. Kaye, B. L. A simplified method for correcting the prominent ear. *Plast. Reconstr. Surg.* 40:44, 1967.
13. Luckett, W. H. A new operation for prominent ears based on the anatomical deformity. *Surg. Gynecol. Obstet.* 10:635, 1910.
14. Mustardé, J. C. The correction of prominent ears using simple mattress sutures. *Br. J. Plast. Surg.* 16:170, 1963.
15. Owens, N., and Delgado, D. D. The management of outstanding ears. *South. Med. J.* 58:32, 1965.
16. Spira, M., et al. Correction of the principal deformities causing prominent ears. *Plast. Reconstr. Surg.* 44:150, 1969.
17. Stenstrom, S. J. A "natural" technique for correction of congenitally prominent ears. *Plast. Reconstr. Surg.* 32:509, 1963.
18. Webster, G. V. The tail of the helix as a key to otoplasty. *Plast. Reconstr. Surg.* 44:455, 1969.

BIBLIOGRAPHY

Elliott, R. A. Complications in the treatment of prominent ears. *Clin. Plast. Surg.* July, 1978.

Elliott, R. A. Otoplasty. In E. H. Courtiss (ed.), *Aesthetic Plastic Surgery: Trouble—How to Avoid It and How to Treat It.* St. Louis: Mosby, 1978.

Furnas, D. W. *Deformities of the External Ear. Clin. Plast. Surg.* July, 1978.

Masters, F. W., and Lewis, J. R., Jr. *Symposium on Aesthetic Surgery of the Nose, Ears, and Chin.* St. Louis: Mosby, 1973.

McDowell, A. J. Goals in otoplasty for protruding ears. *Plast. Reconstr. Surg.* 41:17, 1968.

12. Aesthetic Surgery of the Malar Region

Ulrich T. Hinderer
Juan del Rio Legarreta

The oblique profile of the face is very important in human relationship. This profile has been called the "social profile" by Agban [1]. The shape and size of the malar region dominates this lateral segment of the middle third of the face. High cheekbones are not only a characteristic of some ethnic groups but are considered a mark of beauty in the Western world. In show business, it is common practice to darken the submalar region in order to create the illusion of prominent cheekbones. However, excessively high cheekbones can give a sickly appearance to the face, making the eyes look sunken. In contrast, a flat zygomatic area confers an appearance of a long, thin face. A well-equilibrated malar region is essential for a pleasing harmony of the whole face.

In profileplasty, the preoperative evaluation of the face should include the tridimensional relationship of each segment with respect to the opposite side and to the whole facial unit, both at rest and in active expression. Prominent cheekbones can act as compensation for an exceptionally hypertrophic mandible that would make the face look square if left unbalanced. The prominence or flatness of the zygomatic regions can also affect the nose, giving it a more or less dominant characteristic, and in the same manner influence the width and prominence of the frontal region. Malar implants can compensate for an excessively conspicuous submalar zone as well as for eventual resection of the fat pad of Bichat.

In addition to these advantages, malar implants can be beneficial in the rejuvenation of the aging face as part of a rhytidectomy procedure. In young patients in whom profileplasty is planned, insertion of malar implants permits postponement of rhytidectomy for some time, since they produce not only better facial equilibrium but also a softer face and a younger appearance. If a rhytidectomy is done subsequently, the result is better. Malar implants are also indicated in the treatment of various congenital anomalies, Treacher Collins syndrome, posttraumatic depressions due to fracture or osteomyelitis of the malar, and hypoplasia of the maxilla.

HISTORY

In 1965 and 1967, Hinderer described the subperiosteal insertion of malar prostheses for the treatment of congenital anomalies, asymmetries, and traumatic depressions [3, 4]. In September 1971 Spadafora [14] as well as Hinderer [5] published reports of the correction of flat cheekbones as a purely aesthetic procedure to improve facial aesthetics. Spadafora described the use of polyethylene prostheses, inserted through an oblique preauricular incision and a subperiosteal tunnel along the zygomatic arch. Hinderer [6, 7] subsequently added the insertion through the rhytidectomy and blepharoplasty incision as well as the vestibular approach. In 1974 Jabaley [11] discussed the transoral approach and in the same year Gonzalez-Ulloa [2] placed implants supraperiosteally. Also in 1974 Stark [15] referred to possible damage of the zygomatic ramus of the facial nerve and eventual demineralization of the underlying bone. In 1976 Ribeiro [13] summarized his experience in giving preference to the blepharoplasty approach, which is also the choice of Agban [1].

PREOPERATIVE EVALUATION

The clinical and photographic preoperative examinations place special emphasis on the oblique projection, which defines how much improvement the patient can derive from the procedure. If desired, an x-ray study and cephalometry can be added. A plaster of paris mask can be employed using two reference lines, one from the lateral canthus to the angle of the mouth and the other from the base of the nostril to the tragus. These two lines divide the face into four quadrants. The implant should be placed adjacent to the intersection in the posterosuperior quadrant. This ideal location is traced on the face of the patient immediately prior to surgery (Fig. 12-1).

Figure 12-1. Two lines divide the face into four quadrants. One goes from the lateral canthus to the angle of the mouth. The second goes from the base of the nostril to the tragus. The implant should be placed in the posterosuperior quadrant, just adjacent to these lines.

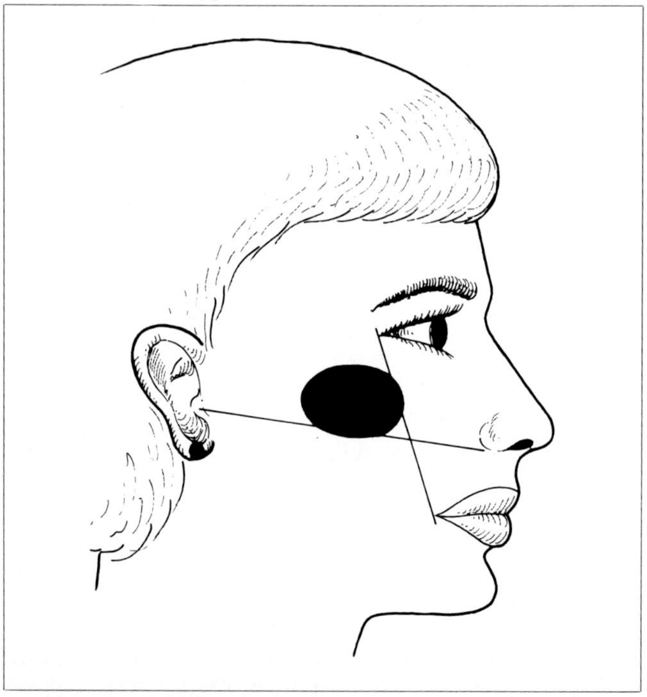

IMPLANT MATERIALS

Although theoretically any tissue-compatible material can be employed—polyethylene, acrylics, bone grafts, cartilage grafts, dermis grafts, fat or composite grafts, etc.—we believe that the ideal material for the implant is silicone [5].

We agree with Spadafora [14] that true bony defects should be corrected only with solid or semisolid materials. From our experience with heterologous bone grafts some 20 years ago, most reabsorbed and were thus inferior to silicone. The same applies to other graft materials. Unfortunately, autogenous tissues have an erratic rate of resorption and they also require additional incisions at the donor site. Besides, they cannot be expected to provide as smooth a surface and as impalpable a contour as the silicone implants. Autogenous grafts tend to leave a "bumpy" or "cobblestone" appearance.

In cases of facial asymmetry, it might be convenient to place implants of different sizes or else to carve the prostheses preoperatively or even intraoperatively in order to provide a perfect fit.

We employ almost exclusively our prosthesis developed by Heyer-Schulte, which is available in two sizes. This range of sizes is quite adequate and the smaller size is by far the more widely utilized. The prosthesis has a concave depth that fits perfectly over the malar bone, and the fit is enhanced by the pliability and consistency of the silicone employed. Alterations in prosthesis shape can be made easily by carving with a scalpel, a file, a rasp, or dermabrasion. The implants come perforated and thus allow an invasion of connective tissue, which occurs a few days after insertion, resulting in complete stability.

SURGICAL APPROACHES

There are numerous incisions that can be used for insertion of malar implants, each with distinct advantages and disadvantages (Fig. 12-2).

Direct Approach

A direct approach with an incision immediately over the malar area is advisable only when there are scars of the malar region that must be corrected simultaneously.

Rhinoplasty Lateral Osteotomy Approach

Although we tried this approach some time ago, we consider it inadvisable because of the proximity of the infraorbital nerve, which can be subject to surgical injuries. At the same time the distance to be tunneled is excessive and makes the procedure cumbersome.

Conjunctival and Blepharoplasty Approach

Agban [1] reported a conjunctival approach, which can be used for the insertion of small prostheses. We prefer to insert the implant through a blepharoplasty incision,

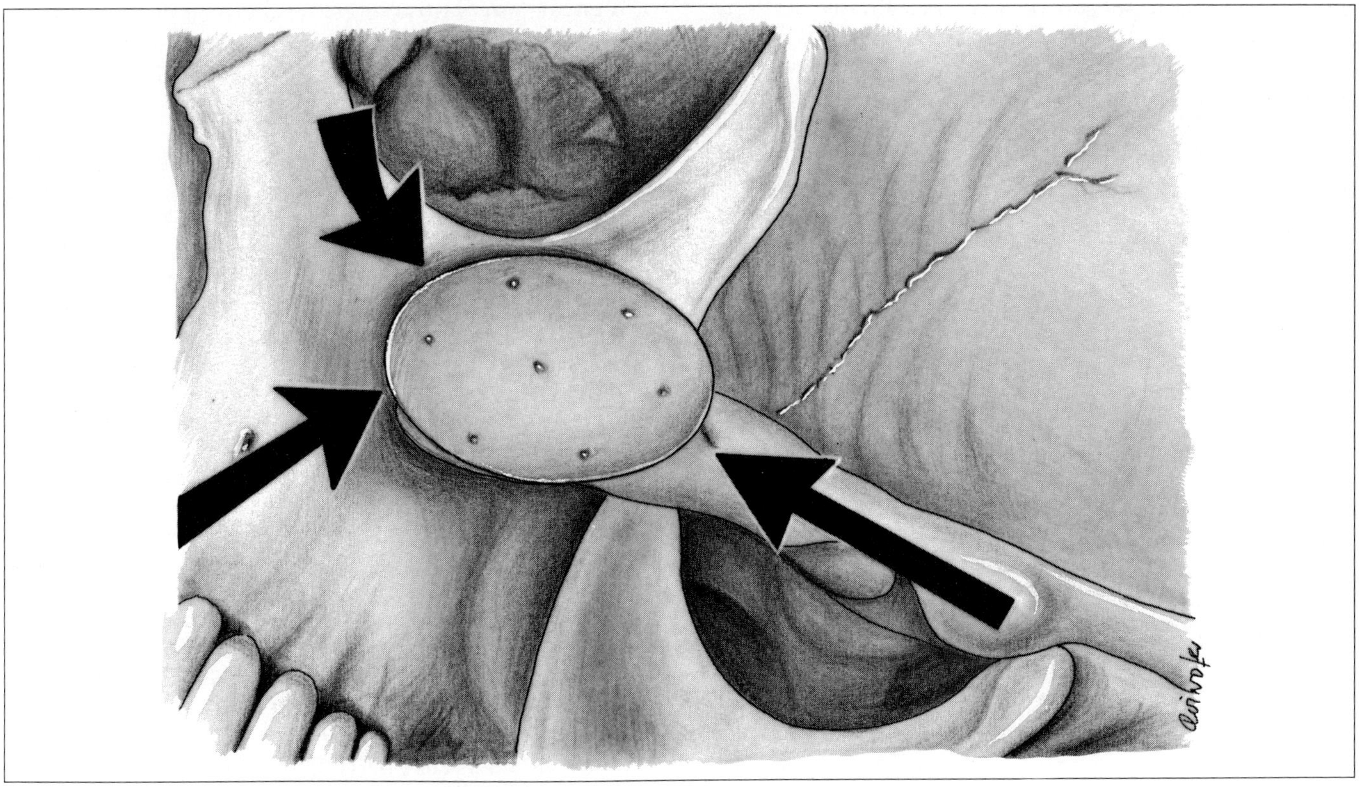

Figure 12-2. The three most commonly used approaches for insertion of malar prostheses are the oral approach, the blepharoplasty approach, and the rhytidectomy approach. The route followed by the implant to reach the correct site is depicted by arrows in the figure.

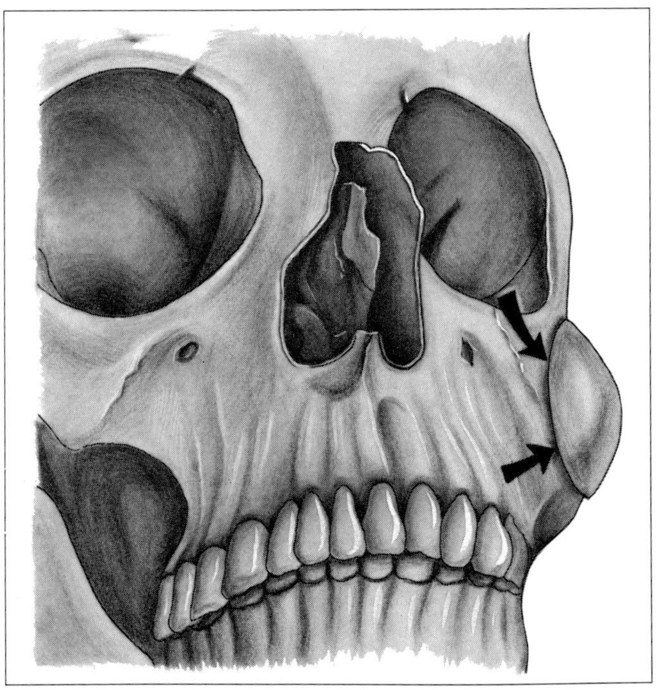

Figure 12-3. Front oblique view of skull with implant in place. Blepharoplasty approach and oral approach are depicted by arrows.

which is easier and offers better exposure. After adequate hemostasis the prosthesis is inserted under direct visual control, using a fiberoptic or other suitable elevator (Fig. 12-3). This incision provides for a wider field and permits the insertion of large implants to increase the volume of the maxillary region and to confer some appearance of depth to the orbit. We advocate this approach in the following cases: (1) when patients are undergoing a simultaneous blepharoplasty; (2) when patients have traumatic sequelae of the lower lid, such as scarring with or without ectropion; and (3) when there are traumatic sequelae of the maxilla.

Rhytidectomy Approach

We prefer this technique whenever a rhytidectomy is performed, with or without a simultaneous blepharoplasty. The rhytidectomy approach is quicker and has greater ease of insertion. We have never observed, up to now, any injury of the zygomatic or frontal branches of the facial nerve.

Oral Approach

Whenever augmentation of the malar area is the only procedure to be performed or when it is related to other profileplasty techniques, such as mentoplasty or rhinoplasty, then the oral approach is preferred.

SURGICAL TECHNIQUE

Blepharoplasty Approach

After a normal subciliary incision, the fibers of the orbicularis muscle are separated by blunt dissection down to the lateral third of the orbital rim. An incision is made on the periosteum, and the implant is inserted folded along its longitudinal axis. Agban [1] designed a custom-molded implant with a shallow furrow at the base. The furrow preserved the infraorbital nerve from damage. The dissection of the subperiosteal pocket should be sufficiently ample for placement of the prosthesis, but not so large as to allow displacement. The tunnel should be just wide enough to permit insertion of the folded implant. This dissection of the periosteum will also elevate the insertions of the quadratus labii superioris and the zygomatic muscle.

Since the entry route to the subperiosteal cavity is narrower than the implant, its position is stable and neither the periosteum nor the orbicularis muscle needs to be sutured. An extremely large periosteal cavity will make the implant excessively mobile. In this event, an external fixation should be provided, a similar implant being placed on the overlying skin and the two prostheses joined through the skin with a 4-0 nylon suture (Fig. 12-4).

If any eyelid skin is to be excised, it should always be done *after* insertion of the implant. Since skin distention is caused by the bulge of the implant and is difficult to predict, the consequent danger of producing an iatrogenic ectropion is very real.

The eyelid skin is then sutured with 6-0 interrupted sutures. Finally, an antiseptic ointment is applied to the lower conjunctival sac and chamomile-soaked gauzes are applied over the eyelid. These gauzes are slightly antiseptic and prevent the formation of crusts. Since the gauzes can be removed momentarily whenever the patient wants to see, the sensation of claustrophobia is also avoided.

Rhytidectomy Approach

After the dissection of the facial skin up to the zygomatic area is completed, the subcutaneous tissue is incised bluntly with delicate scissors, approximately ½ cm lateral to the union of the zygomatic arch and the malar bone (Fig. 12-5). From this point on a tunnel is elevated, going along this arch toward the malar area.

In the rhytidectomy approach direct visual control helps to prevent damage to the branches of the facial nerve. These can be easily identified and protected using blunt elevators. If desired, a nerve stimulator can also be used as well as loupe magnification. The periosteum of the malar bone is raised from its union to the zygomatic arch with sufficient amplitude to accommodate the implant, which is inserted folded on itself. Once the implant is in place, the prosthesis is unfolded. Its position should then be stable enough not to warrant fixation. The results from this procedure can be dramatic (Fig. 12-6).

Oral Approach

A 1-cm incision is made in the vestibular mucosa, immediately below the upper gingival sulcus, at the level of the canine. A tunnel is then dissected bluntly between the quadratus labii superioris and the zygomatic muscle, going first upward and then laterally until the malar bone is reached. Immediately below the mucosa a small branch of the facial nerve can usually be found, running transversely toward the upper lip. This nerve should be dissected carefully. The malar periosteum is then incised, creating a subperiosteal space, and elevated by means of a periosteal elevator (Fig. 12-7). We then insert an Aufricht elevator to permit visualization of the bone surface and to control the width of the subperiosteal space, which must be just wide enough to accommodate the implant. The implant is inserted folded with a Halsted forceps, which is opened once inside. The position is controlled, and the mucosal incision is closed with some 4-0 Vicryl stitches.

Figure 12-4. An excessively mobile implant can be stabilized by suturing a similar one to it through the overlying skin.

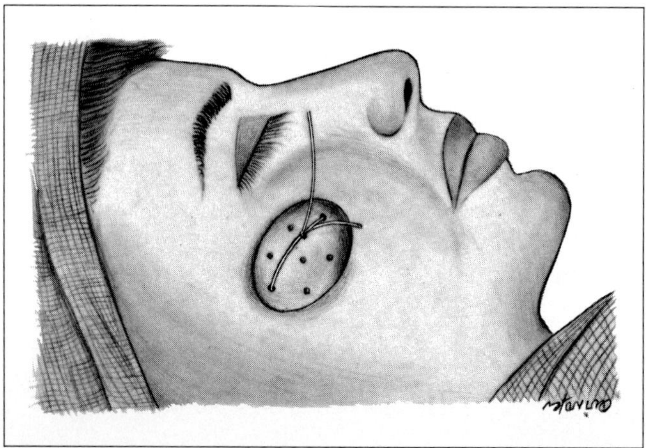

Figure 12-5. After blunt separation of the subcutaneous tissue over the zygomatic arch, a tunnel is dissected over it to the malar area. The implant is inserted folded and then, once in place, unfolded.

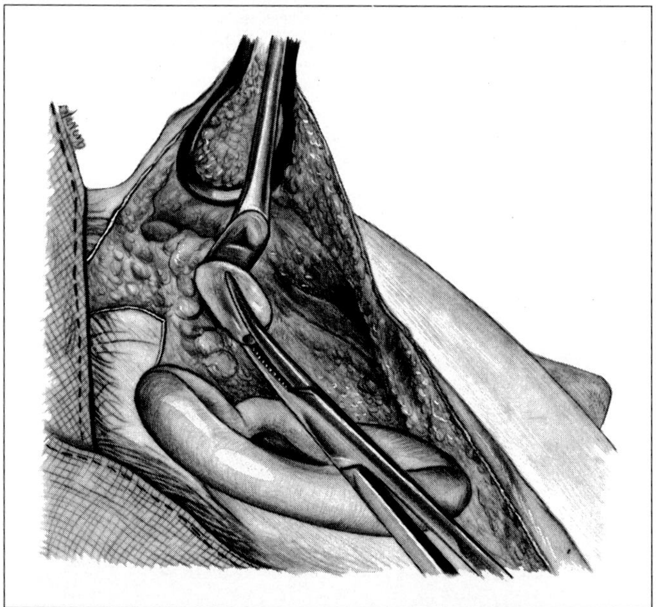

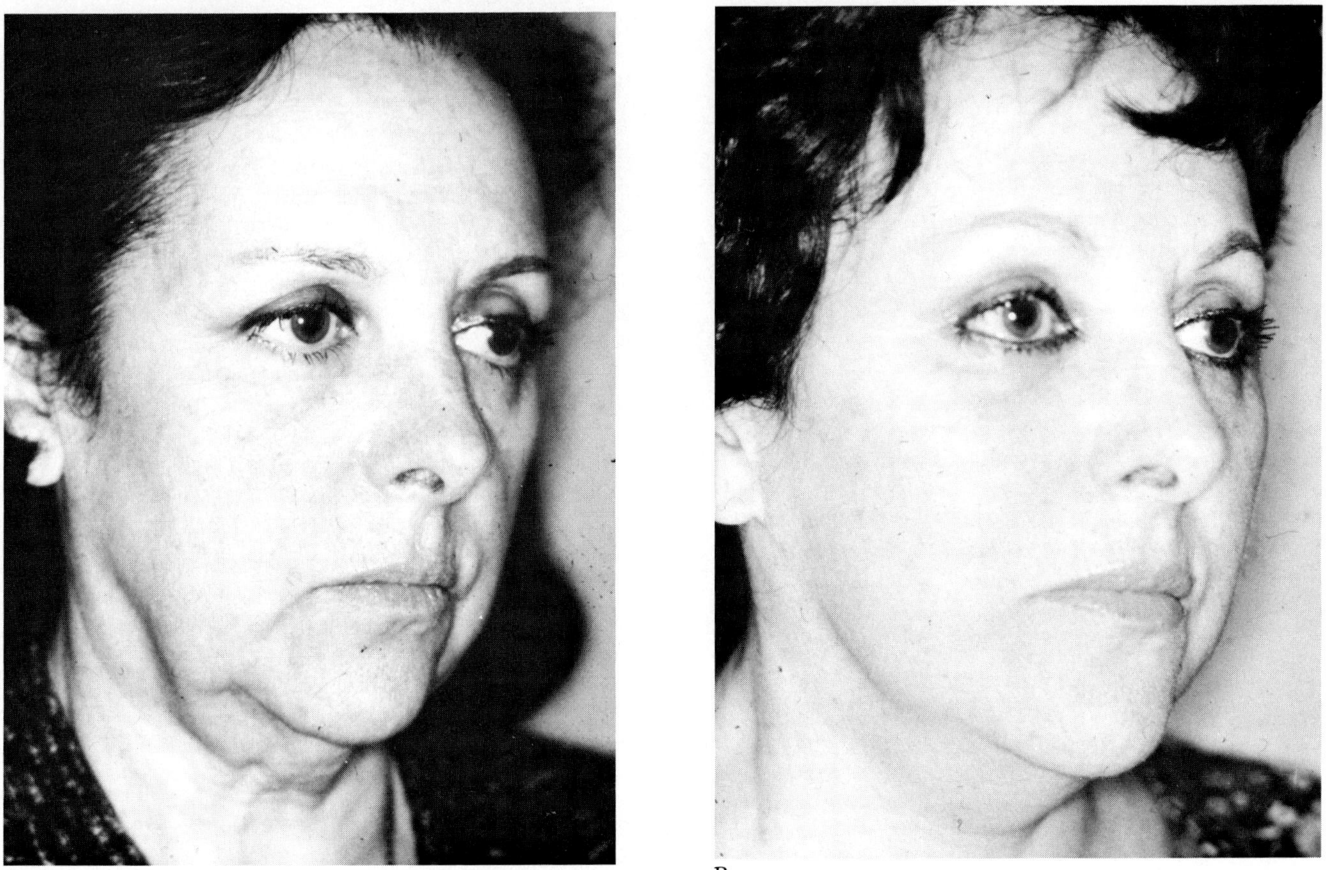

A B

Figure 12-6
A, B. Oblique preoperative and postoperative views of a 50-year-old patient. A rhytidectomy, blepharoplasty, and malar insertion through rhytidectomy approach have been performed. Note change in contralateral malar prominence.

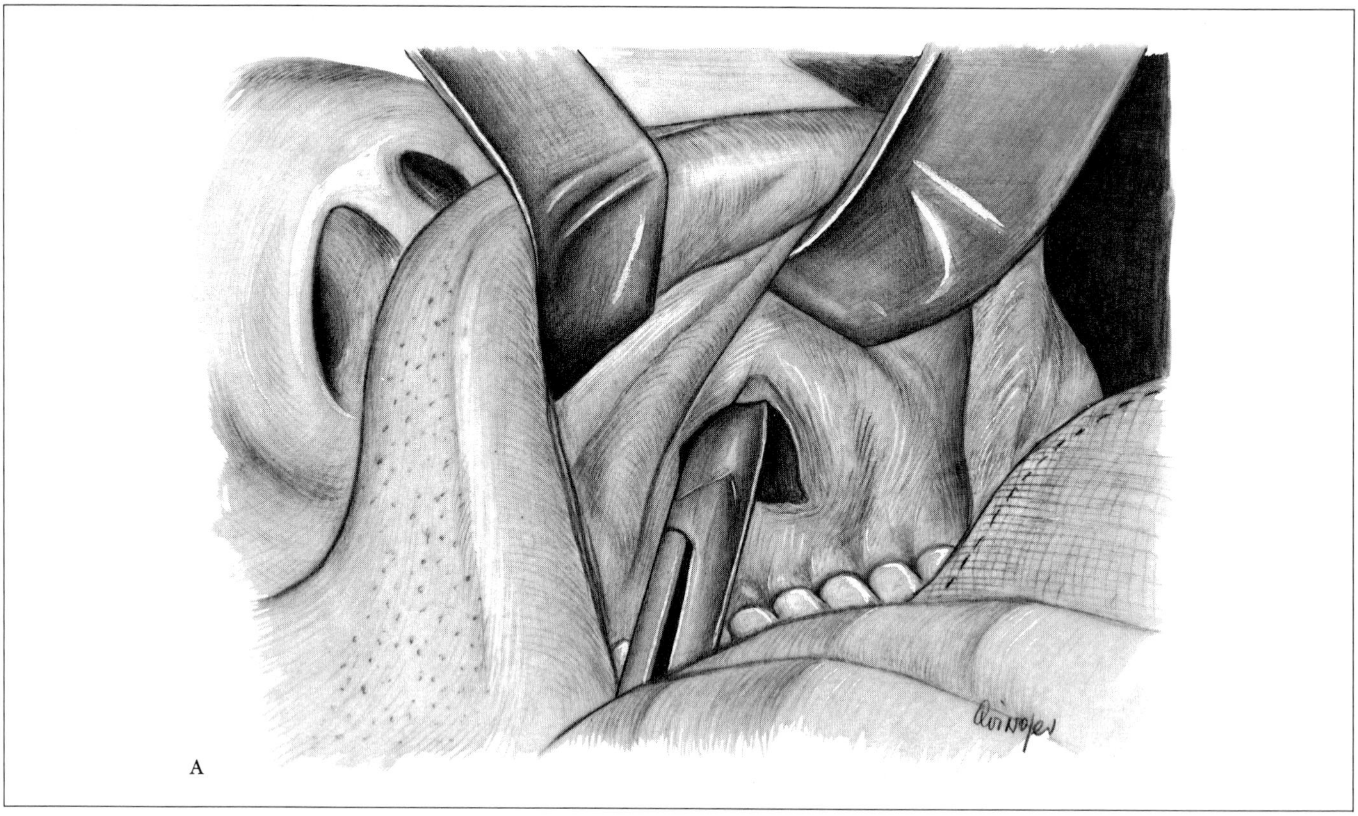

A

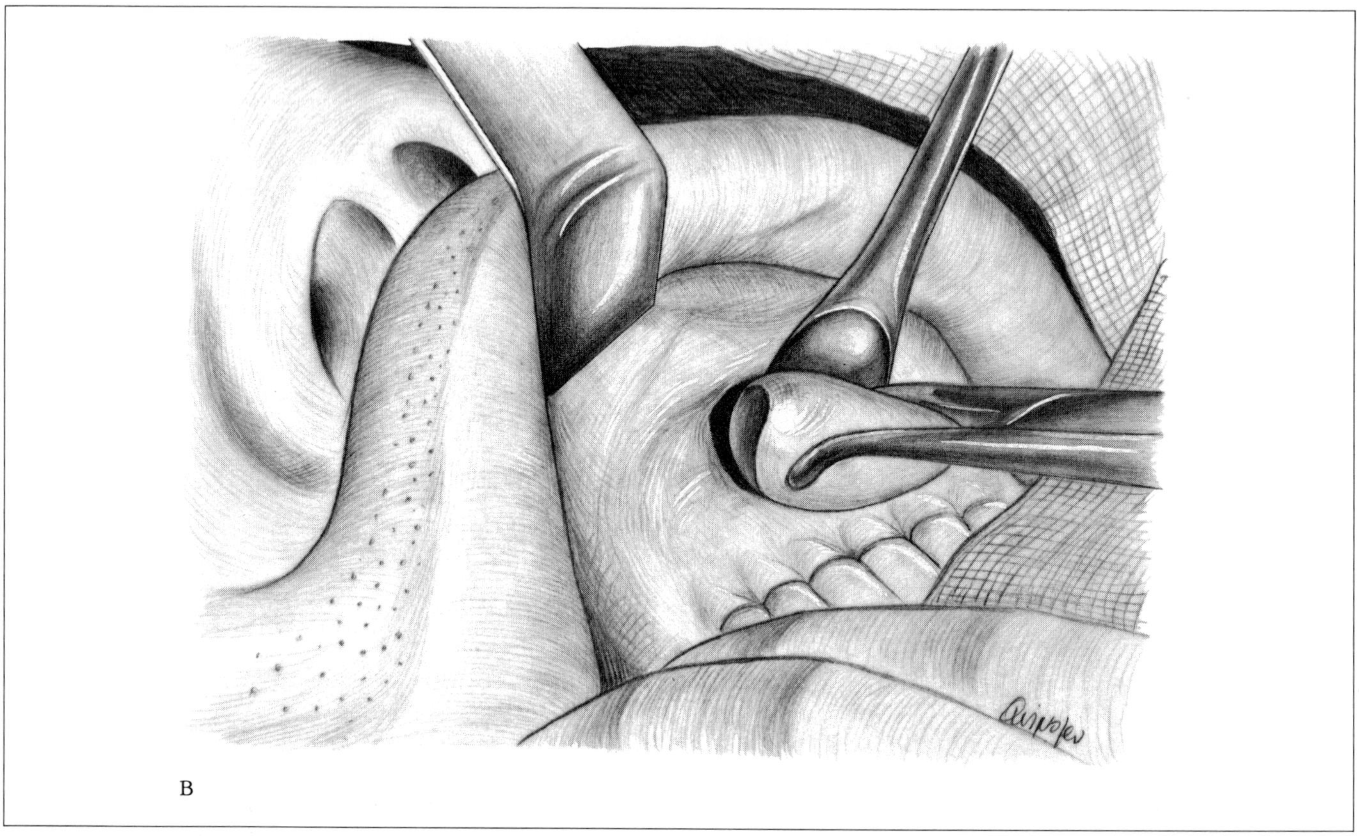

B

Figure 12-7

A. Through an incision in the vestibular mucosa, a tunnel is dissected bluntly, upward and laterally, up to the malar bone.

B. The malar periosteum is incised with a periosteal elevator and a subperiosteal space created. An Aufricht elevator is inserted to permit proper visualization of the cavity. The implant is folded on itself with Halsted forceps.

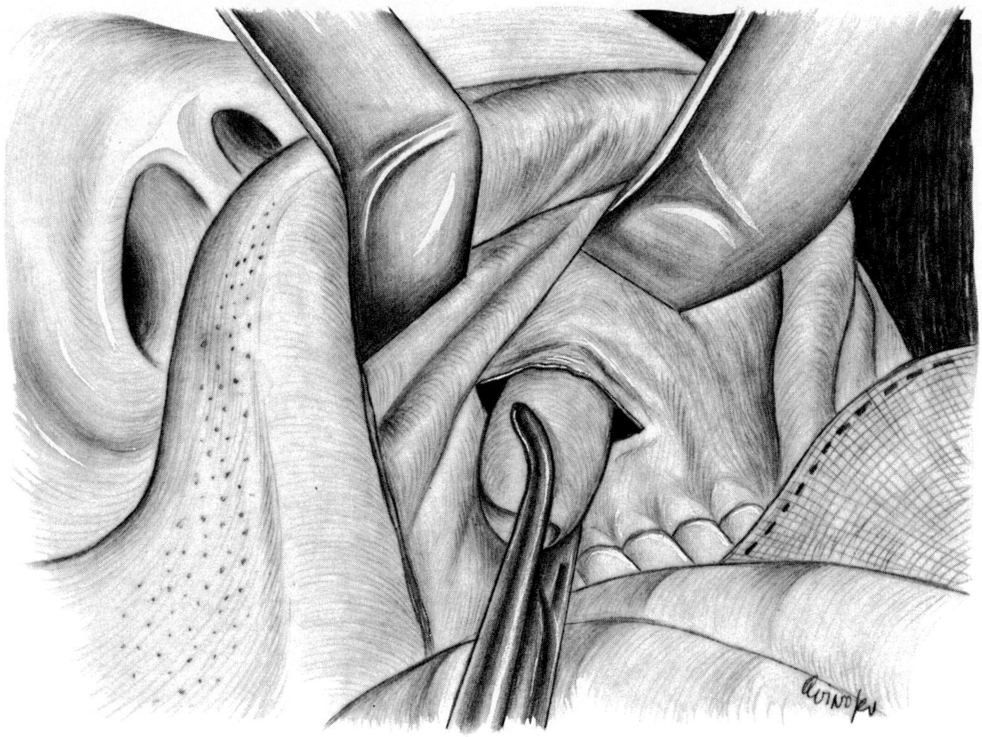

C

Figure 12-7 (continued)

C. The implant is inserted folded on itself and the forceps opened once it is in place. The correct positioning is controlled with the aid of a periosteal elevator. Absorbable sutures are used to close the wound.

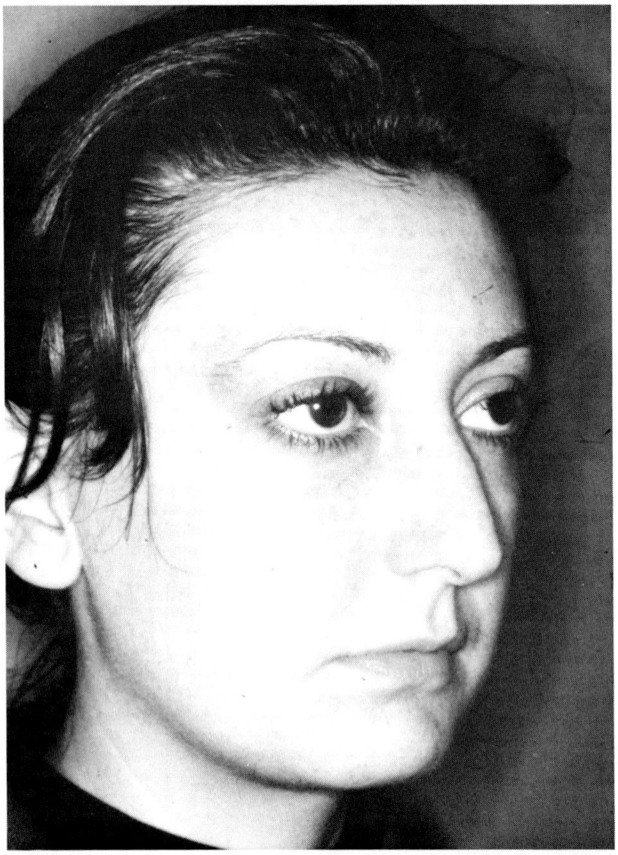

A

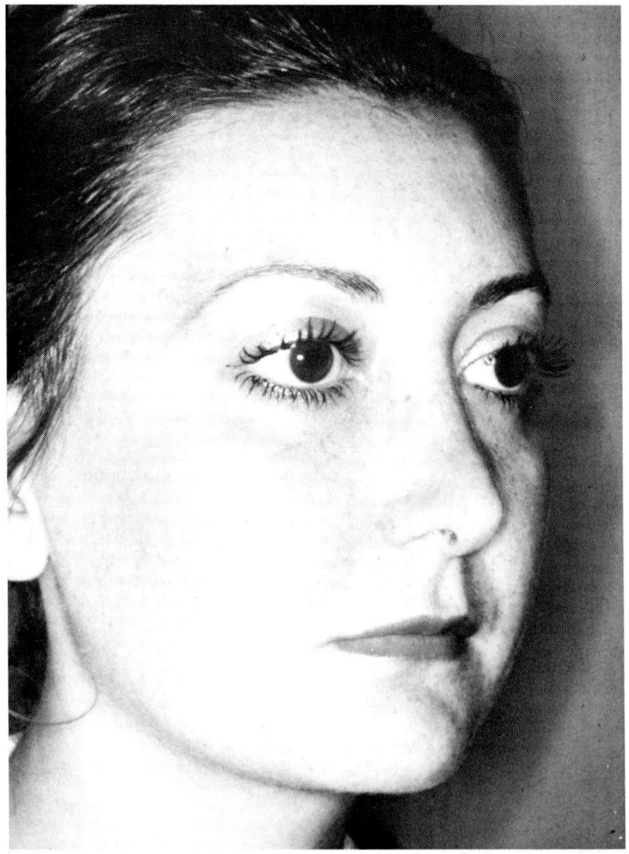

B

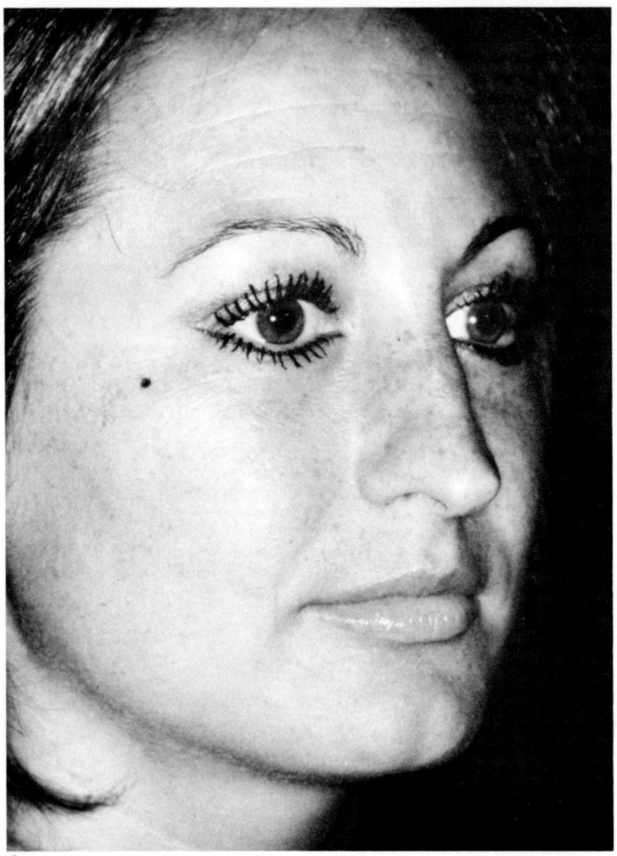

C

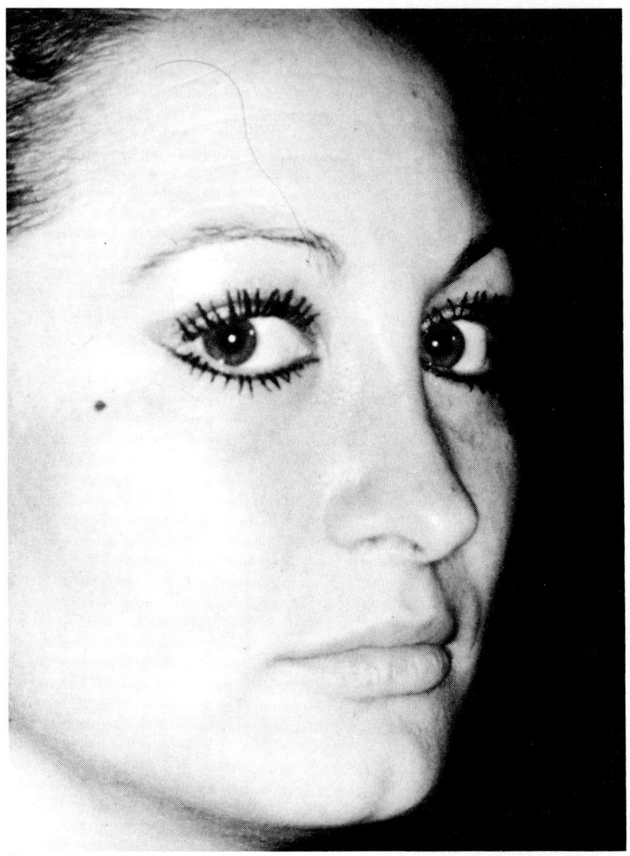

D

Figure 12-8

A, B. Oblique preoperative and postoperative views of a 31-year-old patient. A rhinoplasty and insertion of malar implants through vestibular approach have been performed.

C, D. Oblique preoperative and postoperative views of a 33-year-old patient. A rhinoplasty and insertion of malar implants through vestibular approach have been performed.

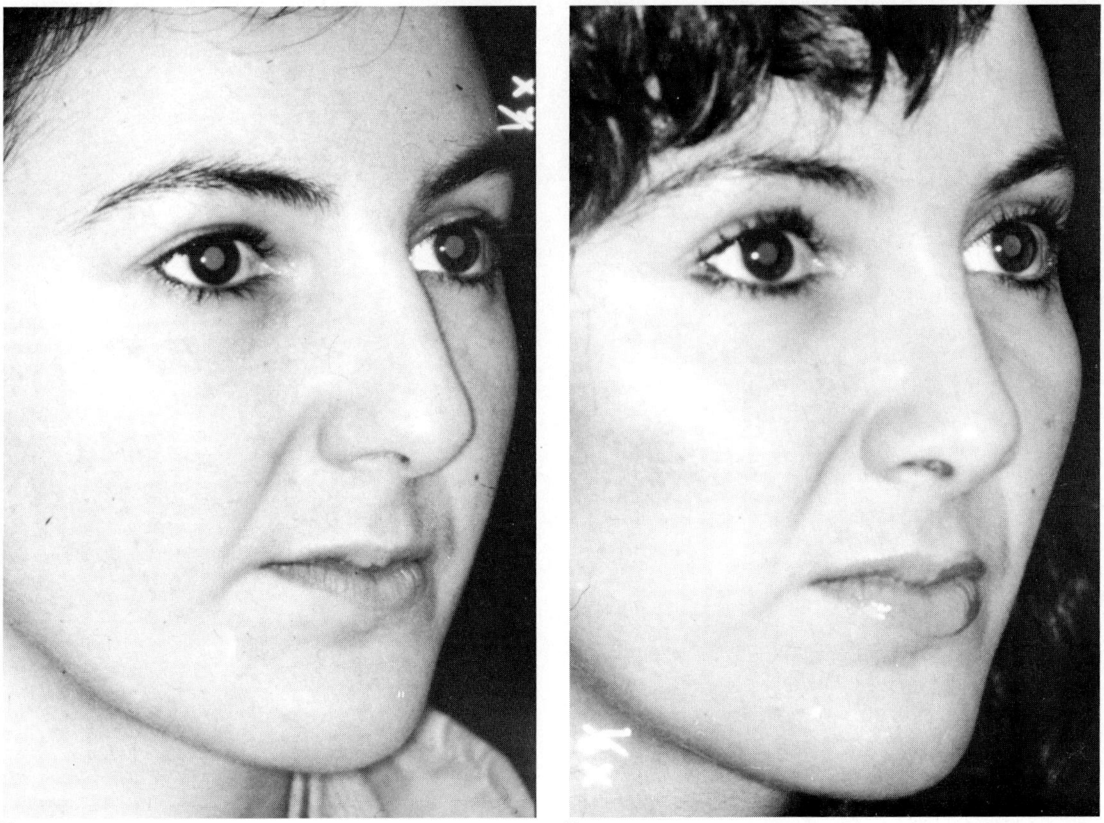

E F

Figure 12-8 (continued)
E, F. Oblique preoperative and postoperative views of a 25-year-old patient. A rhinoplasty and insertion of malar implants through vestibular approach have been performed.

The results are aesthetically pleasing with minimal evidence of surgical intervention (Fig. 12-8).

If the tunnel providing access to the subperiosteal space is narrower than the implant, the latter will be stable. If the tunnel is too large, an external fixation is applied.

POSTOPERATIVE TREATMENT

Special postoperative care is unnecessary following malar augmentation. If external fixation is required, it is left in place for 2 or 3 days and then removed. By the end of 4 or 5 days, the passage of fibrous tissue through the holes in the prosthesis can be detected. After 1 week, it is stable without any sensation of foreign body. The area should then be normal, both to inspection and to palpation. A slight edema is expected for the first few days postoperatively. Although a hematoma can occur in the subperiosteal cavity, it is rare.

COMPLICATIONS

We have inserted more than 350 implants between the years 1964 and 1981 (excluding seven Kiel-Braun heterologous osseous grafts). In approximately 60 percent of these cases the oral approach was used and combined with other profileplasty procedures such as rhinoplasty and mentoplasty. In 30 percent of the cases the rhytidectomy approach was employed, and in 10 percent the blepharoplasty approach was used while 60 percent were put through the oral approach.

Displacement

Only three prostheses placed through an oral approach have undergone immediate postoperative displacement. One patient was reoperated on by another surgeon. In the second case the prostheses were repositioned after 1 week as an outpatient procedure. An infection ensued subsequently but subsided spontaneously 1 week later. The third patient was operated on after 3 months. In a fourth patient the implant was placed frontside backward, being repositioned after 2 weeks through the same oral route. The connective septums, which were already established, had to be severed.

Nerve Injuries

In one patient a traction injury of the buccal branch of the facial nerve caused an asymmetry that resolved spontaneously after 6 weeks. Another patient had an anesthesia of the corresponding half of the upper lip that subsided progressively in 8 weeks. No damage of the zygomatic branches has occurred when the rhytidectomy approach was used.

Miscellaneous Complications

In one patient with sequelae of facial fractures, the implant provided insufficient volume. A second implant was placed over it at a year's interval without any sign of instability or complications. Up to now we have not observed any demineralization of the malar bone or reduction in size. If some were produced, it would undoubtedly be less than in the chin, since the contact area is larger and the muscle pressure significantly less. Even if this might occur, the patient in whom one prosthesis was placed on top of another without any resulting complications can lead us to consider this as a solution for any considerable reduction of the malar prominence. Wilkinson [16] has recently reviewed complications in his series of patients.

TREATMENT OF PROMINENT ZYGOMA

The same considerations that have been presented with respect to the oblique profile in flatness of the malar region apply to the excessively prominent malar region. An excessively bulging malar bone will cause an appearance of sunken orbits and an emaciated face. The cheeks will also appear sunken, and the face as a whole will have a rhomboid or triangular shape.

Prominent zygomata are not frequent in Caucasians but are more often encountered in Orientals. It is therefore natural that the treatment of this anomaly has recently been given emphasis in Asian countries. In 1981 Onizuka and Watanabe [12] first described a method for correction of the prominent zygoma. Preplanning is done and the area of excessive prominence is outlined with pioctanine. An incision is made in the gingival sulcus of the upper lip. A periosteal elevator is introduced subperiosteally over the maxilla and malar bone until wide exposure of the zygoma is obtained. Then the most prominent portion, including the malar prominence, is carved with a broad sharp chisel (Fig. 12-9).

If the chiseled bone block cannot be removed because of ligament fixations, these should be incised with long scissors. Care must be taken not to tear the mucosa of the maxillary sinus. However, if a tear does occur, adequate cover can be provided with the elevated periosteum. The mucosa incision is then sutured, and a bulky pressure dressing is applied over the malar areas. Onizuka and Watanabe [12] consider antibiotic coverage important for avoiding infections. X-ray pictures of the malar areas should be taken preoperatively if a sinusitis of the maxillary sinus is suspected. If it is confirmed, adequate treatment should be prescribed prior to surgery. An x-ray visualization of the maxillary sinus will also prevent any excessive removal with damage to the sinus mucosa.

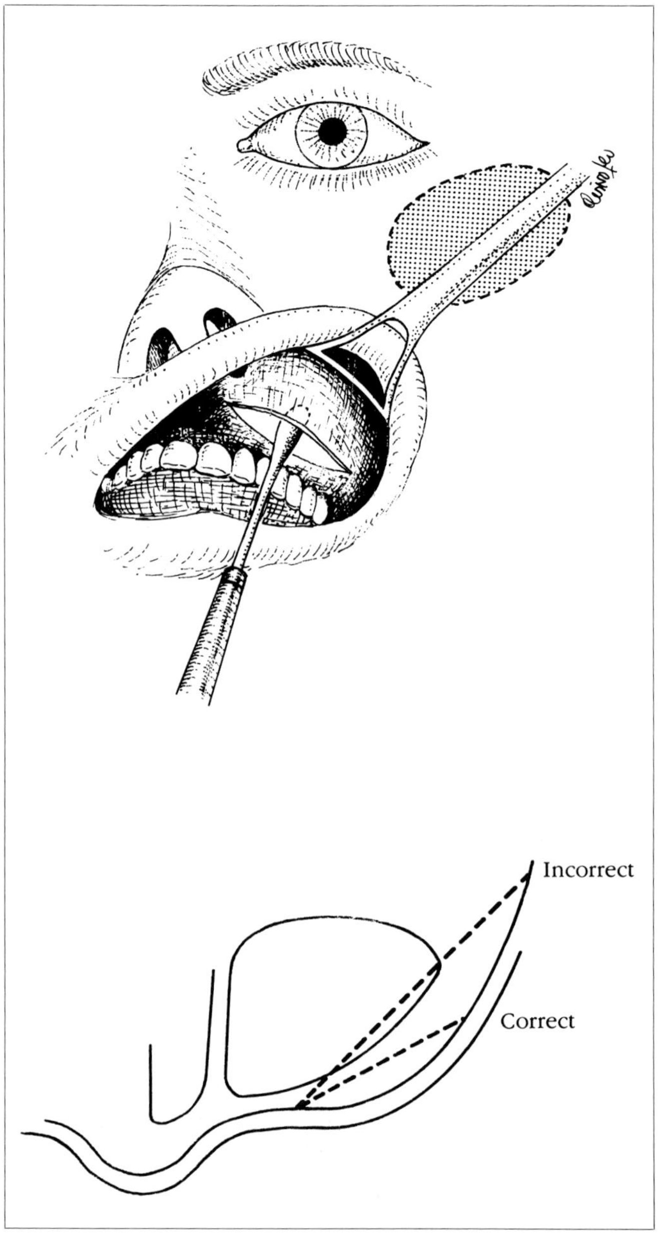

Figure 12-9. Oral vestibular approach for zygomatic reduction. Planes for chiseling. A correct plane respects the maxillary sinus. A too ambitious resection will penetrate the sinus and tear the mucosa.

SUMMARY

Aesthetic correction of flat malar regions contributes to the harmony of the facial proportions, improving the facial oval and especially the oblique or social profile. At the same time it gives a more youthful appearance to the face. Its application extends to the treatment of congenital malformations, asymmetries, traumatic infections, and surgical sequelae of the malar zone.

We have obtained satisfactory results with implants designed by us and distributed by Heyer-Schulte, although implants can be individually carved out of a silastic block. Our implants have perforations that allow invasion of connective tissue and subsequent fixation. Their shape is adaptable to the malar surface. The implant has to be placed subperiosteally. We favor the oral approach when the procedure is done alone or together with other profileplasties. The rhytidectomy approach is advocated if it is part of a treatment of the aging face. The blepharoplasty approach is used when this operation is carried out simultaneously with eyelid surgery or when there are scars to be corrected on the eyelid, or, according to Agban [1], when an augmentation of the maxilla is also indicated. A direct approach is employed only when local traumatic sequelae and scars are to be repaired.

The results have been very satisfactory. The percentage of complications is rather small, and complications usually end in spontaneous resolution should they persist, or, are easy to correct.

REFERENCES

1. Agban, G. Augmentation and corrective malarplasty. *Ann. Plast. Surg.* 2:306, 1979.
2. Gonzalez-Ulloa, M. Building out the malar prominences as an addition to rhytidectomy. *Plast. Reconstr. Surg.* 53:293, 1974.
3. Hinderer, U. Cirugia del perfil de la cara; perfiloplastias. *Ann. Med. Quir. Esp.* 49:3, 1964–1965.
4. Hinderer, U. El injerto oseo heterologo de Kiel en perfilo plastias y depresiones faciales (indicationes y experiencias). *Rev. Lat. Am. Cir. Plast.* 11:158, 1967.
5. Hinderer, U. Profileplasty. *Int. Micr. J. Aesthetic Plast. Surg.* September 1971.
6. Hinderer, U. Profileplasty: Standard and New Personal Techniques. In *Tr. II Cong. European Sect. IPRS* 23 May 1973.
7. Hinderer, U. Rhinoplasty: Routine Stages and Additional Corrections. In *Tr. II Cong. European Sect. IPRS* 23 May 1973.
8. Hinderer, U. Protesis Malar, un Procedimiento para Perfeccionar el Ovalo Facial. In *Tr. II Congr. Soc. Argent. Cir. Est.* 1974.
9. Hinderer, U. Nueva aportacion a la tecnica de blefaroplastia. In *Tr. II Congr. Soc. Argent., Cir. Est.* 1974.
10. Hinderer, U. Malar implants for improvement of the facial appearance. *Plast. Reconstr. Surg.* 56:157, 1975.
11. Jabaley, M. Trans-oral silastic augmentation of the malar region. *Br. J. Plast. Surg.* 27:98, 1974.
12. Onizuka, T., and Watanabe, K. Reduction of prominent zygoma. *Aesthetic Plast. Surg.* 7:228, 1983.
13. Ribeiro, L. Protesis Malares. *13 Congreso Brasileiro de Cirugia Plastica, 1 Congreso Brasileiro de Cir. Est.*, Porto Alegre, Brasil, 1976.
14. Spadafora, A. Pomulos planos (Platizigion) endoprotesis de polietileno insertadas por via subperiostica del arco cigomatico. *Prensa Med. Argent.* 58:1946, 1971.
15. Stark, R. The voice of polite dissent. *Plast. Reconstr. Surg.* 53:469, 1974.
16. Wilkinson, T. S. Complications in aesthetic malar augmentation. *Plast. Reconstr. Surg.* 71:643, 1983.

13. *Eyelids, Periorbital Region, and Forehead-Lift*

Paule Regnault
Rollin K. Daniel

Previously, patients complaining of "baggy" or "heavy" eyelids were often treated by simple blepharoplasty. Bulging fat was removed and redundant skin excised. However, heaviness often remained because of ptotic eyebrows or lateral hooding. In addition, "crow's-feet" were minimally improved. As increasingly sophisticated patients expressed satisfaction with their eyelids but disappointment with the surrounding structures, it became evident that surgical techniques had to be expanded outward to the periorbital region and ultimately onto the forehead. Thus, the eyelids and the influencing periorbital structures must be carefully assessed as one unit. Undoubtedly, a greater number of combined procedures and extended blepharoplasties will be done in the future. The present chapter discusses the classic blepharoplasty, its periorbital extension, and forehead deformities including eyebrow ptosis.

Blepharoplasty

James W. Smith
Fredric Newman

Blepharoplasty is the second most common aesthetic surgical procedure performed in the United States (56,000 procedures in 1981), exceeded in popularity only by breast augmentation (72,000 procedures in 1981). With its genesis in ancient Arabia, eyelid surgery has evolved into a precise procedure with a minimal margin for error. Although technical expertise is important, a detailed knowledge of anatomy and accurate preoperative assessment remain critical in the achievement of a superior result.

HISTORY

Although the origins of eyelid surgery antedate our present efforts by more than 1000 years and are traceable to ancient Arabia, reports of excising excess eyelid skin did not appear in Western literature until the late eighteenth and early nineteenth centuries. Von Graefe [112] is credited with the inception of the word *blepharoplasty* in 1818; however, this was a century of anatomists, and modern eyelid surgery lay dormant for another hundred years.

Early contributors to aesthetic eyelid surgery included Miller [71] and Bourquet [8, 9]. Their emphasis was on skin excision, and it remained for Bourquet [8, 9] in 1929 to advocate the removal of fat in order to attain a more satisfactory contour of the eyelids.

Not until 1951 did Castanares [10] accurately describe the morphologic arrangement of the fat compartments. This work demonstrated the importance of the accumulation of fat beneath the septum orbitale and the improvement that could be obtained with the excision of redundant fat [10–13].

Multitudinous variations in the assessment and solution of problems have led to a gradual evolution of technique in modern blepharoplasty. In 1960 Reidy [92] reported the skin-muscle flap approach in lower eyelid blepharoplasty. Sheen [96, 97] and Flowers [26, 27] have stressed the importance of levator fixation in selected cases while Kay [52–54] has emphasized the forehead-lift as a useful adjunct in upper eyelid ptosis.

More attention has been directed to the orbicularis oculi muscle in refinements of both upper and lower eyelid techniques. Baker et al. [4] excise a strip of excess orbicularis oculi from the upper eyelid (as did Sheen and Flowers) in order to recreate the supratarsal fold. Loeb [61–63] and Furnas [30–32] have demonstrated that in some individuals "baggy eyelids" can be due to an exaggerated development of the palpebral portion of the orbicularis oculi muscle and recommend a conservative excision of the redundant muscle. More recently, as the limits of contour change by the excision of skin, fat, and redundant muscle are approached, Smith [99] and others are redirecting attention to underlying fascial attachments in order to achieve a more satisfying result.

APPLIED ANATOMY

Treatises on eyelid anatomy range in quality from the sublime to the absurd. Accurate knowledge of anatomy continues to be of paramount importance in preoperative assessment of the deformity and intraoperative execution of the procedure in order to attain a superior result with minimal risk of complication.

The nuances of the procedure are clarified by a more sophisticated appreciation of the subtleties of the regional anatomy. The higher incidence of medial fat pad herniation compared to the more lateral pockets may well be explained by the fact that in both the upper and lower eyelids the orbital septum appears to be thicker laterally. In his classic description of the fat pockets Castanares [10] compares the orbital fat to a shock absorber providing, in addition, a smooth surface that permits efficient muscle function.

Exception to Castanares's description of two superior and three inferior pockets is taken by Hugo and Stone [47]. Their dye injection studies were, however, performed on cadaver specimens. Subsequently, Barker [6] has performed in vivo studies confirming the "classic" compartments. Interestingly, Hugo and Stone observed that the amount of intraorbital fat did not appear to be related to body habitus and that the right and left orbits in the same specimen evidenced unequal amounts of fat.

Although the existence of a lateral fat pocket (third pocket) in the upper eyelid remains controversial at best, sometimes a "lateral approach" (see Operative Technique) is necessary to extract the upper "middle" fat collection adequately. Attention during this dissection must be paid to the possibility of encountering a prolapsed lacrimal gland. During the extraction of the white nasal upper lid fat pocket, the muscle-pulley complex of the superior oblique muscle is at risk as the fat pad lies immediately subjacent to this complex.

Penetration of the septum orbitale during the extraction of the upper "middle" fat collection might potentially damage either the superior transverse ligament of Whitehall or the levator mechanism itself. Injury to the levator mechanism, with subsequent ptosis of the eyelid, may also follow the excision of a strip of orbicularis muscle to recreate the supratarsal fold.

Removal of a strip of this muscle from the upper eyelid in the region of the lateral canthus may compromise the nerve supply to the pretarsal portion of the orbicularis. In the lower eyelid, the orbicularis oculi preserves the contact between the eyelid and the globe. Its denervation could jeopardize this relationship and result in epiphora. Finally, injudicious penetration of the septum orbitale during the extraction of lower eyelid fat could damage the inferior oblique.

ANESTHESIA

Adequate premedication consisting of a combination of a narcotic (morphine, 5–10 mg), a phenothiazine (Compazine, 1.5–10.0 mg), and a barbiturate (Nembutal, 50–100 mg) is administered intramuscularly 1 hour preoperatively after a previous intramuscular injection of a barbiturate (Nembutal, 50–100 mg) at least 2 hours preoperatively. Intravenous sedation is obtained with morphine and diazepam (Valium) (in 2.5-mg increments) after an initial intravenous dose (2–4 mg) of lorazepam (Ativan). Local infiltration is obtained using lidocaine, 0.5%, in a solution containing a 1:200,000 dilution of epinephrine. In addition, the supratrochlear nerve is blocked in order to lessen the patient's discomfort when traction is placed on the upper medial fat pad.

OPERATIVE TECHNIQUE

With the patient in the supine position the upper border of the tarsal plate is identified (Fig. 13-1). It serves as the lower border of the segment of skin to be excised. This line is marked with a very fine felt-tipped pen to ensure a precise placement of the incision. The line is carried medially until the medial canthal depression is reached and laterally to extend within the lines of relaxed skin tension as far as is necessary to effect an optimal skin excision.

With the patient in the sitting position and with the eyes closed, the amount of redundant skin is determined. The tissue is grasped in a smooth forceps so that one limb of the instrument lies along the inferior line of excision. The superior line of excision is determined by approximating the two limbs of the forceps until the skin of the eyelid is under slight tension but the lid remains closed. This is done at several different sites along the proposed line of superior excision.

The skin incision for the lower eyelid is placed 2 to 3 mm below the ciliary margin. It extends from the punc-

Figure 13-1

A. Technique for marking incisions for upper and lower eyelid surgery. With the patient in the supine position it is easier to identify the upper margin of the tarsal plate. It lies about 10 mm above the lid margin.
B. With the patient in the sitting position and with the eyes closed lightly, one side of the forceps is placed on the line previously marked and the other side of the forceps above, pinching the skin so that it picks up the major portion of any redundancy that is present. The patient should be able to keep the eyes closed while the excess skin is being pinched. Thus, the amount of skin between the two margins of the forceps should represent the amount that can be excised safely.
C. Remember, the distance between the lid margin and the lower incision should be nearly the same along the entire lid, including the lateral canthus. When there is a marked excess of eyelid skin beyond the lateral canthus, a "hooded" appearance is created. In these cases it is better to extend the line of excision upward and outward so that it includes this extra fold of skin as shown by the dotted line.
D. The lines of incision as they would appear at the completion of marking with the patient sitting and facing the surgeon. The surgeon should look carefully to determine that the markings are symmetric.

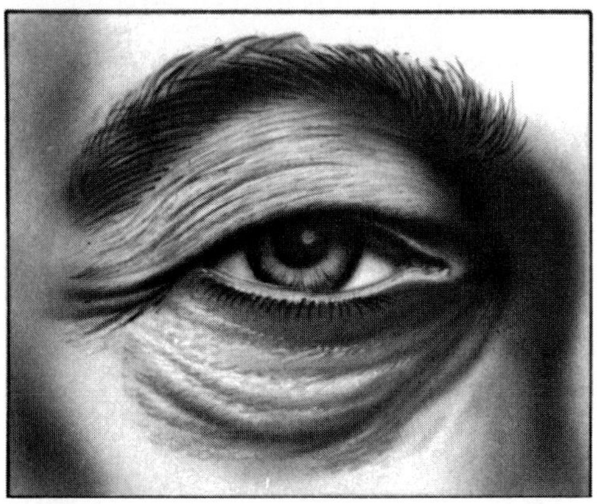
A

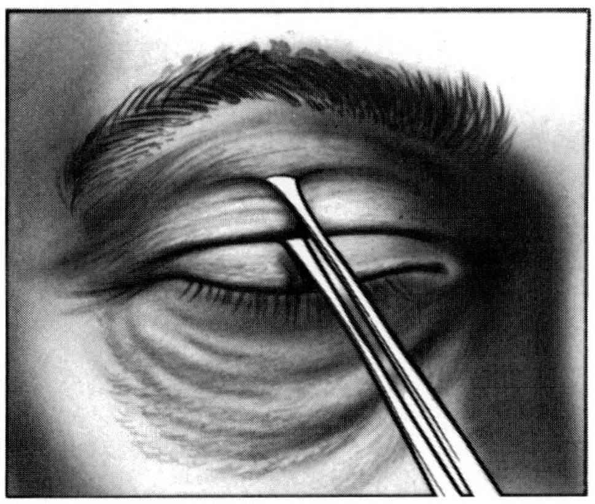
B

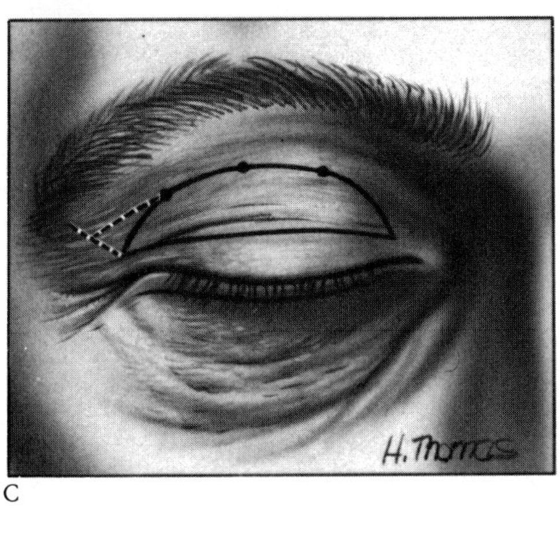
C

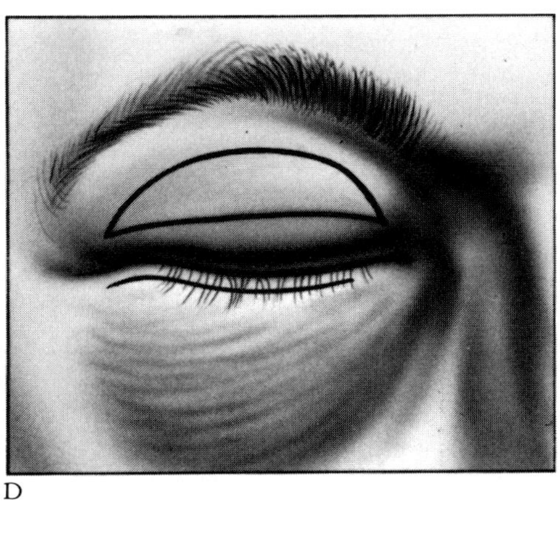
D

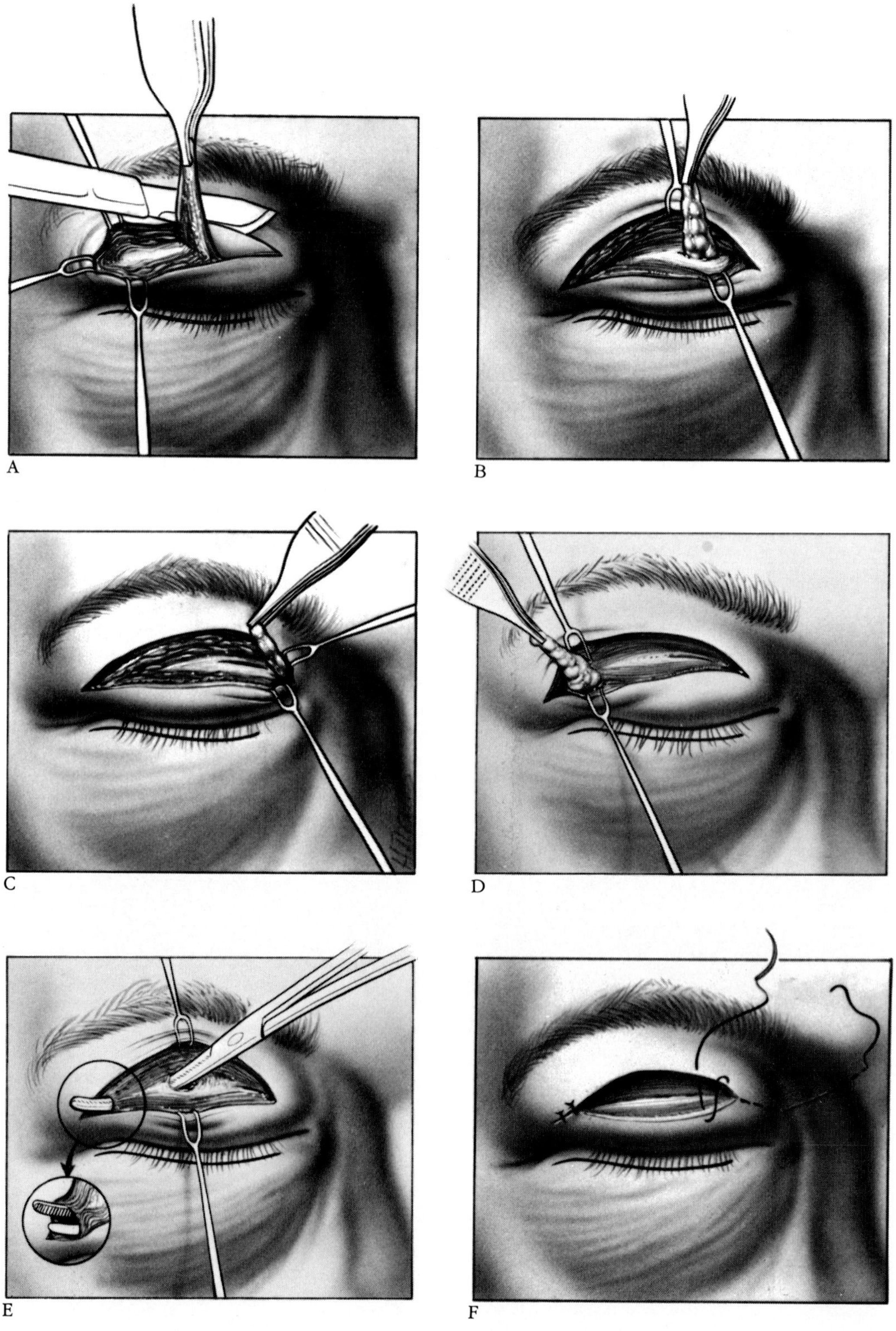
A
B
C
D
E
F

tum medially to the lateral canthus and then continues as a lateral extension within a skin crease. Symmetric excisions are marked in the opposite eyelid with the use of a caliper.

The patient is placed in a supine position with back and head elevated. After satisfactory skin preparation and draping, local infiltration is performed with a 30-gauge needle using 0.5% lidocaine in solution with a 1 : 200,000 dilution of epinephrine.

The plane of injection lies between skin and muscle. Distention of the skin with the injection of local anesthetic is an important adjunct in excision as it increases the stability of the surface for the skin incision.

In the upper eyelid the island of redundant skin is excised (Fig. 13-2). If an increased definition of the supratarsal fold is desired, a 3-mm strip of orbicularis oculi muscle is excised from the center of the site from which the skin has been excised. Hemostasis is obtained with bipolar coagulation.

Definition of the supraorbital fat pads is obtained by gentle finger pressure on the globe. The septum orbitale is incised, and the pockets are divested of fat after the base of each fat pad has been coagulated with the bipolar forceps to help secure potential bleeding sites. Care must be taken to avoid injury to the muscle-pulley complex of the superior oblique muscle to which the medial fat pocket is immediately subjacent. The lateral extension of the upper eyelid fat may be determined by passing a small curved mosquito clamp from the medial portion of the pocket in a lateral direction just beneath the orbicularis muscle. It is necessary to penetrate the fascia laterally in order to obtain adequate exposure. Skin closure is obtained with simple sutures of 5-0 silk in the area beyond the lateral canthus and then a running suture of 6-0 nylon for the remainder.

Correction of the lower eyelid deformity requires even more sophistication in assessment and execution than does the upper eyelid procedure (Fig. 13-3). The incision is made in the first skin crease immediately subjacent to the ciliary margin. The lateral extent of the incision cannot be determined accurately at this point as it varies with the amount of skin to be removed.

Two approaches to the lower eyelid fat compartments are available. A skin flap may be dissected with subsequent sharp penetration of the orbicularis in order to excise the herniated fat, or a skin-muscle flap may be elevated as a more efficient approach to the attenuated septum orbitale, allowing a direct visualization of the fat compartments.

The orbital septum is sharply incised, and redundant herniated fat is removed from each compartment after control of its vascular supply has been obtained with bipolar coagulation. The amount of fat to be removed is determined by gently applying pressure to the globe and excising any fat that protrudes above the infraorbital rim. Excision of too much fat is to be disparaged as the patient will then assume a cadaveric appearance.

The skin-muscle flap is advanced in a superolateral direction to determine the amount of overlying excess tissue. In order to prevent an excessive excision of soft tissue, the patient is asked to look upward and to open the mouth. The overlying skin and muscle are sharply excised after one is certain that a tension-free closure can be attained. A meticulous closure is done with simple sutures of 6-0 silk beyond the lateral canthus and a running suture of 6-0 nylon for the remainder.

Figure 13-2

A. The skin is excised with a portion of the orbicularis oculi muscle usually in the central portion of the skin. This excision effectively accentuates the tarsal fold when it is desirable to do so.

B. A small incision is made to identify the fat in the central pocket. If there is any difficulty in identifying any of the fat pockets in the upper lid, their location can be determined exactly by placing slight pressure on the lower lid. Once the septum orbitale has been incised, the fat freely herniates through it. Picking up the fat with the forceps one can coagulate the base with a bipolar coagulator and then transect it. A great deal of ecchymosis and postoperative edema can be prevented by carefully coagulating all small vessels and by obtaining satisfactory hemostasis before closing the incisions.

C. Fat is then removed from the medial pocket. This pocket is slightly more difficult to locate. Its content can be confirmed because the fat from it has a lighter, less yellow color than does the fat from any of the other pockets.

D. Exposure of the lateral extension of upper eyelid fat may be approached by passing a small curved mosquito clamp directly beneath the orbicularis muscle. Near the outer margin of the area from which the skin has been excised the clamp can be punched through the remaining orbicularis muscle and the area checked for fat.

E. It seems as though in cases where there has been a lot of lateral hooding or sagging of the skin some fat is more likely to be present.

F. We prefer to place two or three sutures laterally to gain accurate closure of the lid margins so that a "dog-ear" is eliminated in the outer portion of the closure. Then the lid is closed with a continuous suture of 6-0 nylon.

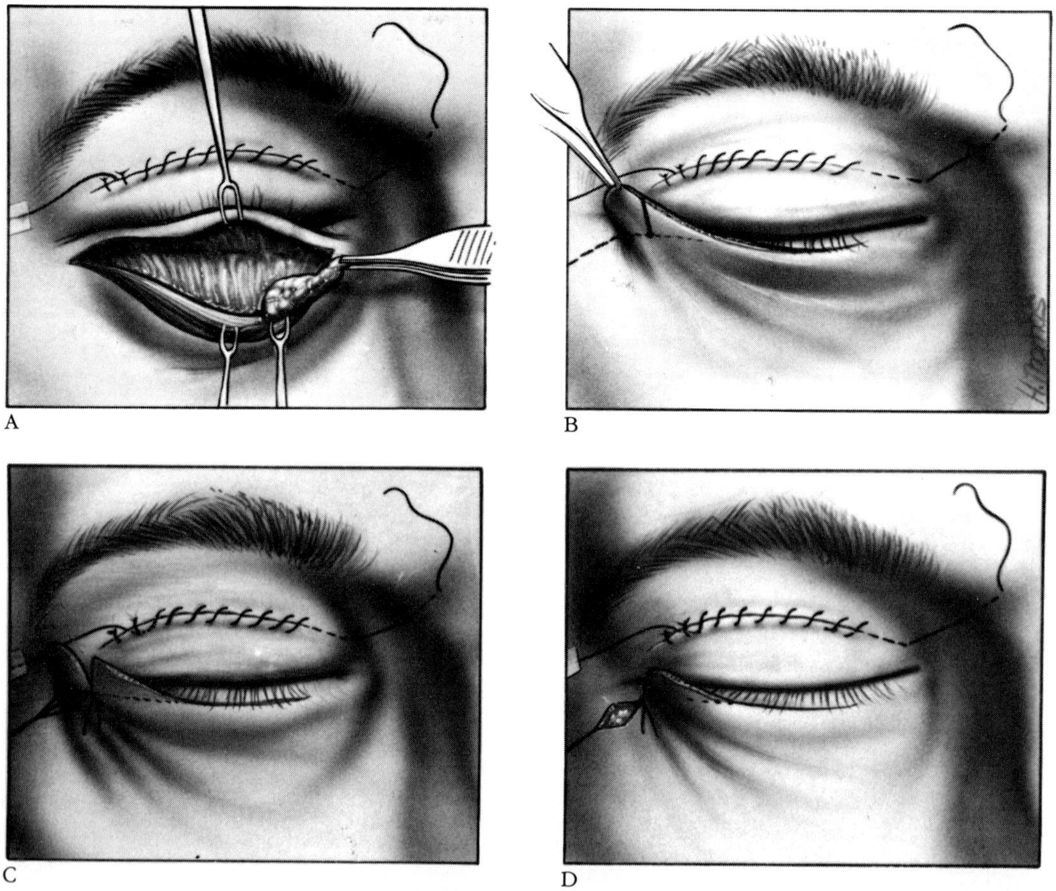

A B C D

Figure 13-3

A. Exposure of the lower lid fat is through a skin-muscle flap. A knife is used to make a short incision in the skin crease extending laterally from the outer canthus. A small pair of straight scissors is inserted into this opening and the skin cut along the line already marked to approximately the level of the lower canaliculus. The skin of the lower lid is separated from the muscle a millimeter or two, and the muscle itself is then incised and opened. With a retractor placed on the lower lid as shown here, forceps can be used to establish the plane between the posterior surface of the orbicularis muscle and the underlying orbital rim. Excess fat is then easily identified and removed. It is important to remove only enough fat to have the surface of the remaining fat parallel the anterior margin of the infraorbital rim.

B. With the patient gazing upward and the mouth open, the amount of redundant skin can be determined. Traction is maintained in a cephalic and lateral direction. An incision is made along the vertical line to a point where the overlap has been eliminated and a suture placed at this location to divide the closure into lateral and medial segments.

C. Once the incision line has been divided into two parts, the lateral excision is completed by removing an ellipse or a diamond-shaped segment from the skin lying obliquely to the original incision. The lateral portion is then closed with several 6-0 interrupted sutures.

D. With the patient gazing upward and the mouth open, the excess amount of skin and muscle of the medial segment may be marked and subsequently removed. Closure is completed with a continuous 6-0 nylon suture.

POSTOPERATIVE CARE

The eyes are irrigated with normal saline and an antibiotic ophthalmic ointment is applied. The eyes may be bandaged for several hours postoperatively, or iced saline compresses may be begun immediately. They are continued for 48 hours.

In order to avoid epithelialization of suture tracks, the skin sutures are removed over a period of 2 to 4 days, and the wounds are supported across lines of tension with Steri-Strips. All scabs are gently removed from the wound at the end of the first week, and women may apply makeup beginning the tenth postoperative day.

COMPLICATIONS OF BLEPHAROPLASTY

Ectropion

The continuum of postoperative lower eyelid deformities ranging from "scleral show" to frank ectropion probably represents the most common untoward sequelae of blepharoplasty. In the immediate postoperative period scleral show may be the result of wound edema and ecchymosis. This generally resolves within a few days and may be hastened by the topical application of steroids.

If excessive skin removal from the lower eyelid is recognized at the time of surgery, a portion of the excised skin can be replaced or the upper eyelid can be used as a donor site for lower eyelid skin. The upper eyelid skin may be transferred to the lower eyelid as a full-thickness skin graft. If these alternatives are not possible or if the problem is first noted in the postoperative period, a conservative approach emphasizing symptomatic treatment is advocated. Additional support may be obtained with the use of skin tapes applied in a superolateral direction. Satisfactory resolution will generally occur over a period of several months. When the wound stabilizes, if ectropion persists, a full-thickness skin graft may be used to resurface the surgically recreated defect.

The failure, preoperatively, to recognize the loss of elasticity of the lower eyelid or tarsal redundancy may also result in ectropion. This is not uncommon in older patients, especially those with a slight drooping of the lateral third of the eyelid (the characteristic "hound dog look"). At the time of surgery a wedge excision lateral to the corneal limbus needs to be performed in addition to the customary procedure.

Dry Eye Syndrome

One of the most commonly written about but nonetheless infrequent sequelae of blepharoplasty is the dry eye syndrome. The fully developed syndrome, keratoconjunctivitis sicca (Sjögren's syndrome), although initially subclinical, may be exacerbated by the surgery because of the slight ectropion and lagophthalmos that can occur during the early postoperative period [49].

Key preoperative symptoms to be wary of include irritation of the eyes, soreness, burning, and a sensation of scratchiness or the presence of a foreign body. On rare occasions, there may be excessive tear production. A Schirmer test may support the diagnosis when positive (normal value: 10 mm/5 minutes). Confirmation is obtained by analysis of tear lysozyme concentration, which is low in patients with keratoconjunctivitis sicca.

If a diagnosis of dry eye syndrome is made preoperatively, a conservative resection and possibly even a staged procedure is indicated. This would involve doing the upper eyelids as the first stage and then, after a suitable period of time, doing the lower eyelids. Postoperative protection and lubrication of the cornea are essential to prevent ulceration. Artificial lubrication consisting of an ointment at night in conjunction with an eyelid-seal dressing and "artificial tears" during the day is required to maintain appropriate corneal lubrication.

Visual Loss

One of the most feared and fortunately one of the rarest of complications is visual loss following elective blepharoplasty [43, 104]. The frequently quoted figure of 0.04 percent from DeMere et al. [19, 20] is difficult to validate because only one-half of the patients in their series had an ophthalmologic examination preoperatively.

It is generally agreed that intraorbital hemorrhage resulting in increased intraorbital pressure with subsequent vascular compromise of the optic nerve or retina is the mechanism of injury. However, considerable controversy exists as to the exact mechanism of insult to the optic apparatus.

Retrobulbar Hematoma

Perhaps the most spectacular complication, retrobulbar hematoma is heralded by the precipitous onset of severe pain, proptosis, and a marked increase in firmness of the ocular globe [108]. Appropriate diagnosis and prompt treatment are essential to prevent permanent visual impairment. Ophthalmologic consultation, with tonometry, fundascopic examination, and close monitoring of visual acuity, is essential. When there are no signs of visual impairment, treatment consists of orbital decompression, which can be accomplished by opening the eyelid suture lines. The condition is frequently self-limiting, and careful assessment of the blood supply to the retina and frequent monitoring of visual acuity are as important as aggressive treatment.

When there is evidence of any compromise in retinal vascularity or diminishing visual acuity, more aggressive treatment is necessary. As before, surgical decompression of the orbit remains of paramount importance. In addition, intraocular pressure may be reduced by the use of intravenous diuretics (mannitol, acetazolamide, and furosemide). Implementation of an oxygen–carbon dioxide mixture is of questionable value. Anterior chamber paracentesis remains a controversial adjunct.

A Potpourri of Postoperative Complications

Pain in the eye in conjunction with the sensation of the presence of a foreign body or "scratch" is often indicative of corneal injury. The cornea should be protected against desiccation during surgery by saline irrigation, and injury by contact with gauze sponges should be avoided to minimize the risk of corneal abrasion.

Hematomas, unless they occur at the time of the operation, are best drained through a stab wound approximately 7 to 10 days postoperatively, at which time the clot has liquefied.

Keloids of the eyelid skin have not been reported although on rare occasions hypertrophic scars can occur. Treatment is usually conservative, and resolution may be accelerated with intralesional injection of steroids.

Milia and inclusion cysts are common after eyelid surgery. Marsupialization or surgical excision results in rapid resolution of the problem.

Enophthalmos may follow the removal of excessive amounts of periorbital fat in a patient with a prominent infraorbital rim. At the time of surgery, if the condition is noted, the fat may be replanted with apparent success. Proper correction at a later date is difficult to achieve.

Damage to the levator aponeurosis may occur during the removal of upper eyelid fat. The resultant ptosis creates an unpleasing asymmetric appearance of the eyelids. If the function of the levator mechanism has been compromised, either primary or secondary repair is mandated.

At the time of fat extraction, the superior oblique and inferior oblique muscles may be damaged, causing extraocular muscle imbalance and diplopia. If the condition persists for more than 6 months, surgical intervention is necessary.

Wound dehiscence can occur although it is extremely unlikely if the wounds are supported with skin tapes. Immediate resuturing may be necessary if the skin tapes prove inadequate.

Infection is mentioned only as a curiosity because it occurs so infrequently. If it does occur, appropriate antibiotic therapy should be instituted.

Periorbital Region

The periorbital area may be arbitrarily divided into inferior, lateral, and superior regions on the basis of frequency of deformities. The medial region is excluded as it is rarely the source of complaints.

INFERIOR REGION

Common deformities in the inferior region include infrapalpebral depressions, malar bags, and festoons.

Infrapalpebral Depression

The presence of a deep groove between the nasal pyramid and lower eyelid is a source of concern to patients, both as an isolated deformity and if accentuated by adjacent bulges. The infrapalpebral depression is an abnormal exaggeration of the natural demarcation between lower eyelid and malar-nasal pyramid (Fig. 13-4). The lower edge of the orbicularis muscle is separated from the adipose tissue overlying the superior portion of the quadratus levator labii superioris muscle.

Since 1975 the following technique has been used in 10 percent of lower blepharoplasties with excellent results [91] (Fig. 13-5). Preoperatively, with the patient sitting, the location of the infrapalpebral depression is outlined as well as a "premark" blepharoplasty. The premarked skin area is excised first, a little less than with a skin-muscle technique, and the skin of the eyelid is undermined 2 mm

Figure 13-4. The cause of an infrapalpebral depression is separation of the orbicularis oculi muscle from the upper portion of the quadratus levator labii superioris. Correction is achieved by approximation of the muscle concurrent with a lower blepharoplasty.

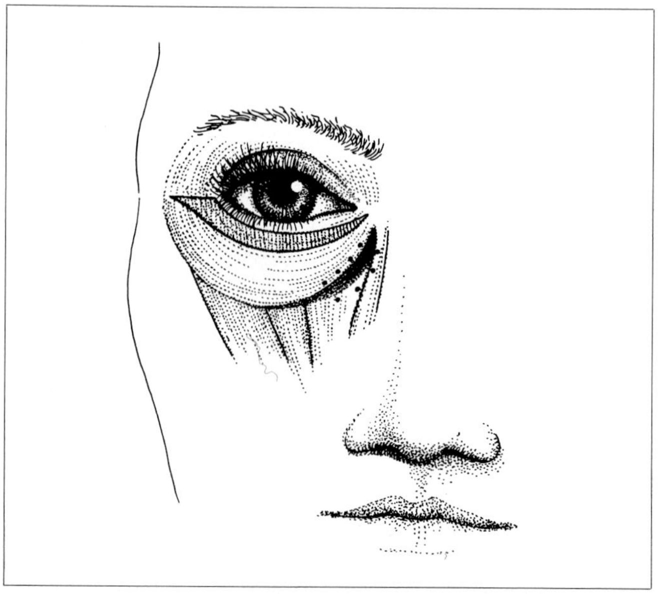

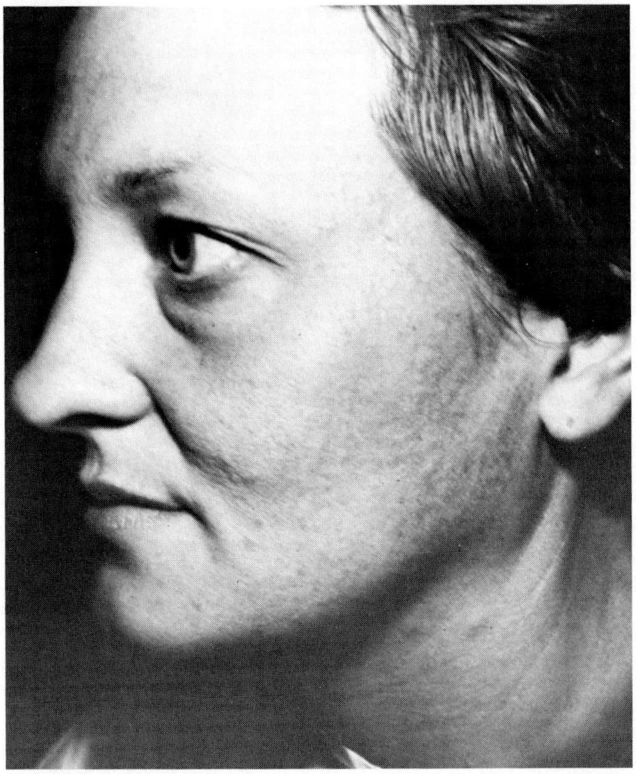

A

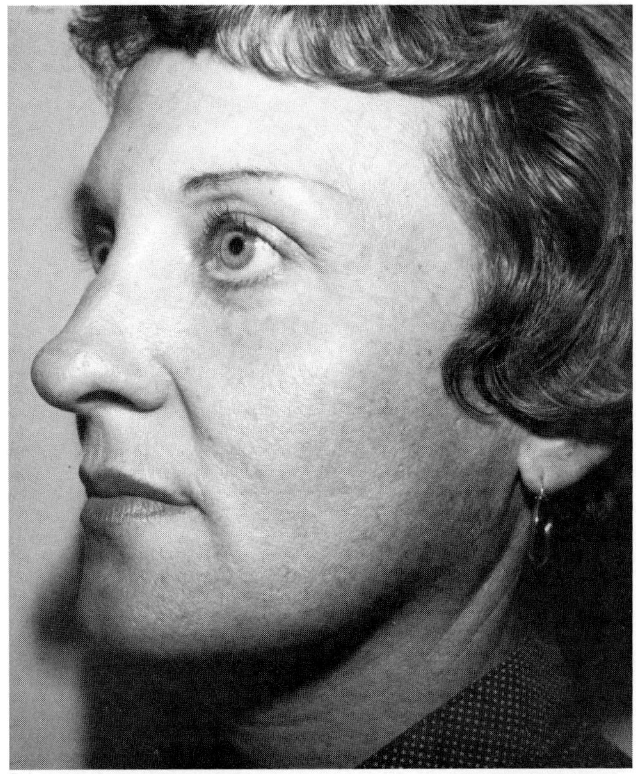

B

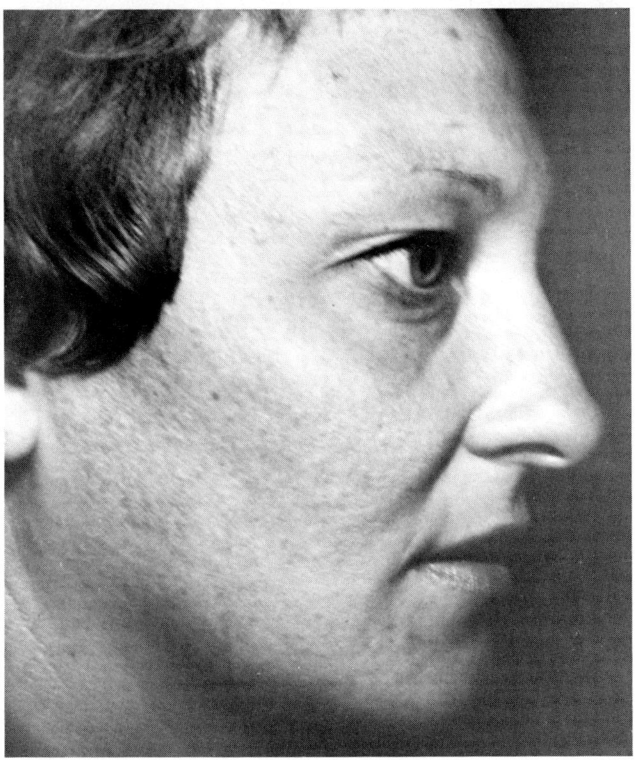

C

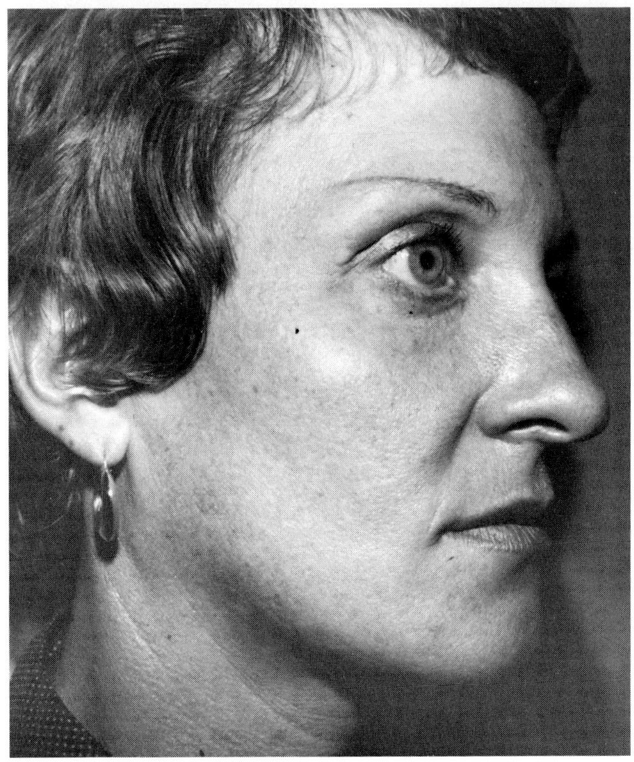

D

Figure 13-5
A, C. Patient with an infraorbital depression accentuated by fat herniation.
B, D. Correction of the deformity by excision of fat from the infraorbital compartments and approximation of the muscles.

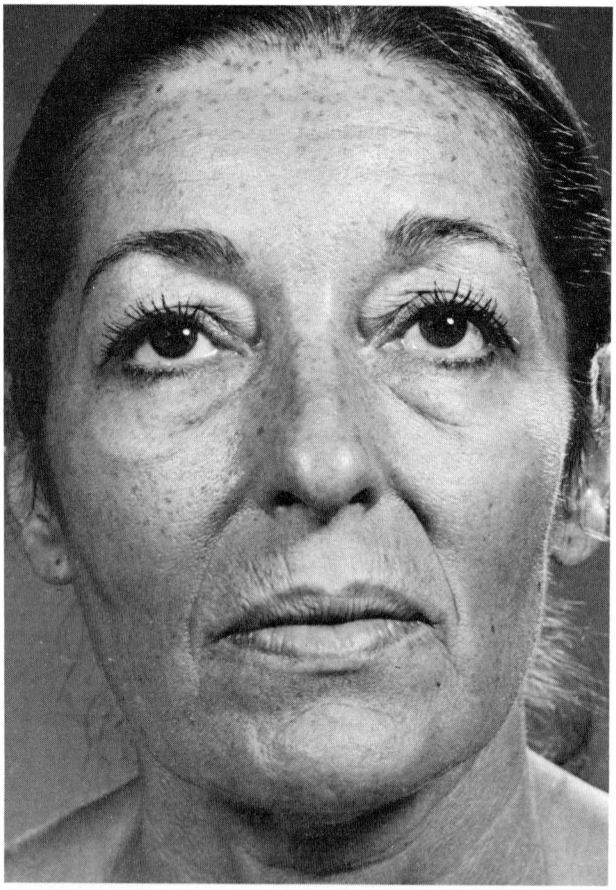

A

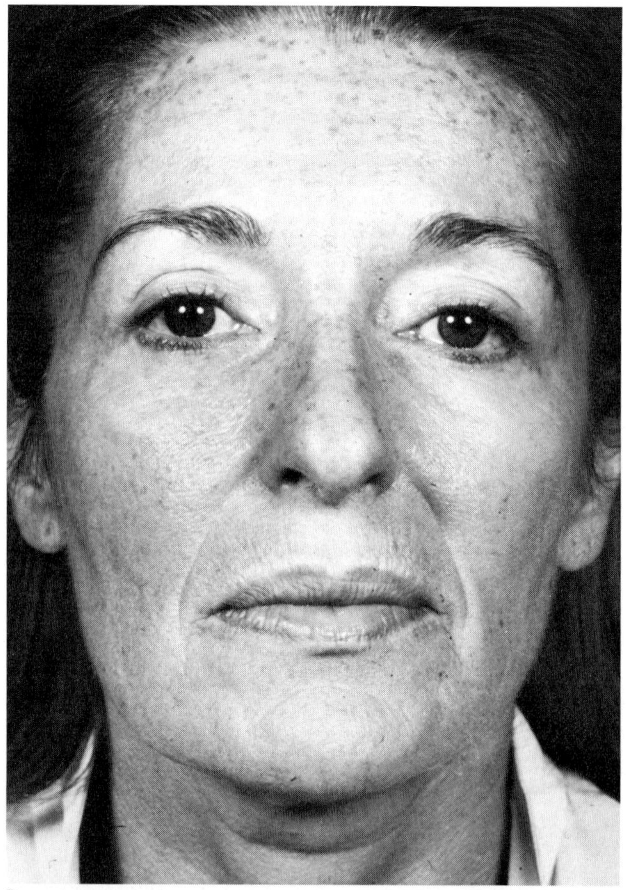

B

Figure 13-6

A. Patient requested blepharoplasty to correct eyelid deformities.

B. Despite detailed preoperative discussion and an otherwise good result, the patient was litigious regarding persistence of the right malar bag.

beyond the lower edge of the depression. The orbicularis muscle is incised, superiorally and the three fat pads are removed. The lower edge of the orbicularis muscle is then approximated to the fascial tissues along the nasal pyramids with two to four interrupted absorbable sutures to close the gap. The skin is approximated with a continuous fine nylon suture, and adhesive strips are placed over the undermined area. Because of the extensive undermining, edema and ecchymosis may persist and minor pulling at the eyelid edge may be present for a few weeks. In a series of 60 cases, correction of the deformity was achieved and ectropion did not occur. In certain severe cases, the depression can be filled with a fat flap taken from above the nasolabial fold. This transposition flap ameliorates the depression while primary closure of the donor site lessens the adjacent fullness.

Infrapalpebral Bulges

Subcutaneous tissue accumulation may be present at the juncture of cheek and eyelid [102]. Laterally, this is subcutaneous fat and may be designated as a malar bag. Centrally, it may be edematous tissue. In the elderly patient, muscle hammocks develop and are called festoons. Furnas [31] has classified festoons of the lower eyelid in three locations: (1) preseptal area, (2) orbital area, and (3) jugal or cheek area. We prefer to differentiate the bulges into two major groups, malar bags and festoons, on the basis of presentation and treatment. In either case, many patients consider them part of the eyelid deformity that will be corrected by a standard blepharoplasty or are not aware of them until they become accentuated postoperatively. Therefore, the deformity must be carefully pointed out preoperatively and the alternative methods of treatment discussed (Fig. 13-6).

Figure 13-7

A. A 57-year-old patient concerned about heavy upper eyelids and infrapalpebral bulges. She did not want either a forehead-lift for ptotic eyebrows or a rhytidectomy.

B. Result following blepharoplasty *alone.* Extensive defatting of the upper lids was done plus excision of subcutaneous tissue in the infrapalpebral region. This result emphasizes that the medial eyebrow can only be elevated by a forehead-lift.

C. Markings demonstrate planned defatting of the lateral upper eyelid and area of fat excision for the infrapalpebral bulge.

D. Dotted area indicates fat beneath the orbicularis oculi muscle requiring excision.

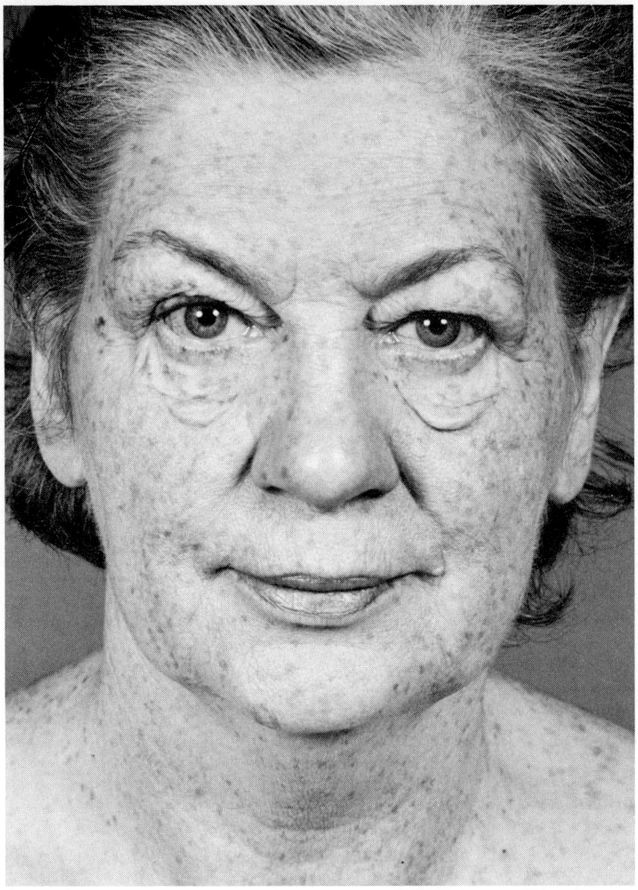
A

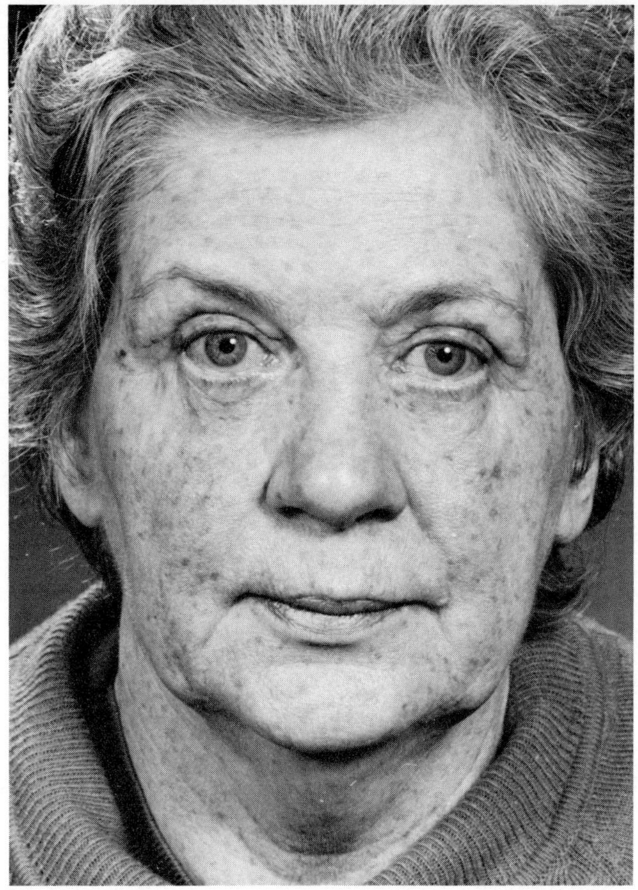
B

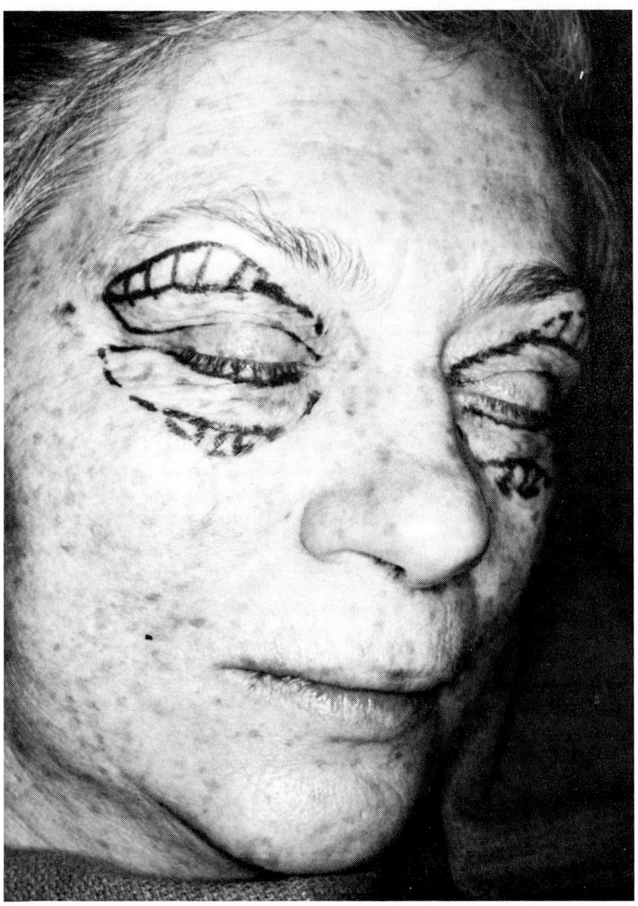
C

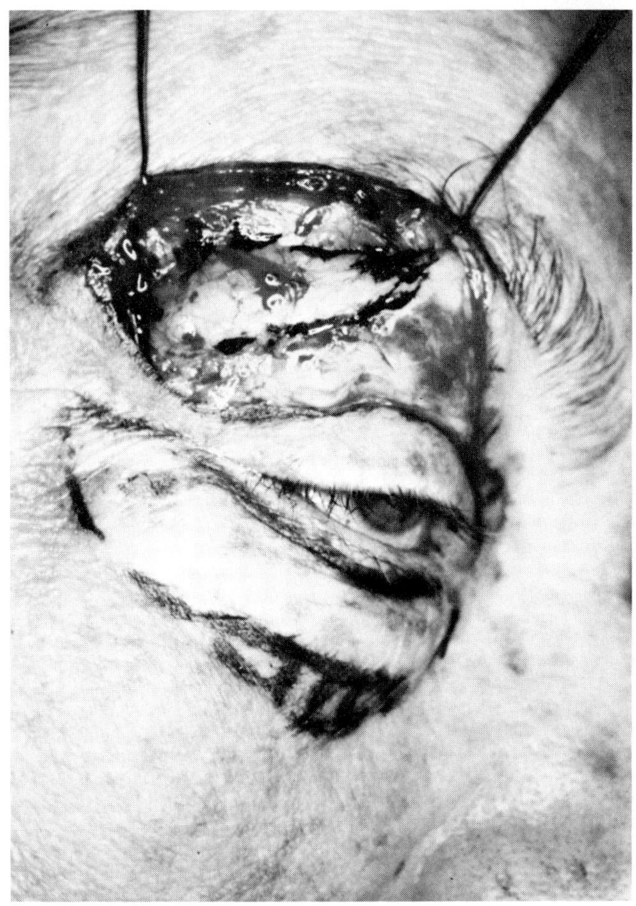
D

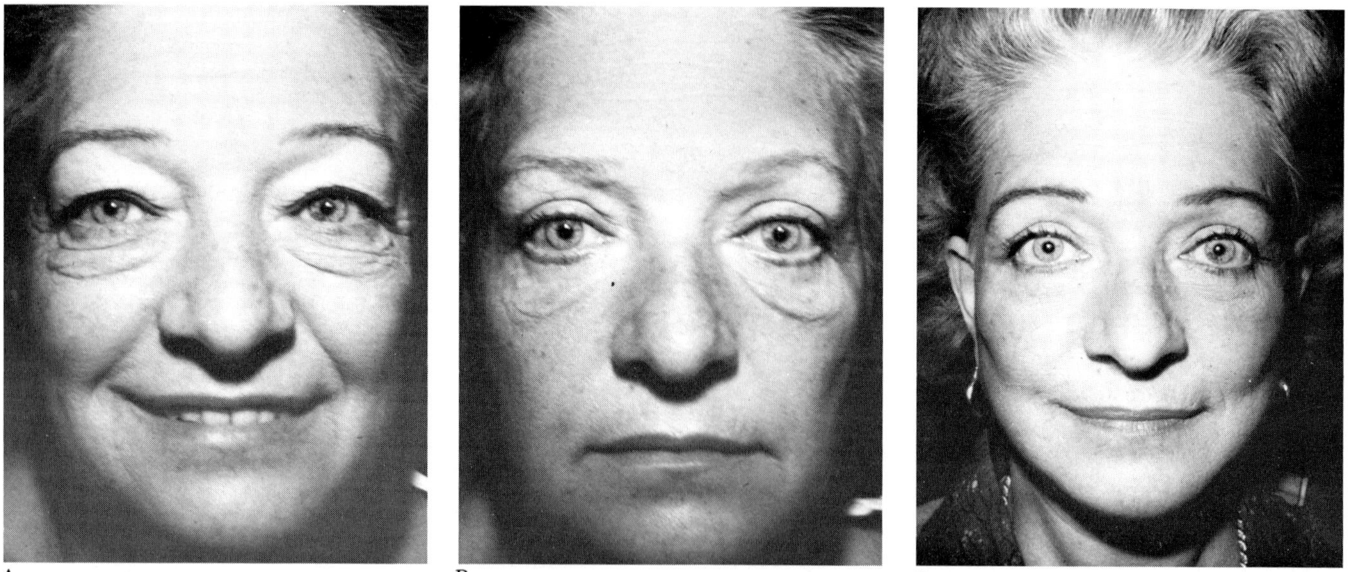

Figure 13-8
A. Patient with heavy eyelids and infrapalpebral bulges.
B. Result following standard blepharoplasty without improvement of the bulges.
C. Secondary revision of the infrapalpebral bulges via the blepharoplasty incision and rhytidectomy.

Although some surgeons consider direct excision of malar bags essential or feel correction is possible only with a rhytidectomy, we have not found it necessary in most cases (Fig. 13-7). Following preoperative markings, the redundant skin-muscle is excised and then the skin widely undermined above the orbicularis oculi muscle. The fat area is excised under direct vision followed by meticulous hemostasis. Resolution of ecchymosis and edema may require many weeks, but the results are usually excellent. In certain severe cases, a combined approach of blepharoplasty and rhytidectomy may be called for (Fig. 13-8). It should be noted that the deformity is often associated with hypoplasia of the malar prominence, which can be corrected by augmentation either simultaneously or secondarily. More central accumulations of subcutaneous fat or edematous tissues can be treated in similar fashion. To differentiate festoons from subcutaneous fat, Furnas [32] uses the "squinch test," in which the patient forcefully screws the eyes shut. If a true festoon is present, it will be effaced as the muscle contracts and will reappear on relaxation. Treatment consists of either muscle plication using muscle-periosteum sutures or muscle-to-muscle sutures via a blepharoplasty incision.

SUPERIOR REGION

In the upper eyelid, deformities include excess skin medially, hollowness centrally, and prominence of subcutaneous tissue or bone laterally. It must be emphasized that the upper eyelid is directly influenced by changes in the upper third of the face and cannot be considered an isolated entity. As noted by Spira [103], a superiorly directed triangle of skin can be added to a blepharoplasty incision for removal of excess skin medially. Excessively wide incisions, especially in the medial third, will result in a visible scar and upward retraction of the lid.

Patients with sunken or hollow eyes often present for blepharoplasty because of redundant skin and bulges. Fat excision must be minimal and confined to specific areas of preoperative concern. The orbicularis oculi muscle is *not* excised, and only small openings are made medially and laterally for fat removal. Previously, the senior author tried fat grafts similar to those recommended by Loeb [63] but discontinued the procedure as the grafts either resorbed or were visible.

Prominence in the lateral third may be either soft tissue or bone. Subcutaneous tissue fullness may be caused by orbicularis muscle as in a festoon, or fat deposits in a lateral fat pad, or descent of the lacrimal gland (see Fig. 13-7). As described by Owsley [77] and later confirmed by Zide [115], a supraseptal submuscular fat pad may be present laterally, contributing to a heaviness of the upper lid. In the younger patient, an upper lid blepharoplasty including excision of a central muscle strip and removal of the lateral fat pad and any laterally displaced central fat pad will produce a marked improvement. In the elderly patient, the incisions are extended laterally out to the eyebrow and any ptosis of the lacrimal gland is corrected by repositioning. Owsley [77] notes that makeup camouflage of the extended scars may be necessary for 6 to 9 months. Ptosis of the lacrimal gland has often been treated by partial excision of one-third to one-half of the gland. However, Scherz and Dohlman [95] reported several cases of keratoconjunctivitis sicca following partial excision. Therefore, Horton et al. [46] advocated repositioning of the gland by creation of a pocket under the orbital rim followed by suturing the gland capsule to the periosteum.

Prominence of the supraorbital ridges can produce a displeasing downward slant of the eyes, which cannot be corrected by excision of the soft tissues. As recommended by Lassus [56], ostectomy can be done through a blepharoplasty or brow incision. Following wide exposure, the area is marked, excised, and rasped. The senior author performs the procedure on occasion using small osteotomes. The patient must be warned that resolution of the edema and ecchymosis may require several months.

LATERAL REGION

The primary deformity is wrinkling, or crow's-feet, in the lateral canthal area, accentuated by skin folds or lateral hooding. Rarely, patients will complain of a downward tilt of the lateral canthus, a deformity correctable with Hinderer's blepharocanthoplasty [44, 45]. Numerous methods of minimizing crow's-feet have been advocated and can be divided into five groups: (1) modification of the lateral portion of blepharoplasty incisions (Lewis [59], Courtiss et al. [17]), (2) combined upper and lower eyelid incisions with direct excision of intervening tissue (Gonzalez-Ulloa and Stevens [38, 39]), (3) forehead-lifts with downward extension to the zygomatic arch, (4) rhytidectomy with upward traction (Regnault [90]), or (5) rhytidectomy combined with modification of the orbicularis oculi muscle (Skoog [98], Aston [1, 2]). In general, most blepharoplasties do not eliminate the underlying cause, contracture of the orbicularis oculi muscle, or excise sufficient skin folds. Thus, the patient must be told preoperatively that little change will be noted in the crow's-feet unless a more extensive procedure is done. An effective treatment is a modified Gonzalez-Ulloa procedure that includes excision of a significant portion of skin from the lateral canthal region. This can be done as an isolated eyelid procedure or extended laterally to effect upward traction on the cheeks. As noted by Rees [86–89], patients must be warned about the extended excision and realize that a more extensive procedure is required.

A forehead-lift can eliminate lateral hooding and decrease "static" crow's-feet but does little to eliminate wrinkling on animation. In a succinct passage from his classic text, Skoog [98] first described adjustment of the orbicularis oculi: "To smooth overlying skin and prevent excessive wrinkling at the lateral canthus, the muscle may be splayed out and sutured in this spread position. The orbicularis oculi may even be split laterally and the cut ends separated without disturbing eyelid function." Following Skoog's presentation of the technique in 1969, the senior author began rearranging the orbicularis oculi muscle during rhytidectomy. In 1980 Aston [1] reported a series of 20 patients who had various orbicularis oculi procedures: (1) isolation and splaying; (2) division of the muscle ring plus separation of the edges; and (3) comparison of the two procedures in the same patient. Division of the muscle ring showed greater decrease in folds and wrinkles. The procedures were done as part of a rhytidectomy, and the muscle was elevated with the skin flap and isolated along the lateral orbital rim. The muscle was then split up to the lateral canthus and sutured outward. Three-year follow-up showed maintenance of the improvement [2]. Su et al. [106] reported their experience in 35 cases using division and suspension of the orbicularis oculi muscle. From the cases presented, it is evident that excellent results can be achieved with blepharoplasty and temporal lift in the younger patient.

Patients complaining of crow's-feet are divided into two groups, those with only eyelid deformities and those in whom the crow's-feet are but part of the problem. The procedures most commonly used are the following: (1) a Gonzalez-Ulloa contiguous blepharoplasty for eyelid-only deformities, (2) a temple-lift plus blepharoplasty with splaying of the muscle in the younger patient, (3) rhytidectomy plus blepharoplasty with splaying of the muscle for the average patient, and (4) upward traction rhytidectomy with a Gonzalez-Ulloa blepharoplasty for maximum correction. The latter three techniques are discussed in Chapter 16.

Gonzalez-Ulloa Blepharoplasty

The fundamental principle of this procedure is that a significant amount of tissue is excised from the crow's-feet area (Figs. 13-9 and 13-10). With the patient sitting, the skin elasticity, redundancy, and area of excision are determined. With the patient recumbent, the skin markings are made and vary little except laterally. The lines of incision from both lids meet at a point 1 cm outward from the lateral canthus, thereby preserving a 1-cm equilateral triangle of lid tissue. The lines of excision meet 2 cm further lateral on a slight 30-degree upward tilt. Skin-muscle excisions are done in the lids but skin only in the lateral canthal area. The fat pads are removed where required. The closure must be meticulous, and the skin triangle must be left in its *normal position and size* as stretching produces a visible purple area whereas compression leads to band formation. The upper eyelid is closed first up to the lateral canthus, and then the lower eyelid is closed extending outward. The procedure is effective in reducing crow's-feet and can be modified to give almond-shaped eyes to those who desire them. The principal disadvantages are a longer scar, which the patient must accept, and a more technically demanding operation [36, 37].

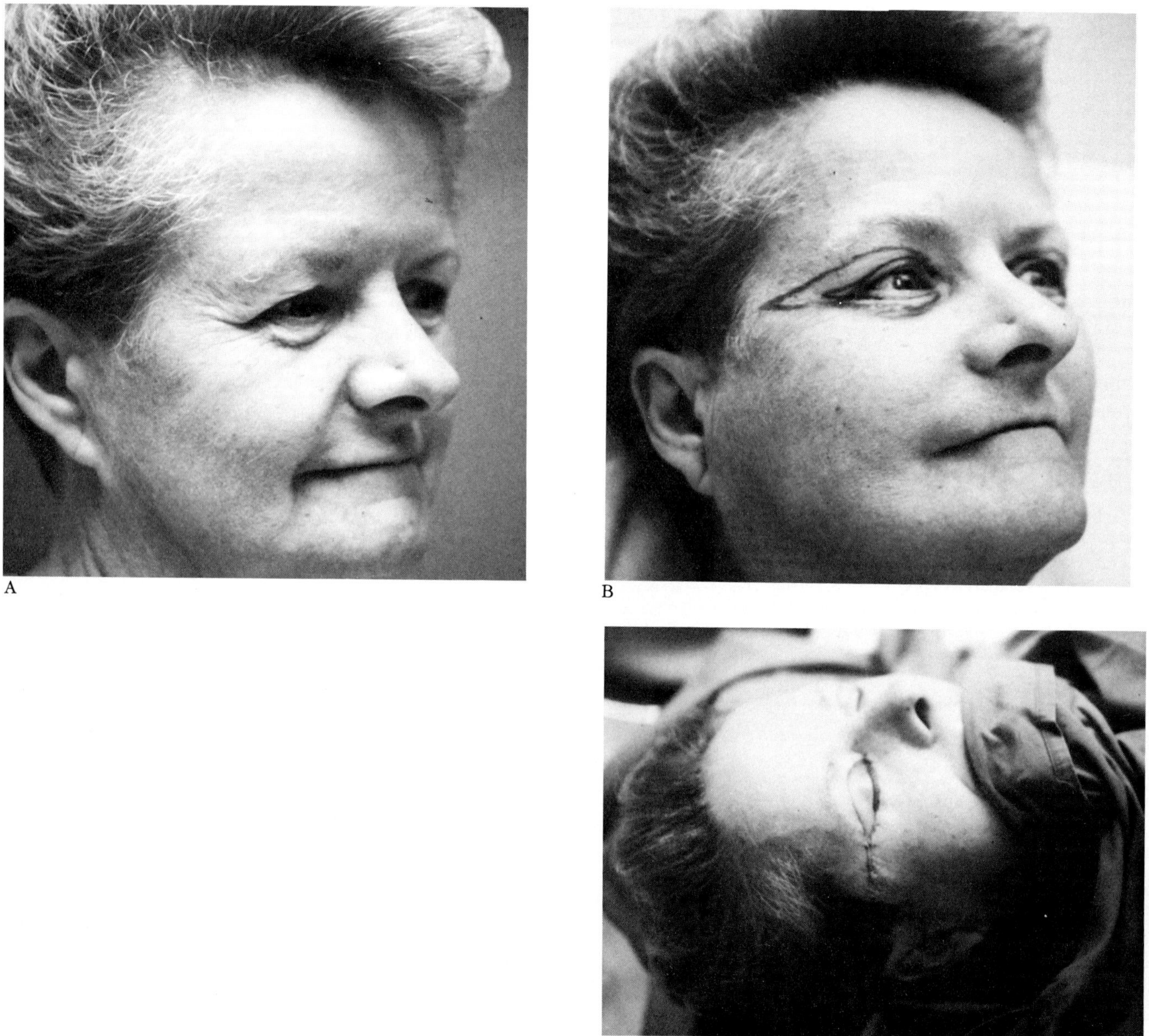

A

B

C

Figure 13-9

A. Patient with heavy lateral hooding and crow's-feet who requested a small local procedure.
B. Markings with the patient recumbent. Note preservation of 1-cm triangle just beyond the lateral canthus.
C. Closure of the wound with desired upward tilt of the eyelid aperture.

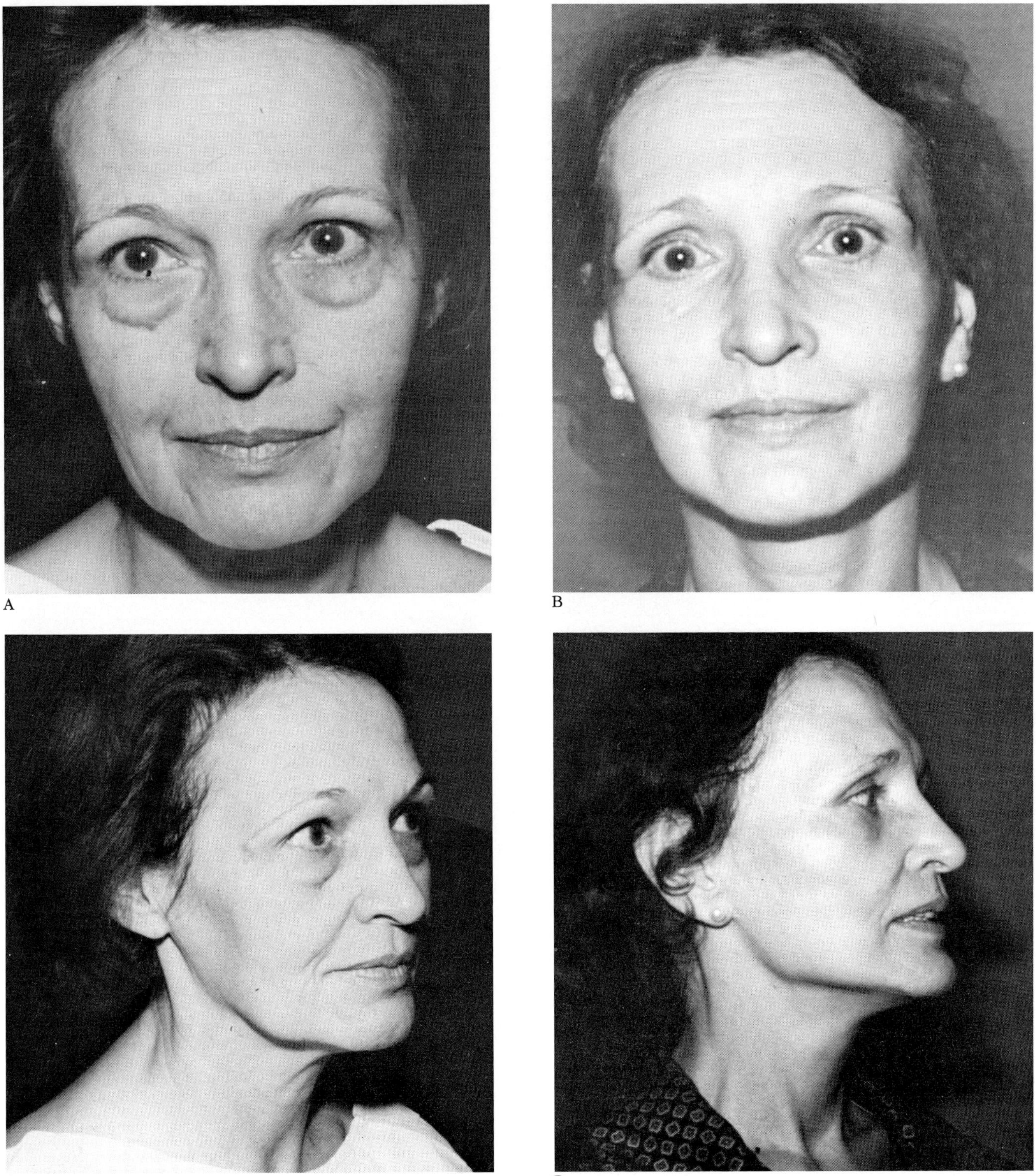

A

B

C

D

Figure 13-10

A, C. Patient with bulging of the lower lids and lateral hooding.

B, D. Result following rhytidectomy plus Gonzalez-Ulloa blepharoplasty. Note significant visibility of the pretarsal skin and absence of lateral hooding without a concurrent forehead-lift. Scar is not significantly visible.

Forehead and Eyebrows

A forehead-lift can achieve the following objectives: (1) elevation of ptotic eyebrows by mobilization and skin resection, (2) improvement in palpebral redundancy and lateral hooding of the upper eyelids, (3) amelioration of glabellar frown lines by resection of the corrugator and procerus muscles, (4) minimization of transverse forehead wrinkles by sectioning of the frontalis muscle, and (5) smoothing of the nasion plus elevation of the nasal tip (Fig. 13-11). As numerous large series have been reported with excellent long-term results, it is evident that the forehead-lift will be done with increasing frequency, thus reducing the need for direct eyebrow and glabellar procedures.

HISTORY

Correction of forehead wrinkles was one of the first aesthetic procedures [60, 105]. Passot [80, 81] used several small elliptic excisions to elevate the eyebrows and minimize crow's-feet. In 1926 Hunt [48] showed extended coronal incisions comparable to today's technique, both prehairline and posthairline, as well as vertical glabellar excisions. During the 1930s Noël [74], Joseph [51], and others routinely performed forehead-lifts with apparently satisfactory results [25]. However, in the 1950s the procedure fell into disrepute because the improvements were considered transitory, with reappearance of forehead wrinkles once edema decreased [5]. The criticism was correct, but only if the action of the frontalis muscle was not interrupted [70]. To overcome this limitation, Edwards [24], Fomon [28, 29], and Castanares [10–13] recommended transection of the frontal branch of the facial nerve. Although this maneuver does eliminate transverse wrinkles, it causes severe ptosis of the eyebrows [16]. Later, Marino [66–68], Vinas et al. [111], and others noted that many rhytidectomy patients were dissatisfied with the aging appearance of their upper face, especially the hooding effect of ptotic eyebrows despite repeated blepharoplasties [110]. The forehead-lift was rediscovered and used for elevation of the eyebrows plus elimination of forehead and glabellar wrinkles [40, 41, 109]. Large series by Vinas et al. [111], Ortiz-Montasterio et al. [76], and Connell [14, 15] have now demonstrated permanence of results, high patient satisfaction, and easy execution as an outpatient procedure often in association with cervicofacial rhytidectomy.

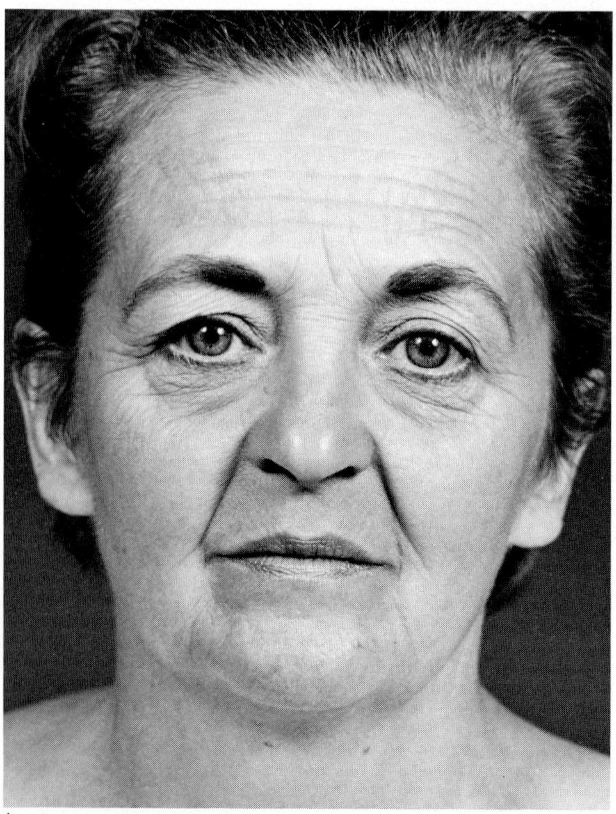

A

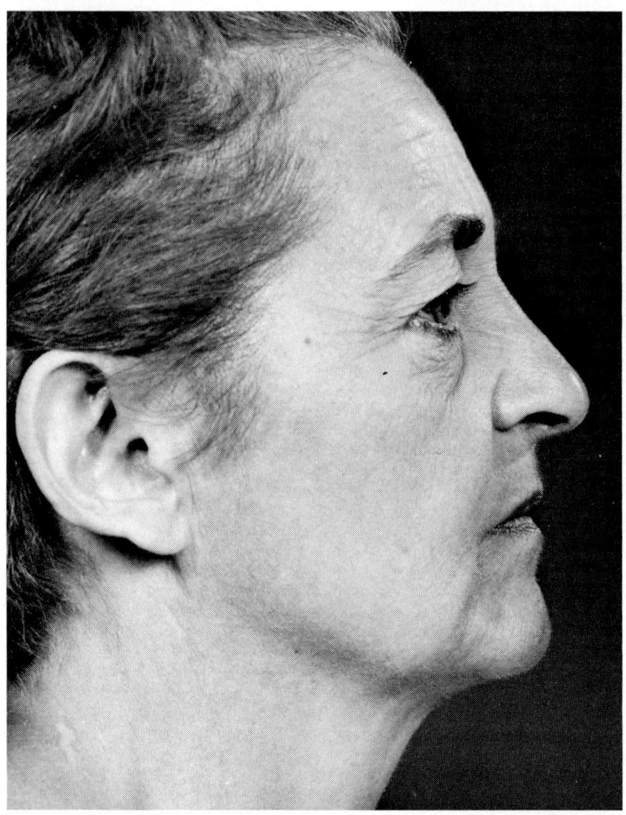

B

Figure 13-11
A, B. A 53-year-old patient with all the indications for a forehead-lift: ptotic eyebrows, lateral hooding, and wrinkles in the glabella, forehead, and nasion.

SURGICAL PROCEDURES

Numerous operations are available for correcting deformities in the upper third of the face. Each has its own indications, advantages, and disadvantages [55, 69, 107].

Bicoronal Forehead-Lift

This is the standard forehead-lift with the anterior incision placed behind or at the hairline and the temporal portion placed within the scalp. The advantages include maximum exposure of structures and concealment of scar. The disadvantages are the extensive dissection and sensory changes. Certain patients prefer a smaller localized procedure.

Hairline Forehead-Lift

In this operation the entire incision is placed at the hairline, including the temporal component. It is considered of value in patients who have had previous rhytidectomy with retrodisplacement of the temporal hair. The primary disadvantage is visible scarring over the temporal area, especially in patients with reddish complexion and multiple telangiectasias. Another variation is a straight-across prehairline incision terminating at the lateral hairline. This operation elevates the eyebrows but does not effect a lateral expansion, thus limiting the result. The authors rarely use this operation, and it should not be confused with the standard forehead-lift.

Temporal Lift

As practiced by Gleason [33–35], the temporal lift consists of paired incisions with a proximal deep dissection and a distal superficial dissection that continues to the lateral orbital fossa. Since there is no muscle resection and the dissection extends only to the center of the eyebrow, the result is truly a lateral eyebrow-lift. It is primarily indicated for the younger patient with lateral orbital hooding who does not require correction of forehead problems. It benefits from scar concealment but risks motor nerve injury and occasional hair loss.

Midforehead-Lift

The incision is placed parallel to the deep forehead wrinkles and may represent a continuation of the rhytidectomy incision. This procedure allows direct interruption of the frontalis muscle and elevation of the eyebrows with optional excision of the medial muscles. Because of the risks of visible scarring, it is primarily restricted to males with deep forehead creases and is used in less than 5 percent of forehead-lifts.

Supraciliary Eyebrow-Lift

In this procedure the eyebrow is elevated by excision of skin immediately above the eyebrow. Although a supraciliary crescent is often shown, Castanares [11] preferred

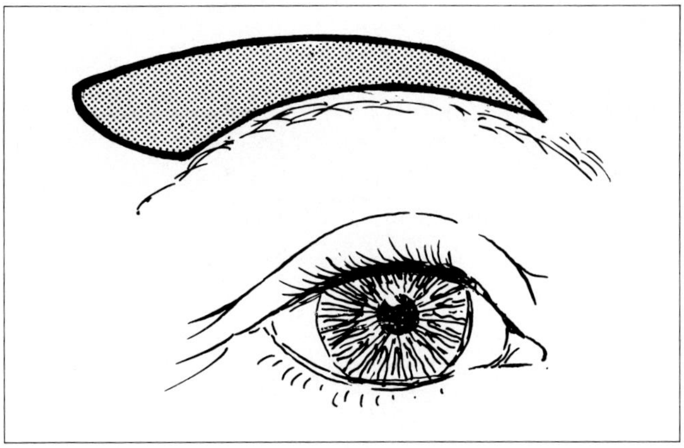

Figure 13-12. A fan-shaped excision for elevation of the ptotic eyebrow. Maximum elevation is lateral.

maximum skin excision laterally to produce an aesthetic eyebrow (Fig. 13-12). The procedure can be combined with a blind medial muscle excision. This relatively simple excision produces dramatic eyebrow elevation and improvement but leaves a *permanent visible scar* that requires daily makeup coverage (Fig. 13-13). Despite claims of universal application by many oculoplastic surgeons, this operation is best restricted to females willing to accept the scar and males with bushy eyebrows.

Transblepharoplasty Eyebrow Suspension

The "internal brow-lift" via a blepharoplasty incision has been advocated by numerous surgeons. Smith [99] and later Spira [103] advocated wide undermining in the supraorbital area followed by basting sutures of 4-0 nylon between the elevated eyebrow and the periosteum. Subsequently, Sokol and Sokol [101] described interdigitating periosteal-subcutaneous flaps, which are sutured in the midlateral position. Despite encouraging results in patients with minimal deformities, failure to modify the corrugators implies continued descent of the eyebrows.

Corrugator Resection

The medial musculature can be resected through short 1.5-cm incisions made in the medial eyebrow (Fig. 13-14). The corrugator-procerus complex between the supraorbital foramina is removed [100]. The procedure is done blindly and is prone to hematoma formation. The limited muscle correction restricts its utilization to younger individuals seeking minimization rather than elimination of their deformity. When performed in older individuals and those with significant forehead wrinkling, it leaves a central island of smoothness within a sea of wrinkles.

Wrinkle Resection

Direct resection of deep glabellar frowns is occasionally done in males and as a secondary procedure in females. Wilkinson [114] uses a combined procedure including

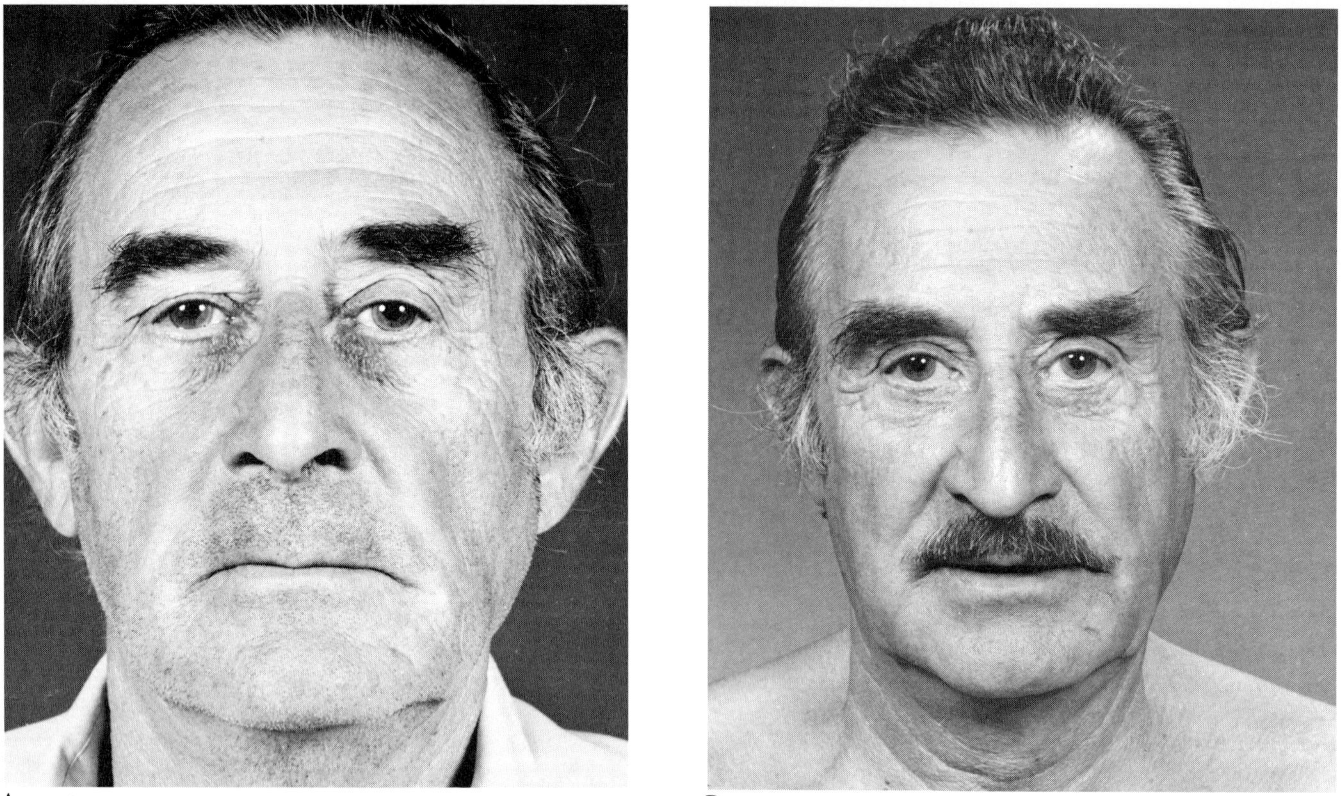

A B

Figure 13-13
A. A 61-year-old male requesting improvement in baggy eyelids.
B. Result at 1 year following blepharoplasty and a supraciliary eyebrow-lift. Despite bushy eyebrows, the scar is visible to the discerning viewer.

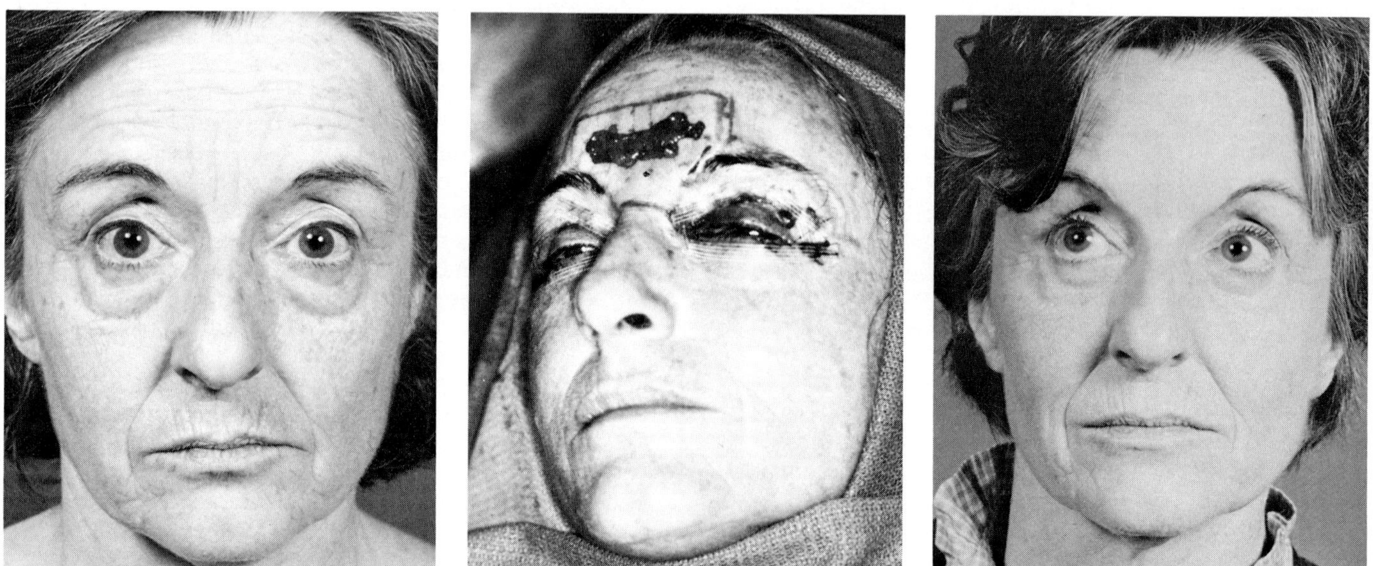

A B C

Figure 13-14
A. A 63-year-old patient requesting blepharoplasty and improvement in glabellar wrinkles. After detailed discussion, patient refused a forehead-lift and insisted on a localized procedure.
B. Intraoperative view of corrugator resection through a short medial eyebrow incision.
C. Result at 1 year. Although there is obvious improvement in the corrugator region, patient is markedly disappointed. Bicoronal forehead-lift as originally proposed is planned.

filling of the depression with fibromuscular tissue and percutaneous section of the corrugator muscles. After 250 cases over 7 years, he considers this ancillary procedure valuable for correcting glabellar frown lines. It would appear to be superior to the direct excisions of Borges [7] or Rosenthal [94].

Injection Therapy

Glabellar frown lines can be reduced by injection of liquid silicone or collagen. The liquid must be placed in the subcutaneous tissue (silicone) or dermis (collagen), primarily beneath the furrow with slight feathering on either side.

Chemical Peel

Depending on the severity of eyebrow ptosis, chemical peel can be used to eliminate early wrinkling or as a secondary procedure to remove persistent wrinkles in sun-damaged skin [3].

ANATOMY

The upper third of the face is bordered superiorly by the scalp and inferiorly by the eyebrows. The intervening skin is subjected to unrelenting muscle contractions that produce severe wrinkling and frown lines, as well as inevitable descent of the eyebrows. Correction of these deformities is predicated on a detailed anatomic knowledge of the underlying facial musculature.

Skin

The forehead skin is the thickest facial skin. The broad expanse of underlying frontal muscle and the absence of significant subcutaneous fat accumulation contribute to its unique characteristics. On the basis of cadaver dissections, Washio [113] found numerous transverse fibrous septums that ran from the frontalis muscle to the dermis. These septums divide the subcutaneous fat into narrow transverse compartments that correspond with the deep forehead lines. Elimination of the overlying furrows requires resection of a segment of frontalis muscle with its associated septums. Any muscle excision must be done carefully as the sensory nerves and blood vessels run within the subcutaneous tissue just superficial to the muscle fascia.

Muscles

The muscles of the forehead are intimately related as to both origin and insertion. The frontalis muscle is the anterior end of the epicranius and is in actuality a paired muscle that blends in the midline. In contrast to the fixed bony origin of the occipitalis, the origin of the frontalis muscle is free, and thus it functions as a weak elevator of the eyelids. Although it is not attached to bone, the frontalis is tethered by its interdigitation with other muscles and its relationship to the galea. The muscle blends with the procerus medially, the corrugator and orbicularis oculi intermedially, and the orbicularis oculi laterally. These attachments are readily confirmed in scalp avulsions where the separation line is below the eyebrows and across the root of the nose. Anteriorly, the galea aponeurotica encloses the frontalis muscle and is intimately associated with the periosteum of the orbit. This fascial attachment prevents scalp hematomas from descending into the eyelids and obscuring vision. Laterally, it continues over the temporalis fascia to the zygomatic arch [72]. If one is to achieve significant lifting, the fascial insertions must be sharply divided both anteriorly and laterally.

The corrugator supercilii arises at the medial end of the eyebrow from the frontal bone near the nasofrontal suture line and passes laterally beneath the frontalis muscle to insert into the skin. Although frequently drawn as a narrow 5- to 10-mm-wide muscle, the corrugator is actually several centimeters in width and covers the supraorbital vessels. It draws the eyebrows downward and medially, thus producing the vertical wrinkles of the glabellar region. In contrast, the procerus is a single small nasal muscle that originates from the upper lateral cartilages, is contiguous with the medial border of the frontalis, and inserts in the forehead skin between the eyebrows. Its contracture produces transverse lines over the nasion.

Nerves

The forehead is innervated by motor and sensory nerves, both of which can be irrevocably injured during a forehead-lift. The course of the facial nerve branches is discussed in detail in Chapter 16. As regards the sensory nerves, the small supratrochlear nerve emerges from the orbit, passes beneath the forehead muscles, and innervates the medial portion of the forehead. The larger supraorbital nerve exits the orbit through a distinct foramen or notch, divides into several branches, and innervates most of the forehead skin back to a line connecting the two external acoustic meatuses. Laterally, the forehead skin is innervated by the zygomaticofacial and zygomaticofrontal branches, which exit through the zygomatic bone. Each of these sensory nerves is closely associated with a specific artery and paired venae comitantes. Because of their close association, blind resection of the corrugator muscle frequently results in severance of the neurovascular bundle with subsequent sensory loss and hematoma formation.

Vessels

The blood supply of the scalp is profuse. The primary supplying artery is the superficial temporal artery, which passes upward from the parotid fascia and divides 4 to 5 cm above the auditory meatus into its frontal and parietal branches. Posteriorly, the occipital artery enters the scalp at the origin of the sternocleidomastoid muscle. These two vessels have numerous interconnections that ensure survival of the scalp provided they are not compressed against the bone by excessive tension. Additional blood supply is from the internal carotid artery via the supraorbital and supratrochlear vessels. The superficial branches course in the subcutaneous tissue above the scalp muscles and galea. The scalp nerves are numerous, parallel the arteries, and have multiple connections with the diploic veins. Their principal drainage is through the jugular system.

Hair Pattern

The height of the forehead is measured from the nasion to the hairline. It may be the classic one-third of the face, or short, on account of encroachment by the anterior hairline, or long, even without any hair loss. Of additional concern is the patient with thinning hair or progressive baldness. The majority of women will undergo some degree of diffuse genetic hair loss, in contradistinction to males, who have a more distinct patterned loss. Thus, the height of the forehead is a relative constant in women, who have a definite opinion on its size, but a changing entity in males with progressive hairline recession. A detailed knowledge of male patterned baldness is of benefit in performing forehead-lifts.

Eyebrows

The eyebrows are composed of numerous hairs resting on a redundant soft tissue base projected forward by bossing of the forehead bone. The eyebrows vary enormously from the totally plucked to the professorial bushy eyebrow. The underlying soft tissue represents the galeal insertion and the thickest portion of the corrugator muscles at their origin and the overlapping orbicularis oculi. Prominent or asymmetric orbital ridges may require correction. Many surgeons consider the eyebrows a fixed anatomic entity. However, few facial features are as dramatically altered as to location and contour. Certain patients pluck their eyebrows severely to decrease their width from 15 to 3 mm. Since their aesthetic objective is to "open the eyes," hair is removed from the inferior portion of the eyebrow, and eyebrow pencil may be used to fill in the completely plucked lateral portion. In severe blepharochalasis, hair follicles may be found overlying the tarsal fold. The shape of the eyebrow is a cultural variable influenced by cosmetic trends, but eyebrows frame the eyes rather than dominate them. Currently, the ideal eyebrow commences above the inner corner of the eye, arches to a point above the outermost portion of the iris, and ends at the lateral orbital contour. It is thicker medially and tapers laterally.

PATHOPHYSIOLOGY AND CLASSIFICATION

In the young patient, the eyebrows are often transverse and parallel the orbital rim, the forehead is creaseless, and vertical glabellar lines disappear on relaxation. During one's thirties, permanence of the glabellar frown lines may become a problem. The eyebrows will begin their descent, usually in the lateral third. In certain women who desire a glamorization of the eyes, complete elevation of the eyebrows may be necessary to complement an advanced blepharoplasty of the upper eyelids. As aging progresses, deep transverse forehead creases persist despite relaxation. Descent of the eyebrows creates a general heaviness of the eyelids and may limit upward gaze.

Classification of the problem involves four local areas: eyebrow, glabella, forehead, and upper eyelid (Fig. 13-15). The location and contour of the eyebrow must be assessed. With the patient sitting and completely relaxed,

Figure 13-15. An evaluation sheet for deformities found in the upper third of the face.

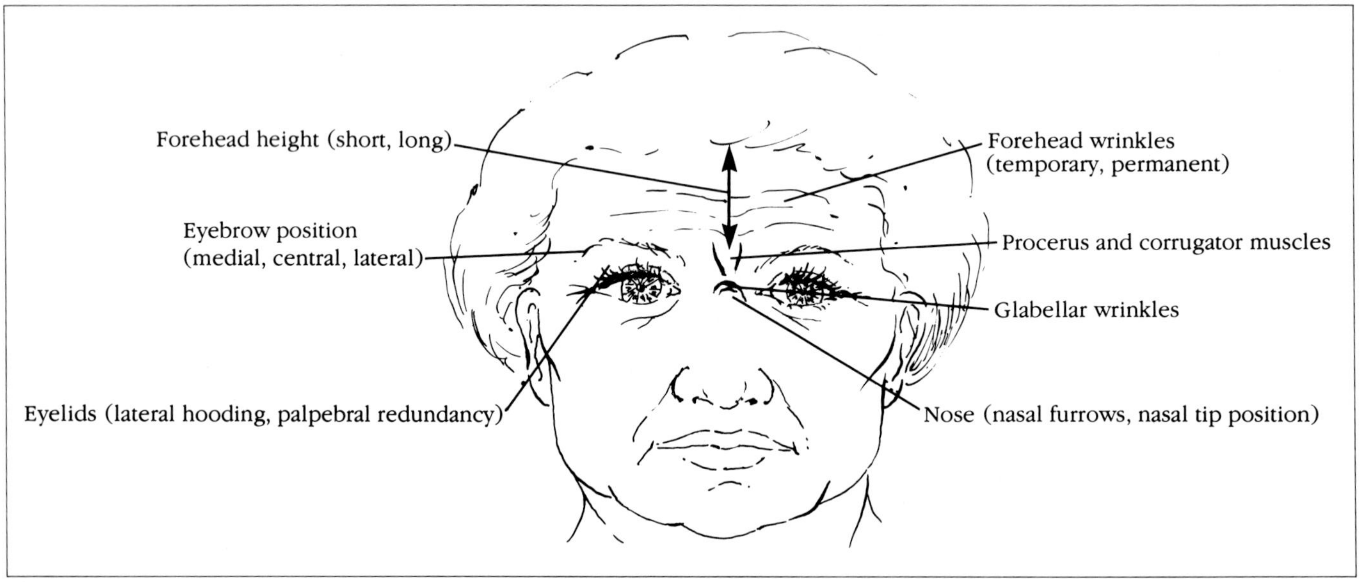

the relationship of the eyebrow to the supraorbital ridge is determined and the distance measured. The contour must be evaluated in thirds: medial, central, and lateral. If the medial eyebrow is lower than the lateral, the patient will look angry or distressed. In contrast, a lower lateral eyebrow gives the patient a concerned or sad appearance. Glabellar frown lines are caused by the corrugator muscles. The severity of the wrinkles is assessed during maximum frowning, normal conversation, and complete repose. One can improve but not eradicate deep wrinkles. Also, the degree of corrugator hypertrophy is estimated as it will guide subsequent resection of the muscles, and the degree of wrinkling in the nasion is checked. Forehead wrinkles are noted on maximum frowning, normal conversation, and repose, to estimate the degree of permanence. The eyebrows are elevated, and the change in upper eyelid redundancy is assessed.

CONSULTATION

Most patients requesting aesthetic surgery want correction of a specific deformity that requires a specific operation; e.g., breast hypoplasia requires breast augmentation. In contrast, patients needing a forehead-lift may be totally unaware of the necessary surgery; e.g., severe eyebrow ptosis in patients requesting blepharoplasty. Alternatively, they may be uncertain about the etiology of the problem, e.g., glabellar frown lines in younger individuals [65]. Therefore, one of the principal purposes of the consultation is to explain the cause of the deformity and to educate the patient as to various methods of correction (Fig. 13-16).

History

After the patient states why she has come and what she wants done, she is asked to point out the problem in the mirror. Frequently, "drooping of the eyelids" becomes hooding of the lateral orbit, and "heaviness of the eyelids" is markedly descended eyebrows. It is important that the surgeon understand the patient's complaint and not interpret a generalized remark. The patient is requested to give a brief review of facial aging: Which lines appeared first? At what age? When did they begin to persist? What bothers her the most? What are her priorities? Next, inquiry is made as to sun exposure and previous facial or cosmetic surgery. Numerous patients have had lesions excised in the forehead region whose scars may be difficult to see but will limit excursion or produce asymmetry. A detailed social history is taken with regard to activities, makeup styles, and normal coiffures. Does she wear lots of eyelid makeup or wear her hair up, away from the forehead? The actual makeup being worn is noted; it is usually a more elegant amount than for everyday wear, but less than the glamorization worn in the evening. Does she consider her forehead short, average, or high? Then a detailed medical history is taken.

Motivation

Patients often present with specific anatomic dislikes or generalized complaints about their expressions and how others perceive their emotional state. Specific dislikes include glabellar frown lines and deep transverse forehead wrinkles. More vaguely, patients will request a change in their expression; they are being told that they look constantly angry, sad, or tired. Older persons who have undergone a rhytidectomy feel that a wrinkled forehead distracts markedly from their more youthful appearance [73]. The psychologic motivation probably varies with age [23]. The younger patient accepts the surgical solution with enthusiasm, whereas the older individual has the secret desires of the face-lift patient and the propensity for postoperative depression.

Physical Examination

After removal of all makeup, the patient is examined in the sitting position. The generalized skin condition, complexion, and facial wrinkling are recorded. The patient is asked to wrinkle the forehead, frown, and look surprised. Any asymmetry is noted. Then a specific examination is done. The location of the eyebrow relative to the supraorbital rim is ascertained. The degree of eyebrow mobility is checked by traction on the forehead skin. The contour of the eyebrow is analyzed in thirds. The lashes of the eyebrows and the extent of depilation are examined. The eyelids are carefully evaluated, especially skin redundancy, lateral hooding, and closure of the upper eyelids. It is essential to determine whether a forehead-lift, a blepharoplasty, or a combined procedure is necessary to eradicate the periorbital problem [21]. Ellenbogen [25] has recently proposed a method of analyzing whether blepharoplasty is indicated based on persistence of blepharoclasis once eyebrow elevation is determined (Fig. 13-17). The reference points of the ideal eyebrow shape are marked and then elevated above the *lower border* of the supraorbital rim. In 75 percent (56/75) of cases, blepharoplasties were done utilizing a tarsal fixation technique after completion of the forehead-lift. The following refinements are proposed: (1) the incision made along the tarsal crease 9–12 mm above the lash line; (2) the levator expansion is identified; (3) the orbicularis overlying the tarsus is sutured to the levator with 6-0 white silk; (4) orbital fat is excised; and (5) the eyes are closed, traction is placed on the upper eyelid skin, and only then is the line of excision determined. With this conservative approach excess skin excision is avoided while an aesthetically pleasing eye is obtained. The glabella and forehead are examined on relaxation, conversation, and frowning. Are the frown lines permanent or transitory? What is the degree of corrugator muscle hypertrophy (mild, moderate, severe) and how far laterally does it extend? Next, the hair and scalp are checked for any thinning or dermatologic conditions. The entire face is examined and the degree of aging noted as well as its potential aesthetic balance [42, 50]. Finally, with skin traction at the hairline, does the patient look better?

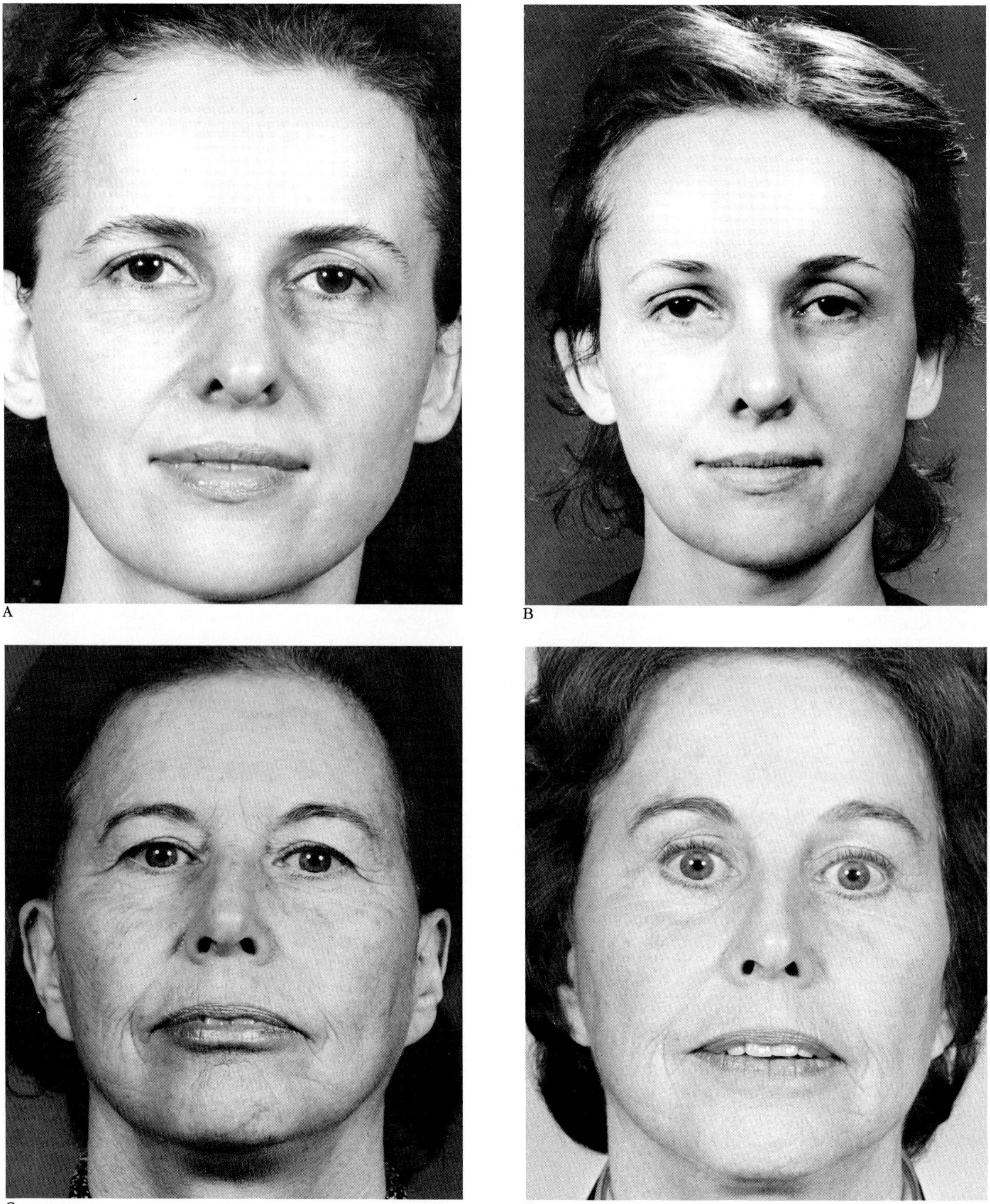

A B C D

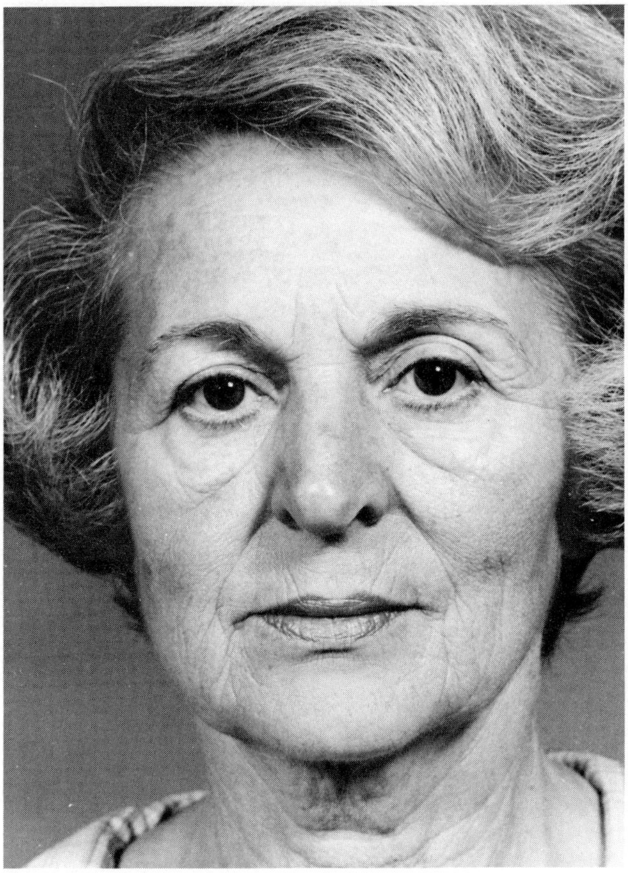

E

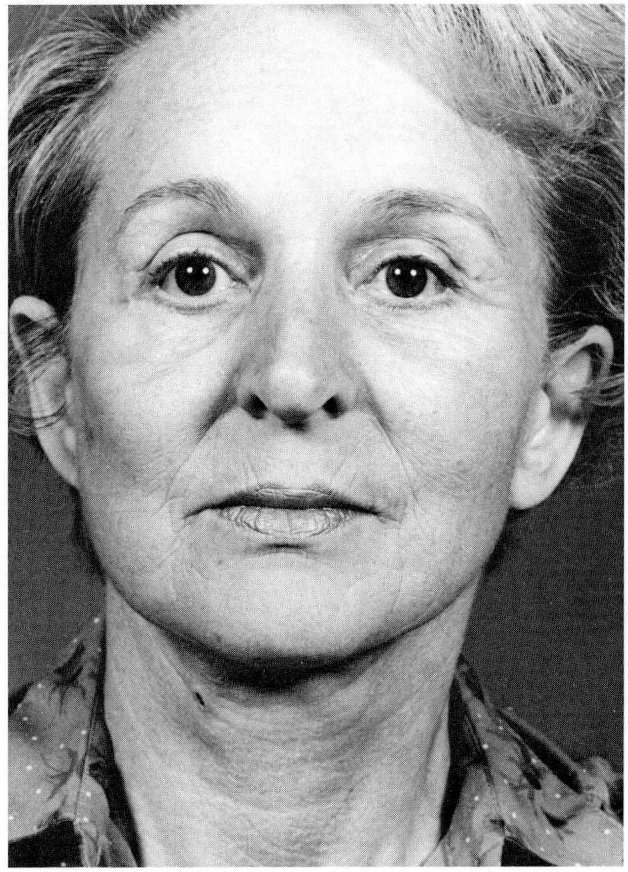

F

Figure 13-16. The interrelationship of forehead-lift and blepharoplasty.

A, B. A 40-year-old schoolteacher complaining of heaviness of the upper lids. On preoperative exam, elevation of the eyebrows corrected the problem and revealed a crisp upper eyelid. Results following forehead-lift *without* blepharoplasty.

C. Six years following rhytidectomy, patient is satisfied with lower facial appearance but wants improvement in the upper third, especially glabellar wrinkles. Severity of deformity warrants both procedures, as a forehead-lift alone would have to be excessive to achieve a smooth upper eyelid, while blepharoplasty alone would neither eliminate lateral hooding and ptotic eyebrows nor rejuvenate the upper face.

D. Result following forehead-lift and upper blepharoplasty.

E. A 63-year-old patient seeking a more youthful appearance. Failure to do a forehead-lift with rhytidectomy and blepharoplasty would leave a conspicuously aged upper third of the face.

F. Result following a discontinuous forehead-lift and rhytidectomy plus four-eyelid blepharoplasty.

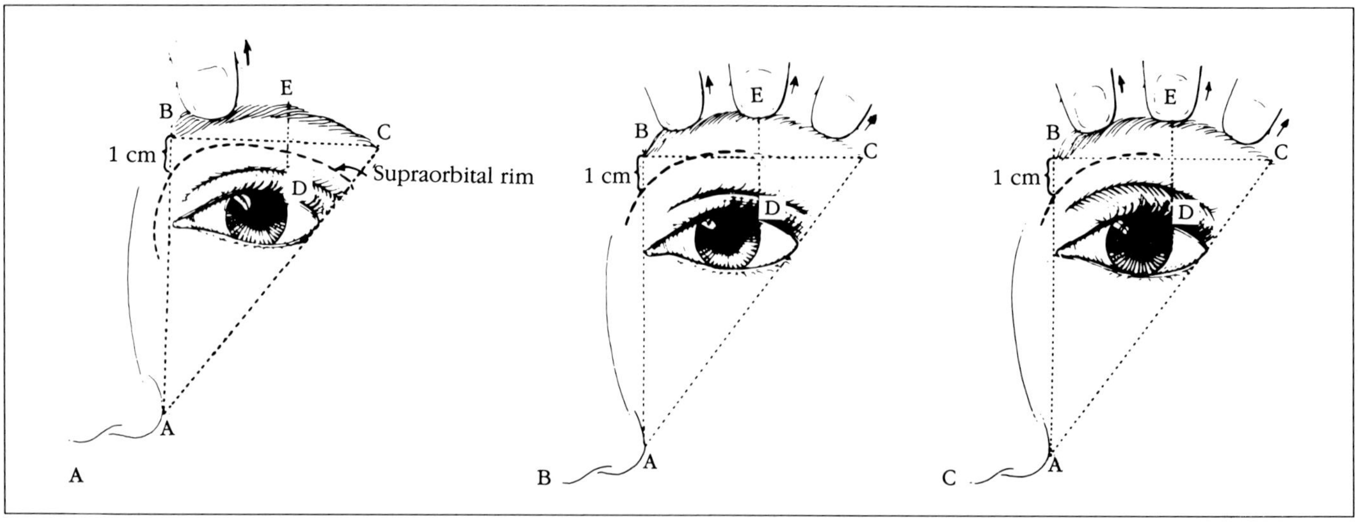

Figure 13-17. Ellenbogen's method of determining whether concomitant upper blepharoplasty is required with a forehead-lift. Westmore's reference marks for eyebrow arch: line *(AB)* from the ala through the medial canthus indicates the medial-most extent of the eyebrow; line *(AC)* from the ala through the lateral canthus determines the lateralmost extent of the eyebrow; *B* and *C* are at the same height; and line *DE* is parallel to *AB* at the temporal limbus of the iris with *E* the highest point of the eyebrow.
A. The test is begun by elevating the caudalmost hairs of the medial eyebrow 1 cm over the supraorbital rim.
B. Then *C* is lifted to the same height as *B* with *E* slightly higher; persistence of blepharoclasis indicates need for blepharoplasty.
C. In contrast, if the crease is distinct without overhang, then blepharoplasty is not done.
(Reprinted with permission from R. Ellenbogen, Transcoronal eyebrow lift with concomitant upper blepharoplasty. *Plast. Reconstr. Surg.* 71:490, 1983.)

Aesthetic Goals

With the patient seated in front of an examination mirror, the surgeon outlines the findings made, beginning with a review of the patient's complaints and how the surgeon analyzes each. Then the method of correction is proposed with the alternatives. At this point many patients will emphasize that their problem is a small one and the solution being offered is major surgery. This dichotomy is best resolved by having the patient face the mirror while the surgeon demonstrates the benefit of lifting the eyebrows by upward traction. Few patients are prepared for the dramatic change that occurs. As the eyebrows return to their supraorbital location, the lateral hooding disappears, and the skin creases are eliminated. If the patient cannot decide between a general or a localized procedure, a second consultation is recommended. Alternative locations for the incision are discussed.

Informed Consent

The various procedures available, the indications for the technique selected, and its potential complications are reviewed as well as features of the favored anesthetic regimen. Specifically, the following points are emphasized for a bicoronal forehead-lift:

1. A permanent scar will be present in the scalp. It will become red and smaller over several months, before fading to a white scar.
2. A feeling of tightness in the scalp and some degree of forehead numbness are to be anticipated for several months postoperatively.
3. Temporary hair loss may occur along the suture line, but hair growth usually returns in several months.
4. The upper forehead is expected to be immobile to ensure permanent removal of the wrinkles.
5. The eyebrows will retain their movement although some minor degree of asymmetry may be present.

Preoperative Preparations

Patients who tint their hair or wear it short are encouraged to have changes done preoperatively. All aspirin-containing medications are discontinued 2 weeks preoperatively. Photographs are taken full-face and oblique, in repose and in animation. The patient washes her hair with pHisoHex daily for 2 days prior to surgery.

SURGICAL PRINCIPLES

The forehead-lift has become one of the most beneficial aesthetic operations, correcting the deformities of the upper face with unparalleled success. During the past 30 years, the senior author has seen it evolve from a relatively simple skin excision to a procedure with more extensive dissection in the orbital region plus muscle resection. On the basis of a personal experience with more than 1500 forehead-lifts, the following principles appear valid.

Markings and Anesthesia

From the preoperative consultation one has determined placement of the incision (prehairline or posthairline) as well as the degree of desired eyebrow elevation and contour. As detailed by Connell [15], eyebrow elevation is done by first marking the location of the orbital ridge on the overlying skin. Then, with the patient looking in the mirror, each third of the eyebrow is elevated over a wide range until the patient indicates the desired position and shape. The skin overlying the orbital ridge is marked again, and the intervening distance determines the requisite elevation. As a useful guideline, the ratio of scalp excision to desired eyebrow elevation is generally 2 : 1, in contrast to supraciliary excisions, which have a 1 : 1 ratio. With the patient sitting, the plan is checked and the areas of muscle excision are marked. The planned incision and excision lines are marked, approximately 1 to 2 cm apart centrally and 2 to 3 cm laterally (Fig. 13-18). Surprisingly, other authors taper their incision laterally, a procedure that we feel limits correction of lateral hooding. In general, limited elevation of the medial eyebrow is required, but maximum lateral expansion is desired. A 2- to 3-cm strip of hair in the area to be excised is cut with scissors (Fig. 13-19). Three reference points, midline and both laterals, are marked to ensure correct orientation at time of closure. Hair along the incision line is matted down with sterile water-soluble petroleum jelly. The posterior hair is held in a ponytail; the anterior hair is divided into two parts and held with hemostats. The initial anesthetic is injected in the supraorbital-supratrocheal region to numb the forehead. Local anesthetic (Xylocaine 0.5% with epinephrine 1 : 200,000) is then injected 1 to 2 cm *behind* the entire incision line; this maneuver reduces blood loss and obviates the need for Rainey clips. The rest of the anterior scalp receives the anesthetic, followed by the areas requiring maximum dissection (supraorbital, temporal) and muscle resection (corrugator, procerus, frontalis).

Dissection

An oblique incision is made (Fig. 13-20). The dissection is done in the subgaleal space with preservation of the pericranium. Uchida [110] favored a subcutaneous dissection above the frontalis muscle, a maneuver that is bloody, ensures sensory loss, and risks skin slough. The initial dissection is done sharply and then bluntly until it is possible to turn the scalp downward. To gain mobility, extension of the incision to the auricles and separation of frontal fascia from temporalis fascia may be necessary. The eyes are covered with a moist gauze and the scalp is everted. Under direct vision, the fibrous corrections are sharply incised and the supraorbital neurovascular bundles identified. The dissection is continued inferiorly below the orbital rims. Common errors in forehead-lift are insufficient dissection and inadequate mobilization.

Muscles

In order to minimize forehead wrinkles, it is necessary to interrupt the action of the forehead musculature. Numerous methods have evolved for minimizing or eliminating muscle action [57]. As practiced by Edwards [24], neurectomy produced a total loss of forehead expression and subsequent ptosis of the eyebrows. Simple skin excision is *unable* to produce a permanent elimination of wrinkles. Of all the modifications that have occurred in forehead-lifts, muscle excision has been the most important. Although others have recommended detachment of muscle origin, simple transection, cross-hatching, or partial excision, permanent correction mandates direct excision of the muscles. Therefore, the corrugator and procerus muscles are excised from their origin outward until subcutaneous tissue is identified (Fig. 13-21). As stressed by Luckey [64], it is the corrugator muscle that causes medial eyebrow ptosis, and failure to interrupt its action cannot be compensated for by scalp resection. Secondary depressions are avoided by complete muscle excision, which prevents prominences, and preservation of the subcutaneous tissues, which prevents depressions. Then a 4-cm-wide transverse strip is excised across the forehead including the superaponeurotic connective tissue, the galea, and the frontalis muscle. This segment is marked preoperatively, usually 2 cm above the supraorbital rims and extending laterally to the temporal region. The remaining frontalis muscle permits animation of the eyebrow. Transection of the galea is necessary to achieve extensibility of the forehead. Although Pitanguy [83–85] favors cross-hatching and Connell [15] recommends partial excision to produce weakening, we feel that total muscle excision is necessary to achieve a long-lasting result.

Currently, temporal fascial grafts to the glabellar region are being suggested as a means of ensuring permanence and preventing depressions [93]. The grafts are inserted between muscles and subcutaneous tissue to serve as scar inducer and filler. Conceptually, a graft may be necessary if one chooses not to excise the muscle. It seems simpler to excise the muscle directly.

Skin Excision and Closure

Following completion of hemostasis, traction is placed on the scalp and the degree of mobility checked. In most cases, excessive eyebrow elevation is possible and one must carefully follow the preoperative plan. A midline alignment suture is placed using 3-0 Vicryl. The two lateral sutures are placed. Small Penrose drains are inserted down to the glabellar region and brought out laterally. The flap is further subdivided and the tension distributed. The redundant scalp is excised. Again, an oblique incision is done to match the incision line. The wound is closed with a continuous 4-0 Vicryl suture. Staples are used by many surgeons because of their speed and the conviction that hair loss is minimized.

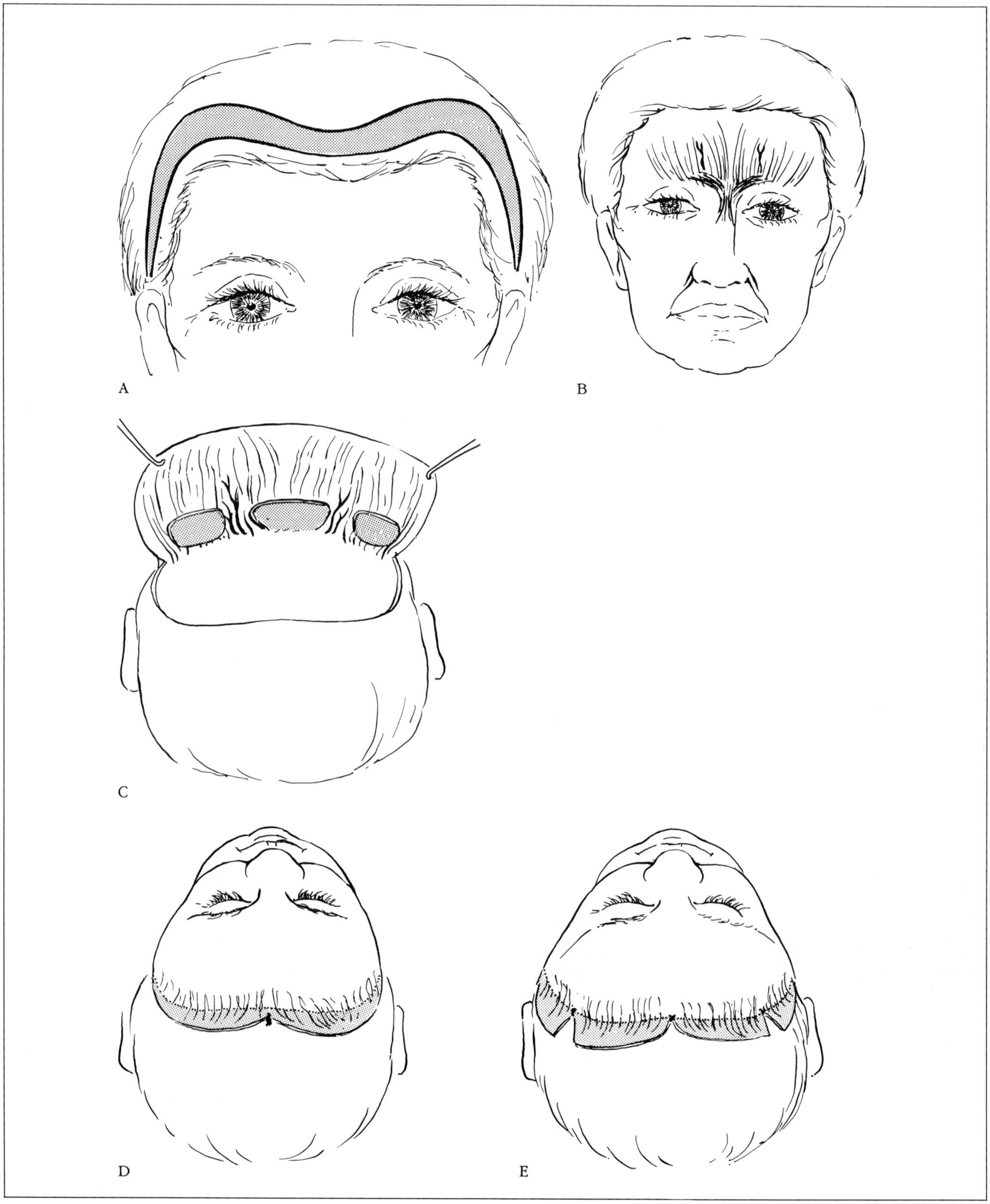

Figure 13-18. Basic steps in a forehead-lift.

A. A bicoronal incision, wider laterally than medially, is used.

B. Muscle division includes the procerus and corrugators as well as resection of frontalis.

C. With the flap reflected, three sections of the frontalis muscle are excised.

D. The flap is brought backward and a midline traction suture placed.

E. Excess skin is split segmentally, sutured, and closed with deep sutures followed by a continuous subcuticular suture.

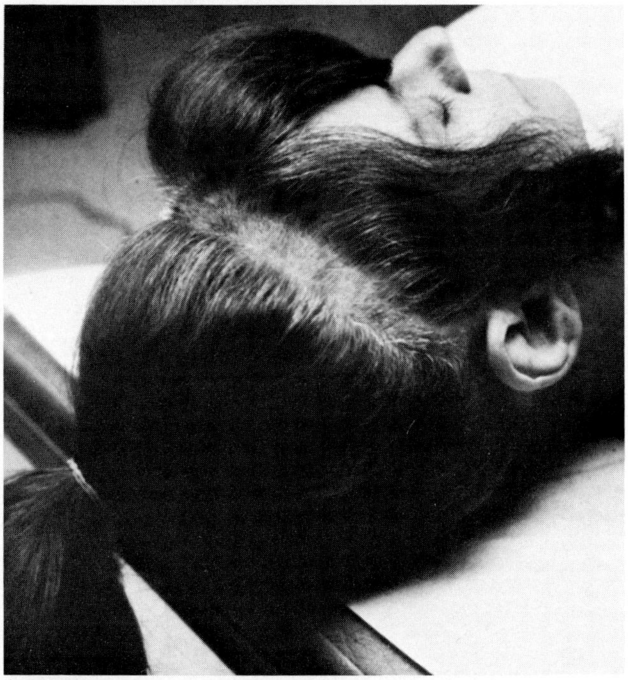

A

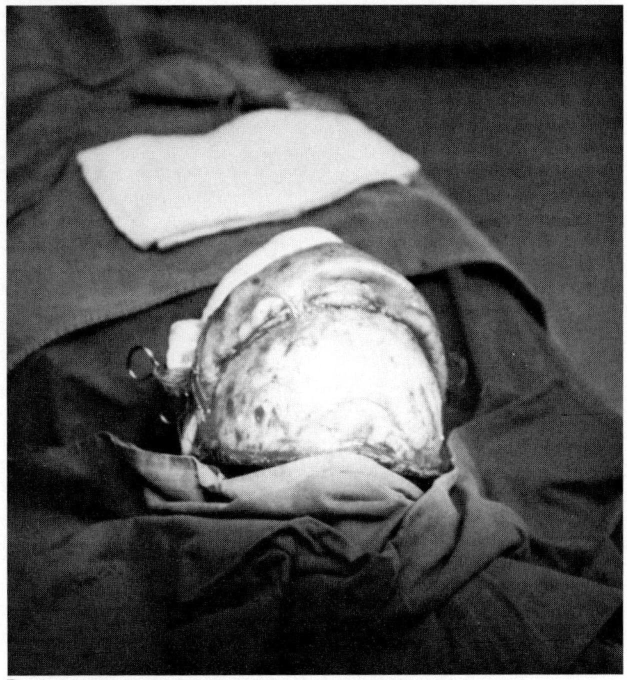

B

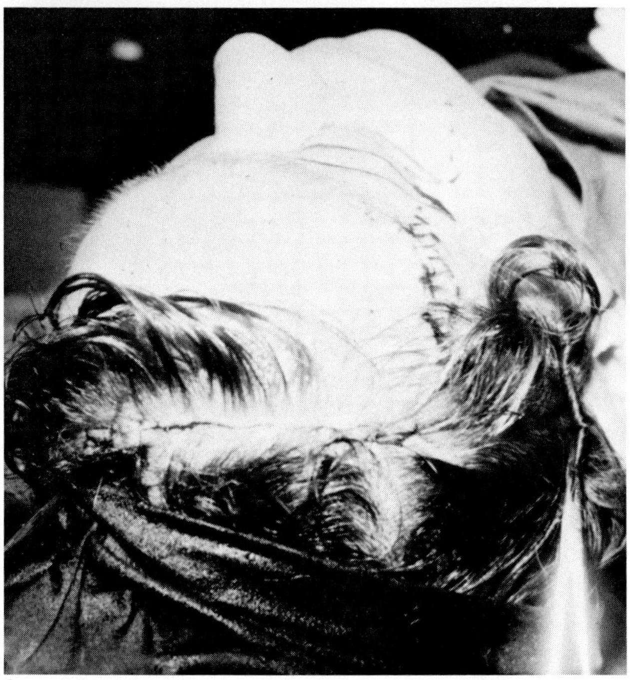

C

Figure 13-19

A. Hair is clipped along the incision line.
B. The scalp is reflected downward with severance of all fascial attachments to the orbital rim, but with preservation of the neurovascular bundles.
C. A two-layer closure is done following muscle and skin resection.

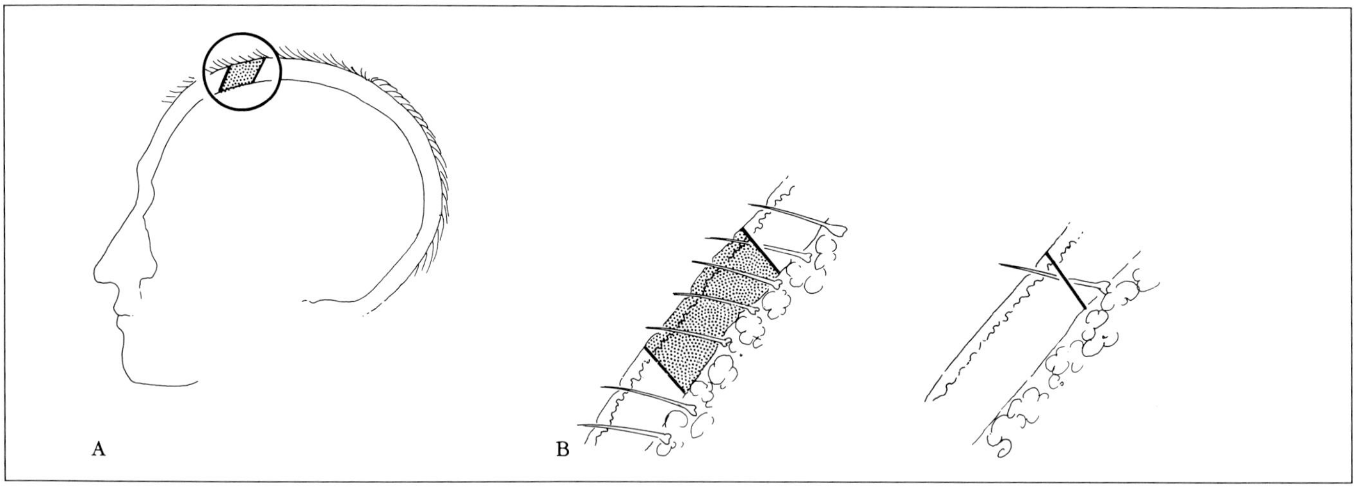

Figure 13-20
A, B. For incisions within the scalp, the lines of incision and excision are beveled posteriorly at a 45-degree angle with the expectation that hair will grow across the closure line and render the scar inconspicuous.

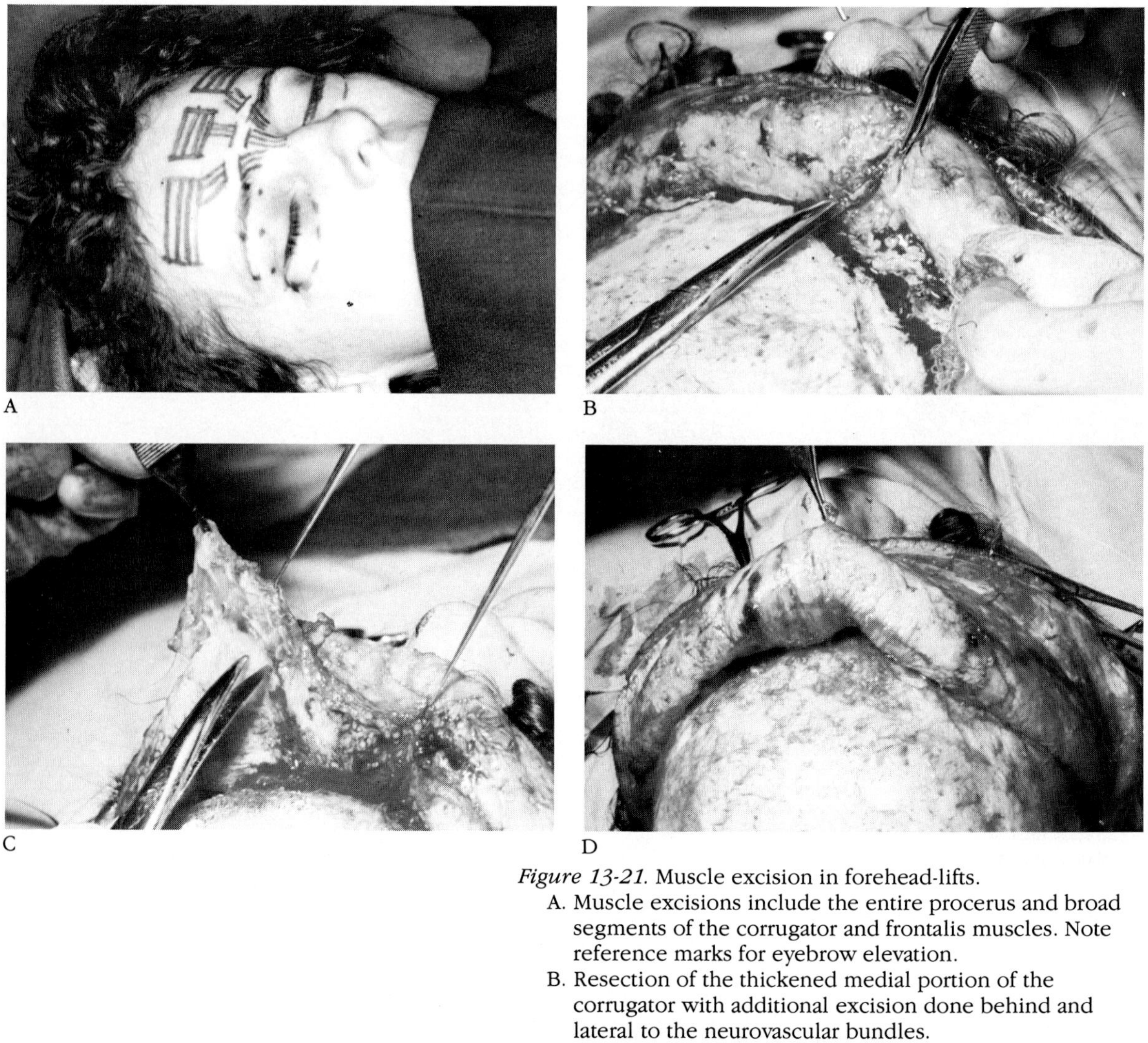

Figure 13-21. Muscle excision in forehead-lifts.
A. Muscle excisions include the entire procerus and broad segments of the corrugator and frontalis muscles. Note reference marks for eyebrow elevation.
B. Resection of the thickened medial portion of the corrugator with additional excision done behind and lateral to the neurovascular bundles.
C, D. Strips of frontalis muscle are extirpated.

Dressing and Postoperative Management

The dressing consists of a 4- × 8-in. petrolatum gauze placed over the forehead. A layer of gauze and then cotton is added and held snugly with a gauze wrap. Ace bandage and tight compression dressings are *not* used. Oral analgesics are given, and the patient is advised to sleep with the head elevated for several days. The patient is warned that eyelid swelling is common and is given ophthalmic ointment if blepharoplasty is performed concurrently. The dressing is removed 48 to 72 hours later, the drains are removed, and the hair is washed. Gentle shampooing and daily showers are permitted. Failure to eliminate crusts and sutures will result in ulceration, localized hair loss, and an unhappy patient.

SURGICAL TECHNIQUES

Bicoronal Incision

Selection of the location for the bicoronal incision should be dictated by the height of the patient's forehead, not by concern for concealment of the resulting scar (Fig. 13-22). Increasing the height of an already high forehead by several centimeters can only produce a dissatisfied patient who must permanently alter hairstyle and appearance. Despite this admonition, most surgeons continue to place the incision 3 to 8 cm behind the hairline, fearing patient dissatisfaction with a visible scar. Males with receding hairlines are routinely discouraged from having a forehead-lift. Is this fear of a visible scar justified?

The senior author employs a hairline incision in one-third of cases. Scar revision has been necessary in only one patient, and only a few patients have complained (Fig. 13-23). Recently, Connell [15] has published his experience with forehead-lifts in patients with male patterned baldness and credits acceptability of the fine scar to localizing tension in a few key points plus wavy incisions. Obviously, each surgeon must be comfortable with the incision selected. However, a single incision cannot be satisfactory for the multitude of deformities encountered. In addition to placement, the type of incision can be either straight or curved, paralleling the hairline (Fig. 13-24). In contrast to middle-aged males with their virtually universal receding hairlines, women of comparable age can have either a straight or curved hairline, dictating different incisions. One need only compare the hairlines of patients in Figures 13-22 and 13-23 to see the difference—one straight, the other curved, but both with high foreheads.

With the patient sitting, the plan is checked, hair is excised, and reference points plus incision-excision lines are marked. Local anesthesia with sedation is used routinely, commencing with a regional block and then infiltration of the area. The entire 45-degree beveled incision is made in one sweep, and hemostats are placed on the major bleeders. The galea is completely separated with straight Metzenbaum scissors. The forehead flap is mobilized initially by sharp dissection with a knife, then bluntly with the thumbs. As the supraorbital ridges are approached, sharp dissection is necessary to avoid avulsing the neurovascular bundles and to ensure division of the galeal fibers. The scalp is then turned downward, a maneuver that may require extension of the skin incision to the zygomatic arch level and dissection in the temporal area. With traction on the everted scalp, the central dissection is continued onto the nasion. A small submucous elevator may be of value in detaching the procerus muscle from the nasal bones. The procerus muscle is then removed from the undersurface of the flap, facilitating visualization of the supraorbital bundles, which is essential prior to muscle resection. By means of blunt scissors, the medial corrugator muscle is dissected away from the neurovascular structures and the underlying subcutaneous tissue. Its origin is detached by vertical stripping. The muscle is excised over as wide an area as possible. Then the corrugator lateral to the supraorbital bundle and even those fibers behind it are excised. Bipolar coagulation of bleeders is recommended to avoid nerve injury. Next, the area of frontalis muscle excision is marked and the passage of the supraorbital nerves noted. Washio [113] commenced frontalis resection 4 cm above the orbital ridges—the point where the sensory nerves penetrate the subcutaneous tissue. As recommended by Kaye [52–54], small bridges of muscle may be left over the nerves for protection, but the galea must be interrupted throughout. Following meticulous hemostasis, mobilization of the flap is checked, especially the lateral component. The medial eyebrow is easily elevated, allowing excessive correction, whereas the lateral eyebrow is more restricted, causing insufficient elevation. Since major muscle resection is central, medial eyebrow placement tends to be permanent whereas lateral descent slowly resumes. Hence, final eyebrow placement is checked from below with traction sutures in place prior to symmetric scalp excision. The excess scalp is then excised segmentally, leaving a slight redundancy that precludes excessive tension. Closure consists of three parts: (1) temporary traction sutures of 3-0 Vicryl inserted in segmental splits to achieve correct orientation and tension, (2) numerous buried 3-0 Vicryl sutures approximating the galea, and (3) a continuous dermal suture with 4-0 Vicryl or staples to approximate the edges.

Combined Forehead-Lifts

The forehead-lift was initially considered an ancillary procedure for improving the final result of a previous rhytidectomy rather than an integral part of total facial rejuvenation [78, 82]. More recently, forehead-lift combined with blepharoplasty has become the method of choice for total correction of periorbital aesthetic problems. When a forehead-lift is combined with other procedures, it must be done first because the elevation and traction dramatically alter their execution, especially upper eyelid blepharoplasty. Ortiz-Montasterio et al. [76] reported a series of 285 bicoronal forehead-lifts, of which 246 were combined with rhytidectomy-blepharoplasty and 39 with blepharoplasty; all forehead-lifts were part of a combined procedure.

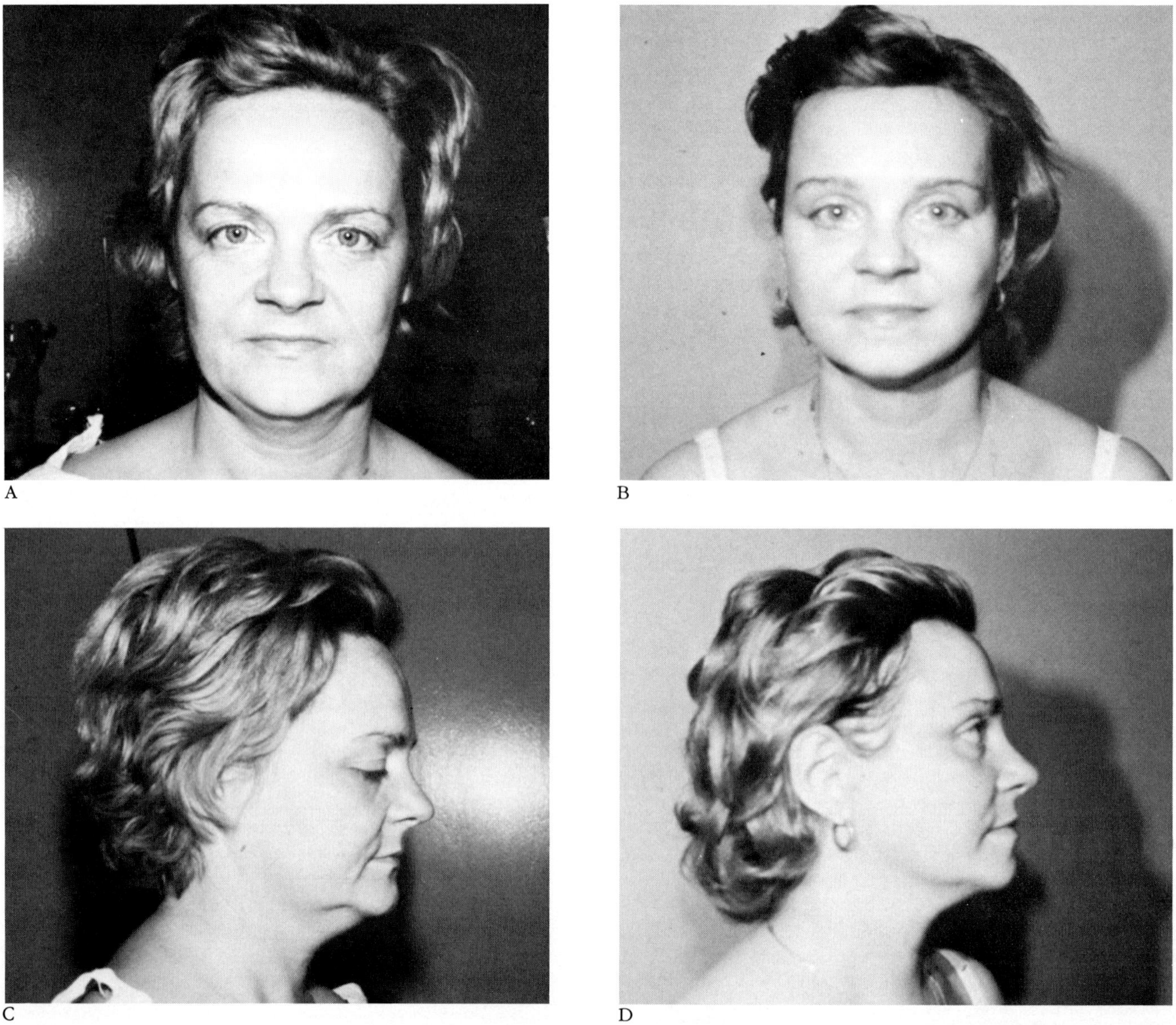

Figure 13-22
A, C. Patient with a high forehead and straight hairline. Placement of the incision in the scalp would only accentuate the high forehead.
B, D. Result following forehead-lift, rhytidectomy, and blepharoplasty. Incision at the hairline does not create a conspicuous deformity. It also decreases the height of the forehead by the amount of excision.

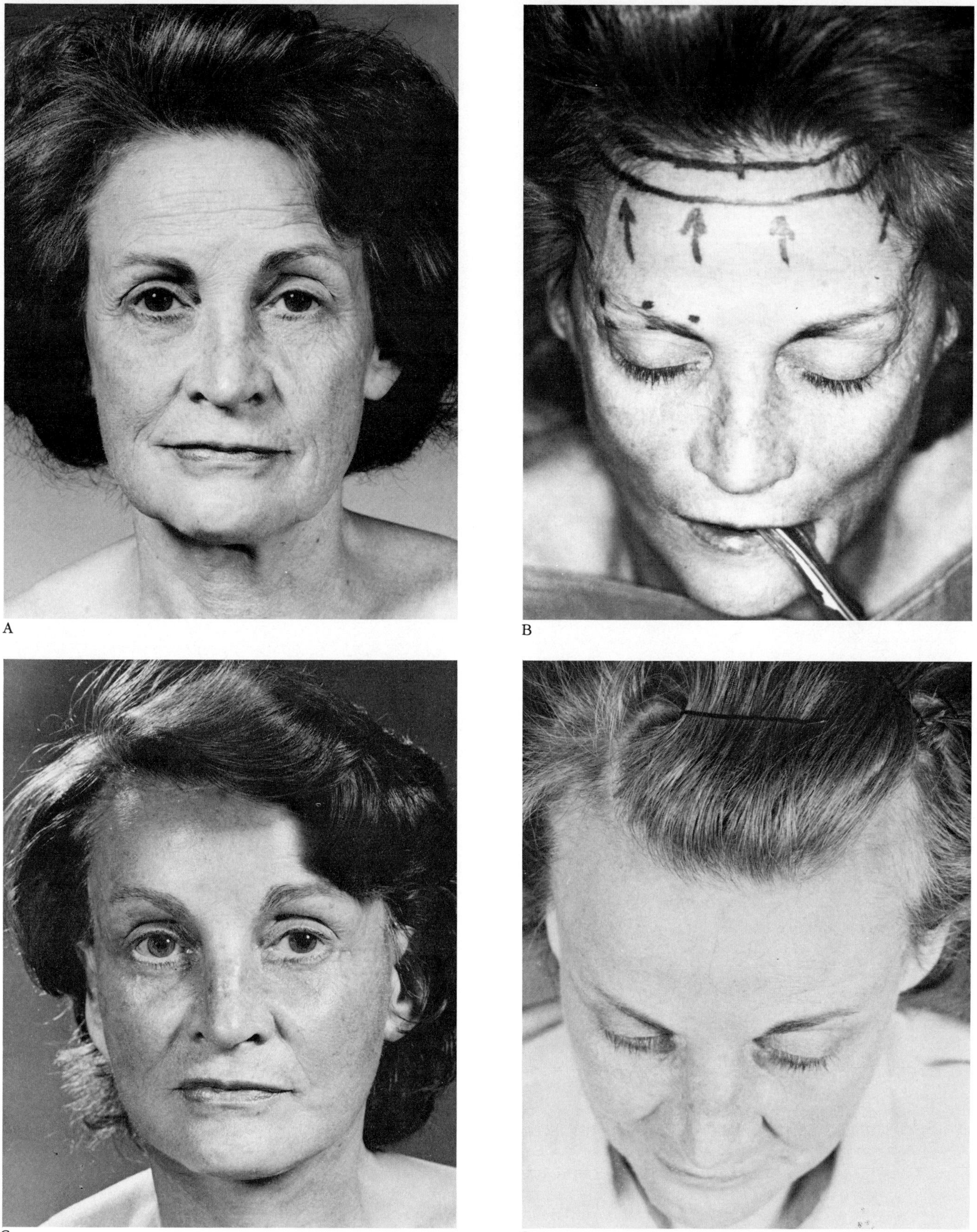

A B C D

Figure 13-23

A. A 53-year-old patient with significant facial wrinkling and posttraumatic nasal deformity.

B. Markings for forehead-lift to be done at the hairline.

C. Result following forehead-lift, lower lid blepharoplasty, and rhytidectomy. Upper blepharoplasty was *not* done. A folded conchal cartilage graft was inserted onto the dorsum of the nose through the forehead incision.

D. Result at 1 year with a virtually invisible scar.

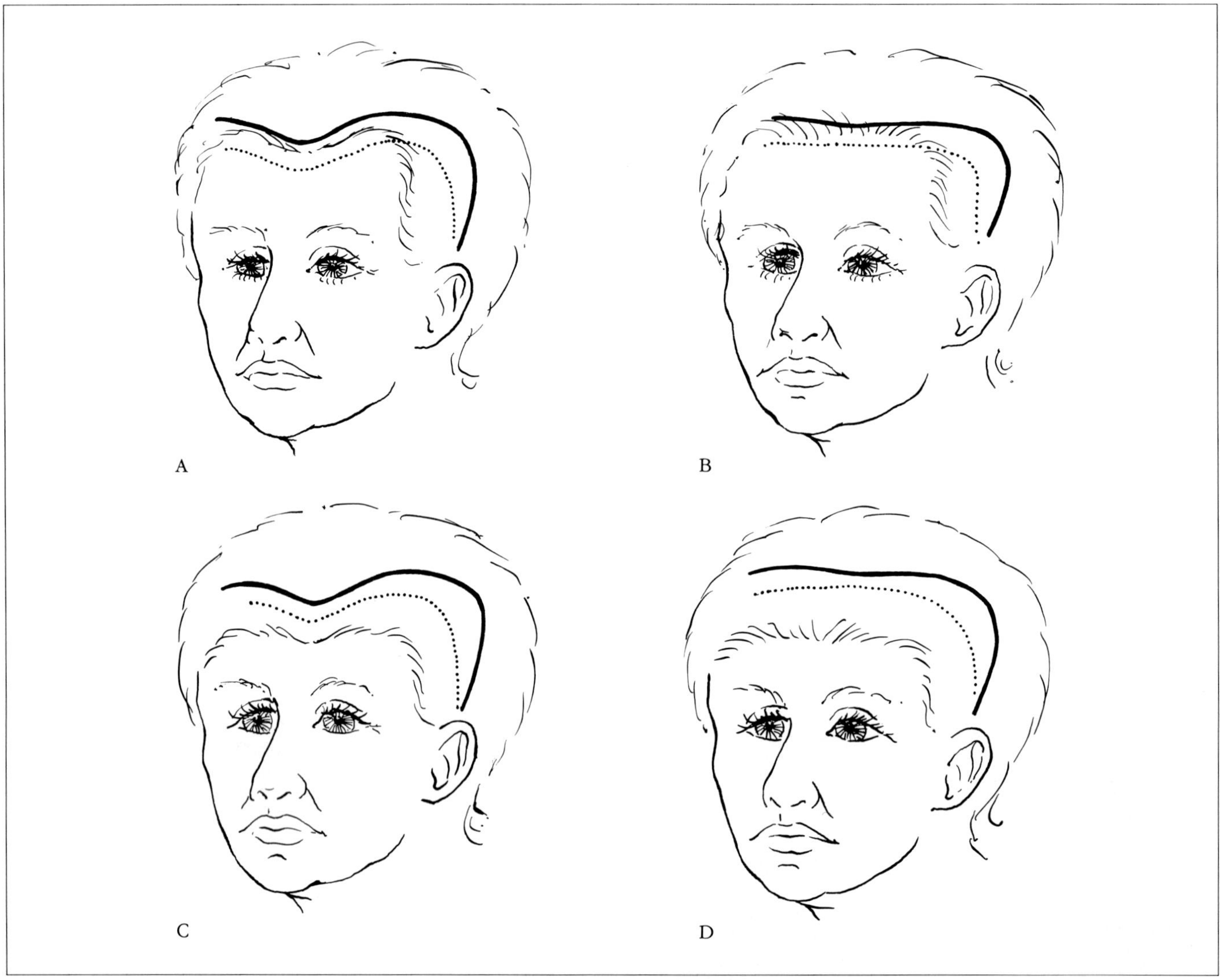

Figure 13-24. The types of incision for bicoronal forehead-lift as indicated by the heavy line and the anticipated excision shown by the dotted line.
A, B. For patients with a high forehead, the incision is placed at the hairline, either curved or straight.
C, D. For patients with a normal or low forehead, the incision is placed in the scalp, either curved or straight.

When a combined forehead-lift and cervicofacial rhytidectomy is planned, one must first decide on the type of incisions (Fig. 13-25). A continuous incision is used in most patients, with a discontinuous incision preferred in those with sparse hair or a receding temporal hairline (Fig. 13-26). There is minimal hairline alteration with a discontinuous incision. If the rhytidectomy incision is in front of the temporal hairline, one can achieve maximum excision and elevation of the facial skin. For anesthetic, hemostatic, and orientation reasons, the forehead-lift is closed prior to commencement of the rhytidectomy.

Since the forehead-lift elevates the eyebrow and decreases palpebral redundancy, it must be done prior to blepharoplasty. Careful preoperative analysis, with the patient sitting and the eyebrows held in the desired location, will allow an *estimate* of the amount of upper eyelid skin to be excised. Before surgery is commenced, the pretarsal incision line for the upper blepharoplasty is marked and the expected excision line is dotted in place. The lower blepharoplasty is unaltered by forehead-lift or rhytidectomy. Occasionally, swelling of the upper eyelids may occur following forehead-lift, forcing postponement of the blepharoplasty for several days.

Male Forehead-Lifts

Since males have heavy eyebrows and rarely pluck the lower border, elevation of the eyebrows is often desirable. However, a receding anterior hairline creates both a high forehead and apparent baldness, thus diminishing the improvements of a forehead-lift. Of further concern is whether the scars will become more visible as baldness progresses. In a remarkable series of cases Connell [15] has demonstrated that males do benefit dramatically from

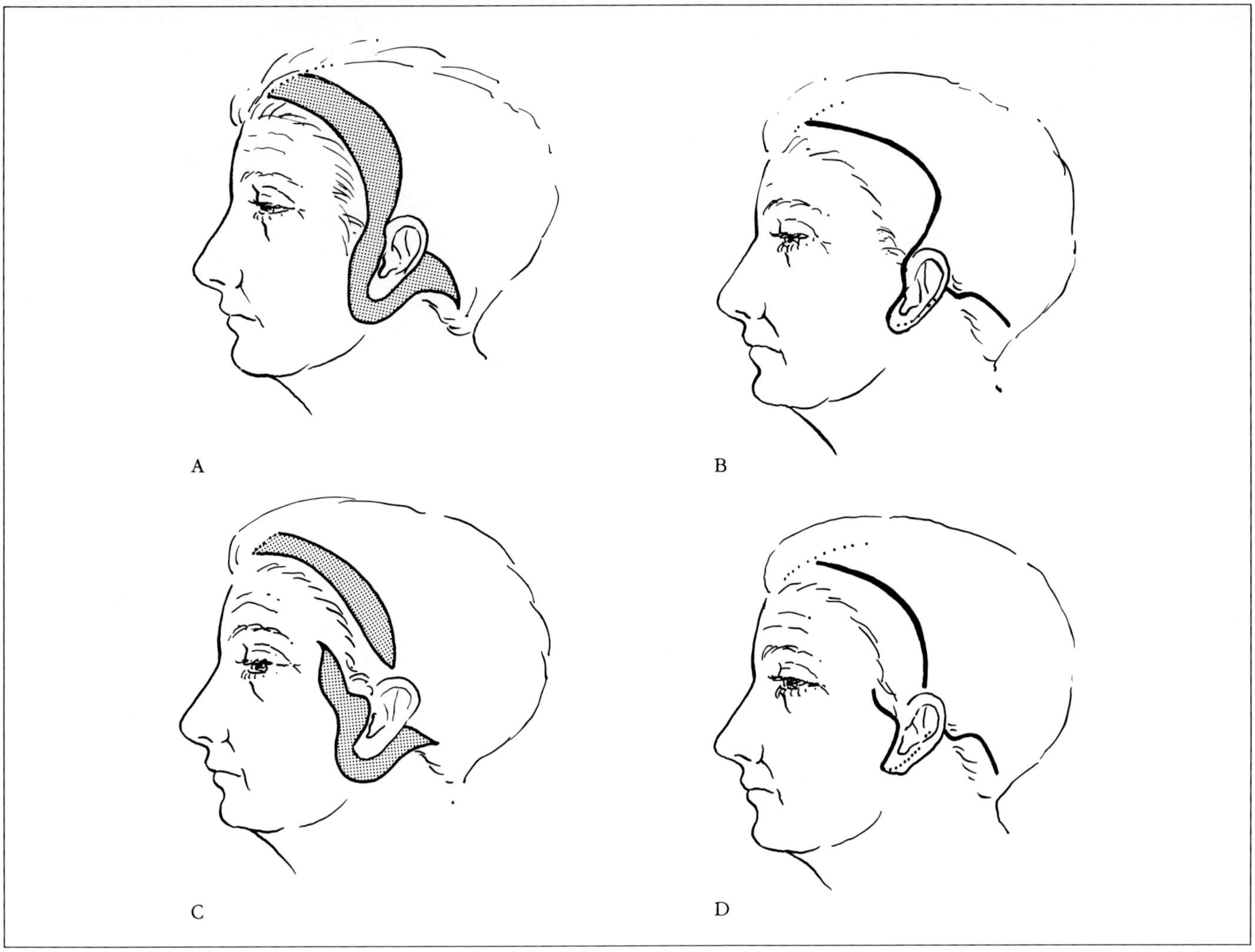

Figure 13-25. Incisions for combined forehead-lift and rhytidectomy.

A, B. A continuous incision is used in the majority of patients.

C, D. A discontinuous incision is used for those with a receding hairline or thinning hair.

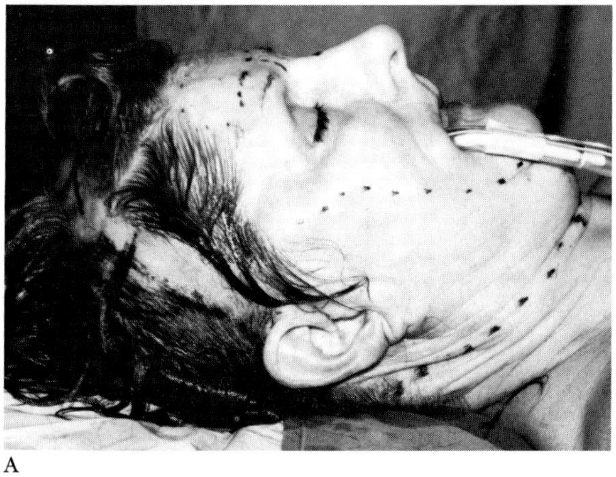

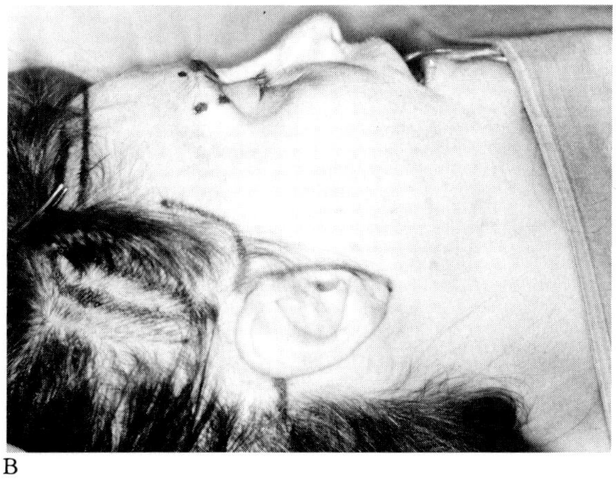

Figure 13-26

A. A continuous incision for a combined forehead-lift and rhytidectomy with area of undermining indicated.

B. A discontinuous incision with the rhytidectomy component in front of the thin receding temporal hair.

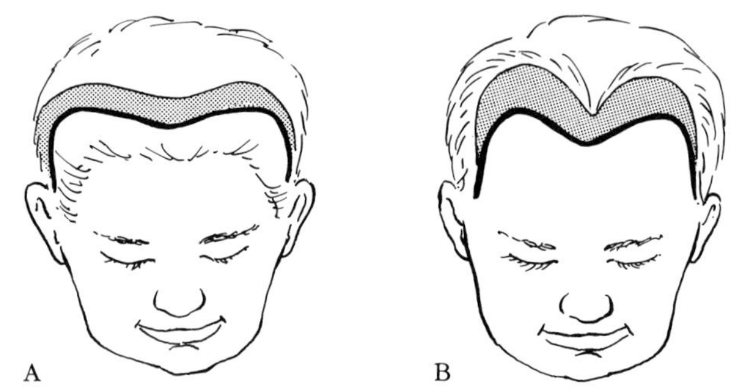
A B

Figure 13-27. Incisions for forehead-lifts in males. A. Behind the hairline in those with adequate hair. B. At the hairline in those with a receding hairline.

forehead-lifts and that the scar can be made acceptable provided a meticulous closure is done. In males with a high forehead, the incision is made at the forehead-hair junction, continuing into the temporal area (Fig. 13-27). This approach reduces the height of the forehead. In males with a receding anterior hairline, the incision is made a few millimeters inside the hair and slightly wavy to replicate a normal hairline. Laterally, the incision passes into the temporal region 3 cm behind the lateral hairline. Tension on the suture line is restricted to key support areas. The remainder of the incision has a 2-mm excess, and closure is accomplished without tension. Patients with red telangiectatic skin may develop a "white scar," and thus a more concealed incision is advocated. As regards progressive exposure of the scar, certain surgeons feel that the baldness pattern is established by age 45 and little progression occurs thereafter. Until one gains sufficient experience, forehead-lifts in balding males should be approached conservatively. For bald patients, Connell [15] uses the most superior forehead crease line rather than the more noticeable bald scalp. On reviewing Connell's writings, one must distinguish between eyebrow-lift procedures, which have virtually no undermining and the more extensive forehead-lifts, which involve wide undermining plus muscle and scalp excision. Although the principles for locating the incisions are similar, the techniques differ markedly.

Supraciliary Eyebrow Elevation

Direct excision of skin above the eyebrow can achieve a dramatic improvement but leaves a permanent scar. The procedure is indicated for males with bushy eyebrows or elderly patients with sufficient wrinkles to hide the scar. O'Neill [75] has emphasized that the procedure can be of particular benefit for the patient with asymmetric eyebrows.

As noted by Castanares [11], a crescent incision paralleling the eyebrow is *not* used as it reproduces the laterally descended eyebrow. The technique of Vinas et al. [111] is employed in which the lateral skin is pinched to determine the desired elevation and the height of the skin excision. Laterally, an ellipse is completed, and medially the excision continues to the head of the brow. All marks are made with the patient sitting, including the expected location of the supraorbital vessels. Under local infiltration, a full-thickness skin excision is done with beveling of the incision to avoid cutting the hair follicles. A strip of frontalis muscle, orbicularis oculi, and lateral corrugator is excised. Wide undermining and excision of the medial corrugator are *not* done. The degree of eyebrow elevation is noted, and further release is undertaken if necessary. The musculature beneath the eyebrow is anchored with 3-0 Vicryl to the frontalis muscle, thereby minimizing skin tension. Next, an everting deep layer of interrupted sutures is used, followed by a running 5-0 Prolene subcuticular suture. Steri-Strips are placed to support the suture.

An interesting variation of this procedure is the infrabrow-lift proposed by Parkes et al. [79]. If eyelid redundancy is present but the eyebrows are at or above the supraorbital ridge, tissue may be excised through an incision located along the inferior border of the eyebrow. It is of particular value in revisional blepharoplasty.

COMPLICATIONS

The incidence and severity of complications with forehead-lifts are quite low, and patient acceptance is quite good provided the patient expects transitory numbness and a significant incision. Virtually all complications are apparent in the early postoperative period.

Hematoma

Because of the avascularity of the dissection plane, bleeding is not a major problem. Significant oozing does occur on resection of the corrugator muscles, and Gleason [34] has recommended cauterization of the muscle stumps. Bleeding from the frontalis muscle resection is controlled with bipolar coagulation. Small Penrose drains are used and allow expression of any clots as they are removed.

Skin Necrosis

Major skin loss has been reported, but usually with extenuating circumstances: hypertension, infected hematoma, or previous scar (Fig. 13-28). Skin necrosis is attributed to excessive tension, which compresses the supraorbital vessels over prominent frontal bossing, or a superficial dissection between the frontalis muscle and skin. Prevention is achieved by limiting the amount of scalp excision and thus required tension. Minor skin loss resulting in small areas of alopecia were present in 13 percent (37 out of 285) of cases reported by Ortiz-Montasterio et al. [76].

Pain

It is quite common for patients to complain of a tightness or a constricting sensation about the head for several weeks postoperatively. Treatment consists in reassurance

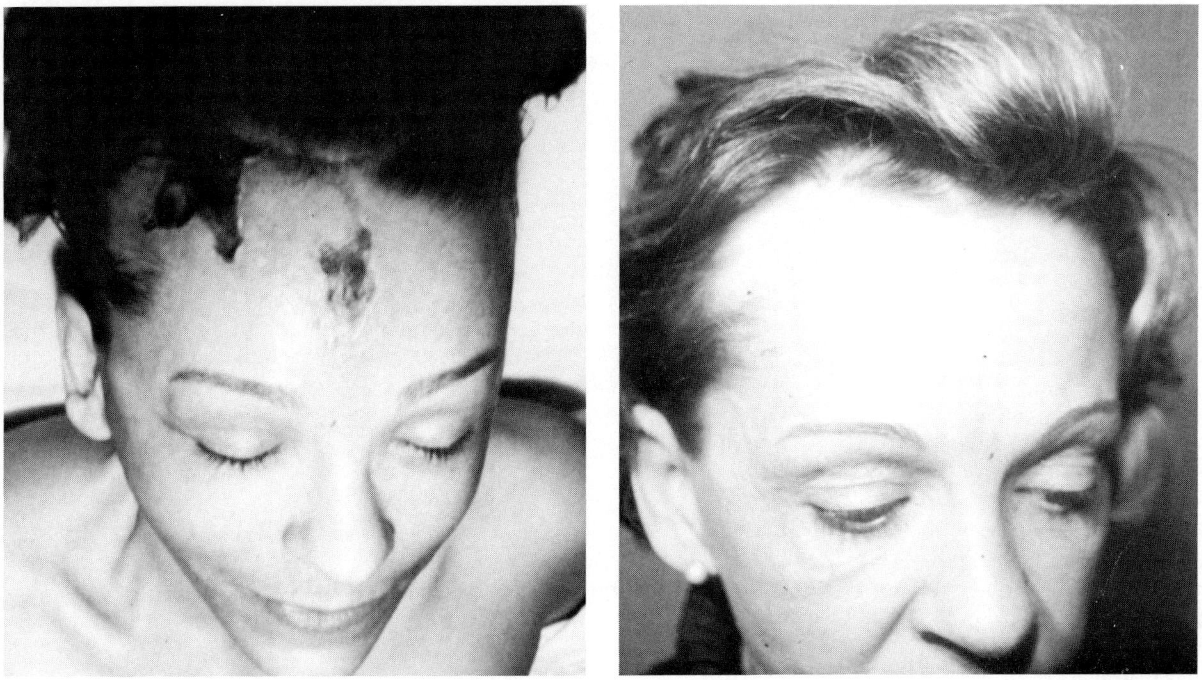

A B

Figure 13-28. Complications of forehead-lifts.
A, B. A skin slough that eventually healed without grafting or revision, as shown at 2 years.

and mild analgesics. Complaints are best minimized by a preoperative warning to expect a tight feeling and postoperative statements that it is a normal occurrence.

Sensory Loss

The immediate loss of sensation in the scalp posterior to the coronal incision that always occurs is due to severance of the supraorbital and supratrochlear nerves. The area of numbness progressively decreases perhaps because of overlap with the posterior occipital nerve supply. Permanent loss of sensation of concern to the patient occurs in less than 5 percent of patients. Although it is unavoidable, the informed patient accepts it as normal while the surprised patient complains bitterly. Numbness of the forehead is due to lower severance of the nerves or even their avulsion along the supraorbital ridges. Transection of the nerves is best avoided by meticulous superficial resection of the frontalis muscle plus bipolar coagulation or preservation of muscle segments over the sensory nerves. Avulsion of the nerves is prevented by blunt pushing dissection medially along the bony orbit with sharp dissection laterally. Sensory loss and patient concern decrease with time.

Motor Nerve Damage

Direct injury of the frontal branch is rare in isolated forehead-lifts but a definite possibility in combined forehead-cervicofacial rhytidectomies. On account of the deep plane of dissection, the frontal branch is protected except when aggressive resection of the lateral frontalis muscle is done. Nerve injury can be minimized by placing the resection at least 3 cm above the bony orbit. Direct severance of the nerve in combined procedures is best avoided by a two-plane dissection technique with careful preservation of a musculoaponeurotic plane in the zygomatic region. If a unilateral paralysis occurs, a conservative regimen with frequent office visits and electromyography (EMG) confirmation is begun. By 6 months, progressive improvement should be evident, but if none has occurred, a selective frontal neurectomy on the opposite side is usually undertaken.

Hair Loss

Most areas of alopecia are quite small and often related to tight anchoring sutures or drain sites. This problem can be avoided by removing the aligning traction sutures once the closure is completed and replacing them with simple coupling sutures. Small areas are treated secondarily by direct excision with closure. Patients with thinning hair should be warned that transitory hair loss of several months may occur. Major alopecia requires sequential resection or reconstruction with scalp flaps.

Scars

Patients with thin hair must be warned that the scar may be visible for several months. Hypertrophic scars are rarely a problem unless wounds are closed under excessive tension (Fig. 13-27). Itching may be a problem requiring direct steroid injections or oral medication. Scars at the hairline are rarely a problem if a beveled incision is made, a two-layered closure performed, and tension minimized. Less than 1 percent of cases require scar revision.

Contour Deformities

Numerous surgeons have reported glabellar depression following resection of large segments of the corrugator muscles. Assuming that subcutaneous tissue is not removed inadvertently, resection of a 1-cm segment of corrugator muscle near its origin should not produce a depression except in extremely thin individuals with hypertrophic muscles. Most depressions are transitory. Minor depressions receive injection therapy whereas a major depression requires a dermal or fascial graft.

Eyebrow Asymmetry

Asymmetry of the eyebrows is often present preoperatively and must be pointed out to the patient. This disparity can be lessened by differential scalp excision, but some asymmetry will persist. Of more catastrophic consequence is iatrogenic eyebrow asymmetry, which occurs if preoperative reference marks are not carefully followed, inadequate dissection is done on one side, or unilateral excessive scalp resection occurs. Once nerve injury is ruled out, treatment should be expectant for several months. Reoperation with mobilization of the entire forehead is preferred to a localized procedure, i.e., direct eyebrow elevation.

Excessive Eyebrow Elevation

Creation of a "surprised" look is unacceptable to most patients and is due to excessive elevation of the eyebrows. It is best avoided by careful preoperative estimation of the amount of eyebrow elevation desired and the skin resection required. Treatment is difficult. The only solution would probably be bilateral temporal scalp flaps rotated into the incision line. Obviously, one should be conservative rather than radical in eyebrow elevation and their position checked from below with traction sutures in place prior to definite scalp excision.

Persistent Wrinkles

As edema decreases over several months, transverse wrinkling may reappear in the forehead. If the wrinkles are deep and active motion of the frontalis muscle remains, inadequate resection of the muscle is the cause. Treatment may be conservative, accepting the benefits of eyebrow elevation or complete reoperation or selective neurectomy. If the wrinkles are superficial and active frontalis motion is absent, a chemical peel may be necessary to eradicate residual fine lines. In the glabellar region, persistent grooves require either injection therapy or, rarely, direct excision.

REFERENCES

1. Aston, S. J. Orbicularis oculi muscle flaps: A technique to reduce crows feet and lateral canthal skin folds. *Plast. Reconstr. Surg.* 65:206, 1980.
2. Aston, S. J. Orbicularis oculi muscle flaps. *Clin. Plast. Surg.* 8:679, 1981.
3. Baker, T. J. The Brow Lift. In D. Goulian, Jr., and G. Courtiss (eds.), *Surgery of the Aging Face.* St. Louis: Mosby, 1978. P. 103.
4. Baker, T. J., Gordon, H. L., and Mosienko, P. Upper lid blepharoplasty. *Plast. Reconstr. Surg.* 60:692, 1977.
5. Bames, H. O. Frown disfigurement and ptosis. *Plast. Reconstr. Surg.* 19:337, 1957.
6. Barker, D. E. Dye injection studies of intraorbital fat compartment. *Plast. Reconstr. Surg.* 59:82, 1977.
7. Borges, A. F. W-plastic glabellar rhytidectomy. *Br. J. Plast. Surg.* 23:386, 1970.
8. Bourquet, J. La chirurgie esthétique de la face. *Concours Med.* Pp. 1657–1670, 1921.
9. Bourquet, J. La chirurgie esthétique de l'oeil et des paupières. *Monde Med.* Pp. 725–731, 1929.
10. Castanares, S. Blepharoplasty for herniated intraorbital fat: Anatomical basis for a new approach. *Plast. Reconstr. Surg.* 8:46, 1951.
11. Castanares, S. Forehead wrinkles, glabellar frown and ptosis of the eyebrows. *Plast. Reconstr. Surg.* 34:406, 1964.
12. Castanares, S. Classification of baggy eyelids deformity. *Plast. Reconstr. Surg.* 59:629, 1977.
13. Castanares, S. Complications in blepharoplasty. *Clin. Plast. Surg.* 5:139, 1978.
14. Connell, B. F. Eyebrow, face and neck lifts for males. *Clin. Plast. Surg.* 5:15, 1978.
15. Connell, B. F. Eyebrow and Forehead Lifts. In E. H. Courtiss (ed.), *Male Aesthetic Surgery.* St. Louis: Mosby, 1982.
16. Correia, P. de C., and Zani, R. Surgical anatomy of the facial nerve, as related to ancillary operations in rhytidoplasty. *Plast. Reconstr. Surg.* 52:549, 1973.
17. Courtiss, E. H., Webster, R. C., and White, M. F. Use of double w-plasty in upper blepharoplasty. *Plast. Reconstr. Surg.* 53:25, 1974.
18. D'Assumpcao, E. A. A new instrument for rhytidoplasty. *Br. J. Plast. Surg.* 23:301, 1970.
19. DeMere, M. Blindness and eyelid surgery. *Aesthetic Plast. Surg.* 2:41, 1978.
20. DeMere, M., Wood, T., and Austin, W. Eye complications with blepharoplasty or other eyelid surgery. *Plast. Reconstr. Surg.* 53:634, 1974.
21. Dingman, R. O., Peled, I., and Izenberg, P. Forehead and brow lifts and their relationship to blepharoplasty. *Ann. Plast. Surg.* 2:32, 1979.
22. Edgerton, M. T. Causes and prevention of lower lid ectropion following blepharoplasty. *Plast. Reconstr. Surg.* 49:367, 1972.
23. Edwards, B. F. Bilateral temporal neurotomy for frontalis hypermotility. *Plast. Reconstr. Surg.* 11:341, 1957.
24. Eitner, E. Weitermitteilungen uber kosmetische Faltenoperationen in Gesicht. *Wien. Med. Wochenschr.* 85:244, 1935.
25. Ellenbogen, R. Transcoronal eyebrow lift with concomitant upper blepharoplasty. *Plast. Reconstr. Surg.* 71:490, 1983.
26. Flowers, R. S. Anchor blepharoplasty. In *Transactions of the Sixth International Congress of Plastic and Reconstructive Surgery.* Paris: Masson, 1976. Pp. 471–472.
27. Flowers, R. S. Belpharoplasty. In E. H. Courtiss (ed.), *Male Aesthetic Surgery.* St. Louis: Mosby, 1982. P. 207.
28. Fomon, S. *The Surgery of Injury and Plastic Repair.* Baltimore: Williams & Wilkins, 1939.
29. Fomon, S. *Cosmetic Surgery: Principles and Practice.* Philadelphia: Lippincott, 1960.
30. Furnas, D. W. Landmarks for the trunk and the temporofacial division of the facial nerve. *Br. J. Plast. Surg.* 52:694, 1965.

31. Furnas, D. W. Festoon of orbicularis muscle as a cause of baggy eyelids. *Plast. Reconstr. Surg.* 61:531, 1978.
32. Furnas, D. W. The orbicularis oculi muscle: Management in blepharoplasty. *Clin. Plast. Surg.* 8:687, 1981.
33. Gleason, M. C. Brow lifting through a temporal scalp approach. *Plast. Reconstr. Surg.* 52:141, 1973.
34. Gleason, M. C. Forehead and Eyebrow Lifts. In E. H. Courtiss (ed.), *Aesthetic Surgery: Trouble—How to Avoid It and How to Treat It.* St. Louis: Mosby, 1978. P. 132.
35. Gleason, M. C. The Temple Lift. In D. Goulian, Jr., and E. H. Courtiss (eds.), *Symposium on Surgery of the Aging Face.* St. Louis: Mosby, 1978. P. 89.
36. Gonzalez-Ulloa, M. Facial wrinkles, integral elimination. *Plast. Reconstr. Surg.* 29:658, 1962.
37. Gonzalez-Ulloa, M. An update on blepharoplasty. *Aesthetic Plast. Surg.* 7:1, 1983.
38. Gonzalez-Ulloa, M., and Stevens, E. F. The treatment of palpable bags. *Plast. Reconstr. Surg.* 27:381, 1961.
39. Gonzalez-Ulloa, M., and Stevens, E. F. Senile Eyelid Esthetic Correction. In. J. W. Smith and J. M. Converse (eds.), *Proceedings of the Second International Symposium on Plastic and Reconstructive Surgery of the Eye and Adnexa.* St. Louis: Mosby, 1967. Pp. 354–361.
40. Griffiths, C. O. The Surgical Management of Forehead Rhytides, Frown Lines, and Ptotic Eyebrows. In J. Conley and J. T. Dickinson (eds.), *Plastic and Reconstructive Surgery of the Face and Neck* (vol. I). New York: Grune & Stratton, 1972. P. 25.
41. Griffiths, C. O. A new approach to the operative management of forehead, brow, and frown rhytidectomies. *Int. Micr. J. Aesthetic Plast. Surg.* 1974B.
42. Guy, C. L., Converse, J. M., and Morello, D. C. Aesthetic Surgery for the Aging Face. In J. M. Converse (ed.), *Reconstructive Plastic Surgery.* Philadelphia: Saunders, 1977.
43. Heinze, J. B., and Hueston, J. T. Blindness after blepharoplasty: Mechanism and early reversal. *Plast. Reconstr. Surg.* 61:347, 1978.
44. Hinderer, U. Treatment of the aging face. *Int. Micr. J. Aesthetic Plast. Surg.* 1974B.
45. Hinderer, U. Blepharocanthoplasty and eyebrow lift. *Plast. Reconstr. Surg.* 56:402, 1975.
46. Horton, C. E., Carraway, J. H., and Potenza, A. D. Treatment of a lacrimal bulge in blepharoplasty by repositioning the gland. *Plast. Reconstr. Surg.* 61:701, 1978.
47. Hugo, N. E., and Stone, E. Anatomy for a blepharoplasty. *Plast. Reconstr. Surg.* 53:381, 1974.
48. Hunt, H. L. *Plastic Surgery for the Head, Face, and Neck.* Philadelphia: Lea & Febiger, 1926.
49. Jelks, G. W., and McCord, C. D. Dry eye syndrome and other tear film abnormalities. *Clin. Plast. Surg.* 8:803, 1981.
50. Johnson, J. P. The problem of the aging face. *Plast. Reconstr. Surg.* 15:117, 1955.
51. Joseph, J. *Nasenplastik und sonstige Gesichtsplastik nebst einen Anhang uber Mammaplastik.* Leipzig: Kabitzsch, 1931. Pp. 507–509.
52. Kaye, B. L. The forehead lift: A useful adjunct to face lift and blepharoplasty. *Plast. Reconstr. Surg.* 60:161, 1977.
53. Kaye, B. L. Forehead and Brow. In. T. Rees (ed.), *Aesthetic Plastic Surgery.* Philadelphia: Saunders, 1980. Pp. 731–748.
54. Kaye, B. L. The Forehead Lift. In R. M. Goldwyn (ed.), *Long-Term Results in Plastic and Reconstructive Surgery* (vol. II). Boston: Little, Brown, 1980. Pp. 654–662.
55. Koechlin, H. Sur la correction des rides intersourcilières. *Ann. Chir. Plast.* 9:140, 1964.
56. Lassus, C. Osteotomy of superior orbital rim in cosmetic blepharoplasty. *Plast. Reconstr. Surg.* 63:481, 1979.
57. LeRoux, P., and Jones, J. H. Total permanent removal of wrinkles from the forehead. *Br. J. Plast. Surg.* 27:359, 1974.
58. Lewis, G. K. Surgical treatment of wrinkles. *Arch. Otolaryngol.* 60:334, 1954.
59. Lewis, J. R. The Z-blepharoplasty. *Plast. Reconstr. Surg.* 60:161, 1977.
60. Lexer, E. Zur Gesichtsplastik. *Arch. Klin. Chir.* 92:749, 1910.
61. Loeb, R. Technique for preservation of the temporal branches of the facial nerve during face lift operations. *Br. J. Plast. Surg.* 23:380, 1970.
62. Loeb, R. Necessity for partial resection of the orbicularis oculi muscle in blepharoplasty in some young patients. *Plast. Reconstr. Surg.* 60:178, 1977.
63. Loeb, R. Fat pad sliding and fat grafting for levelling lid depression. *Clin. Plast. Surg.* 8:757, 1981.
64. Luckey, R. C. The forehead lift. *Plast. Reconstr. Surg.* 68:645, 1981.
65. Macomber, W. B. Symposium on orbital and eyelid surgery. *Clin. Plast. Surg.* 5:4, 1978.
66. Marino, H. Treatment of wrinkles of forehead. *Prensa Med. Argent.* 51:1368, 1964.
67. Marino, H. The Surgery of Facial Expression. In J. Hueston (ed.), *Transactions of the Fifth International Congress of Plastic and Reconstructive Surgery.* London: Butterworth, 1971. P. 1102.
68. Marino, H. The forehead lift: Some hints to secure better results. *Aesthetic Plast. Surg.* 1:251, 1977.
69. Masters, F. W., and Lewis, J. R., Jr. *Symposium on Aesthetic Surgery of the Face, Eyelid and Breast.* St. Louis: Mosby, 1972.
70. Mayer, P. M., and Swanker, W. A. Rhytidoplasty. *Plast. Reconstr. Surg.* 6:255, 1950.
71. Miller, C. C. *Cosmetic Surgery.* Chicago: Oak Printing, 1908.
72. Mitz, V., and Peyronie, M. The superficial musculoaponeurotic system (SMAS) in the parotid and cheek area. *Plast. Reconstr. Surg.* 58:80, 1976.
73. Morel-Fatio, O. Cosmetic Surgery of the Aging Face. In T. Gibson (ed.), *Modern Trends in Plastic Surgery.* London: Butterworth, 1964.
74. Noël, A. *La Chirurgie Esthétique et son Rôle Social.* Paris: Masson, 1926. Pp. 62–66.
75. O'Neill, J. V. Correction of the drooping brow: Analysis of approach. *Laryngoscope* 90:1471, 1980.
76. Ortiz-Montasterio, F., Barrera, G., and Olmedo, A. The coronal incision in rhytidectomy: The brow lift. *Clin. Plast. Surg.* 5:167, 1978.
77. Owsley, J. Q., Jr. Resection of the prominent lateral fat pad during upper lid blepharoplasty. *Plast. Reconstr. Surg.* 65:4, 1980.
78. Pangman, J. W., and Wallace, R. M. Cosmetic surgery of the face and neck. *Plast. Reconstr. Surg.* 27:544, 1961.
79. Parkes, M. L., Kamer, F. M., and Merrin, M. L. Infrabrow lift. *Laryngoscope* 86:1869, 1976.
80. Passot, R. La chirurgie esthétique des rides du visage. *Presse Med.* 27:258, 1919.
81. Passot, R. Quelques généralités sur l'opération correctif des rides du visage. *Rev. Chir. Plast.* 3:23, 1933.
82. Picaud, A. J. Different Forms of Incisions and Techniques in Face-Lifting. In *Transactions of the Fourth International Congress of Plastic and Reconstructive Surgery.* Amsterdam: Excerpta Medica, 1967. P. 1108.
83. Pitanguy, I. Section of the frontalis-procerus-corrugator aponeurosis in the correction of frontal and glabellar wrinkles. *Ann. Plast. Surg.* 2:422, 1979.
84. Pitanguy, I. Indications for and treatment of frontal and

glabellar wrinkles in an analysis of 3,404 consecutive cases of rhytidectomy. *Plast. Reconstr. Surg.* 67:157, 1981.

85. Pitanguy, I., and Silveira Ramos, A. The frontal branch of the facial nerve: The importance of its variations in face lifting. *Plast. Reconstr. Surg.* 38:352, 1966.
86. Rees, T. D. *Aesthetic Plastic Surgery.* Philadelphia: Saunders, 1980.
87. Rees, T. D. Modern trends in blepharoplasty. *Clin. Plast. Surg.* 8:4, 1981.
88. Rees, T. D., and Guy, C. L. Patient selection and technique in blepharoplasty and rhytidoplasty. *Surg. Clin. North Am.* 87:353, 1971.
89. Rees, T. D., and Wood-Smith, D. *Cosmetic Facial Surgery.* Philadelphia: Saunders, 1973.
90. Regnault, P. Complete face and forehead lifting with double traction on "crows-feet." *Plast. Reconstr. Surg.* 49:123, 1972.
91. Regnault, P. Correction of the infrapalpebral depression. *Aesthetic Plast. Surg.* 2:311, 1978.
92. Reidy, J. P. Swelling of eyelids. *Br. J. Plast. Surg.* 13:256, 1960.
93. Robertson, J. G. A handy site for dermal grafts for glabella frown lines. *South. Med. J.* 68:1286, 1975.
94. Rosenthal, S. G. Glabellar rhytidoplasty: A new approach. *Plast. Reconstr. Surg.* 49:361, 1972.
95. Scherz, W., and Dohlman, C. H. Is the lacrimal gland dispensable? *Arch. Ophthalmol.* 93:281, 1975.
96. Sheen, J. M. Supratarsal fixation in upper blepharoplasty. *Plast. Reconstr. Surg.* 54:424, 1974.
97. Sheen, J. M. A change in the technique of supratarsal fixation in upper blepharoplasty. *Plast. Reconstr. Surg.* 59:831, 1977.
98. Skoog, T. *Plastic Surgery: New Methods and Refinements.* Philadelphia: Saunders, 1974. P. 328.
99. Smith J. W. Cosmetic Surgery of the Aging Face. In W. C. Grabb and J. W. Smith (eds.), *Plastic Surgery.* Boston: Little, Brown, 1973.
100. Snow, J. W., and Obi, L. J. Operation to abolish the glabellar frown. *Plast. Reconstr. Surg.* 61:736, 1978.
101. Sokol, A. B., and Sokol, T. P. Transblepharoplasty brow suspension. *Plast. Reconstr. Surg.* 69:940, 1982.
102. Spira, M. Lower blepharoplasty: A clinical study. *Plast Reconstr. Surg.* 59:35, 1977.
103. Spira, M. Blepharoplasty. *Clin. Plast. Surg.* 5:121, 1978.
104. Stasior, O. G. Blindness associated with cosmetic blepharoplasty. *Clin. Plast. Surg.* 8:793, 1981.
105. Stephenson, K. L. The History of Face, Neck, and Eyelid Surgery. In F. W. Masters and J. R. Lewis, Jr. (eds.), *Symposium on Aesthetic Surgery of the Face, Eyelid and Breast.* St. Louis: Mosby, 1972.
106. Su, C. T., et al. Technique for division and suspension of the orbicularis oculi muscle. *Clin. Plast. Surg.* 8:673, 1981.
107. Tenzel, R. R. Correction of brow ptosis. *Ophthalmology* (Rochester) 85:716, 1978.
108. Tenzel, R. R. Complications of blepharoplasty. *Clin. Plast. Surg.* 8:797, 1981.
109. Tessier, P. Ridectomie frontale: Lifting frontale. *Gaz. Med. France* 75:5565, 1968.
110. Uchida, J. I. A method for frontal rhytidectomy. *Plast. Reconstr. Surg.* 35:218, 1965.
111. Vinas, C. A., Caviglia, C., and Cortinas, J. L. Forehead rhytidoplasty and brow lifting. *Plast. Reconstr. Surg.* 57:445, 1976.
112. von Graefe, C. F. *De Rhinoplastice.* Berlin: Reimer, 1818. P. 13.
113. Washio, H. Rhytidoplasty of the forehead—An Anatomical Approach. In *Transaction of the Sixth International Congress of Plastic and Reconstructive Surgery.* Paris: Masson, 1976. P. 430.
114. Wilkinson T. S. A simplified technique for obliteration of glabellar frown lines. *Ann. Plast. Surg.* 3:341, 1979.
115. Zide, B. M. Anatomy of the eyelids. *Clin. Plast. Surg.* 8:623, 1981.

14. Blepharoplasty

Melvin Spira

While *blepharoplasty* describes an operation that may involve a variety of surgical procedures on the eyelids, the term as employed here is used to designate an aesthetic operative technique designed to remove skin or fat from the upper and lower eyelids. The correction of aging eyelids, as in other examples of aesthetic surgery about the face, is dependent on a number of related factors not under the control of the surgeon: age; national origin of the patient; amount, color, and character of eyelid skin; quality of the underlying structures, including tarsal plate and orbicularis muscle; previous sun exposure; and hereditary predisposition to aging as evidenced in the patient's family.

HISTORY

In her thorough historical review, Stephenson [42] described the operation as having its roots in antiquity. Through the ages surgeons have directed their efforts primarily at the excess skin in the upper eyelids. The presence of excess fat was observed by European ophthalmologists about the turn of this century. Merkel [25] observed atrophy of the orbital septum, and Arlt [1] described herniation of orbital fat as ptosis adiposa. Early plastic surgeons in this country, including Miller [26] and Kolle [23], described the incision lines for this operation as designed to remove excess eyelid skin. In 1929 Bourguet [5] reaffirmed the findings of a half century previously and clearly observed the anatomy and described the collection of submuscular fat as a "fatty hernia." He emphasized the need for its removal. It remained for Joseph [20] and his text, published in 1931, to describe the incisions commonly employed today. Castanares's publication [7], in 1951, in the plastic surgery literature is a landmark of clarity, and his technique, which recognized the collection of fat in "pockets," afforded the surgeon an approach to the problem that has stood the test of time. More recent refinements, stemming from the operation to create an upper eyelid sulcus in the Oriental eye (Sayoc [31], Fernandez [11]), have been the techniques proposed to define the upper lid furrow by some type of surgical maneuver (Flowers [12], Sheen [34]) or by simple removal of a strip of orbicularis muscle (Baker et al. [3], Spira [38]). Additional refinements include modifications in the position and shape of the lateral canthal area—either by Z-plasty (Lewis [24]), by reverse V-Y advancement (Gonzalez-Ulloa and Stevens [17]), or by canthal ligament repositioning (Hinderer [19]). These maneuvers are all done to make the eyelid appear more youthful by modifying the antemongoloid slant present.

More recently, Rees [28] has described the effectiveness of ancillary procedures, including the brow-lift, forehead-lift, and excision of glabellar frown lines. Efforts to remove fine wrinkles, as well as to decrease the pigmentation of blepharomelasma, through chemical peeling have been well described.

PATHOPHYSIOLOGY AND CLASSIFICATION

Analysis of the Deformity

The list below is concerned with the terminology used to describe eyelid deformities [9, 41].

blepharochalasis Relatively rare condition occurring primarily in young adults, characterized by bouts of recurrent bilateral edema, mainly in the upper lids, which thins and wrinkles the skin, weakens the septum orbitale, and results in skin redundancy and fat herniation

palpebral dermatochalasis Abnormal relaxation, or looseness, of eyelid skin, with or without herniation of intraorbital fat

"herniation" of intraorbital fat The classic "baggy eyelids" caused by protrusion, or bulging, of fat into a weakened, thinned septum orbitale, also referred to as *ptosis adiposa* and *ptosis lipomatosis*

pachydermatochalasis A pathologic thickening of the lid

blepharomelasma A discoloration of the eyelid skin secondary to hyperpigmentation

periorbital rhytidosis The presence of numerous fine skin wrinkles, or crenulations, which, when prominent in the lateral canthal areas, are commonly referred to as *crow's-feet*

Thus, accurate analysis of the deformity, coupled with the patient's desires, will serve as a guide to the surgeon for selection of the optimal operative procedure. For example, where only skin excess exists, simple elliptic skin excisions will suffice. If excess skin and fat are present, both will need treatment, employing the more common procedure, as described below. Where wrinkles or pigmentations or both are present, a chemical peel can also be considered.

CONSULTATION

The plastic surgeon has a role similar to that of a navigator aboard a ship. He analyzes the present course (physical examination); evaluates past performance of the "vessel" (history); considers distance, the weather, and other factors (patient attitude, realism, medications, etc.); and then elects to chart one or more pathways (operations) for the captain (patient, at the consultation) — directions the captain may or may not choose to travel after being informed of all hazards (informed consent)!

Indications and Contraindications

Gross excess skin or herniated fat in an otherwise healthy patient, not on any routine medication, presents an ideal indication for this surgical procedure. Ideally, the surgeon should employ as his criterion the ability to discern a noticeable *objective* difference between the preoperative and postoperative photographs of the patient. The patient with untreated cardiovascular disease, uncontrolled diabetes, or an abnormal thyroid status presents contraindications, possibly only temporary. Patients with known ocular disease (e.g., unilateral vision loss, cataract[s], glaucoma) or specific ocular conditions (e.g., chronic epiphora, dry eye syndrome) should have ophthalmologic consultation before surgery is considered. Those with negligible skin or muscle excess, those who are unrealistic in their expectations, and those with frank psychiatric diagnoses are a few of the persons in whom blepharoplasty is absolutely contraindicated. The younger patient who exhibits herniated intraorbital fat in the lower eyelid causing bags will be the patient who, following successful removal of this herniated fat, will achieve the longest lasting and most gratifying end result.

Medical History

The patient's general health, with particular reference to thyroid status, should be ascertained. Edema of long standing may result in permanently thickened eyelid skin. Impaired renal or cardiovascular function can cause chronic edema, which may be reflected in the eyelid areas. Long-standing steroid therapy can also cause chronic periorbital edema. Excessive sun exposure and allergic status should be determined and noted. Any change in the patient's vision status, with particular reference to the last ophthalmologic examination, should be recorded. The presence of a dry eye syndrome — keratoconjunctivitis sicca — should be recognized preoperatively. This condition, more common in females, is associated with symptoms of itching, burning, conjunctival irritation, and photophobia; a Schirmer test is indicated (see p. 327). Note should be made of any ocular medications taken on a regular basis, as well as any other medicine, particularly with reference to chronic aspirin ingestion, and hormonal therapy. Any tendency to excessive bleeding should be noted (any problem with a tooth extraction?).

Motivation

The patient who indeed has a degree of eyelid skin excess, with or without bags, who has noted a decrease in upper eyelid "show" with resultant difficulty in the application of makeup, who resents the tired look that eyelid skin redundancy (with or without brow ptosis) causes, and who can place the operation in its proper perspective — a procedure designed to improve appearance and in some instances improve peripheral vision — is a well-motivated candidate for a blepharoplasty. The individual who is motivated by potential socioeconomic gain, is encouraged by well-meaning relatives or friends, and has minimal signs of palpebral dermatochalasis may be sufficiently motivated for the wrong reasons. The properly motivated patient is far better equipped to handle a postoperative complication should it occur. The significance of motivation in preoperative patient evaluation has been well described by Goin and Goin [16].

Physical Examination

The presence, location, and amount of skin redundancy, as well as wrinkling and skin color, are first noted. Where skin redundancy of the upper lid obscures, or obliterates, the superior palpebral furrow, the presence or absence of true ptosis must also be noted. The location of the superior palpebral furrow, with relationship to the upper lid ciliary margin, should be recorded. Fat herniations causing bagginess, particularly in the lower lids, should be recorded, in terms of severity and specific location. Lower eyelid tone, including either presence or absence of ectropion or entropion, should be observed. In contrast to the presence of excess fat, particularly in the upper lids, is the "hollowed eye" appearance noted occasionally in older individuals. The presence of orbicularis oculi muscle festoons, as noted by Furnas [15], should be looked for. Abnormal pigmentations and the presence of "secondary bags"—skin festoons over the malar eminence—should be recorded. Both of these conditions will usually not be corrected by the standard blepharoplasty. Brow position, as well as the presence or absence of glabellar frown lines or crow's-feet in the lateral orbital areas, should be noted. The position of the lateral canthi, in relationship to the medial canthi, should be observed. Consideration can sometimes be given to the correction of the antemongoloid slant. Finally, such special conditions as an eyelid tic, exophthalmos, levator muscle spasm, true unilateral ptosis (in the very elderly, bilateral ptosis), and the presence or absence of eyelid cysts and tumors should be observed. A checklist is sometimes helpful.

Useful Ophthalmologic Tests

SCHIRMER TEAR TEST

This is a test for "dry eye," employing a test strip available, with instructions for use, from the S.M.P. Division of Cooper Laboratories.* The sterile strips, 5 × 35 mm, are made from Whatman No. 41 filter paper and employed as follows: Without topical anesthesia, the rounded bent end of the strip is hung over the lower eyelid border at the junction of middle and nasal third. With the eye either open or closed the strip is maintained in place 5 minutes and the length of moistened area measured. A measurement of 15 mm from the lid margin is regarded as standard for normal tear production. Above the age of 40, normal values may vary from 10 to 15 mm. Measurements below 10 mm in either eye should be given careful consideration and serve as a warning or danger sign to the surgeon considering blepharoplasty. Low measurements are especially significant if the patient has an impending or frank ectropion. Rees and Jelks's [29] discussion of the clinical significance of this test, as it relates to the dry eye syndrome, should be read.

LID DISTENSION TEST

Lower lid laxity can be tested by pinching the skin of the lower lid and pulling the lid margin away from the globe. Stasior [40] advised that a gap of greater than 8 mm suggests impending ectropion and suggested the need to incorporate a tarsal wedge excision with the blepharoplasty. This test is similar to the lower lid retraction test, done by retracting the lower lid down onto the malar and noting the rapidity or slowness of return to normal position.

FLUORESCEIN DYE TEST (FLUOR I STRIP)

The applicator strip is placed in the lower cul-de-sac near the lower punctum on the conjunctiva, and the patient is asked to close the eye over the strip until the desired amount of staining is obtained. The cornea will stain if any abrasion, or any irregularity, is present. Saline irrigations can wash the dye out. Strips are obtainable from the Ophthalmic Division of Ayerst Laboratories, Inc.*

LUEDDE EXOPHTHALMOMETER

This measuring device, employed to estimate the degree of exophthalmos, if present, is an inexpensive, small, rectangular, clear lucite rod. It is graded in millimeters and is placed against the lateral orbital rim to measure the anterior projection of the cornea, as seen through the clear plastic. While not quite as accurate as the Hertel exophthalmometer, it provides a good gauge of the degree and amount of exophthalmos. This instrument is available through Storz Instrument Co.†

SQUINCH TEST

The orbicularis muscle is tightly contracted, or "squinched," and any festoons, or bags, are effaced, only to reappear when the muscle relaxes (after Furnas).

PRIMARY AND SECONDARY DYE TESTS

These tests (after Callahan [6]) are employed to evaluate obstruction to the lacrimal drainage apparatus. A short length of half-inch Nu-Gauze is lightly packed under the inferior turbinate next to the inferior meatus in the nasal fossa on the side being evaluated. In the primary dye test fluorescein solution is instilled into the conjunctival sac, as described above. The test is positive if it runs freely into the nose, generally indicating hypersecretion. Treatment is by locating and removing either a local or general cause and not by operating on the lacrimal outflow. The test is negative if the dye does not run through freely from natural forces. The secondary dye test should then be performed. With a cannula inserted into the common punctum and the patient's head erect or tilted slightly forward, 2 ml of saline solution is instilled. The test is regarded as positive if the saline comes through colored with the dye—and the partial obstruction is probably located in the nasal lacrimal duct. Further diagnostic measures include a detailed examination of the nasal cavity, rhinologic consultation, dacryocystogram, and possible

* San German, Puerto Rico 00753.

* N.D.C. 046-1028, New York, NY 10017.

† 3365 Treecourt Industrial Blvd., St. Louis, MO 63133.

histopathologic examination of mucosa resected from the inferior turbinate. Ultimately, a dacryocystorhinostomy may be required. The test is regarded as negative if fluid coming through contains no dye; obstruction is then generally in the canaliculi. Still other diagnostic measures are probing for canalicular obstructions, and a dacryocystogram with a "canaliculogram." Therapeutic measures involve repeated dilatations. Operative intervention includes increased opening of the canaliculi into the conjunctival sac, or opening of the canalicular lake into the lacrimal sac. Placement of a Jones Pyrex tube may be necessary.

TEXT FOR MÜLLER'S MUSCLE ACTIVITY
Guanethidine, which is a peripheral sympathetic depleter of norepinephrine, acting like a postganglionic blocking agent, is used in determining the role of Müller's muscle in lid retraction associated with hyperthyroidism. The test is best performed with ophthalmologic consultation. If effective in relieving the "thyroid stare" causing lid retraction, secondary to Müller's muscle overactivity, the surgical procedure of levator–Müller's muscle myotomy can be very effective. In the Neo-Synephrine test (10% phenylephrine hydrochloride solution) the function of a sympathetically innervated Müller's muscle on the side of blepharoptosis is assessed by the instillation of several drops of the solution into the conjunctival sac. In some patients with unilateral blepharoptosis the upper lid elevates to the same level as the opposite eyelid or in patients with bilateral blepharoptosis to a cosmetically acceptable level. In these patients the effect of phenylephrine on Müller's muscle can be duplicated by the Fasanella-Servat [10] blepharoptosis procedure or its modification, as described by Putterman and Urst [27]—the Müller's muscle–conjunctiva resection.

TEST FOR LEVATOR ACTION IN THE PRESENCE OF PTOSIS
The brow is immobilized so that it cannot enter into eyelid movement, and the excursion of the lid margin as it travels from the eyes-down to the eyes-up position is measured; a numerical reading is obtained that indicates the degree of levator function. A normal eyelid will usually travel a distance of 15 mm; a ptotic eyelid will travel from 0 to 10 to 12 mm. Superior rectus contraction causes about 2 mm of this excursion.

Aesthetic Goals

The overall objectives of the operation are to restore a more youthful appearance to the eyelids, incur no complications, and satisfy the patient. The specific aims include restoration of, or improvement in, upper eyelid "show" by a well-defined superior palpebral furrow, conservative removal of any bulging fat causing bags in both the upper and lower lids, and correction of an antemongoloid slant, if present, to the palpebral fissure or relief of brow ptosis, if present. The operation will not remove wrinkles or abnormal skin pigmentation unless an adjunctive procedure is performed (chemical peel, etc.).

Preoperative Preparations

TIMING
The author has performed the blepharoplasty operation on individuals as young as 18 years of age and as old as 82. In the younger group obviously the condition of premature bags involving the lower lid only has been the concern.

SEQUENCE
When adjunctive procedures, to include the correction of brow ptosis and cervicofacial rhytidectomy, are planned, it is the author's preference to perform the blepharoplasty first, employing a conservative excision of upper eyelid skin, and then the brow-lift, with the rhytidectomy as the last procedure. On occasion I have performed a blepharoplasty and rhinoplasty together, the blepharoplasty being done first.

SKIN CARE
All cosmetics should be removed the night before surgery and the face washed with soap. No cosmetics of any kind are used the day of surgery.

PHOTOGRAPHY
Patients are photographed with light makeup, using a 105-mm lens at a distance of 2 ft, the eyes in the primary position and looking up.

SURGICAL ANATOMY

The surface anatomy consists of the brow, the eyelids, and the palpebral sulci furrows. The lower lid is separated from the cheek by the sometimes indistinct nasojugal and malar furrows (Fig. 14-1). The furrows, through fascial extensions, are anchored to the periosteum and are barriers to the passage of hemorrhage and inflammation (Fig. 14-2). In the upper lid the superior palpebral furrow

Figure 14-1. Orbicularis muscle in relation to external skin furrows.

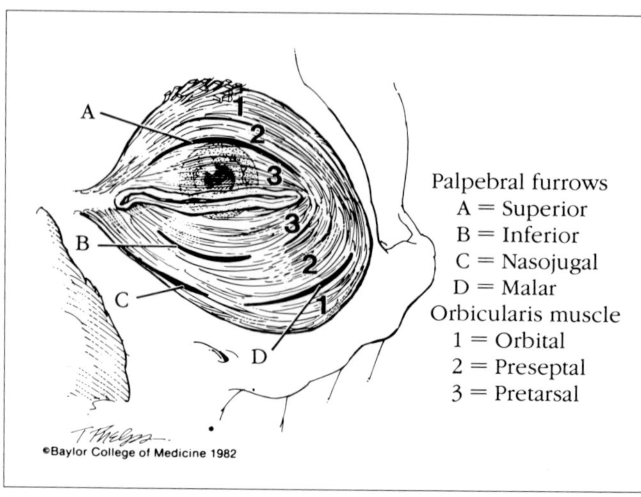

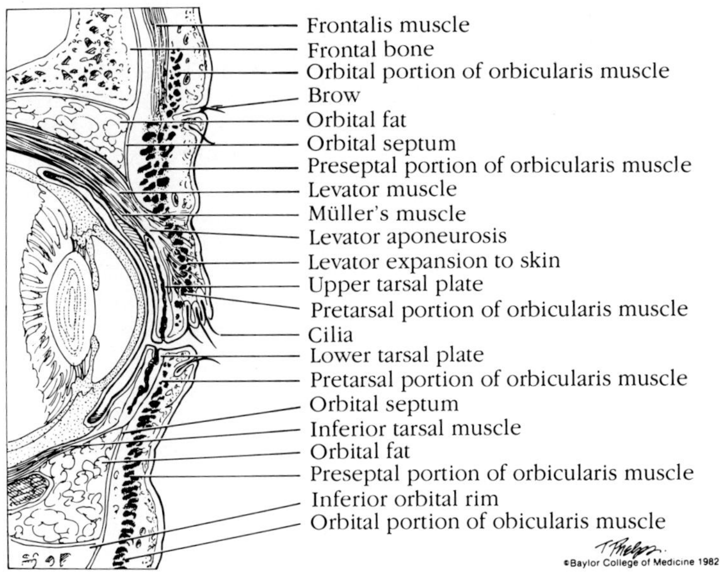

Figure 14-2. Anatomy of the eye and contiguous structures. (See text for details.)

divides the lid into a proximal orbital part and a peripheral tarsal portion. Since most of the levator fascial attachments to skin and tarsus are inferior to the furrow, the skin tends to fold and overhang the furrow as the lid moves up. In the lower lid the inferior furrow is faint. The palpebral fissure, or the opening between the two lids, varies in shape and size with the age and ethnic origin of the patient. In infancy the upper lid margin lies about at the upper limbus but with age it tends to droop and comes to lie halfway between the limbus and the pupillary margin, thus covering the upper 2 or 3 mm of the iris in most adults. The average width of the palpebral fissure, irrespective of age, varies from 7 to 11 mm, most fissures measuring about 9 mm.

The eyelids anatomically are composed of seven layers. Beginning outward and going inward they are (1) skin, (2) orbicularis muscle, (3) orbital septum, (4) levator muscle, (5) Müller's muscle, (6) posterior fibrous septum, consisting of the tarsus and its connections, and (7) conjunctiva with its glands (Fig. 14-2).

The skin of the lids, about the thinnest in the body, is loosely connected to the underlying orbicularis except over the tarsus. The lid margin, about 2 mm in width, is marked in its entire length by a somewhat dark pigmented line, the intermarginal sulcus, or gray line, which separates the skin muscle lamina from the tarsal conjunctival layer of the lid. The orbicularis muscle consists of three main parts—an orbital portion and a lid palpebral portion, consisting of preseptal and pretarsal muscles (see Fig. 14-1). The pretarsal fibers of the palpebral orbicularis cover the tarsus, being separated only by the levator expansion in the lower lid. This muscle unites medially to insert into the medial palpebral ligament behind the posterior lacrimal crest, and laterally the upper and lower segments come together to form a common tendon that inserts into the lateral orbital tubercle. The preseptal fibers lying in front of the orbital septum and under that portion of the skin usually resected (upper lid) have the same origin and insertion as the pretarsal fibers. This segment of orbicularis acts together with fibers of the preseptal portion reflexly to close the eyelids in sleep and in normal blinking and to protect from foreign bodies. The orbital portion and volitional fibers of the preseptal orbicularis are primarily used in voluntary as well as semireflex forced closure of the lid (laughing, sneezing, etc.) [18].

The orbital septum, or tarsal-orbital fascia, has its origin all around the orbital margin and is actually an extension of the dura mater. It fuses with the levator aponeurosis behind it and then extends onto the surface of the tarsus as a joint member. The septum, thick around the bony orbit, becomes thin as it passes forward. The orbital fat always lies *behind* the orbital septum in the preaponeurotic space and hence separates the septum from the underlying levator muscle. For practical purposes the periorbital fat is generally felt to lie in "compartments," the fat in the medial compartment of the upper and lower lids being a bit lighter in color than the more centrally placed fat. The levator and its aponeurosis, the only other muscle with which the surgeon performing the blepharoplasty occasionally must be concerned, originates at the apex of the orbit from the lesser wing of the sphenoid and runs, together with the superior fornix, above the equator of the globe. About 10 mm from the upper tarsal border the muscle splits into two distinct laminas: the posterior lamina (the superior tarsal, or Müller's muscle) and the anterior lamina (a broad fibrous aponeurosis that extends across the width of the orbit and fuses at a transverse ridge of fibrous tissue with the orbital septum, which has extended as a separate membrane from the upper orbital margin). The levator aponeurosis inserts into the lower third of the tarsal plate and, it is thought by many anatomists, gives off fibers that pass through the fascicles of the orbicularis to insert in the pretarsal part of the eyelid skin (Fig. 14-2) [14].

In the upper lid Müller's muscle (superior tarsal muscle) takes origin as a thin sheet of smooth muscle from the undersurface of the levator muscle's anterior border just in back of the fibers of the aponeurosis and is attached anteriorly to the upper border of the tarsus. Despite its intimate connection with the levator it has an entirely different innervation, coming from the sympathetic system. In the lower lid Müller's muscle (inferior tarsal muscle) is a minor counterpart of the muscle of the upper lid. According to Kestenbaum [22], the two muscles have an important function in the control of the width of the palpebral fissure. It is the levator that opens and closes the lid, while the sympathetic tonus of Müller's muscle defines the levator's range of movement. Where sympathetic tone is low, the palpebral fissure will be narrower with relaxation of Müller's muscle, and in cases of excitement or other conditions of high sympathetic tonus it will be wider. Differentiation between the actions of these two muscles is important in the diagnosis and treatment of lid ptosis.

The tarsi are dense fibrous and yellow elastic tissue. In the adult the upper tarsus is about 10 mm wide and the lower about half that. Actually, the tarsal portion of the lid consists of three layers—the levator aponeurosis, the tarsus, and the conjunctiva. The extremities of the tarsi fuse medially and laterally into the medial and lateral palpebral ligaments.

The palpebral conjunctiva is a transparent, highly vascular layer of mucous membrane and separate from the tarsi but loosely attached to the upper adjacent layer of Müller's muscle. Extremely sensitive, it is easily irritated, becoming edematous (chemosis).

The vascular supply of the lids is rich; the arterial supply is mainly from the ophthalmic artery. On the nasal side the superior and inferior medial palpebral arteries pass through the orbital septum above and below the medial palpebral ligament. These anastomose with their counterparts laterally—the lateral superior and inferior palpebral arteries, which are in turn derived from the lacrimal artery to form three tarsal arches, or arcades. The venous system is richer and more complex than the arterial system. A pretarsal group of veins empties into the angular and superficial temporal veins. A deeper retrotarsal group empties into the muscular tributaries of the ophthalmic vein [13].

The motor nerve supply of the lid is from the seventh nerve and from the third cranial nerve to the levator. Sensory supply of the upper lid is mainly through the fifth cranial nerve-supraorbital and supratrochlear nerves frontally and from the infratrochlear nerve medially. Laterally it comes from the lacrimal nerve. The lower lid sensory supply may be from the infraorbital branch of the maxilla and from the infratrochlear nerve medially and the lacrimal nerve laterally. The sensory nerve forms a plexus close to the margins of the orbicularis tarsus [13].

SURGICAL PRINCIPLES

Preliminary Comments on Modern Blepharoplasty Techniques

CASTANARES

This modern oracle or "granddaddy" of present blepharoplasty surgeons [7, 8] pointed the way not only with his descriptions of the various fat compartments associated with baggy eyelids but with his classification of these deformities. He has given us thoughtful, clinically useful guidelines on how to avoid complications associated with this type of surgery. His blepharoplasty technique should be studied by all. This author still follows his basic tenets (Fig. 14-3).

Figure 14-3. Tarsal and modified tarsal fixation techniques.

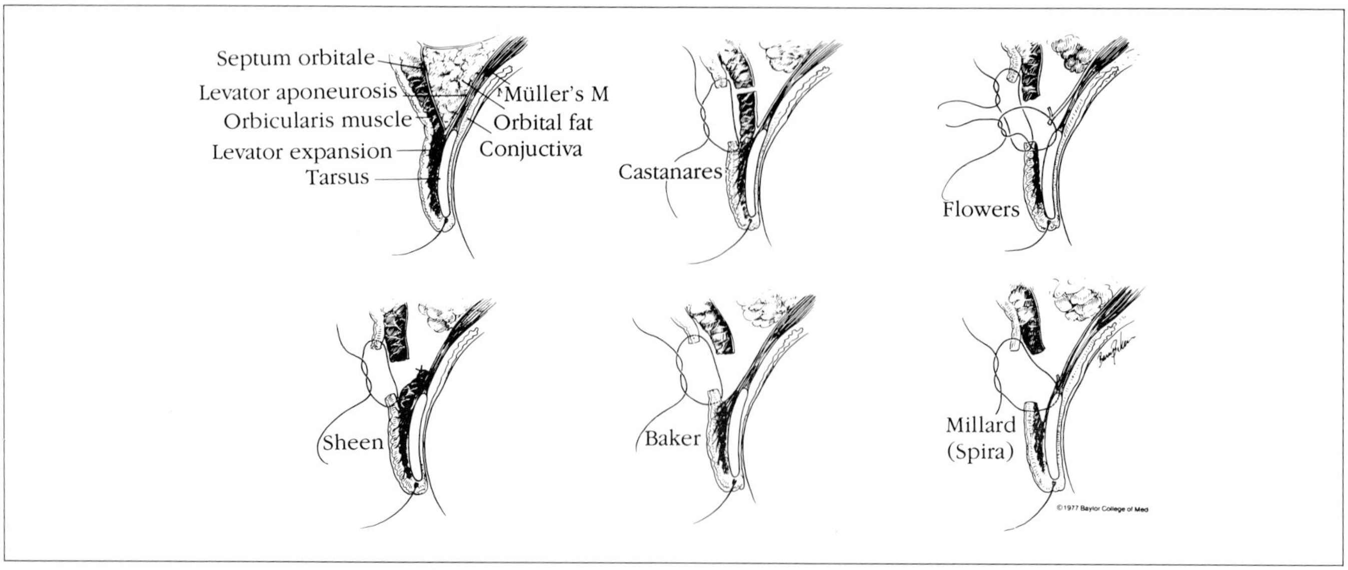

SILVER
Silver's method [35] employs elevation of the upper lid skin, leaving it attached superiorly, and uses multiple vertical incisions in the still attached upper lid skin in an effort better to judge the amount of skin to be removed. The tendency is to undercorrect for skin redundancy on the upper lid. The technique works quite satisfactorily in the lower lid; the skin is left attached inferiorly following undermining.

LEWIS
The use of a Z-plasty [24] laterally, in an effort to elevate the lateral canthal area, has not proved effective in my hands. If the lateral canthus is to be elevated, as in the case of an antemongoloid slant, repositioning of the canthal tendon onto the lateral orbital rim periosteum is required, a method advocated by Hinderer [19].

ASTON
The orbicularis oculi flap approach for the treatment of lateral orbital wrinkles, as originally described by Skoog [36], has been modified and proved effective in Aston's hands [2]. I prefer to utilize a chemical peel postoperatively (3 months) rather than employ the wide undermining as required by this method for improvement of wrinkles, or crow's-feet, in the lateral orbital area.

GONZALEZ-ULLOA
The modification of the V-Y advancement [17] must be used with caution. It is quite possible to end up with visible lateral scars and chronic lid edema (Fig. 14-4).

FLOWERS AND SHEEN
Both of these surgeons have described techniques to improve the position and definition of the supratarsal fold. Flowers [12] sutures the levator expansion to the upper border of the tarsal plate and then to the overlying skin.

Figure 14-4. Variety of incisions employed in blepharoplasty.

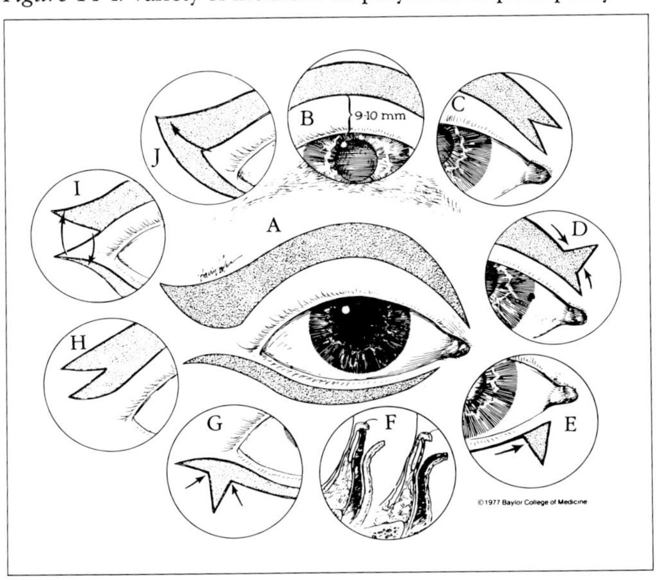

Sheen [33] advances the upper border of the pretarsal orbicularis muscle to the levator expansion at the level of the desired supratarsal fold. Both surgeons close the overlying skin as a separate layer (see Fig. 14-3). Their techniques in their hands give superior results. Most surgeons would agree that these methods, if imperfectly executed, can lead to complications not seen in the usual blepharoplasty.

FURNAS
Furnas [15] has advocated specific treatment for muscle festoons, which are most noticeable when the patient tightly closes or "squinches" the eyelids. He employs a technique combining excision and plication of the orbicularis muscle. I agree that when the problem is present and severe, specific attention should be directed toward it. Furnas's approach is rational but should be preserved for the older patient with severe skin and muscle laxity.

SHEEN—LOWER LID PROCEDURE
In an effort to recreate a more youthful appearing lower eyelid, by restoring pretarsal fullness, the skin-muscle flap is employed to expose the orbital fat [34]. Following removal of the fat, excess skin and muscle are excised and the skin muscle flap is sutured 8 mm from the ciliary edge to the lower border of the inferior tarsal plate with several 7-0 catgut sutures. The flap is *not* sutured in its lateral third. My minimal experience with this flap has not been rewarding although in selected cases Sheen has demonstrated decidedly improved appearance.

BAKER ET AL. AND REES
As alluded to above, tarsal fixation techniques have been advocated for several years. However, these surgeons have shown that basically the same effect can be accomplished by removal of a strip of orbicularis muscle. Baker et al. [3] remove a 5-mm vertical width of orbicularis muscle following skin excision, and Rees [28] removes the skin and underlying orbicularis muscle as a unit. Orbicularis muscle excision is effective in defining the superior tarsal furrow, and now I rarely employ supratarsal fixation for the Caucasian blepharoplasty (see Fig. 14-3).

HINDERER
When an antemongoloid slant exists, only exposure and repositioning of the lateral canthal tendon, as described by Hinderer [19], will truly convert the antemongoloid condition to a more normal slant, with the lateral canthus a little higher than the medial. I have had limited, albeit good, experience with this method. The danger of asymmetry in level of the canthal attachment is a real one.

Caveats to Consider in Blepharoplasty

The following caveats should be well understood by the blepharoplasty surgeon *prior* to surgery.

1. Analyze the deformity.
2. Recognize the presence of associated problems: visual change, eyelid ptosis, tic, etc.

3. Know what the operation will do and what it will not do. Let the operation fit the deformity rather than have an operative procedure looking for a patient.
4. No one technique is applicable to all.
5. Err on the side of conservative skin resection in the lower lid. The admonition to take twice as much skin from the upper lid and half as much from the lower lid, while somewhat oversimplified, should be recognized as one born of an extensive experience with postoperative complications and unhappy patients.
6. Fat in the lateral compartment of the lower lid is frequently missed. It is higher than the middle portion and more difficult to extrude.
7. Symmetry in skin excision and fat removal must be stressed. If you have excess skin that was not, but should have been, excised, hopefully it will present on both sides rather than one. Failure to remove it can be rationalized if this is the case, but no explanation will satisfy the patient if the excess skin is present on only one side.
8. Avoid excessive handling or trauma to the lateral portion of the lower lid skin flap. You may need this tissue.
9. If the patient, under local anesthesia, can close the lid easily at termination of the surgery, you probably have not taken off enough upper eyelid skin.
10. The most dramatic results in blepharoplasties are seen when the primary problem is herniated fat, not skin redundancy or wrinkles.
11. The employment of tarsal fixation techniques may require greater surgical expertise than is possessed by some plastic surgeons. In most patients, simple transverse excision of a 5-mm vertical wedge of orbicularis muscle over and above the superior fourth of the upper tarsal plate will account for the same result.
12. The lower lid incision should be carried slightly lateral to the lateral canthus in a horizontal plane, not downward following the skin crease.
13. Be ultraconservative in your skin and fat excision in secondary and tertiary blepharoplasties.

SURGICAL TECHNIQUES

There are four general types of blepharoplasties performed. They include the following operative procedures:

classic quadrilateral blepharoplasty Removal of excess skin, a strip of underlying orbicularis muscle, and protruding, or herniated, fat in the upper lid; skin and fat excised in the lower lid

bilateral lower lid blepharoplasty Fat removal only, no skin excision

bilateral upper lid blepharoplasty In some cases, fat removal primarily, with minimal skin and muscle excision; in others, as in classic quadrilateral blepharoplasty

"slit" blepharoplasty For herniated intraorbital fat in the lower lid, no skin excision

Adjunctive Eyelid Procedures

In many patients one or more of the procedures listed below are performed, either as a separate operation or with blepharoplasty.

1. Brow-lift
2. Excision of glabella frown lines
3. Periocular chemical peel
4. Ptosis repair
5. Canthal ligament repositioning
6. Kuhnt-Szymanowski procedure for senile ectropion

Standard Blepharoplasty

ANESTHESIA

Local anesthesia is preferred, 2% Xylocaine with epinephrine 1:100,000. If a cervicofacial rhytidectomy is to be performed in conjunction with blepharoplasty, I will do both under general anesthesia at the same operative pro-

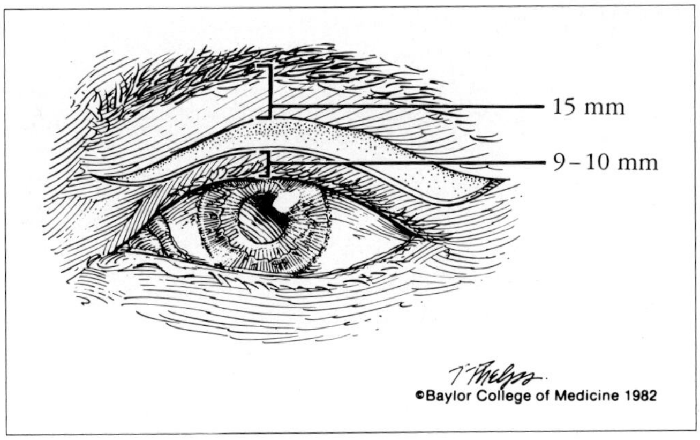

Figure 14-5. In blepharoplasty, the critical factor is how much tissue remains, not how much is excised.

cedure, the blepharoplasty being performed first. If the patient prefers a local anesthetic, I do the blepharoplasty on the first day and the cervicofacial rhytidectomy on the following day.

Most patients are given supraorbital, supratrochlear, zygomatic, temporal, and infraorbital blocks by the deposition of approximately 0.25 to 0.50 ml in each of these areas bilaterally. None of the anesthetic solution is initially deposited at the actual site of the surgery of the eyelids.

MARKING

The markings are then made with brilliant green or methylene blue dye and an appropriate stylus (see Fig. 14-6). The upper lid is marked first, beginning with the superior palpebral furrow, which is generally 9 to 10 mm above the ciliary margin, with the skin on *light upward stretch.* The superior incision line of the upper lid skin excision is marked where the lid skin, or palpebral portion of the lid skin, approximates the orbital portion. Here there is usually a subtle change in pigmentation, as well as thickness, of the skin. As a rule, this point *is never less than 1.5 cm below the midpoint of the brow, measured vertically with the skin on light stretch.* The lateral border of the upper lid excision is marked with the patient's eyes open in the primary position, the lateral excision line being, in essence, a continuation of the upsweep of the ciliary margin of the lower lid (Fig. 14-5). The medial segment is marked out, depending on the amount of skin to be excised. Generally speaking, if a centimeter or so is to be removed, the medial incision can be made as a simple fusiform ellipse; if a 15 mm or more excision is planned (vertical width), the medial and lateral modifications in the incisions are noted (see Fig. 14-4). The excision is *never* carried onto the nose. The lower lid incision is marked out, beginning just lateral to the medial punctum about 2 mm below the ciliary margin, *with the skin on light downward tension,* and carried laterally to the lateral canthus and then horizontally, or slightly upward, *but not downward,* as shown in some of the older texts. It is carried laterally past the canthus about 5 to 7 mm, depending on the amount of skin to be excised. This is determined by gently pinching the skin and marking where excess can be removed without causing obvious ectropion. The marks are rechecked and then nicked in with a No. 15 blade. Outlining the excision lines for the blepharoplasty *before* the patient is taken into the operating room reduces operating room costs and saves time, both for the patient and for the surgeon.

OPERATION

Please refer to Figures 14-6 through 14-8 and accompanying legends.

In the operating room, 2.5 to 5.0 mg of diazepam (Valium) is given intravenously, and the preparation of the facial skin is carried out—usually with a light pHisoHex wash. The conjunctiva and cornea are protected with ophthalmic ointment. The drape is routine. Using a 3-ml syringe, approximately 1.0 to 1.5 ml of local anesthetic is employed for each lid, injected subcutaneously to induce anesthesia, and deposited deep to the muscle in the locale of the fat where fat excision is planned.

A lateral incision is made in the upper lid and the skin

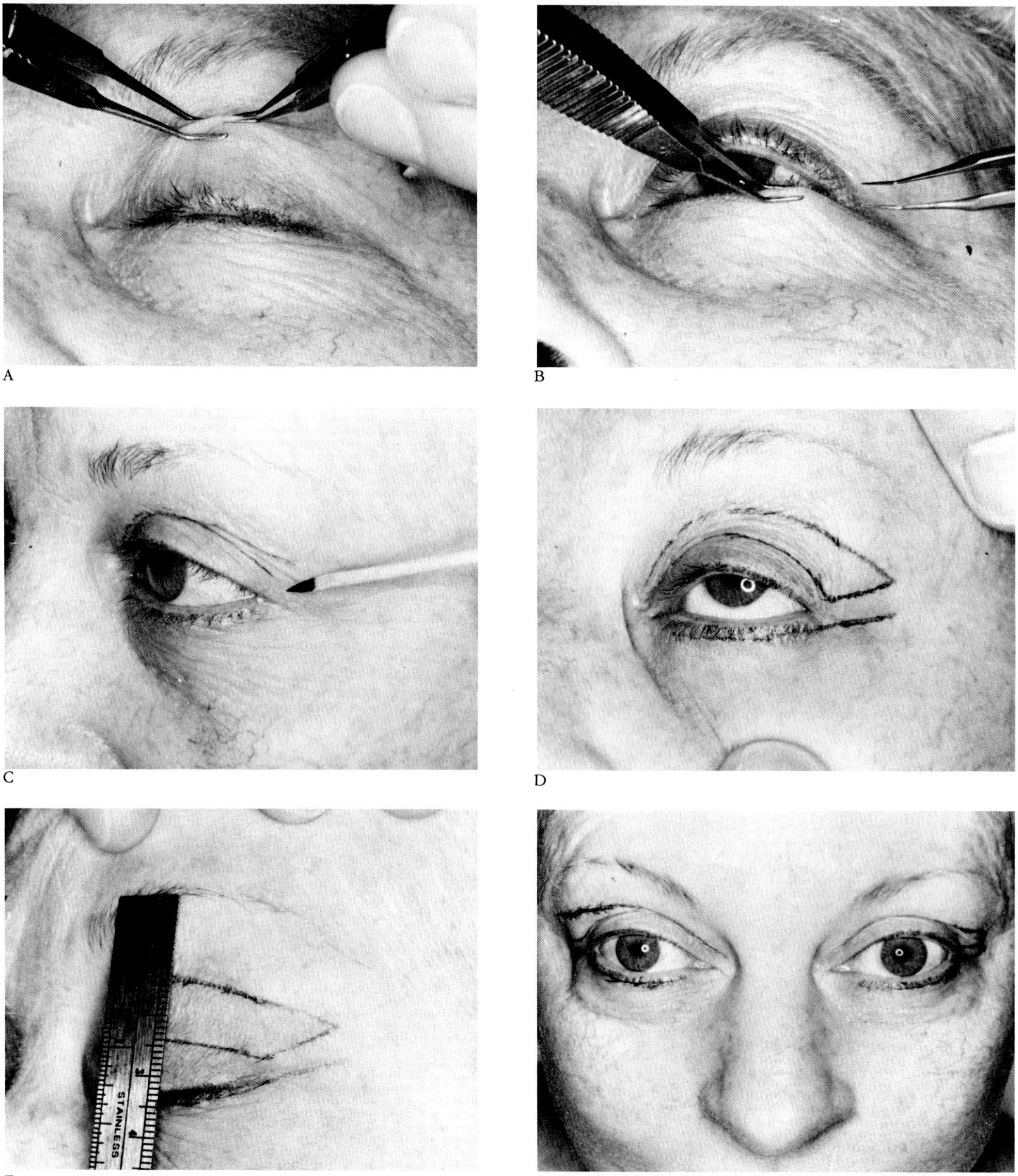

Figure 14-6. Markings for blepharoplasty.
A. Judging amount of skin to be removed from the upper lid.
B. Judging amount of skin to be excised from lower lid.
C. Lateral excision line follows upward sweep of lower lid ciliary margin.
D. Pattern outline of skin excision in upper lid and skin excision in lower lid.
E. Note measurements: It is 9 mm from ciliary margin to new superior tarsal crease; the width of skin excision is 11 mm; the distance between the upper skin excision line and the central brow is 15 mm.
F. Incision lines. Check for symmetry.

undermined rapidly at the subcutaneous level (Fig. 14-7). With the undermining complete, the skin is excised as outlined and any small bleeders encountered are electrocauterized. A strip of orbicularis muscle is removed, sufficient to expose the upper border of the tarsal plate and underlying levator expansion and Müller's muscle. The usual width of muscle excision is approximately 5 mm. With muscle removed and light pressure on the globe, the orbital septum can be observed and is cut transversely. Again, with gentle pressure on the eye, excess fat is removed by teasing the fat from its deeper lie, clamping the obvious excess, excising the fat just above the level of the clamp, and electrocauterizing the superior surface of the clamp. The "medial pocket" is exposed, *generally lying more medially than anticipated.* Again fat that is a little *lighter* in color is extruded and delivered, cross-clamped, excised, and coagulated, as described. Occasionally, in very fatty lids there is some submuscular fat laterally over the orbital rim, and this should be excised. Care should be taken not to remove any portion of the lacrimal gland. Where lacrimal gland ptosis exists, a simple suture of 5-0 chromic catgut can be placed to maintain the lacrimal gland in its position just underneath the orbital rim. Hemostasis is then secured and the incision closed, usually with interrupted sutures of 6-0 black silk. Interrupted sutures of 6-0 black silk may also be used laterally and a running subcuticular suture of 5-0 Prolene employed for the central portion of the lid closure.

Attention is then directed to the lower lid. The lateral portion of the incision is made and the skin undermined at subcutaneous level (Fig. 14-8). This is my usual approach in older patients in whom skin redundancy is the primary problem. When the primary problem is herniated fat and not skin excess, as in some middle-aged and especially younger patients, the lower lid dissection is beneath the orbicularis muscle and the skin is turned down as a skin-muscle flap [37]. In undermining, care is taken not to injure even that portion of the skin planned for excision. Use only hooks on the lower lid skin. Following wide undermining, the skin is incised 2 mm below the cilia with scissors from lateral canthal to almost medial canthal area (stop short of the punctum) and the skin flap turned downward. An incision is then made transversely through the orbicularis muscle and orbital septum, and fat in the middle and medial compartments is exposed and removed, as described above. The herniated fat in the lateral compartment, *usually a little higher* than in the medial compartment, should be searched for, extruded, and removed. This is the most common site for neglect in adequately removing herniated fat, if present. In younger patients or when herniated fat is the primary problem and not skin redundancy, the lower lid is undermined and elevated as skin-muscle flap. In older patients, with impending senile ectropion, a small 3- to 4-mm vertical wedge is generally taken out of the lower lid laterally, in order to tighten up this lid and reduce the incidence of postoperative cicatricial ectropion in a modified Kuhnt-Szymanowski procedure (Fig. 14-9).

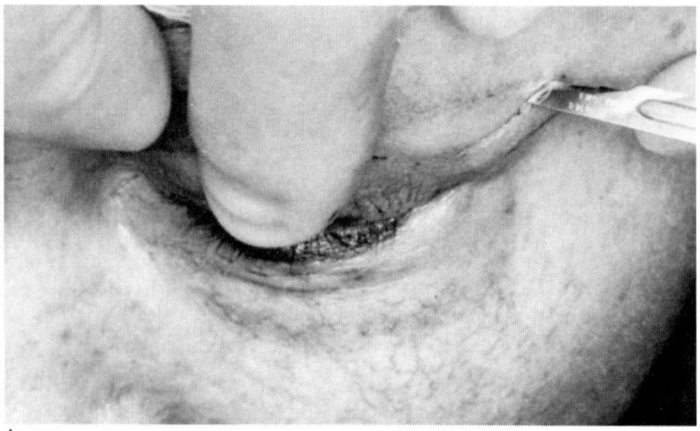
A

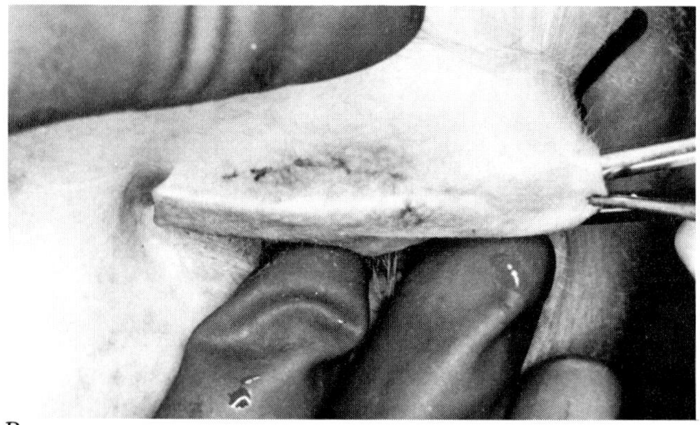
B

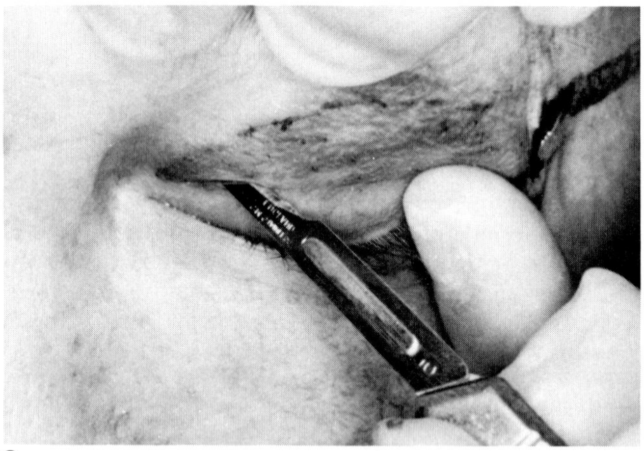
C

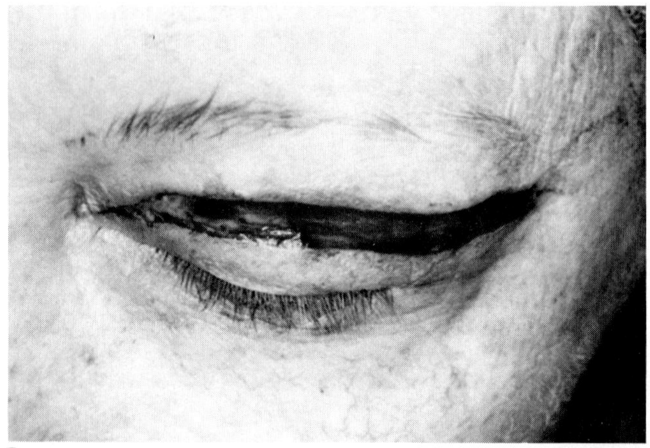
D

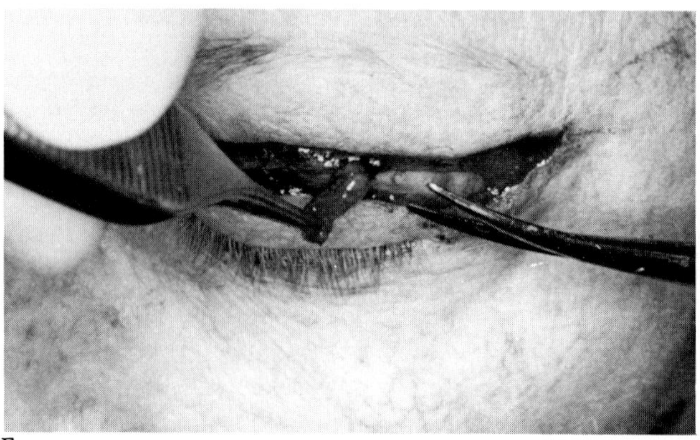
E

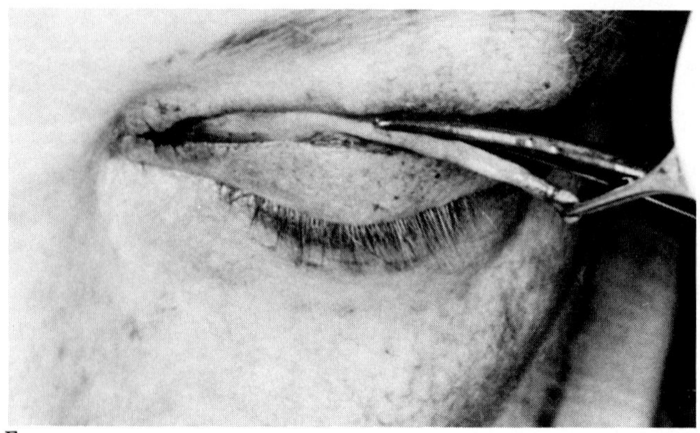
F

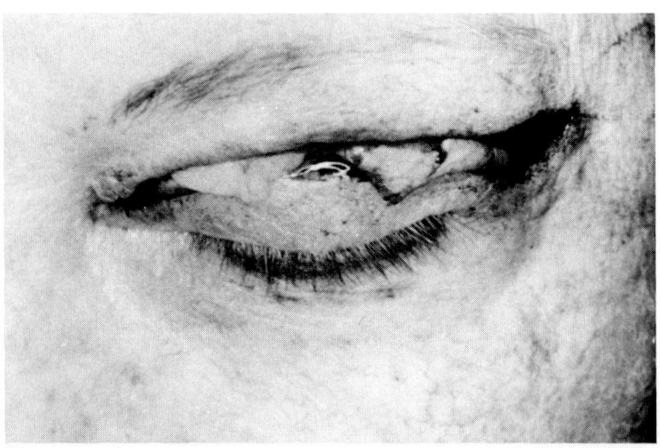
G

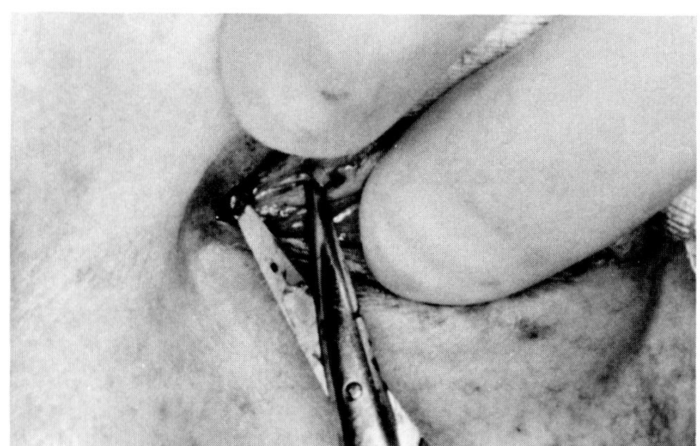
H

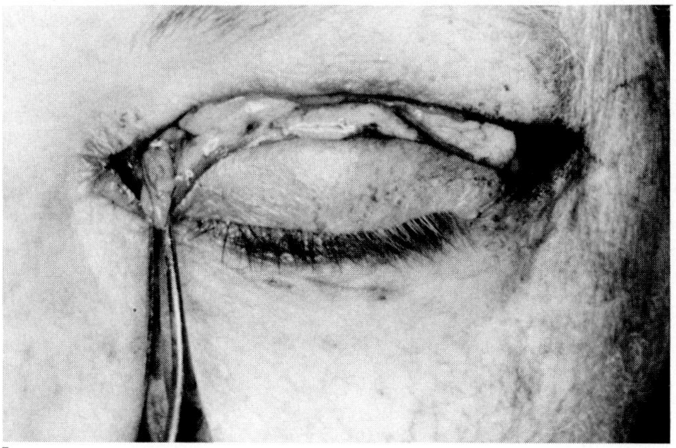

I

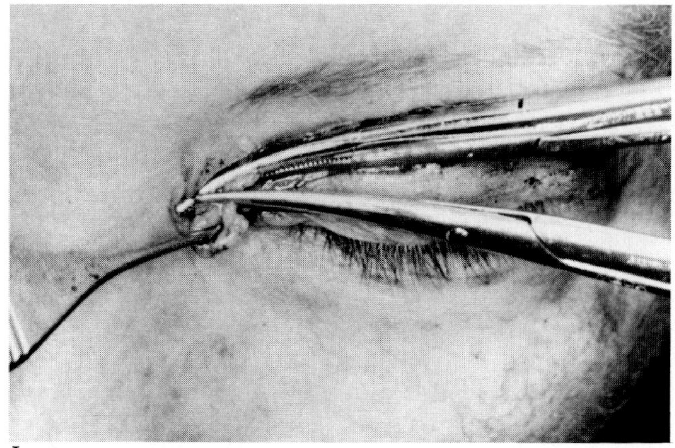

J

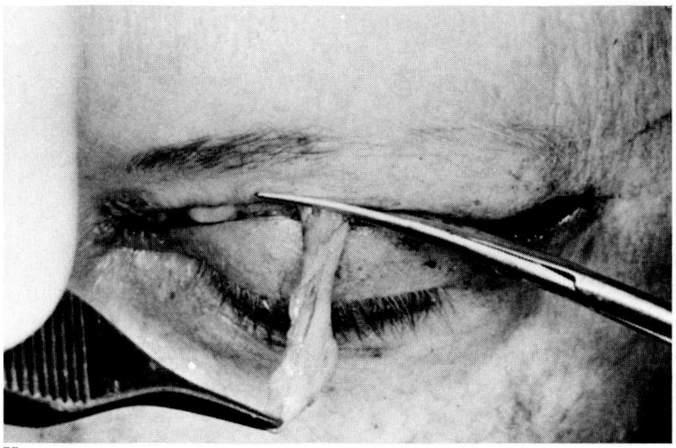

K

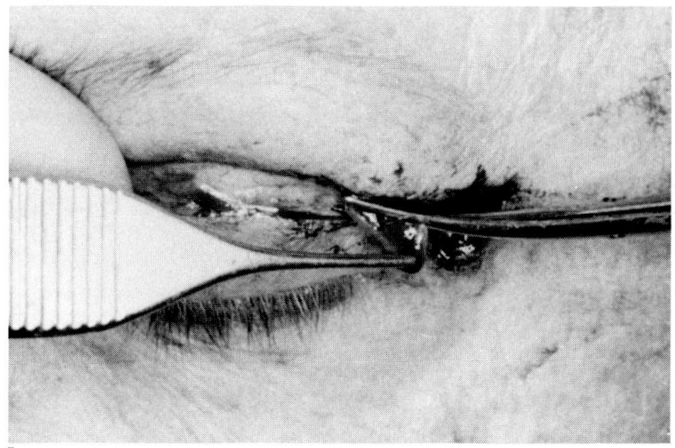

L

Figure 14-7. Upper eyelid blepharoplasty.
A. Lateral incision in upper lid.
B. Upper lid skin totally undermined through lateral incision (curved, blunt-tipped scissors).
C. Skin incised.
D. Skin excision complete.
E. Removing 5 mm vertical width of orbicularis.
F. Excision of septum orbitale.
G. Middle orbital fat exposed.
H. Releasing medial orbital compartment fat.
I. Medial fat exposed.
J. Excising medial compartment fat.
K. Excising middle compartment fat.
L. Additional excision of lateral subcutaneous tissue.

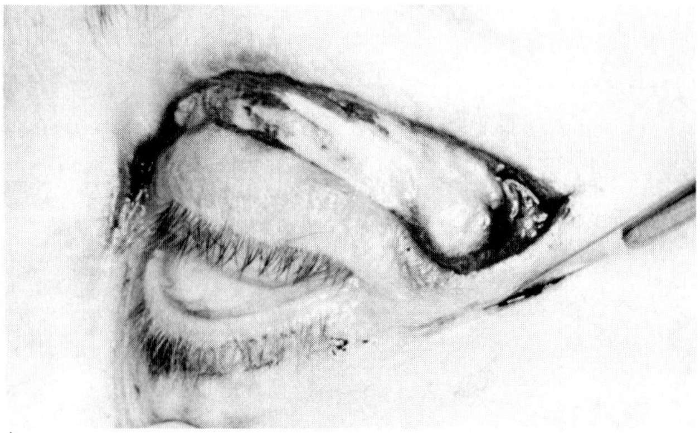

A

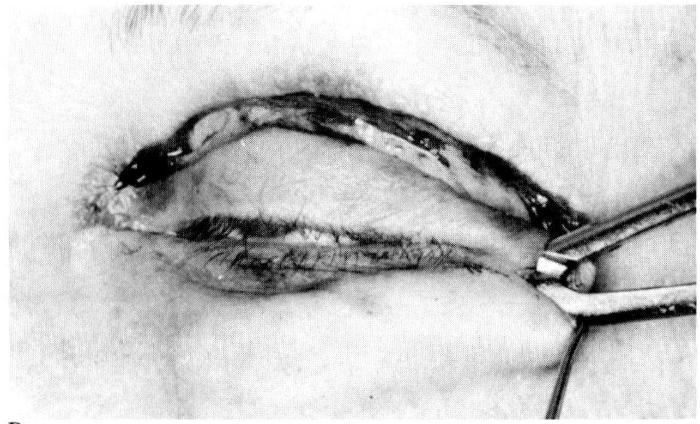

B

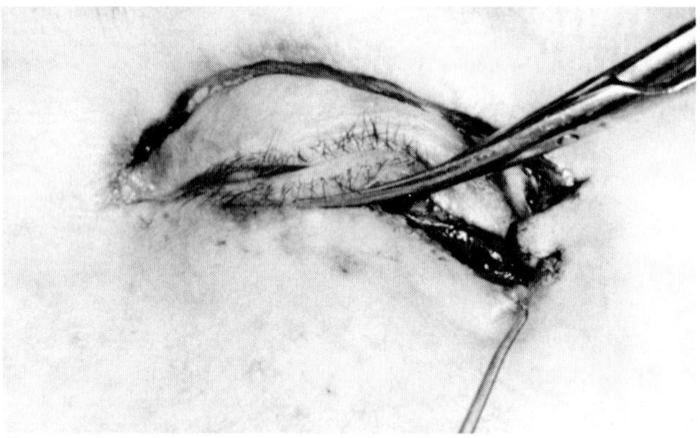

C

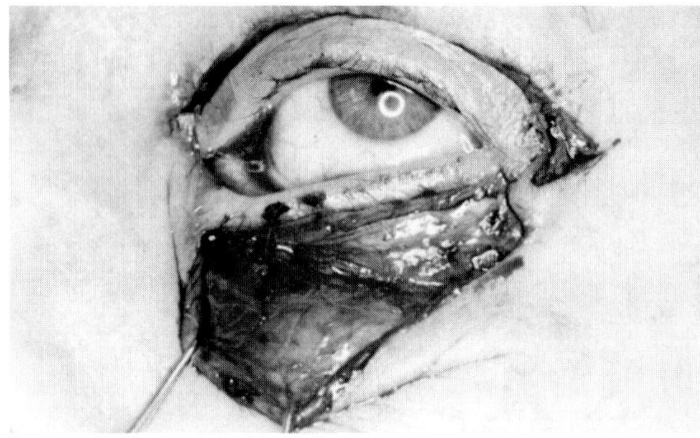

D

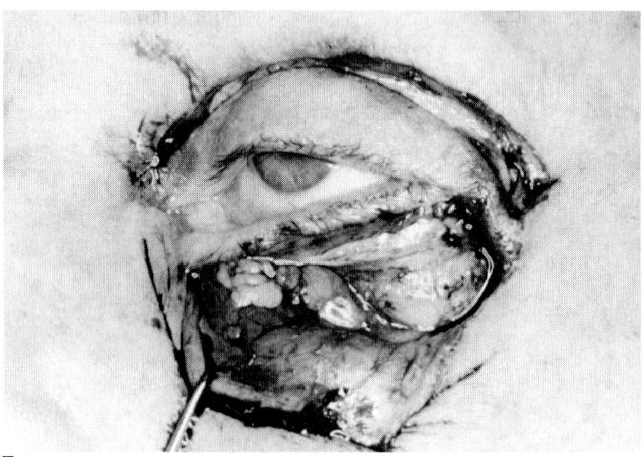

E

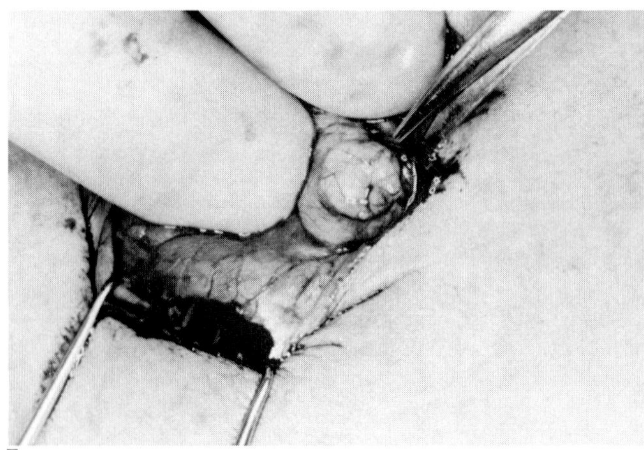

F

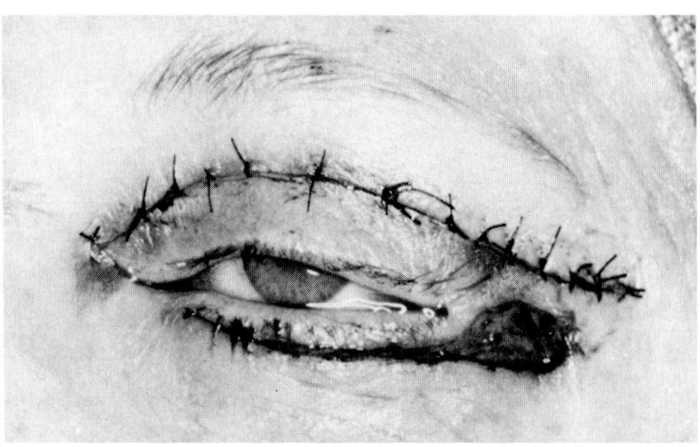

G

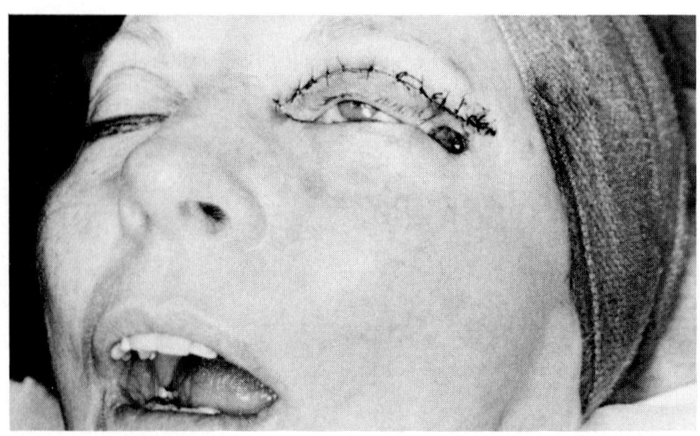

H

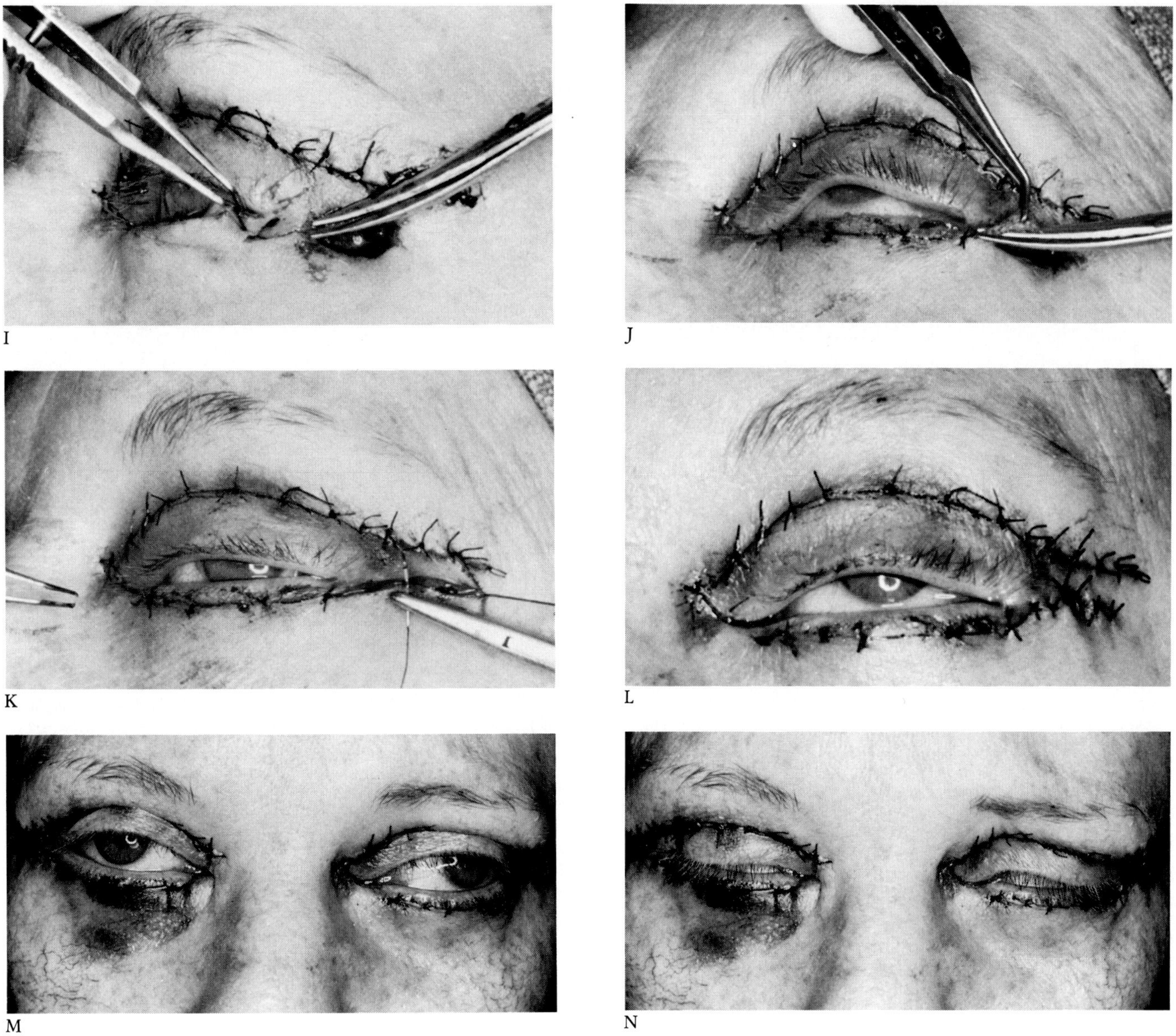

Figure 14-8. Lower eyelid blepharoplasty.

A. Upper lid excision completed, lateral excision made in lower lid.
B. Skin-muscle flap undermined through lateral incision with tenotomy scissors.
C. Lower lid incision completed with scissors.
D. Skin-muscle flap turned down.
E. Herniated fat exposed by cutting through thin attenuated septum orbitale. Fat excised as in medial compartment of upper lid (Fig. 14-7J–M).
F. Lower lid fat at a higher level in lateral compartment than in middle compartment.
G. Upper lid closed with interrupted sutures of 6-0 black silk.
H. Skin excision begun on lower lid with mouth open.
I. Central skin excision with scissors, following tacking suture just below lateral canthus.
J. Final skin excision from lateral margin.
K. Closure completed with 6-0 black silk interrupted sutures.
L. Closure completed.
M. Both eyes at completion of procedure.
N. Inability to close eyes demonstrated.

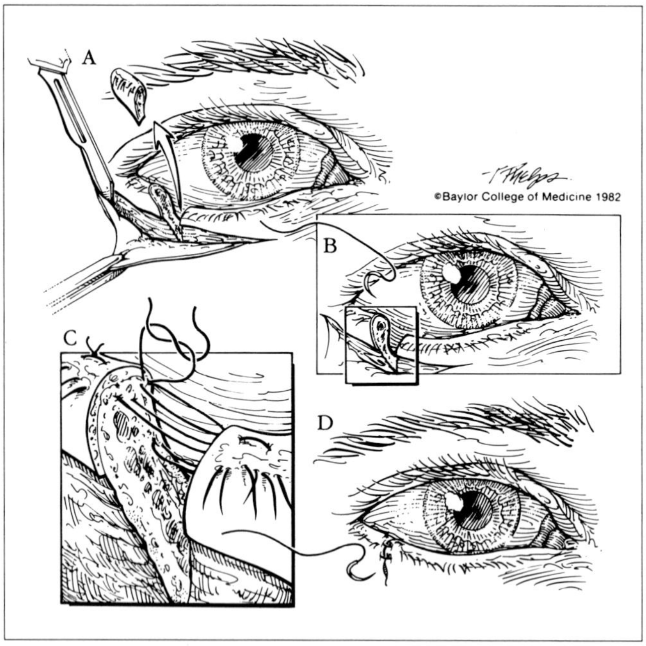

Figure 14-9
A–D. Modified Kuhnt-Szymanowski operation for senile ectropion (see text).

With the patient's mouth open and eyes in a slight upward gaze, the skin is shifted *slightly* laterally and rolled upward with a moistened applicator stick to avoid any "tenting" and the excision is performed. Note that the skin is not excised in toto immediately, but excision is carried from lateral to medial and sutures of 6-0 black silk are employed for the skin closure. If the ciliary margin and lower lid skin do not abut each other and need skin sutures to bring them together, the possibility of having removed too much skin must be considered. If the patient is unable to close the eyes immediately following skin closure in the upper lid, there is no cause for concern. The orbicularis muscle is frequently paralyzed from the anesthetic and its surgical manipulation and does not regain its full tone and activity for several hours. Note again, when excising skin on the lower lids, I prefer a "cut and sew" method to simple amputation of previously judged excess skin, in an effort to avoid excessive excision. In hundreds of blepharoplasties I have replaced approximately 5 mm of upper eyelid skin on one side for a patient on whom I felt that skin excision was excessive at the time of surgery. At a later date I was sorry, as the intraoperative suspicion (skin shortage) was not confirmed postoperatively. However, if the ciliary margin is distorted with the eyelashes rotating up and out, the possibility of excessive skin excision exists, in which case be ultraconservative in lower lid excision.

Light Adaptic gauze strips, impregnated with an antibiotic ointment, are employed on the suture lines, overlaid with a wet Kerlix dressing. The dressing is moistened hourly with saline and removed some 6 hours postoperatively and an eye regimen program of Blinx or Neoflow eyewash, followed by 2 drops of methylose drops (artificial tears—Liquifilm) 3 or 4 times a day, is carried out. A generous amount of ophthalmic ointment is applied at bedtime, particularly where lid closure is not complete. Sutures are removed on the fourth or fifth postoperative day. The patient may wear eye makeup 10 days following surgery and is asked to protect the eyelid skin from excessive sun exposure for 3 months. Sunglasses are helpful during the first few weeks postoperatively, hiding the ecchymosis and edema initially and reducing photophobia symptoms, if present, later.

The Younger Patient. Occasionally, patients present with marked fullness, or hooding, in the upper lid, minimal skin redundancy, considerable fat excess, and a low inset of the levator expansion. In the lower lid we have seen "bags" in individuals as young as 14 or 15 years of age and have operated on them when they were as young as 18. In most young adults, when blepharoplasty is performed it is usually a blepharoplasty of the upper lids for hooding (modified Oriental eye appearance) or of the lower lids where herniated fat is the primary problem, or both. In the upper lid of these patients skin excision is minimal, sometimes only 4 to 5 mm. The author has previously advocated the utilization of tarsal fixation techniques [38]. I now feel that where the inset of the levator expansion is within normal limits simple orbicularis muscle strip excision is adequate and tarsal fixation is unnecessary and at times may be deleterious. In the lower lids of these younger patients a skin-muscle flap is invariably employed, the skin and orbicularis muscle being elevated as a unit from the lateral position and the subciliary incision carried out to develop the skin-muscle flap, which can then be turned downward to expose the underlying herniated fat. Fat removal is then routine, as described above. Skin excision may be unnecessary or limited to only 1 to 2 mm in the vertical dimension. The dressings and postoperative care are in essence the same as in the procedure on older patients. Rarely, where only herniated fat in the medial and middle compartments of the lower lid is the problem, a single 5-mm "slit incision" directly over the central part of the herniation, combined with light pressure on the globe, will permit the surgeon to tease out the excess fat. The fat can be excised and the base cauterized, and two or three 6-0 nylon sutures will complete the closure.

The Older Patient. Where there is marked redundancy of lower lid skin a skin flap is used in the lower lid—not a skin muscle flap, as employing the latter technique may necessitate resection of an excessive amount of already weakened attenuated orbicularis muscle. The need for a Kuhnt-Szymanowski is much greater in the older patient. Furnas's [15] technique of excision of orbicularis oculi muscle festoons, described below, should also be given consideration.

Kuhnt-Szymanowski Procedure. The original procedure involved a splitting of the eyelid at the gray line and a through-and-through vertical wedge excision of tarsal plate and conjunctiva. The commonly accepted modified procedure (Fig. 14-9), usually done in conjunction with the lower lid blepharoplasty, creates a skin or skin-muscle flap, resecting a shield-shaped wedge of tarsal plate and conjunctiva with or without orbicularis muscle. The wound is closed in layers with 6-0 chromic catgut through tarsal plate and conjunctiva and 6-0 black silk to approximate accurately the ciliary margin, with a vertical mattress suture, and then any indicated skin excision and routine closure.

Festoons. Two techniques have been described to remove bagginess in the lower lids when herniated fat is not the prime culprit but festoons are the result of a marked excess of skin and attenuated orbicularis muscle. In the first, a skin-muscle flap is raised and the skin and flap are separated from the muscle laterally. Freeing up the orbicularis muscle above and below permits excision of an appropriate amount judged in excess from the area below and lateral to the lateral canthus. Furnas [15] points to the need for accurate assessment of the amount and localization of the festoons preoperatively. An alternative technique involves plication of the muscle layer lateral to and below the lateral canthus instead of excision.

COMBINED PROCEDURES

Brow-Lift

Where brow-lift is performed at the same operative procedure, the blepharoplasty is done *first,* some downward adjustment being made in the amount of skin removed from the upper lid in view of the impending brow ptosis procedure. Elevation of the brows, where the primary problem is lateral sag, is in the author's hands most easily accomplished through a midtemporal-frontal approach (Fig. 14-10). The usual pattern of this excision takes in an ellipse that begins in the midfrontal forehead skin directly in line with the junction of lateral and middle thirds of the brow at a horizontal level just above the lowest part of the temple hairline. It then extends laterally for about 5 cm and is carried into the hair-bearing scalp. No preoperative shaving of the scalp hair is needed. The central part of the skin ellipse is at least a centimeter wide. The forehead skin is subcutaneously undermined to the brow. Hemostasis is absolute. Hematomas are not uncommon. Two nonabsorbable sutures of 4-0 white Dacron are placed between the dermis of the inferior skin edge and the temporal fascia above, thus elevating primarily the lateral third of the brow where in most cases the ptosis exists. The skin is then closed in layers—5-0 catgut, Dexon, or Vicryl in the subcutaneous tissue and 5-0 and 6-0 nylon in the skin. Where the temporal frontal hairline is high, direct suprabrow excision as a "lazy S"-shaped ellipse of skin is preferred if the patient will accept the trade-off, i.e., a scar that is noticeable for some time. On rare occasions, where the entire forehead is sagging, the coronal approach is employed. I have had very little experience with a frontal hairline excision, and the "internal brow-lift" has not been effective in my hands.

Figure 14-10
A–D. Brow-lift excision sites. Temple excision as depicted in (C) preferred [37].

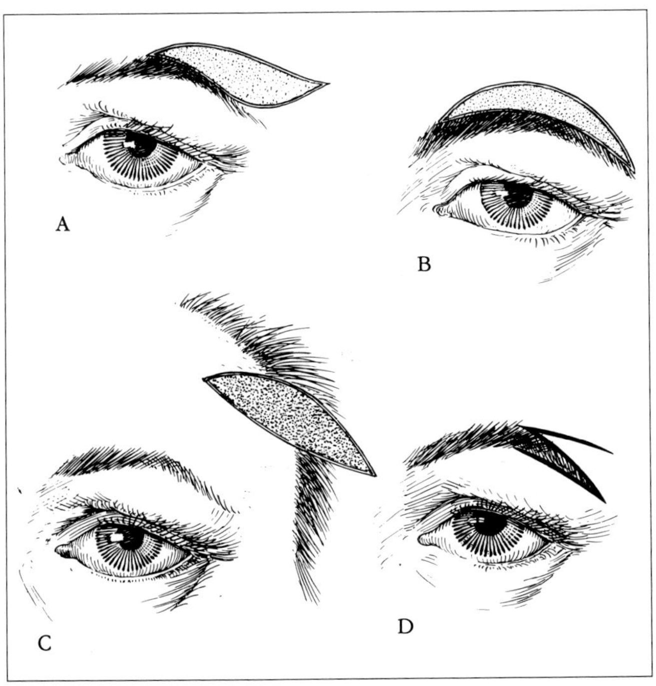

Chemical Peel

Where severe wrinkling is present, some improvement can be afforded the patient by the classic blepharoplasty. However and particularly if the wrinkles are accompanied by any degree of blepharomelasma, the patient is advised that a chemical peel should be considered 3 months after the surgical procedure. Seropian [32] performs the peel at the same time as the primary blepharoplasty. The peel may be localized to the lid and periorbital area, or the forehead and central face, or in some instances a total peel is in the patient's best interest. For the chemical peeling technique a standard solution is used, and taping is not employed to limit penetration of the chemical (tape is applied everywhere except over the tarsal portion of both upper and lower eyelids).

PTOSIS

The normal position of the ciliary margin of the upper lid in the primary position of forward gaze is 2 mm below the limbus. Where a degree of ptosis exists preoperatively, it is imperative that it be discussed with the patient *before* surgery. The condition is sometimes masked by gross skin redundancy, particularly when the skin droops over and obscures the ciliary margin, compounded by ptotic brows. Following blepharoplasty, it will most assuredly be pointed out by the patient and can conceivably be considered a complication of the procedure. The condition may be unilateral or bilateral and usually is of long standing. When of recent onset, it might be an early warning sign of myasthenia gravis. In all but the rarest instances it is of the senile or atonic type, and levator function is good (greater than 10 mm).

Where a degree of ptosis exists, consideration should be given to correction of the ptosis simultaneously with the blepharoplasty operation. Minimal degrees of ptosis (2 mm or less) can be corrected with a Fasanella-Servat procedure [10]. If the ptosis is bilateral, it is usually minimal, with the patient complaining of a "sleepy eye" or "bedroom eye" appearance. The Fasanella-Servat procedure is quite applicable and useful here, and the technique described by Beard [4] is employed.

The procedure is performed after the blepharoplasty is completed. The conjunctiva is topically anesthetized and the lid everted with the underlying cornea protected by appropriate acrylic conformer. Two small, curved, fine-pointed mosquito hemostats are placed 2 to 3 mm over the upper border of the tarsal plate, as shown in Figure 14-11. Beginning in the temporal eyelid skin, a running horizontal mattress suture of 5-0 chromic catgut is passed through the skin to the conjunctiva and then placed 1 mm above the clamps. The tissue above the clamps, including conjunctiva, Müller's muscle, and tarsal plate is excised, and the same suture is used to oversew the edges, as seen in Figure 14-11. It is brought out to the skin and tied to itself. The eye is lubricated, a temporary modified Frost suture is placed, and the eye is patched for a day. When lagophthalmos exists (inability to close the lids fully), the Frost suture is left in place and serves to keep the lids closed at night for at least a week.

When the ptosis is greater than 2 mm, full correction is difficult to achieve without levator expansion with Müller's muscle shortening or imbrication. I prefer to perform a classic shortening of the levator, as described by Fox [13], sufficient to match the opposing lid, although Kahn [21] has successfully employed an imbrication technique. The levator expansion with Müller's muscle is detached from its insertion on the tarsus, under loupe magnification, and dissected superiorly without injuring the conjunctiva. This maneuver is done after skin and orbicularis excision has been carried out. A few drops of local anesthetic injected to balloon out the tissue will be helpful. I prefer to do the procedure under local anesthesia with topical anesthesia for the conjunctiva. The cornea is always protected by corneal-scleral protecting eye conformer during the levator dissection. A Berke muscle clamp facilitates handling of the cut levator muscle. In some instances the lateral medial horns may have to be cut to mobilize the levator fully. Three double-armed sutures of 5-0 chromic catgut are inserted between the muscle and the tarsal plate just above the planned site of resection. The sutures are tightened with a single loop, and lid position is tested. In the presence of good levator function, with minimal ptosis, overcorrection is easily done. It is better to undercorrect than overcorrect in the older patient. When the lid position is as desired, the excess levator expansion with Müller's muscle is excised, the previously placed catgut sutures are appropriately tied, and the blepharoplasty incision is closed per routine. The reader is referred to standard texts for further details [4, 13]. The technique requires a certain amount of judgment, and it might be better for the neophyte plastic surgeon not to attempt correction of both the blepharoplasty problem and ptosis simultaneously.

Figure 14-11. Fasanella-Servat procedure (see text).

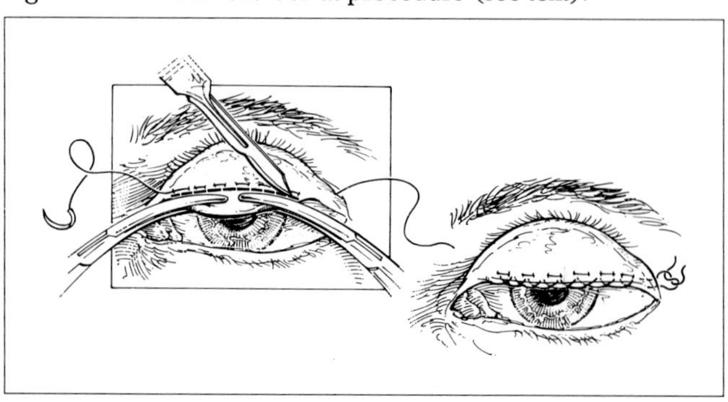

ADDITIONAL NOTES ON POSTOPERATIVE CARE

All dressings, except Adaptic or Steri-Strips, applied at the time of surgery are removed the evening of surgery, so the patient need not have the eyes covered at night (a sometimes distressing situation that can be avoided). The postoperative eye medication regimen has already been referred to. Not rarely, particularly in the older patient, grade "one-half" ectropion occurs laterally in the lower lids. This condition is evanescent and will improve; a program of light massage 3 or 4 times a day is advocated. On rare occasions it is necessary to apply quarter-inch Steri-Strips laterally in the lower lids, taped to the temple skin, in order to maintain the lid in a normal position abutting the globe.

Some degree of lagophthalmos, or the inability to close the lids fully, may be anticipated, particularly where skin resection has been extensive; however, this improves rapidly. The patient is urged to practice forced "squinching" of the lids several times a day, in an effort to improve orbicularis tone. Edema subsides, as does ecchymosis, but in some cases a residual increase in pigmentation may be observed, and this can be managed in one of two ways. Where wrinkling is present, a chemical peel will effect considerable improvement, or, if the patient is not allergic to the medication Eldoquin-Forte, it can be applied twice daily for a 3-month period and will generally bleach out the skin enough to give the patient the desired improvement. Occasionally, a mild degree of conjunctival edema or chemosis is present and as a rule secondary to lagophthalmos or excessive exposure of the conjunctiva and does require particular care. At night the eye should be taped closed, so as to avoid further aggravation of the condition. If patients complain of "dry eye," this is treated by a more prolonged utilization of the methylose drops. If the complaint is diminution of vision, this is usually due to accumulation of ophthalmic ointment. Sometimes milia formations are disturbing; they are evanescent. If of great concern they can be deroofed with a Hyfrecator, or the patient can be taught to open them with a sterile needle and apply a dab of alcohol.

ADDITIONAL COMPLICATIONS

Intraoperative complications such as expanding hematoma and the development of a "hard eye," secondary to a retrobulbar hematoma, are rare. Treatment of the latter is primarily evacuation of any hematoma that is present through a direct approach and *not* any type of anterior chamber incision.

While an expanding hematoma in the early postoperative period is a rarity, treatment is the same as when seen in a rhytidectomy. The sutures are removed, the clot is evacuated, hemostasis is obtained, and the wound is closed. The time required for the ecchymoses to clear up is distressingly prolonged. The use of oral enzymes may shorten it.

The reader is referred to the contributions of Castanares [8], Rees [28], and Stark [39] to the prevention and treatment of complications following blepharoplasty.

RESULTS

Short-Term Results

In the absence of any of the complications just described, the short-term (3 months to 1 year) results are invariably pleasing, to both surgeon and patient. Makeup can be employed in the second postoperative week, and the scars fade rapidly. When the edema has totally subsided, the fine wrinkles and abnormal pigmentations, if present and carefully recorded preoperatively, will return, and the patient will again learn that the routine blepharoplasty is not the answer for these problems. All in all, however, patient satisfaction rates are high, particularly when herniated fat is present preoperatively and has been properly removed. Even the brows remain "up" in the short-term evaluation.

Long-Term Results

While the patient never returns to his or her preoperative status, the aging process is inexorable. One can state categorically that if preoperatively the patients appeared older than their chronologic age, they will age faster postoperatively than patients who appear younger than their stated age, even though the short-term results may be more dramatic in the former. Herniated fat, once successfully removed, does not tend to recur, while skin redundancy does—the skin tends to stretch out and may, particularly in the lateral part of the upper lid, become a cause for concern in the patient. I do not share the enthusiasm of others relative to the long-term results of any of the brow-lift operations. The degree and rate of brow descent is directly proportional to the site of skin excision. Excisions close to the brow (direct suprabrow skin elliptic excisions) are longer lasting than, for example, those involving a coronal incision in the scalp and skin removal next to the coronal suture line. Representative cases of routine blepharoplasties are seen in Figure 14-12.

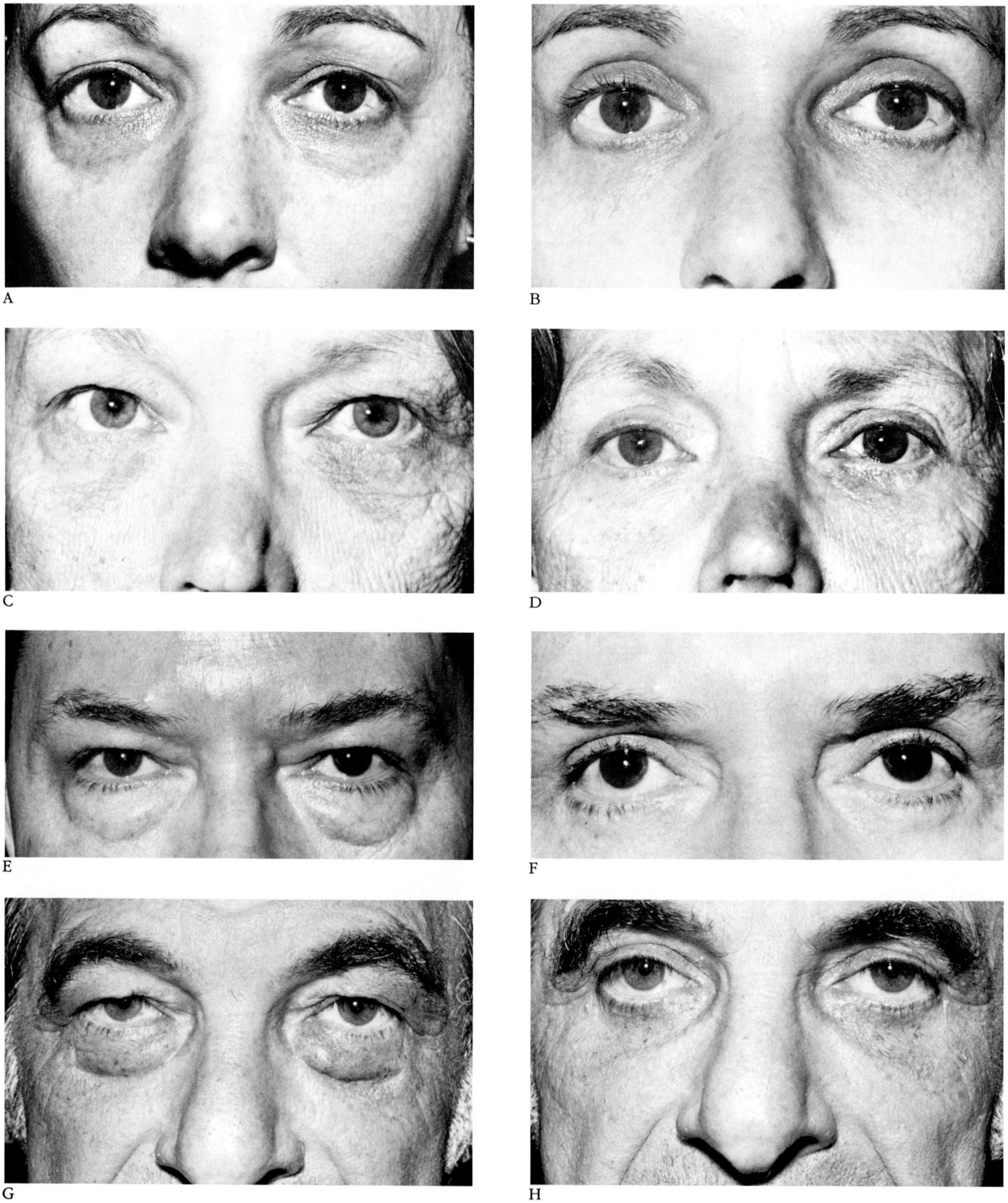

Figure 14-12
A. Preoperative (age 32).
B. Postoperative 10 months (skin-muscle flap).
C. Preoperative (age 70).
D. Postoperative 9 months (skin flap).
E. Preoperative (age 52).
F. Postoperative 22 months (skin-muscle flap).
G. Preoperative (age 59).
H. Postoperative 17 months (skin flap).

REFERENCES

1. Arlt, C. *Graefe-Saemisch Handbuch. Ges. Augenh.* 2:457, 1877.
2. Aston, S. J. Orbicularis oculi muscle flaps: A technique to reduce crow's feet and lateral canthal skin folds. *Plast. Reconstr. Surg.* 65:206, 1980.
3. Baker, T. J., Gordon, H. L., and Mosienko, P. Upper lid blepharoplasty. *Plast. Reconstr. Surg.* 60:692, 1977.
4. Beard, C. *Ptosis.* St. Louis: Mosby, 1969.
5. Bourguet, J. La chirurgie esthétique de l'oeil et des paupières. *Monde Med.* 725, 1929.
6. Callahan, A. *Reconstructive Surgery of the Eyelids and Adnexa.* Birmingham, Ala.: Aesculapius Publishing, 1966.
7. Castanares, S. Blepharoplasty for herniated intra-orbital fat: Anatomical basis for a new approach. *Plast. Reconstr. Surg.* 8:46, 1951.
8. Castanares, S. Eyelid Plasty. In R. M. Goldwyn (ed.), *The Unfavorable Result in Plastic Surgery.* Boston: Little, Brown, 1972.
9. *Dorland's Illustrated Medical Dictionary* (26th ed.). Philadelphia: Saunders, 1981.
10. Fasanella, R. M., and Servat, J. Levator resection for minimal ptosis: Another simplified operation. *Arch. Ophthalmol.* 65:493, 1961.
11. Fernandez, L. R. Double eyelid operation in the Oriental in Hawaii. *Plast. Reconstr. Surg.* 25:257, 1960.
12. Flowers, R. S. Anchor Blepharoplasty. In *Transactions of the Sixth International Congress of Plastic and Reconstructive Surgery.* Paris: Masson, 1976.
13. Fox, S. A. *The Surgery of Ptosis.* New York: Grune & Stratton, 1968.
14. Fox, S. A. Sagittal Section—Eye. In S. A. Fox, *Ophthalmic Plastic Surgery* (5th ed.). New York: Grune & Stratton, 1976.
15. Furnas, D. W. The orbicularis oculi muscle: Management in blepharoplasty. *Clin. Plast. Surg.* 8:687, 1981.
16. Goin, J. M., and Goin, M. K. *Changing the Body: Psychological Effects of Plastic Surgery.* Baltimore: Williams & Wilkins, 1981.
17. Gonzales-Ulloa, M., and Stevens, E. The treatment of palpebral bags. *Plast. Reconstr. Surg.* 27:381, 1961.
18. Gordon, G. Observations upon the movement of the eyelids. *Br. J. Ophthalmol.* 35:339, 1951.
19. Hinderer, U. T. Blepharocanthoplasty with eyebrow lift. *Plast. Reconstr. Surg.* 56:402, 1975.
20. Joseph, J. *Nasenplastik und sonstige Gesichtsplastik nebst einen Anhang uber Mammaplastik.* Leipzig: Kabitzsch, 1931.
21. Kahn, S. Correction of senile (atonic) blepharoptosis during cosmetic blepharoplasty. *Plast. Reconstr. Surg.* 60:925, 1977.
22. Kestenbaum, A. *Applied Anatomy of the Eye.* New York: Grune & Stratton, 1963.
23. Kolle, F. S. *Plastic and Cosmetic Surgery.* New York: Appleton, 1911.
24. Lewis, J. R. The Z-blepharoplasty. *Plast. Reconstr. Surg.* 44:331, 1969.
25. Merkel, F. *Graefe-Saemisch Handbuch. Ges. Augenh.* 1:454, 1874.
26. Miller, C. C. Folds, bags and wrinkles of the skin about the eyes and their eradication by simple surgical methods. *Med. Brief* 35:540, 1907.
27. Putterman, A. M., and Urst, M. J. Muller muscle–conjunctiva resection: Technique for treatment of blepharoptosis. *Arch. Ophthalmol.* 93:619, 1975.
28. Rees, T. D. *Aesthetic Plastic Surgery.* Philadelphia: Saunders, 1980.
29. Rees, T. D., and Jelks, G. W. Blepharoplasty and the dry-eye syndrome: Guidelines for surgery. *Plast. Reconstr. Surg.* 68:249, 1981.
30. Rogers, B. O. Cosmetic blepharoplasty using an electrocauterization technique. *Aesthetic Plast. Surg.* 1:263, 1977.
31. Sayoc, B. T. Plastic construction of the superior palpebral folds. *Am. J. Ophthalmol.* 38:556, 1954.
32. Seropian, O. Personal communication, 1981.
33. Sheen, J. H. A change in the technique of supratarsal fixation in upper blepharoplasty. *Plast. Reconstr. Surg.* 59:831, 1977.
34. Sheen, J. H. Tarsal fixation in lower blepharoplasty. *Plast. Reconstr. Surg.* 62:24, 1978.
35. Silver, H. A new approach to the operation of blepharoplasty. *Br. J. Plast. Surg.* 22:253, 1969.
36. Skoog, T. *Plastic Surgery.* Philadelphia: Saunders, 1975.
37. Spira, M. Lower blepharoplasty: A clinical study. *Plast. Reconstr. Surg.* 59:35, 1977.
38. Spira, M. Blepharoplasty. *Clin. Plast. Surg.* 5:121, 1978.
39. Stark, R. B. *Aesthetic Plastic Surgery.* Boston: Little, Brown, 1980.
40. Stasior, O. Repair of Cicatricial Ectropion. Presented at the Third International Symposium, Plastic and Reconstructive Surgery of the Eye and Adnexa, New York, 1980.
41. *Stedman's Medical Dictionary* (24th ed.). Baltimore: Williams & Wilkins, 1982.
42. Stephenson, K. L. History of blepharoplasty. *Aesthetic Plast. Surg.* 1:177, 1977.

15. Advanced Blepharoplasty

Richard J. Siegel

By heaven, the wonder in a mortal eye!
William Shakespeare

Over the past decade there has been a major evolution in blepharoplasty, from the simple excision of redundant tissues (Figs. 15-1 and 15-2) to complex techniques involving the deepest layers of the eyelid. In the upper lid, techniques that alter the fascial substructure allow the surgeon to raise a low fold permanently, add definition and longevity, correct asymmetry and ptosis, and bring dramatic, crisp detail to aging eyelid tissues (Figs. 15-3 to 15-6). These new techniques, however, are more complicated and demand an extreme degree of precision; there is little margin for technical or aesthetic error.

This chapter emphasizes the diagnostic and technical considerations that are essential in order to clearly understand and *selectively apply* advanced blepharoplasty techniques. No single technique is suggested as routine. Blepharoplasty is the art and craft of eyelid tailoring, *custom tailoring,* because the needs and anatomy of each patient are so different. Since the execution and avoidance of complications with advanced blepharoplasty techniques are predicated on a detailed anatomic knowledge, it is necessary to review the eight major eyelid layers.

ANATOMY

Eyelid anatomy is difficult to study. The many layers of exquisitely thin tissue that glide over each other are easily distorted in anatomic specimens. Thus, *cadaver dissections are often misleading.* The best method for learning the subtleties of eyelid anatomy is to spend the time during surgery to dissect and identify the various layers. Beard recognizes this imperative, stating, "It is often necessary to identify structures by their position and relation to known landmarks, rather than by their appearance" [4]. The anatomic relationships described below have been elucidated during intraoperative dissections on approximately 350 patients over the past 6 years. The identification and relationship of the fascial layers within the eyelid are of particular importance for the aesthetic surgeon (Table 15-1).

I am very grateful to my wife and medical photographer, Patricia McCullough Siegel, for the painstaking accuracy of her photography and for bringing an informed and candid woman's point of view to this work.

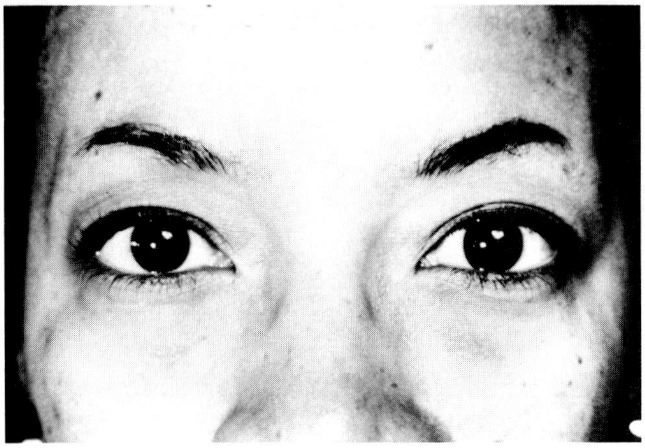

A

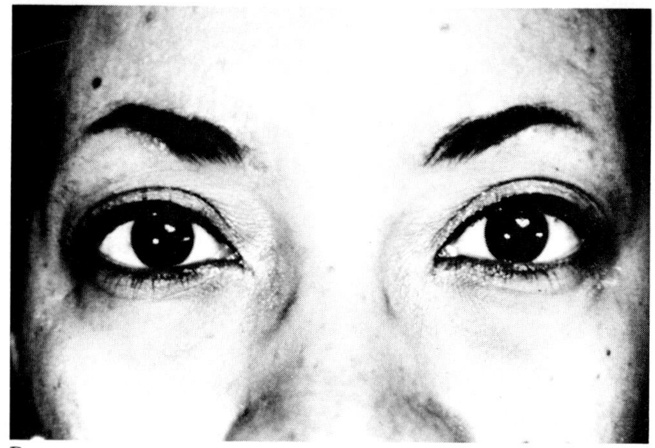

B

Figure 15-1. Good result with basic blepharoplasty.
A. A 37-year-old woman before surgery.
B. Two years after skin-muscle excision upper blepharoplasty.

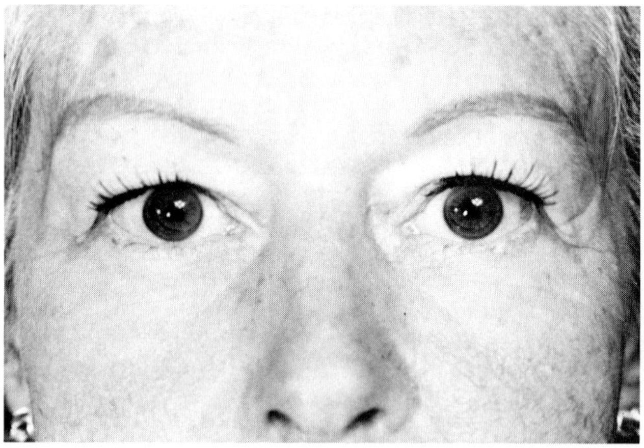

A

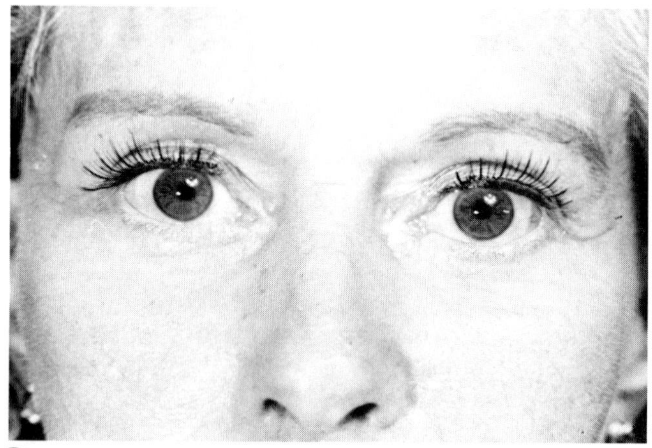

B

Figure 15-2. Poor result with basic blepharoplasty.
A. A 64-year-old woman before surgery.
B. One and one-half years after skin-muscle resection upper lid blepharoplasty. Recurrence of hanging preseptal skin has taken place, and there are multiple pretarsal wrinkles.

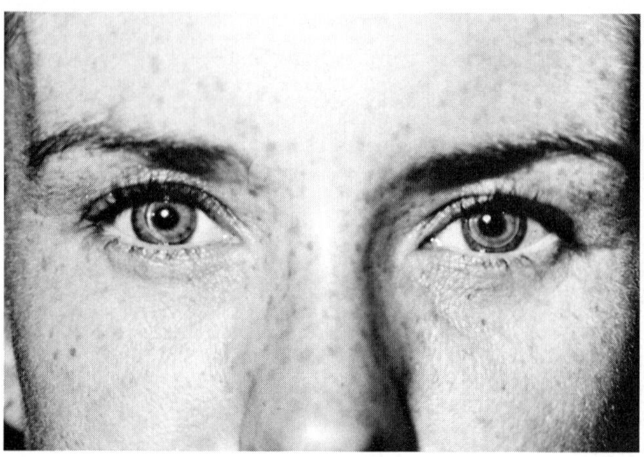

A

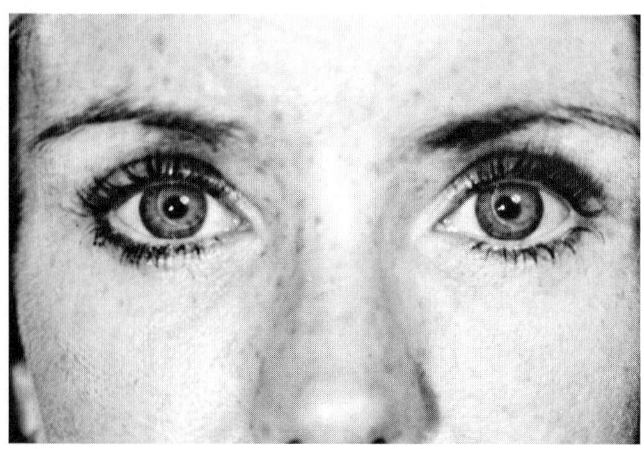

B

Figure 15-3. Good result after advanced blepharoplasty.
A. A 33-year-old woman before surgery.
B. Six months after upper and lower blepharoplasty.

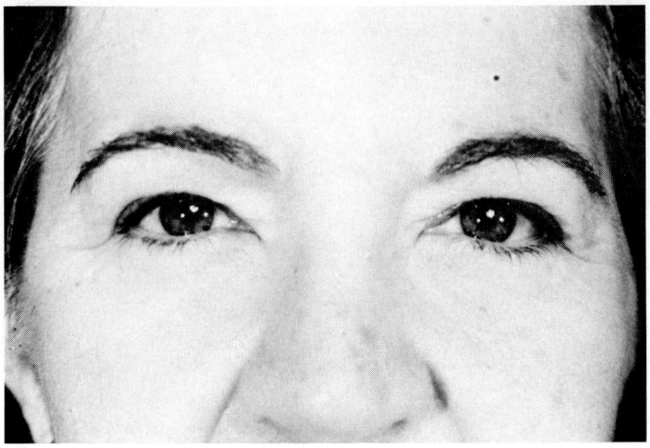

A

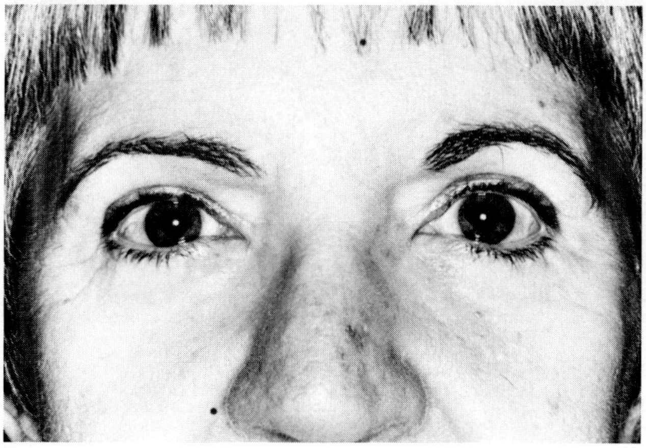

B

Figure 15-4. Conservative secondary blepharoplasty; incision 8 mm above the lashes, low fold height.
A. Preoperative.
B. One and one-half years after surgery. Levator aponeurosis secured to dermis (see Case 3).

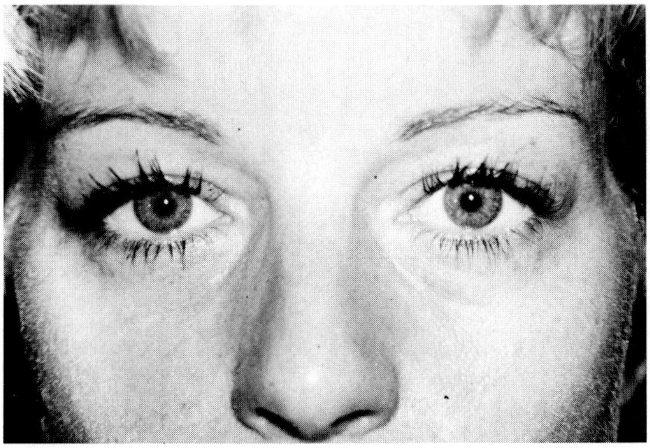

A

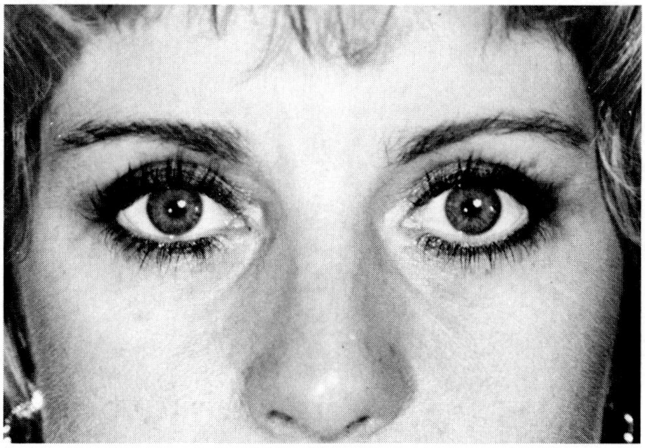

B

Figure 15-5. Intermediate fold height; incision 10 mm above the lashes.
A. A 43-year-old hairdresser before surgery.
B. Three years after advanced blepharoplasty.

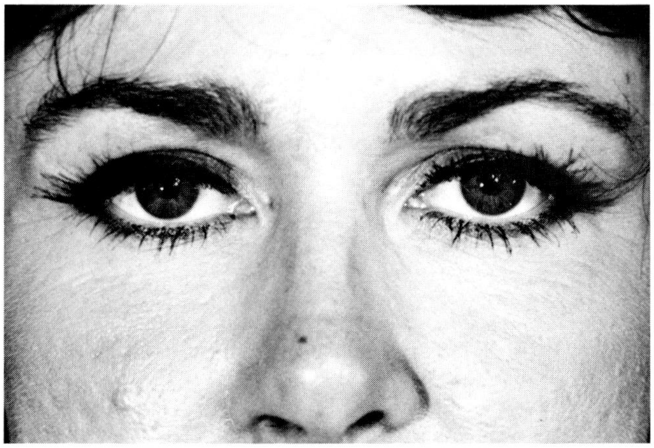

A

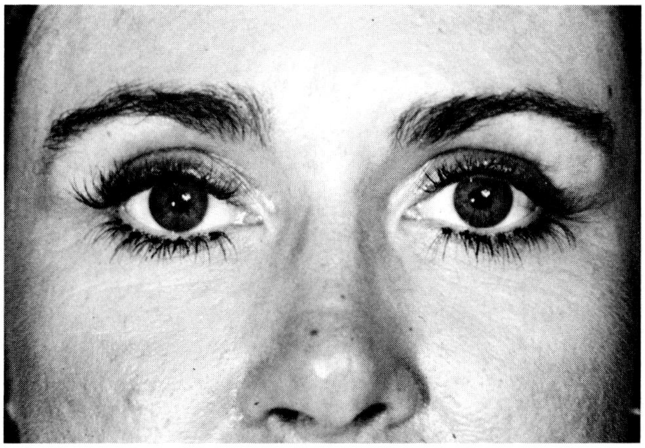

B

Figure 15-6. Dramatic or "high fold" blepharoplasty; incision 12 mm above the lashes.
A. A 46-year-old cosmetologist before surgery.
B. Nine months after advanced blepharoplasty. Extensive resection of preorbital, preseptal, and pretarsal tissues. Fold secured by suturing levator aponeurosis to both upper tarsal edge and inferior edge of dermis.

Table 15-1. Eyelid anatomy

1. Skin	Superficial
2. Muscle	
3. Fascia	
4. Orbital septum	
5. Levator aponeurosis	
6. Müller's muscle	
7. Tarsal plate	
8. Conjunctiva	Deep

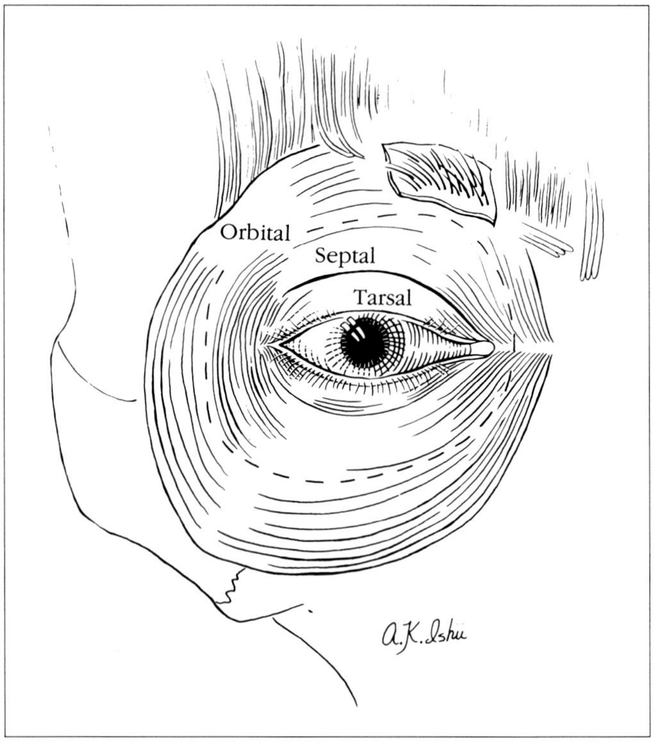

Figure 15-7. Orbicularis oculi muscle. The three major zones: orbital, septal, tarsal. The outermost ring of muscle usually extends far beyond the bony orbital rim.

Skin

The skin of the eyelid is the thinnest in the body and subjected to virtually constant movement, resulting in frequent folding and wrinkling. Subcutaneous fat is usually absent in the Caucasian but may be abundant in the Oriental.

Muscle

The orbicularis muscle fibers are supplied by the seventh nerve and act as the sphincter of the palpebral fissure. There are two main parts, orbital and palpebral.

The *orbital* orbicularis is the most peripheral and consists of the outermost ring of muscle. It usually extends far beyond the bony orbital rim (Fig. 15-7). Superiorly, it fuses partially with the frontalis muscle, while many of its fibers pass anterior to the frontalis, inserting into the eyebrow skin. Laterally it covers part of the temporalis muscle, while inferiorly it extends over the zygoma. This peripheral muscle is responsible for the crow's-feet, the radial wrinkles of eyelid expression.

The palpebral orbicularis can be subdivided into two components: *preseptal* and *pretarsal.* These fibers of the orbicularis muscle are largely responsible for reflex "involuntary" lid closure, as occurs in blinking and sleep. The preseptal fibers arise from the medial canthal tendon and fuse laterally to form a raphe. The pretarsal fibers are more firmly attached to both their overlying skin and subjacent fascia. Laterally, they form the lateral canthal tendon, which "inserts" on the orbital tubercle [15, 33].

Conceptualization of the origin and insertion of the orbicularis oculi sphincter muscle is extremely confusing. Both the medial and lateral canthal tendons are fibrous cords that attach the orbicularis muscle to the orbital bone. These attachments maintain the beautiful shape of the palpebral fissure and allow the muscle vector to be directed to the underlying tarsal plate. They are *not tendinous insertions,* however, as the muscle does not move the bone to which it attaches. Rather, the function of the orbicularis oculi muscle is to move the tarsal plate and thereby control exposure of the cornea. Thus, it is more logical to view the sheet of fascia that attaches orbicularis to tarsus as the major "insertion" of the muscle. This orbicularis fascia is one of the most important and yet rarely considered eyelid layers.

Fascia

The orbicularis "submuscular" fascia is the deep lining of the orbicularis muscle. It is continuous with the galea aponeurotica. Anterior to the tarsus, the orbicularis fascia fuses with the levator aponeurosis to form a *"conjoined" pretarsal fascia* (Fig. 15-8). This critical layer provides the adherent foothold for the pretarsal orbicularis muscle, preventing it from slipping down and away from the tarsus.

The orbicularis fascia is permeated by a rich vascular network, as well as sensory and motor nerves. Traction applied to this layer will be felt superficially and peripherally to the orbital rim and will produce a slight movement of the brow and lower forehead. Also, this tissue will feel more elastic than the orbital septum, which lies just deep to it. Fatty infiltration of the orbicularis fascia plays a key role in many eyelid deformities.

Orbital Septum

The orbital septum is a dense fibrous layer extending from all the edges of the orbital rim. It is an extension of the periosteum and forms the major anterior retaining wall of the orbital fat. Tension placed on this structure during surgery will be felt at the orbital margin or just inside the orbital rim. Unlike the orbicularis fascia, the septum has no "give"—hardly any elasticity or mobility. Inferiorly, it fuses with the levator aponeurosis, forming a "sling" that encloses the orbital fat.

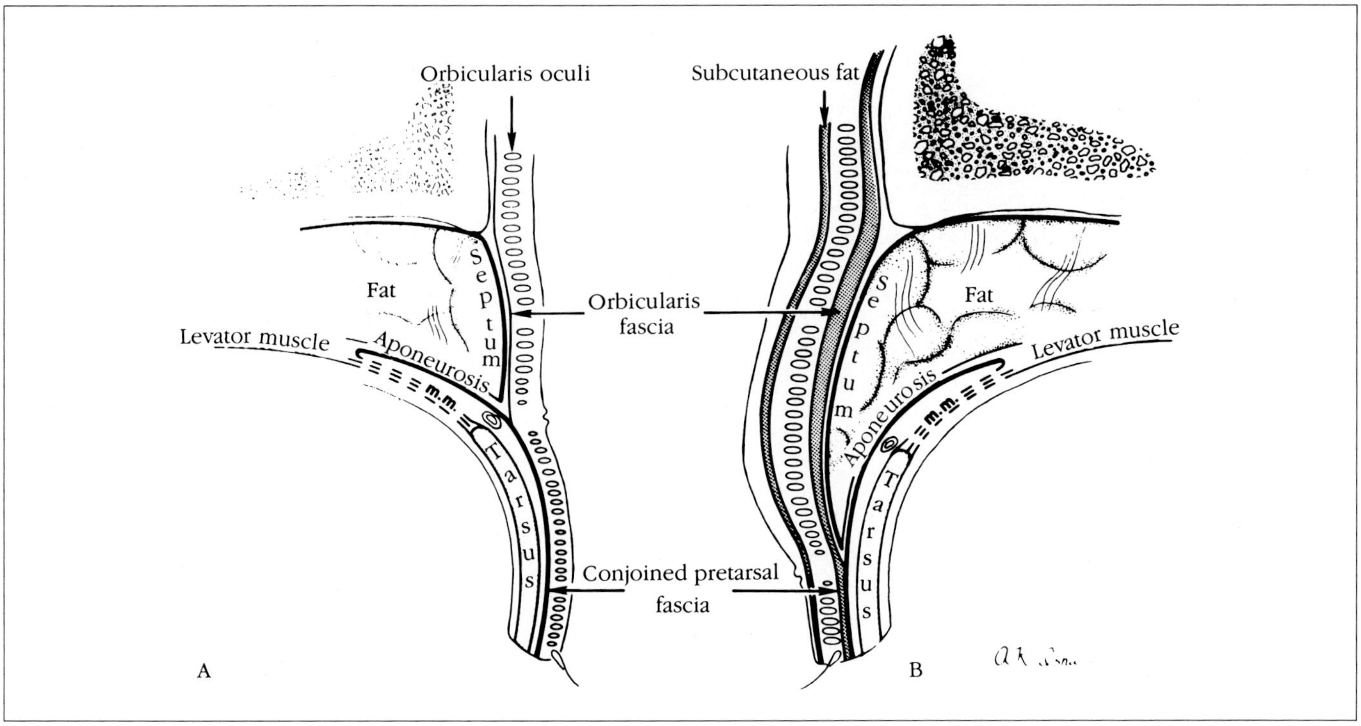

Figure 15-8. Schematic cross section of the upper eyelid.
A. A typical Caucasian eyelid: levator aponeurosis fusing to orbicularis fascia at the level of the upper border of the tarsal plate.
B. An Oriental eyelid. The fusion of the levator aponeurosis and orbicularis fascia occurs lower, closer to the lashes. Fat is often present in many layers.

Levator Palpebrae Superioris

The levator muscle is the last extraocular muscle to develop in the fetus, and the most anomalous. It originates at the apex of the orbit, from the lesser wing of the sphenoid bone. About 4 mm wide at its origin, it gradually increases in width as it passes forward, and eventually overlies nearly all of the superior rectus muscle. Approximately 1 cm superior to the tarsus, the levator *muscle* becomes the levator *aponeurosis.* At this point, it gives origin to Müller's muscle. Thus, the striated levator muscle has two major insertions: an anterior aponeurosis and Müller's muscle. The latter is a fine-adjusting inner arm of smooth sympathetic muscle, a uniquely complex arrangement of striated and smooth muscle in series. Müller's muscle inserts into the upper tarsal edge, but where does the fibrous aponeurosis insert?

Previously, many authors viewed the levator aponeurosis as inserting into the eyelid skin, forming a fold at the level of insertion. But there is little evidence to support this concept [17]. The levator is the opening motor of the eyelid. As the antagonist to the orbicularis, the levator muscle elevates the tarsal plate visor. As with the orbicularis, the *major insertion of the levator is the conjoined pretarsal fascia.* Through this broad, laminated fascial layer the levator moves the tarsal plate, in concert with its posterior muscular insertion at the upper edge of the tarsus.

Above the area where the three fasciae laminate, the eyelid tissues are unattached to the tarsus, so they fold over when the eye opens. In Caucasians, the levator aponeurosis fuses to orbicularis fascia and septum at roughly the level of the upper border of the tarsal plate. The skin therefore forms a crease about 10 mm above the lashes. In Orientals, the fusion is usually lower, over the face of the tarsus (Fig. 15-8). Thus, the Oriental fold appears smaller, or is completely obscured by the preseptal tissues, because the fascial layers are "conjoined" for only a few millimeters above the lashes.

Superior to the fold, the sling formed by aponeurosis and orbital septum contains the orbital fat in the "preaponeurotic space." An eye with a low fold usually appears puffy and thick because the orbital fat wedge comes down over the face of the tarsus. Conversely, when there is an unusually high fusion of levator and orbital septum, the eye appears hollow.

Müller's Muscle

Müller's muscle lies just over the conjunctiva. This sympathetic muscle arises from the underside of the levator muscle and inserts at the upper tarsal edge. About 8 to 12 mm long, Müller's is dissimilar to most muscle bellies, having the appearance of sinuous strands of muscle interwoven with blood vessels and connective tissue. When it is denervated, as in Horner's syndrome, the eyelid droops 2 to 3 mm.

Tarsal Plate

The tarsal plate forms the skeletal foundation of the eyelid. Although it is as stiff as cartilage, it is actually composed of *dense fibrous tissue* containing rows of large Meibomian (sebaceous) glands. It is virtually fused to the conjunctiva, which lines it. Gliding over the globe like a visor, it provides a stiff and stable foundation for the opening and closing motors of the lid. It is shaped like the capital letter D, elongated and lying on its side. The convex upper border measures 9 to 10 mm at the center. Müller's muscle inserts at the upper edge of the tarsal plate. At this same level there is a *major vascular arcade* just anterior to the tarsus and conjunctiva. Because of this constant vascular arcade, bleeding and hematoma formation are major risks when one is placing fixation sutures in or near the upper edge of the tarsus.

Narrowing the tarsal skeleton by resection will predictably raise the level of the eyelid margin on the globe, accounting for the popularity of the Fasanella-Servat operation as a treatment for mild ptosis [30]. A narrowed tarsal skeleton is, however, weaker and more easily deformed. Tarsal resection may thus result in a distorted and peaked eyelid margin, which is very difficult to correct.

Conjunctiva

The conjunctiva is a thin, transparent, highly vascular mucous membrane that connects the globe to the eyelid. At the superior fornix, the bulbar conjunctiva joins with the palpebral conjunctiva. Since the superior rectus and levator muscles send a fascial slip into this fornix, it elevates in concert with movement of the globe and eyelid.

In sum, the deep fascial relationships play a major role in determining the shape and contour of the upper eyelid. It has been noted that *the upper lid folds where the levator aponeurosis fuses to orbicularis fascia and orbital septum.* Whenever possible during surgery, each of these key fascial structures should be identified under direct vision. Traction on the inelastic orbital septum will be felt at the orbital rim, or just inside the rim. If the layer is more mobile and tension is felt beyond the rim, the tension is probably being applied to the submuscular fascia. Traction during voluntary eyelid opening will positively identify the levator aponeurosis.

The safest surgical approach to the levator aponeurosis is via the conjoined pretarsal fascia. With resection of 1 to 2 mm of this fascia, just below the eyelid fold, neither orbital septum nor levator aponeurosis is shortened; wide access is gained into the orbital fat, and a strong free edge of levator aponeurosis is now available for suturing. The importance of freeing the levator aponeurosis from the conjoined pretarsal fascia will be discussed in a later section.

PATHOLOGY OF EYELID DEFORMITIES

Age brings weakening, stretching, and sometimes fatty degeneration to all eyelid tissue. After a lifetime of folding and unfolding, the preseptal skin loses its elasticity and becomes redundant. In addition, there is an apparent excess of orbital fat, producing a fullness behind the orbital septum. The goal of basic blepharoplasty techniques is to correct these twin deformities of redundant skin and bulging orbital fat.

Advanced blepharoplasty aims to correct the pathologic processes affecting the eyelid fascia, for it is often the fascia that defines the deformity. With age and atrophy, three interdependent pathologic processes alter the fascia: displacement, degeneration, and delamination.

Displacement

The relentless contraction of the orbicularis muscle, combined with gravity, causes a progressive downward movement of the peripheral orbicularis muscle and its underlying fascia. Moreover, there is a weakening of the deeper periosteal attachments, resulting in descent of the brow and the orbital skin. The displaced tissues tend to narrow or even obscure the eyelid fold and hide the tarsus from view. The thick orbital skin (as well as muscle and fascia) adds to the heaviness of the lateral hood (Fig. 15-9).

Laterally, there is a centripetal migration of muscle and fascia, causing a "bunching up" of these tissues, which further accentuates the lateral hood and produces "pleats" in the orbital skin, or crow's-feet.

Figure 15-9. Fascial displacement results in downward descent of the eyebrow and orbital tissues. The overhanging tissues hide the tarsus.

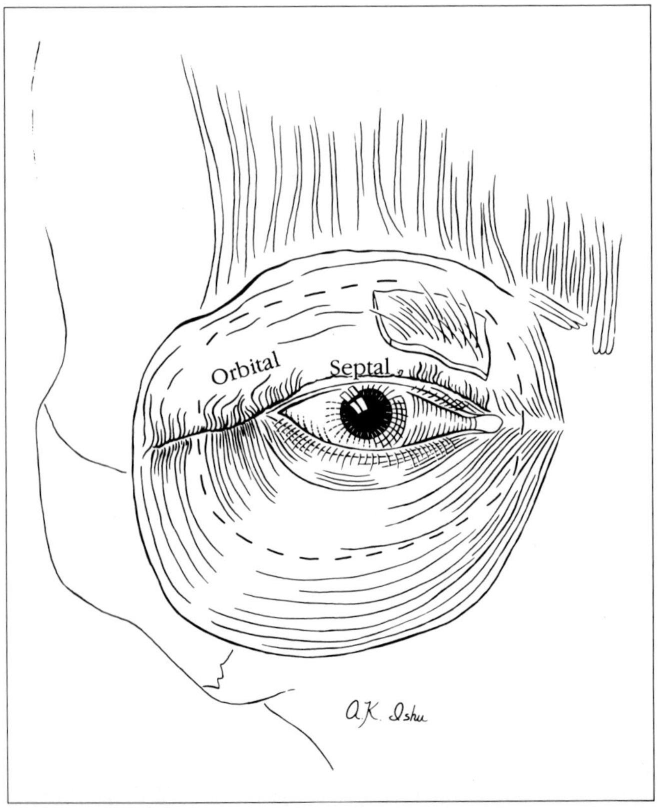

Degeneration

Orbicularis fascia that degenerates often becomes infiltrated with fat. This is a commonly observed major component of the lateral hood. The fat-infiltrated fascia may sometimes appear as a "fat pad," but always *external* to the orbital septum [34].

Pretarsally, the conjoined fascia may also be infiltrated with fat, causing a loss of adherence between the pretarsal orbicularis muscle and the underlying tarsus. When the skin and muscle are heavy, they peel away from the tarsus and join with the already redundant preseptal tissues. As a result, the eyelid fold may appear smaller and smaller. With lighter tissues, there may be *multiple pretarsal folds* (see Fig. 15-2).

Furthermore, the levator aponeurosis may undergo degeneration, with or without fat infiltration. The atrophic aponeurosis stretches, and the excess length results in ptosis.

Delamination

Some patients have one or more demonstrable skin creases above the area where the eyelid folds. In these patients the conjoined fascia has probably separated; there is now an opening of fascial layers that were once fused during youth. Delamination of the conjoined fascia results in a *low fold,* and the internal fascia framework becomes indistinguishable from that of the Oriental. If there is abundant orbital fat, the lid will appear puffy and full, for the fat wedge can now descend lower over the face of the tarsus.

CLASSIFICATION

On the basis of the anatomy and pathology just reviewed, eyelid deformities may be classified as shown in Table 15-2. I have elected to abandon Castanares's classification of "baggy eyelids" [8] because it relies on terms like *blepharochalasis* and *dermachalasis,* words that are confusing and outdated [10, 11].

Table 15-2. Classification of upper lid deformities

I. Orbital
- A. Brow ptosis
- B. Lateral hood
- C. Crow's-feet

II. Septal
- A. Redundant tissue
- B. Bulging fat

III. Tarsal
- A. Multiple folds
- B. Low folds

IV. Aponeurosis
- A. Eyelid ptosis

PATIENT INTERVIEW AND EVALUATION

There is no substitute for getting to know the patient before surgery. Regardless of your aesthetic inclinations, some patients may not want a radical change in eyelid appearance. Thus, preoperative planning must allow not only for peculiarities of anatomy and pathology but also for differences in style and personality.

Fundamental to all aesthetic surgery is insight into *psychologic stability,* often clarified by discussion of family, living, and working situations. Identify friends and relatives who have influenced the patient, pro and con. Caution signs include recent major life change, chronic depression, haste to have surgery, and overly demanding behavior with staff. If there has been prior cosmetic surgery, the patient's description of the experience and judgment of the results are invaluable.

Explore in depth the patient's *goals* for eyelid surgery, which often depend on the patient's ability and desire to use *makeup* and should be in harmony with the patient's *style.* Thus, the glamorous, flamboyant patient may have different needs from those of the elderly matron who simply wants to lighten her heavy eyelids.

Be wary of the patient whose main motivation for surgery is a recommendation from another, either a friend or relative or a physician. The patient must have his or her own personal desire and motivation for surgery. Evaluation by an ophthalmologist is strongly recommended. A general medical review must include a history of thyroid conditions, hypertension, and review of all medications, especially aspirin and antiarthritic drugs. Perhaps most important of all, especially in this era of prerecorded tapes, is the *patient's reaction* to your discussion of the scars, risks, and potential complications of surgery, including blindness. It is particularly helpful to stimulate verbalization of the patient's fears and thus to gain further insight into the strength of motivation for surgery.

Physical examination begins during the interview, with attention to the patient's style, personality, dress, makeup, and general demeanor. An inventory of anatomy would include the following:

1. Observe facial harmony and proportion. Demonstrate to the patient any major asymmetry or unrecognized pathology.
2. Gauge the orbital as well as overall effect of manually elevating the eyebrow. Demonstrate to the patient in the mirror, and discuss the changes produced. Review alternative surgical procedures for brow-lifting.
3. Palpate the orbital bone and its contribution to the eyelid contour, especially as the inferior orbital rim may produce a bulge that sometimes looks like fat.
4. Gauge the extent to which the lateral (preorbital) orbicularis underlying fat and fascia, as well as overlying skin, forms a "hood."
5. Evaluate and discuss the scar potential over the lateral orbital rim.
6. Preseptally, note excess "drapery" and obital fat in front view and in profile.

7. Pretarsally, observe the height of the fold and the relative adherence and fattiness of the pretarsal tissue.
8. Examine extraocular movements carefully, especially an inability to elevate the lid completely and any bizarre movements of the eye and eyelid.
9. Examine for ptosis, including (1) size of palpebral fissures at rest, (2) level of eyelid relative to pupil, and (3) levator excursion while blocking the action of the frontalis muscle.
10. Note orbicularis muscle function and appearance in both gentle and forceful eyelid closure.
11. Finally, review again the patient's goals and expectations in the light of your examination and analysis.

PRINCIPLES OF BLEPHAROPLASTY

There are five principles underlying all techniques of advanced upper eyelid blepharoplasty:

1. Raise the sagging foundation.
2. Resect redundant tissue.
3. Smooth pretarsal and preorbital wrinkles.
4. Elevate the ptotic lid margin.
5. Secure the surgical fold.

Raise the Sagging Foundation

In the upper eyelid, the fascial attachments in the area of the brow form the supporting foundation for the eyelid tissues below. Ptosis of the eyebrow is only the most visible sign of the fascial displacement that is occurring more internally. When the brows descend, the thick orbital skin and the underlying muscle are displaced to the septal region below, adding to the heavy hooded appearance of the eyelid. The coronal approach to the brow and forehead is the most satisfactory to correct and elevate the sagging foundation. It is discussed in detail in Chapter 13. The older supraciliary approach [7] is still occasionally useful but nearly always leaves a noticeable scar.

In general, the brow should rest above the lid margin by a distance equal to at least 2 times the visible eyelid fold. In the young, in males, and in patients for whom glamour is not the primary goal, elevating the brow may not be necessary for a satisfactory result. But for the majority of elderly patients seeking glamorous eyelids, raising the brows is an essential component of blepharoplasty. The patient who needs a brow-lift, but because of expense or other reason elects to have only a blepharoplasty, must be willing to accept a less than optimum result because in this case part of what appears to be redundant septal tissue is actually displaced orbital tissue. Attempting to resect all of this redundancy will tend to further lower the brow. Even worse, if the patient later elects to have a brow-lift, the scar from the prior blepharoplasty may rise above the upper lid sulcus and become visible. So it is difficult to overemphasize the importance of raising the foundation and elevating the ptotic brow.

Resect Redundant Tissue

A crucial aspect of all aesthetic blepharoplasty is the accurate tailoring of redundant preseptal *skin,* and the removal of excess orbital *fat* from behind the septum [6]. Until recently, little attention was paid to *redundant muscle.* In 1955 Millard [18] reported his experience with Oriental blepharoplasty, noting that trimming of subcutaneous tissue and orbicularis muscle fibers allowed the thick eyelid curtain to fold where the tissues were thinned.

PRESEPTAL RESECTION

In 1977 Baker et al. [3] reported their experience removing a 2- to 5-mm strip of preseptal orbicularis muscle as part of upper blepharoplasty in Caucasians. They were able to "deepen the sulcus and adequately expose the pretarsal skin." Other surgeons have since confirmed the value of resecting a strip of orbicularis muscle across the entire width of the lid [9, 10, 22, 31, 34]. Since orbicularis and its fascia form the "lining" of the redundant preseptal skin, tailoring of these deeper tissues should logically match the skin excision. This simple resection has proved extremely effective in contouring this area of the upper lid and has become a fairly routine addition to nearly all aesthetic blepharoplasty.

PREORBITAL RESECTION

In the region of the lateral orbit a thickened hood is often present. Returning the brow to an attractive level usually helps this situation somewhat but seldom corrects most of the hooding. Some direct contouring is usually necessary in addition to raising the brow.

In most cases of thick lateral hooding, bulky soft tissue is responsible for the fullness. This usually results from *overlapping folds of orbicularis muscle, thickly padded with multiple layers of fat-infiltrated submuscular fascia.* Owsley [22] recently described resecting a fat pad from under the lateral orbicularis muscle in selected cases. However, a discrete "pad of fat" is only rarely present, as the offending tissue is usually fat-infiltrated fascia. For access to the heavy lateral hood, the blepharoplasty excision is continued over the orbital rim to the brow, within a natural skin crease (Fig. 15-10). A wedge of orbicularis is excised, usually matching or slightly larger than the skin excision. In patients with chronically exaggerated orbicularis use, larger and more aggressive resections may be necessary. Once the muscle is removed, the underlying fat and fascia is resected, leaving at least one "slippery" layer over the periosteum. The cut fascial edges are approximated, thus reestablishing the muscle ring and preventing a depressed scar over the orbital rim. Caution is advised in patients with thick, large-pored sebaceous skin, as the scar over the orbit may remain permanently visible (see Fig. 15-6).

The direct contouring of the lateral hood does little to change the peripheral wrinkling often referred to as crow's-feet. Nor would we expect it to, since the most peripheral orbicularis extends far beyond the orbital rim. In an occasional case in which there are severe crow's-feet and the patient is willing to accept the scar, as well as the

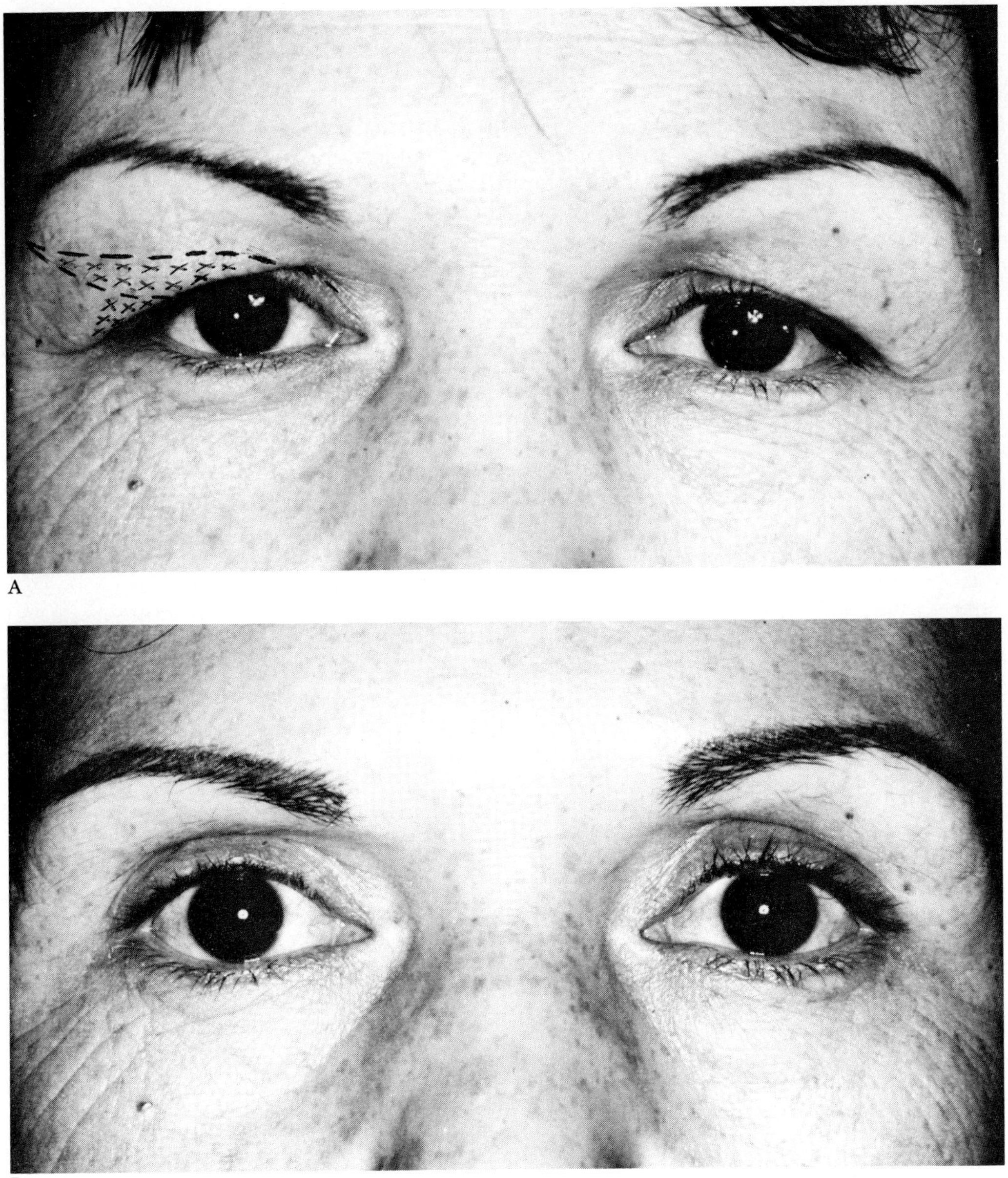

A

B

Figure 15-10. Heavy lateral hood in a 46-year-old woman.
A. Blepharoplasty excision extended to the brow, as indicated in preoperative photograph by dashed line on patient's right side. The resection of the underlying orbicularis muscle and fat-infiltrated fascia is represented by the area shaded in Xs.
B. Two years postoperative.

possibility of frontalis palsy, excision can be extended beyond the brow to the temple hairline. In case 1 (see Fig. 15-14) it was performed unilaterally (on the patient's left side) to evaluate whether this simple excision of skin, redundant muscle, and fascia could improve the wrinkling (in repose) and tighten the orbicular muscle ring.

Smooth Pretarsal and Preorbital Wrinkles

Resecting preseptal orbicularis and the underlying fascia (in addition to skin) removes the "drapery" overhanging the fold and thereby helps to expose the pretarsal area of the eyelid when the eyes are open. But sometimes the tissues over the anterior surface of the tarsus are also loose and wrinkled, with multiple irregular folds. Occasionally this area appears fatty, with thick layers of subcutaneous or submuscular fat.

There are two ways to smooth the pretarsal wrinkles. The most effective and long lasting involves resecting the pretarsal conjoined fascia, and occasionally the orbicularis muscle. This will allow the skin over the tarsus to adhere more closely to the underlying tarsus and will restore a smooth appearance to the pretarsal visor. Of course, the vascular plexus just beneath the skin must be resected, and at least a small bundle of orbicularis should be left above the eyelash follicles to allow reflex eyelid closure. The second method for smoothing pretarsal wrinkles is to place the conjoined fascia under tension as the final step of the blepharoplasty. This provides some improvement but usually lacks the longevity produced by resecting the offending tissue.

The preorbital crow's-feet wrinkles may be substantially reduced by mobilizing and splaying out the displaced orbicularis muscle and its fascia. Reviving a technique originally described by Skoog [29], Aston [1] approaches the lateral orbital orbicularis muscle subcutaneously from the temple, as in a face-lift. The lateral muscle ring is separated from skin and temporalis fascia and then sutured with catgut in a splayed-out position. For a more dramatic effect, the muscle ring is divided before the splaying and suturing. Although this maneuver clearly places the temporal nerve branch supplying the frontalis muscle at risk, Aston's results are impressive, and the technique appears promising.

Elevate the Ptotic Lid Margin

Assuming that there is good levator function, ptosis can be readily corrected during a blepharoplasty. After the levator aponeurosis is separated from the septum and conjoined fascia, shortening it 1 mm will usually elevate the lid a similar amount relative to the globe. Furthermore, resecting pretarsal orbicularis muscle (as well as conjoined fascia) will reduce some of the orbicularis antagonism to the levator [9], producing approximately 0.5 mm of lid elevation postoperatively. After the aponeurosis has been sutured to the pretarsal tissues, voluntary eyelid opening allows a fairly precise evaluation of eyelid level relative to the globe.

Secure the Surgical Fold

All techniques of advanced blepharoplasty in Caucasians that utilize a suture to create or reestablish a fold owe their origin to surgery on Orientals. Therefore, even if one rarely operates on Orientals, it is important to understand the basic techniques of Oriental blepharoplasty, often known as transforming a "single" into a "double" eye.

Many Orientals are born with a "single eye," a slang expression meaning an eyelid without an obvious fold. At one time this was considered beautiful, but since the introduction of Western culture to the Orient the standard of beauty has become the "double eye," an upper lid that forms a fold when the eyes are open. Many operations have been devised to transform the foldless eyelid, and the "new" techniques for Caucasian blepharoplasty are actually modifications of older operations originally designed for Orientals.

The simplest approach to the transformation of the single to the double eye requires neither incision nor excision. Instead, sutures are placed through the entire thickness of the eyelid, from conjunctiva to skin; there are many varieties of suture types and knot placements [21]. This rapid "beauty salon" technique is widely practiced in the Orient and when the tissues are suitably thin will produce an acceptable fold. However, when the stitches are removed or resorbed, the scar tracks soon disappear, along with the fold. This technique has been used by some ophthalmologists in the West [23] but is rarely used by plastic surgeons.

"Open" surgical techniques produce more distinct permanent folds and provide access for contouring and tailoring of fatty and redundant tissue. In 1954 Sayoc [25] was among the earliest to describe an open technique in Western literature. He excised a full-thickness wedge of tissue down to the anterior surface of the tarsus and then sutured the dermis of the lower margin to the tarsal surface [26]. Uchida [32] used a similar pretarsal excision but placed chromic mattress sutures through conjunctiva, tarsus, and skin. Millard [19] aimed at primarily contouring the Oriental lid, resecting both pretarsal and preseptal orbicularis muscle, as well as removing the "excess fatty padding." His skin suture included bites of the tarsal plate and were removed within a week.

In 1960 Fernandez [13] described two operations for Oriental eyelids, which he termed "simple" and "radical." In the "simple" approach, an ellipse of skin was excised 5 to 7 mm above the lashes. Then an *incision* was made through orbicularis muscle and orbital septum until the levator aponeurosis was reached. The aponeurosis was sutured to dermis with buried white nylon sutures. No fat or muscle was resected. In the "radical" operation, skin resection was followed by resection of orbicularis muscle, fascia, orbital septum, and fat. The inferior edge of the levator aponeurosis was *"dissected free across the lid"* before being sutured to the lower dermis with buried nylon sutures (Fig. 15-11). Fernandez described two operations because he observed that no one appearance, and therefore no single technique, could be applied to all patients. He used one technique for a soft superficial fold and the other for patients wanting a deeper, more Caucasian type of lid fold.

Regardless of the technique used to form a fold, the *height of the fold* must be carefully considered for each patient desiring blepharoplasty. Although a patient may express a desire for a Caucasian type of eyelid fold, a short Oriental patient with a round face would look quite unnatural if a fold measuring 13 to 14 mm were created in the upper lids. Suffice it to say: *Orientals rarely desire a Caucasian eyelid. They seek a more youthful and more beautiful appearance, but not the elimination of their ethnic background.* For this reason, measurement and creation of folds in all eyelids, but especially in those of Orientals, must be done with great conservatism. For the same reason, epicanthal modifications are seldom performed, as the epicanthus is a uniquely Oriental structure and is a part of Oriental beauty.

Sheen [27] has modified an Oriental "double eye" technique to improve results in Caucasian blepharoplasty. He noted that when the natural fold was low, in a Caucasian, persistent hooding or redundancy eventually recurred, even after an "adequate" skin excision blepharoplasty. His revised technique of "supratarsal fixation" [28] is similar to the "simple" technique of Fernandez, but Sheen sutured aponeurosis to orbicularis muscle instead of to dermis. It is important to note that Sheen did not dissect the levator aponeurosis prior to suturing. Thus, in the attempt to form an extremely high fold, the lower (pretarsal) margin was

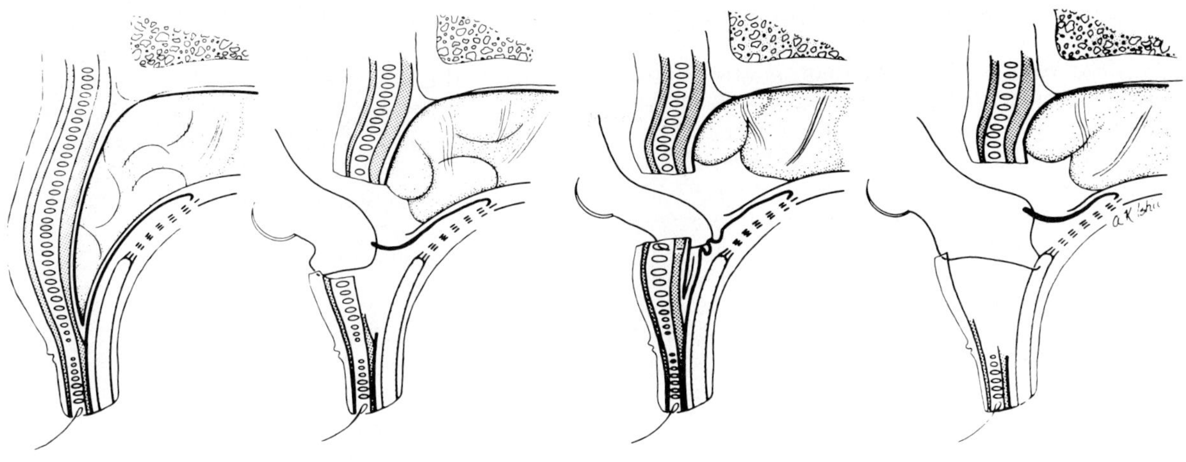

Figure 15-11. Sagittal view of techniques for suturing levator aponeurosis to pretarsal tissues (see text for details).

sutured high on the aponeurosis, and levator dysfunction occasionally resulted [12].

Like Sheen, Flowers [14] has been a vigorous proponent of the application of Oriental techniques to Caucasians. Flowers's "anchor blepharoplasty" is an extension of Fernandez's "radical" technique, combining substantial tissue resection with the levator aponeurosis being dissected free prior to suturing. In a manner similar to Boo-Chai's [5], Flowers further contours the lid by clearing the pretarsal space of fat and fascia. To maximize the depth and definition of the fold, he uses buried sutures to attach the free edge of the levator aponeurosis to *both* the upper edge of the tarsus and the pretarsal dermis.

Which procedure should be used to raise the low fold or secure a "double eye"? Nearly all patients requesting blepharoplasty have an "apparent" low fold, as one of the earliest signs of age is redundant preseptal tissue that hangs down and obscures the pretarsal area. If the tissues are thin and there is a single, sharp skin crease at the level of the upper tarsal border when the patient looks down, there is probably no pathology of the lid fold itself. In other words, the relationship of the underlying fasciae is probably normal. In these cases, a conservative "basic" blepharoplasty with the lower incision placed in the natural skin crease will usually restore a youthful, attractive, and natural appearance to the eyelid.

In patients with thick, heavy tissues, however, the drooping of the preseptal tissues will tend to recur in a few years after blepharoplasty. These patients need additional internal support to add longevity to their youthful appearance. One way to add some support is to resect wide strips of preseptal orbicularis muscle, as strongly advocated by Baker [2, 3]. This tends to lighten and thin the eyelid, allowing it to adhere to the underlying orbicularis fascia. The resulting lid fold can be extremely high, especially if substantial orbital fat is removed, but may be superficial, and barely invaginated, and lacking in definition. Multiple pretarsal wrinkles may rapidly return.

The issue now becomes one of aesthetic preference. I prefer a more defined and invaginated fold, but *not necessarily a very high fold,* as the latter will often look unnatural or overdone, especially when little makeup is worn. To obtain more longevity, precision, and definition, I feel there is no substitute for the permanent attachment of the levator aponeurosis to the pretarsal tissue. Nevertheless, this is currently a debatable area for Caucasian patients with a fairly normal fold, and each surgeon must come to his or her own conclusions. When there is a truly "low fold," the levator aponeurosis meets septum and orbicularis fascia down over the face of the tarsus. In my opinion, no amount of muscle resection will alter the pathology of the fascial substructure. Changing the relationship between the levator aponeurosis and the pretarsal tissue is mandatory in these cases. But which technique? Suturing the undissected aponeurosis in the manner of Sheen is helpful only to *define* or slightly raise a fold. As we have noted, using this technique to substantially raise the fold places the sutures high on the levator aponeurosis. It is like doing a "tuck" of the aponeurosis and tends to shorten it, thereby raising the lid margin relative to the globe.

To safely secure more major change in the eyelids, and whenever the pretarsal tissues are loose or fatty, the levator aponeurosis must be dissected free from both the orbital septum and conjoined fascia. To dissect the aponeurosis safely, the surgeon must *preserve its physiologic length,* usually at the junction with the orbital septum and orbicularis fascia. This step is most easily accomplished by resecting a small strip of conjoined fascia just below the area where aponeurosis and orbicularis fascia fuse. The result is a free edge of aponeurosis, which is then available to secure a new fold.

The next decision in fold making is how to attach this flap of aponeurosis securely to the pretarsal visor. Fernandez's [13] attachment to dermis with 6-0 clear nylon (or polyglycolic) is simple and reliable. Alternatively, Flowers's technique of suturing to both dermis and tarsus produces a slightly deeper and crisper fold. But tarsal sutures have two risks: Cyst formation if a Meibomian gland is violated, and bleeding and hematoma formation if the supratarsal arcade is injured. There is nothing disastrous about the resulting hematoma (which may involve Müller's muscle as well as the tissues anterior to the tarsus) but it prevents the surgeon from judging the precise height of the lid on the globe.

Whichever approach is used to attach the levator aponeurosis to pretarsal tissues, the effect on eyelid function and appearance must be tested before the operation is completed. With the patient's eyes open, the folds must appear smooth and symmetric, with no lash eversion. The eyelid must be at the correct level on the globe, 1 to 2 mm below the limbus of the cornea. Before the skin is closed, it is simple to remove and replace the fixation sutures to accomplish these objectives.

LOWER EYELID BLEPHAROPLASTY

In comparison to the upper lid, the anatomy of the lower eyelid is much less complex. The lower lid is a nearly static structure, does not form a fold when the eye is open, and is not burdened by the weighty tissue displacement associated with a drooping forehead and eyebrow. It usually follows, therefore, that correcting lower eyelid deformities is a much simpler task than correcting deformities of the upper eyelid.

Although the lower eyelid lacks some of the complexity of the upper lid, the relationship of the various layers is quite similar. Deep to the skin lies the orbicularis muscle, fascia lines the muscle, and the orbital septum is found just deep to the fascia. The septum is continuous with the lower orbital rim periosteum and fuses with the orbicularis fascia at or near the lower border of the tarsal plate. The tarsus in the lower lid is narrower than that in the upper, about 4 to 5 mm at the center.

The lower eyelid tissues are deformed by the same pathologic factors that affect the upper lid. The skin, muscle, and fascia become redundant, while fatty fullness and fascial weakening combine to produce the palpebral "bag." Fascial displacement and degeneration (with fat infiltration) may occur, but it is not clear what role they play in the most common lower eyelid deformities. Thus, the major surgical principle that applies to the lower eyelid is *resect the redundant tissue:* skin, muscle with fascia, and orbital fat. In some very elderly patients, however, the tissues are so lax that gentle approximation of the redundant tissue (see below) will draw the eyelid margin down and away from the globe. For these patients, a wedge resection of tarsus and pretarsal tissues is needed [24]. This secures a firm foundation for the lower lid blepharoplasty and reduces the risk of postoperative ectropion.

I employ an extremely simple surgical technique to resect redundant lower eyelid tissues. The skin and muscle excess is precisely measured and marked *preoperatively,* the unsedated, unanesthetized patient *sitting erect* on the operating table. A very fine-tipped felt marker with "permanent" ink is used to mark the subciliary incision 2.0 to 2.5 mm below the lashes. In the very elderly the incision is placed slightly lower, to keep the downward vector farther away from the lid margin. The incision extends only slightly beyond the canthi and turns downward at each end (Fig. 15-12). Then the excess tissue is gently elevated and approximated between delicate toothless forceps until the eyelashes *just begin* to turn downward. The excess is measured and marked at four or five points across the lower lid. Until one is confident that the surgical prep will not remove the markings, it is advisable to record the measurements, in case they are later washed away.

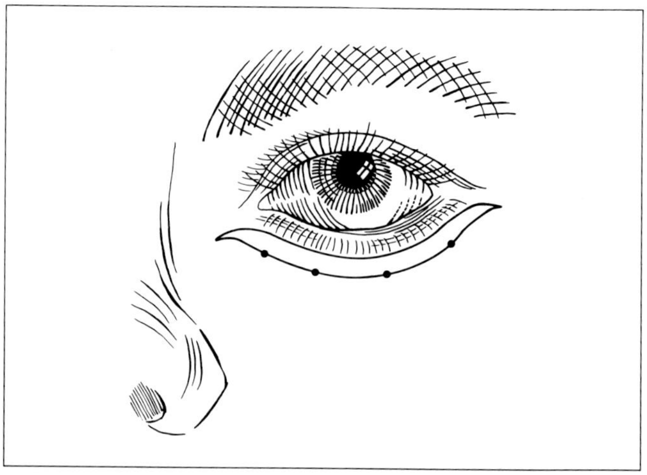

Figure 15-12. Measuring and marking the lower eyelid incision.

It is important to emphasize that measurement of tissue excess is *not* approximate. The tissue excision as marked preoperatively is the tissue excised during surgery. Only in the erect, unsedated patient can the ultimate effect of the proposed tissue excision be precisely gauged, for only at this point are all the vector forces clearly evident. In most techniques of lower blepharoplasty [16, 20, 24, 31] the tissue excess is approximated as one of the last steps of the operative procedure, when virtually none of the ultimate vector forces are evident. At the end of surgery the tissues are edematous, the patient is supine, dissected flaps may later retract, and opening the patient's mouth and asking him or her to look up may bear little resemblance to the effects of gravity. Suffice it to say that the essence of lower lid blepharoplasty is precision tailoring, requiring the most accurate measurements made under the most natural conditions.

After analgesia is established intravenously, local anesthetic is deposited in the fascial layer, and occasionally subcutaneously to facilitate the use of scalpel for the incisions. The point of a 15c blade is used to deeply score and preferably completely incise the skin. After subcutaneous hemostasis is achieved, resection of the orbicularis muscle and fascia (as planned preoperatively) is accomplished by grasping with forceps and trimming with Kaye serrated scissors. Careful hemostasis is always necessary for the relatively large blood vessels found in the orbicularis fascia, especially in the lateral one-third of the eyelid. With an assistant retracting the lower margin, one approaches the fat pockets by a single incision across the orbital septum. The fat is teased out and carefully cauterized. The skin is now redraped directly *upward* or slightly nasally and will invariably fit precisely. If the lower margin is slightly thicker than the upper, an additional sliver of muscle or fascia is removed and hemostasis again secured. A very slight horizontal excess of lower margin skin, compared to the subciliary, is eliminated by distributing this excess across the incision. Only the skin is sutured, with four to eight interrupted 6-0 Surgilon sutures. *There is no undermining.* The redundant tissues have been simply and rapidly excised.

This technique of lower blepharoplasty has been used for the past 5 years, in approximately 200 patients, without a single incidence of lower lid ectropion. Early in the series, however, aggressive resection did result in lowered lid margins and scleral show, especially in patients with firm heavy tissues. As experience was gained, lid retraction was avoided, but it soon became evident that a slight postoperative lid retraction was sometimes quite attractive, and therefore desirable in selected patients. Thus, when patients complain of small eyes and their lower lid rests at least 1 mm above the limbus of the cornea, I now intentionally seek a slight postoperative lid retraction to help widen the palpebral fissure (see Fig. 15-4).

SURGICAL TECHNIQUE

Analgesia

No oral or intramuscular premedication is used. All medication is given intravenously, in small doses. Blood pressure is automatically monitored every 15 minutes and continuously recorded. In lower lid blepharoplasty, the unsedated patient is placed sitting upright, and the precise amount of redundant tissue is defined by gentle approximation between toothless forceps. Phenergan (5–10 mg) followed by 1- to 2-mg increments of morphine and Valium produces a tranquil patient. For hypertensive or talkative patients, Thorazine (5–10 mg) is often added.

Markings

A fine pen (Storz N5840) and accurate caliper are mandatory. Since precision and symmetry are critical, imperfect marks are frequently removed. Gentian violet (1%) is a good ink that erases completely with alcohol. Measurements must be precise—to the half millimeter.

The *lower incision line is critical!* This line determines the shape and height of the upper eyelid fold when it is later attached to the levator or tarsus; great care is required for its measurement and marking. The upper line determines the amount of intervening skin and underlying tissue to be excised. To measure the lower incision, elevate the eyebrow until the eyelid skin is just taut, with the lashes just beginning to turn upward (Fig. 15-13A). Medially, the line tapers sharply and stays relatively low (Fig. 15-13B). Laterally, it sweeps upward, often extending to the eyebrow itself. Preseptal redundancy is then gathered gently between toothless forceps to determine the placement of the upper excision line (Fig. 15-13C). It is helpful to use dots first, medially and laterally, checking the symmetry of contour before completing the markings. *Be conservative when choosing a fold height.* Except for women who wear heavy makeup (and others such as models and actors) the fold height should rarely exceed 8 to 9 mm in Orientals and 10 to 12 mm in Caucasians. In Orientals, the medial incisions must taper very sharply and should be made continuous with the epicanthal fold. As mentioned above, until much experience is gained with Oriental blepharoplasty, do not attempt to modify the epicanthus.

Anesthesia

Local anesthesia is used exclusively. A few milliliters of 1% lidocaine with 1 : 100,000 epinephrine is deposited with a 1-in. 30-gauge needle in the plane of the suborbicularis fascia. This small amount of local anesthetic will often suffice for the entire surgery, although small additional doses may be required for fat removal, especially in the medial fat pocket.

Instruments

The point of a 15c blade allows great precision for medial incisions (Fig. 15-13D). Castroviejo forceps (Storz E1805-WH) and Kaye serrated scissors (Storz N5066) maintain control in resection of small superficial strips of slippery eyelid tissue. Bipolar cautery is strongly recommended, as it offers the safest and most precise hemostasis.

Contouring

As noted earlier, the redundant preseptal skin is lined by a matching excess of muscle, often with fat-infiltrated fascia just deep to the muscle. Without undermining, these tissues are grasped with forceps and resected (Fig. 15-13E). Now the conjoined fascia is approached by resecting a very narrow strip of tissue just at the edge of the lower incision (Fig. 15-13F). This exposes the face of the tarsus but may leave the aponeurotic-septal sling still intact, just retracted slightly upward (Fig. 15-13G). Another snip across this junction and the entire preaponeurotic fat compartment is exposed (Fig. 15-13H). The pale yellow fat of the medial compartment is usually separate and should be conservatively teased out and resected to avoid a hollow appearance. Every vessel should be cauterized, within and around the fat, whether bleeding or not. Once the fat is resected, the levator aponeurosis becomes highly visible, especially over the lateral two-thirds of the lid (Fig. 15-13I). Anterior to the tarsus, fatty, loose or edematous tissue should be resected, but, as previously noted, the subcutaneous vascular plexus must be carefully preserved, along with some orbicularis fibers just above the lashes.

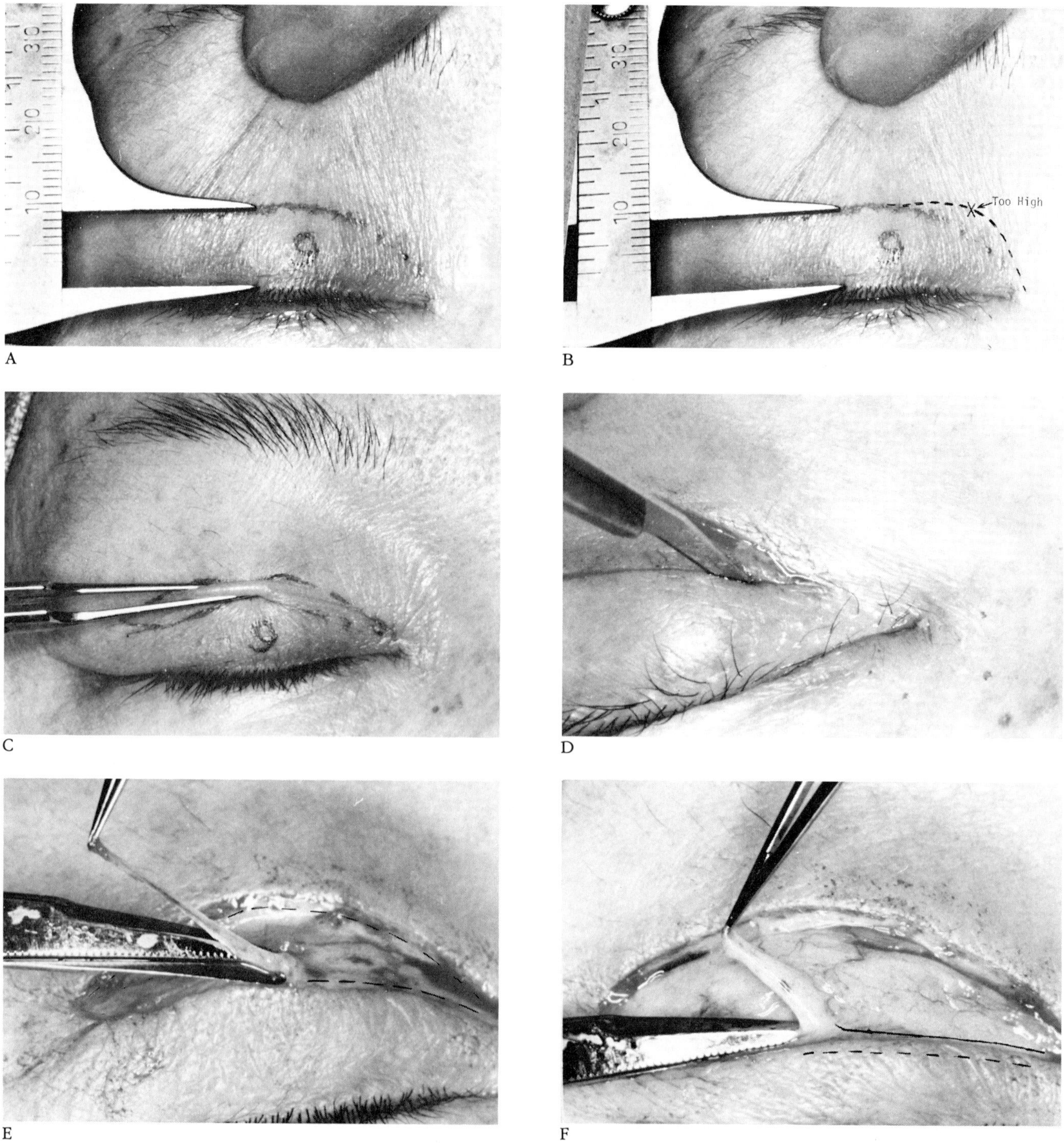

Figure 15-13. Technique of upper eyelid blepharoplasty.

A. The lower incision is measured while the brow is elevated and the lid tissues are just taut; the eyelash is barely turning upward.
B. The incision is kept low medially and tapers sharply.
C. Redundancy is gathered with toothless forceps and marked.
D. The point of a 15c blade is used to incise the skin.
E. Resection of orbicularis muscle and fascia usually matches the skin excision.
F. Conjoined fascia is resected below the edge of lower incision.

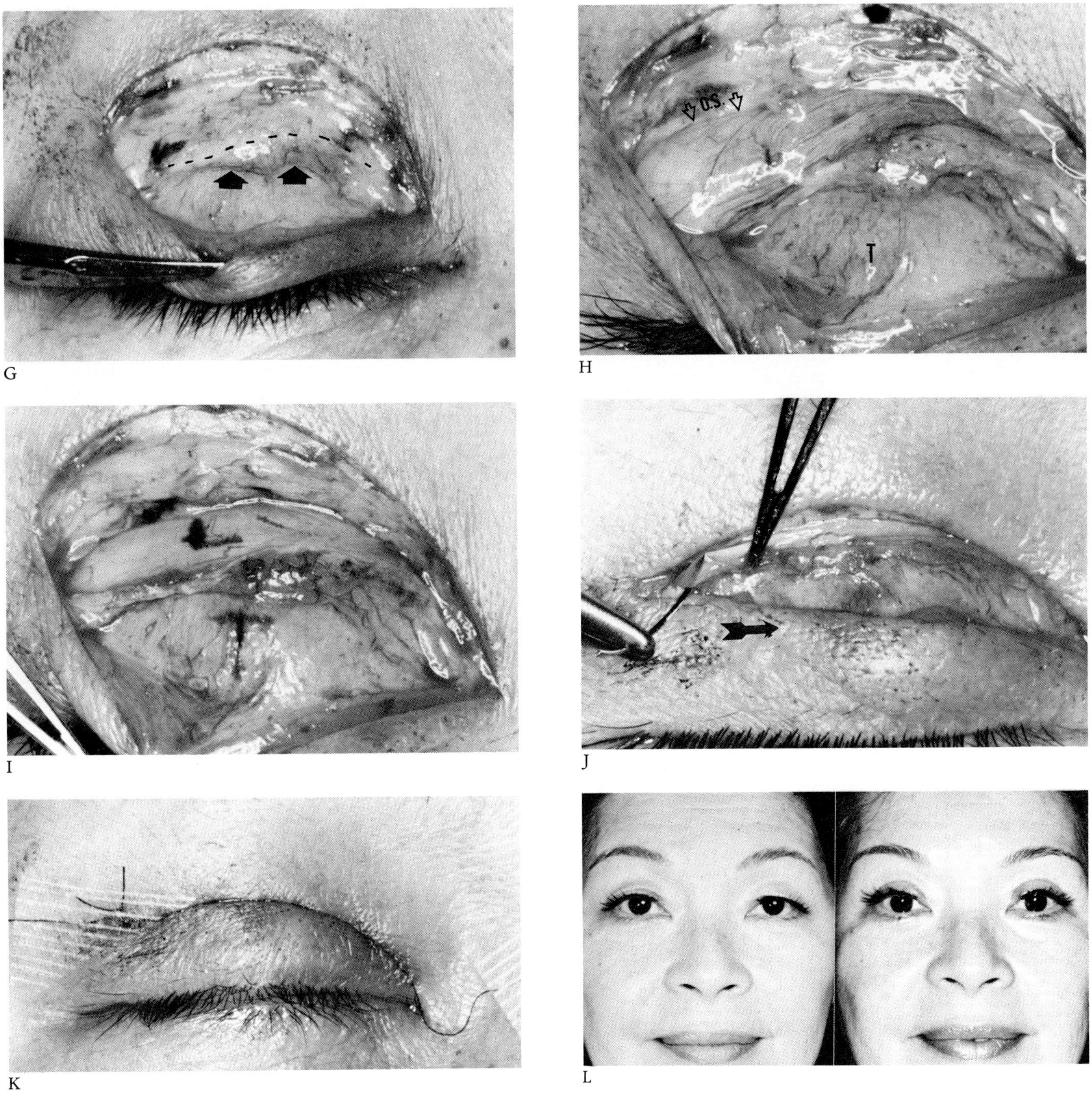

Figure 15-13 (continued)

G. Levator aponeurosis–orbital septum junction is still intact, just retracted slightly superiorly. It is identified by the dashed line. Arrows indicate the supratarsal vascular arcade.

H. After snipping across the aponeurosis-septum junction, the orbital fat spills out.

I. The dense aponeurosis is highly visible. Note how little it retracts above the tarsus, even though separated from fascia and septum.

J. The pretarsal tissues must be advanced medially *(arrow)* prior to suturing to levator aponeurosis.

K. Skin suture is with a running subcuticular 6-0 braided nylon.

L. A 48-year-old part-Oriental woman before *(left)* and 4 months after the upper blepharoplasty shown in the previous photographs.

Suturing

When the conjoined fascia is resected, and especially after aggressive pretarsal contouring, the remaining pretarsal tissues tend to sag laterally. This lower skin must be readvanced medially before the aponeurosis is sutured to the lower dermal edge (Fig. 15-13J). I prefer 6-0 clear nylon for securing levator aponeurosis to dermis or to the tarsus. When suturing to the tarsus, the use of two-power loupes helps to avoid nicking a blood vessel, and relatively small superficial "bites" avoid the possibility of penetrating the tarsus and irritating the underlying cornea. The skin closure can be performed according to preference, but the tissues should fit precisely, without tension. I like to close the palpebral skin with a subcuticular braided 6-0 nylon (Fig. 15-13K), adding a few interrupted sutures over the orbital rim closure. The braided nylon seems preferable to the monofilament variety because it is soft and gentle.

Dressings

Eye pads dipped in extremely cold water are used as intraoperative compresses. After surgery, two layers of ice-cold wet eye pads are applied to each eye, followed by a dry pad and a single piece of tape placed from forehead to cheek. A small ice bag keeps the wet pads very cold. Patients are advised to use these cold wet compresses for up to 3 days postoperatively, as they are very effective in reducing swelling and ecchymosis in the postoperative period.

CLINICAL EXAMPLES

Case 1. A 66-year-old retired actress desired more youthful and dramatic eyes. Her skin was thick and deeply wrinkled, with marked crow's-feet lines (Fig. 15-14). Multiple pretarsal skin creases were present, from 6 to 10 mm above the lashes, with a heavy hood of excess tissue hanging over the tarsus and lateral orbital rim. Mild brow ptosis was evident. Because the patient desired a dramatic change, a high fold was chosen, 12 mm above the lashes. With the eyelid tissues elevated until just taut, and the lashes beginning to turn upward, the lower incision was marked at 12 mm bilaterally. Gentle approximation of the excess presep-

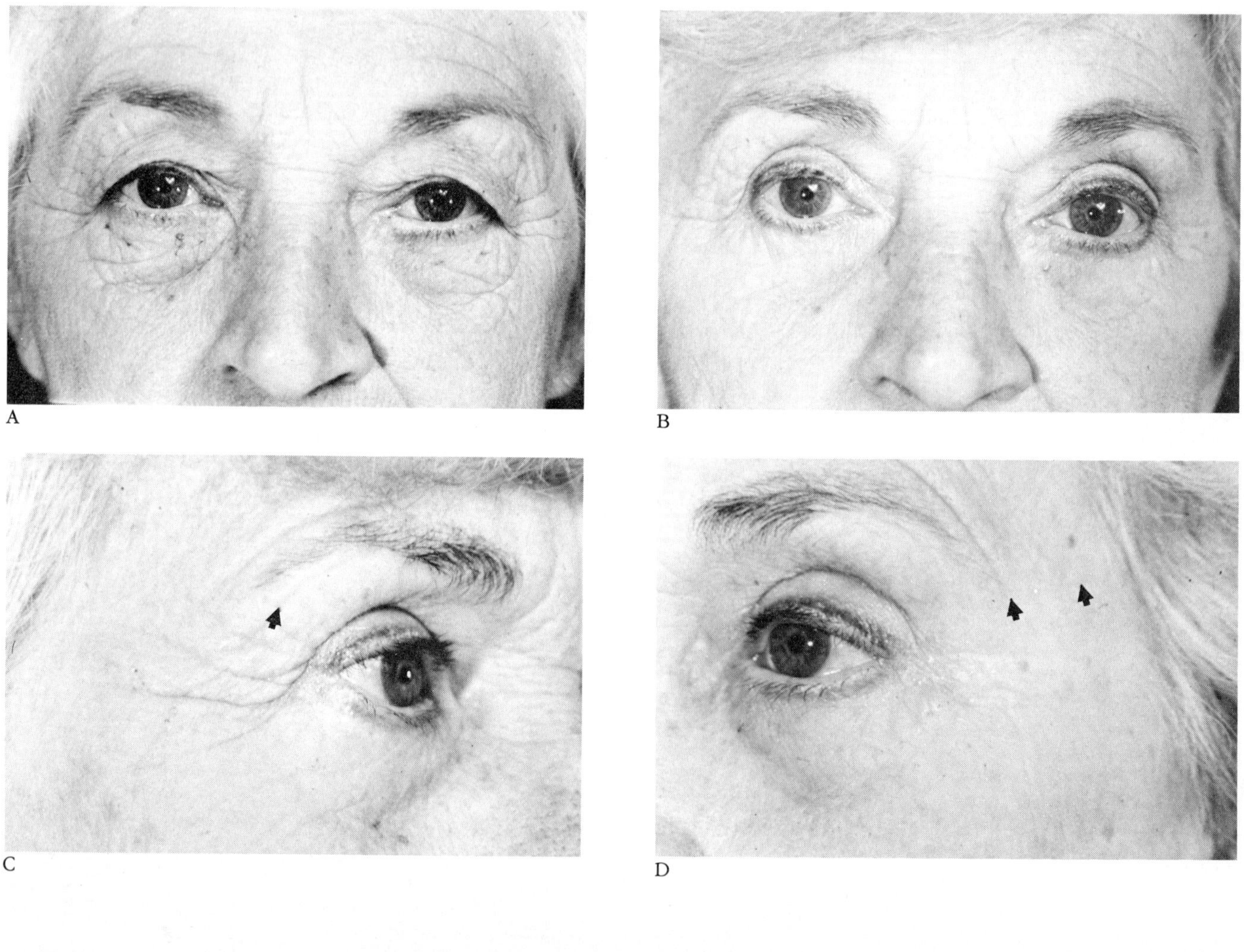

Figure 15-14. Case 1.
A. A 66-year-old actress before surgery.
B. One year after upper and lower blepharoplasty. There is a marked difference in the degree of preorbital wrinkling postoperatively, evidenced in comparing the right side (C) to the left (D).

tal tissues determined the upper excision line. Because of the heavy lateral hood, the excision was continued upward and laterally to the eyebrow on the right. On the patient's left side, the excision was continued past the brow to the temple hairline. This was done on only one side to evaluate the effect on the crow's-feet of resecting a wedge of the most peripheral ring of the orbicularis muscle and fascia, as well as carrying the skin resection farther laterally. The outlined skin, muscle, and orbicularis fascia was excised bilaterally, followed by removal of the orbital fat. To achieve a smooth pretarsal appearance, the pretarsal fascia was excised bilaterally, producing a free edge of levator aponeurosis to secure the new eyelid fold. To evaluate whether the fixation altered the appearance of the fold, on the right side the levator aponeurosis was sutured to the pretarsal *dermis* with three 6-0 clear nylon sutures (Fernandez technique). On the patient's left, three clear nylon sutures were placed through the edge of the aponeurosis, the upper edge of the *tarsus, and then* through the *dermis* and tied (Flowers technique). The lower lid blepharoplasty was performed as described above.

Figure 15-15. Case 2.
A. A 62-year-old schoolteacher with "baggy eyes" before surgery.
B. Nine months after upper and lower blepharoplasty.

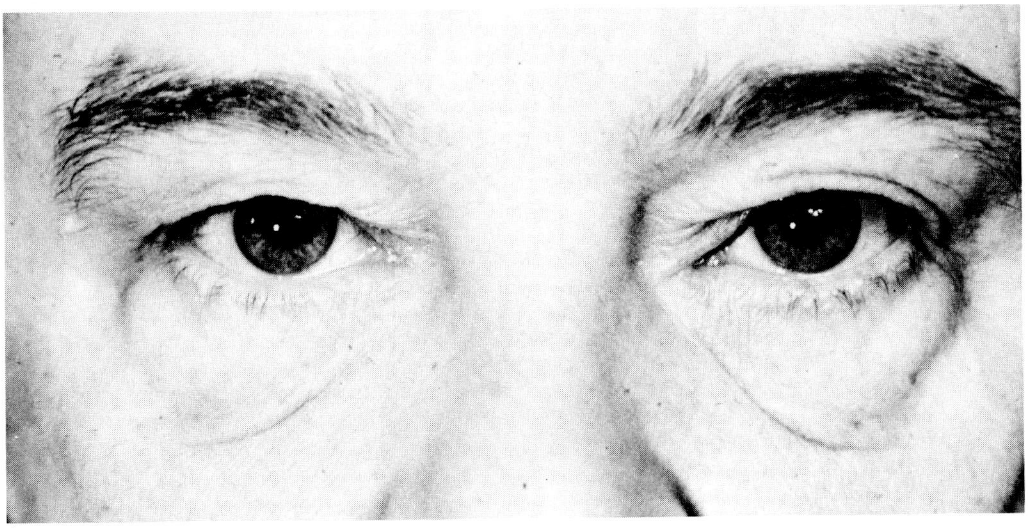

A

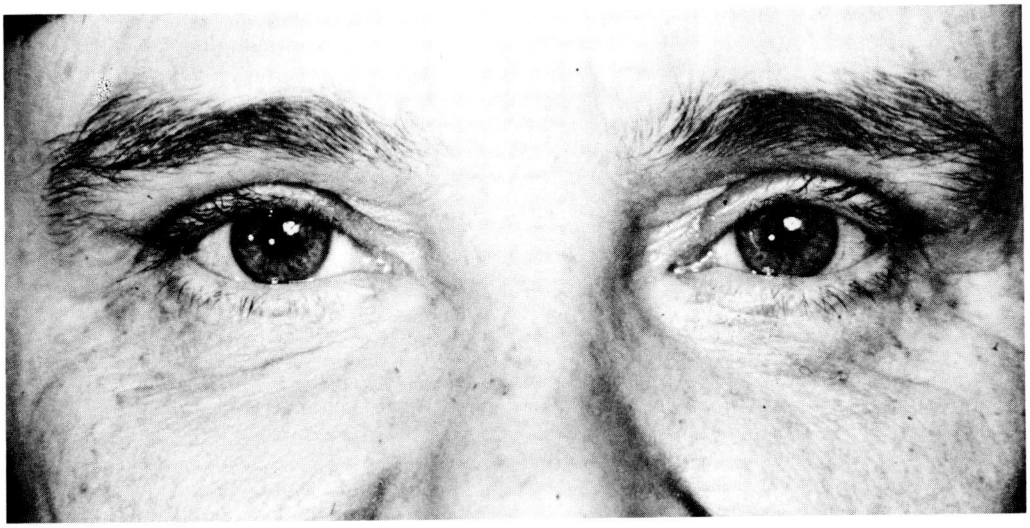

B

At 1 year postoperative, the folds appear identical in spite of the different types of fixation used, but there is a marked difference in the appearance of preorbital wrinkling, as the more peripheral resection of skin and underlying tissue substantially lifted the heavy tissues on the patient's left (Fig. 15-14D) in comparison to the right side (Fig. 15-14C). In the lower eyelids, there is a slight retraction evident in the lateral third of each eyelid.

Case 2. A 62-year-old schoolteacher requested a blepharoplasty because she was constantly teased by her pupils about "baggy eyes" (Fig. 15-15). She had never worn makeup and had no interest in appearing glamorous. In spite of very ptotic eyebrows, she declined a brow-lift. With her eyes closed, she had a natural crease 9 mm above the eyelashes, but with her eyes open, nearly all the pretarsal skin hung down, along with the preseptal. Her pretarsal conjoined fascia had degenerated, so the pretarsal skin and muscle were no longer adherent to the tarsus. In addition, her eyes appeared baggy because the fascia had delaminated and the fat wedge descended over the tarsus. Preoperatively there was a skin crease visible within the overhanging excess tissue of the left lid. This crease represented the area where the three fasciae had once met during youth, but now marked the junction of orbital septum and orbicularis fascia. The aponeurosis had separated off, meeting orbicularis fascia lower down on the lid, a few millimeters above the eyelashes.

At surgery, a lower incision was placed 9 mm above the eyelid margin. A substantial excision of redundant preseptal skin, muscle, fascia, and orbital fat was performed. The pretarsal fascia, heavily infiltrated with fat, was widely excised bilaterally to promote adherence of the pretarsal tissues postoperatively. Because the patient wore no makeup, a soft, slightly full appearance of the pretarsal visor was sought. Therefore, no pretarsal orbicularis muscle was excised, and the free edge of the levator aponeurosis was sutured to the upper edge of the pretarsal orbicularis muscle. In the lower eyelids no undermining was needed to excise the redundant tissues and produce a natural-looking result.

Case 3. A 66-year-old nurse-anesthetist had had a standard blepharoplasty and meloplasty by a plastic surgeon 7 years previously. Her main complaint was that her "small eyes" had returned about a year after her first blepharoplasty. In addition, the hanging upper lid skin smudged her makeup. She dressed conservatively and did not desire another meloplasty. In spite of moderate brow ptosis, she declined a brow-lift.

Her old incisions were marked in the preoperative photograph (Fig. 15-16A) to show the downward migration of her scars. Her pretarsal tissues were lax but not fatty. A moderately heavy lateral hood was present. The old upper lid incision was 8 mm above the lashes when the tissues were held taut. At surgery, the previous incision was used over the tarsus but laterally swept upward to the eyebrow, to gain access for resecting the underlying orbicularis and fat-infiltrated fascia. Moderate orbital fat was removed. No pretarsal dissection was done except at the upper tarsal edge, where a 2-mm resection of the conjoined fascia provided a free edge of the levator aponeurosis. The levator aponeurosis was shortened by 1 mm to raise the lid margin slightly relative to the globe. The aponeurosis was sutured to the pretarsal dermis, smoothing and stretching the pretarsal tissues. In the lower eyelid, only a small amount of fat was excised. Precise skin and muscle excision produced a slight lid retraction to help widen the palpebral fissure and eliminate the "small-eyed" appearance (Fig. 15-16B).

Case 4. A 44-year-old journalist wanted to eliminate the puffy appearance of her eyes. Short (5 feet) and moderately obese (145 pounds), she rarely wore makeup and dressed conservatively. She had asymmetric brow ptosis, more severe on the right (Fig. 15-17A). Her natural upper eyelid crease was 6 mm above the lashes, with extremely fatty and poorly adherent pretarsal tissues. An asymmetric coronal brow-lift was performed to raise her sagging eyelid foundation. A conservative fold height of 8 mm was chosen to match her style and relatively small, round features. Aggressive excision of fatty pretarsal and lateral hood tissues was necessary to add definition. After excision of the fat-infiltrated conjoined fascia, most of the fatty pretarsal orbicularis muscle was also resected to further smooth and define the pretarsal visor. Then the free edge of the levator aponeurosis was sutured to the lower margin dermis. But lash eversion was noted, so these sutures were removed and replaced by levator-tarsus-dermis sutures. No lower lid blepharoplasty was performed.

Case 5. A 15-year-old Japanese student with a "single eye" (Fig. 15-18A) desired a natural-appearing "double eye." She rarely wore makeup and was quiet and shy. A conservative fold height of 8 mm was chosen. The excess preseptal tissues were excised and substantial orbital fat resected. A small excision of the conjoined fascia just below the lower incision provided a free edge of levator aponeurosis. This was sutured to the pretarsal dermis with three 6-0 clear nylon sutures. Although the conjoined pretarsal fascia appeared very fatty at surgery, it was *not* resected. Leaving it in situ achieved a soft, slightly full and natural appearance (Fig. 15-18B).

Case 6. A 56-year-old Japanese clerk desired glamorous eyes. She loved to wear false eyelashes and longed to be able to apply eye makeup as she had in her youth. She had experienced progressive drooping of her eyelids for about 5 years preoperatively. She gave a history of having a low eyelid fold as a young adult, which has gradually disappeared and been replaced by a single fatty eyelid. She presented with bilateral ptosis, no evidence of an eyelid crease, and extremely loose and fatty pretarsal and preseptal tissues (Fig. 15-19A). At surgery, a new fold was planned 9 mm above the lashes. Excision of the substantial excess of preseptal tissues was followed by radical excision of the pretarsal fat, fascia, and fat-infiltrated pretarsal orbicularis muscle. The levator aponeurosis was shortened 2 mm and sutured to the lower dermis. Postoperatively, the appearance of her lids is substantially improved, but 1 mm of ptosis persists on the right (Fig. 15-19B).

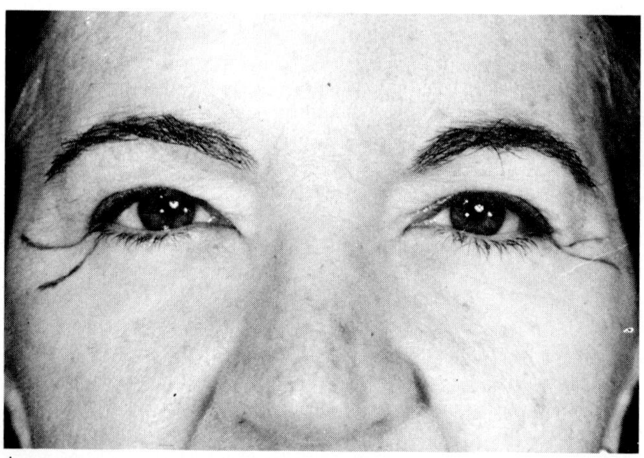

A

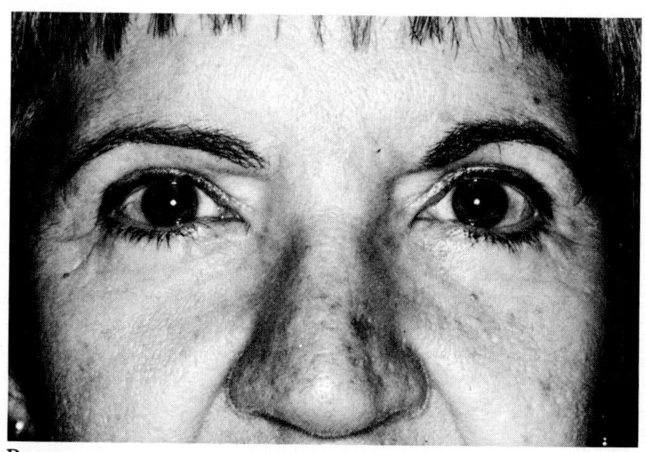

B

Figure 15-16. Case 3. Patient complained of "small eyes" 7 years after a primary "basic" blepharoplasty.
A. Before surgery.
B. One and one-half years after secondary upper and lower blepharoplasty.

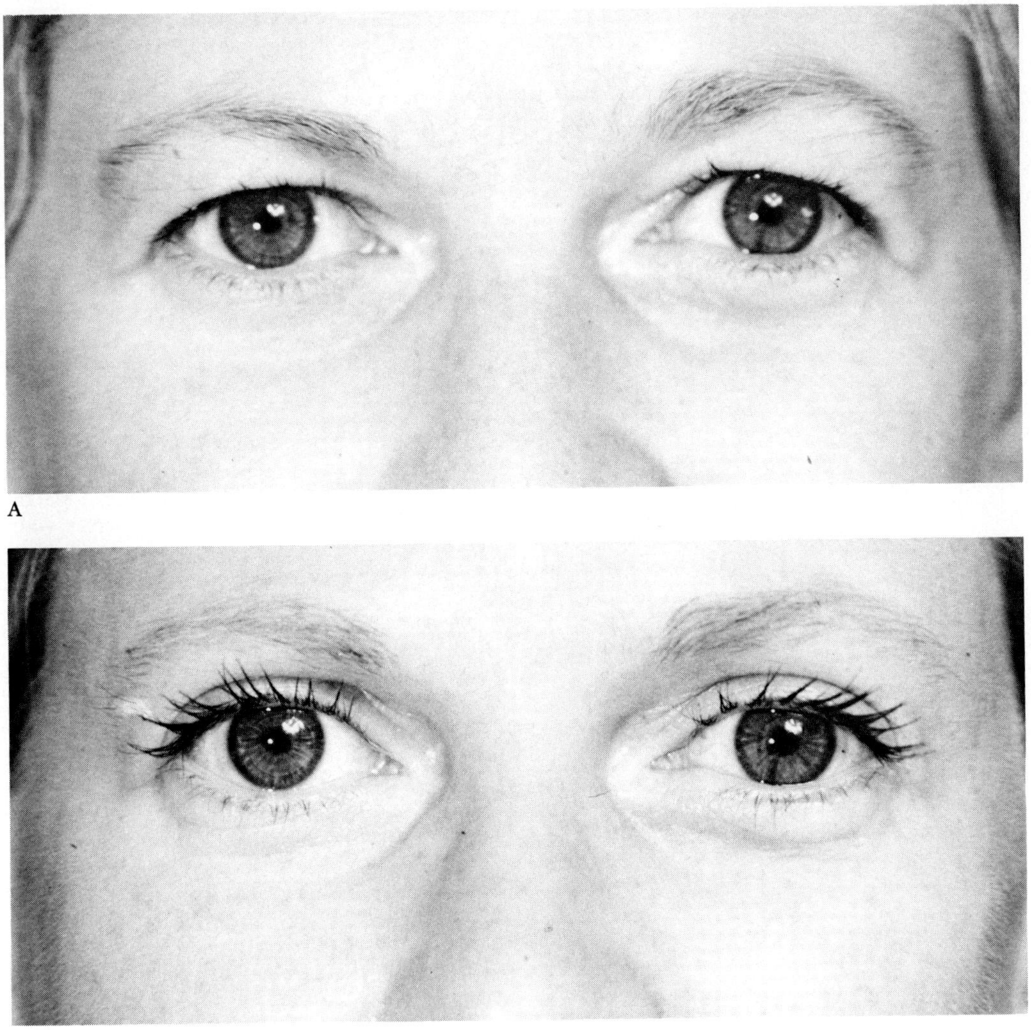

A

B

Figure 15-17. Case 4.
A. A 44-year-old journalist before surgery.
B. One year after upper lid blepharoplasty and asymmetric coronal brow-lift.

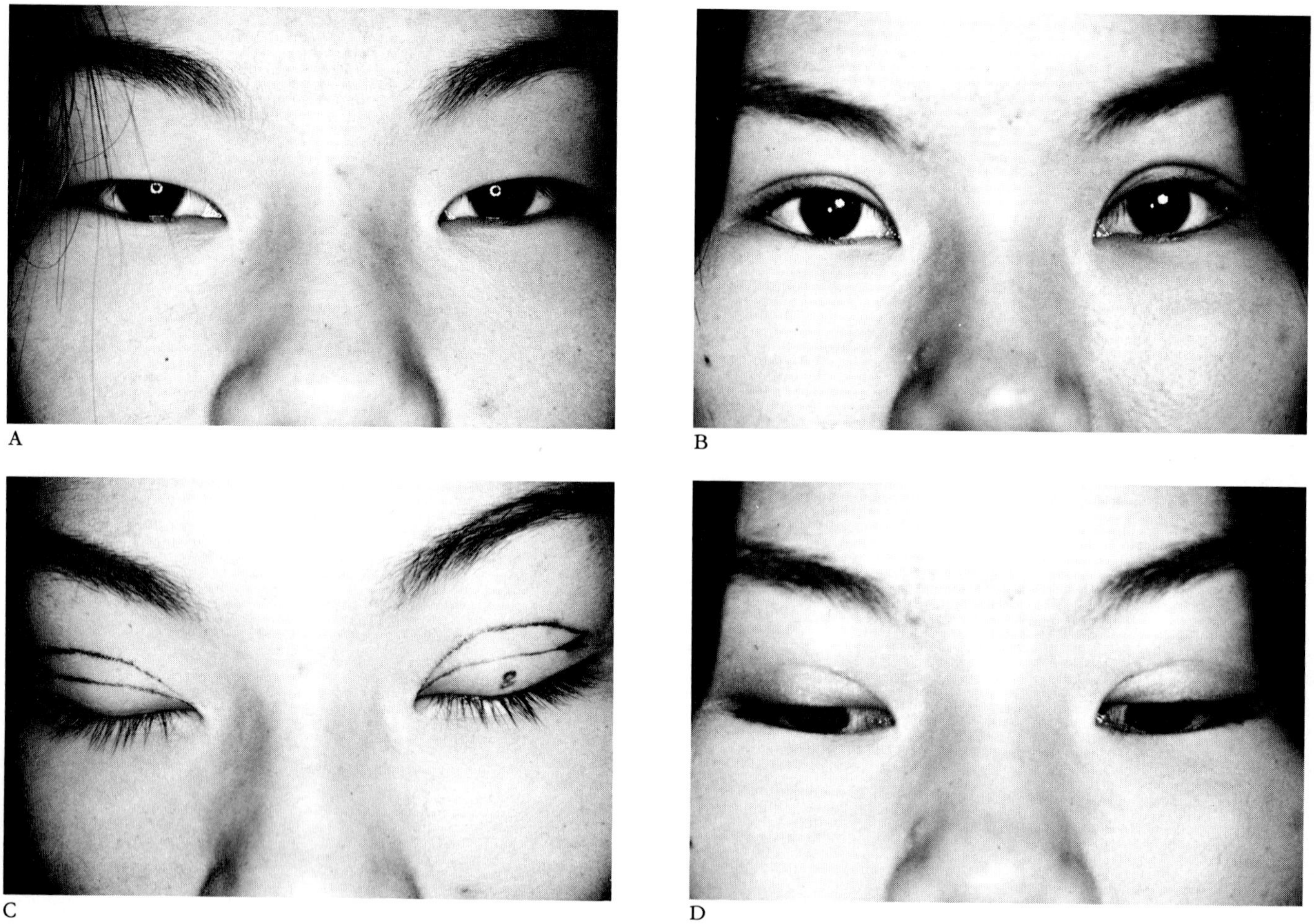

Figure 15-18. Case 5.

A. A 15-year-old Japanese female with "single eye" before surgery.
B. One and one-half years after upper lid blepharoplasty.
C. Intraoperative photograph to demonstrate sharp taper of the medial incision.
D. The "double eye" scar is always fairly evident in downgaze.

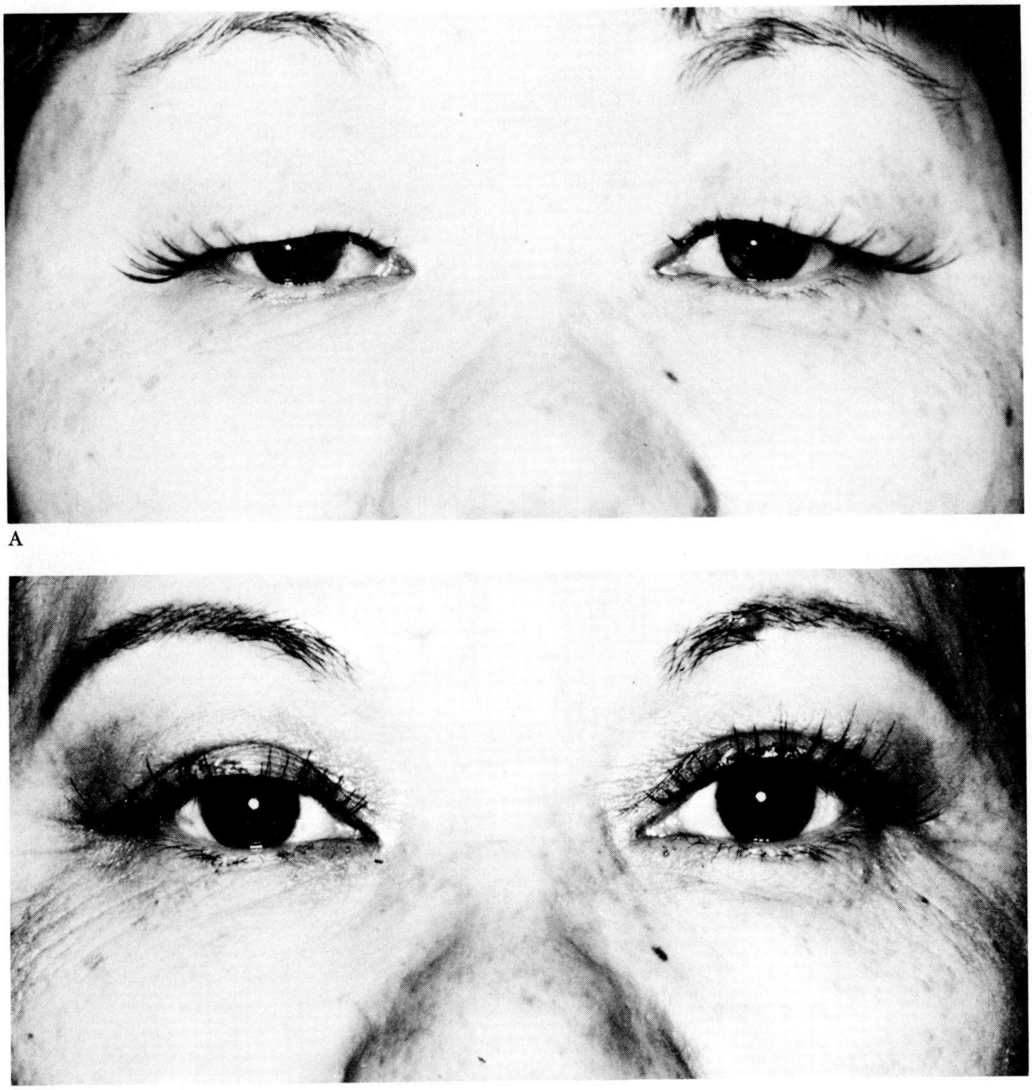

A

B

Figure 15-19. Case 6.
A. A 56-year-old Japanese clerk with ptosis and extreme fattiness of eyelid tissue.
B. Ten months after upper lid blepharoplasty.

REFERENCES

1. Aston, S. J. Orbicularis oculi muscle flaps: A technique to reduce crow's feet and lateral canthal skin folds. *Plast. Reconstr. Surg.* 65:206, 1980.
2. Baker, T. J. Upper blepharoplasty. *Clin. Plast. Surg.* 8:635, 1981.
3. Baker, T. J., Gordon, H. L., and Mosienko, P. Upper lid blepharoplasty. *Plast. Reconstr. Surg.* 60:692, 1977.
4. Beard, C. *Ptosis.* St. Louis: Mosby, 1981.
5. Boo-Chai, K. Plastic construction of the superior palpebral fold. *Plast. Reconstr. Surg.* 31:74, 1963.
6. Castanares, S. Blepharoplasty for herniated intraorbital fat. *Plast. Reconstr. Surg.* 8:46, 1951.
7. Castanares, S. Forehead wrinkles, glabellar frown and ptosis of the eyebrows. *Plast. Reconstr. Surg.* 34:406, 1964.
8. Castanares, S. Classification of baggy eyelids deformity. *Plast. Reconstr. Surg.* 59:692, 1977.
9. Cies, W. A., and Bayliss, H. I. Surgical revision of the upper eyelid fold. *Am. J. Ophthalmol.* 80:1019, 1975.
10. Courtiss, E. H. Alternatives in esthetic blepharoplasty. *Clin. Plast. Surg.* 8:739, 1981.
11. Dupuis, C., and Rees, T. D. Historical notes on blepharoplasty. *Plast. Reconstr. Surg.* 47:246, 1971.
12. Ellenbogen, R. Correction of the too-high supratarsal fixation. *Ann. Plast. Surg.* 2:341, 1979.
13. Fernandez, L. R. Double eyelid operation in the Oriental in Hawaii. *Plast. Reconstr. Surg.* 25:257, 1960.
14. Flowers, R. S. Blepharoplasty. In E. H. Courtiss, *Male Aesthetic Surgery.* St. Louis: Mosby, 1982.
15. Jones, L. T. Anatomy of the upper eyelids. *Am. J. Ophthalmol.* 57:943, 1964.
16. Klatsky, S., and Manson, P. Separate skin and muscle flaps in lower-lid blepharoplasty. *Plast. Reconstr. Surg.* 67:151, 1981.
17. Kuwabara, T., Cogan, D., and Johnson, C. Structure of the muscles of the upper eyelid. *Arch. Ophthalmol.* 93:1189, 1975.
18. Millard, D. R. Oriental peregrinations. *Plast. Reconstr. Surg.* 16:319, 1955.
19. Millard, D. R. The Oriental eyelid and its surgical revision. *Am. J. Ophthalmol.* 57:646, 1964.
20. Mladick, R. A. The muscle-suspension lower blepharoplasty. *Plast. Reconstr. Surg.* 64:171, 1979.
21. Mutou, Y., and Mutou, H. Intradermal double eyelid operation and its follow-up results. *Br. J. Plast. Surg.* 25:285, 1972.
22. Owsley, J. Q. Resection of the prominent lateral fat pad during upper lid blepharoplasty. *Plast. Reconstr. Surg.* 65:4, 1980.
23. Pang, H. G. Surgical formation of upper lid fold. *Arch. Ophthalmol.* 65:434, 1965.
24. Rees, T. D., and Tabbal, N. Lower blepharoplasty. *Clin. Plast. Surg.* 8:643, 1981.
25. Sayoc, B. T. Plastic construction of the superior palpebral fold. *Am. J. Ophthalmol.* 38:556, 1954.
26. Sayoc, B. T. Surgery of the Oriental eyelid. *Clin. Plast. Surg.* 1:156, 1974.
27. Sheen, J. H. Supratarsal fixation in upper blepharoplasty. *Plast. Reconstr. Surg.* 54:424, 1974.
28. Sheen, J. H. A change in the technique of supratarsal fixation in upper blepharoplasty. *Plast. Reconstr. Surg.* 59:831, 1977.
29. Skoog, T. *Plastic Surgery.* Philadelphia: Saunders, 1975.
30. Souther, S. G., Corboy, J. M., and Thompson, J. B. The Fasanella-Servat operation for ptosis of the upper eyelid. *Plast. Reconstr. Surg.* 53:123, 1974.
31. Spira, M. Blepharoplasty. *Clin. Plast. Surg.* 5:121, 1978.
32. Uchida, J. A surgical procedure for blepharoptosis vera and pseudoblepharoptosis orientalis. *Br. J. Plast. Surg.* 15:271, 1962.
33. Wolff, E. *Anatomy of the Eye and Orbit.* Philadelphia: Saunders, 1961.
34. Zide, B. M. Anatomy of the eyelids. *Clin. Plast. Surg.* 8:623, 1981.

IV. Face-Lift

16. Rhytidectomy

Paule Regnault
Rollin K. Daniel

A rhytidectomy, or face-lift, lessens facial folds and wrinkles, creating a more youthful appearance. The incisions are placed in areas of concealment, the redundant skin is excised, and tension is taken in the scalp. Traditionally, the results were acceptable in carefully selected patients, but with restricted application and efficacy. Recent advances in surgical technique have broadened the range of applicability, expanded the deformities that can be ameliorated, and extended the duration of improvement. The key to this revolution has been modification of deeper structures including the fascial network (superficial musculoaponeurotic system — SMAS), the facial muscles (platysma, orbicularis oculi), and excision and contouring of fat deposits. Although the number and variety of procedures have increased arithmetically, the combinations available for the individual patient have expanded geometrically. Therefore, careful analysis of the patient's deformities and desires is essential for selection of the optimal operation. In addition, the surgeon must be highly skilled in a broad range of surgical procedures.

HISTORY

During the early 1900s, aesthetic surgery for correction of facial wrinkles and folds began to flourish in America and Europe. The initial procedures consisted of multiple elliptic skin excisions located at the temporal hairline, preauricular and postauricular areas, and neck [3]. All of these operations were performed under local anesthesia in an office operating room. In 1908 C. C. Miller [156] of Chicago published the first text on cosmetic surgery. As reviewed by Rogers [186], numerous surgeons claimed credit, often in retrospect, for pioneering the face-lift procedures. During the 1920s, surgical approaches became more extensive, with coalescing of the ellipses to form larger excisions, and direct attacks on deeper structures. The contributions of Miller [156], Kolle [127], Lexer [139], Passot [166], and Joseph [117] frequently overlapped as comparable solutions for common problems occurred. In 1928 the state of the art was first illustrated in a text to include preoperative and postoperative photographs written by Mme A. Noël [162]. By the 1930s, aesthetic facial surgery had reached such a state that subsequent evolution has consisted only of "variations and improvements in the operation of their predecessors" [18, 148].

Despite this admonition, the 1960s saw a reawakening of interest in rhytidectomy and especially ancillary procedures [164]. The forehead-lift, eyebrow elevation, plication of parotid fascia, excision of platysma borders, and removal of submental-submandibular fat were all rediscovered [8, 25, 26, 36, 37, 43, 45, 114, 173]. This technical base formation permitted the explosive growth of facial surgery, which was fueled by a youth-oriented society and widespread public acceptance [76, 82, 110, 138]. The 1970s were a renaissance for rhytidectomy [111, 137, 180]. The numerous complications associated with extensive skin undermining forced development of new techniques. Skoog [193] advanced the deep structures of the face and neck, allowing correction of deformities without recourse to extended dissection. Mitz and Peyronie [157] focused attention on the SMAS and its interrelation with the facial musculature. Peterson [168], Guerrero-Santos [100–102], Connell [51–53], and others emphasized the role of platysmal flaps and SMAS traction for rejuvenation of the aging face. Such advances resulted in dramatic correction of neck deformities, a more certain improvement in a larger percentage of cases, and greater persistence of improvements. With this evolution and an aging population, it appears that the golden age of cervicofacial rhytidectomy is now at hand.

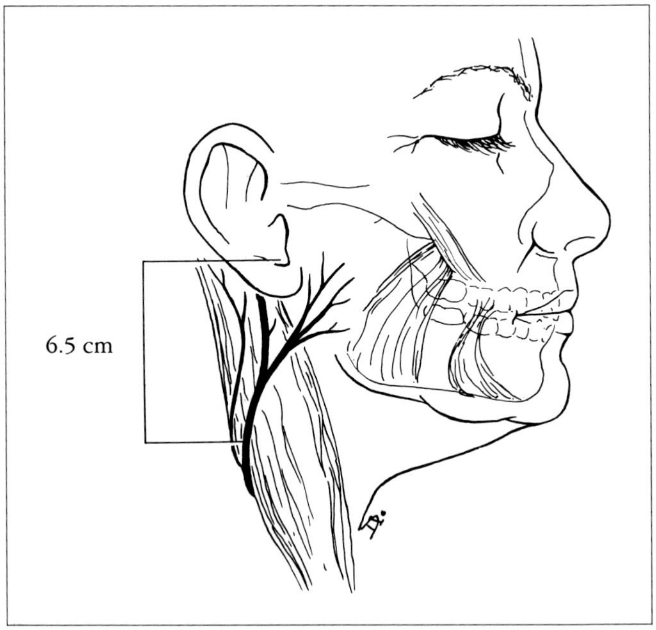

Figure 16-1. The greater auricular nerve crosses the sternocleidomastoid muscle 6.5 cm below the external auditory canal.

ANATOMY

Nerves

The nerves of the face have either a pure sensory or a motor function. The fifth cranial nerve has three major divisions whose foraminal branches (supraorbital, infraorbital, and mental) provide sensation to the face. The seventh cranial nerve controls the muscles of facial expression. The present review emphasizes their surgical anatomy, functional importance, and possible areas of injury during rhytidectomy.

SENSORY NERVES

The greater auricular nerve originates principally from the third cervical root, passes around the posterior border of the sternocleidomastoid muscle, crosses the muscle at a 45-degree angle, and ascends toward the angle of the jaw. It terminates in multiple small branches that innervate the ear and the anterior and posterior auricular area. It is vulnerable as it passes over the sternocleidomastoid muscle. At this point, the SMAS blends with the fascia of the sternocleidomastoid muscle and the skin is very thin, with little subcutaneous fat. Since the face is often turned to the opposite side during dissection, the muscle is tensed, thereby forcing the nerve to become more superficial. In 75 patients, McKinney and Katarana [151] found that the greater auricular nerve trunk crosses the sternocleidomastoid muscle 6.5 cm below the external auditory canal (Fig. 16-1). Also, the external jugular vein was parallel and 0.5 cm anterior to the nerve at this point. If the dissection is kept superficial and the nerve identified, the lateral border of the platysma muscle can be raised without risk. The lesser occipital nerve runs 1 cm behind and parallel to the greater auricular nerve. It innervates the upper posterior one-third of the auricle.

MOTOR NERVES

Following its emergence from the stylomastoid foramen, the facial nerve provides three branches (posterior auricular, posterior belly of digastric, and stylohyoid) before entering the parotid gland. Within the gland, the nerve bifurcates into temporal and cervical divisions, which in turn provide the classic five terminal branches [57, 64] (Fig. 16-2). The temporal division contains 5 to 7 branches with only one branch to the frontal area (rendering it a terminal branch in 85–90% of cases), several branches to the zygomatic area, which is the largest, and a few to the buccal area. The cervical division is smaller, with one branch to the buccal area, three branches to the mandibular area, and one to the cervical region. Since both divisions provide innervation to the buccal region, the area is rarely denervated. Topographically, the facial nerve and its divisions are protected by the parotid gland. The temporal, zygomatic, and buccal branches lie beneath the SMAS, while the mandibular and cervical branches are usually covered by the platysma. Since the nerves are often accompanied by parallel blood vessels, coagulation risks damage, and bipolar coagulation is therefore used. The nerves approach the muscles from the lateral side and innervate them on their deep surface. However, a detailed knowledge of the course of each branch is critical for the execution of the newer rhytidectomy procedures.

Frontal (Temporal) Branch. Topographically, one can mark the expected course of the frontal branch from 0.5 cm below the tragus to a point 1.5 cm above the lateral eyebrow [172]. It terminates in the frontalis and corrugator muscles. Although anatomically constant, it is frequently injured because of its transition from a relatively deep subcutaneous plane in the cheek to a suprafascial location at the zygomatic arch before subsequent termination in the forehead muscle [143]. As noted by Mitz and Peyronie [157], the frontal branch lies deep to the SMAS, but its

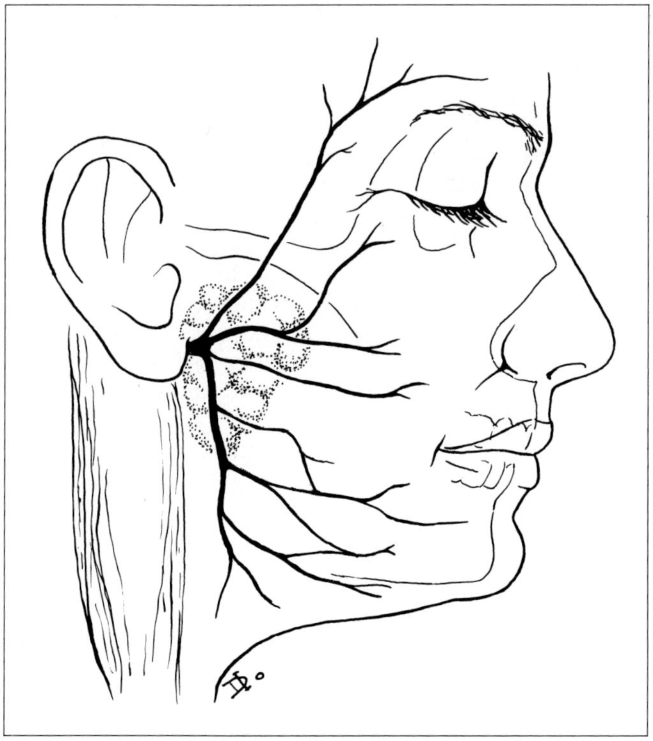

Figure 16-2. The branches of the facial nerve.

close apposition makes dissection at the zygomatic arch extremely precarious. During a conventional rhytidectomy, the temporal skin is elevated in the subcutaneous plane, maintaining visualization of the hair bulbs. As one approaches the zygomatic region, the dissection is done with a sponge-covered finger to avoid sharp severance of the frontal branch. The importance of anatomic location is clearly emphasized at the time of simultaneous forehead-lift and rhytidectomy [183]. Dissection in the cervical-temporal area is done in the areolar space deep to the galea, whereas the cheek is dissected more superficially in the subcutaneous plane. If the two planes are joined anteriorly, the frontal branch will be severed. For this reason, two separate planes are maintained, a deep temporal one and a superficial cheek dissection.

Zygomatic Branch. The zygomatic branch passes along a line drawn from the tragus through the malar prominence with subsequent termination in the orbicularis oculi at the lateral angle of the eye. As it passes over the malar prominence, the nerve is felt to be at risk, and dissection should be performed bluntly. This branch is considered the least subject to injury, and any loss is difficult to detect. Furnas [80] states that several rami of the temporal branch subdivide into numerous interconnecting filaments, ensuring innervation despite division of the orbicularis oculi muscle in crow's-feet procedures.

Buccal Branch. The buccal branches are several in number, with contributions from both divisions and numerous interconnections. These branches exit from the anterior border of the parotid gland onto the surface of the masseter muscle and they are covered by the SMAS. Anterior to the masseter, the nerve branches pass on top of the buccal fat pad. The distribution of the buccal branches is extensive, ranging from the lower eyelid over to the nose and down to the mouth. The nerve is most easily injured anterior to the parotid fascia, especially on elevation of an extensive SMAS flap or defatting of the cheek.

Mandibular Branch. Because of increasingly frequent use of facial lipectomy and platysmal flaps, the mandibular branch is subject to greater risk of transection. Although often considered a single structure, this branch most often consists of two or three separate filaments, which are easily identified with a nerve stimulator during parotid removal or radical neck dissection. Dingman and Grabb [68] used the facial artery at its crossing of the mandible as a landmark for recording the course of the mandibular branch. Posterior to the facial artery, the nerve was above the mandible in 81 percent of dissections and below in 19 percent while anterior to the artery it was above the mandible in 100 percent of dissections. Although subsequently confirmed by others, these cadaver dissections do not correlate directly with clinical cases, in which the tissues are more lax and extension of the neck forces the structures lower. For these reasons, division of the platysma muscle should be done at least 4 to 5 cm below and parallel to the mandibular border. The mandibular branch passes through the platysma to lie beneath the depressor anguli oris before innervating muscles of the chin and lower lip.

Cervical Branch. This branch passes forward and downward beneath the platysma muscle, which it innervates. Although the consequences of its severance are rarely noted, Ellenbogen [71] has reported two cases of pseudomandibular branch paralysis. Specifically, patients with a "full-denture" smile lost the ability to expose the lower teeth because of transection of the platysma and its terminal cervical branch innervation. Although symmetry returned, full exposure of the lower teeth did not. The cervical branch should be preserved whenever possible.

Muscles and SMAS

Embryologically, the muscles of facial expression as well as the platysma and epicranius are all derived from the second pharyngeal arch and innervated by the same nerve. Although our emphasis is on facial expression, these muscles do function collectively as simple sphincters and dilators for the various sense organs and facial orifices. Equally important is the functional interrelationship between the muscles and their fascia, the latter acting as a distributor of muscle contraction. A brief review of the structures is presented here with an in-depth description provided by Lemmon in Chapter 17.

PLATYSMA MUSCLE

The platysma is a broad, flat skin muscle that originates from the fascial covering of the pectoralis major and del-

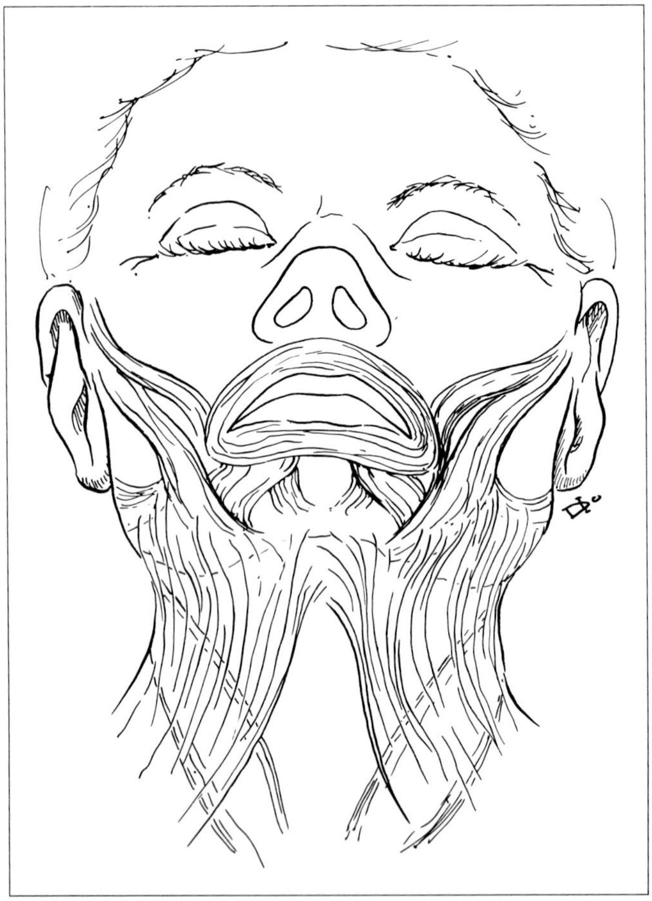

Figure 16-3. The platysma muscle. Separation of the anterior borders will create visible folds.

toid muscles (Fig. 16-3). It passes upward and medially along the side of the neck. The posterior border has an S configuration and covers the mandibular angle in all cases. Medially, the fibers interlace with those of the opposite side, forming an inverted V whose vertex varies from the chin to the thyroid cartilage. From dissecting 100 hemifaces, Cardoso de Castro [41] reported three basic variations of the medial mingling of the two platysma muscles: type I, medial fibers interlace 1 to 2 cm below the chin (75%); type II, fibers interdigitate at the level of thyroid cartilage (15%); and type III, fibers are totally separate (10%). Superiorly, the platysma muscle inserts onto the mandible, SMAS, and skin while blending with the muscles of the mouth and interdigitating behind the mentalis with fibers of the opposite platysma. The muscle is innervated by the cervical branch and functions as a depressor-retractor of the lower lip.

FRONTAL MUSCLE

This muscle is an integral part of the epicranius, which consists of two muscle bellies (occipital and frontal) interconnected by an aponeurosis, the galea. The frontal muscle has *no* bony attachment but originates from a large number of facial muscles. The medial muscle fibers are attached to the procerus, intermediate fibers to the corrugator and orbicularis oculi, and lateral fibers to the orbicularis oculi. The medial margin represents a mingling of fibers from the two sides while the lateral margin is continuous with the temporozygomatic fascia. The muscle is innervated by the frontal branch and functions as an elevator of the eyebrows. This muscle and its attachments are discussed more extensively in Chapter 13.

SMAS

The superficial musculoaponeurotic system or SMAS is the critical interconnecting link between various facial muscles and is recognized now as an important surgical structure (Fig. 16-4). Although it was carefully detailed by anatomists, the true functional and surgical importance of the SMAS went unrecognized until the work of Skoog [193] and its subsequent culmination in the classic anatomic paper of Mitz and Peyronie [157]. The SMAS is a fibromuscular network located between the more superficial dermis and the deeper facial muscles. This broad fibrous sheath is an integral component of the cervicocephalic fascia extending vertically from the frontalis to the platysma muscle and transversely from the pretragal area into the perioral dermis. It is thickest over the parotid fascia, so that easy elevation is possible, and thinnest anteriorly, where its terminal fibers attach to the dermis. Anatomically, the subcutaneous fat superior to the SMAS can be safely excised as the facial nerve branches pass beneath it. Functionally, the SMAS serves as a distributor of facial muscle contractions and facilitates the graded response characteristic of facial expression. Surgically, traction on the SMAS serves to tighten the fascial envelope of the face, thereby improving appearance without recourse to excessive skin tension.

PATHOPHYSIOLOGY AND CLASSIFICATION

Although the aging process is inevitable and universal, it induces an individualistic response (Fig. 16-5). For certain patients, crow's-feet may be of greater concern than jowls whereas the reverse is true for others. Any classification of the myriad deformities must take into account numerous factors based on obvious pathologic changes that occur in each component tissue.

Skin

Patients complain most frequently of wrinkles, which are the superficial manifestation of underlying muscle contraction [60]. These lines are usually perpendicular to the course of the facial muscle and occur in predictable locations—crow's-feet (orbicularis oculi), frown lines (corrugator and procerus), worry lines (frontalis). Additional fine facial wrinkles include cross-hatching, found in the malar and cheek region, and lip lines. It is tempting to attribute the former to chronic sun exposure and the latter to atrophy of subcutaneous tissues. Many patients also

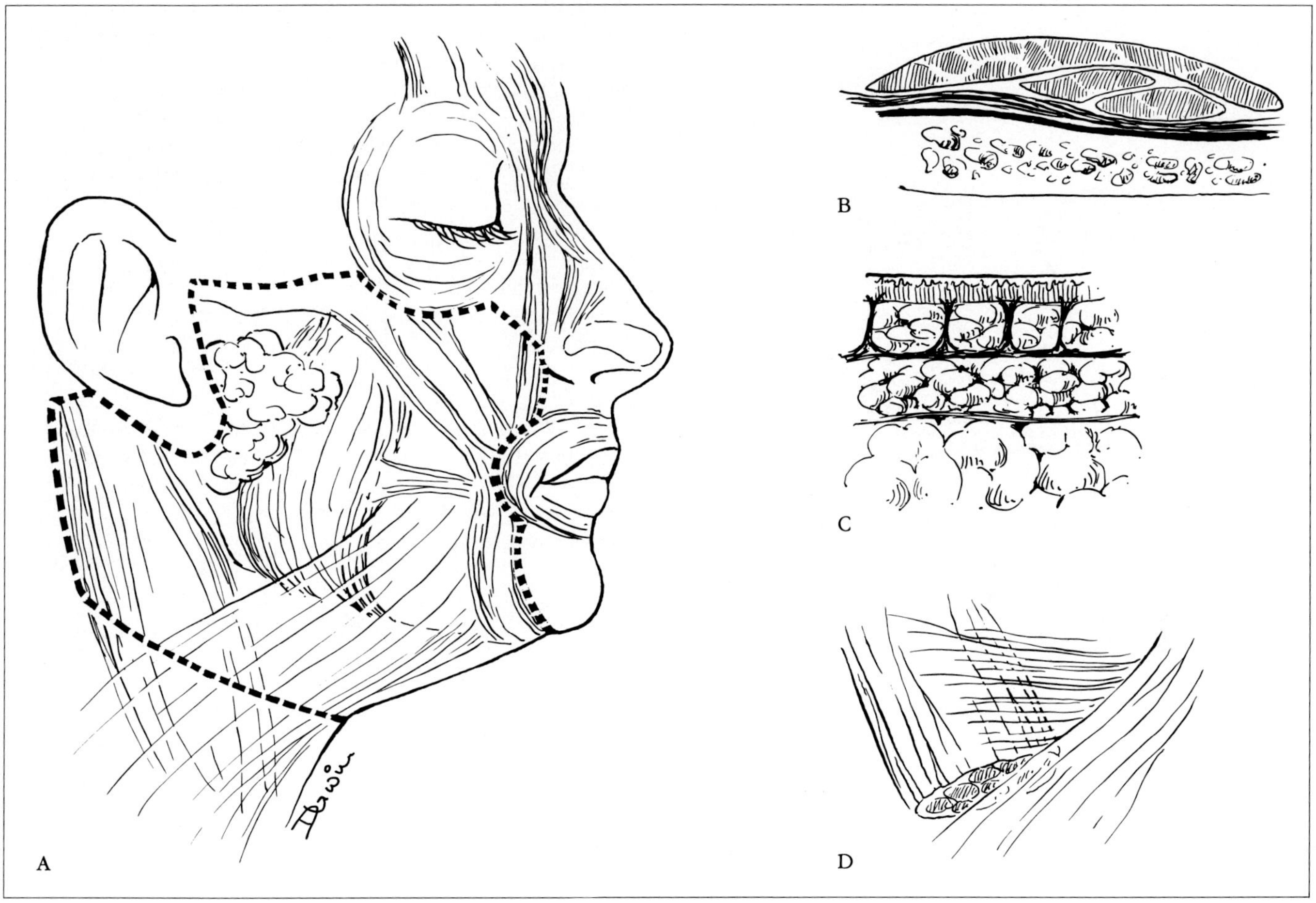

Figure 16-4
A. The extent of the SMAS is outlined by the dotted line.
B. The SMAS continues with the frontalis muscle fascia over the zygomatic arch.
C. In the cheek area, the SMAS separates the subcutaneous fat into two levels, with the upper layer divided by vertical septa that insert into the dermis.
D. The posterior border of the SMAS blends with the fascia of the sternocleidomastoid fascia.

complain of distinct "lines" in the nasolabial regions and jowls, which ultimately progress to heavy sagging folds.

With the passage of time, skin undergoes a definite atrophy process with epidermal thinning and fragmentation of elastic fibers [79, 81, 97, 124]. The subcutaneous fat and muscles are equally affected, thereby accentuating the wrinkles and aging appearance [105, 189]. Many surgeons feel that reabsorption of the bony prominences compounds the problem [91, 118]. Because of decreased sweating, the skin texture becomes dryer and glossier [116]. The cumulative effect of sun exposure is manifested by an increased incidence of epidermal lesions and irregular pigmentation. To determine the skin texture, one must examine the face without makeup and inquire specifically about sun exposure and previous dermatologic problems, especially acne.

Subcutaneous Fat

The subcutaneous fat is present in varying amounts and locations. As noted by Aufricht [11], significant deformities result from ptosis of the subcutaneous tissues, which must be corrected directly at the time of rhytidectomy. These accumulations are most noted in the cheek and submandibular regions. Mitz and Peyronie [157] showed that the SMAS divides the subcutaneous fat into two layers, a superficial layer enclosed by vertical fibrous septa and a deeper layer located between the deep facial muscles. In the submandibular region, the subcutaneous fat is superficial to the platysma muscle except for occasional accumulations medially. From cadaver studies, there is no indication that a distinct submental fat pad exists, but rather there is a continuous sheet of subcutaneous fat all along the lower border of the mandible.

Quantitatively, the patient may have insufficient fat, which results in skeletonization of the neck, or excessive fat, which may be of the firm obesity type or flabby with displacement. The subcutaneous fat may be asymmetrically or unaesthetically placed, as manifested by jowls or submental fullness. Lipomas may be seen occasionally beneath the platysma muscle. Jowls can be accentuated by ptosis or hypertrophy of the submandibular glands. The adequacy of support for these glands by the digastric and platysma muscles is assessed by palpation.

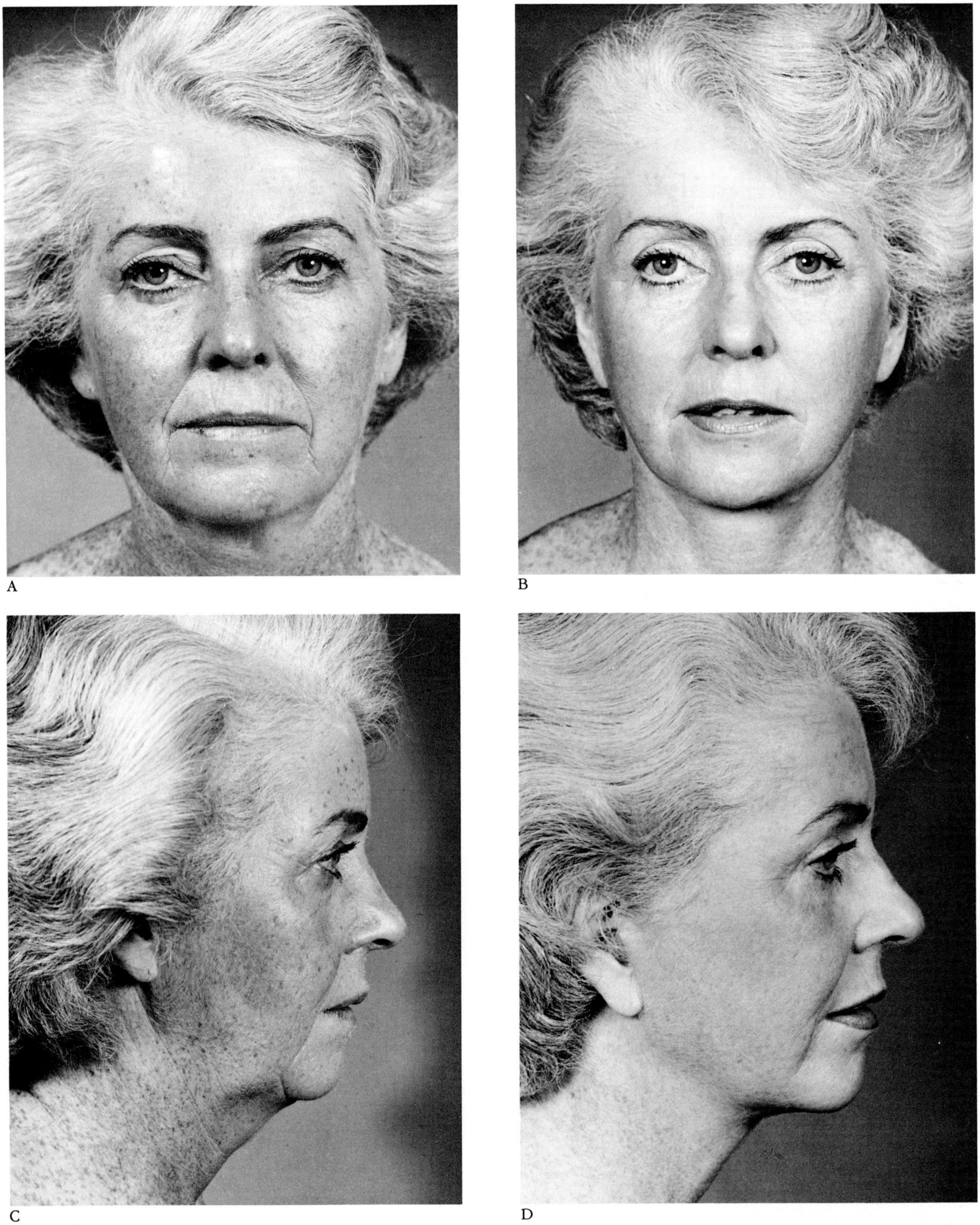

Figure 16-5.
A, C. A 47-year-old patient sought improvement in facial appearance because of "looking old," especially with regard to heavy redundant eyelid skin, laxity of neck, and early jowl formation.
B, D. Result at 18 months, following cervicofacial rhytidectomy with platysmal traction, lipectomy, and four-eyelid blepharoplasty.

Muscles

The primary muscle deformities are those of the platysma. Souther and Vistnes [197] attribute vertical neck bands to the free medial margin of the platysma muscle, a problem that was corrected by the plication of the muscle edges. Aston [8] described eight platysma muscle deformities that could be divided into variations of three problems: borders, bands, and laxity. The medial borders may be quite hypertrophic, requiring direct excision, or separated, requiring approximation. The appearance of vertical bands within the muscle requires midline approximation and full-width platysmal flaps. Laxity or separation of the platysma muscle is treated by approximation and advancement of partial-width flaps.

Bone

The bony configuration of the face is determined during development but is accentuated during the aging process [210]. Descent of the soft tissues aggravates flattening of the malar region and drooping of the nasal tip. Mandibular contours are altered by alveolar reabsorption. A receding chin is emphasized by fullness of the adjacent jowls and fat accumulation.

The obtuse cervicomental angle is one of the best examples of the interrelationship between pathologic changes in the various tissues (Fig. 16-6). As defined by Ellenbogen and Karlin [72], the youthful neck is characterized by five features: (1) a distinct inferior mandibular border with no jowl overhang, (2) a subhyoid depression, (3) a visible thyroid cartilage bulge, (4) a visible anterior border of the sternocleidomastoid muscle, and (5) a cervicomental angle of 105 to 120 degrees. As noted by Peterson [168], an obtuse cervicomental angle consists of a low-positioned hyoid, microgenia, and cervical kyphosis and results in roughly parallel anterior and posterior cervical profiles. To correct these problems, a cervicofacial

Figure 16-6

A, B. Comparing normal to obtuse cervicomental angle. Note all structures above the lips are identical on the two figures.

C, D. The obtuse cervicomental angle is created by microgenia, a low hyoid position, and excess fat accumulation.

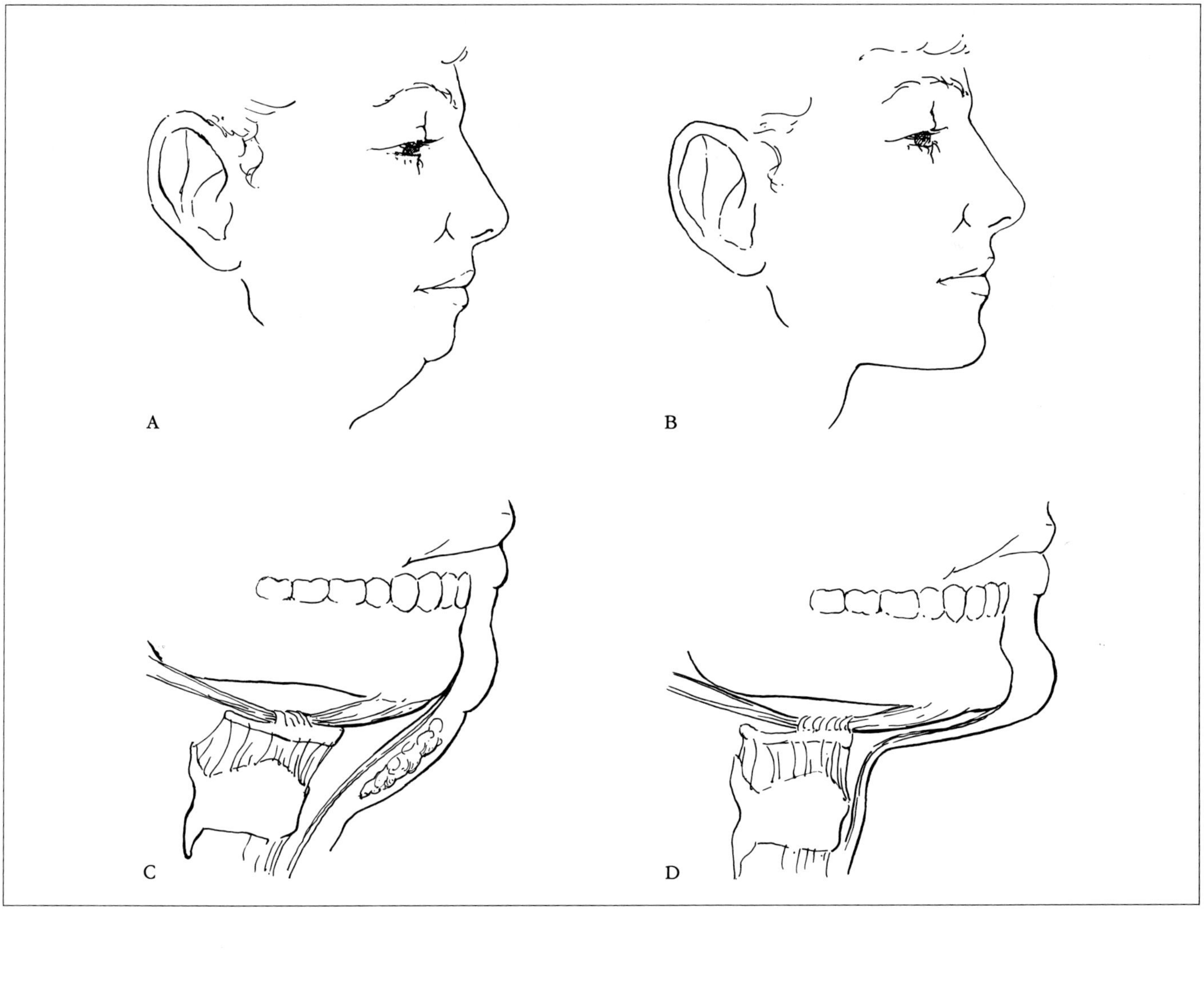

rhytidectomy with extensive submandibular lipectomies and platysmal flaps is required plus consideration of chin modification.

The pathologic changes that occur in each of the tissues can be classified as to location and age with certain variations according to sex and previous surgery. Although treatment can be either surgical or medical, surgical techniques are grouped as to extent (temporal, cervicofacial, or complete including forehead), tissues altered (skin, subcutaneous fat, SMAS and platysma, or bone augmentation), and additional procedures (blepharoplasty, septorhinoplasty, direct excisions).

Location of Deformities

Classically, the face is divided into equal thirds: the upper third extending from hairline to nasion, the middle third from nasion to nasolabial angle, and the lower third from nasolabial angle to chin. To these divisions of examination the plastic surgeon must add the neck and specific regional areas as well as the skin itself. One can modify the examination sequence of Fredericks [78] to ensure that each factor is assessed. However, the principal features that patients complain of are neck deformities, jowls, nasolabial folds, perioral lines, deep forehead lines, and eyelid deformities [205].

Age Determinants

Even 20- to 35-year-old patients complain of looking old. Often they are unable to define precisely what causes their dissatisfaction, but after an in-depth discussion it is usually related to either bone or fat deformities. Microgenia associated with cervical fat accumulation produces an obtuse cervicomental angle whereas hypoplasia of the malar prominences combined with low cheeks provides a tired look. If the nose droops sufficiently to close the nasolabial angle, the impression of aging is created. Also, herniation of orbital fat in the lower eyelids may become manifest in late adolescence as well as dermatochalasis of the upper eyelids. One must be receptive to the patient's problem and try to ascertain its causes.

In the 35- to 45-year age group, patients begin to complain of nasolabial folds, crow's-feet, fine wrinkles, and eyelid deformities, in addition to the defects previously described [47, 136]. Most are concerned about the onset of aging stigmata and wonder whether it is too soon to have a face-lift [74]. Many can be improved sufficiently with blepharoplasty alone, but those wishing to obtain optimal improvement will require a rhytidectomy and blepharoplasty.

The mean age for rhytidectomy occurs in the fifties, and patients in the 45- to 65-year age group often request an extended cervicofacial rhytidectomy plus blepharoplasty. Although their concerns may be localized to certain areas, they normally want the complete effect of looking younger and better. In individuals over 65, one must include the forehead in order to achieve a total improvement.

Surgically, one should develop the optimal operative plan to fit the patient's specific deformities, whether this requires isolated or combined procedures including blepharoplasty, mentoplasty, septorhinoplasty, and cervicofacial rhytidectomy. The rhytidectomy itself may be divided into four broad categories, which can be simplistically associated with various age groups: (1) regional lift including temporal, meloplasty, or cervical (25–35), (2) cervicofacial rhytidectomy (35–45), (3) extended cervicofacial rhytidectomy (45–60), and (4) complete rhytidectomy (60 and over).

CONSULTATION

Prospective rhytidectomy patients require in-depth evaluation and establishment of a supportive patient-doctor relationship [178]. Goin et al. [85, 86] analyzed 117 consecutive face-lift consultations; 50 patients had the procedure, 37 were accepted by the surgeon but did not schedule surgery, and 30 were rejected by the surgeon. It is interesting to note that, of the 30 rejected, 14 were obese, 10 were poor medical candidates, and 6 were psychologically unstable. Of concern, the majority of patients (54%, 27 of 50) developed some degree of depression during the postoperative period, yet most (94%, 47 of 50) rated their result good to excellent.

Indications and Contraindications

The basic indication for cervicofacial rhytidectomy is the presence of wrinkles and folds that can be improved by traction in the preauricular region or of a significant neck deformity correctable by skin resection, platysmal modification, or defatting procedures. Judgment is required to determine whether the anticipated change justifies a major procedure. Obviously, the patient with well-developed jowls and hanging platysma borders will be improved. In contrast, the patient with a full face, early jowl lines, and only a few wrinkles that are not significantly improved by preauricular skin traction is told that it is "too early" and scheduled to return for reassessment in a year. Rhytidectomies are also indicated for treatment of acne, facial paralysis, and facial asymmetries due to trauma or previous surgery.

Contraindications are numerous. The emotionally high-risk group includes patients with a previous psychiatric history, those currently undergoing therapy or recovering from a severe life crisis, and individuals with continuing depression. Emotional stability is a primary prerequisite and an absolute necessity for surmounting any postoperative complication. The patient with unrealistic expectations or total perfectionist tendencies must be "educated" [126]. Certain patients are unwilling to accept the fact that a face-lift is major surgery with inherent permanent scars and significant risk of complications. A second visit is often necessary. Despite recent advances in correcting the obtuse cervicomental angle, the obese patient remains a difficult problem. Since the wrinkles, folds, and bony structure of the face are obscured by fat, correction is often disappointing to both patient and surgeon.

History

The patient is asked which aspects of aging and which facial features are the most bothersome and requested to rank them in order of severity thus setting the priorities. A three-way mirror is invaluable for the discussion. During this preliminary analysis, the inherent technical limitations in certain areas (lip lines, nasolabial folds, crow's-feet) are pointed out. A detailed social history regarding employment, marriage, family, psychologic condition, previous cosmetic surgery, leisure-time activities, and sun exposure is obtained. A brief review of systems should concentrate on previous facial surgery, Bell's palsy, cardiorespiratory problems, metabolic diseases, and drug regimen ranging from hypertensive medication to tranquilizers.

Motivation

Most patients have considered surgery for some time but take action only after an unflattering remark or a change in socioeconomic circumstances [145–147]. The optimal motivation is an internal one: to feel better about oneself rather than attempting to influence others or to obtain material gain [15]. From reading the popular press, most patients know the "correct" response: "I want to look as young as I feel. People are always telling me how tired I look. I want to look better for myself." Although most patients consider these to be their true motivations, Goin et al. [85, 86] have found different subconscious desires, including the following: (1) to *feel* physically younger, thereby avoiding abandonment because of their aging, (2) to develop a more intimate relationship with their spouse or to find a new mate, and (3) to get a better job because of improved appearance. Since these motivations were never disclosed to the surgeon and were revealed only postoperatively to an empathetic psychiatrist, it is obvious that the surgeon must detect patients with significant psychologic problems, unrealistic expectations, or instability to handle the postoperative period [69].

Physical Examination

The patient is examined in the sitting position with the face and neck exposed, under good lighting. The entire face is examined without makeup from top to bottom, both in repose and with expression. The examination period is the surgeon's opportunity to identify the pathologic changes, to classify the deformities, and to select the optimal operative plan.

The abundance of hair (thick, thin, balding) and hairline (low, high) are noted, and inquiries are made about recent hair loss. Forehead and glabellar wrinkles are assessed plus any eyebrow ptosis. The eyelids are evaluated for redundancy, ptosis, and fat herniation. The presence of crow's-feet is observed at rest and on forced smiling. With skin traction over the parotid area, the degree of skin laxity is determined—especially how much the traction decreases wrinkles and folds. The skin is inspected for previous incisions, acne scars, and dermatologic conditions. Next, the quantity and distribution of subcutaneous fat are determined, generalized or localized to specific areas including buccal, submandibular, and submental. The position of the submandibular gland and its relation to the jowls are observed. The platysma muscle is evaluated as to its borders, bands, and laxity both in repose and on forced clenching of the teeth [10]. The cervicomental angle and its hyoid-mental component are assessed, as is the mandibular configuration. As the final plan is formulated, one checks for any asymmetry and facial nerve weakness.

Aesthetic Goals

The surgeon reviews the patient's priority list, comments on the feasibility of correction, and then presents a proposed surgical plan based on the physical deformities. In many instances, the patient will want the desired result but with less surgery or will casually say, "Well, you decide, you're the doctor." The surgeon must stress that, while it is the surgeon's responsibility to analyze which deformities are correctable and what the associated risks are, the patient must make the final decision.

Next, the operative plan and possible complications are described in detail. While the patient looks in the mirror, the surgeon demonstrates the location of the incisions and the degree of expected correction. The difference between moderate and excessive traction is shown, as well as the effect on skin folds under realistic traction. Any asymmetries are pointed out. Sitting next to the patient, the surgeon draws incision lines in the chart, lists major complications (hematoma, nerve injury, skin slough, hair loss, too great an expectation), and explains each in simple terms. The patient is given the choice of anesthesia (local or general) and location (office or hospital) [4–6, 23, 29, 66, 67, 115, 123, 192, 199, 208, 209]. A complete medical workup, including appropriate preoperative tests, is requested from the patient's personal physician [61].

Informed Consent

Patients must realize that a rhytidectomy will make them look better and more rested. The improvement can be interpreted as a younger appearance, as evidenced by the amelioration of neck bands, jowls, and wrinkles. However, patients must accept the following risks:

1. Hematoma formation or bleeding is a very real possibility. Reoperation may be required for drainage. Minor accumulations will be aspirated if they occur although their resolution may take several months.
2. Scars are permanent and occasionally visible. Every effort will be made to minimize their occurrence, but revision may be necessary.
3. There will be a loss of sensation over the cheeks and possibly the lower ear for several months. Sensation should return in 3 to 6 months.
4. Delayed healing or minor loss of skin may be present behind the ear. Transitory loss of hair sometimes occurs in the temporal area.

5. Some degree of facial asymmetry is present preoperatively in all patients and will often remain postoperatively.
6. Normal postoperative swelling will mask many fine wrinkles and lessen deep folds for several months. A return of normal expression lines must be expected by 3 to 6 months [191].
7. Rhytidectomy is a major operation with all its attendant risks [187].

Patient Instructions

Preoperative photographs are a medicolegal necessity and a useful adjunct as many rhytidectomy patients have not scrutinized their appearance for several years. All aspirin- and estrogen-containing medications are stopped at least 2 weeks prior to surgery. If hair tinting is used, it is done preoperatively and not before 6 weeks postoperatively. The patient is encouraged to shampoo with pHisoHex for 3 days prior to surgery. Antibiotics are given only when a silastic chin implant is inserted.

SURGICAL PRINCIPLES

Although each patient deserves an individualized operative plan to correct a specific deformity, certain principles are common to all rhytidectomies (Fig. 16-7). The key decisions are whether to include a particular step (lipectomy, platysmal flaps), how extensive a dissection to make, and what incisional variations to use (hairline, previous operations).

Preparation

The patient is placed on a comfortable, well-padded operating table with the upper end elevated approximately 20 degrees. Fredericks [77, 78] recommends a contoured narrow head support that allows simultaneous suturing of both sides while other surgeons prefer a cerebellar headrest. The hair is clipped with scissors in the postauricular and temporal regions as required.

The planned incision line, area of dissection, and appropriate reference points are drawn. The standard reference lines include the midline over the chin, the submental crease, the upper cervical line, which represents the direction of pull, and the anterior border of the sternocleidomastoid muscle. The planned incision is then marked (patterns are not used) [99, 133]. The extent of dissection is drawn, usually extending transversely across the neck at the level of the thyroid cartilage and up to the end of the posterior scalp incision. Superiorly, the dissection line extends from a point 2 cm lateral to the eyebrow downward to the lateral border of the malar prominence, then across the cheeks to the nasolabial fold, continuing along the jowl line and ending in the submental crease. The hair is matted with sterile water-soluble lubrication jelly, which obviates the need for rubber bands, hair clips, or aluminum foil. The face is prepped with a clear sterile solution and then injected with local anesthetic. A copious amount (150–200 ml) of *dilute* Xylocaine with epinephrine (1 : 200,000) is injected with a long No. 25 spinal needle [96]. If a submental dissection is planned, the neck region is injected first and then the right hemiface. Extensive injection produces "hydrostatic dissection," which is particularly valuable in the retroauricular area.

Incisions

Factors in the selection of the incision line must include the patient's desires, hairline, and normal coiffure and the surgeon's recommendation (Fig. 16-8). In the *temporal* region, the classic incision is located within the hair. It is crescent shaped, extending in a slightly posterior direction before curving anteriorly, with the termination point about 2 cm above the lateral eyebrow. This incision is coupled with a crescent excision of scalp, which tightens the temporal region. Alternatively, a temporal incision anterior to the hairline is used for the following patients: (1) those with a receding hairline who do not wish further elevation of the hairline, (2) those with sparse hair, (3) younger patients (less than 45) who may be candidates for a secondary lift, and (4) those with significant crow's-feet. Although this anterior incision is condemned by certain surgeons for being too conspicuous, it is often accepted by patients provided the alternatives are presented preoperatively and the permanence of the scars is emphasized. The senior author employs this incision in approximately one-third of rhytidectomy cases. Where upward lifting is desired and a great deal of excess skin must be excised, a transverse temporal incision is added.

In the *preauricular* area, the choice is between a pretragal and a posttragal incision, the latter originally proposed by Joseph [117]. Classically, the straight-line incision has given way to a curvilinear modification with a small indentation above the tragus to prevent any longitudinal scar contracture. Advocates of the posttragal incision stress concealment of the scar whereas its critics note deformation of tragal projection as well as loss of the pretragal crease [106]. The authors generally prefer the pretragal incision as it is rarely visible and minimizes possible tragal deformities. The earlobe is generally detached with a small 2-mm cuff of facial skin at its base. This maneuver ensures preservation of the natural contour and avoids subsequent traction that will create satyr-ears.

In the *retroauricular* area, the classic incision was just below or in the groove. Unfortunately, all incisions in this area tend to migrate inferiorly. Therefore, placement within the cephaloauricular groove risks subsequent visibility, difficult suturing, and hygienic problems [95]. For these reasons the incision is brought onto the posterior concha approximately 3 to 4 mm above the groove.

In the *scalp* area, the classic incision went straight back and then downward along the hairline. The upper transverse scar tended to be hypertrophic while the lower descending scar was usually visible. Consequently, the scalp incision has been modified. On a line with the tragus, the incision passes back into the scalp, but with creation of a small superiorly based triangular flap in the

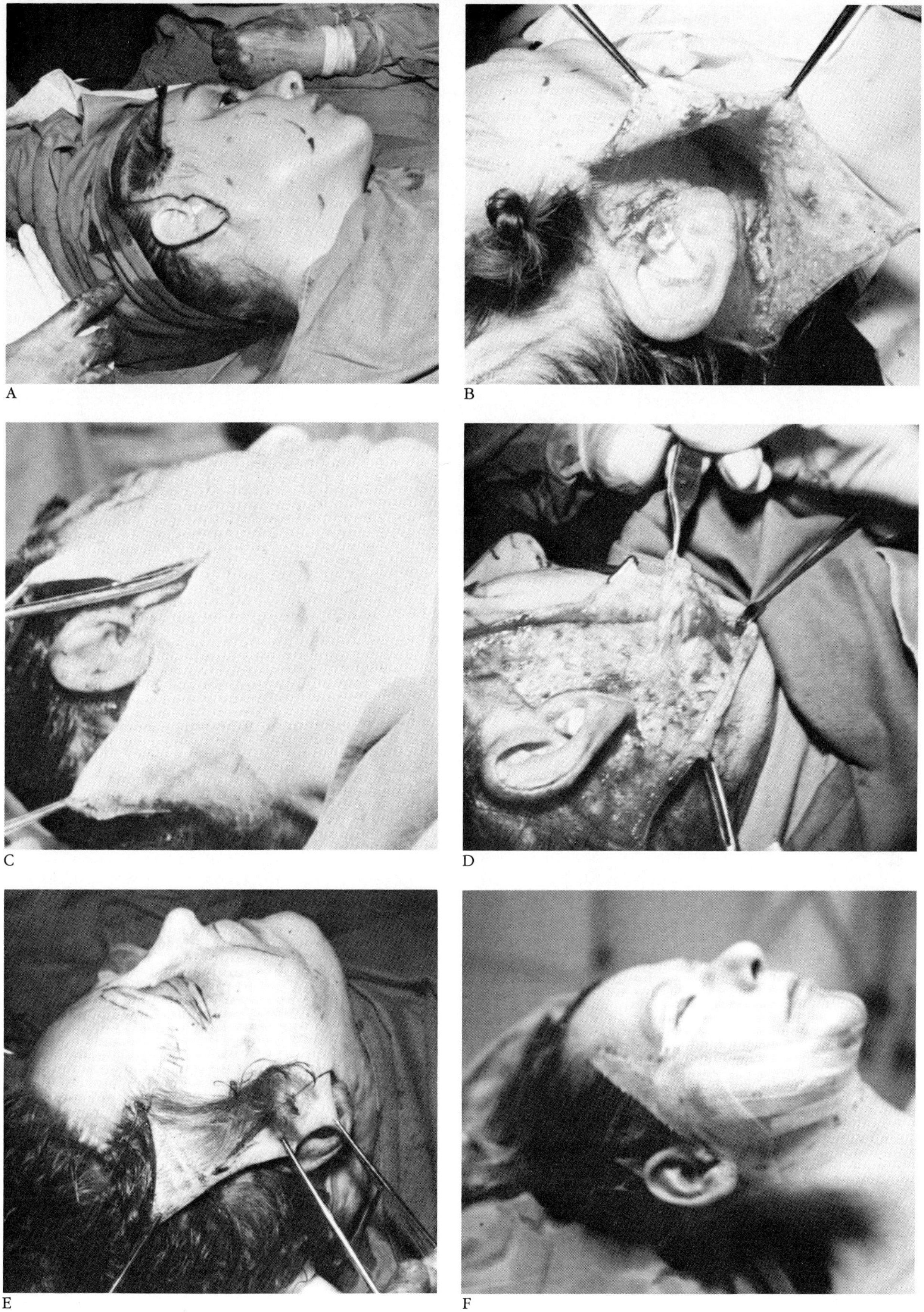

Figure 16-7. Rhytidectomy technique.

A. Incision consists of an L-shaped temporal extension, a curved pretragal portion, retroauricular prolongation with extension on the concha, and backward passage into the scalp.

B. The skin is undermined.

C. With traction on the flaps, the skin is partially split to facilitate vision and modification of the deep structures.

D. Platysma and SMAS traction flaps are done as well as lipectomies.

E. With traction on the flaps, the excess tissue is excised.

F. Following closure, the dressing is applied.

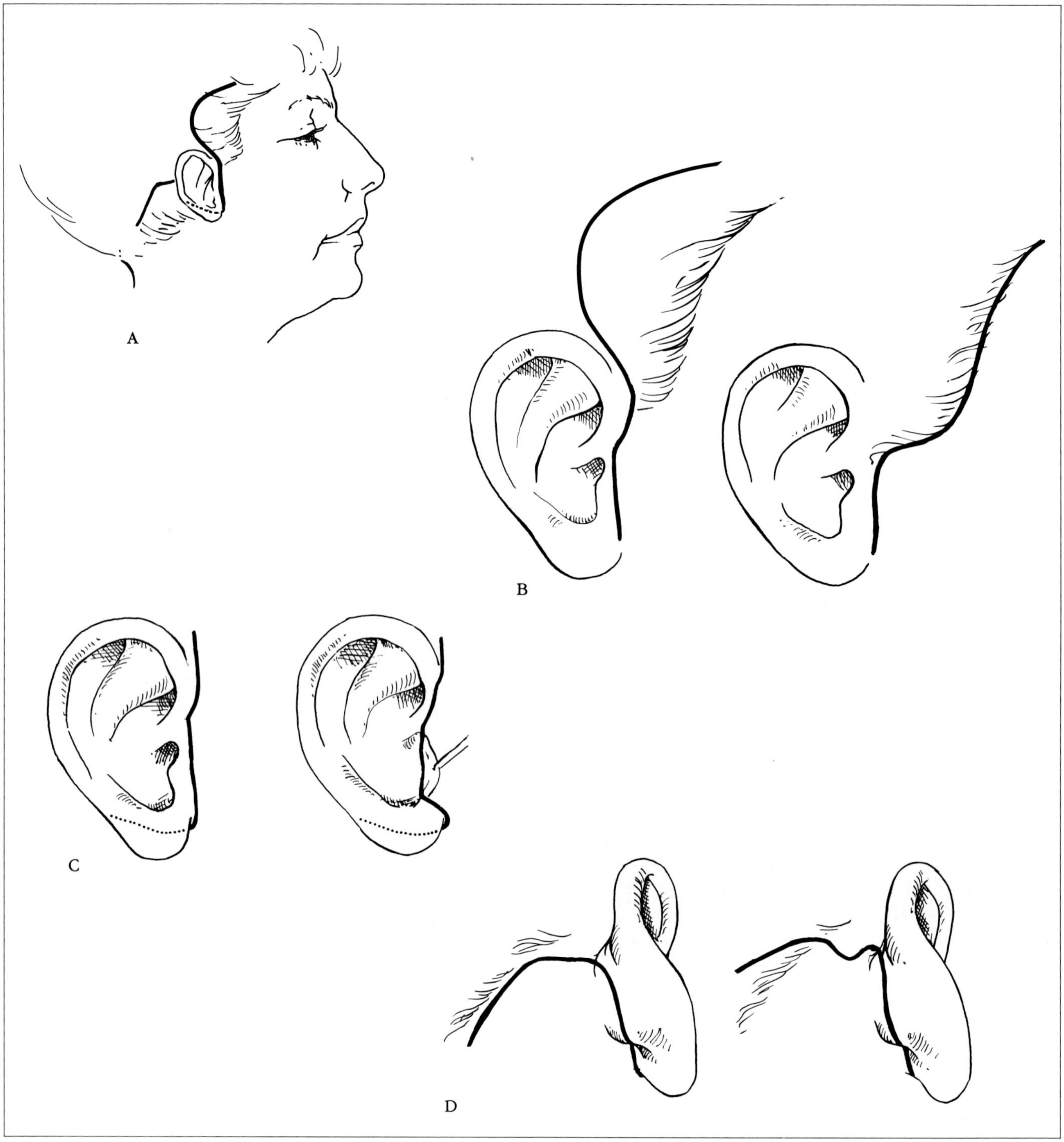

Figure 16-8. Variations in rhytidectomy incisions.

A. The standard incision has four components: temporal, preauricular, retroauricular, and posterior scalp.

B. In the temporal region, the choice is either behind or in front of the hairline.

C. The preauricular incision may be in front of or behind the tragus.

D. The retroauricular incision is always placed on the concha and usually back into the scalp, rather than the classic incision at the hairline.

mastoid area [152]. This dart of skin serves to break the straight-line contracture and minimize the incidence of hypertrophic scars. Prolongation of the scalp incision beyond 6 cm is infrequent, and continuation to the posterior midline is rarely necessary [122]. Thus, the incision we use most frequently consists of four parts: (1) temporal, depending on the patient's hairline, (2) a preauricular curvilinear pretragal location, (3) retroauricular, on the concha, and (4) a transverse continuation into the scalp with a superior triangular dart of skin (Fig. 16-9).

Undermining

Questions regarding dissection include its extent, sequence, depth, and instrumentation [94]. The extent of undermining varies with each patient, but it must go beyond the folds and wrinkles one is trying to correct. Advocates of subfascial techniques would defend a more limited skin dissection as they believe that correction of the foundation will eliminate their more superficial expression [132]. The depth of dissection varies in each region: (1) in the posterior scalp, deep to the hair follicles, (2) over the mastoid and sternocleidomastoid, very superficial, (3) over the parotid region, through the subcutaneous fat, and (4) in the temporal region, deep to the hair follicles (Fig. 16-10). In general, the dissection is begun with a knife, but once skin elevation is achieved, one switches to straight round-tipped serrated scissors. In contrast to the blind push technique, we prefer to dissect under direct vision. Initial hemostasis is with a standard cautery, but a bipolar cautery is used more distally where the risk of injuring the nerve branches is greatest. The use of a lighted retractor is beneficial.

Dissection begins in the mastoid area because it is the most dependent, least painful, and easiest for determining the surgical plane. If one has injected liberally, dissection with serrated scissors is simple; otherwise, knife dissection is necessary to separate the rigidly adherent skin. Flap elevation over the sternocleidomastoid muscle must be superficial to avoid penetrating the muscle, thereby increasing bleeding and risking severance of the greater auricular nerve. At this point, the extent of dissection is comparable to that in many of the classic face-lifts. Hemostasis is achieved.

Traction is placed on the skin flaps in the temporal and retroauricular regions in the direction of the anticipated lift. The elevated skin flap is then split, often for a distance of 1.5 to 2.0 cm. This maneuver opens the skin flap and offers better visualization. The dissection is resumed, completing the flap elevation over the cheek area out toward the nasolabial folds. Once the anterior border of the parotid is passed, accidental descent into the fat pad of Bichat must be avoided. The cervical region is approached from the sternocleidomastoid muscle, leaving sufficient subcutaneous fat on the skin. Too superficial a dissection along the dermis results in adherence to the platysma; too deep a dissection risks penetration of the platysma. The dissection is carried anteriorly and joins with the submental dissection. Hemostasis is again obtained.

SMAS and Platysma

Although SMAS and platysma procedures are not new, resurgence of interest has occurred as they appear to offer improvement of difficult deformities (jowls, neck bands) as well as longer-lasting results. Platysma surgery begins submentally where the anterior borders may be resected or partially divided but are always plicated. The SMAS may be either plicated or converted to a distinct flap. In 1960 Aufricht [11] described a two-layer rhytidectomy procedure with suspension of the loose areolar tissue by plication to the parotid fascia. He used it for correction of nasolabial folds and jowls but emphasized that the improvement might be transitory. Subsequently, Skoog [193], Peterson [168], and others drew attention to the SMAS as a distinct entity that could be handled by traction procedures, plication, and specific flaps. Tipton [207] and later Rees and Aston [176] performed comparison rhytidectomy studies employing skin-only procedures on one side and plication or subfascial traction on the opposite side. No significant difference was noted at 1 year. In these studies, traction was placed on the lateral border of the platysma muscle, which was then sutured posteriorly. Since neither the cervical skin nor the platysma muscle was completely undermined and a distinct platysmal flap was not created in all patients, comparison to current procedures is of limited value. It should be noted that despite finding little difference in their initial 25 patients Rees and Aston [176] have subsequently become strong advocates of modern platysmal and SMAS flaps in selected patients. The value of these procedures is dramatically illustrated in patients who remain dissatisfied following skin-only rhytidectomy. Many problems can be corrected with deep procedures that should have been done at the original operation (Fig. 16-11).

It is our opinion that SMAS plication and SMAS flaps are different procedures [13]. It is our custom to plicate the SMAS in 80 percent of cases, either in a superolateral direction to ameliorate the jowls or in a vertical direction to tighten the cheeks (Fig. 16-12) [24]. Distinct SMAS flaps are used by the junior author in 20 percent of cases to improve the nasolabial folds or jowls (Fig. 16-13). As described by Peterson [168], the SMAS flap is made 4 mm below and parallel to the zygomatic arch and 4 mm anterior to the preauricular incision line before it is continued along the posterior border of the platysma muscle. The flap is raised first over the parotid gland, whose dimensions are palpated, and then divided superiorly [119]. The platysma muscle is completely elevated and a partial-width muscle flap created. Then, with upward traction, the excess SMAS is excised and sutured to the zygomatic fascia with 4-0 Vicryl. The platysmal flap is anchored to the mastoid fascia. We have not seen regrowth of the platysma [73]. Because of the close proximity of the facial nerve branches and major vessels beneath the platysma, caution and surgical expertise are required. The admonition of Adamson and Toksu [2] is realistic: "This operative technique is not for the occasional or self-taught cosmetic surgeon, but must be reserved for those well-trained and significantly skilled in reconstruction in this area."

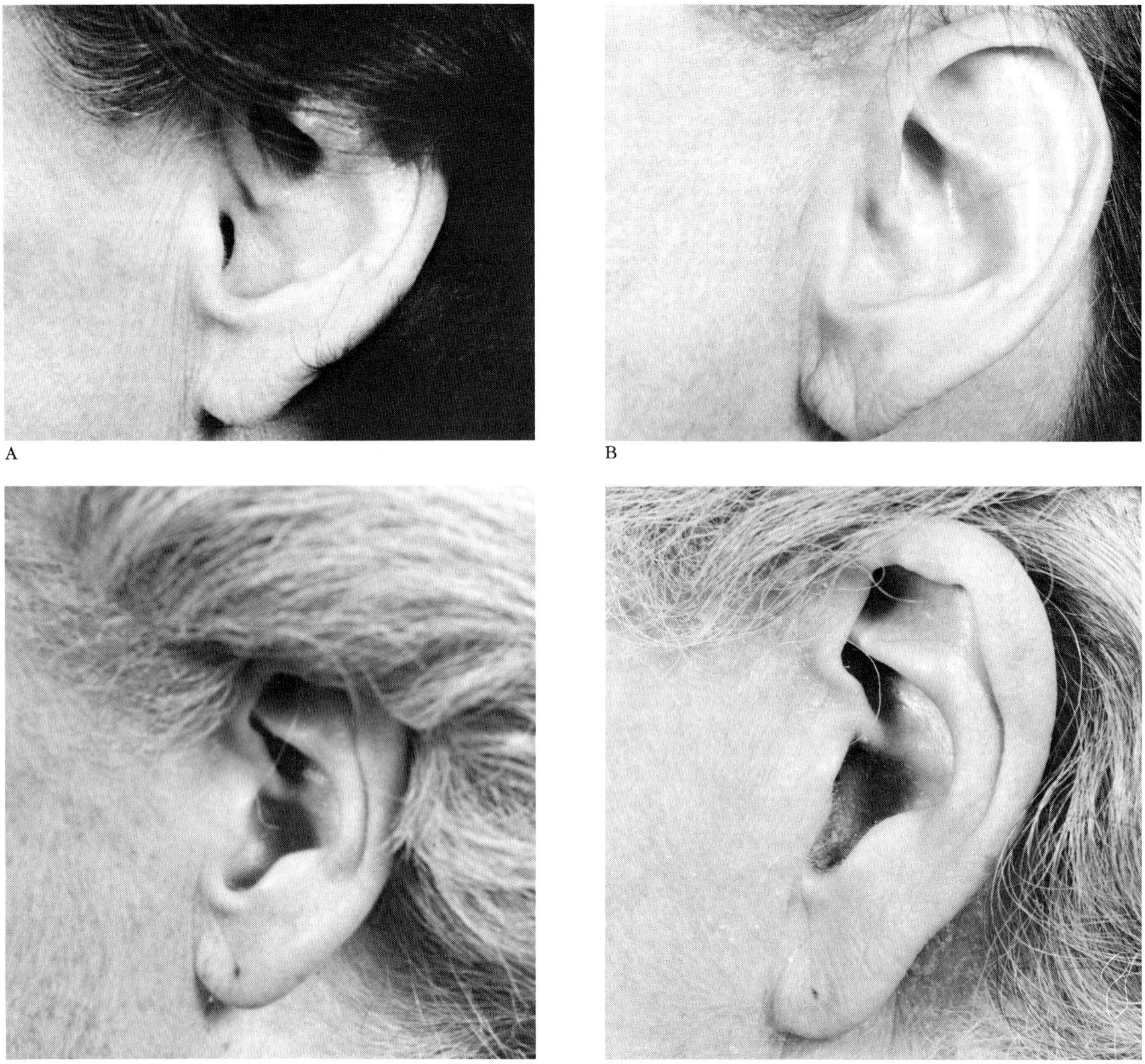

A B C D

Figure 16-9. Rhytidectomy incisions.

A, B. Preoperative and postoperative condition following rhytidectomy with virtually invisible preauricular incision as well as temporal incision at the hairline.

C, D. Preoperative and postoperative condition following rhytidectomy with posttragal incision. Note obscuring of the infratragal notch.

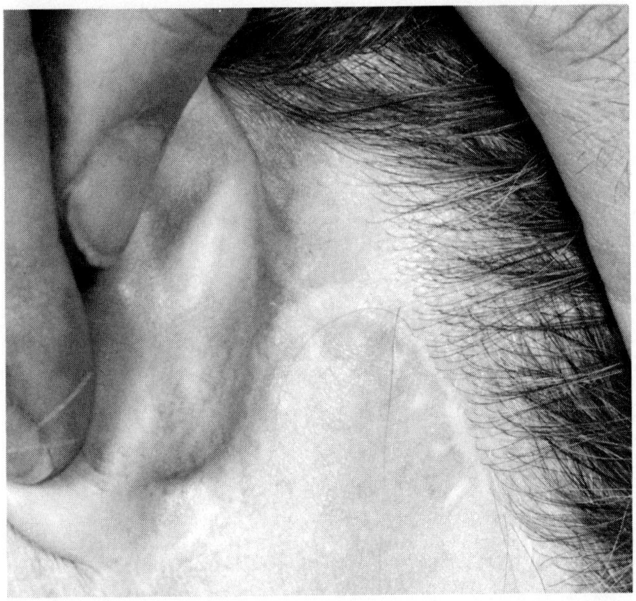

E

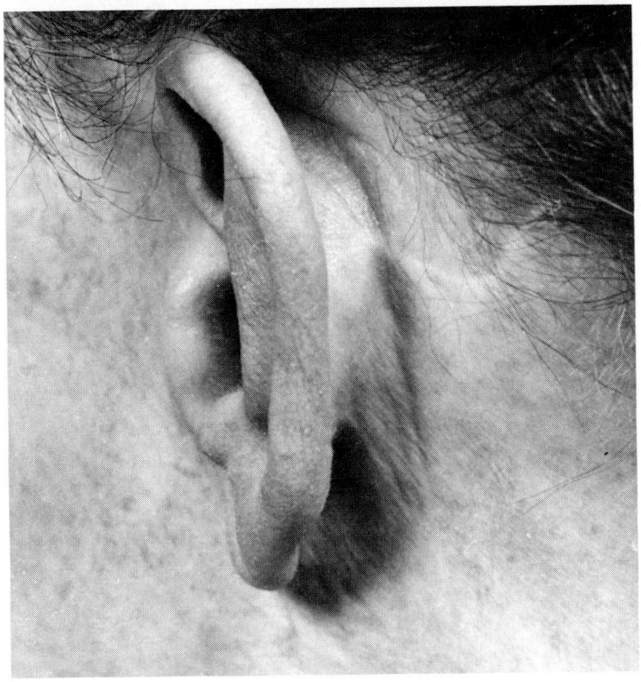

F

E. Classic retroauricular incision with descent below the groove and marked visibility at the hairline.

F. In contrast, the recommended incision is on the ear, incorporates a dart to prevent contracture, and reestablishes the hairline.

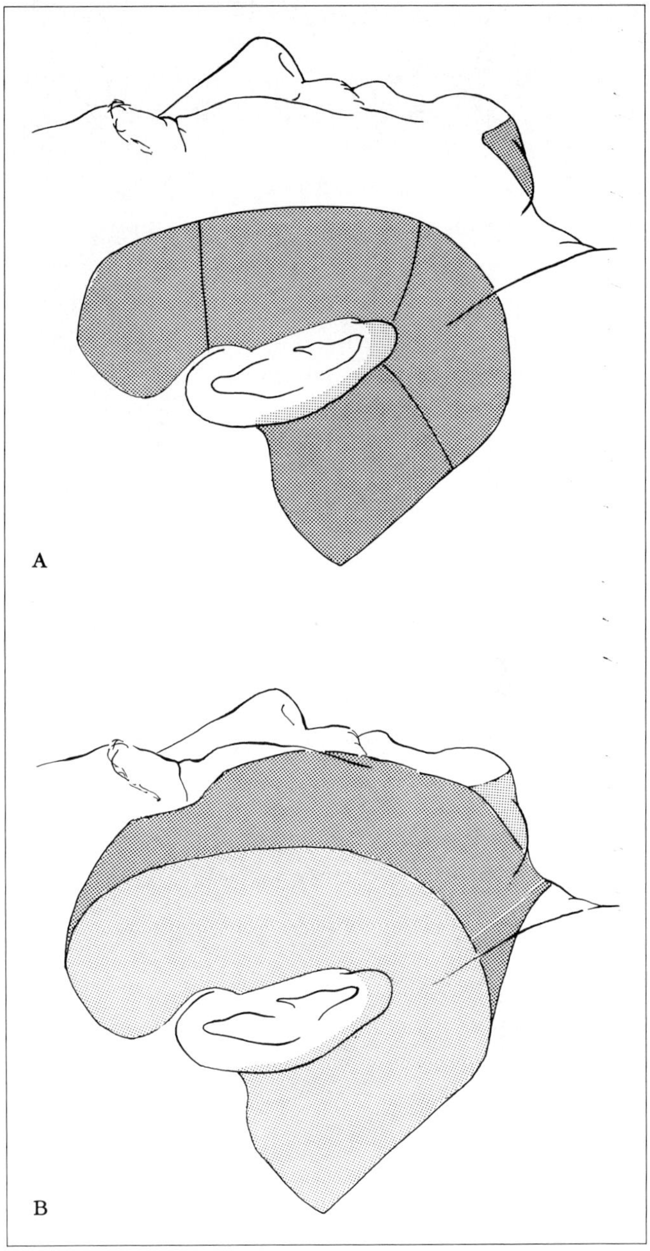

Figure 16-10. In the extended cervicofacial rhytidectomy, the dissection is done in three steps. First, the submental area is defatted and the platysmal borders are plicated.

A. Second, the flaps are elevated in the posterior scalp, sternocleidomastoid, preauricular, and temporal regions.

B. Third, the dissection is continued anteriorly following an initial split of the cheek flap.

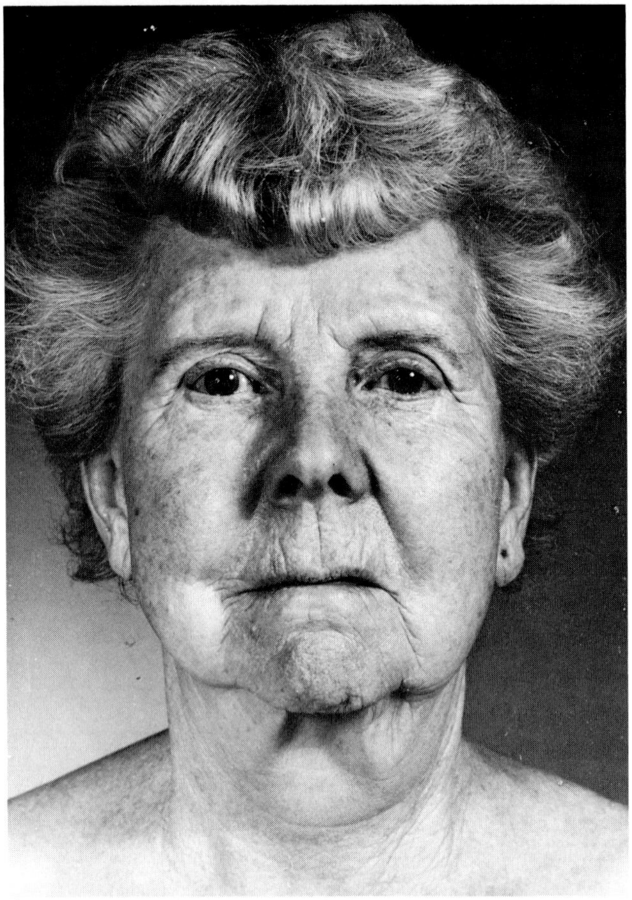

A

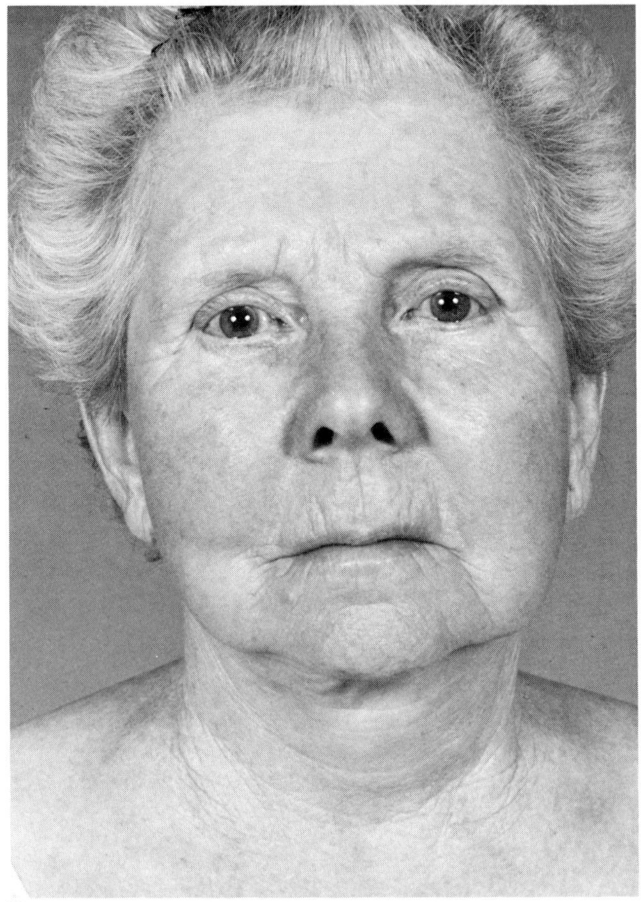

B

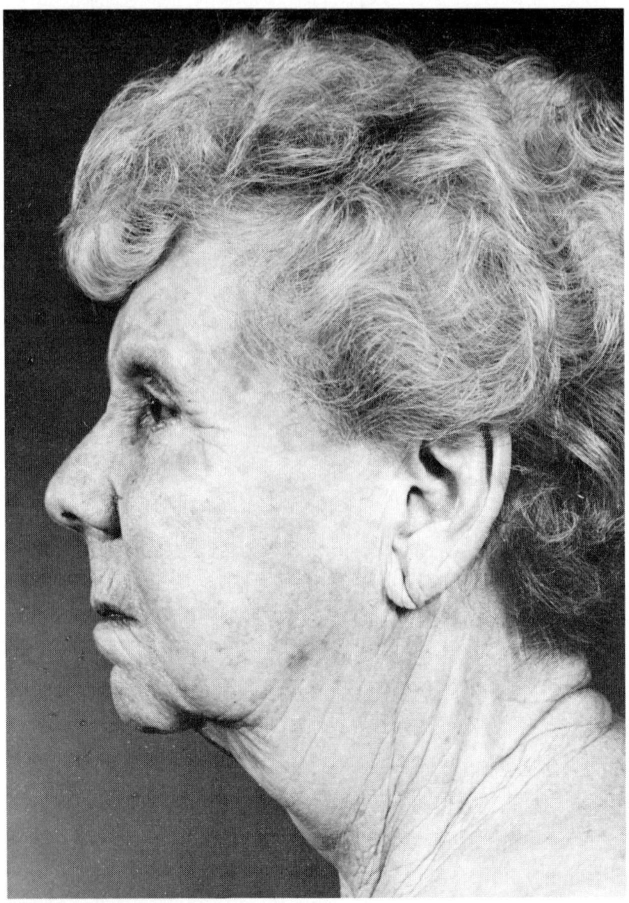

C

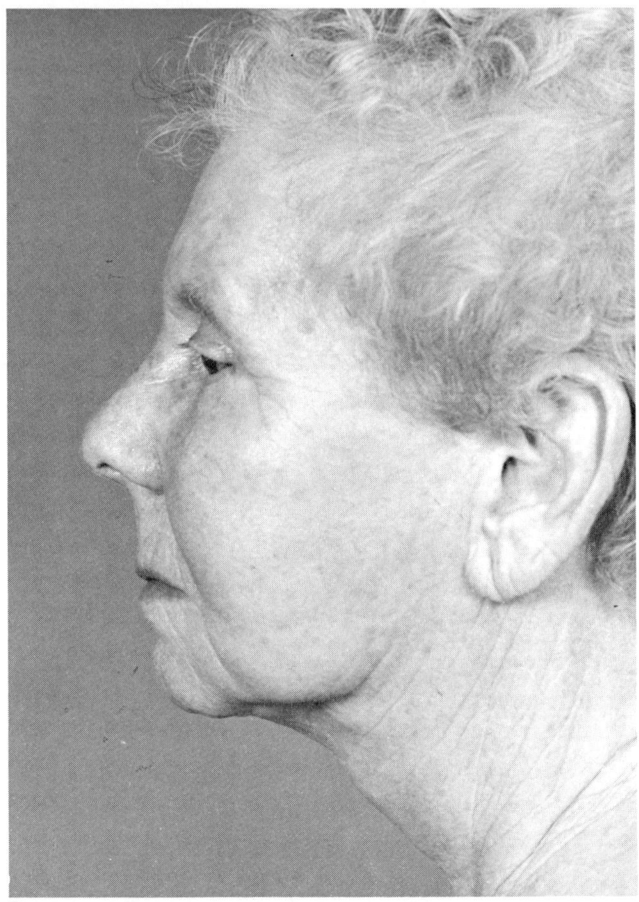

D

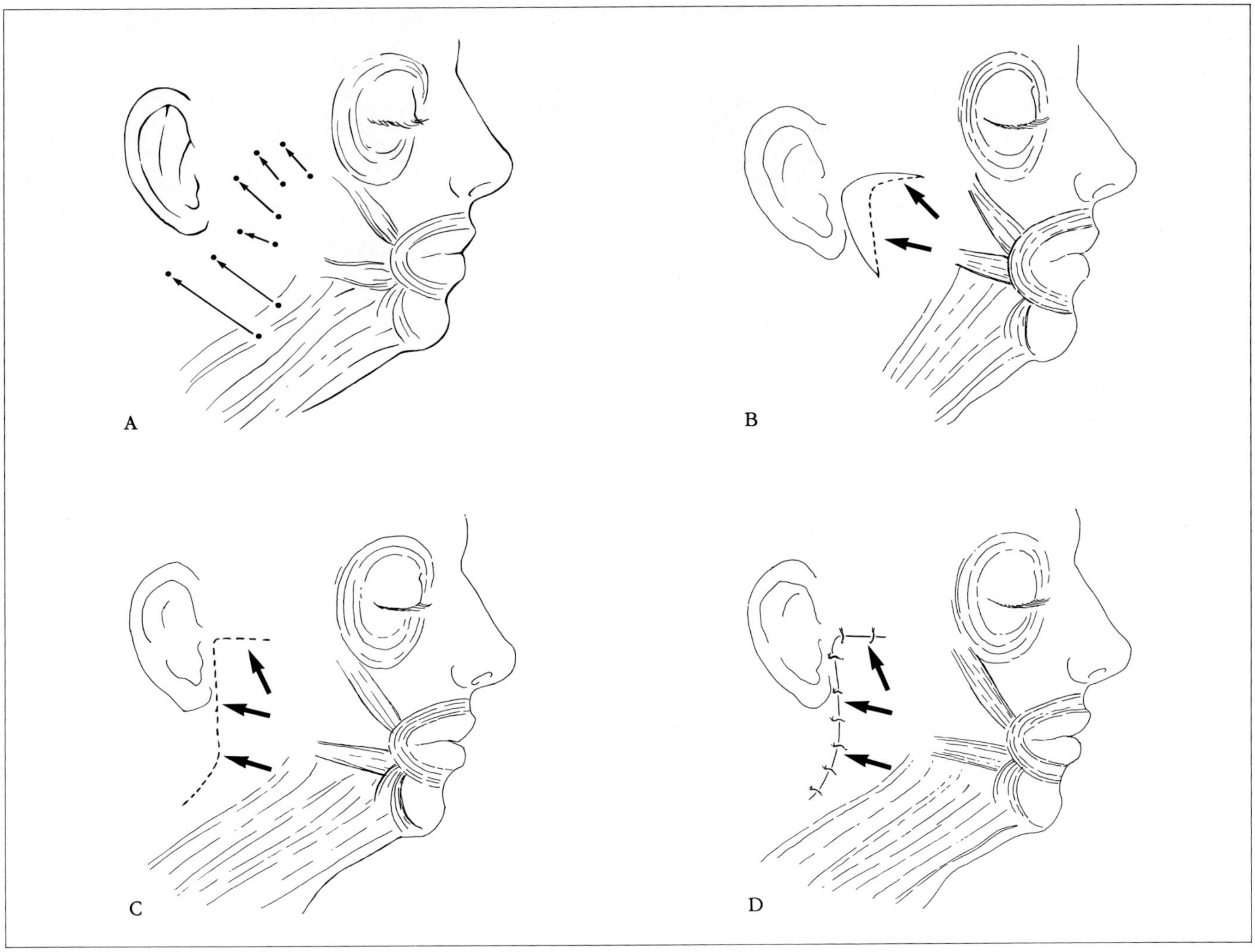

Figure 16-12. Alterations of the SMAS may be achieved by either plication or a flap.

A. SMAS plication is done at numerous points, tightening the soft tissues.

B. A localized SMAS flap can improve jowls and lessen the nasolabial folds.

C. Alternatively, the SMAS flap can join with the posterior border of the platysma.

D. Upward traction on the SMAS smooths the jowl area whereas posterior traction on the platysma tightens the neck.

Figure 16-11. The need for platysmal surgery.

A, C. Six months following skin-only rhytidectomy done elsewhere, patient complained of little improvement.

B, D. Result following medial platysma plication, partial platysmal flaps, SMAS plication, and lipectomy. Additional correction of the jowls would have required an upward traction rhytidectomy. No significant skin excision.

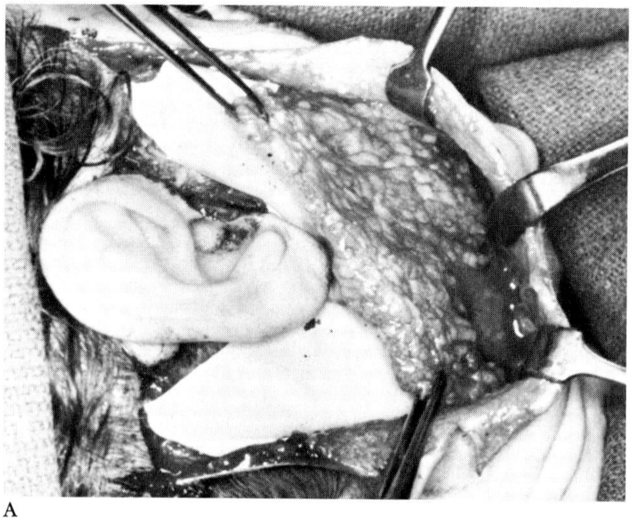

A

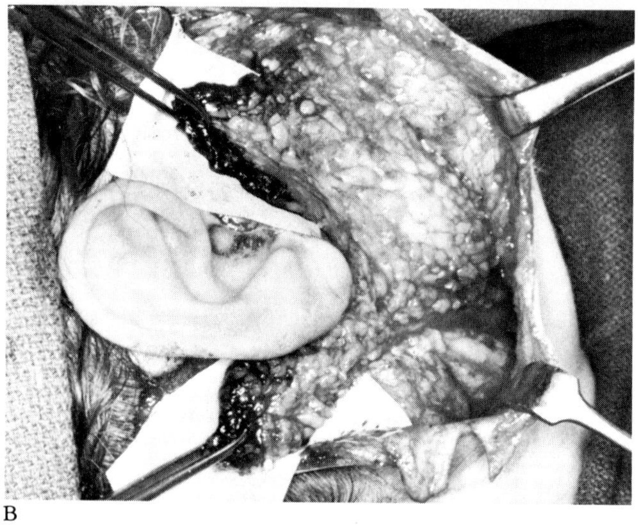

B

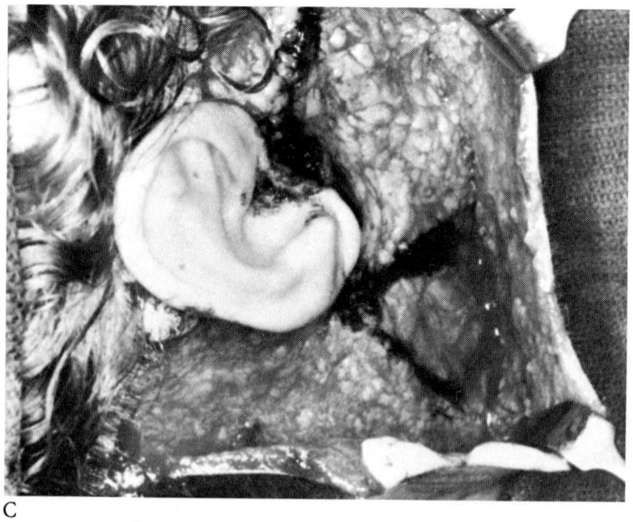

C

Figure 16-13
A. The SMAS flap is outlined at the level of the zygomatic arch, several millimeters in front of the preauricular incision, and often continued inferiorly along the posterior border of the platysma. With traction on the flap, the face is literally elevated and tightened.
B. The flap is divided into a superior SMAS flap and an inferior platysmal flap. Note that the platysma will not be defatted until all elevation is completed.
C. The excess SMAS flap is excised and sutured into position. The platysma is anchored to the mastoid and then defatted.

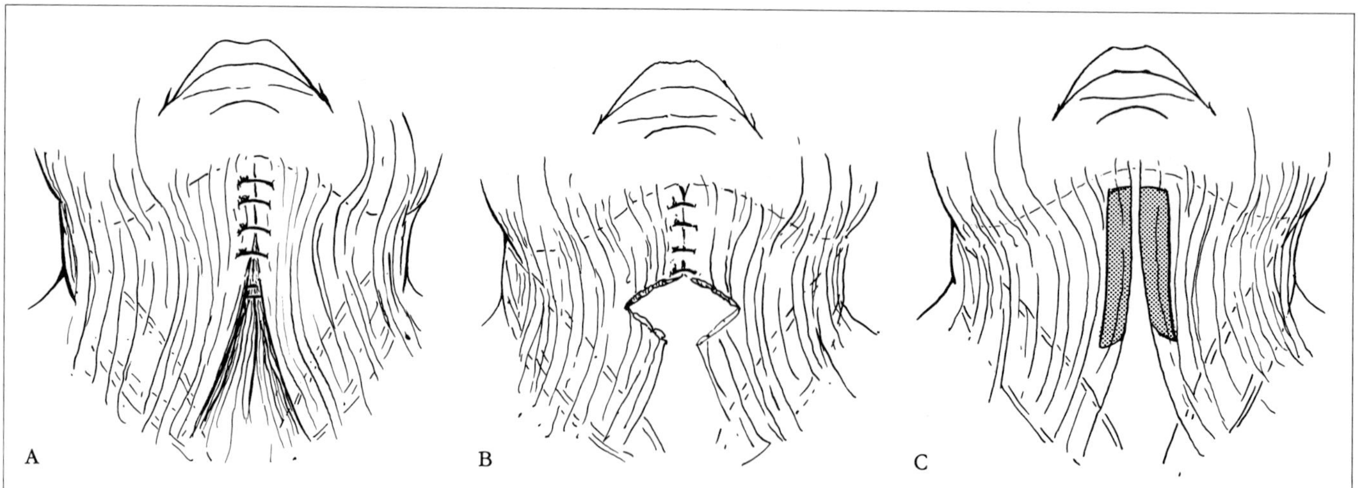

Figure 16-14. Medial modifications of the platysma muscle.
A. Most often, the anterior borders are separated, and it is necessary to reapproximate them by direct suturing.
B. If distinct bands are present, partial-width transection is done followed by plication.
C. If heavy anterior borders exist, they are excised followed by plication.

As noted previously, surgery on the platysma muscle is not new, but the percentage of cases and surgeons attempting it has risen dramatically [163]. Anteriorly, heavy redundant anterior borders are best excised whereas widely separated borders are reapproximated (Fig. 16-14). Partial medial transection is done to ensure division of obvious anterior bands and to facilitate approximation. In *all* cases, the anterior borders are approximated with 3-0 Dexon sutures, and those without significant separation are reinforced. The goal is to create a continuous hammock that can be elevated, thereby achieving a more definite cervicomental angle. Laterally, the platysma border is freed over a distance of 5 cm, and then the muscle is separated from its deep connections by blunt dissection. At this point, we perform one of the following: (1) traction with fixation to the mastoid fascia, (2) partial transection with superolateral suspension, or (3) complete transection (Fig. 16-15). Once the platysma has been *undermined* to the midline, the lateral border is stretched toward the mastoid area. If it moves easily, traction sutures are inserted [153]. If the muscle is thick and immobile, it is partially divided and a flap created. Complete transection is done only in patients with short, thick necks where a distinct separation of face and neck is desired. Any patient having platysma surgery must be warned preoperatively that a feeling of tightness about the throat may be present for several weeks postoperatively. Occasionally, the platysma may be a thin insubstantial structure precluding flap traction.

Figure 16-15. Lateral modifications of the platysma muscle.
A. Traction on the lateral border.
B. Partial-width platysmal flaps for increased traction.
C. Complete division of the platysma muscle is done only in patients with short, fat necks.

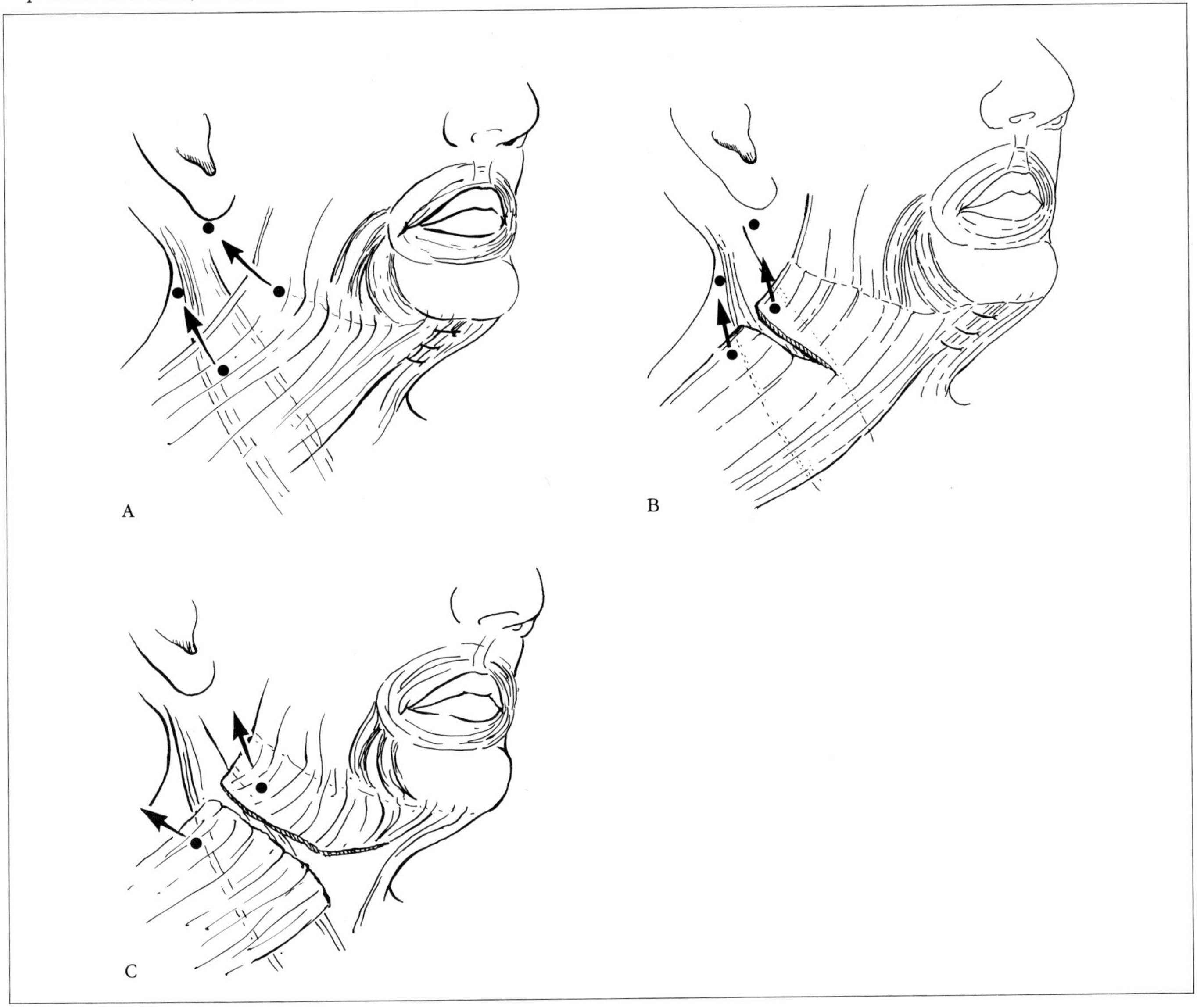

Lipectomy

Discrete fat resection or lipectomy has gradually been extended to include "fat contouring" procedures [154,

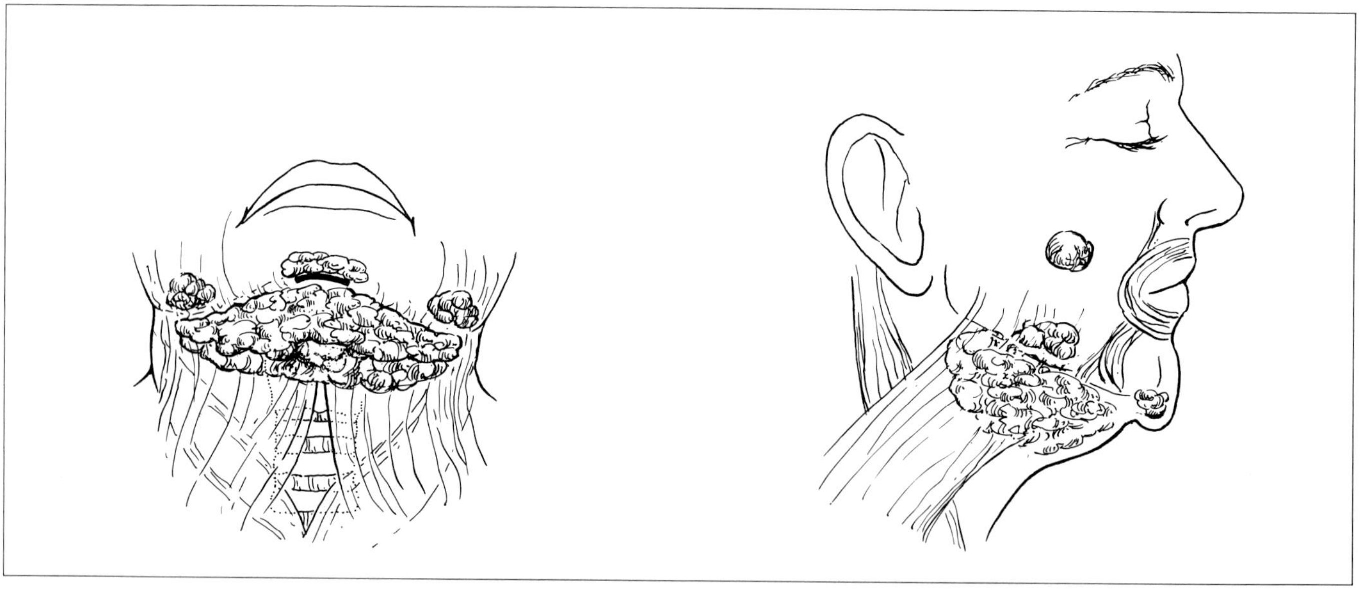

Figure 16-16. Facial lipectomies are performed as indicated including the entire submental-submandibular area, the chin, the cheeks, and the buccal fat pad.

155]. The goal is to give definition to the mandibular border and to recreate a sharp cervicomental angle. The need for fat contouring is determined preoperatively with each deposit carefully evaluated (Fig. 16-16). Actual excess fat is defined as that remaining on top of the platysma muscle once the overlying skin with a 2- to 3-mm subcutaneous fat layer has been elevated (Fig. 16-17). Following modification of all the deep structures, the fat is removed in a strip 4 to 5 cm wide extending across the entire neck. Both edges must be carefully beveled or distinct ridges will be palpated postoperatively. As noted by Gonzalez-Ulloa [88, 89, 91, 92], fat can be rotated to areas of bony hypoplasia to restore facial contour. Submental fat can be used to build up a receding chin, submandibular fat to augment a pencil-thin mandible, and buccal fat to restore a malar prominence [167, 184].

Traction, Excision, and Closure

Once undermining is completed, all deep procedures are performed, and hemostasis is achieved, the final skin resection can be determined. The face is derotated from the lateral to the vertical position, and clamps are applied to the flaps in the temporal and postauricular area. The skin flaps are advanced in a superolateral direction, thereby elevating the face and neck. If the flaps are elevated too much superiorly, the hairline will be raised and hairless preauricular skin will be inserted into the temporal region. If the flaps are pulled too far posteriorly, correction cannot occur. Under traction, the overlapping skin is split up to the scalp margin, and key tension sutures are inserted (Fig. 16-18). When the degree of lifting is satisfactory, excess skin is excised segmentally. Traction and excision are two separate steps; traction determines the degree of lifting while excision varies segmentally and objectively (Fig. 16-19). The temporal incision can be extended transversely and the flap rotated superiorly to minimize hair excision or posterior displacement of the temporal hairline. The preauricular skin is brought directly posterior and resected with *minimal* tension on the flap. In the postauricular region, the scalp is rotated anteriorly, thereby reestablishing the postauricular hairline and avoiding a step deformity [112]. The retroauricular skin flap is excised conservatively to minimize tension on the flap, but sufficiently to avoid creases. With experience, the excess skin can be accurately estimated and excised en bloc, and then a single subcuticular suture closure can be performed with 4-0 Vicryl [213]. Measurement of the excised skin is not necessary [135, 204]. Drains of split silicone tubing are regularly employed. The dressing consists of paper tape strips placed from zygoma to zygoma, thus supporting the neck, followed by petrolatum gauzes, multiple cotton gauzes, then cotton pads and a gauze dressing. An elastic bandage is not used.

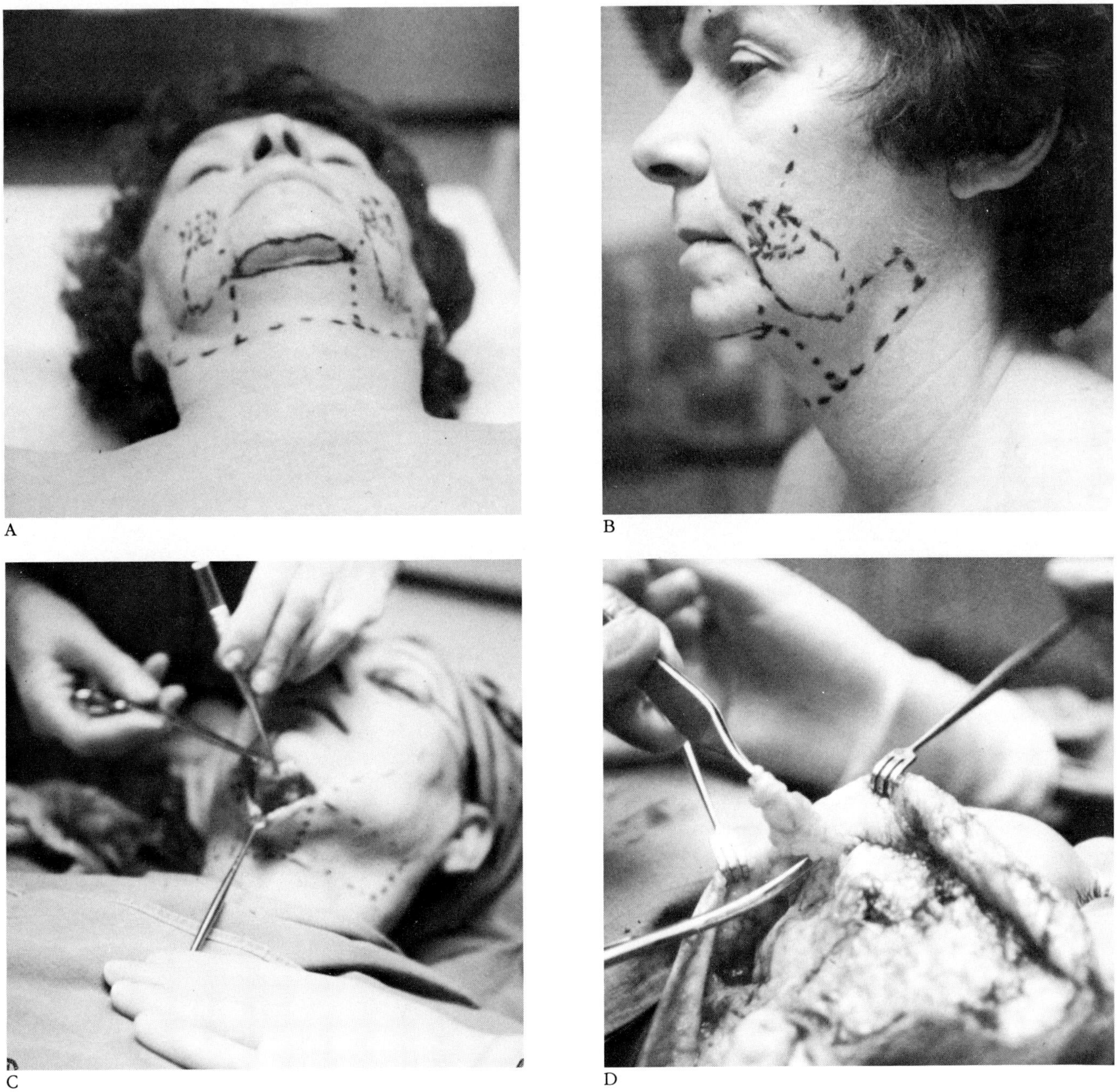

Figure 16-17
A, B. Patient undergoing extended cervicofacial rhytidectomy with lipectomy and correction of chin ptosis.
C. The initial resection is through a submental incision.
D. The submandibular fat is excised off the platysma muscle through the lateral flap.

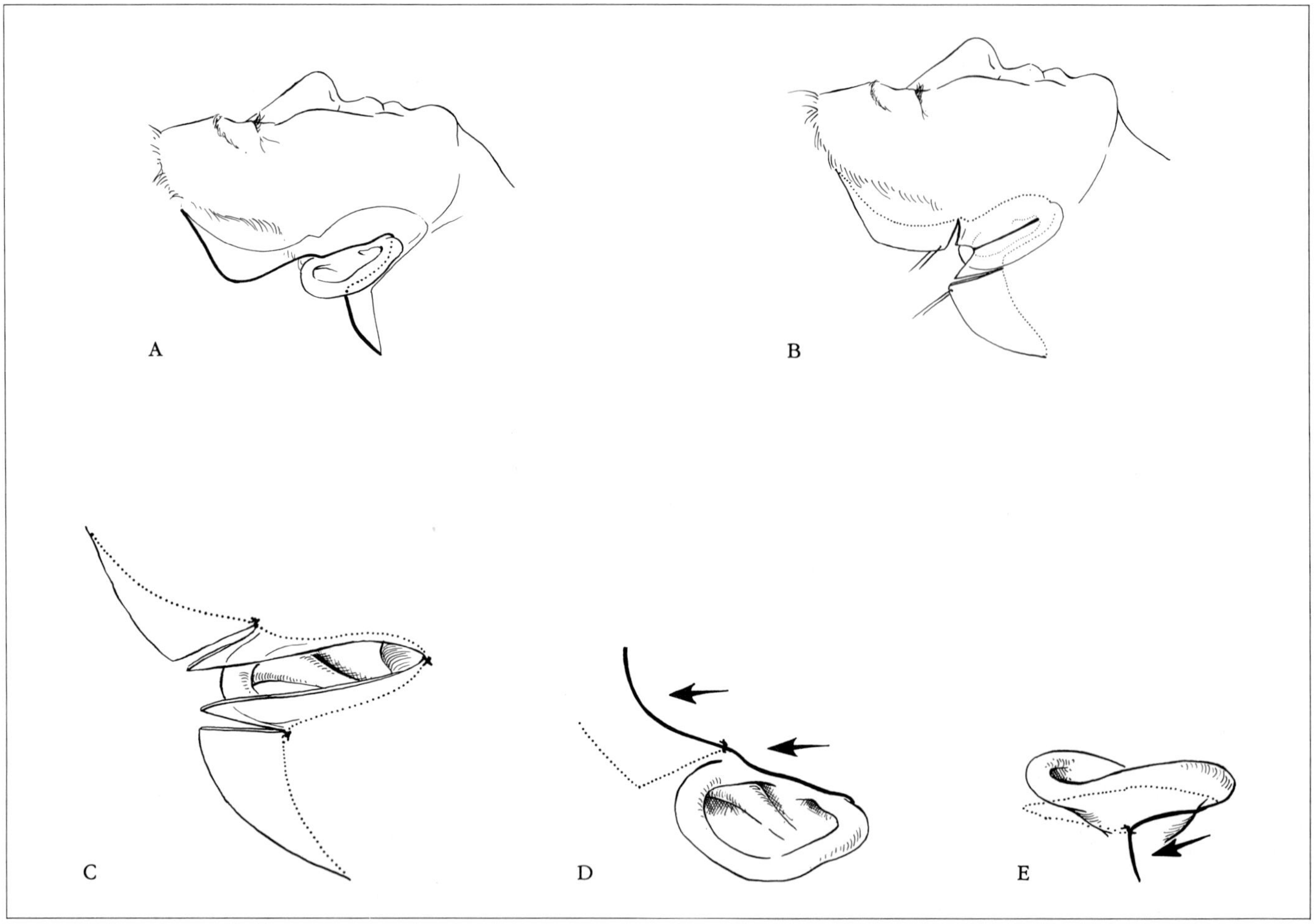

Figure 16-18. Traction and skin excision.

A. Traction is placed on the flaps.

B. The overlapping flaps are split in the temporal and retroauricular areas.

C. Key traction sutures are inserted.

D, E. Arrows indicate direction of advancement.

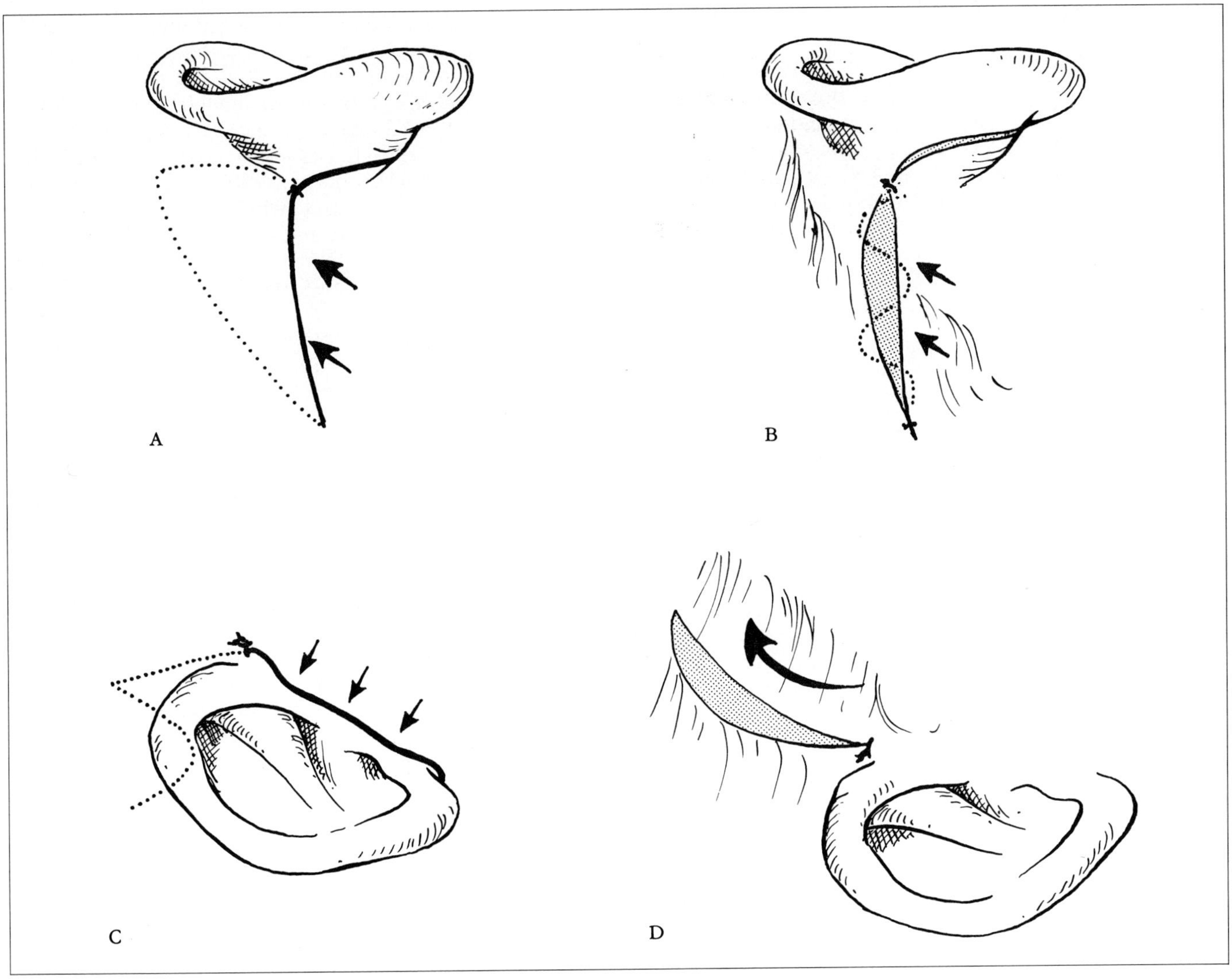

Figure 16-19. Wound closure usually progresses from posterior scalp to temporal region.

A, B. Posteriorly, excess skin is excised and rotated to reestablish the hairline, thus avoiding a step deformity.

C. The preauricular skin is approximated without tension.

D. The temporal flap is rotated superoanteriorly to avoid pulling the hairline too far back.

SURGICAL TECHNIQUES

The selected surgical technique varies according to the patient's priorities, previous surgery, preference for incisions, modification of deep structures, and ancillary procedures. Overall, the operations represent a spectrum beginning with regional lifts, then the standard cervicofacial lift, and ultimately the extended cervicofacial lift [22, 56].

Regional Lifts

With an increasingly sophisticated population, patients are requesting and having aesthetic surgery at younger ages. This trend implies that a greater number of regional procedures will be done, both primarily and secondarily. For example, a woman in her midthirties may have her crow's-feet corrected by an extended temple-lift with modification of the orbicularis oculi muscle plus four-eyelid blepharoplasty. Five years later, amelioration of the jowls in the presence of normal neck contour may warrant only a classic skin rhytidectomy with SMAS plication rather than a complete cervicofacial rhytidectomy. It must be stressed that regional lifts differ markedly from "minilifts" as the undermining is more extensive and alterations of the deep structures ensure a more prolonged benefit.

TEMPLE-LIFT

The temple-lift, which extends from the temporal to the preauricular area, is indicated for patients concerned about their eyes, especially crow's-feet and lateral hooding, but without descent of the medial eyebrow. In most cases, the patient requests a blepharoplasty but emphasizes the crow's-feet and aging around the eyes (Fig. 16-20). As described by Gleason [83, 84], the skin in the lateral canthal area is elevated off the orbicularis oculi muscle, but the muscle is not altered. In order to rearrange the muscle, the incision must be extended downward at least to the tragus to gain the necessary exposure. Thus, one is not doing a minimal direct excision, but rather wide undermining of the lateral third of the face plus alteration of the deep structures [20, 201].

Preoperatively, the degree of desired eyebrow elevation is estimated. In most cases, a posthairline incision is used, but a prehairline incision may be necessary for patients with a previous rhytidectomy or thinning hair. The expected course of the frontal nerve branch, a line going from the earlobe to a point 1.5 cm above the lateral eyebrow, is marked. The area of undermining and the scalp are infiltrated with dilute local anesthetic. The forehead dissection is done first in the avascular subgaleal plane and continued below the orbital rim to release the fascial attachments. Next, a superficial subcutaneous dissection is completed over the cheeks and zygomatic area passing above the orbicularis oculi muscle. In contrast to Aston [10], who elevates the muscle with the skin flap, we prefer to leave the muscle in situ and splay it out with 4-0 Dexon sutures. Originally, the senior author divided the muscle along the lateral raphe and expanded it but found little advantage over outward traction. Division of the muscle does lead to more bleeding and occasionally a lateral depression, which can be filled with the excess SMAS flap in more extended procedures. It would appear prudent to use a graded approach: splaying of the muscle in minor and moderate cases, with complete division reserved for severe cases. Hemostasis is done with a bipolar coagulator to avoid damaging the frontal nerve branch. We have not found it necessary to divide the intervening tissue between the two dissection planes as recommended by Gleason [83, 84]. With upward traction on the skin flap, the degree of eyebrow elevation is checked, and then tacking sutures are inserted through splits in the anterior flap. Redundant tissue is excised flush with the incision line to avoid tension and alopecia. The wound is closed with a running 4-0 subcuticular Dexon suture. Blepharoplasties, both upper and lower, are then performed as indicated.

MELOPLASTY

The classic skin-only rhytidectomy is indicated for the patient whose deformity is confined to wrinkling of the cheeks, minor accentuation of the nasolabial folds, and early jowl formation (Fig. 16-21). If significant cervical problems are present, a more extensive procedure is required. This classic procedure is done in less than 5 percent of patients. The skin incision is in the temporal hairline, continuing behind the tragus, then above the sulcus, and ending in the scalp (Fig. 16-22). The dissection extends toward the nasolabial fold, along the jowls, downward across the mandibular border, and in the neck for several centimeters [209]. Hemostasis is then achieved. A SMAS flap and plications at several points in an upward direction are done to minimize heaviness in the jowl area. Since the dissection does not extend far onto the neck, platysmal traction is not possible nor should it be indicated if the patient was properly selected. Skin traction is exerted in a superolateral direction, with tension taken in the supraauricular and retroauricular areas.

Figure 16-20

A. Reduction of crow's-feet utilizing a temple-lift, four-eyelid blepharoplasty, and modification of the orbicularis muscle, either outward splaying or partial division.

B, D. A 34-year-old patient who complained of heavy eyelids, crow's-feet, and a tired appearance.

C, E. Result following a temple-lift plus anchor blepharoplasty. Note crispness of the upper eyelid fold and eradication of lateral hooding.

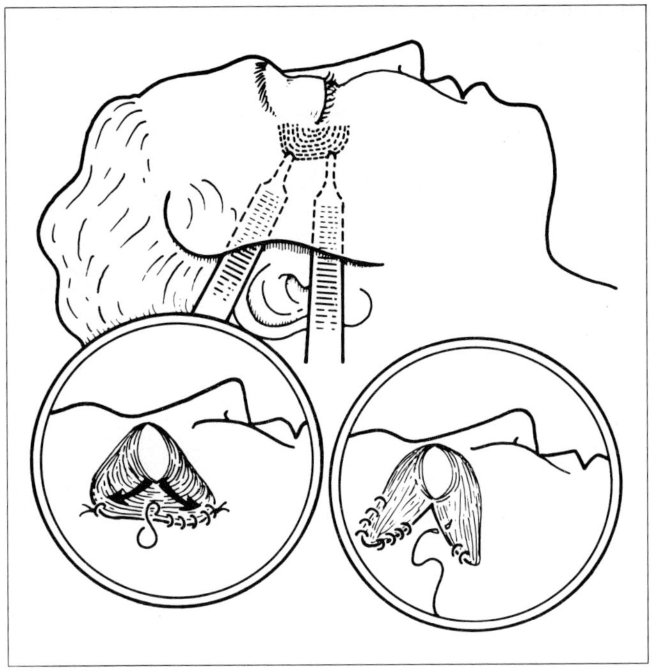

A

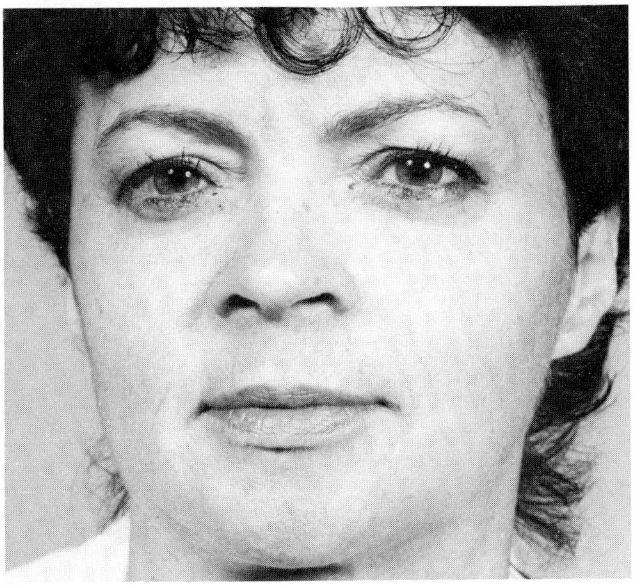

B

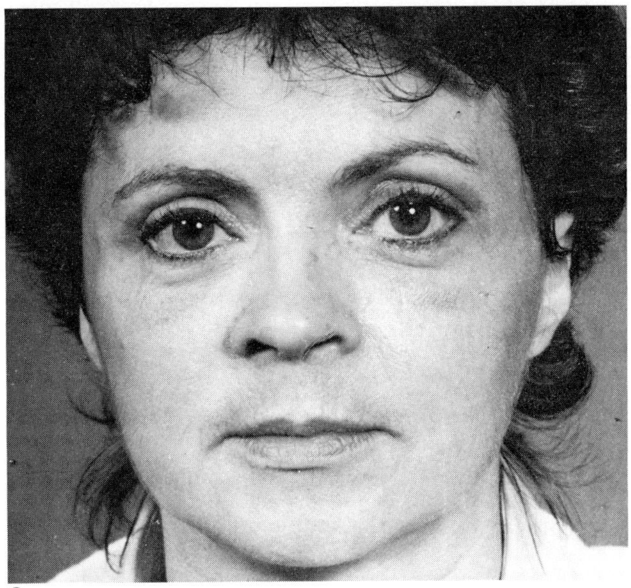

C

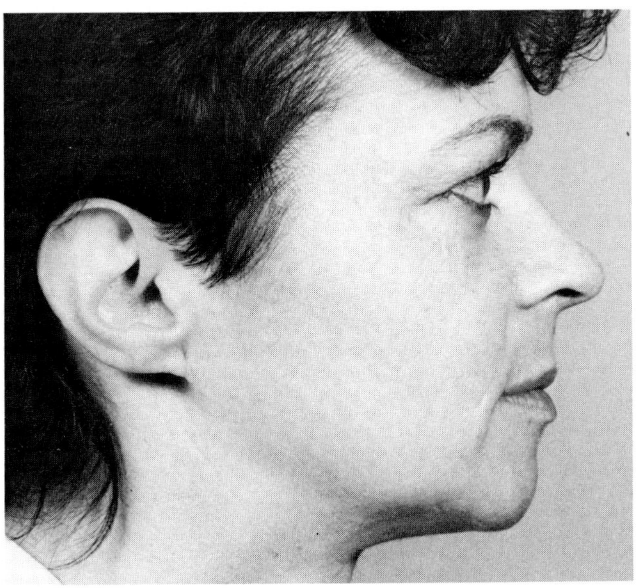

D

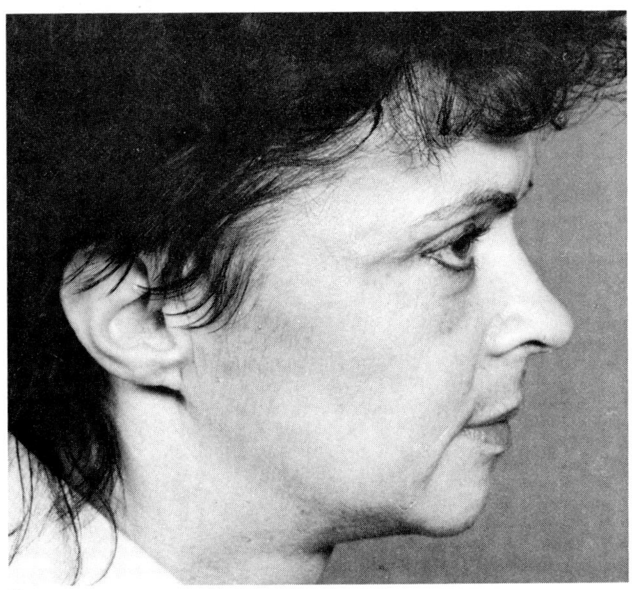

E

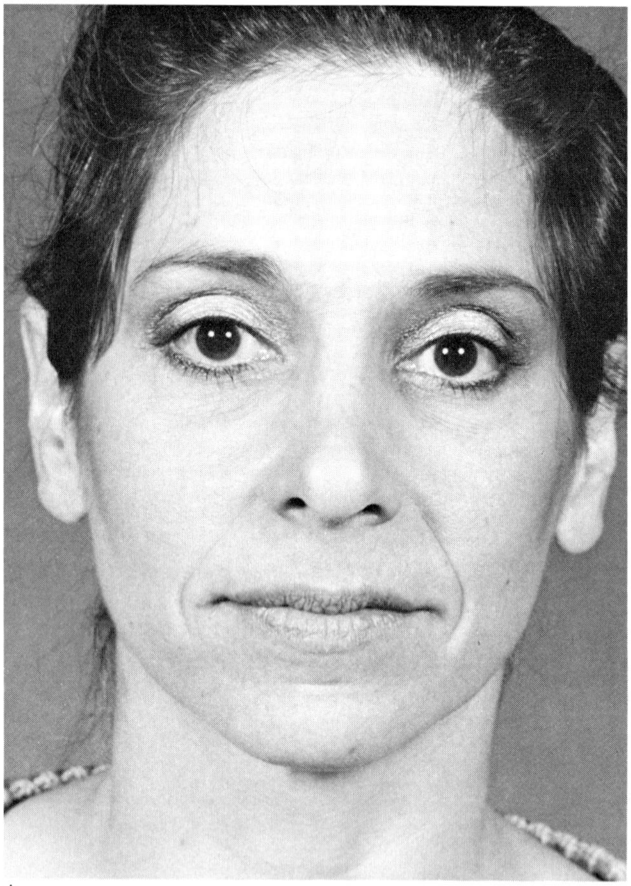

A

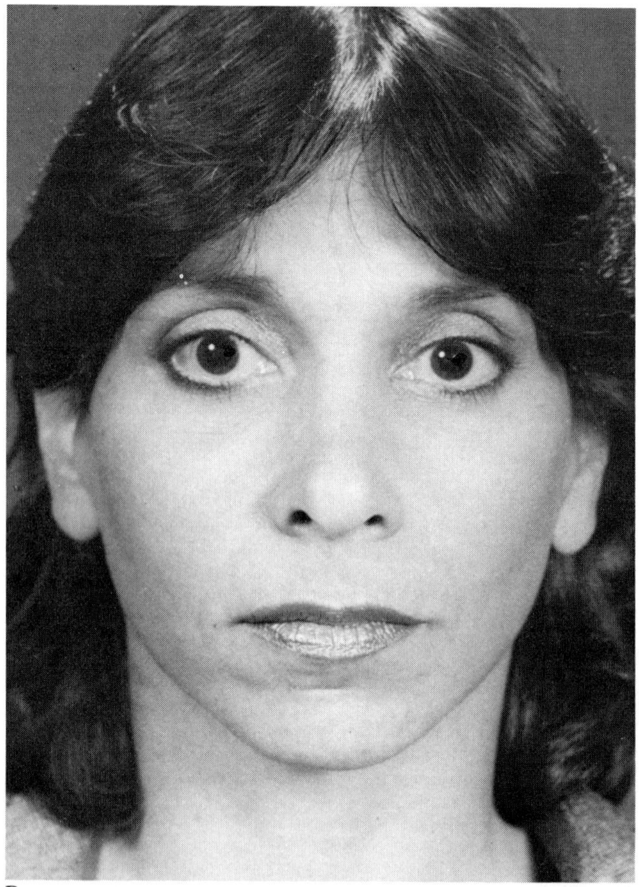

B

Figure 16-21

A. A 39-year-old patient who sought improvement of early aging signs, especially heavy nasolabial folds.

B. Result at 9 months following a limited meloplasty, including the SMAS flap procedure shown in Figure 16-22.

Figure 16-22

A. Limited meloplasty with SMAS flap in a 39-year-old patient. A posttragal incision will be used.

B. Extent of dissection.

C. Following creation and traction on the SMAS flap, the SMAS is plicated at multiple points.

D. Dotted lines indicate SMAS flap, while *X*s indicate SMAS plication points.

E. Skin traction followed by excision of 2 cm of skin circumferentially.

F. Closure. Result shown in Figure 16-21.

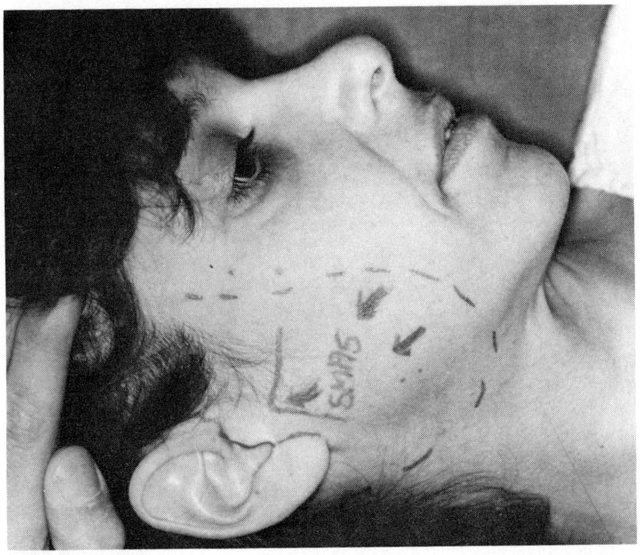

A

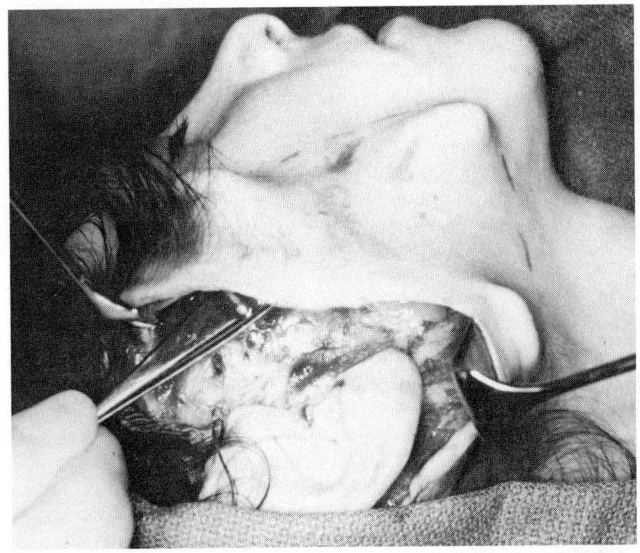

B

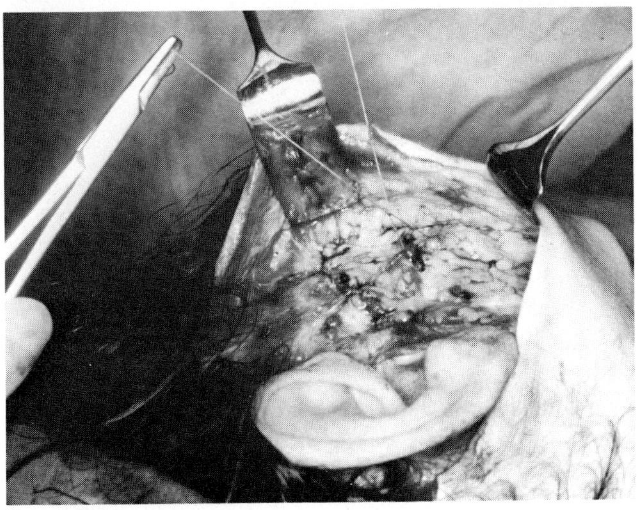

C

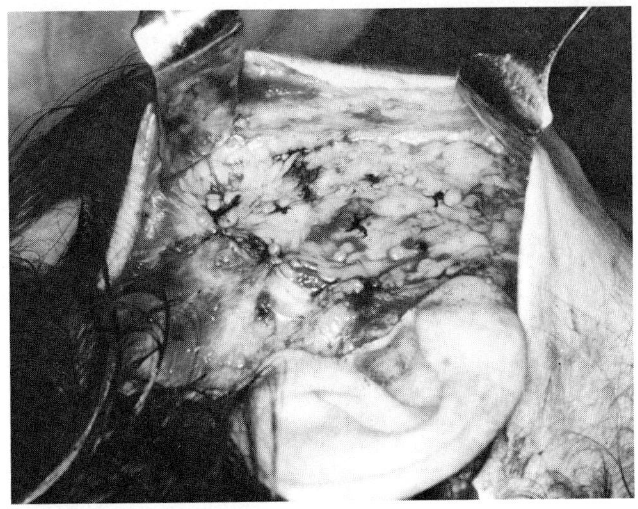

D

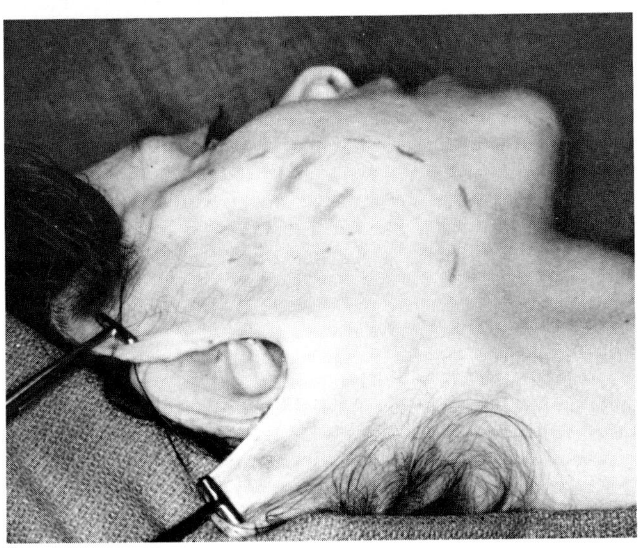

E

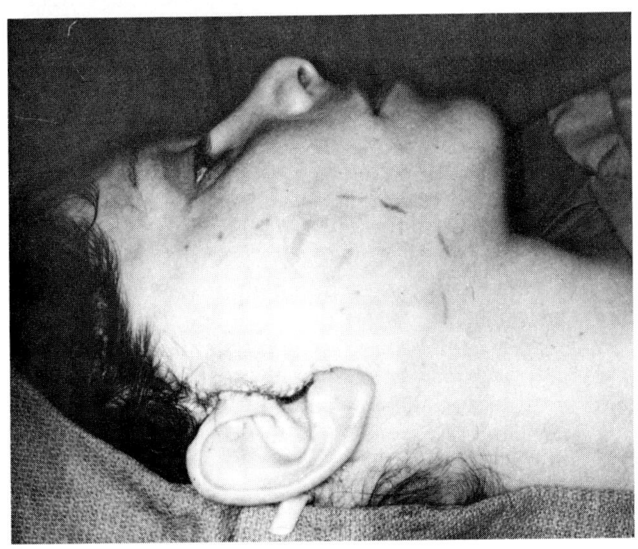

F

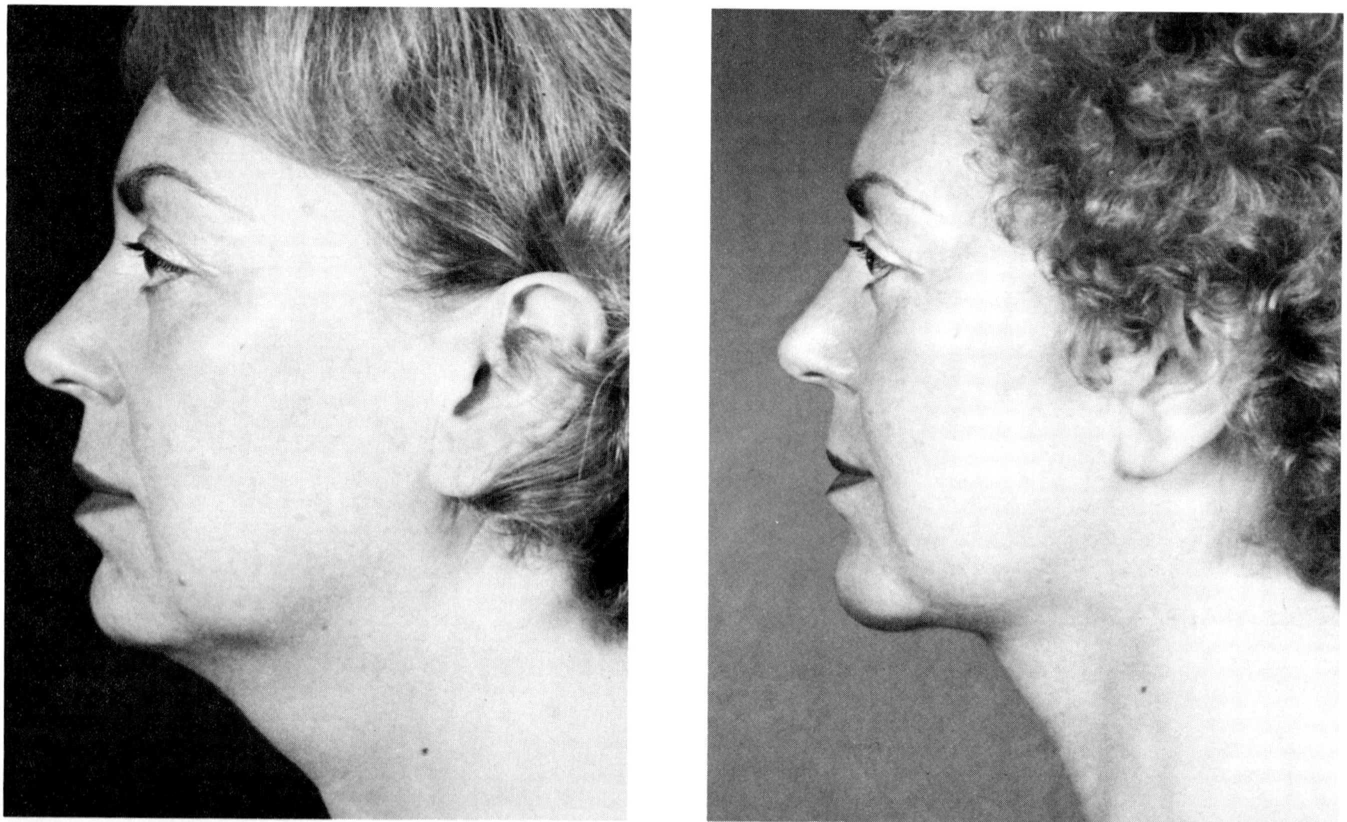

A

B

Figure 16-23
A. A 35-year-old patient, modestly overweight, with an obtuse cervicomental angle.
B. Result at 1 year following limited rhytidectomy, submandibular lipectomy, platysmal flap traction, and a small silastic chin implant. Despite obesity, a relatively ideal neck has been achieved.

NECK AND CHIN

Localized neck procedures are indicated for the younger individual with an obtuse cervicomental angle or persistence of a platysmal deformity following rhytidectomy (Fig. 16-23). In the younger patient (below 35), one must decide whether the deformity is localized to the submental area or affects the entire neck [38, 65]. In the former, a chin implant coupled with a contoured fat excision plus platysmal plication will suffice. Where the entire neck is involved, a cervical lift through a limited rhytidectomy incision will be necessary. As noted by Ellenbogen and Karlin [72], one must carefully evaluate preoperatively each of the anatomic structures that contribute to the ideal neck and decide on their modification: (1) position of the hyoid bone, (2) degree and location of adiposity in the neck, (3) jowl formation, (4) platysma borders and bands, and (5) chin projection. The operation begins in the submental region, where the fat is excised, the platysma approximated, and the chin implant inserted [165]. Next, the cheeks and neck are undermined completely. The posterior border of the platysma is partially divided and plicated posteriorly except in the patient with a short, thick neck, in whom full-width platysma division is carried out. The SMAS is plicated in a superior direction to minimize jowl formation. Then an extensive lipectomy is done to define the mandibular border.

In older persons the deformity is routinely compounded by skin laxity, platysmal bands, and significant jowl formation. The solution is an extended cervicofacial rhytidectomy rather than a localized procedure. Numerous authors have advocated direct excision of skin, subcutaneous fat, and muscle followed by various flap closures to conceal the scar [1, 35, 62]. Inevitably, the scars are visible and must be accepted as a permanent sequela by the patient. For this reason we do not advocate local excisions except in the very elderly. Of greater concern are the errors of commission (too much excision) and omission (failure to alleviate the jowls) that can produce a noticeable submental depression, thereby in effect swapping one deformity for another [109]. To correct surgical sequelae, Wilkinson [211] used a technique of digastric muscle plication and buried dermal flaps in five cases.

Rhytidectomy

The standard face-lift consists of three major areas of undermining (temporal, cheek, and posterior neck) plus modifications of deeper structures (SMAS plication, partial-width platysmal flap) (Fig. 16-24). It is indicated for the patient with facial wrinkles and folds including early jowl formation, but without significant submental problems. It is done in approximately 45 percent of patients seeking rhytidectomy (Fig. 16-25). The preoperative

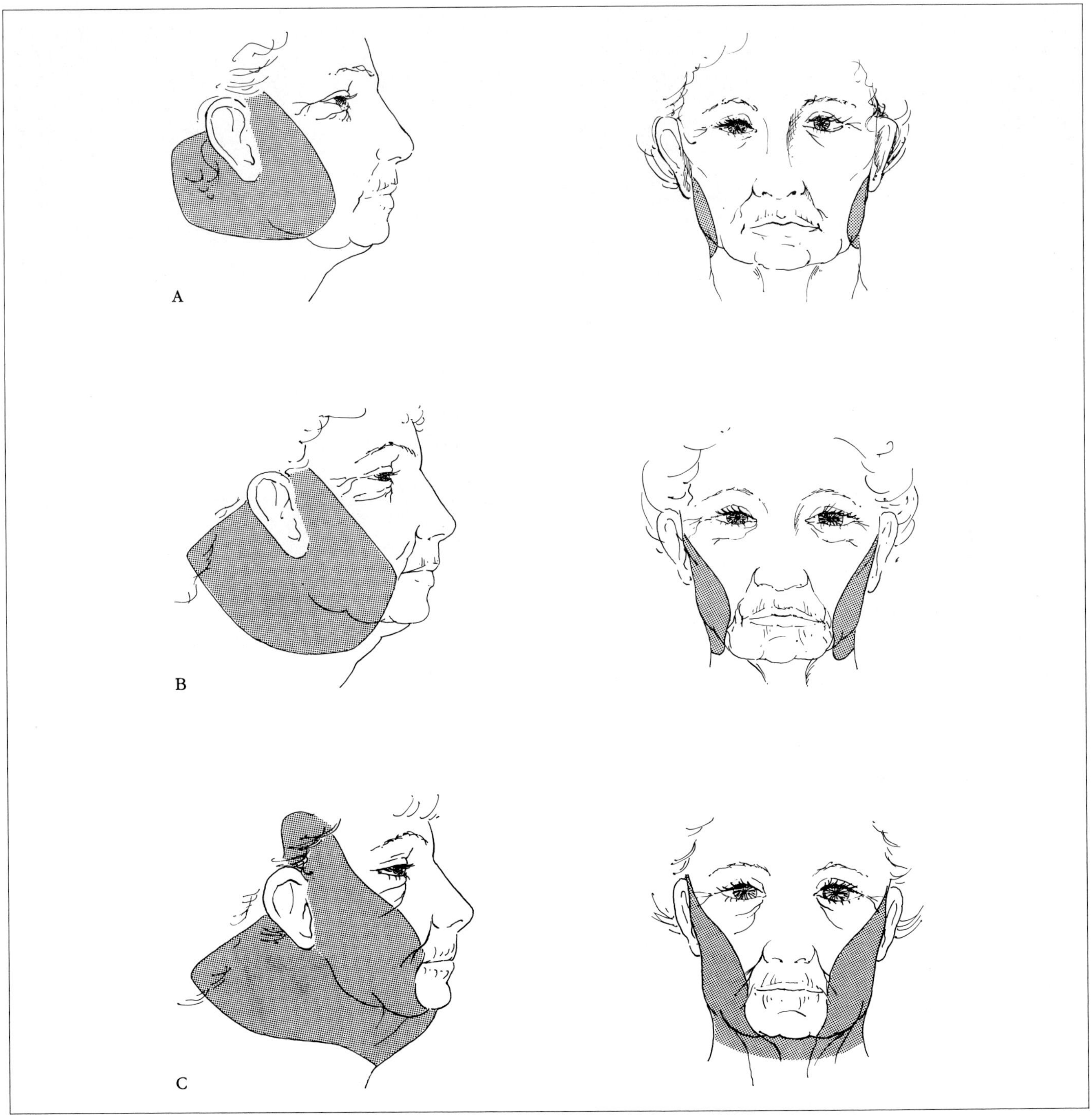

Figure 16-24

A. The classic meloplasty with its dissection limited to the cheeks.

B. The standard rhytidectomy, which extends across the jowl line and into the upper neck.

C. The cervicofacial rhytidectomy, which extends completely across the neck.

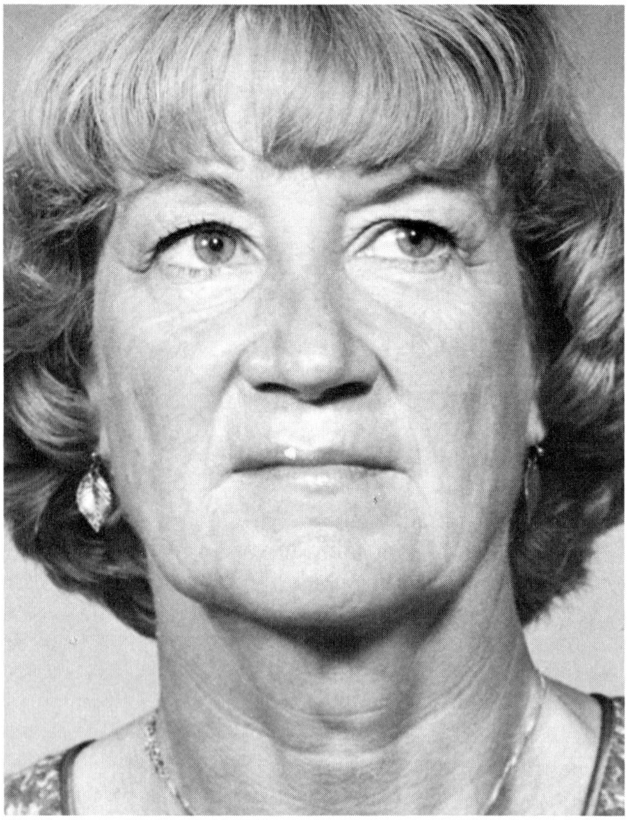

A

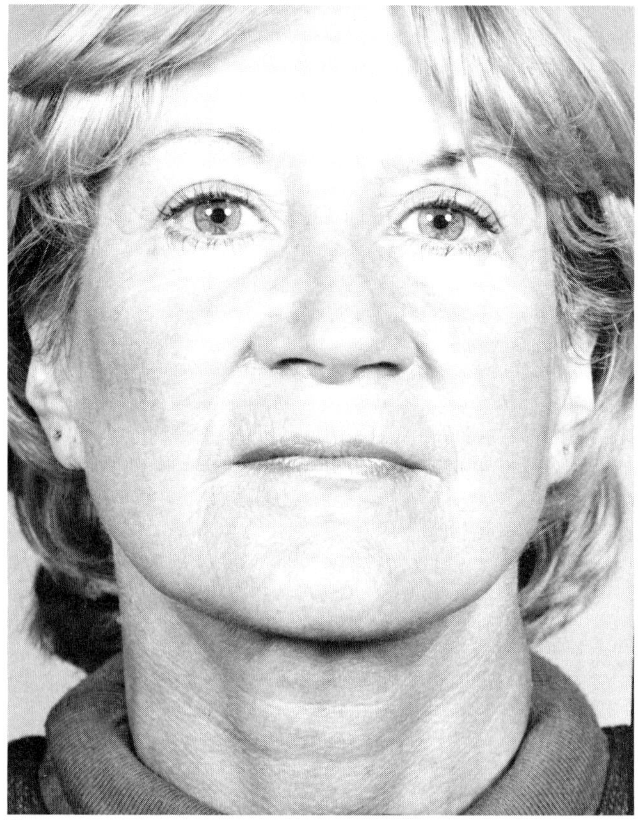

B

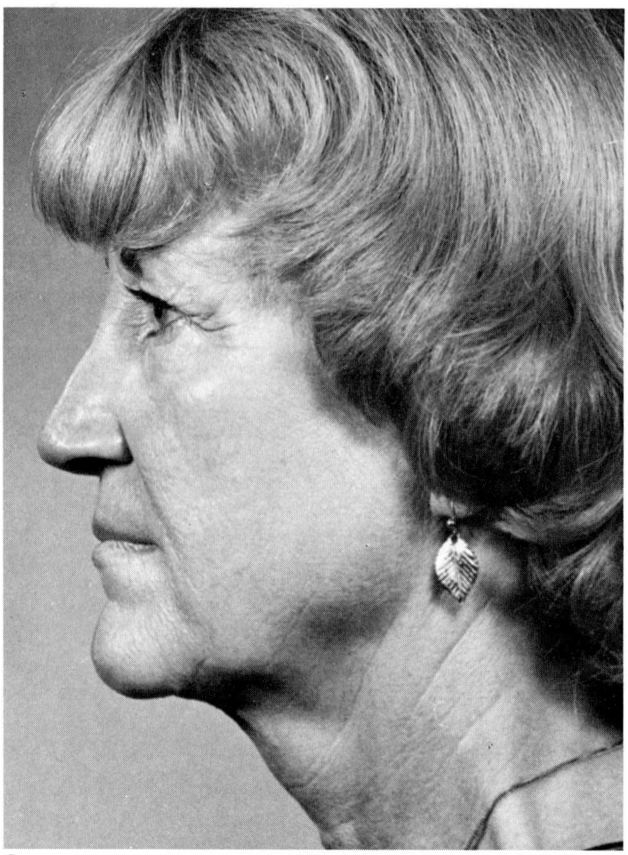

C

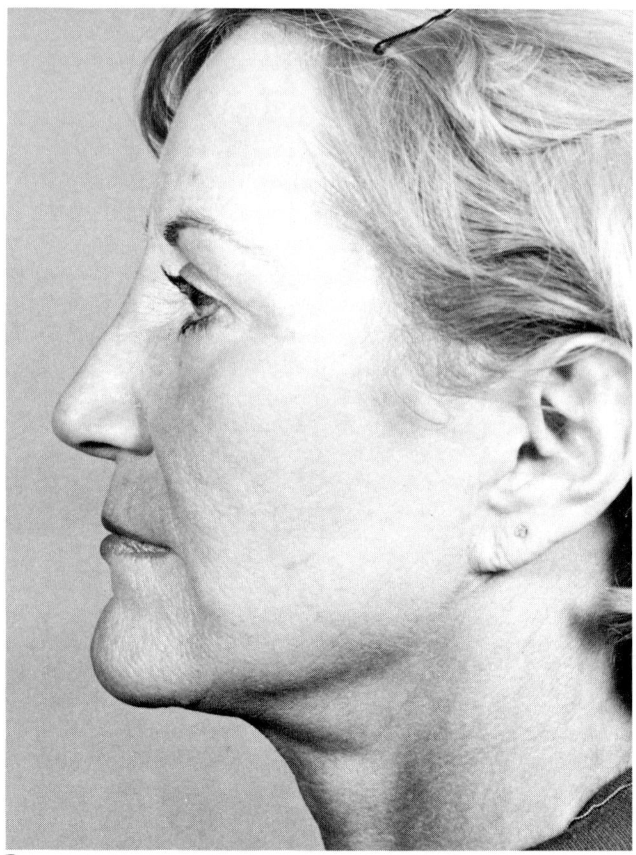

D

Figure 16-25

A, C. A 52-year-old woman seeking improvement in facial appearance.

B, D. Result at 1 year following standard rhytidectomy and blepharoplasty. Improvement in the lateral hooding is attributed to ***prehairline*** temporal incision allowing greater traction without a significantly visible scar.

preparations, infiltration, incision, and dissection have been previously discussed. The undermining continues to the nasolabial folds, beneath the jowls, and across the upper neck for 4 cm. It is then brought posteriorly in an upward direction and anchored with 3-0 Dexon sutures to the mastoid fascia at several points. Next, the SMAS is plicated with 4-0 Vicryl sutures superolateral to elevate the jowls and lessen the nasolabial folds. Any skin puckering is eliminated by further skin undermining while additional plicating sutures are added to eradicate any furrows. Once the deep procedures are completed, skin excision is done with the face turned back to the vertical position. The key sutures are inserted, the excess skin is excised, and a continuous subcuticular closure is done with 4-0 Dexon. The results are quite good in the carefully selected patient and include improvement in lateral hooding, smoothing of the cheeks, lessening of the jowls, and tightening of the neck.

Cervicofacial Rhytidectomy

Arbitrarily, a cervicofacial rhytidectomy may be defined as undermining of the face and upper neck (Fig. 16-26). The dissection is extended to the orbicularis oculi muscle, across the malar prominence, beyond the nasolabial fold, beneath the jowls, and across the neck from the posterior border of one sternocleidomastoid muscle to the other at the level of the thyroid cartilage. A submental incision is required to gain access to the anterior neck. It varies in accordance with the procedures done on the deeper structures. It represents a flexible approach to a set of highly variable problems.

CERVICAL DEFORMITIES

In the older individual of normal weight, common deformities of the neck include loose skin, platysmal bands, and loss of mandibular definition. With the face vertical, a submental incision is made and the anterior neck skin elevated over a wide area. The subcutaneous fat overlying the platysma is excised, avoiding excessive resection between the muscle bellies. A common error is failure to extend the excision down to the thyroid cartilage or sufficiently lateral. The degree of platysma muscle desiccation is then evaluated and any heaviness of the anterior borders is excised in a vertical direction. In virtually all cases the platysma edges are sutured together or reinforced with 3-0 Dexon simple sutures. The rhytidectomy is then performed with the face turned in the lateral position. The temporal area is widely undermined and, if crow's-feet are a problem, the orbicularis oculi muscle is splayed out. The skin is elevated over the malar prominences, especially in older patients. Significant complications have not been noted. Extension beyond the nasolabial folds is necessary, especially in males. The postauricular area and entire neck skin are elevated. The posterior border of the platysma is penetrated, the platysma widely undermined, and a partial-width flap created 5 cm below the mandibular border. The platysmal flap and SMAS plication are accomplished in the usual fashion. In general, full-width platysmal flaps are not used for fear of "skeletonization" or "masculinization" of the neck. Large amounts of skin may be excised, necessitating triangular darts in the temporal area.

CERVICOFACIAL LIPECTOMY

Facial lipectomy is done whenever indicated, either as an ancillary procedure or in combination for the patient with an obtuse cervicomental angle [41, 195]. The majority of facial lipectomies consist of complete excision in the submental and submandibular area and contouring of the cheek over the mandibular border [113, 161]. Occasionally, patients will require the entire gamut of maneuvers: (1) excision and contouring of submental and submandibular fat, (2) beveling of cheek fat overlying the mandible, (3) excision of the fat pad of Bichat, (4) plication of the platysma muscle anteriorly plus its full-width division and lateral advancement, (5) chin augmentation, and (6) redraping of the cervical skin with lateral resection of the excess skin (Fig. 16-27).

The submental incision is made first, and the skin is widely elevated with careful preservation of 2 to 3 mm of fat on its undersurface. Fat is removed en bloc and the intraplatysmal area carefully checked for excess fat accumulation. Once the face-lift flaps are elevated, a submandibular lipectomy is done but only after suturing of the platysmal flap. If fat is excised prior to platysma or SMAS plication, contour deformities above the mandible can occur. The fat is excised in a single wide sheet using Metzenbaum scissors with the tips upward and with gentle traction. One must avoid excision or penetration of the platysma muscle. The fat pad of Bichat is palpable anterior to the masseter muscle and is exposed by being spread transversely to avoid injuring the neurovascular structures. As noted by Tenta et al. [205], the buccal space contains Stensen's duct, the buccal nerve branch, and the external maxillary artery and vein. The fat pad may be rotated superiorly to augment the facial skeleton or may be excised. Primary excision is always done subcutaneously, with the perioral route used for isolated deformities or secondary correction. Lower cheek defatting is done tangential to the facial aponeurosis and measures $2 \times 2 \times 1$ cm.

Peterson [168] considers the problem more complex because these patients often have cervical hypoplasia, low placement of the hyoid, and hypoplasia of the chin. Despite the more extensive procedures, rhytidectomy is not universally successful in the obese patient, and weight loss prior to surgery is stressed. As with lower extremity surgery, patients with skin flaccidity will do better than those with tense, firm adiposity.

A more isolated problem is the "witch's chin." It is basically a chin fat ptosis that is accentuated by a deep submental crease (Fig. 16-28). It is corrected by elliptic excision that includes the crease. The excision is placed 1 mm beneath the crease but much higher on the chin side (Fig. 16-29). The fat can be either excised if sufficient anterior projection is present or rotated upward to increase projection.

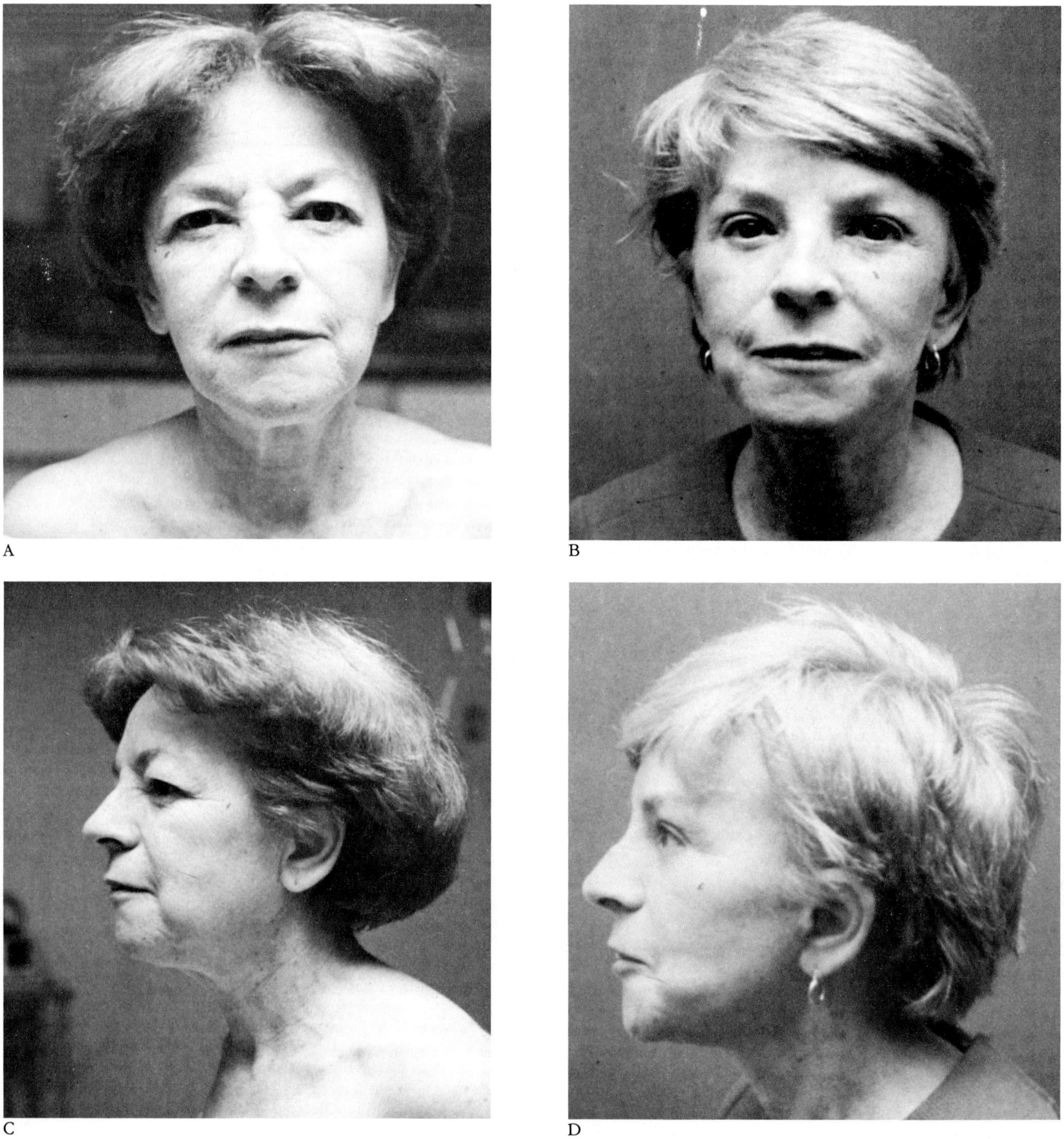

Figure 16-26
A, C. Patient complaining of sagging of the face and neck.
B, D. Result following cervicofacial rhytidectomy, forehead-lift, and blepharoplasty.

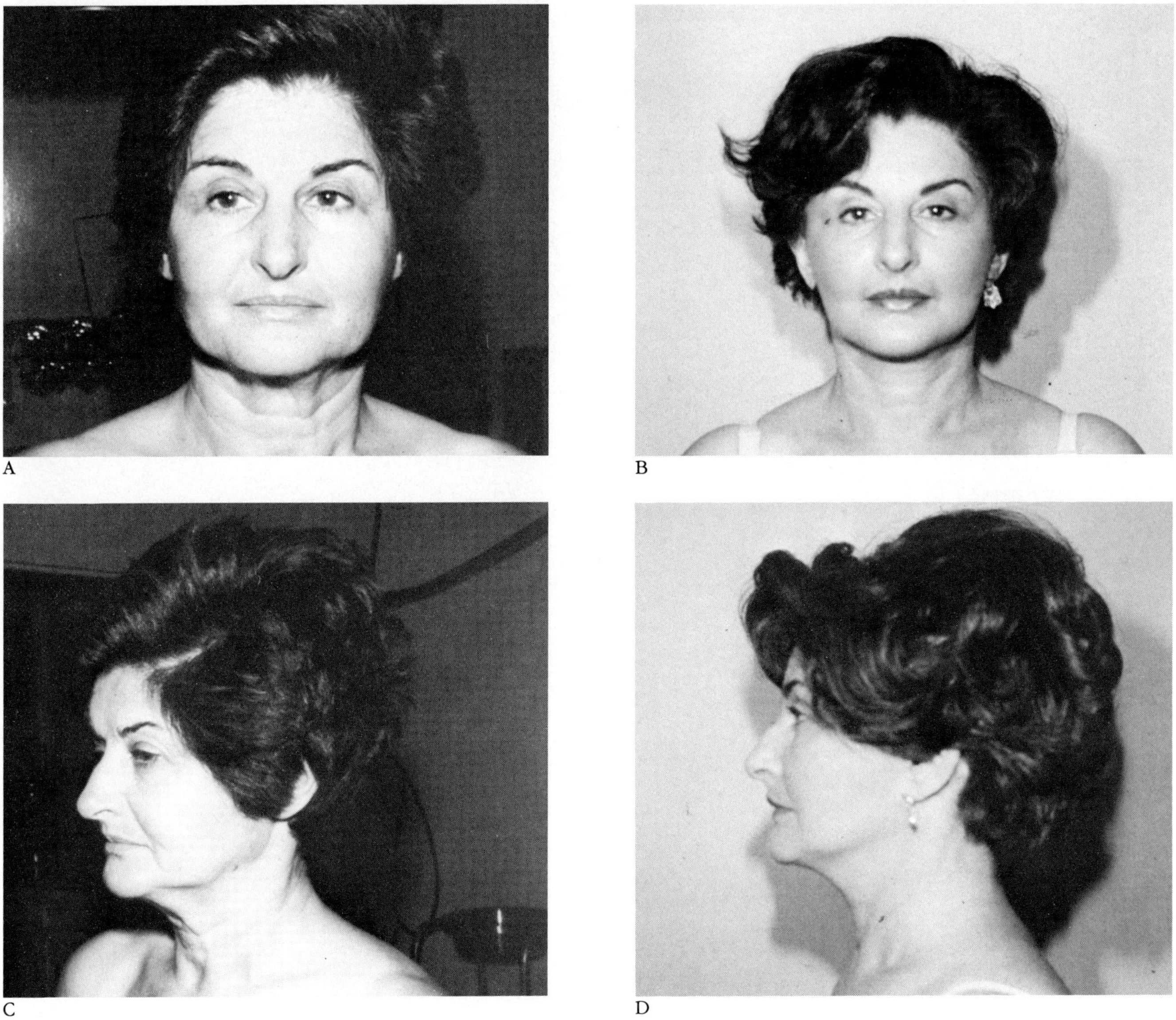

Figure 16-27
A, C. Patient with platysmal bands, jowl formation, and facial heaviness.
B, D. Result at 2½ years following cervicofacial rhytidectomy with lipectomy.

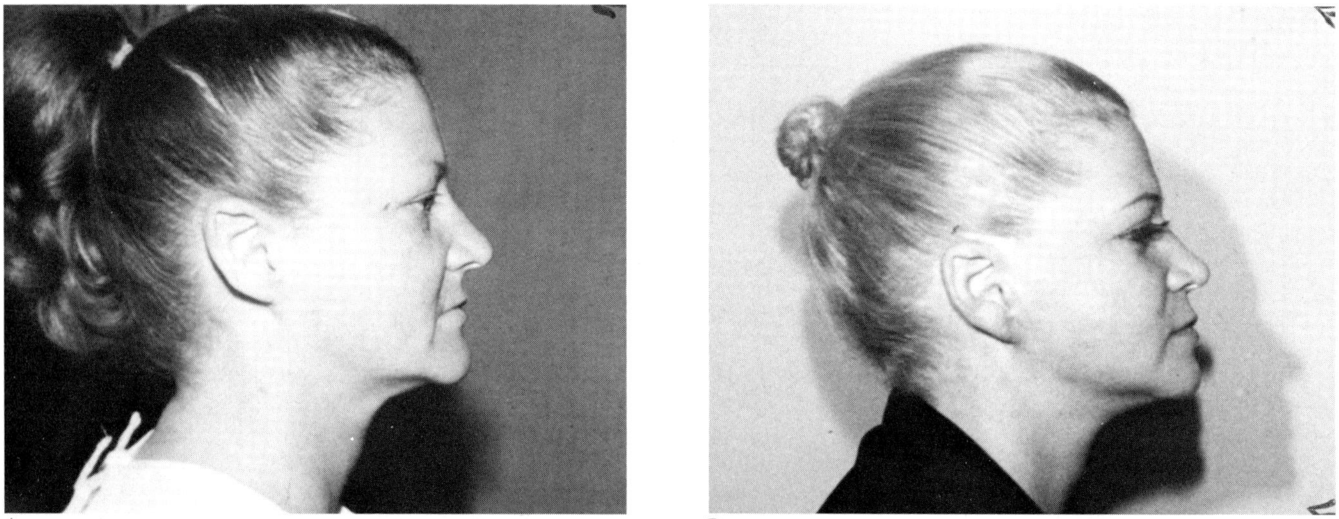

A B

Figure 16-28
A. Patient with a "witch's chin" deformity.
B. Result at 3 years following rhytidectomy plus elliptic excision of the submental crease and defatting.

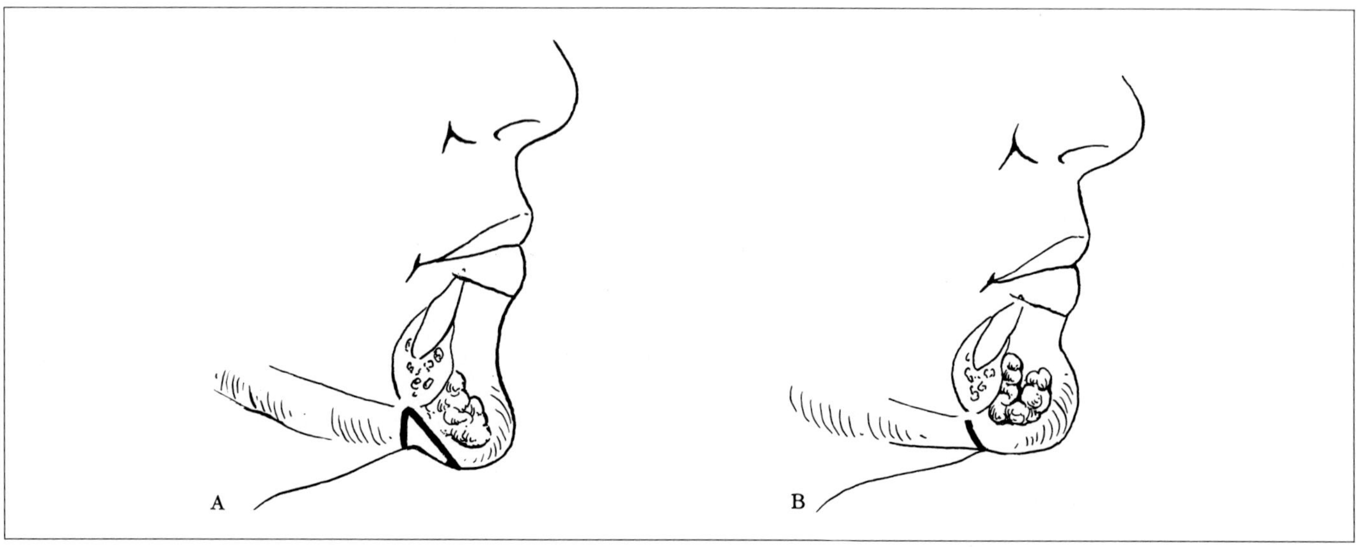

Figure 16-29. Correction of the "witch's chin" deformity.
A. Excision of the deep submental crease wider on the chin side.
B. Fat is either excised or flapped upward to increase anterior projection.

SEVERE SKIN LAXITY

Excess skin of the neck represents a significant problem in certain patients, especially those with marked wrinkling or those requiring extensive lipectomy. The dilemma is what to do with the skin as upward traction would result in vertical folds while posterior traction distorts the hairline markedly. Certain authors accept the fact that skin redistribution is impossible and the end result is compromised [175]. For this reason the senior author devised the upward traction rhytidectomy, which is distinguished by removal of a wide wedge of skin at the level of the lateral canthus [181]. The incision is placed in front of the hairline. The rhytidectomy, with modification of deeper structures and lipectomy, is done in the standard fashion. With the usual skin traction, the key sutures are inserted and excess skin is resected. Next, an incision is made along the upper crow's-feet connecting the prehairline incision and the lateral canthal region. The facial flap is completely dissected and upward traction placed on it. The excess skin is resected conservatively, and tension is minimized. The incision is closed with a few deep sutures to achieve approximation followed by a running subcuticular suture (Fig. 16-30).

When blepharoplasty is done, the wedge of tissue to be removed is determined by the excision lines of the blepharoplasties [90]. Careful preservation of the lateral triangle is important, and closure at the lateral canthus is done prior to resection of cheek skin. Another variation occurs in elderly patients with an infinite number of wrinkles in very fine skin (Fig. 16-31). Rather than doing an extensive undermining, one may simply resect the skin and achieve a satisfactory result with minimal morbidity.

COMBINED PROCEDURES

Most major rhytidectomies are combined procedures, usually including blepharoplasty and perioral chemical peels or dermabrasion [14, 17, 21, 42, 169]. Increasingly, a forehead-lift or mentoplasty is added. Septorhinoplasty, malar augmentation, and other procedures are done occasionally. Currently, persistent small folds and furrows can be ameliorated by injection therapy and depressions improved by grafts and minor excisional procedures [31, 48, 49, 129]. The frequency of combined procedures reflects the sophistication of the population and the type of practice. With wider acceptance of aesthetic surgery, blepharoplasty will be done undoubtedly as an isolated procedure in younger patients (30–40), thus leading to more frequent incidence of forehead-cervicofacial rhytidectomy with the former correcting any palpebral redundancy. Another factor is the increased number of males seeking rhytidectomy [13, 18, 59, 104]. Combined procedures call for consummate surgical skill and flawless execution [63, 142]. Courtiss's admonition is well remembered: "Combined procedures are additive, but their complications are geometric."

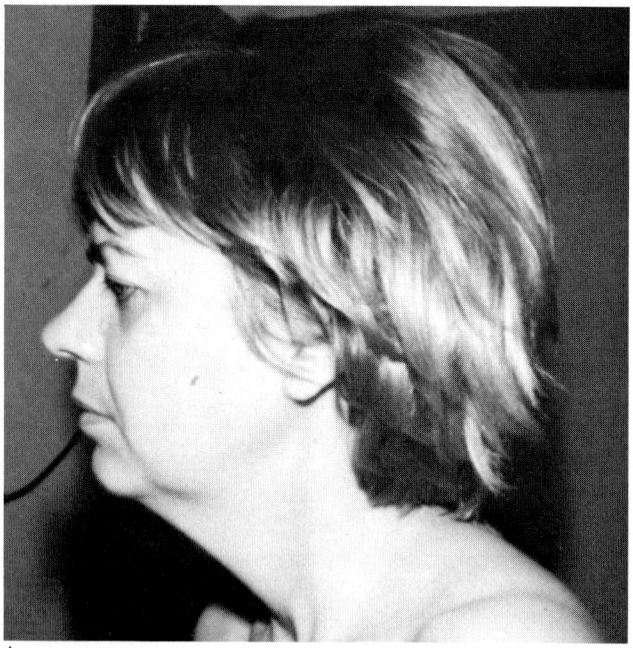

A

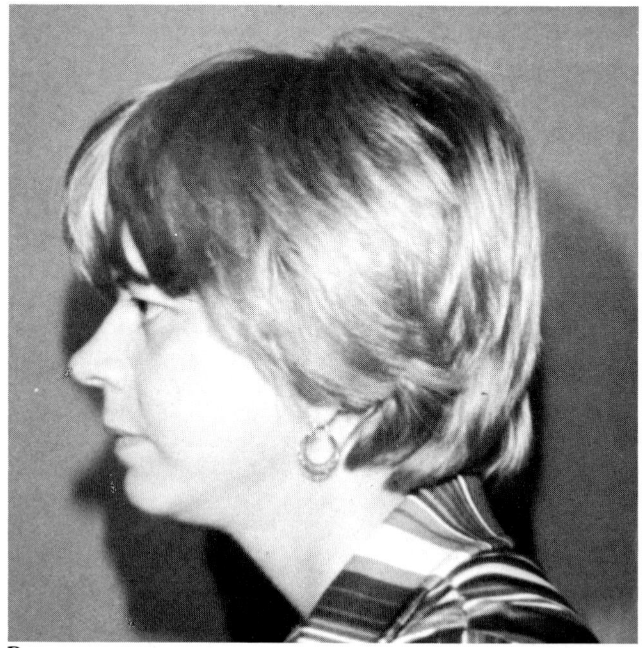

B

Figure 16-30. The upward traction rhytidectomy.
A. Young patient with an obtuse cervicomental angle and jowl formation.
B. Result following an upward traction rhytidectomy with cervical lipectomy, but without blepharoplasty.

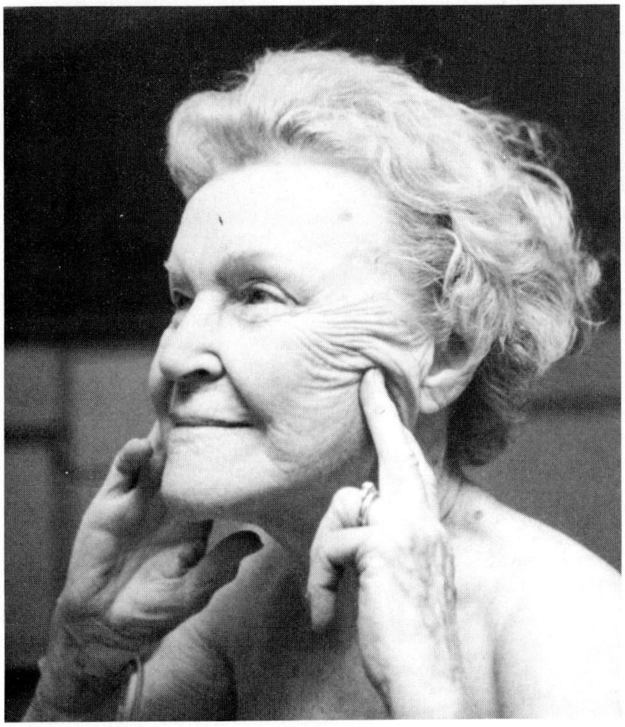

A

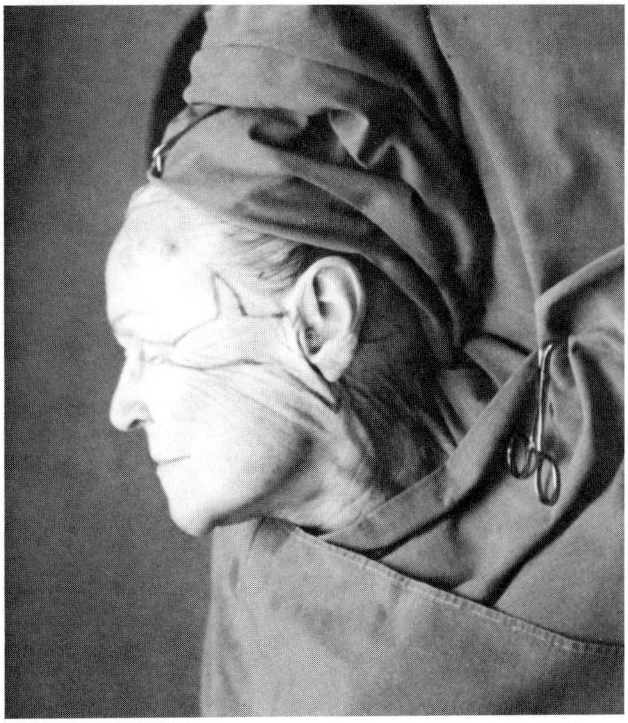

B

Figure 16-31. Upward traction rhytidectomy with blepharoplasty.
A. An elderly patient with multitudinous wrinkles demonstrating the desired result, but also the problem of excess skin.
B. Technique of combined upward traction rhytidectomy and blepharoplasty. No undermining is done.

COMPLICATIONS

As rhytidectomy procedures become more extensive and variable, the incidence of certain complications will increase and new ones will appear [14, 58]. However, renewed emphasis on hemostasis and meticulous dissection under direct fiberoptic illumination may compensate [75]. At the present time, the overall complication rate is certainly acceptable and has perhaps decreased from what was reported in the 1970s (Table 16-1) [125, 131, 200, 206].

Intraoperative Complications

During the operation, the principal concerns are hematoma, profuse bleeding, and nerve transection. Following closure of the first side, one will occasionally encounter a hematoma on that side prior to application of the dressing. Although compression of the venous system by forced turning of the neck has been implicated, the cause is most logically inadequate hemostasis. Surprisingly, some surgeons favor evacuation followed by compression rather than the recommended exploration with hemostasis.

Rarely, profuse bleeding with repeated hematoma formation will occur [175]. It is signaled by significant bleeding from the blepharoplasty incisions. Transfusion with whole fresh blood and liberal application of Avatet may stanch the flow, but secondary exploration 4 to 6 hours later may be necessary. Inadvertent nerve severance should be repaired immediately with loupe magnification and epinural technique using 8-0 nylon. Although recovery may not occur because of the patient's age and other factors, the repair may minimize painful neuroma formation, especially in sensory nerves.

Early Complications

The vast majority of early complications are related to technical problems: hemostasis (hematoma), dissection (nerve injury), and tension (skin slough, dehiscence, pigmentation) [32, 150].

HEMATOMA

Accumulation of blood may be a major or a minor event, the former requiring operative evacuation and the latter treated by expression or aspiration. A major expanding hematoma is signaled by pain, swelling, discoloration of the oral mucosa, and patient agitation (Fig. 16-32). If left untreated, the overlying skin flap can slough on account of compressive tension or marginally survive with subsequent desquamation, pigmentation, and persistent induration. Since early reoperation will prevent these sequelae, it is in the best interest of *both* the patient and the surgeon to treat the problem definitively [171]. Under general anesthesia, the flaps are elevated, the clot is removed, the wound is irrigated, and any bleeding points are coagulated. Minor hematomas of 2 to 20 ml of blood may be obvious at the first dressing change and should be evacuated by pressure toward the incision line or aspiration. If a minor hematoma is not apparent until edema decreases, evacuation is delayed until liquefaction occurs, at 7 to 10 days. Because of anesthesia of the flaps, aspiration with a 16-gauge needle is easily done but may have to be repeated every 2 days in larger hematomas. If minor hematomas are not treated, the patient will note the firm indurated area and subsequent skin puckering.

The cause of hematomas has been attributed to inadequate hemostasis, bleeding dyscrasias secondary to aspirin ingestion, medical problems (especially hypertension), general anesthesia, and postoperative agitation [7, 27, 30, 149, 202]. A detailed preoperative history and physical examination plus an admonition to avoid aspirin-containing compounds will help identify potential problems. Rees et al. [177, 179] demonstrated that hypotensive anesthesia did not lessen the incidence of hematomas. Spira et al. [198] advocate lowering the patient's head prior to closure to facilitate identification of bleeding points. Berner et al. [33] noted that the patient's blood pressure rises significantly 3 hours postoperatively because of loss of sedation and analgesia. During this period the problem may be compounded by nausea or restlessness due to inhalation anesthetic agents. A review of multiple rhytidectomy series performed in the late 1960s but reported in the 1970s shows a major hematoma rate of 3 to 8 percent, with minor hematomas in 10 to 15 percent of cases. Recent series of extended rhytidectomies indicate a comparable incidence of hematomas but a more diverse location. Thus far, the only practical method advocated for lowering the incidence of hematoma is the "second-look" concept of Baker and Gordon [16]. Essentially, one side is completed, with the anchoring sutures inserted, then the opposite side is done, then one returns for a second look

Table 16-1. Rhytidectomy complications

	Thompson and Ashley [206]	Pitanguy [170]	Smith et al. [194]
Early complication	922 (1971–76)	2934	114 (1972–74)
Hematoma	1.7/3.4	7	2.6/2.6
Skin necrosis	14	2.5	0.9/12.2
Infection and wound dehiscence	2	1.6	3.5
Nerve injury			
Motor	—	—	
Sensory	—	—	4.4
	17.7%	11.1%	11.4%

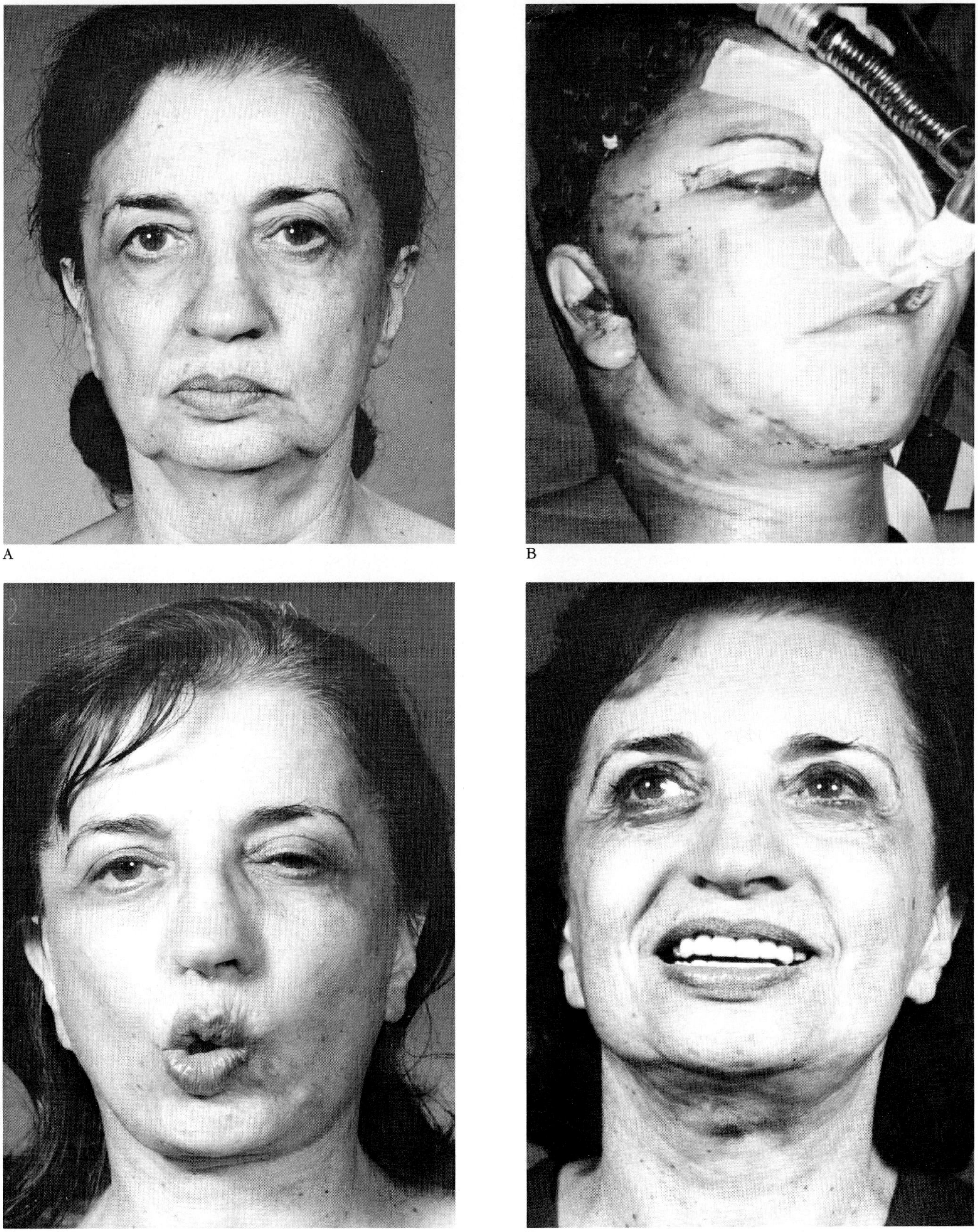

Figure 16-32. Complications in rhytidectomy.

A. A 56-year-old patient with jowl formation and hanging neck.

B. Patient at 6 hours following rhytidectomy and blepharoplasty complicated by massive bilateral hematoma requiring reoperation.

C. Significant *weakness* of multiple right facial nerve branches rather than total paralysis, perhaps due to compression secondary to the hematoma.

D. Result at 1 year is obviously less than desired, but fortunately complete recovery of muscle strength occurred.

at the original side. Following adoption of this maneuver, Schnur et al. [190] reported a significant decrease in the incidence of both expanding and small hematomas.

SKIN NECROSIS

Skin sloughs are most often associated with untreated major hematomas. Conservative treatment of a skin slough with sequential debridement and eventual epithelialization of a contracted area is recommended. Occasionally, skin grafts will be required with scar revision at 1 year. It is anticipated that the 2 percent incidence of retroauricular sloughs will decrease with newer techniques that place tension on deep structures. Also, patients should avoid smoking in the early postoperative course.

INFECTION AND WOUND DEHISCENCE

Infections occur in less than 1 percent of cases. Small pustules occasionally develop along the suture line, which require unroofing and application of topical antibiotic ointment. More severe infections including cellulitis or chondritis require systemic antibiotics. Wound dehiscence is rare, and healing will occur by secondary intention, often with acceptable scarring.

NERVE INJURY

The most common nerve injuries are sensory (greater auricular and lesser occipital), with motor nerve damage infrequent (frontal branch and marginal mandibular) [44, 147]. Damage to the greater auricular nerve results in loss of sensation over the lower ear and earlobe whereas injury to the lesser occipital results in pain over the posterior scalp. Transection of sensory nerves can be prevented by a detailed knowledge of their course, a superficial dissection in the auricular area, and early identification of the main trunk prior to platysma surgery. As noted by McKinney and Katarna [151], the greater auricular nerve trunk can be found 6.5 cm beneath the external auditory canal and the terminal branches spared by superficial dissection after extensive infiltration. With this approach, injury of the greater auricular nerve will decrease from the reported high of 5 percent [134]. Transient numbness, due to severance of terminal fibers, should ameliorate by 3 months, and damage to superficial branches should improve by 6 to 12 months. However, recovery from complete transection of the trunk is rare. Secondary surgery is not done except for painful palpable neuromas, which are directly excised. Patients who complain of numbness are reminded of their preoperative consultation during which numbness of the cheeks for 3 months was discussed. Certain patients will be unable to wear clasp earrings and are encouraged to wear earrings designed for pierced ears.

Injuries of motor nerve branches range from weakness to complete motor paralysis. Damage to the facial nerve is best avoided by detailed anatomic knowledge, use of bipolar cautery, spreading dissection beneath the SMAS and platysma, and limited dissection in the temporal region. Avoidance of facial nerve injuries is mandatory, and the reader is referred to the excellent work of Baker and Conley [12]. The incidence of motor nerve injury ranges from 0.3 to 2.6 percent with frequency variable but including temporal, buccal, and mandibular plus the spinal accessory. When a patient complains of weakness or paralysis, the surgeon should acknowledge the problem in a direct manner. The patient with weakness should be told that it is probably temporary and may be caused by a variety of factors (cautery, anesthesia, dissection, edema, etc.). If it does not improve or the patient has a complete paralysis, electromyography (EMG) is done at 6 weeks and serially thereafter. The patient is told that recovery as manifested by improved symmetry is probable and should begin within 3 months and continue over a period of 1 to 2 years. Surprisingly, few papers discuss management of motor nerve injuries following rhytidectomy.

The temporal branch can be damaged inadvertently by trunk transection during combined forehead-rhytidectomy procedures or its terminal branches injured in superficial dissections anterior to the hairline. The former is best avoided by creation of a two-plane dissection at the juncture of the forehead (deep) and rhytidectomy (subcutaneous) while the latter is minimized by dissection with a sponge-covered finger in a peeling motion rather than a pushing motion or sharp dissection. The result of temporal nerve injury is asymmetric drooping of the eyebrow and loss of forehead creases on the injured side. If recovery does not occur by 2 years, a neurectomy of the temporal branch on the opposite side will produce symmetry but may cause drooping of the eyebrows. In rhytidectomy-only patients, an alternative is to perform a forehead-lift with frontal branch neurectomy, thereby correcting the problem and giving the patient an improved appearance [70].

The buccal nerve is most commonly injured by transection of its trunk anterior to the masseter muscle in the fat pad of Bichat or by damage of its branches in the nasolabial fold area. Paralysis of the buccal branch results in drooping of the upper lip and marked facial asymmetry. It is best avoided by a superficial dissection and limited elevation of the SMAS anterior to the parotid. Recovery is generally the rule, and only rarely is neurectomy of the contralateral side through a buccal incision considered [46].

With recent emphasis on platysma surgery, damage to the marginal mandibularis has become a major concern. The nerve trunk can be transected as one passes beneath the lateral border of the platysma, and its terminal branches can be damaged in the mental region at the anterior extent of the subcutaneous dissection [188]. Complete transection produces drooping or flattening of the lower lip that rarely improves with time [158]. In contrast, weakness will improve and may occasionally be due to loss of platysma function following its complete transection. Damage to the mandibular branch is best avoided by careful subcutaneous dissection over the neck without penetration of the platysma followed by subplatysmal dissection commencing at a point at least two fingerbreadths below the mandibular border. Complete transection of the platysma is done at least 5 cm below the mandibular border.

EDEMA

Significant facial swelling will occasionally occur, usually in the multiple-procedure patient. If a distinct venous etiology is not evident, it is assumed to be a transitory lymphatic obstruction that will ameliorate by 3 to 6 weeks. A conservative course of diuretics or steroids has been recommended. A case report by Zaworski and Noriega [212] demonstrates convincingly the occurrence of facial edema in the absence of hematoma formation.

Late Complications

Most late complications are attributed to excessive tension or nonspecific events (edema, pain) [55]. However, the greatest time investment will be with the dissatisfied or demanding patient. It must be considered part of the service, accepted with equanimity and given as required.

SCARS

Hypertrophic scars occasionally occur in 1 to 2 percent of patients, with the retroauricular segment prone to painful scars and the temporal segment associated with hair loss. Development of hypertrophic scarring is attributed to excessive tension, probably justified as visible scars in the preauricular area are exceedingly rare [40]. Retroauricular problems are best avoided by insertion of a small superiorly based triangular skin flap that prevents contractural webbing. Intralesional injection of triamcinolone at 6 to 12 months postoperatively is recommended for retroauricular scars, but direct excision with hair-bearing flap advancement is the choice for the temporal region [98]. Short transverse submental scars are seldom a problem unless an extensive skin resection is done that produces tension. However, large Z-plasty and thyroid-level scars are often visible and require surgical revision.

EARLOBE DEFORMITIES

Tension on the earlobe can produce a variety of malformations including downward or anterior displacement [50]. These problems are best avoided by conservative splitting of the skin flap to the level of the antitragus and then custom-tailoring the flap once the key tension sutures are inserted [107, 140, 144]. If the problem is compounded by visible scars passing anteriorly from the earlobe, early revision will be necessary. Rich et al. [182] correct the pixie earlobe by direct excision, creating a rounded lobule and closing the excised cheek triangle directly. For more severe problems, one can undermine skin and do a "second lift," bringing the excised area behind the auricle and thereby avoiding an anterior scar. In addition, minor preoperative size abnormalities can become major disproportions—too small or too large. Patients with large earlobes may be *particularly* disappointed postoperatively as the smooth skin and mandibular contour emphasize the deformity. Therefore, a discrete preoperative discussion is often necessary, and an operative solution offered [144].

CONTOUR DEFORMITIES

These problems range from localized residue of small hematomas (nodules, skin puckering) to the deforming sequelae of neck contouring (platysmal rolls, submental hollowness, skeletonization) (Fig. 16-33). If small hematomas cannot be drained at time of detection, frequent warm compresses are recommended and repeat attempts at aspiration are made. Chronic complaints of nodularity

Figure 16-33

A. Patient seen in consultation following rhytidectomy plus direct excision of redundant neck skin.

B. Extensive fat and skin removal has created a "blast effect" beneath the chin.

C. Any statement that these scars are not visible is difficult to accept.

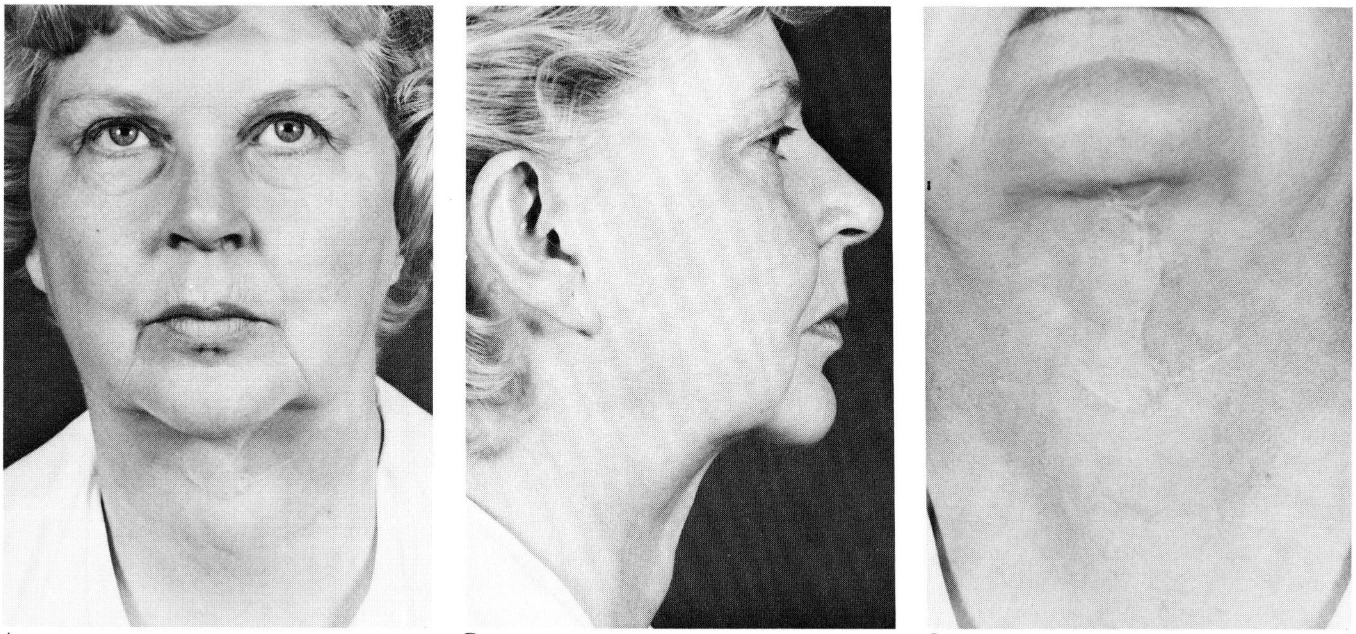

A B C

and visible puckering of the skin are treated by frequent massaging and reassurance. Ultimately (6–12 months) the problem will resolve but with a disappointed patient rather than a happy one. Major contour deformities result from high transection of the platysma without beveling of the edges, excessive removal of submental fat often without plication of the platysma, or transection of the platysma in thin patients. Each of these problems is best avoided by careful preoperative planning and intraoperative dissection. Secondary correction may require a repeat rhytidectomy with selective grafting.

PIGMENTATION
Hyperpigmentation of the skin is attributed to persistence of iron pigment at sites of postoperative edema in patients with skin sensitivity. The only preoperative warning sign is a history of easy bruisability. The most severe postoperative pigmentation is seen in skin areas that marginally survive ischemic insults as manifested by crusting. Coverage with a dark liquid foundation is the best method of treatment, and improvement may require 1 year. Conversely, the patient with a reddish complexion and multiple telangiectasia may suffer accentuated pigmentation.

HAIR LOSS
Areas of alopecia are distressing to the patient, particularly as they often occur in persons with thinning hair. Small areas are often seen along incision lines and are due to excessive tension [174]. In most cases, hair loss is a temporary phenomenon, with recovery by 3 to 4 months. If large alopecic areas are seen in the temporal area, the hair loss may be relative or absolute, the former being due to posterior displacement of the hairline or upward migration of preauricular skin. Absolute hair loss may be due to transection of the hair follicles or tension. Definitive treatment can be accomplished by rotation of a small scalp flap [120, 130].

PAIN
As previously noted, acute pain is usually associated with hematoma formation, chronic pain with sensory nerve neuromas, and early discomfort with platysma tightening. The latter two conditions require initial reassurance, with surgery indicated only for localized neuroma pain at approximately 9 months [54].

PATIENT DISSATISFACTION
According to senior surgeons, the objective dissatisfaction rate dropped significantly following introduction of the more extended cervicofacial rhytidectomies. Fewer patients present postoperatively who feel that "nothing has been done" or state, "I don't see any improvement." Although many surgeons have advocated a two-stage rhytidectomy, it is rarely necessary [108, 121]. An exception is a preplanned two-stage procedure beginning with a rhytidectomy followed by a chemical peel [141, 160, 185]. However, a small percentage of patients will persist with a series of minor nonspecific complaints including pain, numbness, or swelling. Often these problems are related to ongoing life stresses that were not solved by a rhytidectomy as the patient had secretly wished [39]. Goldwyn [87] has emphasized that the surgeon must project an open and available attitude, prepared to accept the patient's hostility and concerns.

RESULTS

Any evaluation of the efficacy of rhytidectomy must integrate the preoperative condition, surgical technique, and postoperative factors. It is generally accepted that the thin patient in her late thirties can achieve a striking youthful beauty whereas the overweight woman in her midfifties will be improved marginally. Following the introduction of platysma surgery, patients with significant cervical deformities have obtained dramatic improvements (Fig. 16-34). Postoperatively, even the best results will be adversely affected by marked fluctuation in weight, continued sun exposure, and severe life crises.

Short-Term Results

If properly prepared, the patient will accept the bruising, swelling, and discomfort of the first postoperative week. Early referral to an aesthetician for assistance with makeup and hairstyling improves the patient's spirits. At 1 month, many patients will benefit from comparing themselves in the mirror with the preoperative photographs, thereby being reassured that the result was well worth the effort. As the edema slowly disappears, fine skin wrinkles and nasolabial folds return, a situation accepted by the informed patient but a major crisis for the perfectionist who fears that her "face has fallen." At one year, 85 percent of patients consider the objective physical improvement good or excellent.

Long-Term Results

Since the aging process continues unabated, it is inevitable that skin laxity and facial changes will occur. Morgan [159] reported that the conservative skin excision rhytidectomy gave a beneficial result of only 1 to 2 years whereas the addition of plication techniques extended it to 3 to 4 years. The most obvious sequelae were cervical bands and fine wrinkles, which can be improved by platysma surgery and chemical peel respectively. With the more radical rhytidectomies being performed currently, it is expected that smoothing of the cheek and jowl areas will last 3 to 5 years and the cervical improvement 5 to 7 years for average

Figure 16-34. Short- and long-term results of rhytidectomy.
A, B. Patient with heavy eyelid deformities and early jowl formation.
C, D. Result at 1 year following forehead-lift, blepharoplasty, and rhytidectomy. Note forehead-lift was done at the hairline.
E, F. Result 9 years later with maintenance of a smooth forehead and mandibular border.

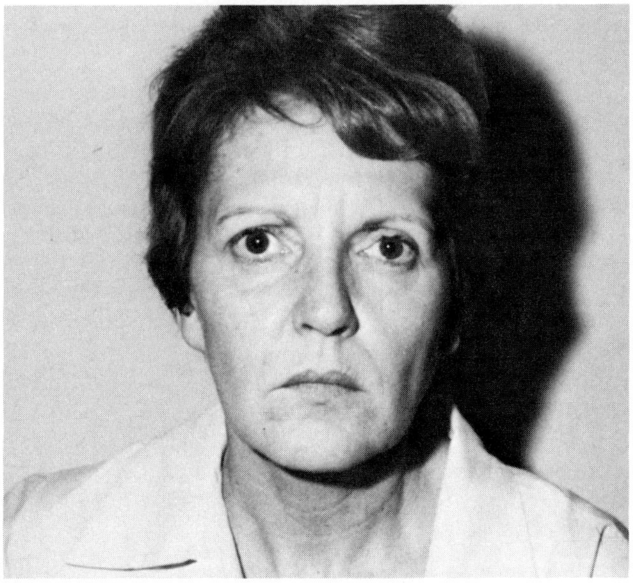
A

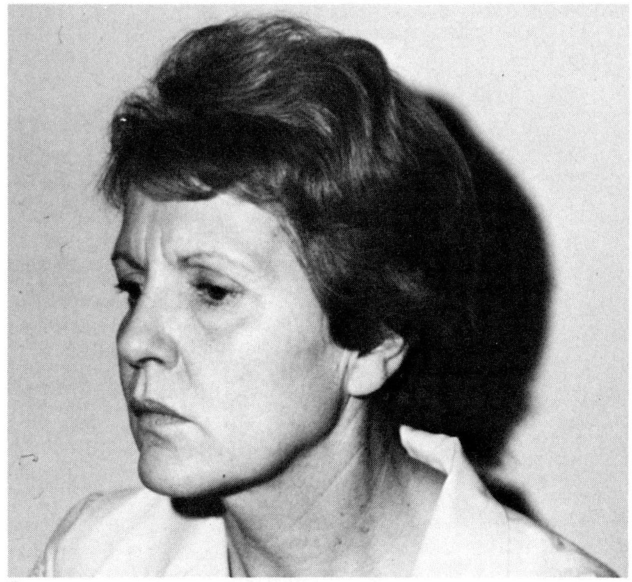
B

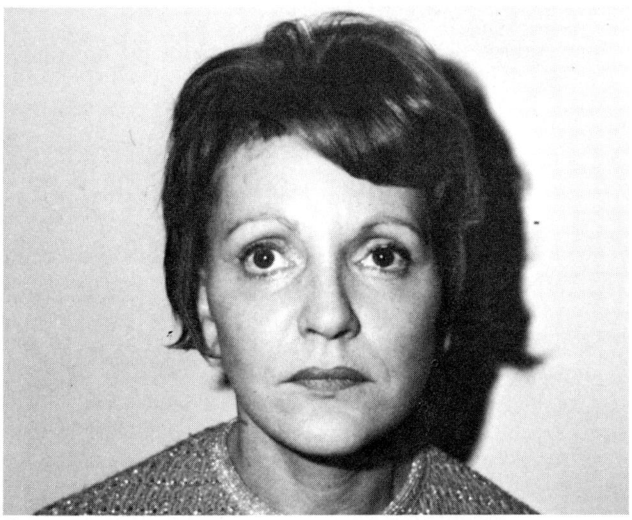
C

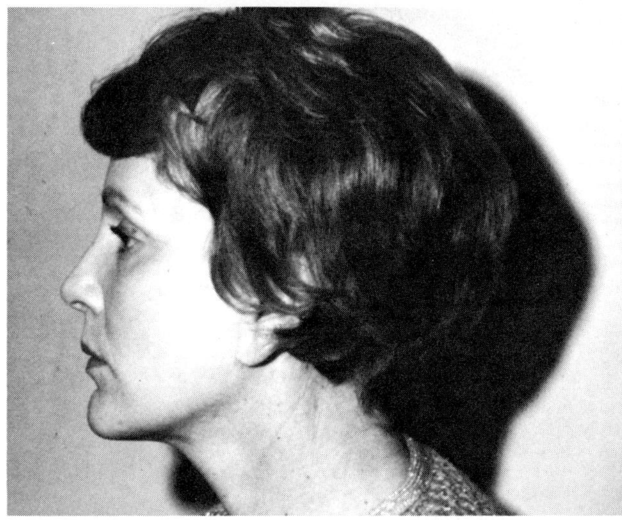
D

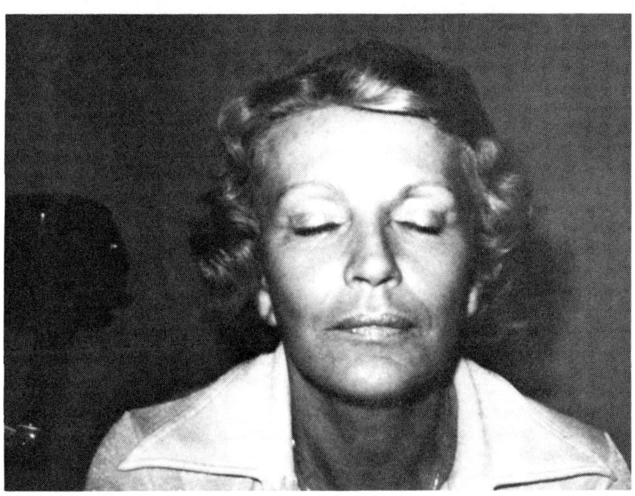
E

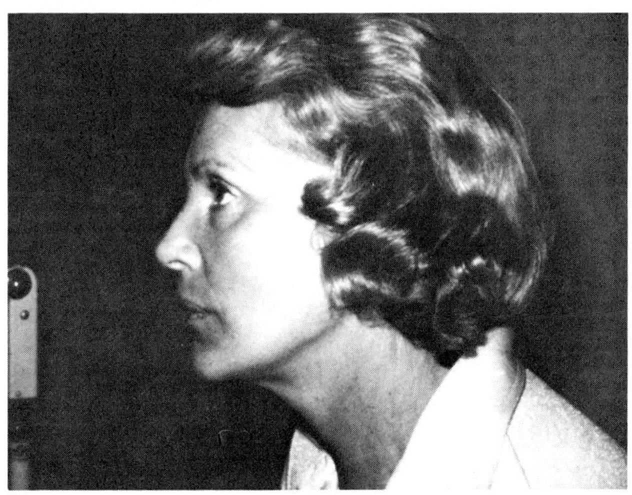
F

patients in their fifties. Patient satisfaction with the final result is adversely influenced by the occurrence of complications, especially bothersome scarring, hair loss, or permanent numbness. Berry [34] observed that only 52 percent (21 out of 60) of patients who had rhytidectomy alone would repeat the procedure compared to 79 percent (11 out of 14) of patients having rhytidectomy plus blepharoplasty. In certain patients, especially in the 50 to 60 age bracket, one must consider the total approach of forehead-lift, cervicofacial rhytidectomy, and eyelid blepharoplasty with optional chemical peel at a later date. However, final satisfaction depends on how well the surgeon achieved the *patient's* expectations based on a careful preoperative evaluation with selection and execution of the optimal operative procedure.

SECONDARY SURGERY

Even after an excellent result from the initial procedure, a secondary rhytidectomy may be done because the patient wants to keep a younger-looking face. It is not uncommon for certain individuals to have three to five face-lifts during a lifetime. However, in certain cases reoperation may have to be done early after the primary surgery because of an inadequate first procedure or because of complications.

Secondary Rhytidectomy After Initial Complications

The main complications giving a permanently poor result are visible scars, skin slough, deformities of the face and neck, asymmetry, and paralysis.

Although hypertrophic scars may be related to the patient's intrinsic wound-healing capabilities, they are most often associated with tension. Often one can excise or conceal the previous scars and reduce their recurrence by modifying the fascial foundation to secure improvement without recourse to skin tension.

When an extensive skin slough has occurred after the first operation, a very large subcutaneous undermining is necessary at the second procedure to remove as much scar as possible. In the temporal area, a transverse scalp flap can be transferred to replace the area of alopecia with primary closure of the donor site. In the retroauricular and mastoid areas, a very extensive neck dissection usually provides enough skin to cover even the largest sloughs. Skin loss in the preauricular area is the most difficult to remove completely as it often resulted from excessive skin tension. Serial excision may be necessary.

Facial and cervical irregularities following rhytidectomy may be due to uneven lipectomy, skin resection, or traction on deep structures. Once the origin of the deformity is diagnosed, treatment is obvious and corrected at secondary rhytidectomy. Prior to infiltration of local anesthetic, the location for either more extensive removal or shifting of deep structures is marked precisely. A common deformity is traction on the earlobe, which becomes triangular on descent. It is corrected by reducing the skin tension and attaching the lobe upward to the concha. The occipital and temporal skin flaps are redraped to avoid displacement of the earlobe. Asymmetry of the face and neck may also be due to unequal fat removal, unequal tension on the platysma or SMAS, and unequal skin removal. A second rhytidectomy should correct all existing deformities by careful analysis of the trouble, very precise planning, and meticulous execution.

Terminal branches of the nerve branches may be injured by a sharp transection during dissection below the platysma or around the lips, and by inadvertent coagulation, an event that is lessened by use of bipolar coagulation. When the paralysis has lasted for more than a year, it is usually permanent. The patients may get used to it and, if minor, compensate for it voluntarily. However, significant deformities are rarely accepted. A second face-lift can help correct the neural asymmetry by plicating the deep structures more extensively on the paralyzed side, or by contralateral sectioning of the nerve branch, which is often the best solution.

Secondary Rhytidectomy After an Inadequate Primary Operation

An inadequate primary result may be due to failure of platysma of SMAS modification, lipectomy, or insufficient skin resection. Diagnosis of the problem is accomplished by examining the patient's face and neck, palpating the deep structures, and testing the skin elasticity. The patient's dissatisfaction is often exaggerated in order to influence the surgeon's decision to perform a second procedure. Before a year, reoperation is rarely indicated. Those with definite indications should be reassured that a correction is possible and the result will be better after 1 year.

The skin incision follows the same rules as apply to any secondary rhytidectomy. A submental incision in the natural crease is done whenever submental defatting is required. In selected cases, a direct submental defatting may be indicated, with submental skin excision; otherwise the undermining must be more extensive than the first time. When the platysma was left untouched, it is treated as in a primary operation. If it was dissected, it may be redissected and split transversely to create a definite flap. The anterior borders may need to be reduced as well as sutured together. The cheek SMAS may be redissected and pulled upward, or a simple plication may be done. The skin excision is minimal at the earlobe but may be quite large in the preauricular, temporal, and occipital areas. The result of a second rhytidectomy after an insufficient first one is usually quite satisfactory when performed correctly.

Secondary Rhytidectomy

The timing of a secondary rhytidectomy following a good primary procedure varies according to the case. The durability of the result depends on both the surgical technique and patient factors including skin characteristics, skin care, aging factors, and life-style. Normally, a 5- to 10-year period separates the two procedures. However, for persons with fine skin or those who abuse their skin with heavy makeup, sun exposure, or smoking, the durability can be shortened.

With the classic skin-stretching rhytidectomies, it was often said that a second face-lift would be necessary after 1 or 2 years; the additional stretching would offer a much longer durability. Now that the fascial foundation is being modified, a significantly greater amount of skin is resected at the primary operation. Therefore, the first procedure often lasts more than 7 years, and most secondary face-lifts last almost the same period of time. Third and fourth ones persist for a somewhat shorter time. Preoperatively, it is critical to separate the procedure into two parts: (1) rhytidectomy (previous scars influence incisions, omissions determine selection, previous steps modify selection) and (2) additional procedures (both primary and secondary). For example, analysis of certain candidates for secondary rhytidectomy may reveal the following: (1) temporal incision with retrodisplacement of scalp, therefore a hairline incision; (2) failure to do a lipectomy, therefore extensive submandibular lipectomy; (3) previous SMAS plication, therefore a repeat plication; (4) initial blepharoplasty but persistent eyebrow ptosis and crow's-feet, therefore a forehead-lift plus orbicularis oculi modification; and (5) repeat chemical peel of the perioral region.

The technique of a second face-lift is influenced by the first one. Any visible scars should be removed. The temporal hairline, which has often been elevated by the first procedure, should not be further displaced. Thus, the temporal incision at the hairline is used. When the temporal scalp scar is wide, it is corrected by reducing the temporal skin excision. The periauricular excision is modified according to the tension on the earlobe, and sometimes no skin is removed, only the scar. In the mastoid and occipital areas, the incision is placed in the scalp in the preferred manner. When the previous scar is at the posterior hairline, it is better not to follow the same line but to stay above it in the scalp. Thus, removal of some scalp causes the previous scar to be elevated.

Undermining in a second face-lift must be more extensive than in the first one and advance beyond the fibrotic subcutaneous area. In contrast to what is stated in most articles, there is little bleeding and only the capillary oozing in the predissected area. Dissection or redissection of the platysma and the SMAS over the cheeks is followed by the appropriate plication or flaps. However, if these structures were considerably modified at the first operation, a simple plication is done in one or two layers and is considered more effective than a repeat dissection. Modification of deep structures is the most important step in obtaining a good secondary result. It is more critical in a secondary face-lift than a primary one because of the reduced skin elasticity that follows excision of the initial face-lift.

The skin excision varies according to the skin elasticity and to the initial excision. Five years after the first operation, skin elasticity may be virtually normal and a large quantity of skin can be removed, especially in the occipitomastoid area. However, skin excision is always reduced in the earlobe and preauricular areas.

Subsequent rhytidectomies after the first and second operations do not require significant undermining of the skin, as modification of the platysma and SMAS is limited to plication. It is often advantageous to perform an upward type of face-lift, removing the greatest part of the skin both in the temporal area by direct transverse excision and in the occipital area by plication of the deep structures at the same level. The results of tertiary face-lifting are of shorter duration than with the first two, and after multiple procedures the value of ancillary procedures increases dramatically, i.e., chemical peel, brow-lift, cheiloplasty, or collagen injections.

In summary, secondary cervicofacial rhytidectomy is an excellent way of bringing more rejuvenation and of correcting errors or complications, but it requires very careful diagnosis and planning. Detailed explanation of the procedure to the patient, as well as the expected results and limitations, is essential.

REFERENCES

1. Adamson, J. E., Horton, C. E., and Crawford, H. H. The surgical correction of "turkey gobbler" deformity. *Plast. Reconstr. Surg.* 34:598, 1964.
2. Adamson, J. E., and Toksu, A. E. Progress in rhytidectomy by platysma-SMAS rotation and elevation. *Plast. Reconstr. Surg.* 68:23, 1981.
3. Alibert, J. L. *Monographie des Dermatoses ou Précis Théorique et Pratique de la Peau.* Paris: Daynac, 1832. P. 795.
4. Anderson, J. R. The facelift operation and the otolaryngologist. *Laryngoscope* 81:866, 1971.
5. Anderson, J. R. The tuck-up operation: A new technique of secondary rhytidectomy. *Arch. Otolaryngol.* 101:739, 1975.
6. Anderson, J. R. Some tips on face-lifting. *Otolaryngol. Head Neck Surg.* 87:522, 1979.
7. Apfelberg, D. B., Maser, M. R., and Lash, H. Use of Trendelenburg position to reveal open blood vessels and prevent hematomas in face lifts. *Plast. Reconstr. Surg.* 63:419, 1979.
8. Aston, S. J. Platysma muscle in rhytidoplasty. *Ann. Plast. Surg.* 3:529, 1979.
9. Aston, S. J. Orbicularis oculi muscle flaps. *Clin. Plast. Surg.* 8:679, 1981.
10. Aston, S. J. Cervicofacial Rhytidoplasty. In E. H. Courtiss (ed.), *Male Aesthetic Surgery.* St. Louis: Mosby, 1982.
11. Aufricht, G. Surgery for Excess Skin of the Face and Neck. In G. M. Wallace (ed.), *Transactions of the Second Congress of the International Society of Plastic Surgery.* Baltimore: Williams & Wilkins, 1960. Pp. 495–502.
12. Baker, D. C., and Conley, J. Avoiding facial nerve injuries in rhytidectomy. *Plast. Reconstr. Surg.* 64:781, 1979.
13. Baker, D. C., et al. The male rhytidectomy. *Plast. Reconstr. Surg.* 4:514, 1977.
14. Baker, D. C. Complications of cervicofacial rhytidectomy. *Clin. Plast. Surg.* 10:543, 1983.
15. Baker, T. J. Patient selection and psychological evaluation. *Clin. Plast. Surg.* 5:3, 1978.
16. Baker, T. J., and Gordon, H. L. Complications of rhytidectomy. *Plast. Reconstr. Surg.* 40:31, 1967.
17. Baker, T. J., and Gordon, H. L. Adjunctive aids to rhytidectomy. *South. Med. J.* 62:108, 1969.
18. Baker, T. J., and Gordon, H. L. Rhytidectomy in males. *Plast. Reconstr. Surg.* 44:219, 1969.

19. Baker, T. J., and Gordon, H. L. Chemical face peeling and dermabrasion. *Surg. Clin. North Am.* 51:387, 1971.
20. Baker, T. J., and Gordon, H. L. The temporal face lift ("mini-lift"). *Plast. Reconstr. Surg.* 47:313, 1971.
21. Baker, T. J., and Gordon, H. L. Chemical peeling as a practical method for removing rhytides of the upper lip. *Ann. Plast. Surg.* 2:209, 1979.
22. Baker, T. J., Gordon, H. L., and Mesienko, P. Rhytidectomy. *Plast. Reconstr. Surg.* 59:24, 1977.
23. Baker, T. J., Gordon, H. L., and Whitlow, D. R. Our present technique for rhytidectomy. *Plast. Reconstr. Surg.* 52:232, 1973.
24. Balch, C. R. Superficial musculoaponeurotic system suspension and buccinator plication for facial nerve paralysis. *Plast. Reconstr. Surg.* 66:769, 1980.
25. Bames, H. Truth and fallacies of face peeling and face lifting. *Med. J. Rec.* 126:86, 1927.
26. Bames, H. Frown disfigurement and ptosis of the eyebrows. *Plast. Reconstr. Surg.* 19:337, 1957.
27. Barker, D. E. Prevention of bleeding following a rhytidectomy. *Plast. Reconstr. Surg.* 54:651, 1974.
28. Baroudi, R., Keppke, E. M., and Carvalho, C. S. Rhytidectomie: Etude analytique des incisions. *Ann. Chir. Plast.* 21:137, 1976.
29. Beekhuis, G. J. Anesthesia for facial cosmetic surgery: Low dosage ketamine-diazepam anesthesia. *Laryngoscope* 88:1709, 1978.
30. Beekhuis, G. J. Facelift: Postoperative hematoma, prevention and management. *Laryngoscope* 90:164, 1980.
31. Berger, R. A. Use of silicone injections in facial defects. *Arch. Otolaryngol.* 101:526, 1975.
32. Berman, W. E., and Monell, C. M. Complications in blepharoplasties and face lift operations. *Otolaryngol. Clin. North Am.* 7:87, 1974.
33. Berner, R. E., Morian, W. D., and Noe, J. M. Postoperative hypertension as an etiologic factor in hematoma after rhytidectomy. *Plast. Reconstr. Surg.* 57:314, 1976.
34. Berry, E. P. Subjective evaluation of the face-lift and eyelid operations. *Plast. Reconstr. Surg.* 46:429, 1970.
35. Biggs, T. M., Jr. T-Z-plasty for the male "turkey gobbler" neck. *Plast. Reconstr. Surg.* 65:238, 1980.
36. Bourguet, J. La chirurgie esthétique de la face. *Concours Med.* 43:1657, 1921.
37. Bourguet J. La chirurgie esthétique de l'oeil et des paupières. *Monde Med.* 39:725, 1929.
38. Brennan, H. G., and Parkes, M. L. Submentoplasty: Classification and theoretical outline of management. *Arch. Otolaryngol.* 95:24, 1972.
39. Burgoyne, R. W., Goin, J. M., and Goin, M. K. Intraoperative psychological reactions in face-lift patients under local anesthesia. *Plast. Reconstr. Surg.* 60:582, 1977.
40. Cameron, R. R., et al. Use of dermal flaps for attachment of rhytidoplasty flaps. *Plast. Reconstr. Surg.* 51:596, 1973.
41. Cardoso de Castro, C., and Aboudib, J. H., Jr. Extensive cervical and lower face lipectomy: Its importance and anatomical basis. *Ann. Plast. Surg.* 4:370, 1980.
42. Carlin, G. A., and Gurdin, M. M. Ancillary procedures for the aging face and neck. *Surg. Clin. North Am.* 51:371, 1971.
43. Castanares, S. Forehead wrinkles, glabellar frown and ptosis of the eyebrows. *Plast. Reconstr. Surg.* 34:406, 1964.
44. Castanares, S. Facial nerve paralysis coincident with, or subsequent to rhytidectomy. *Plast. Reconstr. Surg.* 54:637, 1974.
45. Claoue, C. La ridectomie cervico-faciale: Correction de la ptose cutanée cervico-faciale par accrochage parieto-temporo-occipital et resection cutanée. *Acad. Natl. Med. Bull.* 109:257, 1933.
46. Clodius, L. Selective neurectomies to achieve symmetry in partial and complete facial paralysis. *Br. J. Plast. Surg.* 29:43, 1976.
47. Conley, J. *Face-Lift Operation.* Springfield, Ill.: Thomas, 1968.
48. Conley, J., and Baker, D. C. Thread augmentation for facial rhytides. *Ann. Plast. Surg.* 3:118, 1979.
49. Conley, J. J., and Clairmont, A. A. Subdermal fascial augmentation. *Arch. Otolaryngol.* 103:44, 1977.
50. Conley, J. J., and Clairmont, A. A. The significance of the earlobe in rhytidectomy. *Laryngoscope* 88:880, 1978.
51. Connell, B. F. Cervical lift: Surgical correction of fat contour problems combined with full width platysma muscle flap. *Aesthetic Plast. Surg.* 1:355, 1978.
52. Connell, B. F. Contouring the neck in rhytidectomy by lipectomy and a muscle sling. *Plast. Reconstr. Surg.* 61:376, 1978.
53. Connell, B. F. Eyebrow and Forehead Lifts. In E. H. Courtiss (ed.), *Male Aesthetic Surgery.* St. Louis: Mosby, 1982.
54. Conway, H. Factors Underlying Prolonged Pain Following Rhytidectomy. In *Transactions of the Fourth International Congress of Plastic and Reconstructive Surgery.* Amsterdam: Excerpta Medica, 1967. Pp. 1120–1122.
55. Conway, H. The surgical face lift–rhytidectomy. *Plast. Reconstr. Surg.* 45:124, 1970.
56. Conway, H., and Lacy, G. M. Analysis of 325 consecutive rhytidectomies. *N.Y. State J. Med.* 67:790, 1967.
57. Correia, P. de C., and Zani, R. Surgical anatomy of the facial nerve as related to ancillary operations in rhytidectomy. *Plast. Reconstr. Surg.* 52:549, 1973.
58. Courtiss, E. H. *Aesthetic Surgery: Trouble—How to Avoid It and How to Treat It.* St. Louis: Mosby, 1978.
59. Courtiss, E. H. *Male Aesthetic Surgery.* St. Louis: Mosby, 1982.
60. Cox, H. T. The cleavage lines of the skin. *Br. J. Surg.* 29:234, 1941.
61. Crikelair, G. F., and Wolf, C. E. Preoperative work-ups and near catastrophes. (Letter to the Editor.) *Plast. Reconstr. Surg.* 53:216, 1974.
62. Cronin, T. D., and Biggs, T. M. The T-Z plasty for the male "turkey gobbler" neck. *Plast. Reconstr. Surg.* 47:534, 1971.
63. Davis, P. K. B., and Jones, S. M. The complications of silastic implants: Experience with 137 consecutive cases. *Br. J. Plast. Surg.* 24:405, 1971.
64. Davis, R. A., et al. Surgical anatomy of the facial nerve and parotid gland based upon a study of 350 cervicofacial halves. *Surgery* 102:385, 1956.
65. Dedo, D. D. A preoperative classification of the neck for cervicofacial rhytidectomy. *Laryngoscope* 90:1894, 1980.
66. Desnoyers, Y., et al. Anaesthesia for facial rhytidectomy. *Can. Anaesth. Soc. J.* 26:222, 1979.
67. Dicker, R. L., and Syracuse, V. R. Local anesthesia in facial plastic surgery. *ORL* 86:461, 1978.
68. Dingman, R. O., and Grabb, W. C. Surgical anatomy of the mandibular ramus of the facial nerve based on the dissection of 100 facial halves. *Plast. Reconstr. Surg.* 20:266, 1962.
69. Edgerton, M. T., et al. Surgical results and psychosocial changes following rhytidectomy. *Plast. Reconstr. Surg.* 33:503, 1964.
70. Edwards, B. F. Bilateral temporal neurotomy for frontalis hypermotility. Case report. *Plast. Reconstr. Surg.* 19:341, 1957.
71. Ellenbogen, R. Pseudo-paralysis of the mandibular branch of

the facial nerve after platysmal face-lift operation. *Plast. Reconstr. Surg.* 63:364, 1979.
72. Ellenbogen, R., and Karlin, J. V. Visual criteria for success in restoring the youthful neck. *Plast. Reconstr. Surg.* 66:826, 1980.
73. Ellenbogen, R., and Karlin, J. V. Regrowth of platysma following platysma cervical lift: Etiology and methodology of prevention. *Plast. Reconstr. Surg.* 67:616, 1981.
74. Ellis, D. A. F. The development of the aging face. *Can. J. Otolaryngol.* 2:231, 1973.
75. Fodor, P. B. Platysma-SMAS rhytidectomy. *Aesthetic Plast. Surg.* 6:173, 1982.
76. Fomon, S. *Cosmetic Surgery: Principles and Practice.* Philadelphia: Lippincott, 1960.
77. Fredericks, S. The lower rhytidectomy. *Plast. Reconstr. Surg.* 54:537, 1974.
78. Fredericks, S. Rhytidectomy. In E. H. Courtiss (ed.), *Aesthetic Surgery: Trouble—How to Avoid It and How to Treat It.* St. Louis: Mosby, 1978.
79. Fry, P., Harkness, M. L., and Harkness, R. D. Mechanical properties of the collagenous framework of skin in rats of different ages. *Am. J. Physiol.* 206:1425, 1964.
80. Furnas, D. W. The orbicularis oculi muscle: Management in blepharoplasty. *Clin. Plast. Surg.* 8:687, 1981.
81. Gibson, T., and Kenedi, R. M. Biochemical properties of skin. *Surg. Clin. North Am.* 47:279, 1967.
82. Gillies, H., and Millard, D. R. *Principles and Art of Plastic Surgery.* Boston: Little, Brown, 1957.
83. Gleason, M. C. The Temple Lift. In D. Goulian and E. H. Courtiss (eds.), *Symposium on Surgery of the Aging Face.* St. Louis: Mosby, 1978. P. 89.
84. Gleason, M. C. Forehead and Eyebrow Lifts. In E. H. Courtiss (ed.), *Aesthetic Surgery: Trouble—How to Avoid It and How to Treat It.* St. Louis: Mosby, 1978.
85. Goin, M. K., Burgoyne, R. W., and Goin, J. M. Face-lift operation: The patient's secret motivations and reactions to "informed consent." *Plast. Reconstr. Surg.* 58:273, 1976.
86. Goin, M. K., et al. A prospective psychological study of 50 female face-lift patients. *Plast. Reconstr. Surg.* 65:436, 1980.
87. Goldwyn, R. M. The Dissatisfied Patient. In D. Goulian and E. H. Courtiss (eds.), *Symposium on Surgery of the Aging Face.* St. Louis: Mosby, 1978. P. 81.
88. Gonzalez-Ulloa, M. Facial wrinkles. *Plast. Reconstr. Surg.* 29:658, 1962.
89. Gonzalez-Ulloa, M., and Flores, E. S. Sectional rhytidectomy. *Int. Surg.* 56:266, 1971.
90. Gonzalez-Ulloa, M., and Stevens, E. The treatment of palpebral bags. *Plast. Reconstr. Surg.* 27:381, 1961.
91. Gonzalez-Ulloa, M., and Stevens, E. F. Senility of the face: Basic study to understand its causes and effects. *Plast. Reconstr. Surg.* 36:239, 1965.
92. Gonzalez-Ulloa, M., et al. Symposium sur le traitement chirurgical des rides et ptoses cutanées faciales. *Ann. Chir. Plast.* 16:97, 1971.
93. Gordon, H. Rhytidectomy. *Clin. Plast. Surg.* 5:97, 1978.
94. Goulian, D. The need for extensive undermining in face-lifting operations. *Br. J. Plast. Surg.* 26:387, 1973.
95. Goulian, D., and Courtiss, E. H. (eds.). *Symposium on Surgery of the Aging Face.* St. Louis: Mosby, 1978.
96. Grabb, W. C. A concentration of 1:500,000 epinephrine in a local anesthetic solution is sufficient to provide excellent hemostasis. (Letter to the Editor.) *Plast. Reconstr. Surg.* 63:834, 1979.
97. Grahame, R., and Holt, P. J. The influence of aging on the in vivo elasticity of human skin. *Gerontologia* 15:121, 1969.
98. Griffith, B. H. The treatment of keloids with triamcinolone acetonide. *Plast. Reconstr. Surg.* 38:202, 1966.
99. Griffith, B. H. A simplified technique for marking the line of excision in rhytidectomy. *Br. J. Plast. Surg.* 27:276, 1974.
100. Guerrero-Santos, J. Muscular lift in cervical rhytidoplasty. *Plast. Reconstr. Surg.* 54:127, 1974.
101. Guerrero-Santos, J. The role of the platysma muscle in rhytidoplasty. *Clin. Plast. Surg.* 5:29, 1978.
102. Guerrero-Santos, J., Espaillat, L., and Morales, F. Muscular lift in cervical rhytidoplasty. *Plast. Reconstr. Surg.* 54:127, 1974.
103. Habal, M. B. Parotid retention cysts as a complication of rhytidectomy. Case report. *Plast. Reconstr. Surg.* 61:920, 1978.
104. Hamilton, J. M. Rhytidectomy in the male. *Plast. Reconstr. Surg.* 53:629, 1974.
105. Hayflick, L. The biology of human aging. *Plast. Reconstr. Surg.* 67:536, 1981.
106. Hernandez, A. The post-tragal face lift incision. *Br. J. Plast. Surg.* 31:362, 1978.
107. Hirshowitz, B. A modification in the face-lift incision to facilitate suturing around the earlobe. *Plast. Reconstr. Surg.* 55:368, 1975.
108. Hirshowitz, B. The two-stage face lift. *Br. J. Plast. Surg.* 31:159, 1978.
109. Hoffman, S., and Simon, B. E. Complications of submental lipectomy. *Plast. Reconstr. Surg.* 60:889, 1977.
110. Hollander, M. M. Rhytidectomy: Anatomical, physiological and surgical considerations. *Plast. Reconstr. Surg.* 20:218, 1957.
111. Horton, C. E., et al. Cosmetic surgery. *Br. J. Plast. Surg.* 31:566, 1974.
112. Horton, C. E., et al. Postauricular skin excision in rhytidectomy. *Plast. Reconstr. Surg.* 62:128, 1978.
113. Hugo, N. E. Rhytidectomy with radical lipectomy and platysmal flaps. *Plast. Reconstr. Surg.* 65:199, 1980.
114. Hunt, H. L. *Plastic Surgery of the Head, Face and Neck.* Philadelphia: Lea & Febiger, 1926. P. 198.
115. Johnson, H. A. Comparison of 0.25% Marcaine with 0.50% Xylocaine as local anesthetic agents (both with 1:200,000 epinephrine). *Plast. Reconstr. Surg.* 65:375, 1980.
116. Johnson, J. B., and Hadley, R. C. The Aging Face. In J. M. Converse (ed.), *Reconstructive Plastic Surgery.* Philadelphia: Saunders, 1964. Pp. 1306–1342.
117. Joseph, J. Verbesserung meiner Hangemangenplastik (Melomioplastik). *Dtsch. Med. Wochenschr.* 54:567, 1928.
118. Jost, G. *Atlas of Aesthetic Plastic Surgery.* Paris: Masson, 1975.
119. Jost, G., and Lamouche, G. SMAS in rhytidectomy. *Aesthetic Plast. Surg.* 6:69, 1982.
120. Juri, J., Juri, C., and DeAntueno, J. Reconstruction of the sideburn alopecial after rhytidectomy. *Plast. Reconstr. Surg.* 57:304, 1976.
121. Kamer, F. M. The two-stage concept of rhytidectomy. *Otolaryngol. Head Neck Surg.* 87:915, 1979.
122. Kaye, B. L. The extended neck lift: The "bottom line." *Plast. Reconstr. Surg.* 65:429, 1980.
123. Kaye, B. L., and Kruse, J. C. General anesthesia for rhytidectomy. A review of 100 consecutive cases. *Plast. Reconstr. Surg.* 60:747, 1977.
124. Kirk, J. E., and Chieffi, M. Variation with age in elasticity of skin and subcutaneous tissue in human individuals. *J. Gerontol.* 17:373, 1962.
125. Klein, D. R., and Rosenberg, A. A comparison of complications between in-hospital patients and outpatients for aes-

thetic surgical procedures: A ten-year study. *Plast. Reconstr. Surg.* 67 : 17, 1981.

126. Knorr, N. J., Edgerton, M. T., and Hoopes, J. E. The "insatiable" cosmetic surgery patient. *Plast. Reconstr. Surg.* 40 : 285, 1967.
127. Kolle, F. S. *Plastic and Cosmetic Surgery.* New York: Appleton, 1911.
128. Lagarde, M. Nouvelles techniques pour le traitement des rides de la face et du cou. *Arch. Franco-Belg. Chir.* 31 : 154, 1928.
129. Lassus, C. Thickening the thin lips. *Plast. Reconstr. Surg.* 68 : 950, 1981.
130. Lauzon, G. Transfer of a large, single temporo-occipital flap for treatment of baldness. *Plast. Reconstr. Surg.* 63 : 369, 1979.
131. Leist, F. D., Masson, J. K., and Erich, J. F. A review of 324 rhytidectomies, emphasizing complications and patient dissatisfaction. *Plast. Reconstr. Surg.* 59 : 525, 1977.
132. Lemmon, M., and Hamra, S. T. Skoog rhytidectomy: A five-year experience with 577 patients. *Plast. Reconstr. Surg.* 65 : 283, 1980.
133. Letterman, G., and Schurter, M. A pattern for the postauricular incision in rhytidectomy. *Plast. Reconstr. Surg.* 51 : 697, 1973.
134. Lewin, M. L., and Tsur, H. Injuries of the great auricular nerve in rhytidectomy. *Aesthetic Plast. Surg.* 1 : 409, 1978.
135. Lewis, C. M. Method for immediate measurement of skin removed during rhytidectomies. *Plast. Reconstr. Surg.* 69 : 614, 1982.
136. Lewis, G. K. Surgical treatment of wrinkles. *Arch. Otolaryngol.* 60 : 334, 1954.
137. Lewis, J. R. *Atlas of Aesthetic Plastic Surgery.* Boston: Little, Brown, 1973.
138. Lewis, J. R. Surgical face lift. *South. Med. J.* 72 : 914, 1979.
139. Lexer, E. Zur Gesichtsplastik. *Arch. Klin. Chir.* 92 : 749, 1910.
140. Lindgren, V. V., and Carlin, G. A. Preventing a pulled-down or deformed earlobe in rhytidectomies. *Plast. Reconstr. Surg.* 51 : 598, 1973.
141. Litton, C. Chemical face lifting. *Plast. Reconstr. Surg.* 29 : 371, 1962.
142. Litton, C., Fournier, P., and Capin, A. A survey of chemical peeling of the face. *Plast. Reconstr. Surg.* 51 : 645, 1973.
143. Loeb, R. Techniques for preservation of the temporal branches of the facial nerve during face-lift operations. *Br. J. Plast. Surg.* 23 : 390, 1970.
144. Loeb, R. Posterior aricular nerve preservation, double chin leveling, and earlobe reimplantation during neck lifts. *Clin. Plast. Surg.* 10 : 405, 1983.
145. Macgregor, F. C. Some psychological hazards of plastic surgery of the face. *Plast. Reconstr. Surg.* 12 : 123, 1953.
146. Macgregor, F. C. Selection of cosmetic surgery patients: Social and psychological considerations. *Surg. Clin. North Am.* 51 : 289, 1970.
147. MacGregor, M. W., and Greenberg, R. L. Rhytidectomy. In R. M. Goldwyn (ed.), *The Unfavorable Results in Plastic Surgery.* Boston: Little, Brown, 1972.
148. Maliniac, J. W. Is the surgical restoration of the aging face justified? *Med. J. Rec.* 135 : 321, 1932.
149. Mara, J. E., and Baker, J. L. Hypertension and haematomas: Prophylaxis with Apresoline. *Br. J. Plast. Surg.* 30 : 169, 1977.
150. McDowell, A. J. Effective practical steps to avoid complications in face-lifting. *Plast. Reconstr. Surg.* 50 : 563, 1972.
151. McKinney, P., and Katarna, D. J. Prevention of injury to the great auricular nerve during rhytidectomy. *Plast. Reconstr. Surg.* 66 : 675, 1980.
152. McKinney, P., and Maywood, B. T. Camouflage of the postauricular scar in rhytidectomy. *Plast. Reconstr. Surg.* 69 : 352, 1982.
153. Meyers, A. D. Submandibular platysmal plication flap. *Laryngoscope* 89 : 1706, 1979.
154. Millard, D. R., Pigott, R. W., and Hedo, A. Submandibular lipectomy. *Plast. Reconstr. Surg.* 41 : 513, 1968.
155. Millard, D. R., et al. Submental and submandibular lipectomy in conjunction with a face lift, in the male or female. *Plast. Reconstr. Surg.* 49 : 385, 1972.
156. Miller, C. C. *Cosmetic Surgery. The Correction of Featural Imperfections.* Chicago: Oak Printing Co., 1908.
157. Mitz, V., and Peyronie, M. The superficial musculo-aponeurotic system (SMAS) in the parotid and cheek area. *Plast. Reconstr. Surg.* 58 : 90, 1976.
158. Moffat, D. A., and Ramsden, R. T. The deformity produced by a palsy of the marginal mandibular branch of the facial nerve. *J. Laryngol. Otol.* 91 : 401, 1977.
159. Morgan, B. L. The aftercare of rhytidectomies with the "no dressing" technique. *Plast. Reconstr. Surg.* 51 : 576, 1953.
160. Mosienko, P., and Baker, T. J. Chemical peel. *Clin. Plast. Surg.* 5 : 79, 1978.
161. Mullin, W. R., and Millard, D. R. Meloplasty, with Emphasis on the Neck. In E. H. Courtiss (ed.), *Male Aesthetic Surgery.* St. Louis: Mosby, 1982. P. 263.
162. Noël, A. *La Chirurgie Esthétique: Son Rôle Social.* Paris: Masson, 1926.
163. Owsley, J. Q., Jr. Platysma-fascial rhytidectomy. *Plast. Reconstr. Surg.* 59 : 843, 1977.
164. Pangman, W. J., and Wallace, R. M. Cosmetic surgery of the face and neck. *Plast. Reconstr. Surg.* 27 : 544, 1961.
165. Parkes, M. L., and Kanodia, R. Helpful hints in augmentation mentoplasty. *Laryngoscope* 90 : 1740, 1980.
166. Passot, R. La chirurgie esthétique des rides du visage. *Presse Med.* 27 : 258, 1919.
167. Pennisi, V. R., and Capozzi, A. The transposition of fat in cervicofacial rhytidectomy. *Plast. Reconstr. Surg.* 49 : 423, 1972.
168. Peterson, R. The Role of the Platysma Muscle in Cervical Lifts. In D. Goulian and E. H. Courtiss (eds.), *Symposium on Surgery of the Aging Face.* St. Louis: Mosby, 1978. P. 115.
169. Pitanguy, I. Ancillary procedures in face-lifting. *Clin. Plast. Surg.* 5 : 51, 1978.
170. Pitanguy, I. *Aesthetic Plastic Surgery of Head and Body.* Berlin: Springer, 1981.
171. Pitanguy, I., and Ceravolo, M. P. Hematoma postrhytidectomy: How we treat it. *Plast. Reconstr. Surg.* 67 : 526, 1981.
172. Pitanguy, I., and Ramos, A. S. The frontal branch of the facial nerve: The importance of its variations in face lifting. *Plast. Reconstr. Surg.* 38 : 352, 1966.
173. Pollet, J. Les rides de la patte d'oie. *Ann. Chir. Plast.* 18 : 191, 1973.
174. Rafaty, F. M. Surgical management of temporal alopecia following face lift operation. *Laryngoscope* 89 : 1175, 1979.
175. Rees, T. D. *Aesthetic Plastic Surgery.* Philadelphia: Saunders, 1980.
176. Rees, T. D., and Aston, S. J. A clinical evaluation of the results of submusculo-aponeurotic dissection and fixation in face lifts. *Plast. Reconstr. Surg.* 59 : 851, 1977.
177. Rees, T. D., and Aston, S. J. Complications of rhytidectomy. *Clin. Plast. Surg.* 5 : 109, 1978.
178. Rees, T. D., and Guy, C. L. Patient selection and techniques in blepharoplasty and rhytidoplasty. *Surg. Clin. North Am.* 51 : 353, 1971.
179. Rees, T. D., Lee, Y. C., and Coburn, R. J. Expanding hema-

toma after rhytidectomy. *Plast. Reconstr. Surg.* 51:149, 1973.
180. Regnault, P. Face and forehead lifting with double traction on "crow's feet." *Plast. Reconstr. Surg.* 49:123, 1972.
181. Regnault, P. Facial and submandibular lipectomy with upward rhytidectomy. *J. Maxillofac. Surg.* 4:199, 1981.
182. Rich, J. D., Gottlieb, V., and Shesol, B. F. A simple method for correction of the pixie earlobe. *Plast. Reconstr. Surg.* 69:136, 1982.
183. Robbins, T. H. The protection of the frontal branch of the facial nerve in face-lift surgery. *Br. J. Plast. Surg.* 34:95, 1981.
184. Robertson, J. G. Chin augmentation by means of rotation of double chin fat flap. *Plast. Reconstr. Surg.* 36:471, 1965.
185. Robertson, J. G. Rhytidectomy combines with chemical peeling of the superficial cutaneous tissues. *Int. Surg.* 47:576, 1967.
186. Rogers, B. O. A brief history of cosmetic surgery. *Surg. Clin. North Am.* 51:265, 1971.
187. Rose, E. H., Laub, D. R., and Avakoff, J. Cardiac asystole secondary to carotid sinus compression in the face-lift operation. *Plast. Reconstr. Surg.* 59:252, 1977.
188. Rubin, L. R. The anatomy of a smile: Its importance in the treatment of facial paralysis. *Plast. Reconstr. Surg.* 53:384, 1974.
189. Rudolph, R., and Woodward, M. Ultrastructure of elastosis in facial rhytidectomy skin. *Plast. Reconstr. Surg.* 67:295, 1981.
190. Schnur, P. L., Burkhardt, B. R., and Tofield, J. J. The second-look technique in face lifts—does it work? *Plast. Reconstr. Surg.* 65:298, 1980.
191. Seltzer, A. P. Wrinkles around the mouth. *ORL* 82:106, 1976.
192. Singer, R., and Lewis, C. M. Rhytidectomies in office operating rooms. *Plast. Reconstr. Surg.* 63:173, 1979.
193. Skoog, T. *Plastic Surgery.* Philadelphia: Saunders, 1975.
194. Smith, G. A., et al. Risks of facial plastic surgery in an otolaryngology program. *Arch. Otolaryngol.* 104:137, 1978.
195. Snyder, G. B. Cervico-mentoplasty with rhytidectomy. *Plast. Reconstr. Surg.* 54:404, 1974.
196. Snyder, G. B. Submental rhytidectomy. *Plast. Reconstr. Surg.* 62:693, 1978.
197. Souther, S. G., and Vistnes, L. M. Medial approximation of the platysma muscle in the treatment of neck deformities. *Plast. Reconstr. Surg.* 67:607, 1981.
198. Spira, M., Gerow, F. J., and Hardy, S. B. Cervicofacial rhytidectomy. *Plast. Reconstr. Surg.* 40:551, 1967.
199. Spoerel, W. E., and McFarlane, R. M. Anesthetic techniques for operations about the face. *Anesth. Analg.* 45:170, 1966.
200. Stark, R. B. A rhytidectomy series. *Plast. Reconstr. Surg.* 59:373, 1977.
201. Stephenson, K. L. The "mini-lift," an old wrinkle in face lifting. *Plast. Reconstr. Surg.* 46:226, 1970.
202. Straith, R. E., Raju, D. R., and Hipps, C. J. The study of hematomas in 500 consecutive face lifts. *Plast. Reconstr. Surg.* 59:694, 1977.
203. Tardy, M. E., and Becker, O. J. Surgical Correction of Facial Deformities. In J. J. Ballenger (ed.), *Diseases of the Nose, Throat, and Ear.* Philadelphia: Lea & Febiger, 1977.
204. Tegtmeier, R. E. Intraoperative measurement in cosmetic surgery of the face. *Plast. Reconstr. Surg.* 68:608, 1981.
205. Tenta, L. T., Tardy, M. E., and Pastorek, N. J. Buccal Lipectomy. In J. Conley and J. T. Dickinson (eds.), *Plastic and Reconstructive Surgery of the Face and Neck.* Stuttgart: Thieme, 1972. P. 22.
206. Thompson, D. P., and Ashley, F. L. Face-lift complications. *Plast. Reconstr. Surg.* 61:40, 1978.
207. Tipton, J. B. Should the subcutaneous tissue be plicated in a face lift? *Plast. Reconstr. Surg.* 54:1, 1974.
208. Webster, G. V. The ischemic face-lift. *Plast. Reconstr. Surg.* 50:560, 1972.
209. Webster, R. C., et al. Conservative face lift surgery. *Arch. Otolaryngol.* 102:657, 1976.
210. Whitaker, L. A., and Pertschuk, M. Facial skeletal contouring for aesthetic purposes. *Plast. Reconstr. Surg.* 69:245, 1982.
211. Wilkinson, T. S. The repair of a submental depression occurring after rhytidectomy. *Plast. Reconstr. Surg.* 57:33, 1976.
212. Zaworski, R. E., and Noriega, C. J. Massive postoperative facial edema in a rhytidectomy. *Plast. Reconstr. Surg.* 62:622, 1978.
213. Zide, B. M., and Laub, D. R. Variations of technique in the face-lift operation. *Ann. Plast. Surg.* 2:114, 1979.

17. Superficial Fascia Rhytidectomy

Mark L. Lemmon

An elective, aesthetic operation should be as free of complications as possible while producing as long lasting a result as possible within tissue limitations. The face-lift techniques that are performed by a wide elevation of the skin at the level of the subdermis and the subcutaneous fat meet the first criterion but not the second. The reason the subcutaneous face-lift does not meet the second criterion is the failure to repair all the tissues of the face and neck, both anatomically and functionally, contributing to the changes in appearance in this region that are characteristic of aging. The proximity of the facial nerve and the fear of an increased rate of complications because of it have inhibited the development of techniques to restore the anatomic and functional relationship of the deeper tissues.

Skoog, with the assistance of Ellenby [12], began in the 1960s to consider the anatomy of the superficial fascia of the face and neck and its relationship to the facial nerve and the skin. Subsequently, Skoog [32–34] described a "two-layer shift" of the cervical region and the elevation and advancement of "the complex morphologic unit" of the face. The "two-layer shift" of the cervical region (based on the adherence of the platysma muscle to the skin), with the elevation and advancement of the superficial fascia (platysma muscle) of the cervical region, relieved the skin and muscle folds of the anterior region of the neck. The "complex morphologic unit" advancement corrected the tissues of the face that subsequently were described by Mitz and Peyronie [27] as the superficial musculoaponeurotic system (SMAS).

The technique of elevating the superficial fascia of the head and neck was based on the relationship of the fasciae of the head and neck and the location of the facial nerve deep to the deep fascia of the head and neck. Skoog believed that the technique produced a more lasting result and that the incidence of complications was no greater than with the more limited techniques to correct the appearance of aging in the face and neck. His approach to the correction of the changes of the face and neck that are characteristic of aging opened a new era in face-lift surgery.

Peterson [30, 31] recognized and advocated the advantages of the advancement of the SMAS and the platysma muscle as an adjunct to a subcutaneous rhytidectomy. Owsley [28] in 1977 and Lemmon and Hamra [20, 21] in 1978 and 1980 agreed that a superficial fascia rhytidectomy was a longer-lasting procedure. However, Lemmon and Hamra concluded the more lasting result of the advancement of superficial fascia of the face and neck was limited to the face and that the characteristics of the tissues (platysma muscle) of the neck required techniques other than an advancement to produce a more enduring result in the neck. Several adjunctive procedures were superimposed on the technique of Skoog in an effort to manage

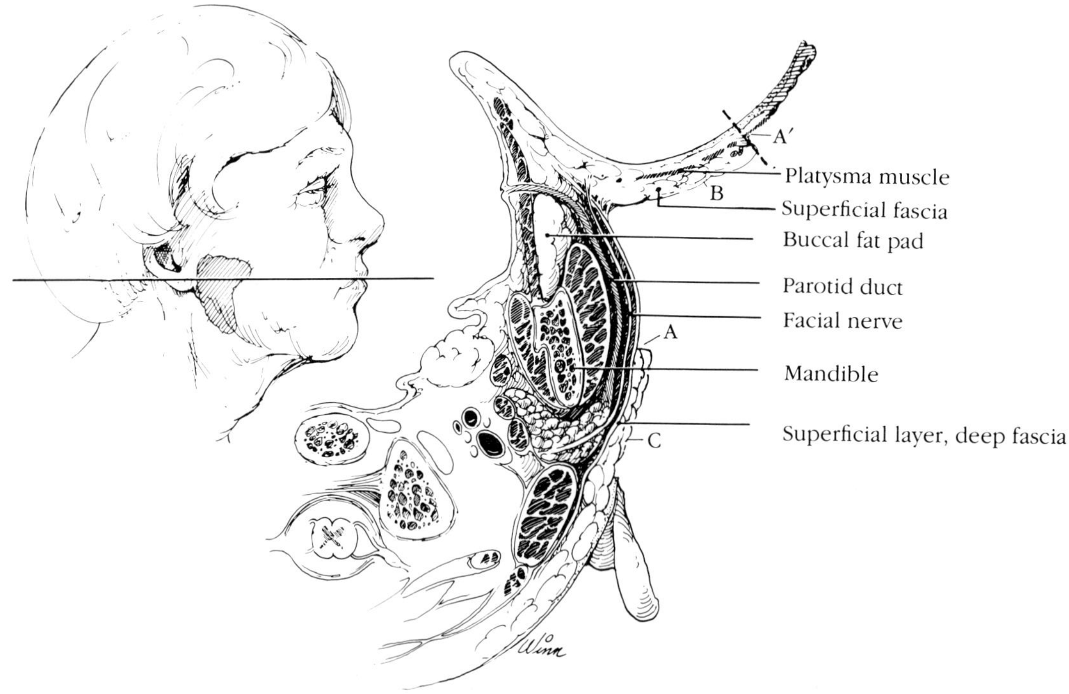

Figure 17-1. Anatomic cross section of the cheek. Elevation of the SMAS. Points A and A′ are the site of the penetration of the superficial fascia of the face (3.5 cm anterior to the preauricular skin incision). Point B is a point selected on the deep surface of the superficial fascia (sub-SMAS), which, when advanced to point A, will provide maximum advancement of the skin of the cheek and the SMAS to point A with minimal tension. The relationships of the deep fascia of the face to the branches of the facial nerve and to the parotid duct are shown.

the early recurrence of the changes of the anterior region of the neck, and the advancement of the superficial fascia of the face and neck and a transection of the platysma muscle as proposed by Connell [5, 6] appeared to afford the best result.

This exposition presents a concept of the restoration of the anatomy and the function of the SMAS as it relates to the young face. A technique of the repair of the superficial fascia of the face and neck that restores anatomy and function of the SMAS and manages the changes of appearance of the cervical region caused by the platysma muscle and the fatty tissue is offered. The technique fulfills the criterion of freedom from unacceptable levels of complication and equals or reduces the incidence of complications of subcutaneous rhytidectomy. Further, improvement can be expected to be maintained for the greatest period of time possible. The complications experienced in the development of the standard technique of superficial rhytidectomy and their prevention are included to emphasize the freedom of the present procedure from these complications.

ANATOMY

The ability to perform a superficial fascia rhytidectomy with confidence and safety depends on an understanding of the deep fascia of the head and neck and its relationship to the facial nerve (Fig. 17-1) whereas an understanding of the anatomy of the superficial fascia is related to its reconstruction (Figs. 17-1 and 17-2). The anatomy of the nerves, muscles, and blood vessels of the face and neck has been described and can be reviewed in standard anatomy texts [13, 18].

The young face reveals a relationship of functional dynamics and contour. The face and neck are unique as the musculature attaches to the skin (muscles of facial expression) or is relatively adherent to the skin (platysma muscle) of the neck. This musculature is superimposed on the deep or investing fascia of the face and neck, which serves as the platform for facial expression.

The surgeon may visualize the soft tissue of the face as a tectonic plate covering the deep fascia of the head and neck. The tectonic plate is composed of the skin, subcutaneous fat, facial muscles, and their fascia (SMAS). Underlying the tectonic plate is the "core" of structural tissue, which is covered with a static but stronger fascia, the deep fascia of the head and neck. Although the deep (investing) fascia relaxes with the passage of time, it is better developed and provides strength for support. But because it is better developed and is a support fascia, it relaxes at a slower rate or maintains its strength longer than the less well-developed superficial covering. By middle age, the more rapid relaxation of the tectonic plate (SMAS and platysma muscle) produces excess skin, wrin-

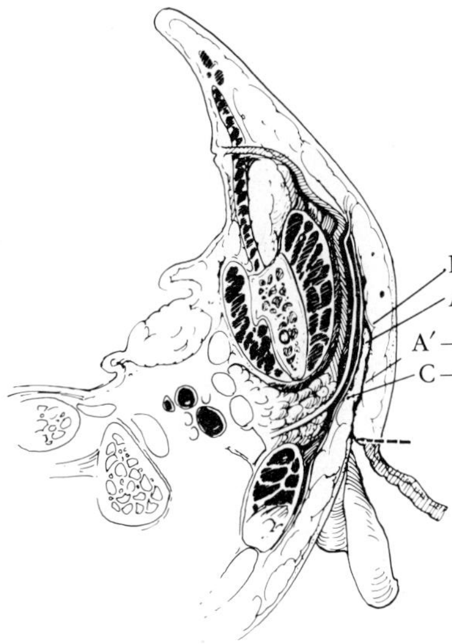

Figure 17-2. Restoration of anteroposterior dimension of superficial fascia and SMAS of face. Points A (and A′) are the site of the penetration of the superficial fascia of the face (3.5 cm anterior to the preauricular skin incision). The imbrication of the superficial fascia approximates the relaxed and elevated superficial fascia (point B) to the superficial fascia (point A) (anterior row of sutures). The overlapped portion of the superficial fascia (point A′) is sutured to subcutaneous tissue (point C) to complete the imbrication (posterior row of sutures).

kling of the face, and anterior platysma muscle folds of the neck.

As stated, a thorough knowledge of the deep fascia of the head and neck is necessary to prevent an injury to the facial nerve. A brief description of the deep fascia of the area of the head and neck that is visualized with superficial fascia rhytidectomy follows. The anterior, or superficial, layer of the deep fascia of the head and neck cephalad to the hyoid bone and ventrad divides and embeds the submandibular gland. There is no distinct submandibular gland capsule, and the septum of the gland fuses with the anterior layer of the deep fascia [18]. Cephalad and posterior to the submandibular gland, the investing or deep fascia thickens and is attached to the inferior margin of the mandible. In the parotid region, it again splits into two laminas to incorporate the parotid in the same fashion as the submandibular gland; that is, the septum of the gland extends into the fascia. Anterior to the parotid gland, the laminas fuse and cover the masseter muscle. Above (cephalad) the parotid gland, the external layer of the superficial layer of the deep fascia attaches to the zygoma while the deep layer is attached to the temporal bone.

Below the hyoid bone and lying ventrally, the anterior or superficial layer of the deep fascia splits and encloses the sternocleidomastoid muscle and the strap muscles of the neck, fusing to form the anterior triangle of the neck. The external jugular vein perforates the superficial layer of the deep fascia just above and at the midportion of the clavicle. It is external to the deep fascia of the neck and deep to the platysma muscle or superficial fascia.

The superficial fascia of the face may vary considerably in its development and adherence to the deep fascia of the face and neck. Hollinshead [18] states that "there is no generally accepted definition as to how dense connective tissue must be before it can be regarded as forming a fascia." The deep fascia over the fat pad of Bichat is very thin, and branches of the facial nerve may be visualized through the fascia. The most adherent zone of the superficial and deep fascia of the face is in the region of, and just anterior to, the fat pad of Bichat (Fig. 17-3, zone B). Below the level of the fat pad of Bichat (Fig. 17-3, zone C), the superficial fascia is usually thinner and loosely adherent to the deep fascia, perhaps because of its relationship with the platysma muscle in the face and the gliding mechanism of the muscle. Cephalad to the fat pad of Bichat and extending over the malar prominence, the superficial fascia is better developed and more adherent to the deep fascia (Fig. 17-3, zone A). The superficial fascia below the inferior border of the mandible in the submandibular region is tightly adherent (Fig. 17-3, zone D). Below the cervicomental angle, the superficial fascia is less adherent (Fig. 17-3, zone E) and the excursion of the platysma muscle on the deep fascia is more extensive.

When an individual is overweight and there is a large amount of fat in the face, the superficial fascia of the face may be poorly defined and obscured by the fatty tissue, which is superficial and deep to the superficial fascia and permeates the tissues of the SMAS. It should be emphasized, however, that once the proper plane is determined in relation to the deep fascia, no matter what the thickness or the definition of the superficial fascia is, its elevation can be completed safely.

This macroconcept of the "sliding tectonic plate" (compound morphologic unit of Skoog or SMAS), rather than a total cellular basis for redundancy of the skin and tissues of the head and neck, suggests that the slippage of

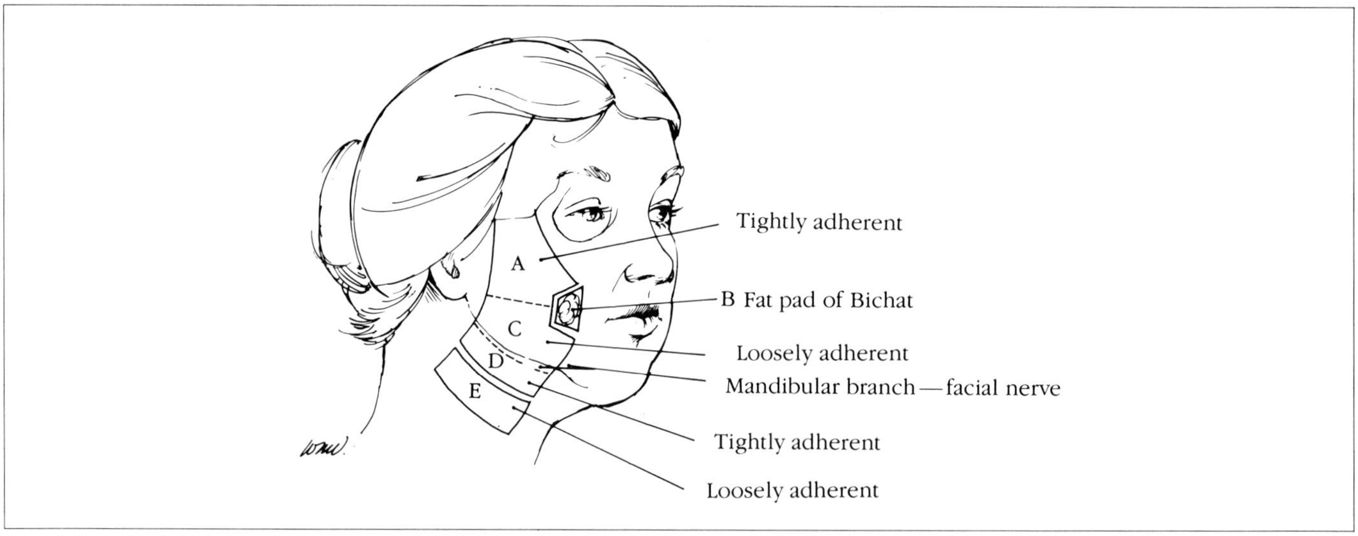

Figure 17-3. Anatomic variation in adherence of superficial to deep fascia of the head and neck. Adherence of zones A and B is firm, and sharp dissection is required to separate the plane. Zones C and E are loosely adherent, and zone D is tightly adherent. Release of superficial fascia in zone B is difficult as the deep fascia of the face over the fat pad of Bichat is thin and the branches of the facial nerve are just deep to it (see Fig. 17-1).

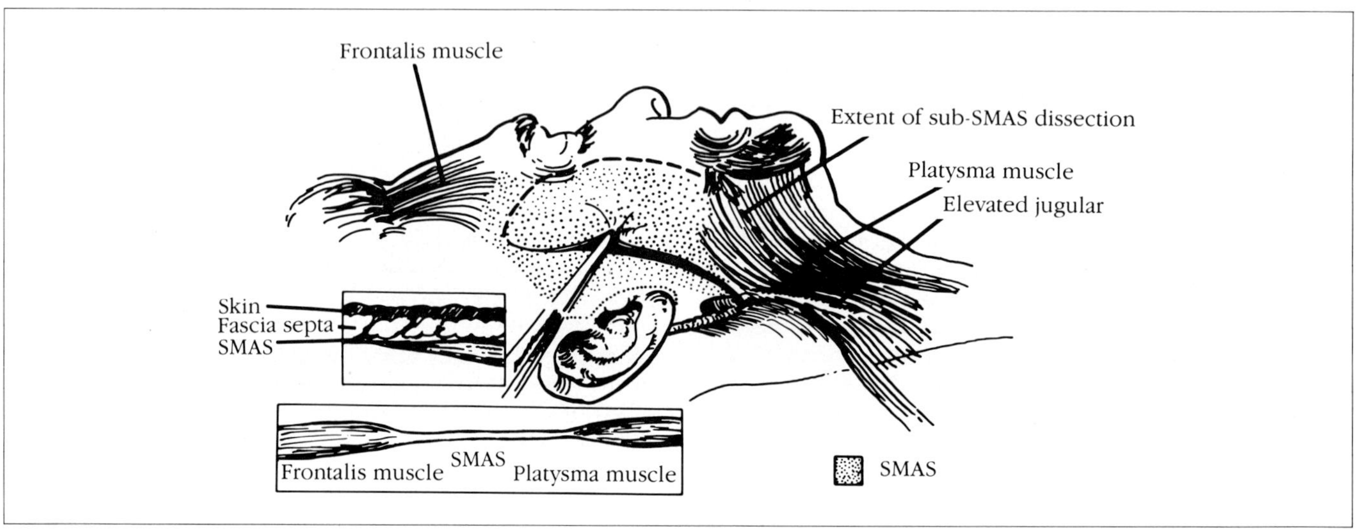

Figure 17-4. Superficial musculoaponeurotic system (SMAS). Continuity of SMAS with posterior portion of frontalis muscle and platysma muscle. (Lower inset) Schematic of the continuity of SMAS and frontalis and platysma muscles that provide tension on the SMAS. (Upper inset) Fibrous tissue septa of subcutaneous fat superficial to SMAS, which connects the SMAS and the dermis of the skin and transfers the contraction of facial muscles.

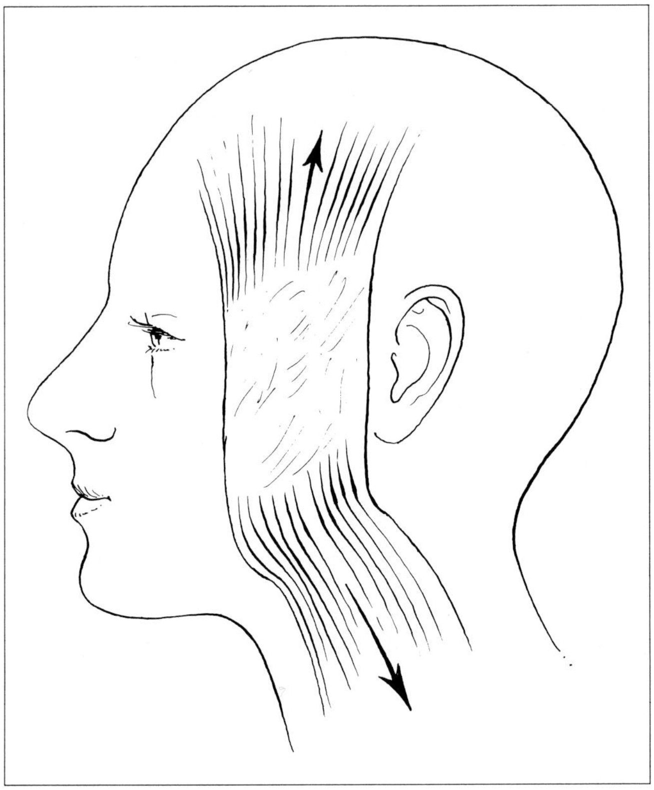

Figure 17-5. Tension of platysma and frontalis muscle on SMAS at age 20 years. Tension of SMAS amplifies and distributes facial muscle contractions to the skin.

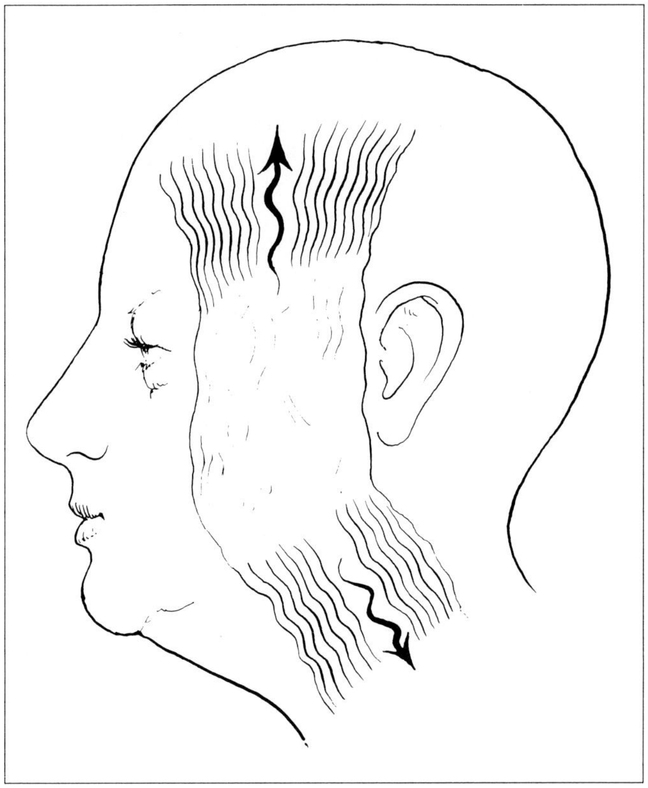

Figure 17-6. Tension of platysma and frontalis muscle on SMAS at age 50 years. Loss of elasticity and fibrosis of the SMAS. Attenuation of the anteroposterior dimension diminishes the tension on the SMAS, which reduces the distribution and amplification of facial muscle contractions.

the tectonic plate on a stronger "core" be repaired by shortening it to the dimensions of an earlier year. It is assumed that the sliding or slippage will then take a longer time to return than if the tectonic plate had been held by a tissue (skin) of lesser strength than the superficial fascia of the face.

Mitz and Peyronie [27] described the superficial musculoaponeurotic system (Fig. 17-4). At 20 years of age, the platysma muscle and the frontalis muscle maintain a continuous tone on an elastic superficial fascia of the face (SMAS) (Fig. 17-5). At 50 years of age, the vector force of the muscle tone is relaxed and the SMAS has become an inelastic and fibrotic tissue and has increased in its anteroposterior dimensions (Fig. 17-6). The appearance of the face and neck at middle age is a reflection of the relaxation of the superficial fascia (SMAS and platysma muscle). The soft tissues of the face and neck (SMAS and platysma muscle) are relaxing on the deep fascia, and, with the slippage of the soft tissue of the face and neck, there is not only loss of contour but a reduction in function. The objective of a superficial fascia rhytidectomy is to restore the soft tissue of the face to a position on the "core," or deep platform, that was present during a younger age and, at the same time, to reestablish some tension on the SMAS to improve the distribution and amplification of facial muscle contracture (Fig. 17-7).

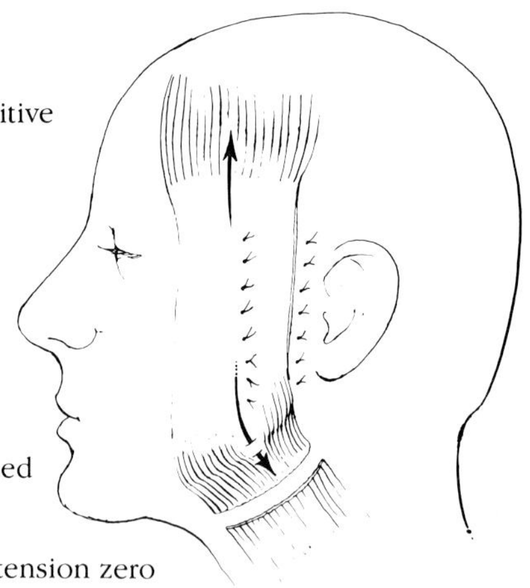

Figure 17-7. Restored SMAS and superficial fascia of the face. Imbrication of the SMAS and the platysma muscle above the cervicomental angle improves the tension and the transmission of facial muscle contraction (dynamics). Fibrous tissue septa between SMAS and dermis are intact. Platysma muscle below the cervicomental angle adapts to the deep structures of the neck.

ANESTHESIA

Anesthesia of the face and neck is accomplished by a regional nerve block of the infraorbital and the mandibular branches of the trigeminal (fifth) nerve and the cervical cutaneous plexus. A total of 10 ml of Marcaine 0.25% (infraorbital foramen, 2 ml; pterygoid fossa, 4 ml; cervical subcutaneous plexus, 4 ml) is administered. This produces a satisfactory and prolonged block of the sensory nerves of the face and cervical region. In some cases it is necessary to augment the block over the temporal region at the level of the outer canthus of the eye or the malar region.

The submental-submandibular area and the line of incisions are infiltrated with Marcaine 0.25% with epinephrine (1:600,000). Approximately 6 to 8 ml of the anesthetic solution is placed in the submental and submandibular region and approximately 6 ml in the line of incisions.

There have been no complications or permanent nerve anesthesia as a result of this technique.

If the surgeon prefers infiltration of the tissues of the head and neck with an anesthetic agent, this may be utilized.

Table 17-1. Operative pathway of superficial fascia rhytidectomy with complete transverse segmental resection of the platysma muscle

1. Skin and subcutaneous fat elevation, submental and anterior submandibular area
2. Anterior transverse segmental resection of platysma muscle at level of cervicomental angle (actual or proposed)
3. Controlled lipectomy (location and depth) of submental and anterior submandibular area
4. Preauricular and postauricular skin flaps elevated
5. Superficial fascia, face and neck, elevated (orbit to cervicomental angle)
6. Skin and subcutaneous fat elevation in cervical region (mandible to cricoid cartilage)
7. Transverse segmental resection of the posterior portion of the platysma muscle, completing anterior-to-posterior transection
8. Imbrication (posterior advancement) of superficial fascia of the face and neck
9. Controlled (location and depth) cervical lipectomy
10. Skin closure with minimal tension

TECHNIQUE

The operative pathway of the restoration of the cervicofacial dynamics (function and contour) is outlined in Table 17-1.

The initial step in the procedure is performed on the anterior region of the neck through a submental incision at the level of the mentum and neck crease. The skin and subcutaneous fat are elevated from the platysma muscle* to a point about midway long the border of the mandible and in a caudal direction to at least the level of the cricoid cartilage (Table 17-1, step 1) (Fig. 17-8C). The anterior border of the platysma muscle caudad to the cervicomental angle is elevated from the deep fascia of the neck and to the posterior extent of the skin and subcutaneous fat elevation in the neck. A segment of the anterior border of the platysma muscle (approximately 1.0–1.5 cm) (Table 17-1, step 2) is resected in a transverse direction at or just below the cervicomental angle (Fig. 17-8A, B). The anterior border of the platysma muscle is approximated from the mentum to the cervicomental angle (or a proposed cervicomental angle) (Fig. 17-8D).

* Suggested by S. T. Hamra, M.D.

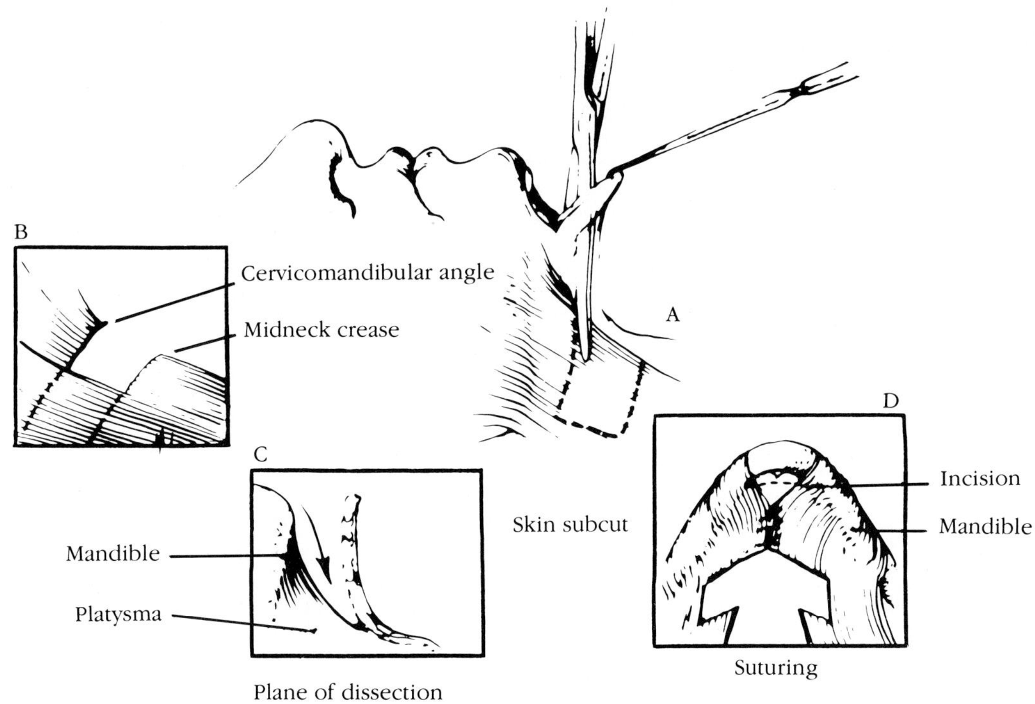

Figure 17-8. Superficial fascia rhytidectomy, submental region.
A, B. Transverse segmental resection (anterior portion) of platysma muscle at the level of the cervicomental angle.
C. Elevation of skin and subcutaneous fat at level of platysma muscle.
D. Closure of the anterior borders of the platysma muscle from mentum to cervicomental angle.

The skin and the subcutaneous fat flap (Table 17-1, step 3) are trimmed in the location and to the depth desired (Fig. 17-9). The details of the technique of lipectomy will be described subsequently.

On completion of the anterior region of the neck, the incisions of the skin are made in the temporal, preauricular, postauricular, and occipital regions. The incisions are of the usual type. The occipital limb of the incision is placed at the level of the anterior (inferior) crus of the anthelix of the ear and extends posteriorly for approximately 5 cm in a horizontal direction or at right angles to the preauricular incision.

The skin is elevated at the subdermal level and is extended anteriorly approximately 3.5 cm in the preauricular region and caudally over the mandible (Table 17-1, step 4). The occipital skin flap is mobilized at the subdermal level and elevated caudally to the level of the cricoid cartilage and anteriorly to the posterior border of the platysma muscle.

The preauricular skin flap is placed under tension, and, in the region of a change of the subcutaneous fat to a more lobular character, the superficial fascia is penetrated to its deep surface (Fig. 17-10). The area of the penetration of the superficial fascia is in a safe location in relation to the facial nerve. In the region of the orbit, it is anterior to the temporal branch of the facial nerve. The orbicularis oculi muscle is in the superficial fascia and is readily visualized for orientation deep to the superficial fascia. Caudad to this area, the parotid gland is easily identifiable prior to penetration to a level of the facial nerve. The platysma muscle in the cervical region is easily recognized. All these anatomic features assure the operator that the correct plane has been identified and that the dissection is external or superficial to the deep fascia and the facial nerve (see Fig. 17-1).

Utilizing these anatomic landmarks, the superficial fascia is penetrated slightly cephalad to the zygoma at the level of the outer canthus of the eye. With blunt and sharp dissection, the superficial fascia is penetrated in a tangential or slightly external direction until the shiny, smooth, deep surface of the superficial fascia of the area and the fibers of the orbicularis oculi muscle are identified. With the deep surface of the superficial fascia identified, the dissection is continued in a caudal direction, penetrating anteriorly beneath the superficial fascia for a distance of approximately 0.5 to 1.0 cm until the deep surface of the superficial fascia is exposed from the temporal to the cervical area (Table 17-1, step 5) (Fig. 17-11).

With the proper plane established, the dissection can proceed anteriorly, separating the superficial fascia from the deep fascia. The dissection is both blunt and sharp. The blunt dissection should not be done forcibly or with wide separation of the blades of the scissors. The sharp release of fibrous or areolar tissue bands between the superficial and deep fascia of the face and neck is carefully performed at the most posterior attachment of these bands

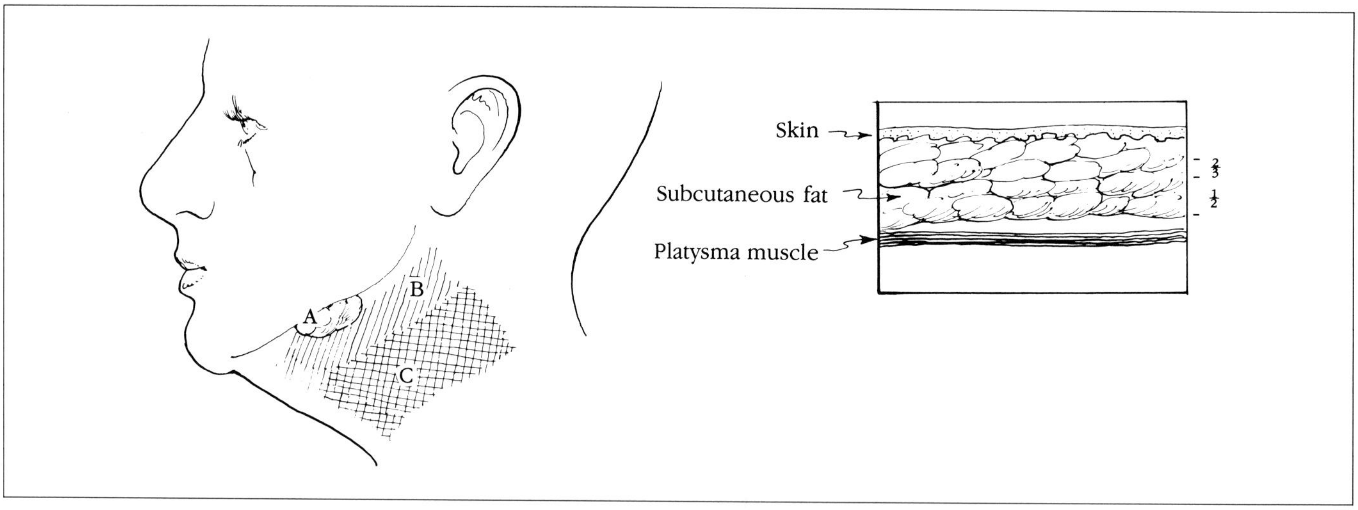

Figure 17-9. Technique of cervical lipectomy. Excision of fatty tissue is controlled in location (submental region, area A, B, or C, or all areas, if indicated) and depth from one-third to two-thirds thickness, with removal of subcutaneous fat from a deep to a more superficial level.

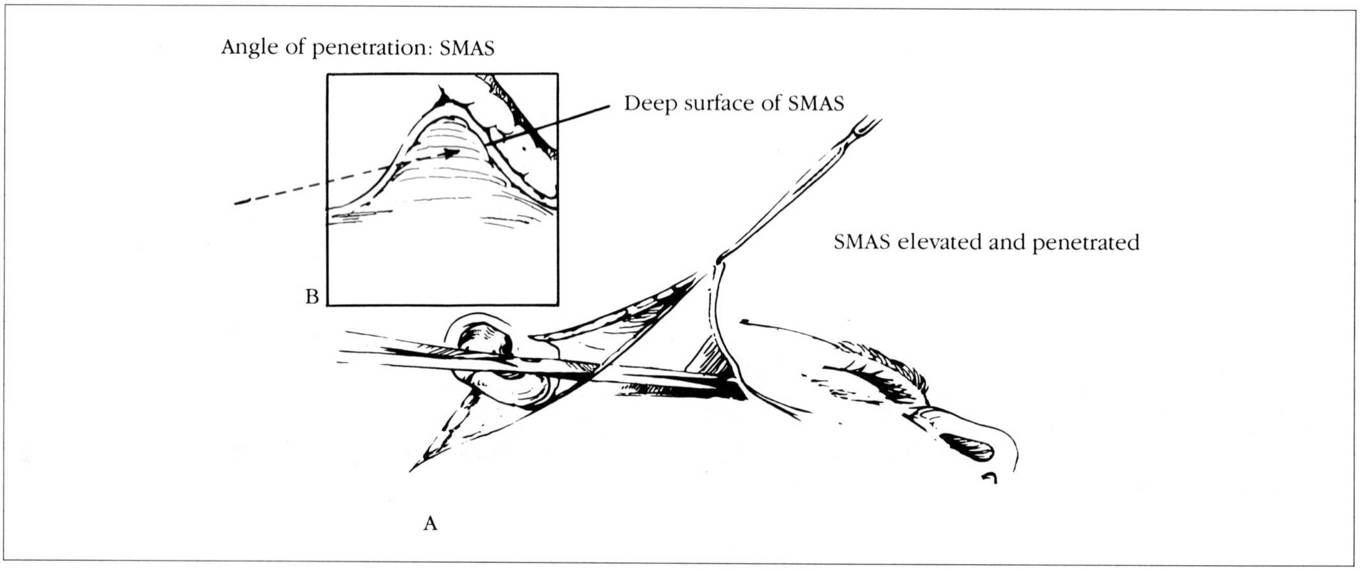

Figure 17-10. Identification of the plane between the superficial and deep fasciae of the face and neck.

A. Scissors are held in a tangential plane or are angled superficially.
B. Subcutaneous tissues are tented and penetrated from zygoma to cervicomental angle 3.5 cm anterior to preauricular incision and in region of the thick deep fascia of the parotid area.

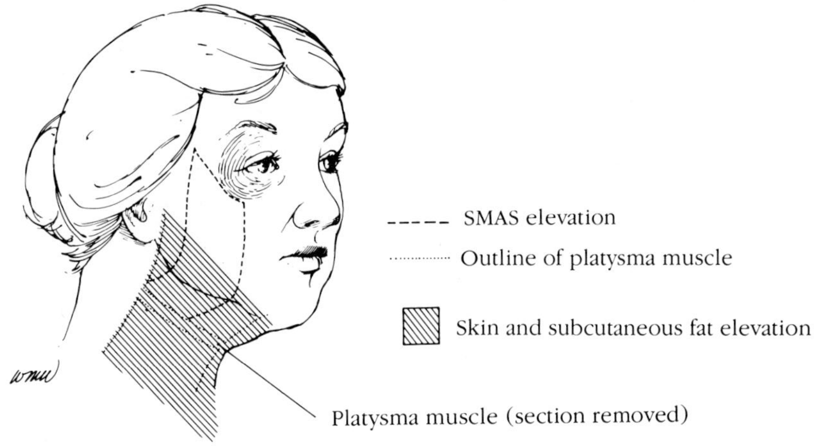

Figure 17-11. Relationship of the elevation of SMAS and the skin and subcutaneous fat flap. Dashed line indicates the elevated area of the superficial fascia of the face and neck to the level of the cervicomental angle. Parallel hatching indicates the area of the skin and subcutaneous fat elevation at the level of the platysma muscle. The preauricular area and the area posterior to the sternomastoid region and postauricular skin flap are elevated at the subdermal level.

and as closely approximating the superficial fascia as possible.

The anterior extent of the elevation of the superficial fascia of the face can be varied, depending on the appearance of the nasolabial fold. Skoog [34] recommended advancing the dissection scissors in the cheek to the nasolabial fold in an "easily separated" plane. If the nasolabial folds are deep and a prominent feature of the aging process of the face, the superficial fascia can be elevated as described by Skoog. To enhance the elevation and provide the maximum results in the central part of the face, the superficial fascia should also be released over the malar prominence, or the superficial fascia caudad to the malar prominence, which has been elevated to the nasolabial fold, is restricted in its posterior advancement by the area of the superficial fascia over the malar prominence that has not been released.

When the nasolabial folds are not a prominent feature of the aging process of the face, the superficial fascia should be elevated anteriorly to a point that permits its posterior advancement without tension on or a rolling of the deep tissues. Thus, a smooth redraping of the superficial fascia or implantation in a more posterior position on the deep fascia is permitted.

The most difficult area of separation of the superficial and deep fascia of the face is the tightly adherent area in the region of and just anterior to the fat pad of Bichat (see Fig. 17-3, zone B). When the plane between the superficial and deep fascia is established cephalad and caudad to the adherent zone in this region, the plane of dissection can be continued and the layers of the fascia can be separated by sharp dissection. Approaching the adherent zone first from the cephalad and then from the caudal direction and vice versa and utilizing just the tips of the scissors for very small sharp advancement, one can separate the two layers of fascia and establish the plane between the fascial layers. Anterior to this zone the superficial and the deep fasciae are not so adherent and can be easily separated. Unless considerable caution is exercised in the anterior region of the fat pad of Bichat—and the deep fascia in this region is thin—the scissors can penetrate deep to the adherent zone of the superficial and deep fasciae, and an injury to the buccal branches of the facial nerve may occur (see Fig. 17-1).

After the superficial fascia has been elevated from the temporal region to the level of the cervicomental angle, the skin and subcutaneous fat is elevated from the platysma muscle in the cervical region (Fig. 17-11). The posterior border of the platysma muscle is identified over the mandible, and the skin and subcutaneous fat is released from the platysma muscle. This dissection is continued anteriorly to join the elevation of the skin and subcutaneous fat from the platysma muscle in the anterior neck.

The draping of the cervical skin and subcutaneous fat flap is improved if the flap is elevated from the platysma muscle beginning at a level approximately 2.5 cm above the lower border of the mandible. As the skin and subcutaneous fat flap dissection continues anteriorly, it should be angled in a caudal direction, reaching the lower border of the body of the mandible anterior to its midpoint. Figure 17-11 (Table 17-1, step 6) outlines the cephalad extent of the elevation of the skin and subcutaneous fat of the neck and lower face. The caudad extent of the skin and subcutaneous flap elevation of the cervical region is at least to the level of the cricoid cartilage, and lower if necessary.

At this juncture, the superficial fascia of the face and neck (cephalad to a level corresponding to a line drawn transversely on the neck at the level of the cervicomental angle) is elevated, and the cervical skin and subcutaneous fat flap are elevated from the level of the cricoid cartilage to above the lower border of the mandible (Fig. 17-11).

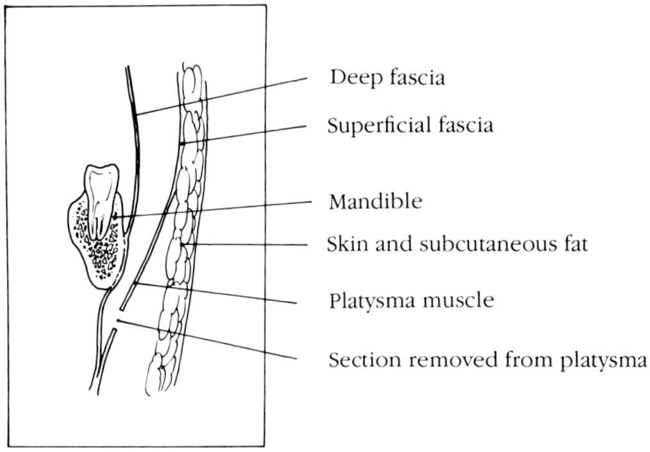

Figure 17-12. Cross section of the relationship of the elevation of the SMAS and the skin and subcutaneous fat flap. Superficial fascia elevated to level of cervicomental angle (section removed from the platysma muscle). Skin and subcutaneous fat of the cervical region elevated from platysma muscle cephalad to the mandible in posterior half of the body of the mandible to the level of the cricoid cartilage. The overlap of the elevated superficial fascia and the skin and subcutaneous fat flap permits the maximum posterior advancement of the superficial fascia and a cephalad advancement of the cervical skin.

The result is an overlap of the release of the elevated cervical skin and subcutaneous fat and the elevated superficial fascia of the face and neck in the region of the posterior half of the body of the mandible (Fig. 17-12). This permits the optimum draping of the cervical skin and subcutaneous fat and the posterior advancement of the superficial fascia of the face and neck to the level of the cervicomental angle.

With completion of the elevation of the superficial fascia of the head and neck to the level of the cervicomental angle and the skin and subcutaneous fat over the cervical region at the level of the platysma muscle, a transverse segment of the platysma muscle is removed. The posterior border of the platysma muscle (superficial fascia) is elevated from the deep fascia of the neck at the level of the cervicomental angle. At this level on the platysma muscle, a 1.0- to 1.5-cm tunnel extending from the posterior border of the platysma muscle to the anterior transverse segmental resection of the platysma muscle is developed. After the muscle is released from the deep fascia of the neck, a segment of the platysma muscle is resected to join the anterior resection of the platysma muscle (Table 17-1, step 7) (Fig. 17-13), thus completing the transverse segmental resection of the platysma muscle from anterior to posterior border.

The superficial fascia of the face and neck above the level of the complete transverse segmental resection of the platysma muscle (cervicomental angle) is imbricated (Table 17-1, step 8). The first, or anterior, row of sutures of the imbrication is placed at the line of penetration of the superficial fascia of the face (point A) approximately 3.5 cm anterior to the preauricular skin incision. A point (point B) (Figs. 17-1, 17-2, and 17-14) is selected on the deep surface of the elevated superficial fascia of the cheek,

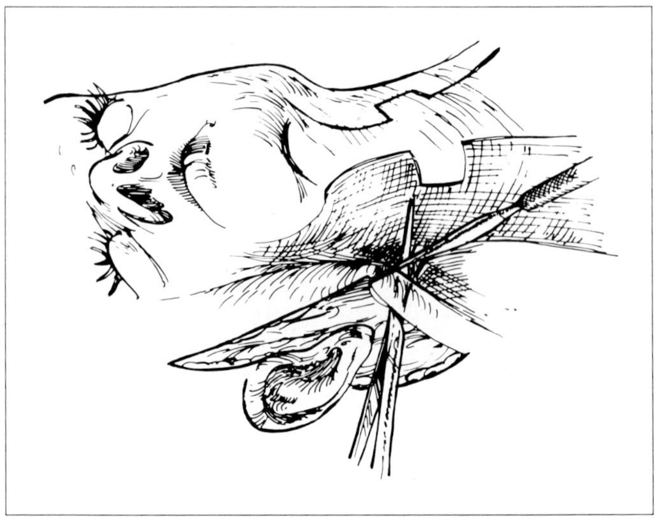

Figure 17-13. Resection of a transverse segment of the platysma muscle, posterior portion. Elevation of the superficial fascia (and SMAS) from the zygoma to the cervicomental angle and the skin and subcutaneous fat flap (see Figs. 17-11 and 17-12) is completed. The platysma muscle is elevated from the deep (investing) fascia of the neck, and the posterior segment (1.5 cm) of the muscle is resected to join the resected anterior portion of the platysma muscle (see Fig. 17-8).

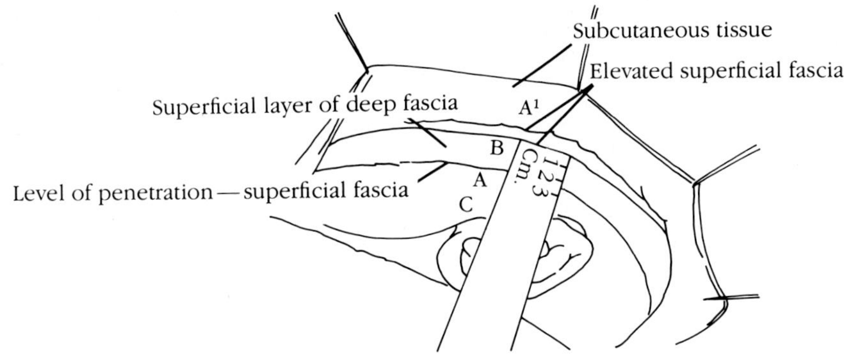

Figure 17-14. Elevated superficial fascia of the face and the neck from the level of the zygoma to the level of the cervicomental angle. Points A and A′ were the original site of the penetration of the superficial fascia to its deep surface. Point A′ (originally at point A) is the elevated superficial fascia. Point B (see Fig. 17-2), on the deep surface of the superficial fascia, when advanced to point A, provides maximum advancement of the SMAS with minimal tension, reducing the anteroposterior dimension of the SMAS approximately 2.0 to 2.5 cm and permits placement of a row of sutures in an area of the restoration that is more proximate to the relaxation of the central face. The posterior row of sutures approximates the superficial fascia (point A′) and a point on the subcutaneous tissue of the preauricular region (point C).

which, when advanced to point A (the site of the penetration of the superficial fascia), will permit the maximum advancement of the superficial fascia. The closure of the superficial fascia (point B) to the superficial fascia of the cheek (point A) commences at the level of the zygoma and proceeds in a caudal direction to the cephalad border of the platysma muscle transection at the level of the cervicomental angle. Absorbable synthetic suture material (4-0 Vicryl) is used.

The second, or posterior, row of sutures approximates the deep surface of the advanced superficial fascia (point A) to the subcutaneous tissue anterior to the preauricular skin incision (point C). The closure of the superficial fascia to the subcutaneous tissue commences at the level of the cervicomental angle and proceeds cephalad, including the posterior border of the platysma muscle in the cervical region (points A′ to C). This second row of sutures is the closure described by Skoog, in which a single row of sutures is inserted to maintain the advanced superficial fascia of the face and the neck.

When the superficial fascia of the submandibular area (cephalad to the cervicomental angle) is imbricated and the anterior border of the platysma muscle is approximated from the mentum to the cervicomental angle (actual or proposed), the cephalad stump of the transected platysma muscle produces a "drawstring" effect (Fig. 17-15). With healing, the scar tissue of the cephalad stump of the platysma muscle and the intervening gap created by the resection of a transverse segment of the platysma muscle from its anterior to posterior border maintain the improvement in the cervicomental angle.

The posterior cervical portion of the controlled (location and depth) lipectomy (Table 17-1, step 9) (see Fig. 17-9) is performed, if indicated, to adjust the depth of the subcutaneous fat in the posterior cervical region to a level corresponding with that removed in the anterior region of the neck or sufficiently to improve the contours of the mandible and sternomastoid muscle.

The skin and subcutaneous fat flap is draped and tailored. The skin is closed under minimal tension.

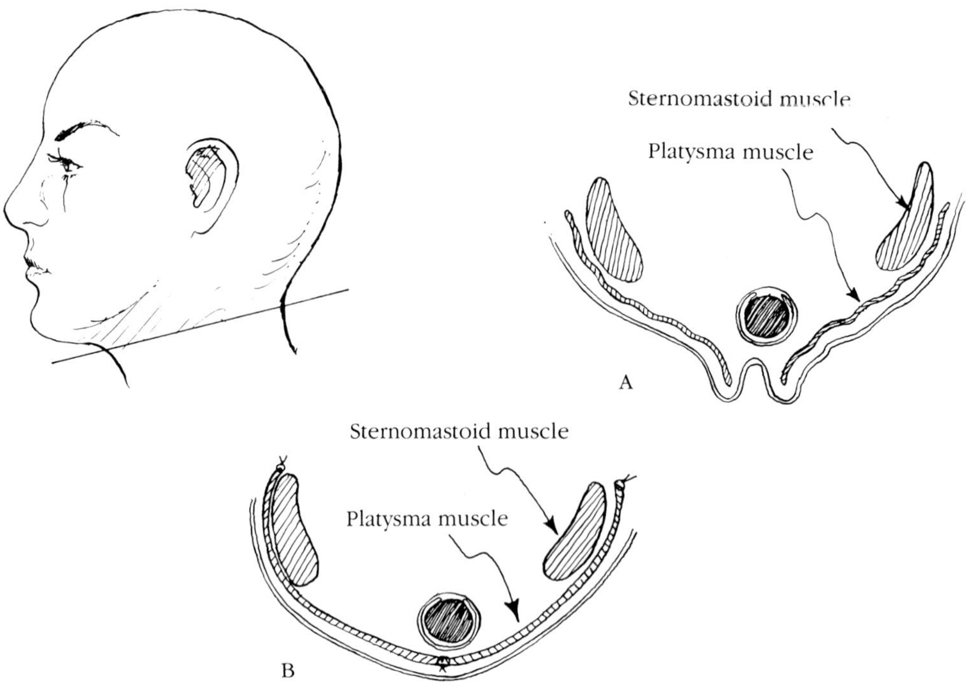

Figure 17-15. Cross section of the neck at the level of the resection of a transverse segment of the platysma muscle (cervicomental angle).
A. Relaxation of the platysma muscle creates the platysma muscle and skin folds of the anterior region of the neck.
B. Closure of the anterior borders of the platysma muscle between mentum and cervicomental angle, and posterior advancement of the superficial fascia of the neck (platysma muscle) cephalad to the cervicomental angle with suturing to the sternomastoid fascia. The continuity of the cephalad stump of the platysma from sternomastoid to sternomastoid muscle assists in creating, or maintaining, an improvement in the cervicomental angle.

COMPLICATIONS

The major complications of superficial fascia rhytidectomy, as described, and their incidence are listed in Table 17-2.

The incidence of complications was determined from a total of 648 patients* who were operated on in the years 1979 to 1981 by superficial fascia rhytidectomy combined with transection and resection of a segment of the platysma muscle, elevation of the skin and subcutaneous fat of the cervical region from the platysma muscle, and, if indicated, lipectomy of the skin and subcutaneous fat from the deep surface of the cervical skin and subcutaneous fat flap to a more superficial level in the location required.

The facial nerve was not injured.

Temporary dysfunction of the lower lip occurred in 13 of 648 patients for an incidence of 2 percent. Permanent lower lip dysfunction occurred in 1 of the 648 patients (0.15%). Table 17-3 lists the incidence of temporary and permanent lower lip dysfunction by year. The year 1979 was a transition year, and some patients operated on in its early months by techniques other than described in the section on technique are included. The incidence of 0.15 percent compares favorably with the incidence of facial nerve injury of 0.12 percent reported by Baker and Conley [3] in a subcutaneous rhytidectomy.

A major hematoma, requiring surgical removal to evacuate the blood, occurred in 2 of the 648 patients (0.3%). Both hematomas developed in males and involved the lateral region of the neck on the right side. Expansion of

* Combined patients of Drs. Lemmon and Hamra.

Table 17-2. Complications of superficial fascia rhytidectomy with platysma muscle transection and lipectomy (648 cases, 1979–1981)

Type	Number	Percent
1. Facial nerve injury (temporary, permanent)	0	0
2. Lower lip dysfunction (temporary)	12	2.0
3. Lower lip dysfunction (permanent)	1	0.15
4. Hematoma	2	0.3
5. Skin slough > 2.5 cm	0	0
6. External jugular vein injury	0	0
7. Skin, fascia, muscle adhesion	0	0
8. Infection (localized)	6	0.9

Table 17-3. Incidence of temporary and permanent lower lip dysfunction (648 patients, 1979–1981)

Year	Total patients	Total lip dysfunction	Percent	Temporary dysfunction	Permanent dysfunction	Percent permanent dysfunction
1979	204	12	5.9	11	1	0.15
1980	220	2	0.9	2	0	0
1981	224	0	0	0	0	0
Total	648	14		13	1	0.15

the hematomas was confined to the lateral region of the neck although the entire cervical region had been elevated across the midline of the neck. The hematomas developed in hospital patients within 8 hours of operation. Skin flap viability was not impaired, and wound healing was not delayed.

No major skin slough (greater than 2.5 cm) occurred in this period nor has it occurred since superficial fascia technique was adopted in 1973. Wound healing is usually uneventful. Rarely, there are some minimal alterations in the viability of the skin at the cephalad point of the postauricular flap.

No injury to the external jugular vein occurred.

Skin adhesions to the deep (investing) fascia of the neck and the submandibular region or to the platysma muscle did not occur with the transection-resection of 1.0 to 1.5 cm of the platysma muscle at the level of the cervicomental angle.

Wound infection occurred in 6 of the 648 patients (0.9%). All the infections occurred in the lateral region of the neck (3 left, 2 right, 1 not stated), and all developed on the fifth to the ninth day except for one, which developed on the third day. Infections were limited in size and were well localized under the skin flap. In three patients the organism cultured was *Staphylococcus aureus.* In the remaining three patients the organisms cultured were beta-hemolytic streptococci, *Escherichia coli,* and *Klebsiella,* respectively. The infections responded rapidly to antibiotic therapy. Stab wound incision and drainage were performed in three of the six patients. In one patient, a drain was inserted through the postauricular skin incision. There were no residua.

Table 17-4. Complications of superficial fascia rhytidectomy* (1449 patients, 1979–1981)

Type	Number	Percent
1. Facial nerve injury (permanent)	2	0.14
2. Lower lip dysfunction (permanent)	3	0.21
3. Combined 1 and 2	5	0.35
4. Hematoma	8	0.55
5. Skin slough > 2.5 cm	0	0
6. External jugular vein injury	0	0
7. Skin-fascia-muscle adhesion	16	1.10
8. Infection (localized)	6	0.41

* Including all variations in technique to manage the platysma muscle and lipectomy.

Table 17-4 lists the complications of superficial fascia rhytidectomy in 1449 patients* who were operated on between 1973 and 1981. Except for the years 1979 to 1981, various techniques were combined with the superficial fascia rhytidectomy in an attempt to control the recurrence of the skin and platysma muscle folds of the anterior region of the neck and to contour the cervical region with extensive subdermal lipectomy. As the technique of the management of the platysma muscle and the contouring of the fat of the cervical region was expanded, reaching a peak in 1978, the incidence of complications increased.

Table 17-5 lists the method, or combination of methods, utilized to manage the platysma muscle and the relationship of the technique to the incidence of permanent lower lip dysfunction from 1973 to 1981. Lower lip dysfunction ("pseudoparalysis") [10] (Fig. 17-16) may develop with the wide undermining, a high transection, or the removal of a wide strip of the platysma muscle (Table 17-5). In the years 1973 to 1981, exclusive of 1978, temporary lower lip dysfunction occurred in 22 of 1225 patients (1.8%) (Table 17-6). The incidence of permanent lower lip dysfunction was 0.5 percent (1 of 1225 patients).

The incidence of lower lip dysfunction rises dramatically when the platysma muscle is elevated from approximately 1.5 cm below the inferior border of the mandible to the midneck crease and from its posterior to its anterior border and when a large segment of the elevated platysma muscle is resected. In 1978, 37 of 224 patients (16.5%) (Table 17-6) had a temporary lower lip dysfunction and 2 of 224 patients (0.9%) had a permanent lower lip dysfunction.

Table 17-7 lists the location of the dysfunction of the lower lip in 59 patients in the years 1973 to 1981.

The degree of the dysfunction of the lower lip may vary considerably. An arbitrary classification of maximum, moderate, and minimum was utilized in an effort to predict the recovery of the lower lip dysfunction (Table 17-8). With maximum dysfunction there was no movement of the affected side. Partial movement was observed with moderate dysfunction. Minimum dysfunction presented as only a slight loss of movement.

The records of the 59 patients with lower lip dysfunction in 1973 to 1981 were reviewed and classified on the basis of the historical description (Table 17-8). According to this classification, 19 patients had maximum lower lip dysfunction, 13 had moderate lower lip dysfunction, and 27 had minimum lower lip dysfunction (Table 17-9).

* Combined patients of Drs. Lemmon and Hamra.

Table 17-5. Relationship of platysma muscle dysfunction of the lower lip to technique of platysma muscle management

Year	Extensive elevation platysma	Transection	Resection: Radical	Resection: 1.5-cm strip	Number of patients	Percent permanent lower lip dysfunction
1. 1973–1977	X				505	0
2. 1973–1977	X	X			72	0
3. 1978	X	X	X		224	0.9
4. 1978	X	X		X	204	0.5
5. 1979		X		X	220	0
6. 1981		X		X	224	0

Table 17-6. Incidence of temporary and permanent platysma muscle dysfunction of the lower lip (1499 patients, 1973–1981)

Year	Total patients	Total lip dysfunction	Percent	Temporary dysfunction	Permanent dysfunction	Percent permanent dysfunction
1973–1977	577	8	1.4	8	0	0
1978	224	37	16.5	35	2	0.9
1979	204	12	5.9	11	1	0.5
1980	220	2	0.9	2	0	0
1981	224	0	0	0	0	0
Total	1449	59	4.1	56	3	0.21

Figure 17-16. Permanent dysfunction of the lower lip after extensive elevation of the platysma muscle with a resection of a wide transverse segment from the anterior to the posterior border of the platysma muscle and from 1.5 cm below the mandible to the midneck crease.
A. Postoperative smile.
B. Slight inability to depress the left lower lip when asked to show the teeth.

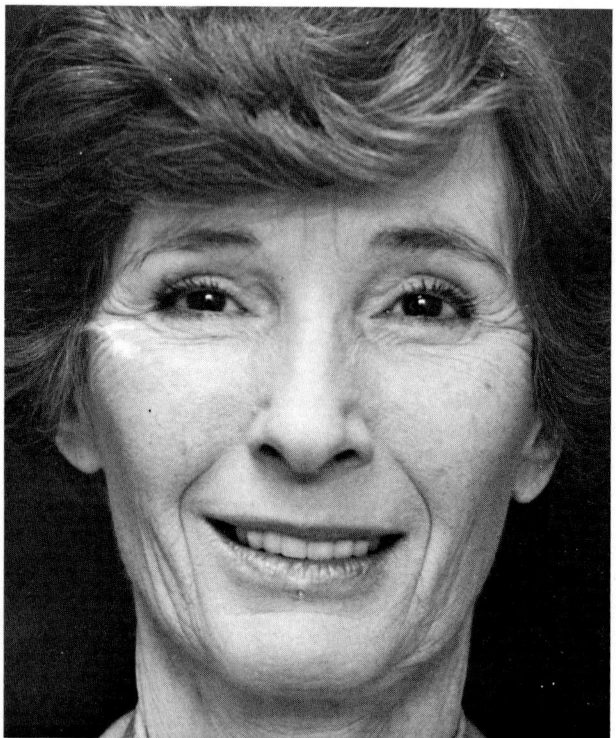

A

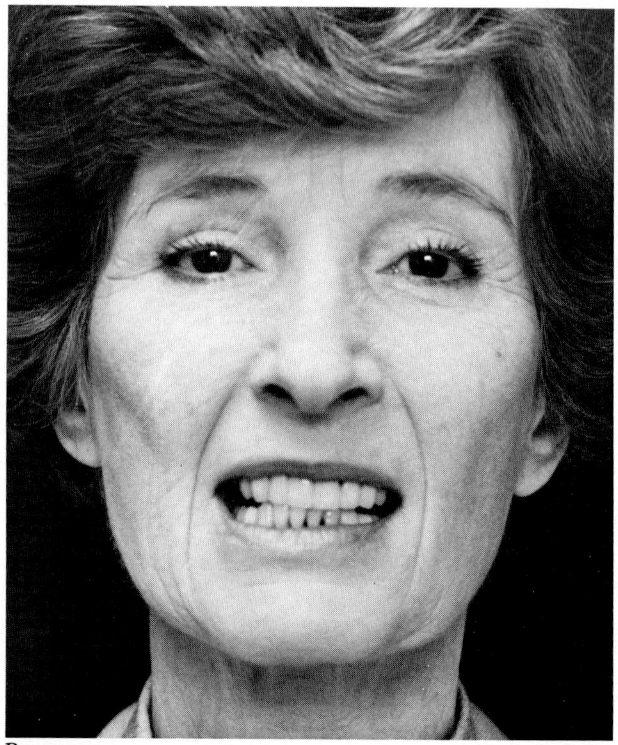

B

Table 17-7. Location of lower lip (platysma muscle) dysfunction (59 patients, 1973–1981)

	Temporary				Permanent		
Year	Right	Left	Both	Not stated	Right	Left	Both
1973–1977	6	2	0	0	0	0	0
1978	19	14	0	1	2	0	0
1979	6	5	0	1	0	1	0
1980	1	1	0	0	0	0	0
Total	32	22	0	2	2	1	0

Table 17-8. Classification of lower lip dysfunction

1. Maximum—no movement
2. Moderate—partial movement
3. Minimum—slight lag

Table 17-9. Type of lower lip (platysma muscle) dysfunction (59 patients, 1973–1981

	Dysfunction		
Year	Maximum	Moderate	Minimum
1973–1977		2	6
1978	15	8	13
1979	4	3	6
1980	0	0	2
1981	0	0	0
Total	19	13	27

Table 17-10. Relationship of degree of temporary lower lip (platysma muscle) dysfunction to recovery of normal function (56 patients, 1973–1981)

Lip dysfunction	Total patients	Average recovery time (months)	Range (months)
Maximum	19	3.75	1–10
Moderate	13	2.9	1–10
Minimum	27	1.5	1–3

Table 17-11. Recovery time of temporary lower lip (platysma muscle) dysfunction (56 patients, 1973–1981)

	Recovery time		
Year	<3 months	3–6 months	>6 months
1973–1977	8	0	0
1978	26	6	2
1979	11	1	0
1980	2	0	0
1981	0	0	0
Total	47	7	2

Fifty-six of the patients (94.9%) had a temporary lower lip dysfunction. Table 17-10 classifies them and relates the degree of dysfunction to the recovery time. If there was maximum dysfunction, the recovery time averaged 3.75 months. With a moderate or a minimum dysfunction, the average recovery time was 2.9 months and 1.5 months, respectively.

The ability to predict a recovery of the lower lip is not enhanced by classifying the dysfunction. The reason is that the range of time for a moderate dysfunction of the lip to recover may be as long as that of a lip with maximum dysfunction (no movement).

A better indicator of whether the dysfunction of the lower lip is temporary is related to the period of time required for the return of normal function of the lip. Table 17-11 demonstrates that 47 of 56 patients (83.9%) with a temporary dysfunction of the lower lip in 1973 to 1981 recovered in less than 3 months. Fifty-four of 56 patients (96.4%) with a temporary dysfunction of the lower lip recovered in less than 6 months.

Subdermal lipectomy of the cervical region may cause a variety of defects. These include a skeletonized appearance of the neck and mandible, defects of the contour of the neck and the inferior border of the mandible, and skin adhesions to the transected platysma muscle or, with extensive resection of the platysma muscle in the submandibular region, adherence of the skin and the deep cervical fascia.

The skin and subcutaneous fat of the cervical region and lower face may camouflage some anatomic features that should not be accentuated. In an attempt to achieve an improvement in contour of the cervical and submandibular regions, the removal of even small amounts of fat may unveil the feature, and the result may be a skeletonized appearance (Fig. 17-17).

Care should be exercised with respect to the amount of fat removed even though there is a thick layer of fat. If the consistency of the fat is firm, a lipectomy may cause a depressed or "scooped out" area in the site of the fat removal. Also, if this type of subcutaneous fat is encountered and the lipectomy is extended too close to the inferior border of the mandible, it may result in a defect of the mandible contour when the skin is advanced cephalad and draped for closure (Fig. 17-18).

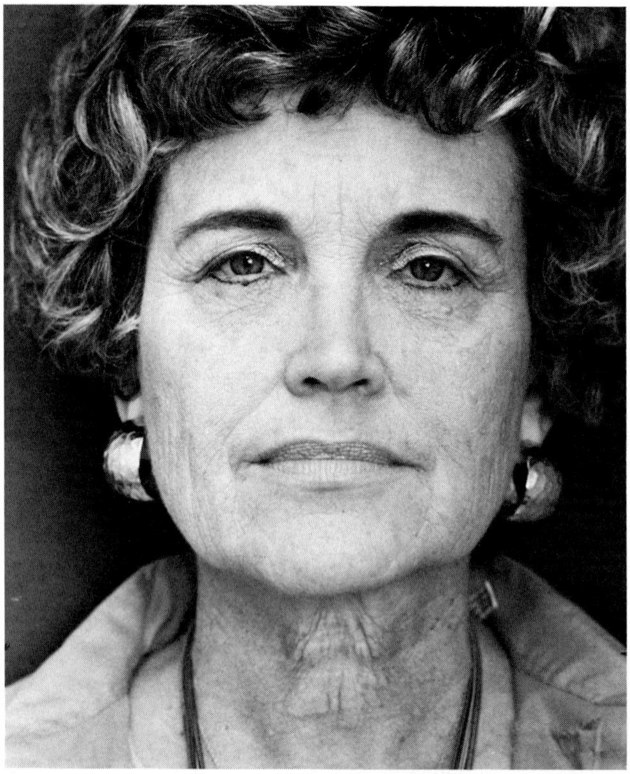
A

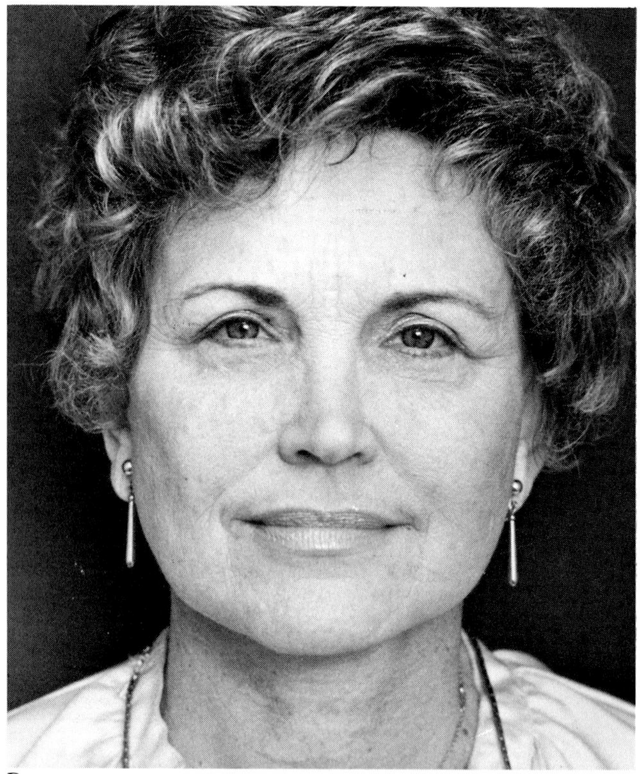
B

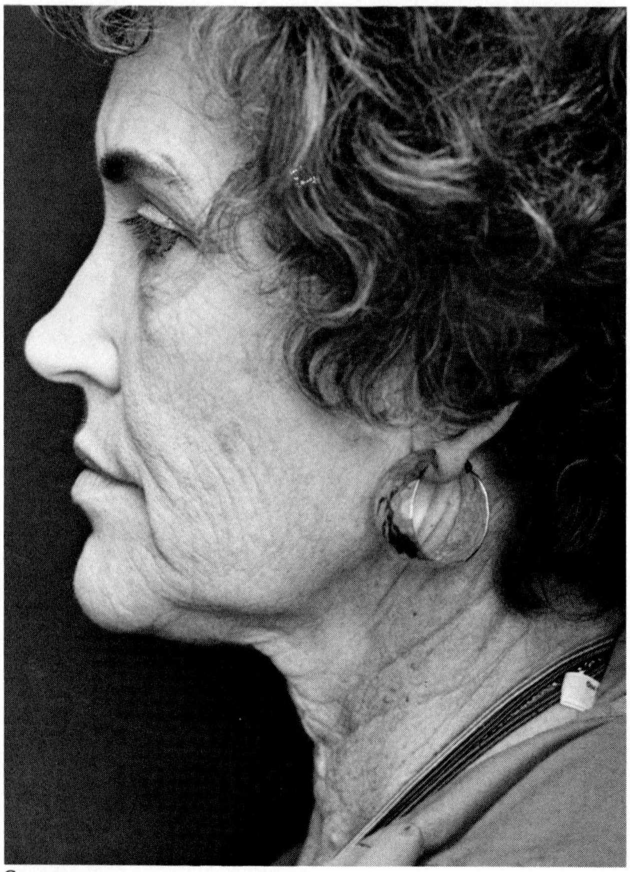
C

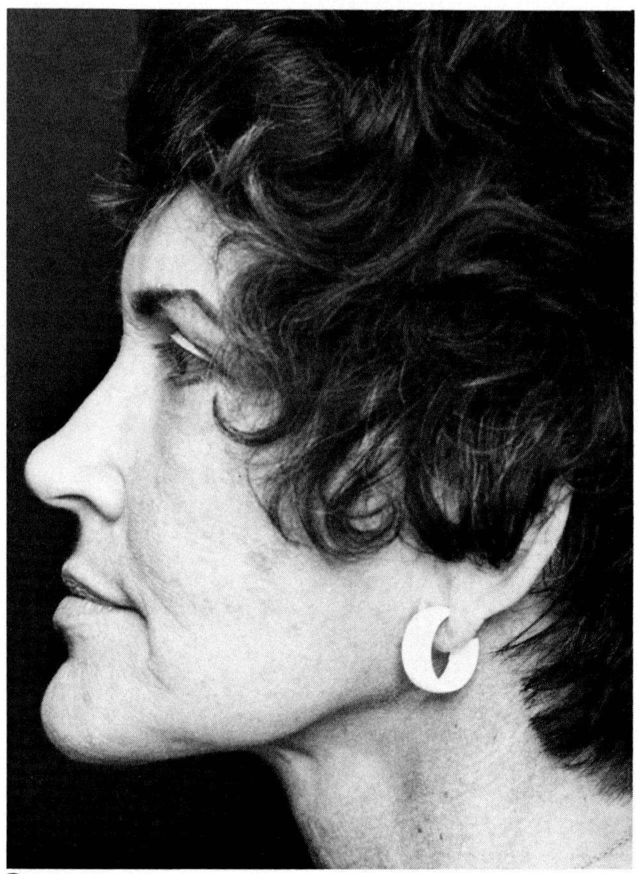
D

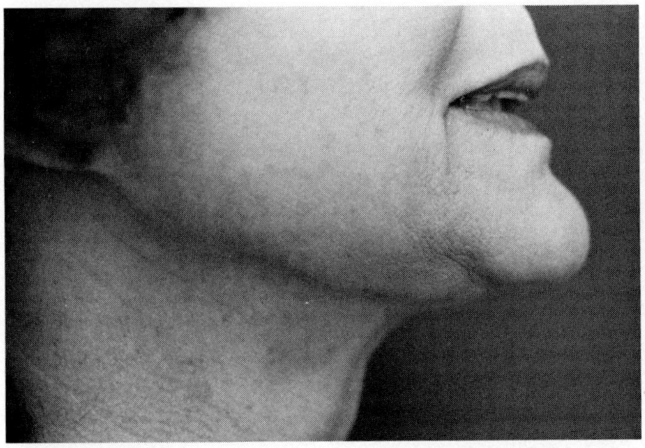

Figure 17-18. Cervical lipectomy and resection of a strip of platysma muscle (described in Fig. 17-17). When the skin is elastic and the subcutaneous fat of the cervical region is firm, a minimum amount of subcutaneous fat (one-third depth) should be removed to prevent the "scooped out" appearance in the area of the lipectomy. The level of the removal of subcutaneous fat in the submandibular area should be maintained well below the inferior border of the mandible, or upon rotation of the skin and subcutaneous fat flap of the cervical region there will be a depressed area over the mandible.

Figure 17-17. Superficial fascia rhytidectomy with resection of the platysma muscle from anterior to posterior border and from 1.5 cm below the lower border of the mandible to the midneck crease and subdermal lipectomy (patient's age, 58 years, 7 months after operation).

A, C. Preoperative views. The changes in the skin of the face and neck reflect the relaxation of the SMAS and the platysma muscle. The contours of the cheeks, inferior border of the mandible, and cervicomental angle are altered. The subcutaneous tissue is uniform in depth. The contour of the cervicomental angle in the profile is satisfactory, although relaxed.

B, D. Postoperative views. The front view of the patient presents a good result in the restoration of the cheeks (SMAS) and neck (platysma muscle), and the contour of the mandible is good. The profile reveals a "skeletonized" appearance of the mandible that creates a relative prognathism (no chin implant).

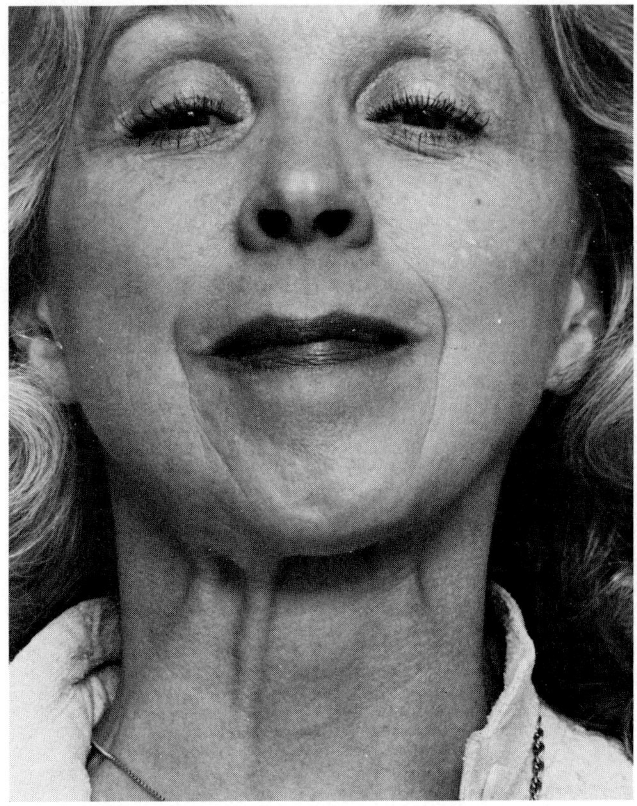

Figure 17-19. Transverse resection of a segment of the platysma muscle from anterior to posterior border. On animation, some fibers of the platysma muscle are seen to be intact. With a "blind" or direct exposure technique of transverse resection of the platysma, the fibers of the platysma muscle may be left intact (scissors penetrate muscle body like a shuttle) or the posterior sheath of the platysma muscle remains intact with a thin layer of muscle fibers attached and the bands of muscle tissue regenerate.

When the platysma muscle is transected, the dissection scissors may weave in and out of the fibers of the muscle in the fashion of a shuttle so that not all the fibers are transected (Fig. 17-19). If the deep fascia of the platysma muscle and some fibers that are attached to it remain intact, the platysma muscle may regenerate and present an appearance similar to an incomplete transection [11].

Skin and platysma muscle adhesions (Fig. 17-20) may develop, particularly if the transection of the platysma muscle is too high. The removal of a wide transverse segment of the platysma muscle after an extensive subdermal lipectomy may result in adhesions of the skin and platysma muscle or in the adhesion of the skin and the deep cervical fascia (Fig. 17-21).

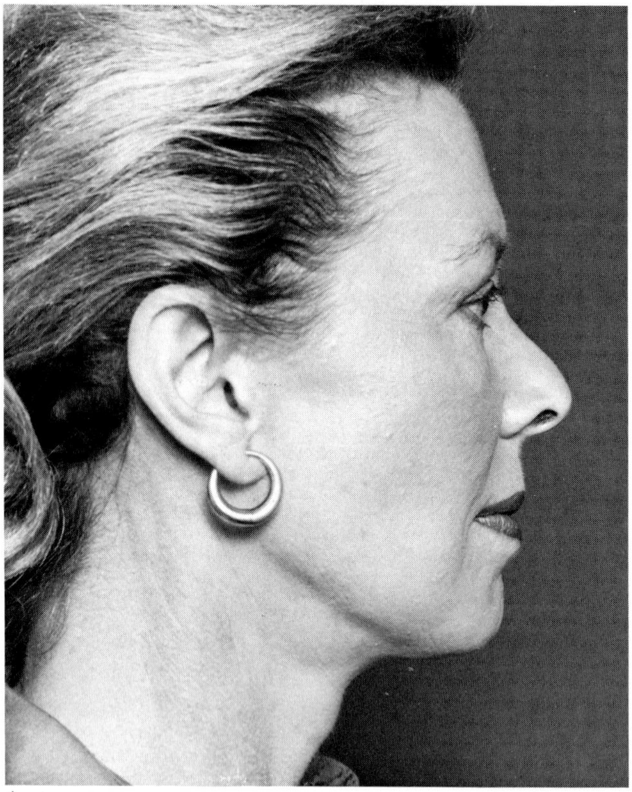

A

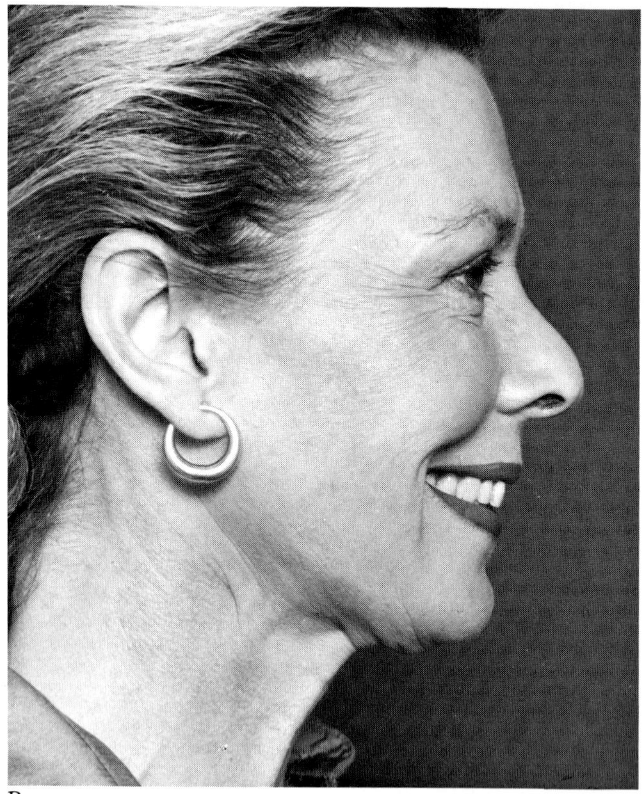

B

Figure 17-20. Transection of the platysma muscle (patient's age, 44 years).
A. Postoperative profile in repose.
B. On animation, the cephalad stump of the transected area of the platysma muscle is found to be adherent to the skin and creates a retracted fold, or dimpling of the skin in the adherent area. The fibers of the platysma muscle in the anterior region of the neck and in the region of the submandibular gland are intact or have regenerated.

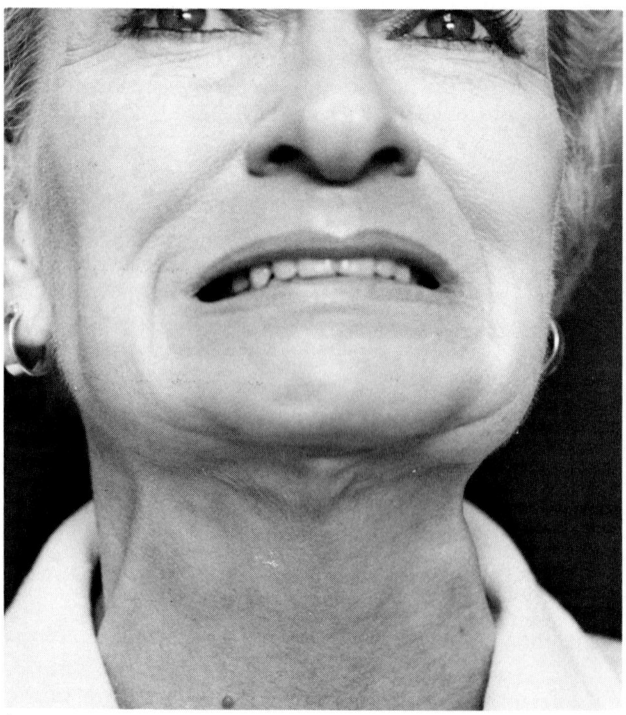

A

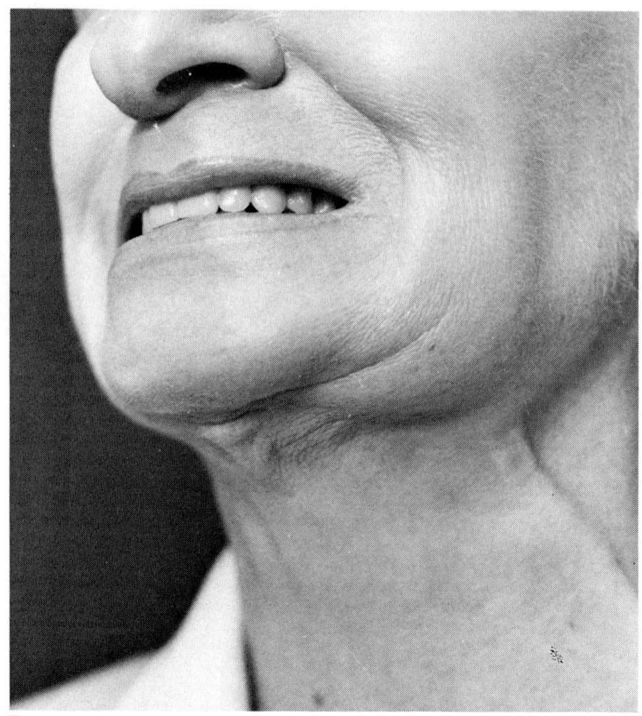

B

Figure 17-21
A, B. Subdermal lipectomy in the submental and submandibular region (lower border of the mandible to midneck) and resection of a wide transverse strip of the platysma muscle (described in Fig. 17-16). Skin is adherent to the cephalad stump of the platysma muscle and to the deep cervical fascia.

DISCUSSION

The soft tissues of the face (muscle, fascia, subcutaneous fat, skin) take 40 to 50 years to develop an appearance that displeases the individual and emphasizes the aging process. The changes of the face characteristic of aging are visible in the relaxation of the skin, platysma muscle folds of the anterior neck, and fat redistribution or lipodystrophy in the heavy neck.

The model for a face-lift is the young face, the appearance of which is a relationship of function and contour. Ideally, a successful anatomic restoration should reestablish the appearance of the model including both contour and function (dynamics). To approximate this, it is necessary to restore as much of the anatomy as possible and, where restoration is not possible, to alter the tissues that contribute to the defect in order to maintain the offending tissues (fat and muscle) in the corrected state for as long a time as possible. The restoration of the contours of the neck requires an alteration of the platysma muscle and the elimination of the subcutaneous fat in the areas where youthful contours have been modified over time. The restoration of the function (dynamics) of the face requires a reconstruction of the SMAS to dimensions and tensions that may have been present at an earlier age.

To reestablish some of the criteria of the young face (model), the superficial fascia and the associated tissues (SMAS) of the face and neck cephalad to the cervicomental angle are elevated, advanced posteriorly, and imbricated. The advanced superficial fascia (platysma muscle) of the neck cephalad to the cervicomental angle contributes to facial expression and, at an earlier age, acts in concert with the frontalis muscle to provide the "guy wire" tension for the efficient mechanical function of the SMAS (see Fig. 17-4). The posterior advancement and imbrication of the superficial fascia of the neck (platysma muscle), after approximation of the anterior borders of the platysma muscle and resection of a transverse segment of the platysma muscle from its anterior to posterior borders at the level of the cervicomental angle, may improve the efficiency of the dynamic portion of the platysma muscle above the cervicomental angle. At the minimum, the transection-resection of a segment of the platysma muscle eliminates the countertraction of the platysma muscle below the cervicomental angle and, when placed at the level of the cervicomental angle, directly contributes to a more lasting result in this region.

The platysma muscle below the transection at the level of the cervicomental angle is the "true" rudimentary portion of the platysma muscle. When relaxed, it contributes to the appearance of the anterior platysma muscle and skin folds of the anterior neck. The transection of the platysma muscle at the cervicomental angle permits this portion of the platysma muscle (caudad to cervicomental angle transection) to adapt to the contour of the deep structures of the neck, eliminating the "bowstring" of the anterior border of the platysma muscle between the mentum and the midneck. If the function (imbrication of the superficial fascia of the face and neck to the cervicomental angle level of the platysma muscle) and the contour (cervicomental angle tightening of the cephalad stump of the transected platysma muscle and controlled lipectomy) restoration is satisfactory, the cervical skin and subcutaneous fat flap need only be redraped under minimal tension and the wound closed after tailoring of the redundant skin.

To achieve the most successful restoration of the superficial fascia and the associated tissues (SMAS) of the face, the superficial fascia is elevated anteriorly to an extent that permits the advancement of the superficial fascia and the SMAS without traction on or a rolling of the deeper structures of the apex of the elevation of the superficial fascia and the deep fascia. The objective is to release the superficial fascia sufficiently to correct the appearance of the cheek by advancing and implanting it in a more posterior position on the deep fascia of the face. If the superficial fascia is elevated and on posterior advancement there is a rolling of the deep tissues, release of the superficial fascia is not sufficient. Under these circumstances, the surgeon is requiring the advanced tissue to support the anterior face rather than elevating the relaxed tissues and redistributing them over a new foundation.

To provide the maximum advancement of the SMAS and the most satisfactory result in the appearance of the face, one should advance the superficial fascia in a posterior direction. A significant cephalad rotation of the superficial fascia is not possible, and it is the maximum anteroposterior reduction in the superficial fascia that achieves the increased tension and better mechanical advantage of the SMAS. This "tectorial" realignment restores the superficial fascia to an anteroposterior dimension that existed at some earlier age and provides a more youthful appearance of the face, both in contour and in mechanical function.

The restoration of the anteroposterior dimensions of the SMAS and the implantation of the superficial fascia of the cheek over a broad area and in a more posterior position on the deep fascia of the cheek has not altered the morphologic unit (SMAS) of the cheek. Mitz and Peyronie [27] demonstrated the relationship of the musculoaponeurotic system and the fibrous tissue septa of the subcutaneous fat of the cheek in the transmission of normal facial expression. Superficial fascia rhytidectomy preserves this relationship. It also reduces postoperative swelling, and the cheeks appear normal and "soft" early in the postoperative period.

The ability of the platysma muscle to glide on the deep fascia of the neck varies in different locations depending on the adherence of the superficial fascia (platysma muscle) to the deep fascia. In the region of the lower half of the face (see Fig. 17-3, zone C), it is loosely attached and can be elevated easily from the deep fascia of the face over the masseter muscle and the mandible. The superficial fascia of the neck (platysma muscle) is more adherent to the deep fascia of the neck from the lower border of the mandible to approximately the cervicomental angle (see Fig. 17-3, zone D) and is more difficult to separate from the deep fascia in this region. Below the cervicomental angle (see Fig. 17-3, zone E), it is less adherent to the deep fascia of the neck than it is over the submandibular area.

As a result of this variation in the adherence of the platysma muscle (superficial fascia) to the deep fascia of the neck, there seems to be a variation in the extent of the excursion of the platysma muscle on the deep fascia. Below the cervicomental angle, the platysma muscle (superficial fascia) has a wide excursion. It can be easily advanced posteriorly a considerable distance with a minimum release of the muscle from the deep fascia of the neck. With an equal release of the platysma muscle in the submandibular region, the ability to advance the platysma muscle in this more adherent area above the cervicomental angle is more limited. Also, the force of the countertraction is greater as the more adherent platysma muscle does not have the same excursion as elsewhere. The more adherent portion of the platysma muscle in the submandibular region, while mobile, may provide a point of functional attachment of the SMAS, or the "tie down" for the caudad extent of the SMAS described by Mitz and Peyronie [27]. Moreover, the platysma muscle above the cervicomental angle is to a variable extent an integral part of the function of the lower lip, and this more adherent area may assist in the segmental contraction of the platysma muscle in its role as a depressor of the lower lip.

The transection-resection or "break" in the platysma muscle at the cervicomental angle and the closure of the anterior border of the platysma muscle between the mentum and the cervicomental angle eliminates the anterior platysma muscle folds in the submental region. The advancement of the posterior border of the SMAS and the superficial fascia (platysma muscle) above the cervicomental angle creates a tightening of the cephalad stump of the platysma muscle transection (see Fig. 17-15). With healing, the scarring of the cephalad stump of the platysma muscle acts as a "drawstring," accentuating the cervicomental angle or helping to create one where very little or none existed. This provides a more lasting result in the neck and even with the passage of time usually does not approach the preoperative appearance.

The technique of accomplishing the division between the functional and rudimentary positions of the platysma is critical to the maintenance of the cervicomental angle. If the platysma muscle is only transected, particularly by a subcutaneous tunneling in the cervical region, it may not be completely transected or it may regenerate some of the fibers [11]. In these circumstances, the platysma muscle folds of the neck redevelop or there may be a regeneration of bands of the platysma muscle, which creates a most unpleasant appearance in the neck when the patient is animated (see Fig. 17-19). To ensure a complete transection of the platysma muscle, the transection is performed by direct vision. This is obtained by the elevation of the skin and subcutaneous fat flap from the platysma muscle. The strip of muscle that is to be removed is elevated from the deep fascia of the neck, and the posterior segment is eliminated. Thus, along with the anterior segment removal the transection is completed (see Fig. 17-13). Surprisingly, even with good exposure it is possible to leave the posterior platysma muscle sheath with a thin layer of the platysma muscle fibers intact. The transverse resection of a segment of the platysma muscle of approximately 1.0 to 1.5 cm assists in determining whether an intact muscle sheath and muscle fibers exist and reduces the chance of a regeneration of the muscle fibers.

When the contours of the submental, submandibular, or mandible area are altered by excess subcutaneous fat, a lipectomy of the involved area is indicated. A lipectomy should eliminate the offending fat and improve the contour of the area but leave an adequate thickness of the subcutaneous fat, which is characteristic of the young face. If a subdermal elevation of the skin of the cervical region is performed, the bulk of the subcutaneous fat remains attached to the platysma muscle. As the lipectomy proceeds from a superficial level to a deeper one, it is difficult to determine the amount and the location of the offending fat to be removed. When the skin and subcutaneous fat are elevated at the level of the platysma muscle, all the subcutaneous fat of the cervical region is attached to the skin. Consequently, the surgeon can both visualize and palpate the thickness of the subcutaneous fat and have greater control of the depth and location of the lipectomy (see Fig. 17-9). Furthermore, irregularities of contour frequently seen with a superficial to deep lipectomy are preventable.

It is of great significance that a lipectomy that removes fat from the deep level to a more superficial one requires less fat removal to achieve a desired result. The reason appears to be the complete mobilization and redistribution of the skin and subcutaneous fat of the cervical region.

The extent of the lipectomy of the skin and subcutaneous fat flap also depends on the type of skin and subcutaneous fat in the neck. In a thin neck with a minimal subcutaneous fat layer, the elevation of the skin and subcutaneous fat flap from the platysma muscle and the redraping may be sufficient to remove the small fat deposits that interfere with contour of the mandible. When the skin and subcutaneous fat flap are advanced over the sternomastoid muscle in this type of neck, the fat posterior to the sternomastoid muscle can be thinned to the subdermal level to preserve the contour of the sternomastoid muscle.

A heavy layer of subcutaneous fat of the cervical region that is pliable can be thinned to approximately half thickness with a good result in the contouring. If the neck has a heavy appearance with a thick layer of firm subcutaneous fat and the skin has good elasticity, removal of the fat should be limited to approximately one-third depth or a "scooped out" appearance may result (see Fig. 17-18). With this type of subcutaneous fat, the redraping of the skin and subcutaneous fat flap after a minimal lipectomy produces the desired contouring and preserves the appearance of a thick, firm subcutaneous fat layer that is seen over other areas of the face.

The submental area and the angle produced in the submandibular area by the junction of the mandible and the sternomastoid muscle are the most consistent areas requiring lipectomy. In almost all cases, the subcutaneous fat located in the region of the junction of the mandible and the sternomastoid muscle must be removed, or, with mobilization and advancement of the skin and subcutaneous fat flap, the fat located more anteriorly and inferiorly in the cervical region will produce a thickening over the sternomastoid muscle and obscure the angle produced by the junction of the mandible and the sternomastoid muscle. To emphasize the contours of the junction of the mandible and the sternomastoid muscle, the fat in this area should be trimmed after a trial draping of the advanced skin and subcutaneous fat to prevent any deformity of contouring that may occur from an overzealous lipectomy in an area to be advanced to a new location.

The complications of the technique of superficial fascia rhytidectomy, which has been the standard procedure for 3 years, are not significantly different from those observed in a subcutaneous rhytidectomy (Table 17-12). Injury of the facial nerve has not been experienced with the technique described (648 patients, 1979–1981). One of 648 patients (0.15%) had a permanent dysfunction of the lower lip. Table 17-3 indicates the incidence of the lower lip dysfunction by year. The reduction in the extent of the elevation of the platysma muscle and the lowering of the transection of the platysma muscle to the level of the cervicomental angle have been responsible for the diminished incidence and subsequent absence of dysfunction of the lower lip.

Baker and Conley [3], reviewing the reported incidence of facial nerve paralysis after all types of rhytidectomy in the years 1970 to 1979, found the incidence of temporary injury of the facial nerve to be 0.7 percent (50 cases in 6500 face-lifts). The incidence of permanent facial nerve injury was 0.1 percent (7 cases in 6500 face-lifts). If the one patient with a lower lip dysfunction is considered to have an injury of the facial nerve (rather than a dysfunction of the platysma muscle), the incidence of facial nerve injury in superficial fascia rhytidectomy is 0.15 percent (see Table 17-3). The risk of this complication should not be the justification for utilizing a less complex procedure as this outcome compares with the results reported for subcutaneous rhytidectomy (Table17-12).

With subcutaneous rhytidectomy the incidence of hematomas that require the removal of sutures of the skin to evacuate the blood ranges from 2.8 to 8.1 percent (Table 17-12). With superficial fascia rhytidectomy, in the years 1979 to 1981, 2 of 648 patients (0.3%) had a hematoma requiring reentry into the wound. The technique, as described, has a minimum amount of subdermal skin elevation (3.5 cm in the preauricular and postauricular region extending into the cervical region to the posterior border of the platysma muscle), and bleeding in these areas is visible and managed easily. The remaining tissue elevated is the superficial fascia and the skin and subcutaneous fat flap of the cervical region. In the cheek and the neck, the elevation of the superficial fascia and the skin and subcutaneous fat flap encounters perforating blood vessels, which again can be managed adequately. Another factor, no doubt, is use of the regional block anesthesia and minimal use of infiltration anesthesia of the tissues. In addition, when infiltration is utilized, the concentration of epinephrine (1:600,000) is sufficient to reduce the bleeding but not sufficient to mask any significant bleeding. As a result of this combination of the technique and the anesthesia, small hematomas of the cheek are practically nonexistent and large hematomas requiring evacuation are a rarity.

Superficial fascia rhytidectomy virtually eliminates skin slough. Once the surgeon is confident that the technique of anatomic restoration of the superficial fascia will provide more lasting support of the face, closure of the skin under minimal tension almost excludes skin sloughs of any size (Tables 17-2 and 17-4). Table 17-12 shows the range of skin sloughs reported with a subcutaneous rhytidectomy.

Superficial fascia rhytidectomy has numerous other advantages for both patient and surgeon. The postoperative course is usually uneventful. The swelling and bruising of the face are minimal. Wound healing is rapid and uneventful, and, as a result of a skin closure that requires minimal tension, the scars are usually very fine throughout the closure. Facial swelling subsides rapidly, but, perhaps more significant, the skin has a normal appearance. As there is minimal skin edema, the skin looks pliable and "soft" soon after the operation. This appearance has a profound effect on the patient's attitude but perhaps impresses acquaintances even more, and they comment frequently on the natural aspect of the face, in both the early and the late period of recovery.

With the restoration of the SMAS, the fat in the cheek is relocated to a region that is consistent with the appearance of a younger face. This maneuver relieves some of the hollowness of the cheeks associated with aging.

Severe wrinkling of the cheeks seen in some patients can be relieved for many years by a superficial fascia rhytidectomy. It is generally believed that only an exten-

Table 17-12. Comparison of the incidence of complications of superficial fascia and subcutaneous rhytidectomy

Complication	Superficial fascia		Subcutaneous
	1973–1981 (1449 patients, all techniques) (%)	1979–1981 (648 patients, technique described) (%)	Reported range (%)
1. Facial nerve injury or dysfunction of lower lip (permanent)	0.35	0.15	0.06–1.0
2. Hematoma	0.55	0.3	2.8–8.1
3. Skin slough > 2.5 cm	0	0	0.3–2.44
4. Skin-fascia-muscle adhesion	1.1	0	Not reported
5. Infection (localized)	0.4	0.9	1.0

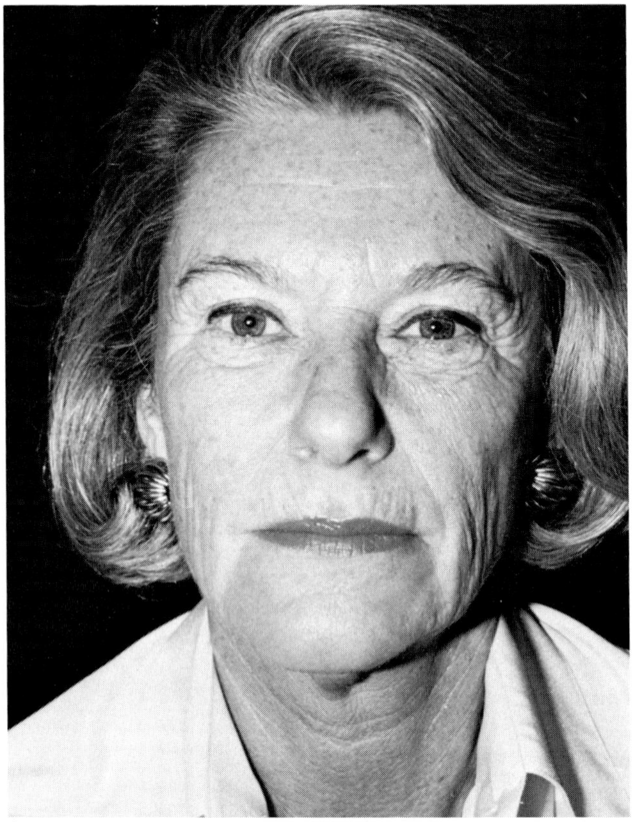

A

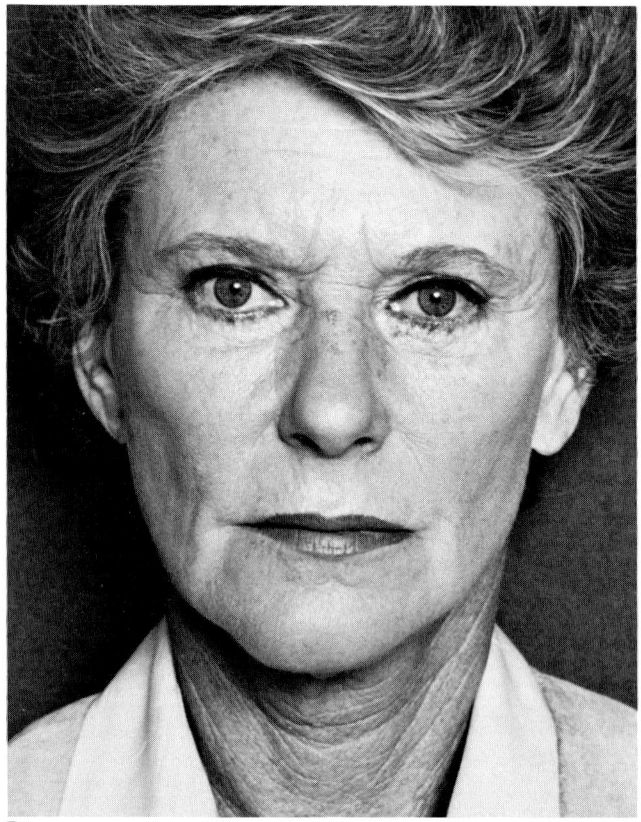

B

Figure 17-22. Superficial fascia rhytidectomy (Skoog technique) with submentoplasty and chemical peel of perioral region (no chemical peel or undermining of the skin of the cheeks) (patient's age, 59 years).
A. Before operation. Fair complexion with history of long exposure to solar radiation. Relaxation of SMAS and marked wrinkling of skin of cheeks.
B. Six years after operation. Correction of the appearance of the cheeks, the central face, and the contour of the mandible remains satisfactory.

sive elevation of the skin at the subcutaneous level will release the skin sufficiently to correct this change of the cheeks. The morbidity associated with such elevation can be considerable as the bruising of the area resorbs slowly and at times will leave permanent spots of pigmentation in the cheeks. Figure 17-22 illustrates the effectiveness of a superficial fascia advancement of the cheeks (without skin undermining at the subdermal level) in the control of severe wrinkles of the face.

Improvement in the appearance of the nasolabial folds (central face) is another advantage of superficial fascia rhytidectomy. Preoperative appraisal of the midface in the individual with deep nasolabial folds indicates that it will be necessary to elevate the superficial fascia extensively (Fig. 17-23). As described, the operation includes release of the superficial fascia over the malar process. The wide release and advancement of the superficial fascia improves the appearance of the nasolabial folds and produces a more lasting correction. Morbidity is not increased.

If there are questions or complaints in the postoperative period, they are usually concerned with a dimpling of the cheeks and with tenderness and tightness in the region of the transection of the platysma muscle. If the superficial fascia is advanced under too much tension or there is considerable facial swelling (e.g., with a chemical peel of the perioral region), the sutures of the imbrication of the superficial fascia will create a dimple. This resolves as the facial swelling diminishes and does not become a permanent problem.

The tenderness or tightness of the neck in the region of the transverse segmental resection of the platysma muscle and the "drawstring" advancement of the platysma muscle at the level of the cervicomental angle also subsides rapidly as wound healing progresses. Some patients will experience recurrent tightness in the neck with vigorous exercise or on becoming excited or extremely warm. This too resolves with the maturation of the wound and has not been a prominent complaint.

Removal of the subcutaneous fat in the cervical region produces a permanent contour and therefore must be performed judiciously. When a successful lipectomy (depth and location) is superimposed on the transverse segmental resection of the platysma muscle, the result in the contour of the cervicomental angle is very good. The patient can be assured that although there will be relaxation of the skin, subcutaneous fat, and underlying muscu-

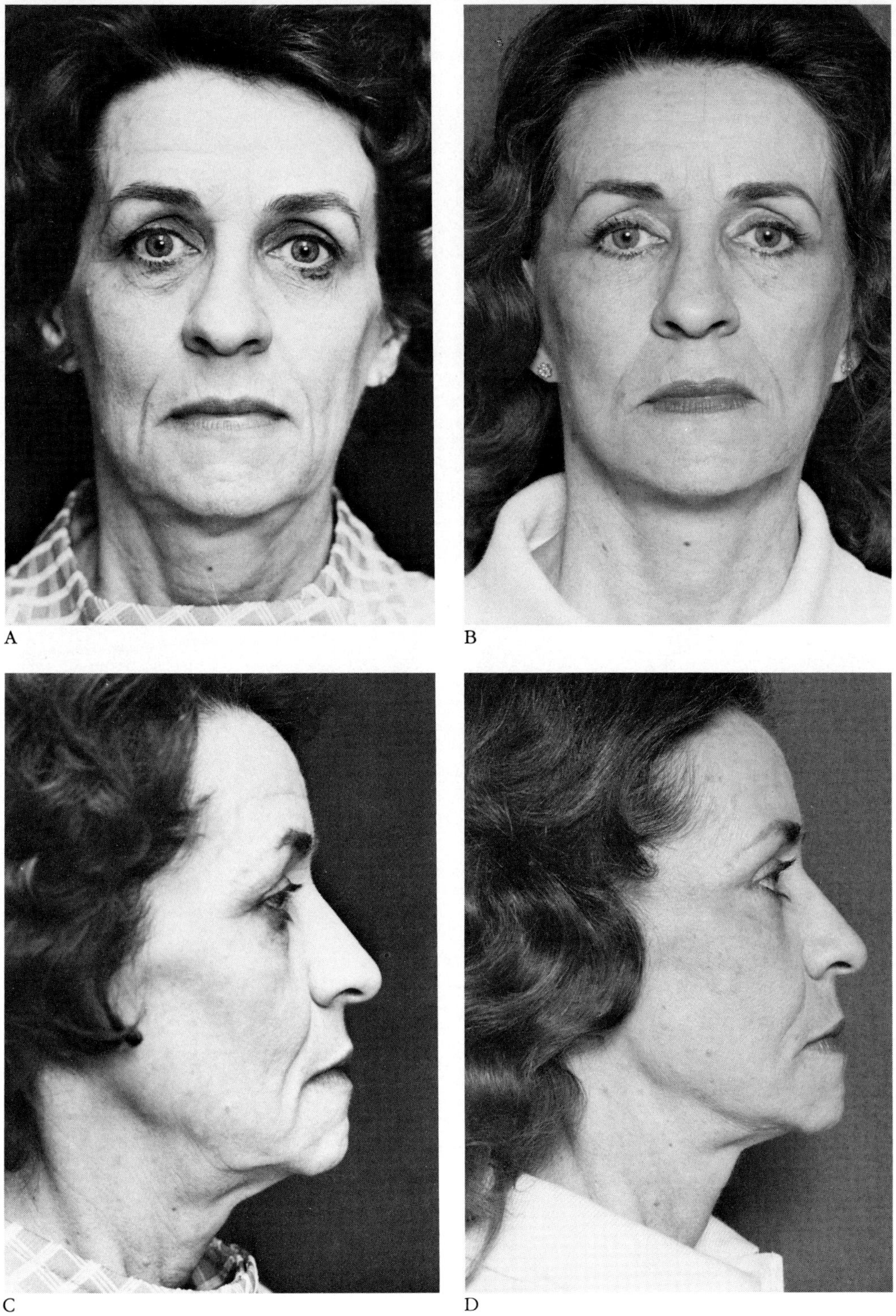

Figure 17-23. Superficial fascia rhytidectomy with resection of a transverse segment of the platysma muscle (patient's age, 52 years).

A, C. Preoperative views. Redundant skin of face and neck with prominent nasolabial folds extending below the angle of the mouth, a fold of skin extending from the angle of the mouth, and redundant skin of the inferior border of the mandible that interrupts the contour of the mandible.

B, D. Postoperative views after 4 years. Restoration of the SMAS has provided a satisfactory long-term correction of the features that are characteristic of aging.

lature over a period of time, the contours will remain very good. If the jowl fat or submental fat, or fat in other regions, is removed, it will not develop in the future. The same thing applies to subcutaneous fat defects from an overzealous fat removal. If a defect results, it is a permanent contour.

Once the surgeon is familiar with the anatomy of the superficial and deep fascia in vivo and confidently relies on the relationship of the superficial and the deep fasciae to the branches of the facial nerve, the technique will become standardized. A superficial fascia rhytidectomy is a more exacting procedure than a subcutaneous face-lift. However, it is like all procedures in that it is most demanding in the early learning period and becomes less so as knowledge and confidence in the technique are gained. The procedure requires approximately 3 hours of operating room time. The submental area and the anterior region of the neck take 15 to 30 minutes and each side of the face from 1 to 1¼ hours. Table 17-12 reflects the safety of the superficial fascia rhytidectomy as presented. Superficial fascia rhytidectomy with a transverse segmental resection of the platysma muscle at the level of the cervicomental angle and lipectomy, as described and if indicated, will yield an optimum result. The patient positively can be assured that after the initial period of the maturation of the wound (6 months) the outcome can be expected to remain satisfactory for the greatest period of time possible with this type of surgery (Figs. 17-24 and 17-25).

Figure 17-24. Superficial fascia rhytidectomy with resection of a transverse segment of the platysma muscle (patient's age, 50 years). Adjunctive procedures: chemical peel of forehead and perioral region, small chin implant, blepharoplasty.
A, C. Before operation. Redundant skin of cheeks and neck with loss of the contour of the mandible. Deep skin folds of nasolabial region and lateral to angle of the mouth over the mandible.
B, D. Postoperative views after 1 year. Restoration of the SMAS and cervicomental angle. The appearance is characteristic of a young face.

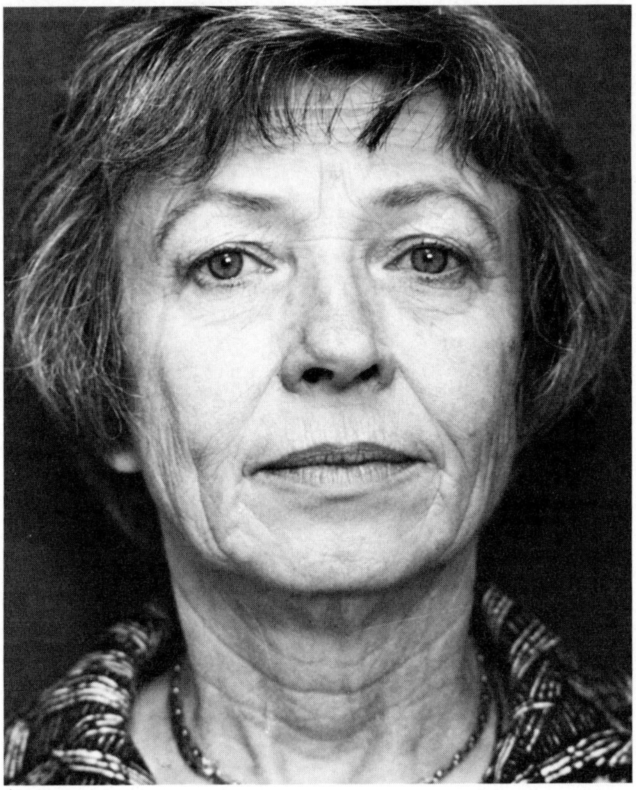

A

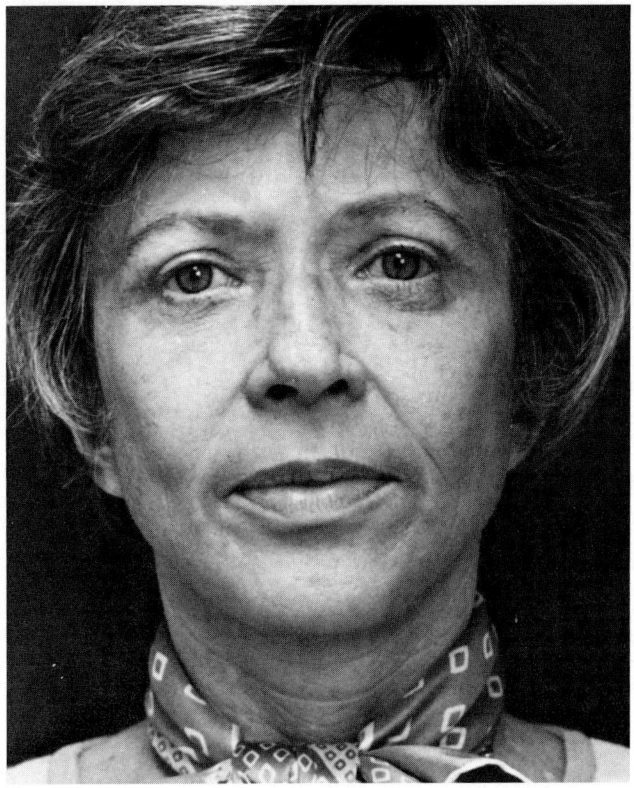

B

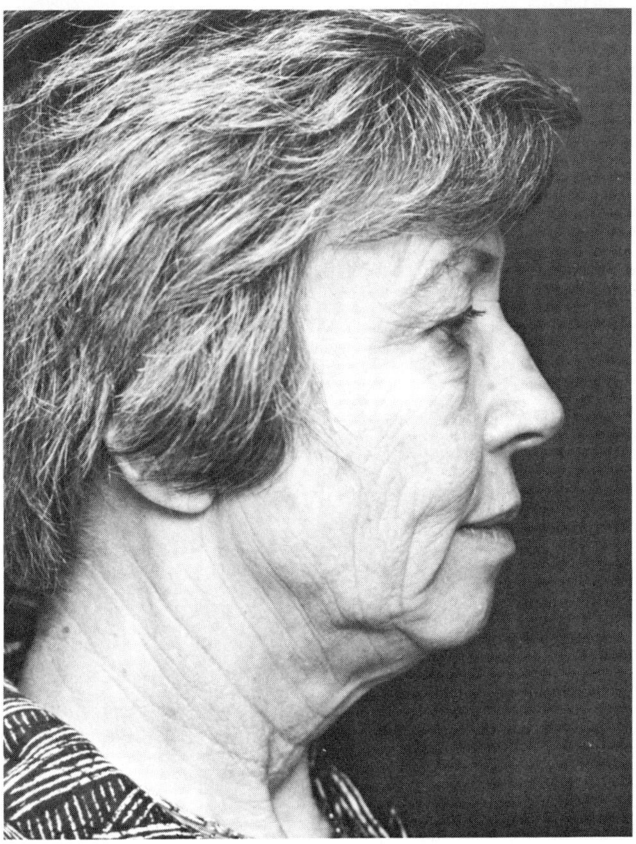

C

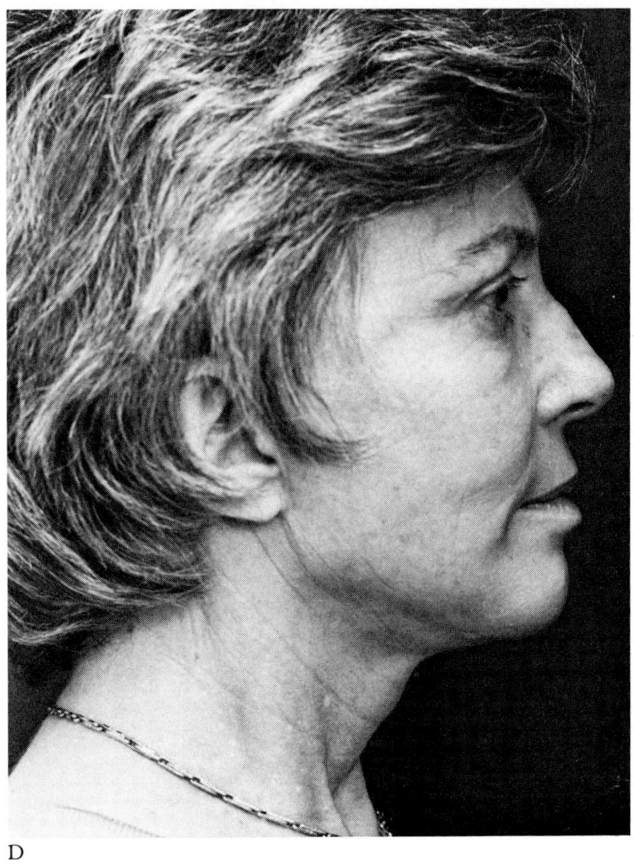

D

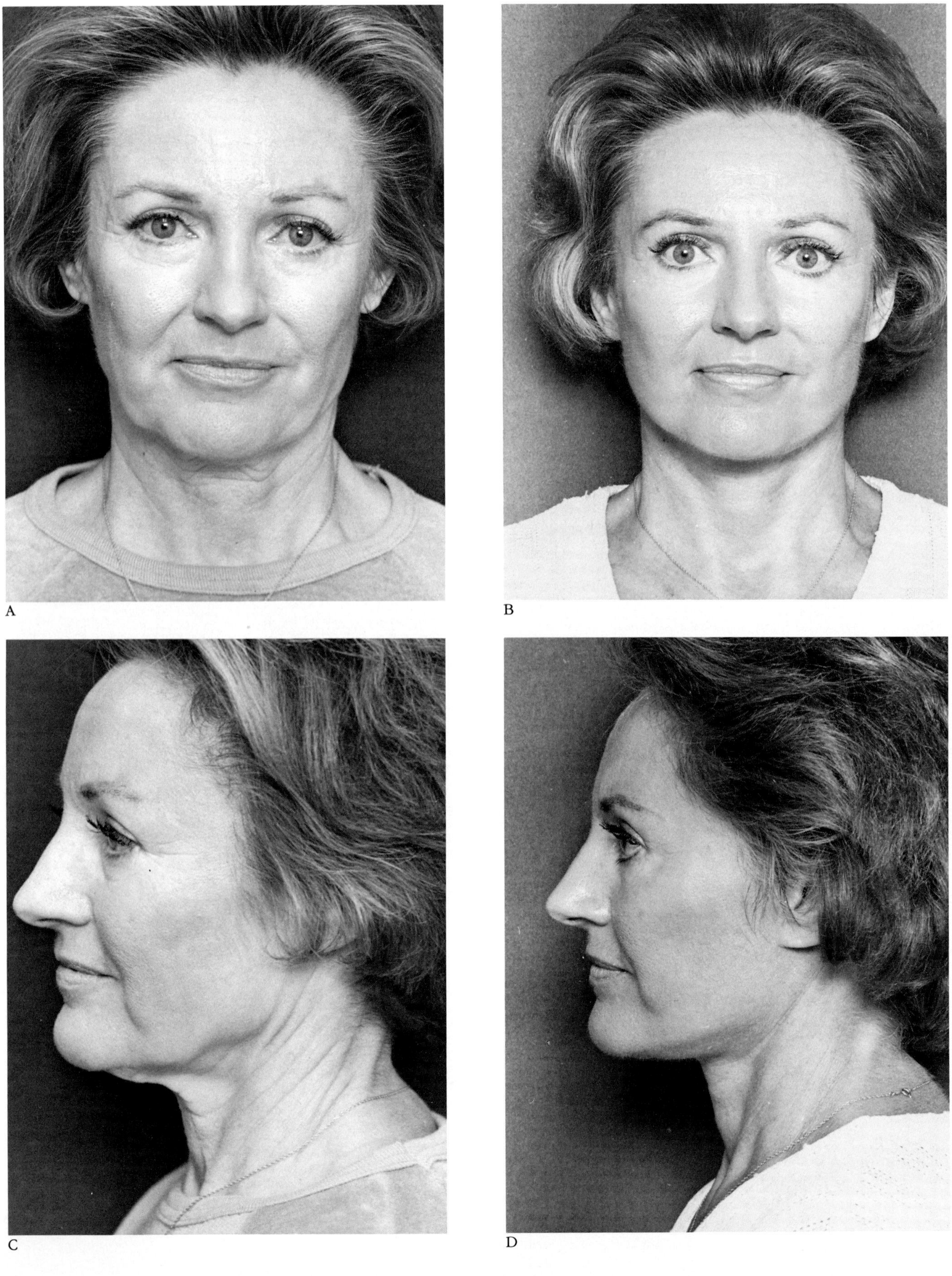

A B C D

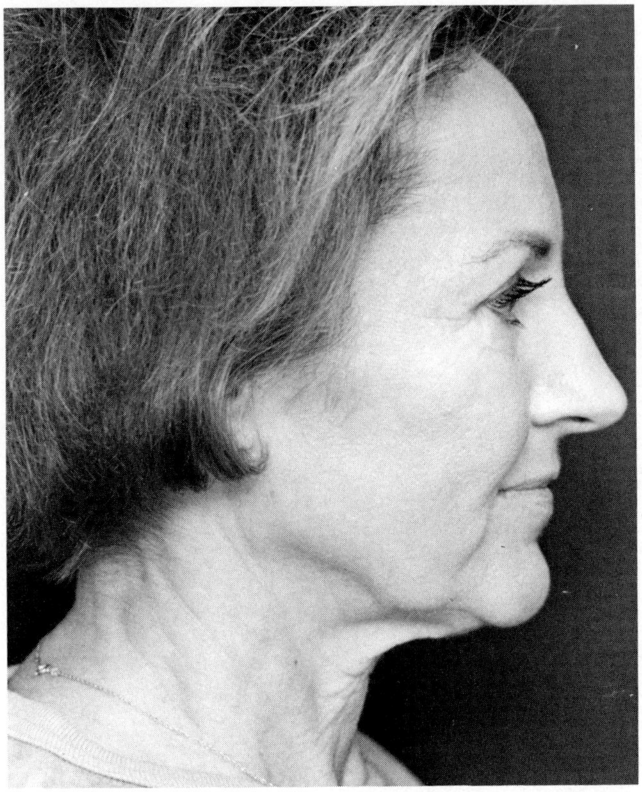

E

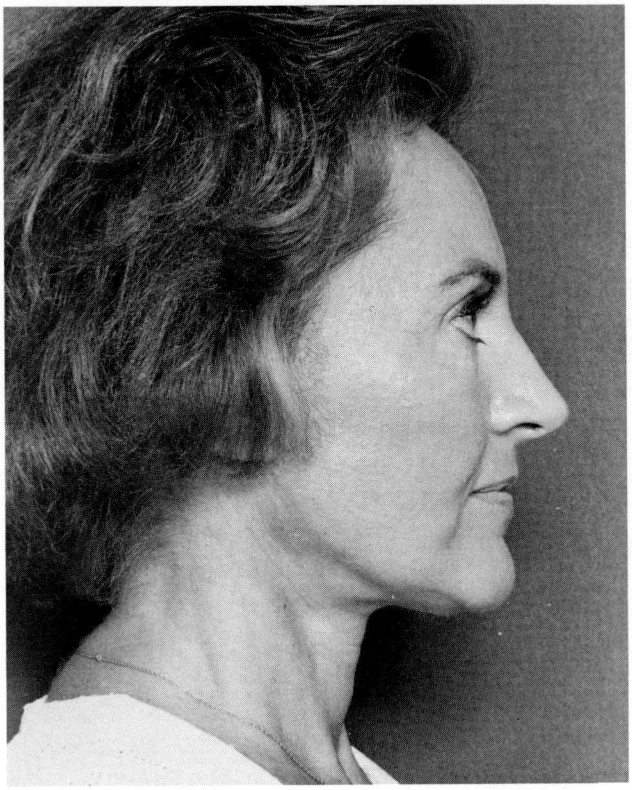

F

Figure 17-25. Superficial fascia rhytidectomy with a transverse segmental resection of the platysma muscle from anterior to posterior border at the level of the cervicomental angle (patient's age, 55 years).

A, C, E. Preoperative views. Relaxation of the SMAS and the platysma muscle and the skin resulting in deep nasolabial folds, redundant tissue of the cheeks, jaw, and skin, and platysma muscle folds of the anterior region of the neck.

B, D, F. Postoperative views after 2 years. Restoration of SMAS and platysma muscle cephalad to the cervicomental angle to the anteroposterior dimension and tension, respectively, of a former age. Cephalad stump of the platysma muscle assists in maintaining the cervicomental angle.

SUMMARY

To fulfill the criterion of restoration of an anatomic defect, all of the tissues that contribute to the defect should be corrected. If a replacement of the tissues in their normal anatomic relationships is not maintained by the repair, the tissues that cannot be maintained in the correct relationship must be altered. Superficial fascia rhytidectomy restores the anatomic relationship of the SMAS and improves the tension of the SMAS and the platysma muscle. The change is reflected in the patient's appearance in repose and in animation and is more lasting in the face and the contour of the inferior border of the mandible.

An alteration in the tissues of the neck (platysma muscle and subcutaneous fat) is necessary to maintain the contours of the neck (cervicomental angle). Transection of the platysma muscle, resection of a transverse segment of the platysma muscle at the level of the cervicomental angle, and, if indicated, lipectomy of the subcutaneous fat proceeding from the level of the platysma muscle (deep) to a more superficial level in the location required produce a longer-lasting result in the cervical region.

The anatomy, anesthesia, technique, complications, and advantages of superficial fascia rhytidectomy are described and discussed. The results of the technique are compared with those of superficial fascia rhytidectomy combined with various forms of management of the platysma muscle and lipectomy and subcutaneous rhytidectomy.

REFERENCES

1. Adamson, J. E., Horton, C. E., and Crawford, H. H. Surgical correction of the "turkey gobbler" deformity. *Plast. Reconstr. Surg.* 34:589, 1964.
2. Baker, D. C., et al. The male rhytidectomy. *Plast. Reconstr. Surg.* 60:514, 1977.
3. Baker, D. C., and Conley, J. Avoiding facial nerve injuries in rhytidectomy. *Plast. Reconstr. Surg.* 64:781, 1979.
4. Baker, T. J., Gordon, H. L., and Mosienko, P. Rhytidectomy. *Plast. Reconstr. Surg.* 59:24, 1977.
5. Connell, B. F. Cervical lifts: The value of platysma muscle flaps. *Ann. Plast. Surg.* 49:385, 1978.
6. Connell, B. F. Contouring the neck in rhytidectomy by lipectomy and a muscle sling. *Plast. Reconstr. Surg.* 61:376, 1978.
7. Converse, J. M., McCarthy, J. G., and Littler, J. W. *Reconstructive Plastic Surgery* (2nd ed.). Philadelphia: Saunders, 1977. P. 1920.

8. Conway, H. The surgical face lift: Rhytidectomy. *Plast. Reconstr. Surg.* 45:124, 1970.
9. Cronin, T. D., and Biggs, T. M., Jr. The T–Z plasty for the male "turkey gobbler" neck. *Plast. Reconstr. Surg.* 47:534, 1971.
10. Ellenbogen, R. Pseudo-paralysis of the mandibular branch of the facial nerve after platysmal face-lift operation. *Plast. Reconstr. Surg.* 63:364, 1979.
11. Ellenbogen, R. Regrowth of platysma following platysma cervical lift: Etiology and methodology of prevention. *Plast. Reconstr. Surg.* 67:616, 1981.
12. Ellenby, J. D. Personal communication, 1981.
13. Gray, H. *Anatomy of the Human Body.* Philadelphia: Lea & Febiger, 1959.
14. Guerrero-Santos, J. Muscular Flap in Cervical Rhytidoplasty. Presented at the Annual Meeting of the American Society of Plastic and Reconstructive Surgeons. Hollywood, Fla., October 1973.
15. Guerrero-Santos, J. Face-Lift Surgical Technique. Presented at the Annual Symposium on Aesthetic-Plastic Surgery. Guadalajara, Mexico, October 1974.
16. Guerrero-Santos, J. The role of the platysma muscle in rhytidoplasty. *Clin. Plast. Surg.* 5:29, 1978.
17. Guerrero-Santos, J., Spaillat, L., and Morales, F. Muscular lift in cervical rhytidoplasty. *Plast. Reconstr. Surg.* 54:127, 1974.
18. Hollinshead, W. H. *Anatomy for Surgeons: The Head and the Neck* (2nd ed.). New York: Harper & Row, 1968. P. 306.
19. Leist, F. D., Masson, J. K., and Erich, J. F. A review of 324 rhytidectomies, emphasizing complications and patient dissatisfaction. *Plast. Reconstr. Surg.* 59:525, 1977.
20. Lemmon, M. L., and Hamra, S. T. Skoog rhytidectomy: A five year experience with 577 patients. *Plast. Reconstr. Surg.* 65:283, 1980.
21. Lemmon, M. L. Superficial fascia rhytidectomy: A restoration of the SMAS with control of the cervicomental angle. *Clin. Plast. Surg.* 10:449, 1983.
22. McDowell, A. J. Effective practical steps to avoid complications in face lifting: Review of 105 consecutive cases. *Plast. Reconstr. Surg.* 50:563, 1972.
23. McGregor, M. W., and Greenberg, R. L. Rhytidectomy. In R. M. Goldwyn (ed.), *The Unfavorable Result in Plastic Surgery: Avoidance and Treatment.* Boston: Little, Brown, 1972.
24. Millard, D. R. Plastic peregrinations. *Plast. Reconstr. Surg.* 5:26, 1950.
25. Millard, D. R., et al. Submental and submandibular lipectomy in conjunction with a face lift, in the male or female. *Plast. Reconstr. Surg.* 49:385, 1972.
26. Millard, D. R., Pigott, R. W., and Hedo, A. Submandibular lipectomy. *Plast. Reconstr. Surg.* 41:413, 1968.
27. Mitz, V., and Peyronie, M. The superficial musculoaponeurotic system (SMAS) in the parotid and cheek area. *Plast. Reconstr. Surg.* 58:80, 1976.
28. Owsley, J. Q. Platysma-fascia rhytidectomy. *Plast. Reconstr. Surg.* 60:843, 1977.
29. Pennisi, V. R., and Capozzi, A. The transportation of fat in cervico-facial rhytidectomy. *Plast. Reconstr. Surg.* 49:423, 1972.
30. Peterson, R. Cervical-Rhytidoplasty: A Personal Approach. Presented at the Aesthetic Society Symposium on the Aging Face. Denver, October 1976.
31. Peterson, R. The Role of the Platysma Muscle in Cervical Lifts. In D. Goulian and E. H. Courtiss (eds.), *Symposium on Surgery of the Aging Face.* St. Louis: Mosby, 1978. P. 115.
32. Skoog, T. Useful Techniques in Face Lifting. Presented at the meeting of the American Association of Plastic Surgeons. San Francisco, April 1969.
33. Skoog, T. Rhytidectomy: A Personal Experience and Technique. Presented and demonstrated on live television at the Seventh Annual Symposium on Cosmetic Surgery at the Cedars of Lebanon Hospital. Miami, Fla., February 1973.
34. Skoog, T. *Plastic Surgery.* Stockholm: Almquist & Wiksell, 1974. Pp. 300–330.
35. Snyder, G. B. Cervico-mentoplasty, with rhytidectomy. *Plast. Reconstr. Surg.* 54:404, 1974.
36. Stark, R. B. A rhytidectomy series. *Plast. Reconstr. Surg.* 59:373, 1977.
37. Weismann, P. A. Simplified technique in submental lipectomy. *Plast. Reconstr. Surg.* 48:443, 1971.

18. The Male Aging Face

Eugene H. Courtiss

Surgical treatment of the aging face is being undertaken with increasing frequency. Although this fact applies to both males and females, in males the increase is greater in both absolute and relative numbers. Still, males account for only approximately 10 percent of aging face surgery; not long ago the percentage was even less. This chapter focuses on the management of males who undergo surgical treatment of their aging face and neck; the differences between males and females are highlighted also.

Although aesthetic surgery of the forehead, eyebrows, eyelids, chin, and nose will be omitted, its importance in improving the aging face cannot be overstated. As a matter of fact, the simple insertion of a chin implant, the elevation of a drooped nasal tip, or the removal of an eyelid "bag" may be *more important* than the face-neck procedure. Those operations are presented elsewhere; only face- and neck-lifting will be discussed herein.

TERMINOLOGY

A face-lift means different things to different individuals. To the patient, a mystical or magical connotation may be assumed, no doubt because the press, and some surgeons, publicize "miraculous" and "dramatic" results, particularly in the famous (or the infamous). Nonetheless, referring to the procedure as a face-lift is incomplete; as performed at present the operation includes a "lift" of the neck as well as a "lift" of the face.

In an effort to find scientific-sounding names, terms such as *rhytidectomy, rhytidoplasty, meloplasty,* and *facioplasty* have been used. Therefore, examination of their stems [10] is appropriate:

rhytid- (or rhitid-): Greek, *rhytis,* "wrinkle"
-ectomy: Greek, *ektome,* "excision"
-plasty: Greek, *plassein,* "to shape"
facio-: Latin, *facies,* "face"
melo-: Greek, *melon,* "cheek"
cervico-: Latin, *cervix,* "neck"

Because the surgical procedure minimally affects wrinkles, forms that include *rhytid* are inaccurate.

The operation alters more than the cheeks, so forms incorporating *melo* are incomplete. Furthermore, *melo* is a contraction of *melon,* "cheek." Thus, *melonoplasty* would be more accurate. To further complicate matters, *melo* is Greek for "limb." In any case, the awkward term *melonocervicoplasty,* which is poor because it contains both Latin and Greek stems, would be more precise.

Facioplasty, a combination of Greek and Latin stems, is a generic categorization that refers to any plastic surgery of the face.

Perhaps the problem in terminology is due to the fact

that the ancient Greek and Latin cultures did not conceive of current aesthetic surgical practice! Incidentally, the terms *face-lift* and *face- and neck-lift* are not included in a current medical dictionary [10].

ETIOLOGY AND PATHOLOGY

Obviously, aging of the face is part of the total aging process, a poorly understood phenomenon that is basic to all forms of life. The inexorable process begins at the moment of fertilization and continues until cellular death.

Although the *cause* of facial aging is unknown, certain observations are relevant: Racial (hereditary) characteristics are important (the facial skin of blacks appears to age differently from that of whites); men and women age differently (men infrequently develop fine wrinkles, particularly in their bearded area); environment and occupation are important (solar exposure is generally felt to cause fine wrinkles, particularly in women).

Parents may "pile guilt" on their children by statements that the children's failures make them grow old faster, but there is little evidence that such a relationship exists.

CLASSIFICATION OF DEFORMITIES

As aging of the face occurs, certain characteristics develop: Forehead wrinkles form, cheeks sag, jowls develop, vertical neck folds become prominent, and the inferior mandibular border loses its definition. *A* precise *preoperative evaluation of the* individual *patient's* pathologic anatomy *is the key to achieving the best possible result.* Each patient must be categorized as an *individual,* depending on the physical examination (see Physical Examination).

Some authors suggest that the characteristics of aging develop in a predictable sequence. However, it is so variable that such concepts are of little clinical value. Rather, aging occurs subtly and simultaneously in many areas; it cannot be classified, quantitated, or predicted. In addition, some patients, more frequently women than men, are bothered by aging of their face as an abstract concept, but usually certain features (deep "nasolabial" folds, jowls, neck folds, etc.) become points of patient focus. *The procedure planned must be directed to the* patient's *specific complaints.* As currently performed, at best, face-lifting tightens the temples, elevates and firms the cheeks, lessens the jowls, and improves the mandibular and neck contour; however, the "nasolabial" folds are changed minimally, if at all.

Face- and neck-lifting alters the *quantity* and location of tissues; little, if anything, is done to the *quality* of the tissues. Patients who request a change in the quality of tissue (fine wrinkles) should be treated by a chemical face peel or perhaps by a dermabrasion. Experienced aesthetic surgeons [5] note that chemical face peels are rarely done in males. This fact underscores the earlier observation that fine wrinkles rarely occur in males.

The face- and neck-lifting rarely effaces deep nasolabial folds. The residual ones *may* be improved further by collagen injection, a technique that may also benefit glabellar frown lines.

Although some authorities assert that surgery of the aged face rejuvenates ("restores youthful vigor or appearance to") patients, such is not the case. Patients look different and certain features are changed, but the patients' vigor is unaltered and they will not look as they did years previously.

PREOPERATIVE EVALUATION

History

As always, the first question asked by a plastic surgeon should be: "What brings you to see me?" The answer embodies the patient's motivations. Patients who denote a desire to improve certain features and feel better about themselves (internal body image) are acceptable [12]. Patients who wish external (economic, social, or marital) changes are poor candidates. Other poor candidates are those whose family or friends are opposed to the surgery. *If the patient's reason for surgery is to obtain a subsequent change in an* external *situation, the surgery should be postponed or denied.*

Inquiry should be made: "Why now?" If the answer is related to a life crisis (divorce, death, or similar incident), the patient may have psychologic factors that preclude happiness with the result. Finally, if the extent of patient concern exceeds the extent of deformity, the patient is a poor candidate [13].

The patient's past general health (particularly cardiac and vascular) should be ascertained. Patients who have had a heart attack within a year should be delayed; those with hypertension should have their blood pressure controlled. Other medical problems should be evaluated as indicated.

Physical Examination

Starting at the hairline and moving to the clavicle, one should examine the entire face. The forehead, eyebrows, eyelids, face, nose, chin, and neck must be evaluated individually and as they affect the entire face [11]. This assessment forms the basis of the *individual* patient's surgical plan:

- I. Scalp hair
  - A. Pattern (? receding)
  - B. Thick or thin
- II. Forehead
  - A. Configuration
  - B. Wrinkles (? depth)
  - C. Glabella (? frown lines)
- III. Eyes and associated structures
  - A. Eyebrows
    1. Position (? ptosis)
    2. Configuration of hairs

- B. Upper eyelids
  1. Redundancy of skin
  2. Position of upper tarsal fold
  3. Medial, central, and lateral bulges (fat)
  4. Lateral bulging (lacrimal gland)
- C. Lower eyelids
  1. Resting position of lid margin in relation to pupil (? scleral show)
  2. Atony, entropion, ectropion
  3. Medial, central, and lateral bulges (fat)
  4. Muscle (? hypertrophy)
  5. Redundancy of skin (? crow's-feet, ? fine wrinkles)
- D. Globe
  1. Sunken or bulging
  2. Mobility
  3. Dryness
  4. Visual acuity

IV. Cheeks
- A. Scars
- B. "Malar" bags
- C. Preauricular redundancy
- D. "Nasolabial" (actually, cheek-lip) folds
- E. Jowls
- F. Obesity (diffuse or local)

V. Neck
- A. Anterior (or lateral) cervical folds
- B. Cord formation on neck contraction
- C. Definition of jaw-neck line
- D. Fat deposition (diffuse or local)

VI. Skin
- A. Scars (including previous mastoid surgery)
- B. Color (? plethoric or pale)
- C. Texture (? wrinkles)
- D. Size of pores
- E. Hair pattern, density

The anatomic analysis of the patient is the basis for selecting the optimal technique for a given patient. The exact maneuvers required vary from patient to patient. Those affecting the face and neck are discussed here; other deformities are covered elsewhere.

If the patient's general health is good, examination by a family physician or internist is rarely required. The surgeon should be able to decide whether the patient can safely undergo surgery. Routine "screening" by primary physicians is neither medically effective nor cost-effective and it does not preclude intraoperative or postoperative complications. Patients whose general health is questionable should be evaluated by a physician specializing in whatever disease or organ is involved.

Surgeon's Evaluation of Self

After the patient's desires and anatomic configurations are assessed, the surgeon should evaluate his or her own experience, philosophy, and skills. Scant consideration has been given to the *surgeon's* personality and philosophy; however, they may be more important in determining the success of an operation than the patient's desires and anatomy. Some surgeons are conservative, others are radical; some believe in the tried and true, others in the innovative; some look on aesthetic surgery as a challenge, others do it condescendingly; some do the procedures daily, others rarely.

Counseling

Counseling, the mutual interchange between patient and surgeon, begins with a discussion of the goals of the surgery. This must be realistic. This is also a good time to dispel common myths about the operation: Patients look "better," not "younger"; and they do not "have to have it done again." Comments about "minilifts," which are of no value, may be made.

Informed Consent

Patients' unhappiness after surgery is less frequent in those who were well informed prior to the operation. Informed consent is also a legal requirement in most jurisdictions. The fundamentals of informed consent include a discussion of the alternative methods of treatment and the expectations, limitations, and complications of the proposed procedure.

ALTERNATIVE METHODS OF TREATMENT

The various methods of treating the aging face (surgery, chemical peel, dermabrasion, and collagen injections) should be discussed. In addition, the advantages, disadvantages, and *applicability to the individual patient* should be noted.

EXPECTATIONS

The patient's expectations should be detailed. This discussion might begin with the basic mechanism of how the surgery is scheduled, followed by an outline of what happens before the operation (changing clothes, premedication), what happens in the operating room (intravenous injections, monitoring, anesthesia, degree of pain, dressings), and postoperatively (edema, sensory changes, sutures, return to work, time before a "final" result).

LIMITATIONS

Surgery is not magic. It has limitations. These should be noted with precision and clarity (e.g., patients cannot be made to look like anyone else; the operation does not stop the aging process; and scars, which are unpredictable, are always present). The location and characteristics of scars should be reviewed clearly and *in detail.*

The fact that the human body is not symmetric and can never be made symmetric should be noted. Showing the patient his face in a reversing mirror [14] emphasizes this fact.

COMPLICATIONS

Not every complication can or need be addressed. If the most common complications (hematoma and nerve deficit) and the most severe (fatal drug response) are appropriately reviewed, the patient should have sufficient insight into the complexities of the procedure to be properly informed. Most patients are realistic about complications; those who become obsessed with them may be looking for guarantees that cannot be given. Such patients should be refused surgery.

Final Evaluation

After informing the patient of the alternative methods of treatment and the expectations, limitations, and complications of the surgery, and being sure the patient understands them, remain uncommitted and ask for a subsequent consultation or a "second opinion" elsewhere. One of the arts of plastic surgery is determining which patients should *not* have surgery. *It is better to have the patient angry at you for a day for refusing to operate than for a lifetime after having done so.*

SURGICAL PREPARATION

Booklets

Booklets describing the dos and don'ts of the procedure obviate the need for having the patient remember such preoperative instructions as diet, hair care, and arranging for a driver. Furthermore, including such postoperative instructions as positioning, diet, and dressings makes it easier for the surgeon and staff. If the booklet includes the signs and symptoms of hematoma (unilateral pain, swelling on one side, hardness of the cheeks, black-and-blue cheeks or lips), the patient knows what to look for; he is both informed and reassured.

Because of the deleterious effect of smoking on skin circulation, patients who smoke should stop. Unfortunately, this ideal is not always achieved. If the patient persists in smoking, he must understand the risk he is incurring.

Absolute Requirements

1. The patient should *not* take *any aspirin* for 2 weeks before surgery. Aspirin causes bleeding, the most common complication of (plastic) surgery.
2. Good preoperative *photographs* must be taken. Patients who refuse are denied surgery.
3. An *authorization form,* permitting both the surgery and photography, must be signed. Of course, no form precludes subsequent litigation, but it is wise to have a signed release. Having the photo release obviates the subsequent need to track down a patient whose photographs are to be shown in a lecture or publication.
4. *Fees* for aesthetic surgery are payable before the operation. If for no other reason, the patient does not receive a bill when the edema and ecchymosis are already making him depressed or unhappy.

Laboratory Studies

Although many hospitals, and some surgeons, require extensive routine preoperative laboratory studies, in an apparently healthy patient they are neither medically effective nor cost-effective. Furthermore, no study predicts intraoperative problems.

On the other hand, patients in whom *positive* findings of poor general health are made should be properly assessed. Thus, those who appear anemic or have renal, respiratory, bleeding, or other disease should be evaluated appropriately. Patients who take diuretics should have a serum potassium determination or an electrocardiogram if they are to receive a general anesthetic.

Technical Planning

The final phase of the preoperative preparation is planning the technical details of the operation. In the light of the *anatomic* objectives of the surgery, mental (or, better, written) notes should be made of the *precise* technical details. These form the basis for the specific plan to treat the patient's excesses and malpositions.

APPLIED ANATOMY

Skin

The thickness of the skin varies according to its anatomic location (preauricular and postauricular skin is thinner than scalp skin) and the patient's sex. (Male skin is thicker, less elastic, and coarser than female skin.) The skin of males is also more vascular, a fact often used to explain the greater incidence of hematomas [2] in males than in females.

Hair

Hair patterns differ according to gender and individual. In order to visualize the patient's own facial hair pattern, male patients (Fig. 18-1) should not shave for a day or two prior to surgery. Particular attention should be paid to the hair in three areas.

TEMPLE

The incision should be planned according to the present (or perhaps anticipated) pattern of male hair distribution. Some surgeons [15, 16] feel that the pattern of temple hair should not be altered; they place the incision directly back, across the temple, to the ear. Most surgeons, however, prefer to hide the scar within the temple hair (see Operative Technique, Marking).

PREAURICULAR AREA

In males, a hairless area is present in the preauricular area. Most authors agree that it should be preserved or reconstructed. As a result, they [1, 4, 6, 16, 18, 20, 21, 23, 26–28] make their preauricular incision 5 to 10 mm in front of the ear and leave a strip of hairless skin. Others [2, 15] remove

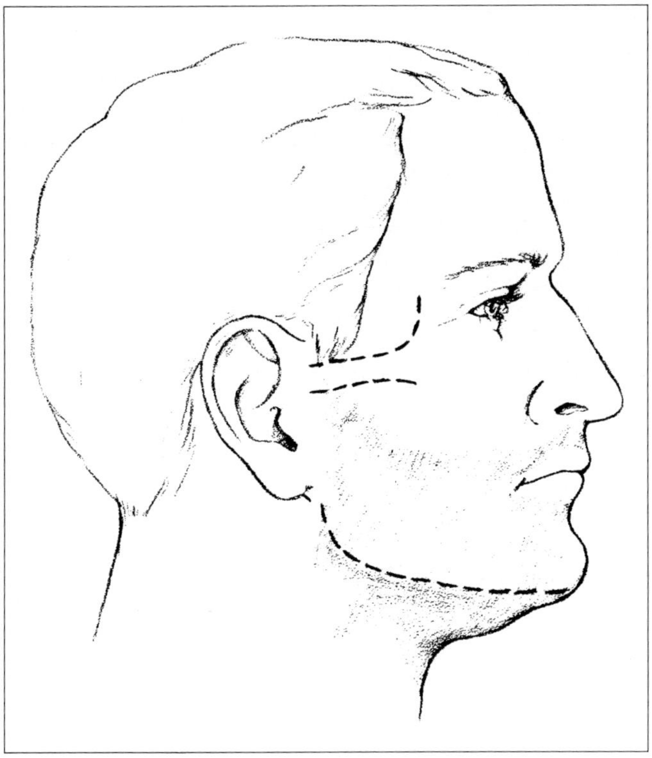

Figure 18-1. Usual male hair pattern. Patient's *own* pattern should be determined.

the strip, bringing hair-bearing skin close to the ear. Still others (including this author) prefer a retrotragal incision, in which case the hair follicles under the flap in the area of the preauricular skin must be removed (see Operative Technique, Marking). All techniques narrow the sideburn, but when the scar is located behind the tragus, the junction of hairless and hair-bearing skin, which is accentuated by the scar (different texture and color), is eliminated.

NECK

As neck skin is advanced posteriorly, hair follicles are simultaneously transposed. However, they should not be advanced onto the ear. Instead, the hair follicles should be excised from the deep side of the flap also.

The gentle curve of the hairline should be preserved. Some surgeons maintain it by locating the neck incision in front of the hairline. Because it shows there, I prefer to go directly into the scalp; then the curve is recreated by adjusting the tension at the time of the closure (see Operative Technique, Marking).

Subcutaneous Fat

Although subcutaneous fat is present beneath the skin of the entire face (except the eyelids), its thickness is variable. It is greater over the cheeks, jowls, and neck regions. Some fat may be excised, but complete excision may cause adherence of the skin to the underlying muscle, an unaesthetic condition.

Superficial Musculoaponeurotic System

Deep to the subcutaneous fat lies the superficial musculoaponeurotic system (SMAS) [19], a clearly defined anatomic layer. The SMAS overlies the parotid gland. Superiorly it is in continuity with the fascia overlying the temporalis muscle and inferiorly it is *in continuity with* the platysma muscle. Anterior to the parotid gland, the SMAS may become thinner. The SMAS is unyielding, and septa connect it to the skin. Therefore, when the SMAS is tightened and repositioned, the force is transmitted to the overlying skin.

Nerves

MOTOR NERVES

The facial nerve and its branches lie within the parotid gland. Anterior to the parotid, the nerves are just under the SMAS, which in that area may be thin. Thus, if the dissection is carried anterior to the parotid, care must be taken lest the nerves be damaged.

Inferior to the parotid, the nerves remain *deep* to the platysma muscle. Thus, dissection *superficial* to the platysma is safe, but that deep to the platysma is risky. Furthermore, if the muscle is perforated or divided, trauma to the nerve may follow, particularly when it occurs 4 cm or less from the mandibular border [3].

Superior to the zygomatic arch, the nerve branches penetrate the SMAS. As a result they become superficial one-third of the distance posterior to the lateral orbital margin [25].

SENSORY NERVES

The great auricular nerve, the main sensory nerve to the ear, lies just under the superficial fascia overlying the sternomastoid muscle. Its location is constant: 6.5 cm inferior to the inferior border of the external auditory canal in the midmuscle belly [17].

SELECTION OF OPTIMAL TECHNIQUE

Temple

If ptosis of the lateral brow is present, the direction of the pull should be adjusted accordingly. Some patients should have a coronal forehead- and brow-lift [8].

Cheeks and Nasolabial Folds

When deep nasolabial folds are present, the underlying SMAS should be elevated and repositioned to afford the most improvement in them. Although patients often say that they "don't want the mask look," it is virtually impossible to create. As a matter of fact, since improvement in these folds is often slight, some surgeons have advocated their direct excision; to me, the resulting scar may be too high a price to pay.

Collagen injections may help by plumping out the folds.

Jowls

Jowl formation may be due to laxity of the skin, which is quite easily treated by the skin flap repositioning. Or it is due to fat accumulation, in which case a local lipectomy may be beneficial. However, when jowl fat is excised, care should be taken to avoid damage to the external facial vessels.

Neck

Vertical folds are due to skin excess, which is managed by rotating and repositioning of the skin flaps. On the other hand, the vertical cords are due to bands of the platysma muscle, which must be divided. Differentiation between skin excess (folds) and muscle bands (cords) should be made preoperatively. (Cords are accentuated when the patient contracts his anterior neck, lower jaw, and lip.)

Submandibular and submental fat accumulations must be excised.

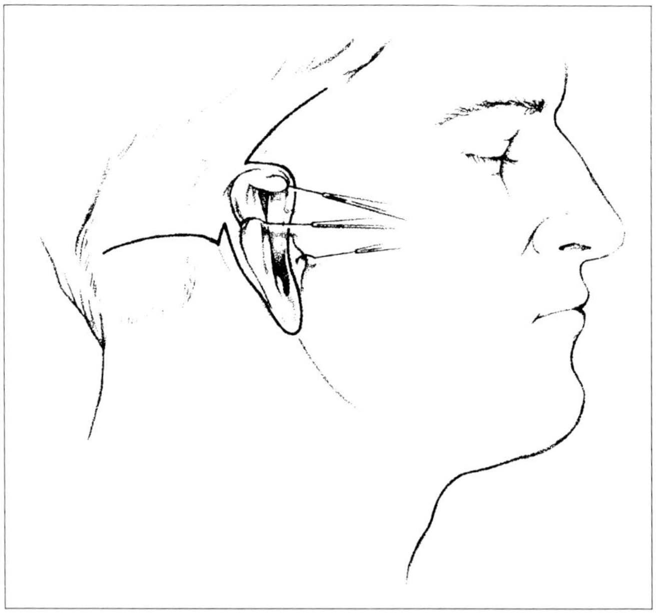

Figure 18-2. Author's face- and neck-lift incision. Same used in males and females. In both, the preauricular segment passes *behind* the tragus. Note "dart" as incision passes from ear to scalp.

OPERATIVE TECHNIQUE

Premedication and Preparation

If desired, the patient may be given a sleeping medication the night before surgery. All other medications may be given intravenously in the operating room. No hair is shaved; rather, it is parted and held in place with surgical lubricant, aluminum foil, and hair clips. A blood pressure cuff and cardiac monitor are applied, and then an intravenous line is started.

Marking

The proposed incisions are marked with marking dye. The following (Fig. 18-2) is my usual incision; alternative incisions have been discussed (see Applied Anatomy). As in females, the proposed incision starts in the temple and runs diagonally, posteriorly and inferiorly, toward the top center of the ear. It continues parallel to the helix and then curves *behind* the tragus, whence it courses into the junction of the cheek and earlobe. After passing just under the earlobe, the incision extends behind the ear going superiorly in the sulcus between the ear and mastoid skin as high as the level of the upper border of the tragus. (In women, in whom the transposition of hair-bearing skin is not a consideration, the incision is brought onto the posterior surface of the ear.) A superiorly based dart (8–10 mm) is placed in the retroauricular sulcus. (This breaks the scar and minimizes subsequent web formation where the scar courses posteriorly from the ear onto the mastoid area.) From the dart, the incision is carried *into* the hair in a gentle posterior and downward curve.

After the center of the chin is marked (to ensure symmetry), the central 2 cm of the submental crease is drawn.

Anesthesia

The operation can be performed under general anesthesia, in which case the anesthesiologist is responsible for the agents used, or local anesthesia with continuous monitoring and intravenous sedation may be employed. Both approaches have their advocates, whose fervor and convictions are based more on emotion than on fact.

Sedation

If local anesthesia with continuous monitoring and intravenous sedation (which I prefer) is used, the patient is given intravenous diazepam (Valium), the dose being determined by what is required to make the patient drowsy. Occasionally 10 mg is required, but the usual dose is 20 mg. Besides its sedative effects, diazepam is proper treatment of the reactions that may follow an overdose of local anesthetic. It also provides 15 to 20 minutes of amnesia (of pain), which is of great value. Then 2 ml (0.1 mg) of fentanyl (Sublimaze) is given, and after a delay of a minute or so the anesthetic is injected. If the patient responds to the pain of the injection and if the systolic blood pressure is less than 150 mm Hg, ketamine (Ketalar, Ketaject), 1 mg *per kilogram,* is injected. Usually both ketamine and fentanyl are used. In all cases, the surgeon should be familiar with the side effects of the agents used (diazepam—muscle relaxation; fentanyl—respiratory depression; ketamine—tachycardia, hypertension).

Local Anesthetic Agents

Lidocaine 0.5% (Xylocaine) works quite satisfactorily, but I prefer 0.25% bupivacaine (Marcaine) because of its longer action. Regardless of the anesthetic agent, *fresh* epinephrine (0.25 ml of 1 : 1000 epinephrine) and 300 NF hyaluronidase (Wydase, Alidase) are added to each 50 ml of anesthetic, producing a solution with 1:200,000 epinephrine and 300 NF hyaluronidase per 50 ml. The total volume of anesthetic injected should not exceed 100 ml. The epinephrine provides hemostasis; the hyaluronidase hastens the anesthetic and vasoconstriction effects.

The interval after injection is utilized for handscrubbing, preparing the patient, and applying the drapes. It also allows the injected agents sufficient time to work.

Incision and Dissection of Skin Flaps

The initial incision is made in the skin of the submental crease. Then the dissection is carried through the subcutaneous fat to the medial borders of the platysma muscle and as far posteriorly as the level of the thyroid cartilage.

The scalp incisions are made with the knife blade held *parallel* to the direction of the hair follicles. By means of Gorney face-lift scissors and push-to-cut and spread techniques, a flap is elevated in the temple and cheek areas. In the temple the dissection should be at the level of the temporalis fascia; in the cheek it is in the subcutaneous plane. Since little is gained by dissecting closer than 2 cm to the nasolabial fold (and further dissection may damage the terminal branches of the facial nerve), the dissection need not be extended. The subsequent submandibular dissection is simplified greatly if the cheek dissection is extended inferiorly into the neck anterior to the sternomastoid muscle.

As in the temple, the retroauricular segment of the incision is started with the knife blade held parallel to the direction of the hair follicles. Then, also with the Gorney face-lift scissors, the flap is dissected from the underlying mastoid and sternomastoid fascia. This requires care because the skin is thin and adherent to the fascia and the subcutaneous fat is meager. The neck dissection is simplified if an "Army-Navy" retractor is placed in the cheek and external countertraction is applied in the neck simultaneously. As the flap is elevated over the sternomastoid muscle, the location of the great auricular nerve (see Applied Anatomy) should be kept in mind. The neck dissection continues anteriorly until it connects with that in the submental region, and it extends 7 to 8 cm inferior to the mandibular border (Fig. 18-3). After preliminary hemostasis, a moistened sponge is placed in the wound. Then the other side is done.

Figure 18-3. Area of undermining shaded.

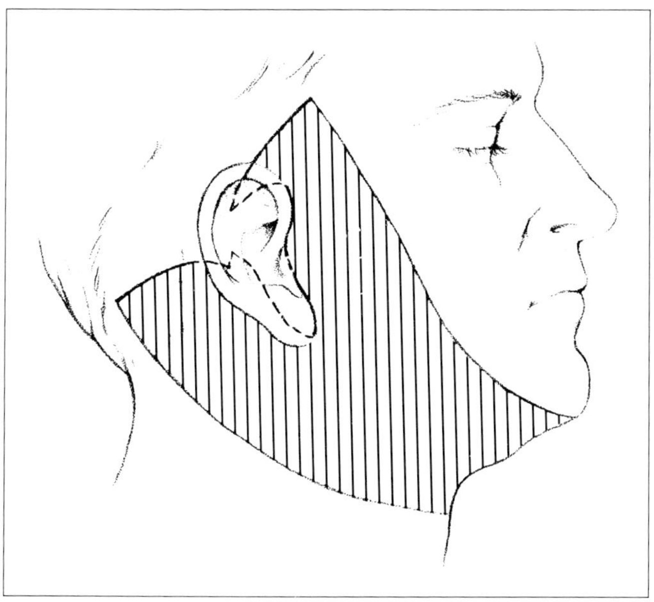

Hemostasis

Since hematoma formation is the most common complication of the procedure, "absolute" hemostasis is important. This admonition applies particularly to males, who are more likely to bleed than females. Monopolar electrocautery is sufficient for most vessels, but when one is near nerves, bipolar coagulation is preferred. Should coagulation of a vessel cause contraction of facial muscles, hemostasis must be achieved chemically; topical epinephrine, microfibrillar collagen hemostat (Avitene), or thrombin solution may be used.

Elevation of Superficial Musculoaponeurotic System

At the lower border of the zygomatic arch and 0.5 to 1.0 cm anterior to the ear, a scissor pierces the SMAS, which is then incised and elevated horizontally for 3 cm. Then another incision is made vertically through the SMAS 0.5 to 1.0 cm anterior to the ear. The SMAS is elevated inferiorly until it reaches the anterior border of the sternomastoid muscle (Fig. 18-4).

Figure 18-4. SMAS-platysma flap held in forceps, being elevated off parotid gland, which is "phantomed" beneath. Parotid "protects" underlying facial nerve, whose peripheral branches have been dotted.

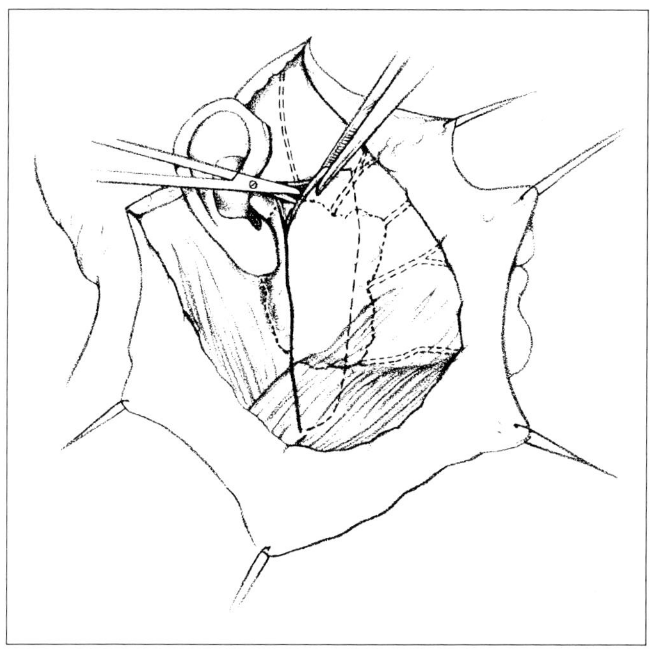

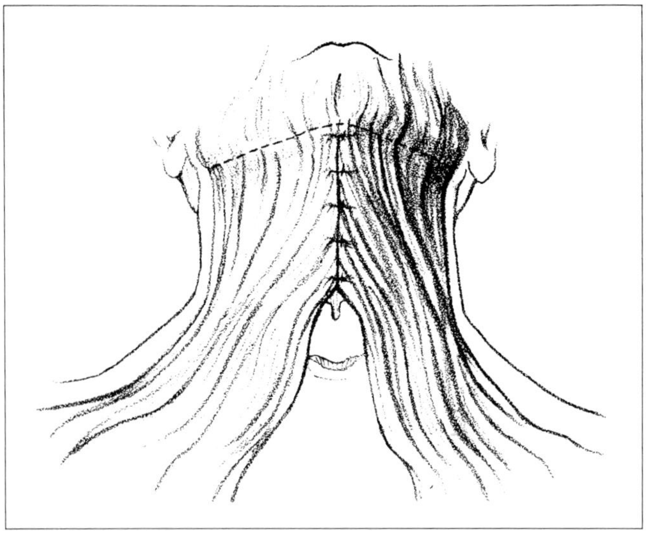

Figure 18-5. Medial borders of platysma sutured (regardless of whether decussation is present).

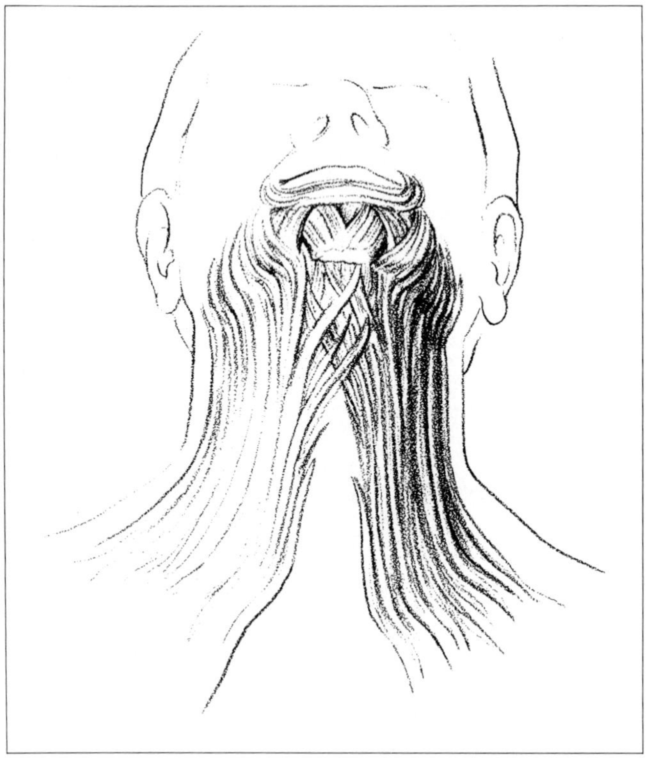

Figure 18-6. Decussation of anterior borders of platysma muscle.

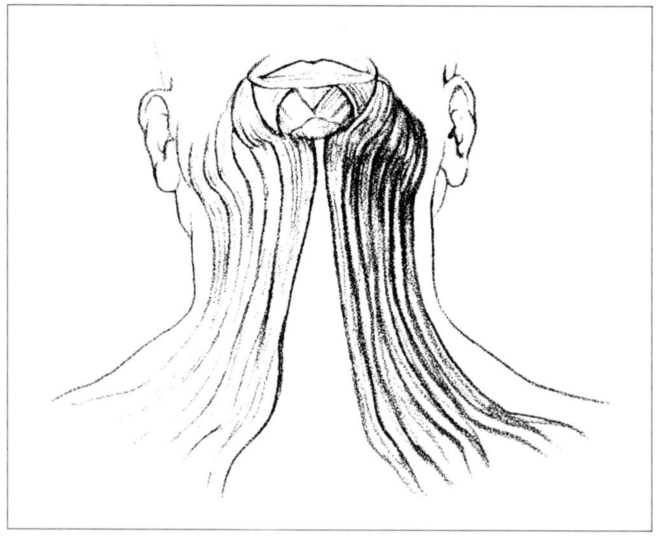

Figure 18-7. Failure of decussation of anterior borders of platysma muscle.

At this level, the SMAS of the cheek becomes *continuous* with the platysma muscle in the neck. If the dissection under the platysma is done *bluntly,* damage to the facial nerve is minimized. As a result of the dissection, the SMAS and platysma are elevated as a sheet from the underlying parotid gland (in the cheek) and deep tissues (in the neck).

Suture and Trimming of the SMAS

Through the submental incision, the medial borders of the platysma muscle are approximated (Fig. 18-5). Because medial stability is essential to obtaining a tight submandibular "sling," medial approximation of the platysma is done whether (Fig. 18-6) (or not, Fig. 18-7) "decussation" [29] of the medial fibers of the platysma is present.

Then, through the cheek flap, the SMAS is pulled up and back as a rotation-advancement flap. The result is a triangle of redundant SMAS [22], which is excised. Next, the SMAS is sutured to itself at the level of the zygomatic arch with 3-0 Vicryl.

The platysma is now pulled up and back. After the excess muscle is trimmed (Fig. 18-8), the platysma is sutured to the mastoid fascia. Finally, sutures are used to close the preauricular part of the SMAS-platysma rotation flap (Fig. 18-9). If the SMAS is sutured first in the zygomatic area, then in the neck, and last in the preauricular area, the neck is not distorted.

Proper management of the SMAS is the key to obtaining the optimal result from a face- and neck-lift.

Lipectomy

After the SMAS has been trimmed and sutured, a lipectomy is performed as required (Fig. 18-10). If the lipectomy is performed *before* stabilization of the SMAS, the lipectomy is more difficult, and denuded platysma may be elevated onto the cheek.

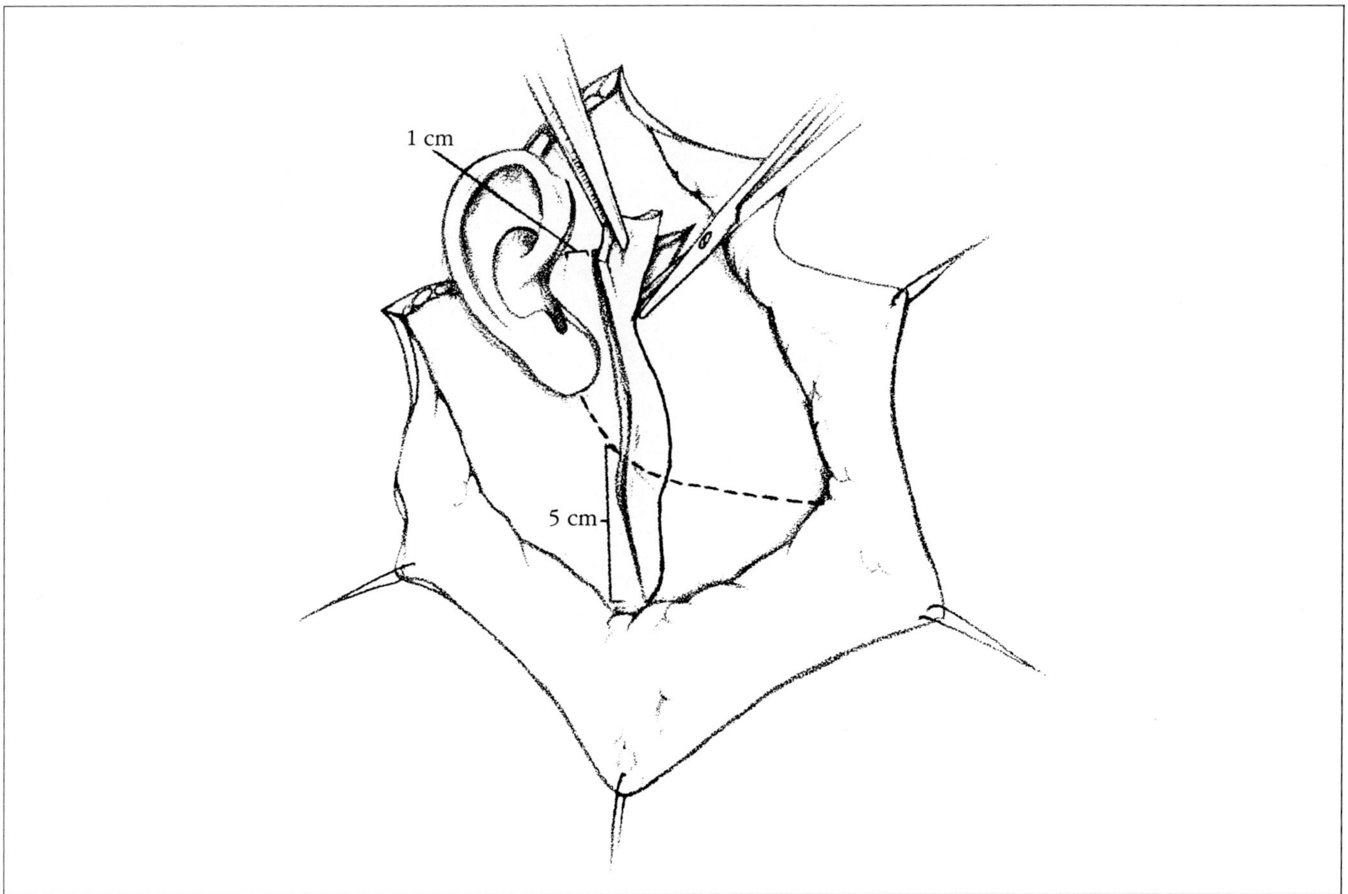

Figure 18-8. SMAS and platysma pulled up and back. Trim of excess started.

Both the submental and face-neck incisions are used to visualize the underlying fat, which is contoured under direct vision. Once one is certain that sufficient fat remains on the skin flap, all fat superficial to the platysma is removed. This maneuver is done across the neck and as far inferiorly as the thyroid cartilage. Superiorly, at the level of the mandibular border, the fat should be beveled.

If the patient has fat accumulation in the jowl area, it may be excised; however, excision of fat above the mandibular border may cause bleeding. In addition, the surgeon should always be aware of the plane of dissection and the plane of the facial nerve branches. Because of these potential problems (bleeding and nerve damage), fat should be excised above the mandibular border only in patients in whom the fat accumulations mar the result.

Skin Excision and Closure

Conceptually, the skin flap is a posterior advancement flap, but with the ear in the way. If two (one anterior and the other posterior) *temporary* mattress sutures are placed, the scalp slides down and the cheek and neck tissue is pulled up. Then the closure tension can be adjusted. *Excessive tension is the enemy of success.* It causes alopecia, poor wound healing, and thickened scars.

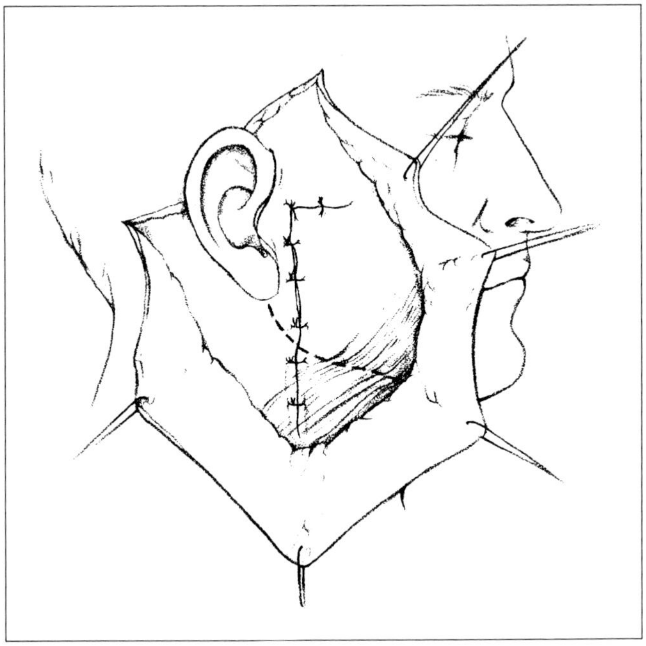

Figure 18-9. SMAS-platysma flap sutured.

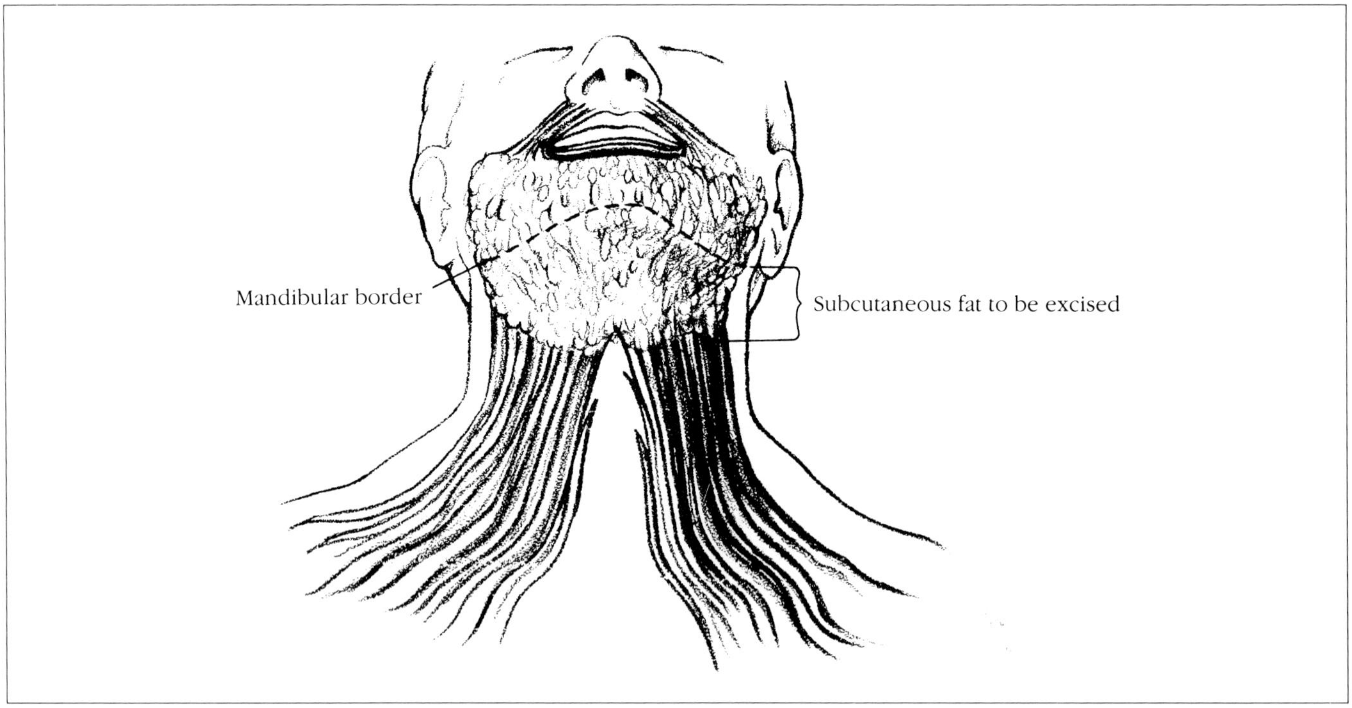

Figure 18-10. Submental and submandibular lipectomy as required.

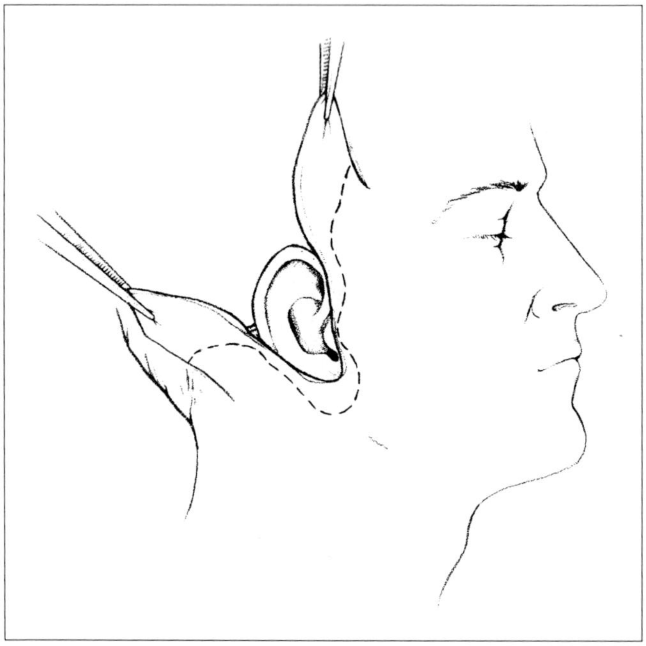

Figure 18-11. Excess skin pulled up and back, then excised.

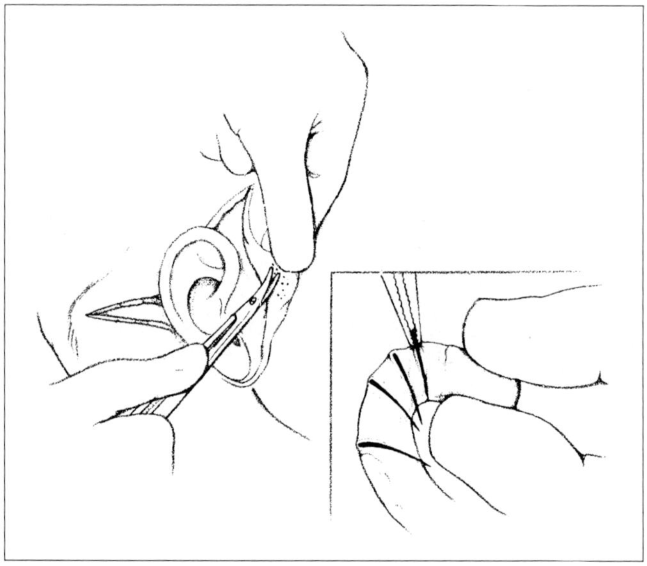

Figure 18-12. Hair follicles excised, then hair shafts plucked (inset).

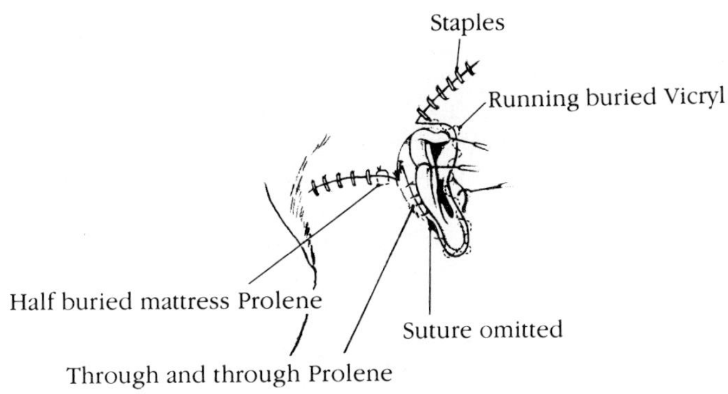

Figure 18-13. Final closure.

After the temporary mattress sutures are placed, the excess tissue is marked. One must be sure that no tension is present on the ear. Then the excess skin is excised (Fig. 18-11).

In *males,* the hairless areas in front, below, and behind the ear are recreated by removing fat, subcutaneous tissue, and hair follicles with scissors and cautery (Fig. 18-12). If a few hairs grow later, epilation by hyfrecation may be employed.

Staples are used to close the temple and mastoid scalp wounds. Then the temporary mattress sutures can be removed.

The final closure (Fig. 18-13) is performed with a running, buried 4-0 Vicryl suture approximating the dermis. Half-buried vertical mattress (Prolene) sutures close the hairless mastoid skin. Through-and-through Prolene sutures are used on the posterior dart and adjacent retroauricular skin.

Drains

Some surgeons use drains. Instead, if two sutures behind the ear and above the earlobe are omitted, any fluid (blood, serum, or liquefied fat) that collects may be evacuated with either a curved mosquito forceps or a Gorney nasal suction dissector. *Neither drains nor dressings prevent hematomas.*

Dressings

Cotton soaked in mineral oil is placed around the ears and under the chin. Then a Kerlix dressing is wrapped around the head and taped in three directions. The purpose of the dressing is to keep the patient's eyes and fingers away from the wounds and to absorb any blood that may ooze from the suture lines.

POSTOPERATIVE MANAGEMENT

Every effort should be made to prevent hematoma formation, which may be caused by an increase in venous pressure (Valsalva maneuver) or arterial hypertension. Venous pressure is lessened if the head of the bed is elevated; besides, a patient breathes easier with the head up. Straining, anxiety, pain, and nausea should be minimized by medication. Hypertension is controlled intraoperatively and postoperatively by chlorpromazine (Thorazine), 2.5 mg given intravenously [7, 9].

If the surgery has been done on an outpatient basis, when alert and stable the patient may be driven home by a "responsible adult," who should remain with the patient that evening. Responsible adults can be better observers than trained nurses, who have never cared for aesthetic surgical patients, have psychologic hangups of their own about "vain" patients, and are often more interested in bowel and bladder function than in the patient's face.

The afternoon of surgery and the next morning either the surgeon or a staff member should telephone to make sure all is well. Besides comforting the patient, the surgeon can be reassured that a hematoma is not forming. If the following questions are specifically asked, and answered in the negative, it is unlikely that a significant hematoma is present: "Are the cheeks hard?" "Is one cheek more swollen than the other?" "Are the lips black and blue?"

Unless otherwise indicated, the patient should return to the office in 2 days, at which time the dressings should be removed (permanently) and any collection of fluid or blood evacuated. At that time the patient may be allowed to wash his hair with 3% hydrogen peroxide, followed by ordinary shampoo.

The staples are removed from the scalp wounds 10 to 14 days after surgery.

COMPLICATIONS: THEIR PREVENTION AND TREATMENT

Distinguishing normal sequelae (postoperative depression, edema, ecchymosis, erythema in scars, hypesthesia of earlobes and cheeks) from complications (hematoma, hair loss, skin slough, nerve deficit, contour deformities) is important. Both should be managed suitably: the former by reassurance, the latter as appropriate.

Hematoma

Hematoma formation is the most common complication of the surgical treatment of the aging face. When large, a hematoma is obvious; when small, it may be missed. Although there is no absolute method of prevention, blood pressure control is essential: Strong evidence [7] indicates that bleeding is greater when the systolic blood pressure is higher than 150 mm Hg. Pain and anxiety cause blood pressure elevation. They must be controlled during and after surgery. Since the venous pressure increases with straining, nausea, and vomiting, prevention and treatment are indicated.

If a hematoma develops, it must be evacuated. Otherwise, at best, fibrosis and distortion will result; at worst, the vascularity of the skin may be compromised. Generally, a fresh, large hematoma requires evacuation in the operating room, under general anesthesia [9]. However, one author [24] feels it can be done in the patient's room.

Later small, liquefied hematomas may be aspirated or expressed through the area behind the ear where the sutures were omitted.

Hair Loss

Hair loss is best prevented by avoiding direct damage to the hair follicles and by not compromising the blood supply to the hair or skin by excess tension.

Treatment is expectant. It may require as long as 1 year before the hair regenerates. If regeneration does not take place, the same techniques used to manage male pattern baldness should be employed.

Skin Slough

A skin slough may be due to excessive tension or a hematoma. In addition, if the patient is a smoker, nicotine may be a major factor. Regardless of the cause, treatment is expectant: Skin grafts are rarely required; better scars usually follow when the wound heals without grafts.

Nerve Deficit

With older methods of face-lifting, motor nerve damage occurred in an average of 0.7 percent of patients [3]. However, the more recent extensive operations may be expected to result in a higher incidence of nerve deficits. The cause is usually cautery or scissor damage to the nerves [3]. Differentiation of direct damage to the marginal mandibular branch, which innervates the depressors of the lower lip, from a weakened platysma, which in some patients is part of a full smile, should be made.

If the surgeon believes that a major trunk of the nerve has been cut, microscopic repair should be performed. On the other hand, if the nerve deficit is more likely to be due to cautery or traction, treatment should be expectant and very supportive.

Contour Irregularities

Contour irregularities may result if fat resection is irregular or excessive, producing an adherence of skin to muscle that is worse on animation. Although treatment is difficult, collagen injections usually bring some improvement.

If the platysma muscle is transected completely, the submaxillary gland may become prominent, a condition without satisfactory treatment.

RESULTS

Although the ecchymosis is usually gone by 2 weeks, the edema lasts a minimum of 1 month and often as long as 3 months. At that time most patients who were originally good candidates are pleased (Fig. 18-14).

The early results following the SMAS-platysma face-neck–lift are excellent, and they persist longer than those following traditional methods. As a matter of fact, I have been performing the described procedure for 5 years and have yet to feel that a secondary procedure was indicated. Of course, the aging process does not stop, but, in contrast to the result with older methods, the face does not seem to "fall so fast."

Male patients rarely obtain as clean a neck-jawline as women. However, men are rarely looking for that outcome.

SECONDARY SURGERY

Secondary procedures may be indicated when the first procedure fails to achieve the desired result or when the patient wishes more improvement. The most common secondary procedure is excision of more submental fat.

In complete secondary face-lifts, scarring from the original procedure decreases the amount of skin that can, or should, be removed. If the SMAS-platysma procedure was done at the first operation, the distorted anatomy should be considered in planning secondary operations.

ANCILLARY PROCEDURES

The *eyebrow* positions should be evaluated preoperatively. Perhaps they should be lifted by a forehead-lift, a temple-lift, or even a suprabrow excision.

Although "bags" of the *eyelids* are due more to hereditary than to aging factors, often a bilateral upper and lower

Figure 18-14. A 56-year-old male before and 1 year after face- and neck-lift and rhinoplasty.
A, C. Preoperative views.
B, D. Postoperative views.

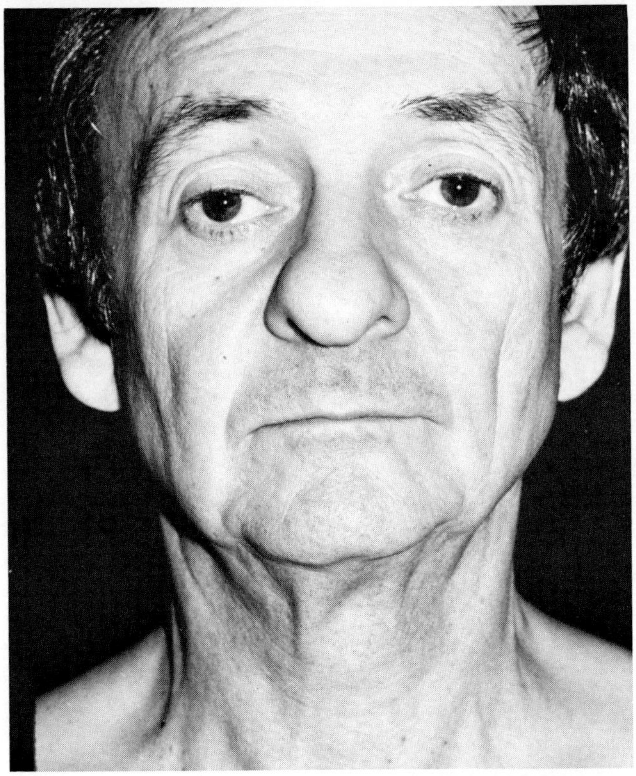

A

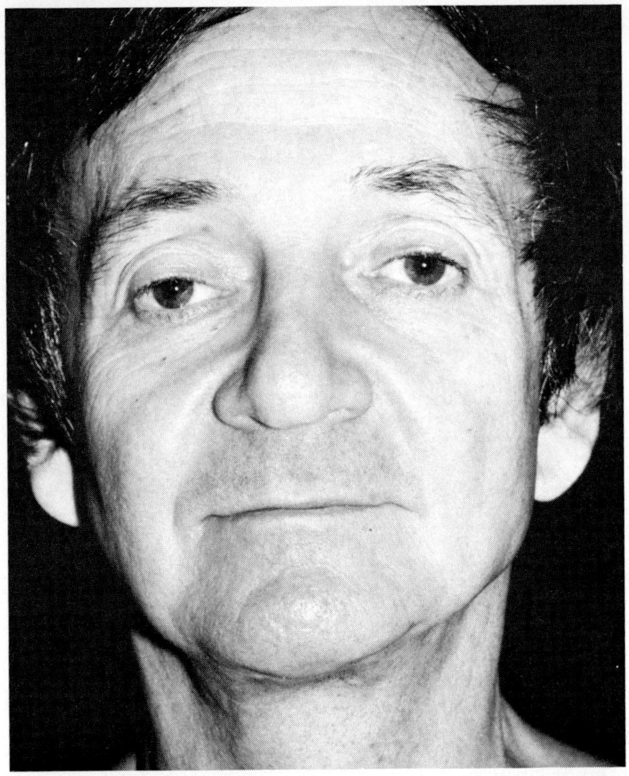

B

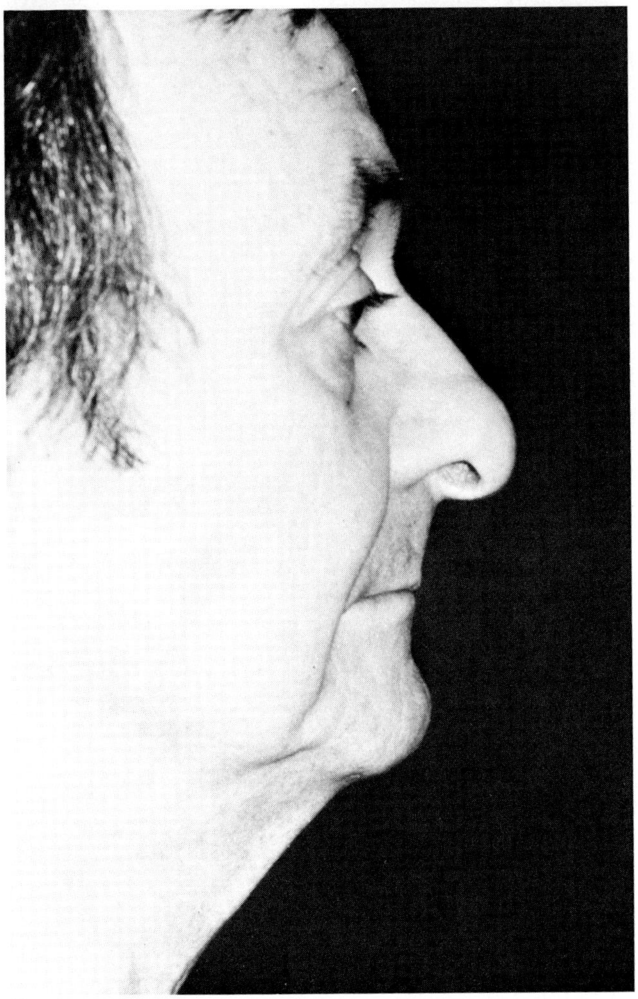

C

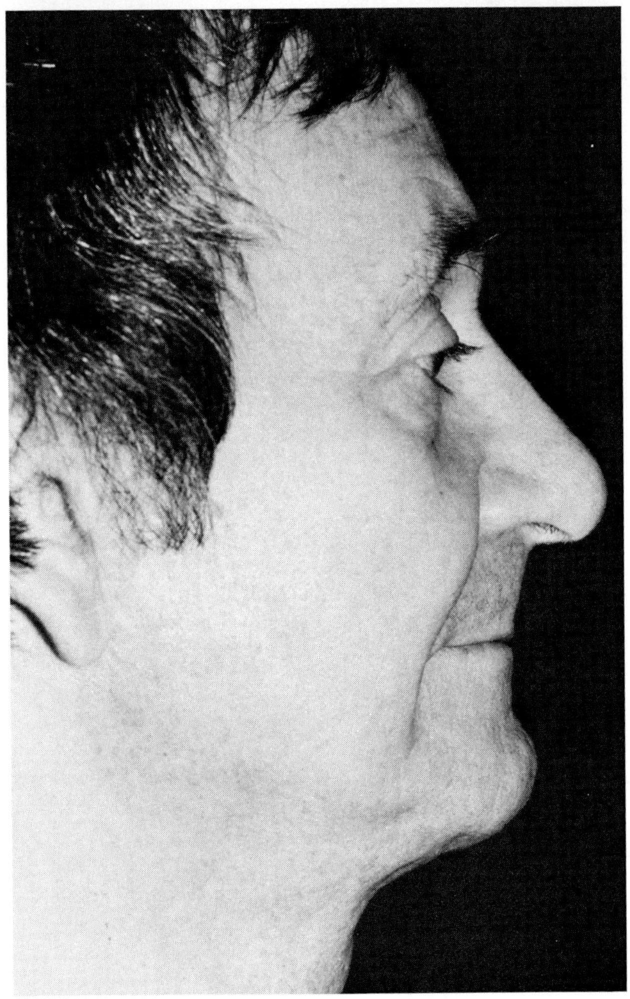

D

blepharoplasty affords the patient a fresher, more rested appearance.

Patients whose appearance is marred by a small *chin* should be offered the benefits of a chin implant, which can be inserted through the submental incision.

Occasionally a drooped *nasal* tip or dorsal hump will bother the patient. It may benefit from simultaneous treatment.

Ancillary procedures should be considered according to the *patient's* desires; they should not be "sold" by the surgeon. When they are done simultaneously, discretion should be used. Performing "all of the above" at one operative session is rarely indicated. *As the number of procedures simultaneously performed increases arithmetically, the complication rate increases geometrically.*

FINAL COMMENT

Males who undergo surgical treatment of the aging face tend to be more satisfied than their female counterparts. Perhaps males are better motivated than females. Perhaps males wish specific corrections. Or perhaps men rarely look to recapture their youth.

REFERENCES

1. Aston, S. J. Cervicofacial Rhytidoplasty. In E. H. Courtiss (ed.), *Male Aesthetic Surgery*. St. Louis: Mosby, 1982.
2. Baker, D. C., et al. The male rhytidectomy. *Plast. Reconstr. Surg.* 60:514, 1977.
3. Baker, D. C., and Conley, J. Avoiding facial nerve injuries in rhytidectomy: Anatomical variations and pitfalls. *Plast. Reconstr. Surg.* 64:781, 1979.
4. Baker, T. J. Rhytidectomy in the Male Patient. In D. Goulian and E. H. Courtiss (eds.), *Symposium on Surgery of the Aging Face*. St. Louis: Mosby, 1978.
5. Baker, T. J. Chemical Peel. In E. H. Courtiss (ed.), *Male Aesthetic Surgery*. St. Louis: Mosby, 1982.
6. Baker, T. J., and Gordon, H. L. Rhytidectomy in males. *Plast. Reconstr. Surg.* 44:219, 1969.
7. Berner, R. E., Morain, W. D., and Noe, J. M. Postoperative hypertension as an etiological factor in hematoma after rhytidectomy. *Plast. Reconstr. Surg.* 57:314, 1976.
8. Connell, B. F. Eyebrow and Forehead Lifts. In E. H. Courtiss (ed.), *Male Aesthetic Surgery*. St. Louis: Mosby, 1982.
9. Courtiss, E. H. Discussion of I. Pitanguy and M. P. Ceravolo, Hematoma postrhytidectomy: How we treat it. *Plast. Reconstr. Surg.* 67:529, 1981.
10. *Dorland's Illustrated Medical Dictionary* (26th ed.). Philadelphia: Saunders, 1981.
11. Fredricks, S. Rhytidectomy. In E. H. Courtiss (ed.), *Aesthetic Surgery. Trouble: How to Avoid It and How to Treat It.* St. Louis: Mosby, 1978.
12. Goin, J. M., and Goin, M. K. *Changing the Body. The Psychologic Effects of Plastic Surgery.* Baltimore: Williams & Wilkins, 1981.
13. Gorney, M. Patient Selection. In E. H. Courtiss (ed.), *Male Aesthetic Surgery*. St. Louis: Mosby, 1982.
14. Gorney, M., and Harris, T. The preoperative and postoperative considerations of facial asymmetry. *Plast. Reconstr. Surg.* 54:187, 1974.
15. Gurdin, M. M., and Carlin, G. A. Aging Defects in the Male: A Regional Approach to Treatment. In F. W. Masters and J. R. Lewis, Jr. (eds.), *Symposium on Aesthetic Surgery of the Face, Eyelid, and Breast.* St. Louis: Mosby, 1972.
16. Hamilton, J. M. Rhytidectomy in the male. *Plast. Reconstr. Surg.* 53:629, 1974.
17. McKinney, P., and Katrana, D. J. Prevention of injury to the great auricular nerve during rhytidectomy. *Plast. Reconstr. Surg.* 66:675, 1980.
18. Millard, D. R., Jr., et al. Submental and submandibular lipectomy in conjunction with a face lift, in the male or female. *Plast. Reconstr. Surg.* 49:385, 1972.
19. Mitz, V., and Peyronie, M. The superficial musculoaponeurotic system (SMAS) in the parotid and cheek area. *Plast. Reconstr. Surg.* 58:80, 1976.
20. Mullin, W. R., and Millard, D. R., Jr. Meloplasty with Emphasis on the Neck. In E. H. Courtiss (ed.), *Male Aesthetic Surgery*. St. Louis: Mosby, 1982.
21. Newsom, H. T. A different incision for rhytidectomy in males. *Plast. Reconstr. Surg.* 60:809, 1977.
22. Owsley, J. Q. Platysma—facial rhytidectomy: A preliminary report. *Plast. Reconstr. Surg.* 60:809, 1977.
23. Peterson, R. A. Variations in Rhytidectomy Technique. In D. Goulian and E. H. Courtiss (eds.), *Symposium on Surgery of the Aging Face*. St. Louis: Mosby, 1978.
24. Pitanguy, I., and Ceravolo, M. P. Hematoma postrhytidectomy: How we treat it. *Plast. Reconstr. Surg.* 67:526, 1981.
25. Pitanguy, I., and Ramos, A. S. The frontal branch of the facial nerve: The importance of its variations in face lift anatomy. *Plast. Reconstr. Surg.* 38:352, 1966.
26. Rees, T. D. The SMAS and the Platysma. In T. D. Rees, *Aesthetic Plastic Surgery*. Philadelphia: Saunders, 1980.
27. Sturman, M. J. Sideburn relationship in the male face lift. *Plast. Reconstr. Surg.* 57:248, 1976.
28. Vistnes, L., and Jobe, R. Rhytidectomy with Emphasis on the Differences Between Males and Females. In E. H. Courtiss (ed.), *Male Aesthetic Surgery*. St. Louis: Mosby, 1982.
29. Vistnes, L. M., and Southier, S. G. The pre-anatomical basis for common cosmetic anterior neck deformities. *Ann. Plast. Surg.* 2:381, 1979.

19. Chemical Face Peeling

Thomas J. Baker
Howard L. Gordon

Chemical face peeling is a procedure that has been investigated by the authors since 1958 [3, 4]. It is a process in which chemicals are applied to the skin that produce alterations in gross and microscopic anatomy of the dermis and epidermis. The indications for the procedure include removal of fine wrinkles in facial skin, pigmentation problems, and other minor skin blemishes. Various synonyms have been applied to this process, such as *chemosurgery, chemerasure, dermapeel, skin peeling,* and *chemical exfoliation.* It has been referred to as *chemical face-lifting* [26], but this term is not accurate, since the face is not actually lifted as in a rhytidectomy. Several agents have been advocated for a chemical peeling, including trichloroacetic acid, salicylic acid, and phenol [2, 25]. They are all keratolytic, and most are weak acids. The agent most frequently used is phenol, C_6H_5OH, commonly referred to as carbolic acid although its formula does not contain the carboxyl group that is characteristic of an organic acid. The hydroxyl group indicates that it is nearer to being an organic base or an alcohol.

HISTORICAL BACKGROUND

The Ebers papyrus (a well-known historical document, circa 1560 B.C.) contains considerable information on cosmetic treatment by early Egyptians. This document discusses methods of removing wrinkles and moles, dying hair and eyebrows, correcting squints, and other procedures for beautifying the body. Mixtures of alabaster, natron, salt, extracts of animal oil, and other items were applied to the skin in an attempt to achieve rejuvenation. Early chemosurgery included the use of certain types of acids on the skin. It is known that exfoliation of the skin was effectuated by poultices from mineral and plant substances directly applied. Agents such as sulfur, mustard, and limestone were used. Indian women are known to have mixed urine with pumice and applied it to the skin to improve their appearance, although there is little scientific evidence of value to substantiate this method. Turkish women used fire to singe the skin and lightly exfoliate it. Despite frequent usage of chemicals and other methods since the beginning of recorded history, little specific information is available on early methods of surgical or chemical treatments for the aging skin. However, we may be reasonably certain that the same oils, creams, and abrasives employed for cosmetic purposes were probably prescribed by the medical men of those times.

During the early part of the twentieth century, chemical face peeling was principally carried out by "lay operators," and considerable publicity was given to these individuals through the news media. Such statements as "The fountain of youth has been found" were seen in print and heard on radio and television. Miraculous results were illustrated in magazine articles with spectacular "before" and "after" pictures exhibited in the advertising by lay clinics. Around 1960, many patients began questioning their physicians about this process. The prospective patients were surprised to learn that little knowledge had been documented in the medical literature about the specifics of the procedure. The clinical results obtained by "lay operators" were obviously an indication for scientific investigation and evaluation of the process [5]. Personal conversation with the operators of lay clinics yielded scant information on their formulas. We undertook some basic animal studies utilizing various chemical solutions—specifically phenol, trichloroacetic acid, and salicylic acid. However, since animal skin does not respond exactly the way human skin does, it was necessary to begin using various formulas on human volunteers. An article published by Bames [17] gave some background clinical observations. Our own initial observations were made by treating small areas of human skin, including the inner aspect of the forearm by one of the authors (TJB). At first the chemical formula was applied to areas of hyperkeratoses ("brown" spots of aging). All the basic experiments seemed to indicate that the procedure was effective and safe for use in clinical trials. Our first experience was with the forehead—the ideal experimental site since the skin is thicker there and it was felt that catastrophic results would be unlikely. Having gained success in this area on several patients, we treated larger areas of facial skin. Subsequently, histologic studies were carried out on a series of treated patients, who have been followed for a period of 18 years [14, 15].

Chemical face peeling should be considered an adjunctive treatment [6] of a problem that confronts all of us in our daily practice—the aging process. If medicine does not supply the answer to the problems of aging in a controlled and scientific way, patients will obviously turn to quacks and charlatans for their solutions.

SELECTION OF PATIENTS

The principal benefactors of chemical peel seem to be (1) individuals with fine wrinkling of the skin (Fig. 19-1), (2) patients with abnormal pigmentation problems (Fig. 19-6), (3) patients with superficial acne scarring (Fig. 19-8), and (4) those with skin damage due to radiation. Perhaps the most knowledge that we have gained in the past 20 years, as far as producing an excellent result is concerned, is in the proper selection of patients. This should be done after the usual psychologic and physiologic surveys are completed. The ideal patient has a fair complexion and has not allowed the elements to abuse the skin, especially by chronic sun exposure. The opposite extreme is the person who has spent many years in the sun, constantly abusing the skin and acquiring a leather-like appearance. Because chemical peeling bleaches the

Figure 19-1

A. A 60-year-old prospective patient for face peeling. Note the fine lines radiating in the perioral area and the mosaic lines in the cheek. This patient had a minimum of facial sagging for her age group and is the ideal candidate for chemical face peel.

B. Four months following chemical face peel. The peel has succeeded in smoothing the facial skin. However, a slight droop in the area of the jowls and neck still exists.

C. Eleven years after chemical peel. This photograph demonstrates that the procedure is long lasting and that the peeling process causes changes in the gross appearance of the skin that are permanent.

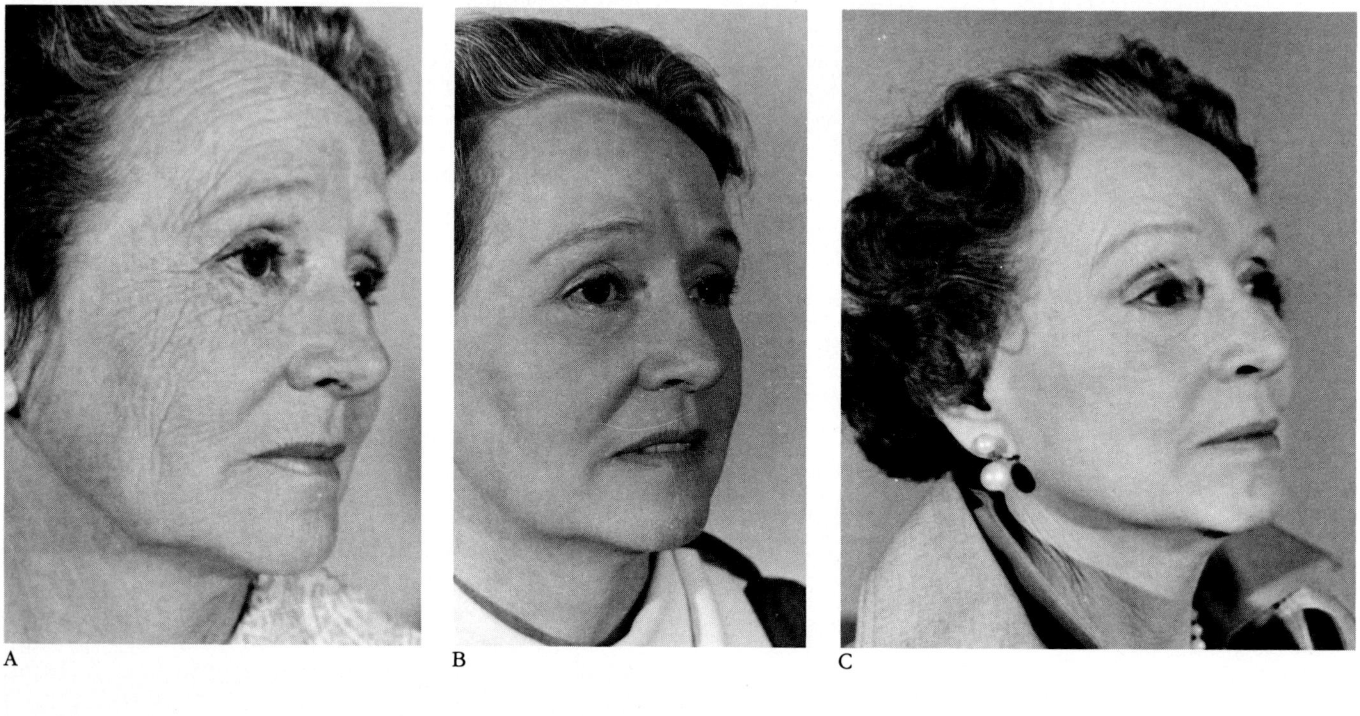

A B C

skin, the darker skin types present problems with color contrasts between treated and untreated areas, especially at the line of demarcation where the treatment terminates. We have had no experience with utilizing chemical agents on the skin of blacks but believe it to be contraindicated. An individual with delicate, thin skin is more likely to have a smooth, natural appearance after face peeling than one with coarsely textured skin that is thick and oily. The latter tends to have less response from the chemical peel and will probably undergo blotchy pigmentation with subsequent exposure to the sun—an undesirable sequela. Patients requesting chemical peel usually have the following complaints:

1. Vertical lines on the upper lip
2. Glabellar frown lines
3. Multiple crow's-feet in the periorbital area
4. Fine mosaic lines in the face
5. Irregular pigmentation of the facial skin

Some patients request treatment for chloasma, ephelides, lentigo, weather-beaten skin, blotchy pigmentation, multiple hyperkeratosis of the face, and, occasionally, superficial acne scarring. Although patients are almost always apprehensive about the prospective treatment, chemical face peeling seems to be more acceptable to the public than the surgical blade of the face-lift. The patient must be counseled prior to the peel in order that all known facts about the procedure be adequately explained. This prior discussion helps greatly in the postpeel phase, and the patient is also more likely to be satisfied with the outcome.

The application of the phenol mixture is relatively simple. However, it is followed by several days of restrictions, discomfort, and inconvenience. For example, the patient is not permitted to eat solid foods or talk for 48 hours, because these activities jeopardize the end results by causing the mask to become separated from the underlying skin. This fact and other aspects of the treatment can create apprehension and lack of cooperation on the part of the patient who lacks a clear understanding of the anticipated events. As in all procedures, patients should be informed of the pros and cons regarding the outcome and of the possible complications. Features that will not be corrected by chemical peel should be carefully stressed. The effects of gravity, which necessitate a rhytidectomy, will not be significantly improved, and it should be made clear that the chemical peel is not a substitute for rhytidectomy [4]. If the patient has sagging skin as well as the fine mosaic lines on the face, and if a rhytidectomy is not done, one only produces smooth skin on a sagging face. Many prospective patients need a rhytidectomy as well as a chemical peel (Fig. 19-2). If the patient has a darker complexion, the line of demarcation between treated and untreated areas must be mentioned and stressed. The patient must also be fully

Figure 19-2
A. A 67-year-old patient who is in need of chemical peel and a rhytidectomy. In this instance, the chemical peel was done first, followed by a rhytidectomy 6 months later.
B. The surgical lift corrected the sagging of the face and neck, while the chemical peel smoothed the fine wrinkling of the skin. This patient was also encouraged to wear a wig and use more care with her makeup.

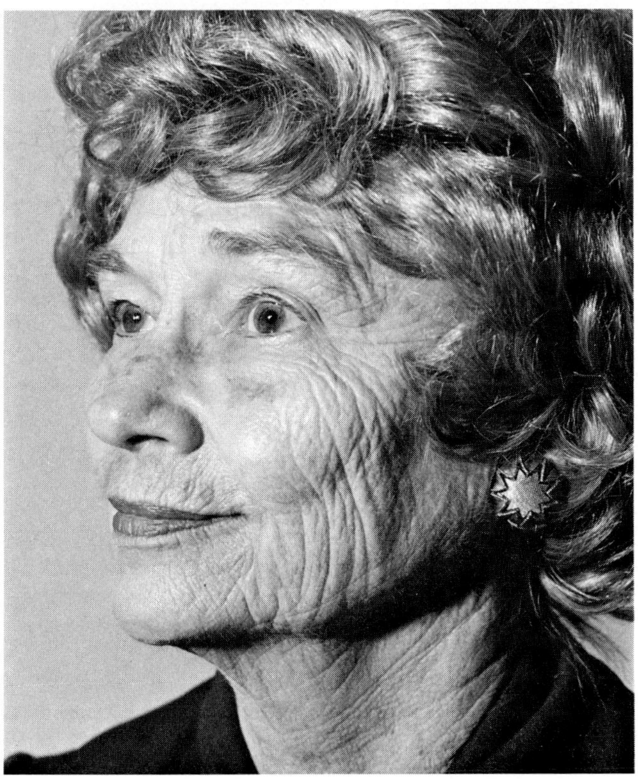

A

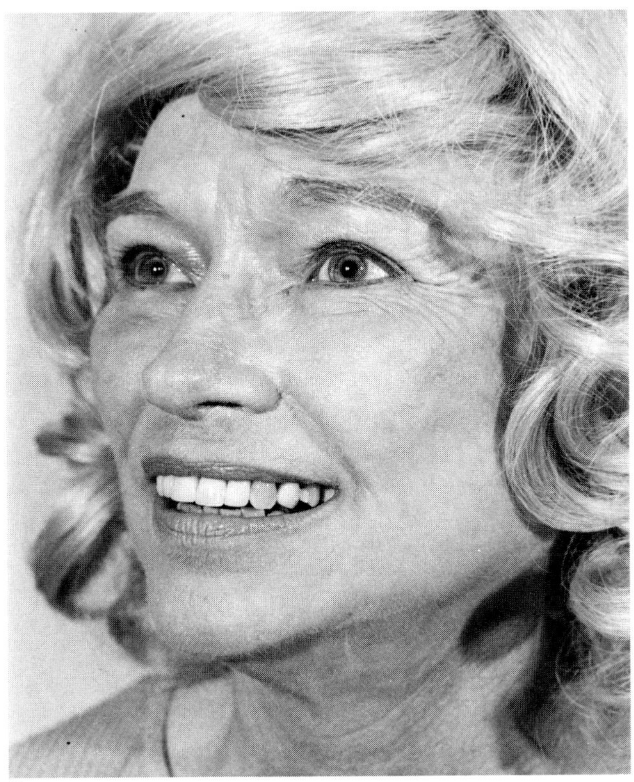

B

aware of the time required for the healing process and must be forewarned about protecting the skin from sun exposure for several months following the treatment. These factors should be fully discussed in order that patients may properly evaluate whether they are willing to make the personal sacrifices to achieve the anticipated end result.

TECHNIQUE

There are many variations described in the literature with regard to the treatment of patients undergoing chemical face peel [1, 2, 19, 25, 34]. However, the technique described here has produced consistently satisfactory results in the hands of the authors and, in our opinion, offers the fewest complications. The procedure should be carried out in a hospital or a clinic properly equipped to handle such patients. During the initial 4 or 5 days of treatment, the management is too complex to warrant treatment on an outpatient basis. It is unnecessary to utilize an operating room, since the treatment can be easily carried out in the patient's own bed. The patient should be completely relaxed and tranquil prior to the application of the chemical mixture, and to enter this state of tranquillity the patient is premedicated approximately 1 hour prior to the treatment, usually with 15 mg of diazepam (Valium) by mouth. A plastic intravenous catheter is placed in an arm vein, and 5% glucose in distilled water is used as an intravenous drip. Subsequent medication is given through this route—usually additional diazepam and sometimes a narcotic if the patient experiences too much of a burning sensation. Supplements of intravenous diazepam and possibly narcotics are usually necessary during the next 6 to 8 hours.

Prior to the application of the mixture, the skin is thoroughly washed with surgical soap followed by a complete cleansing with diethyl ether. The ether is applied on a 4- × 3-in. surgical sponge, and gentle cleansing of the skin removes all superficial oils and debris. Ether is an explosive agent, and other patients in the room must be cautioned not to smoke; adequate protection is necessary so that a spark not be inadvertently created, causing a fire or explosion. Since the ether removes the oils from the skin, effective contact of the phenol mixture and the mask is complete.

FORMULA

The formula is a mixture that is a saponified phenol suspension:

3 ml U.S.P. phenol (C_6H_5OH)
2 ml tap water
8 drops liquid soap (Septisol)
3 drops croton oil (from the seed of *Croton tiglium*)

The mixture is formulated fresh at the time of each treatment in order to be absolutely certain that the ingredients are correct, stable, and fresh. All necessary ingredients for preparation of the formula are kept in individual containers in a small medicine bag along with other necessary materials, such as scissors, tape, gauze, and cotton-tipped applicators. Since the mixture tends to separate, it must be stirred vigorously with the tip of a cotton-tipped applicator immediately before each individual application to the skin.

APPLICATION OF THE MIXTURE

The mixture is applied to the face with ordinary cotton-tipped applicators. It must be spread evenly and uniformly over the entire area and into each wrinkle (Fig. 19-3A). As a matter of habit, the forehead is generally done first. When the mixture comes into contact with the skin, the skin turns pearly white and the patient experiences a mild burning sensation. This sensation subsides within 10 to 15 seconds because of the local anesthetic quality of the phenol. The mixture is carried well into the hairline to minimize the line of demarcation that could exist in that area. Hair follicles are not affected by the peeling process. The applicator is semimoist, rather than saturated with the mixture, to prevent dripping of the mixture into areas of the body where it would not be desirable. The applicator can be lightly rolled on a piece of dry gauze, which absorbs the excess of the mixture, when it is being utilized around the eyelids so that none of the liquid will inadvertently come into contact with the cornea. Application of the mixture around the eyelids must always be done with a semimoist applicator. The mixture is carried to within 2 mm of the ciliary margin of the lower lid. The upper lid is held open until the lower lid has been treated, blotted, and allowed to air dry. Using this meticulous method, we have had no incidents of damage to the surface of the eye. Initially, ointments were applied to protect the surface of the eye; however, it was found that the patients would squint and cause the ointment to spill over onto the skin, thereby making the phenol mixture ineffective and adherence of the tape impossible. It is a good cautionary measure to keep an irrigating syringe full of water close at hand in case some of the mixture inadvertently comes into contact with the surface of the eye. We have never had to use it, but it does add insurance. The upper eyelids are treated to and including the tarsal plate, but not to the margin of the eyelid, so as to prevent unnecessary edema of the upper eyelid. The mixture should be carried into the eyebrows, but no tape is applied over the eyebrows, since a temporary loss of hair results when the tape is later removed. Because most earlobes are wrinkled, they are usually treated at the same time as the face peeling.

The mixture is applied over the entire face down to a line 1 or 2 in. below the inferior margin of the mandible (Fig. 19-3B). If a natural skin crease is present in the upper area of the neck, this is a logical line to terminate the peeling process. If there is no obvious crease in the upper

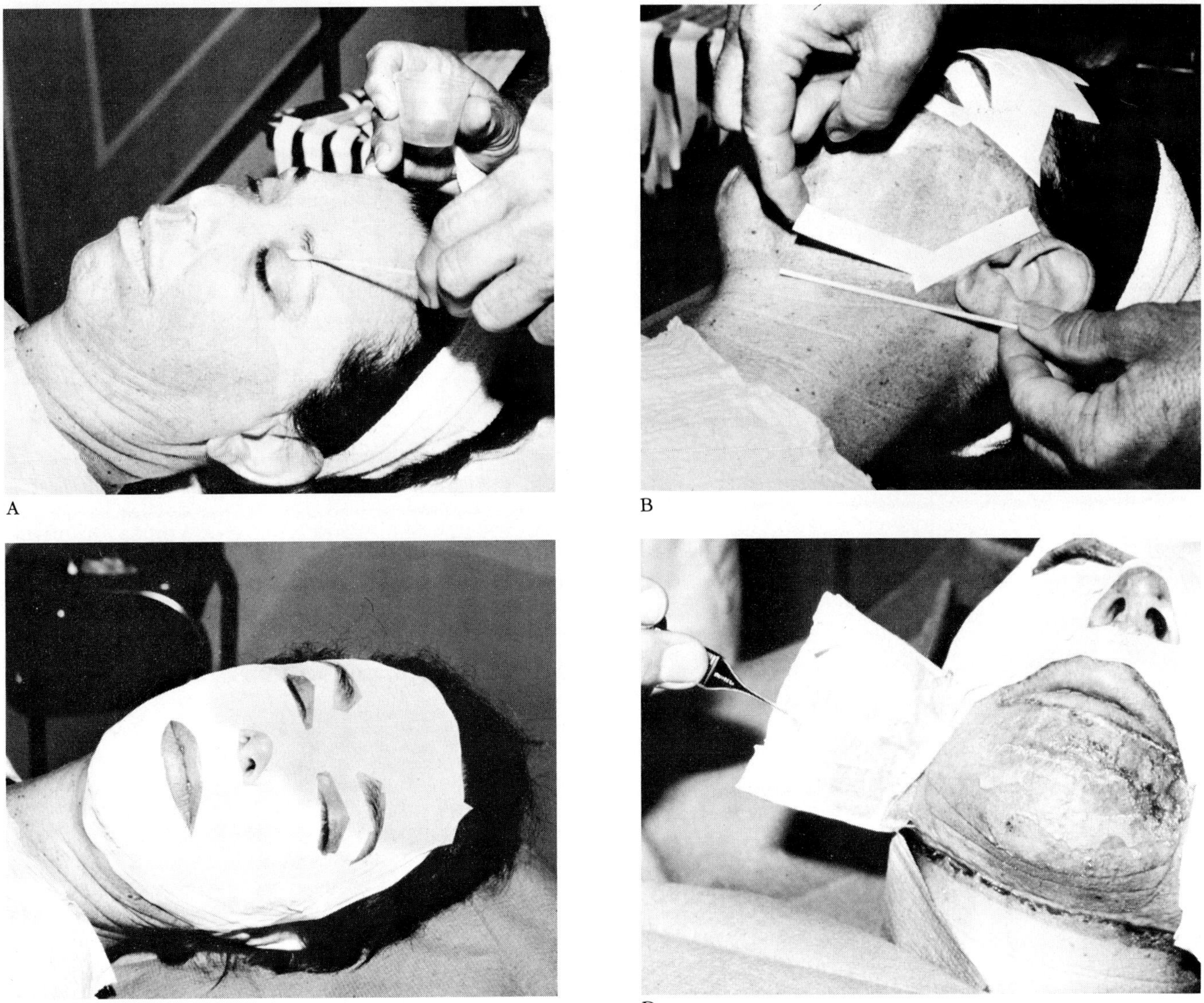

Figure 19-3

A. The mixture is applied evenly with a cotton-tipped applicator. Here the mixture is being carried down to, but not over, the tarsal plate. Extreme caution must be taken to prevent the mixture from coming into contact with the surface of the eye.

B. The mixture has been carried down to a level just below the mandibular border. The tape is not brought as far down as the mixture has been applied. Thus, there is a transition zone, allowing a small margin beyond the mask to be treated, but not occluded with the adhesive tape.

C. The mask has now been completed. Note that the eyebrows are not covered and that the nose and mouth are left exposed. This mask will remain in place for approximately 48 hours.

D. Removal of the mask is carried out in about 48 hours. The surface is weeping, and punctate hemorrhages may be seen. The epithelium can be seen adhering to the undersurface of the mask, and most of the epithelium is removed along with the mask.

portion of the neck, the mixture extends onto the neck only far enough to camouflage the treated area as well as possible. Around the mouth, care is taken to apply the mixture at least to the vermilion border, but preferably slightly onto it. Thus, the vertical wrinkles of the upper lip can be entirely eradicated, especially the smaller ones that radiate from the vermilion border (most patients are women, and they complain that their lipstick migrates into these creases, giving an objectionable appearance).

The timing of the application of the mixture should be over a period of approximately 2 hours, allowing a longer time for the absorption of the phenol through the skin and thereby reducing the chances of systemic toxicity. Our usual procedure is to do the forehead first, then apply the tape to this area. After an interval of 30 to 45 minutes the right cheek application is carried out, followed by another 30- to 40-minute period, when the remainder of the mixture is applied and the mask completed (Fig. 19-3C). The entire procedure occupies approximately 2 hours, and in scheduling the technique in this manner we have had no problems with systemic toxicity whatsoever.

APPLICATION OF THE WATERPROOF MASK

After each segment of the face has been completely covered with the chemical mixture, a mask of Johnson & Johnson waterproof adhesive tape is applied directly to the skin. The eyes, eyebrows, nostrils, and mouth are left exposed. The initial layer is made up of short pieces of ½-in. tape, carefully overlapped so that good adhesive contact is made with the entire surface. For the difficult areas, such as the lower eyelids, nostril rims, and upper lips, small lengths of ¼-in. strips are used for better adhesion. After the initial layer has been applied, it is overlaid with 1-in. tape to ensure total coverage. The palm of the hand is utilized for gentle pressure so that absolute and complete contact is made between the tape and the skin. After the entire face has been taped, all areas are rechecked to be sure that adequate adherence of the tape has been achieved to all areas of treated skin.

During the initial 6 to 8 hours after the application of the mask, the face becomes edematous, and the eyelids may be swollen shut, making it difficult for the patient to see. Also, during this time the patient will experience discomfort from the burning sensation, and it is usually necessary to administer narcotics. Once this 6- to 8-hour period has passed, the patient no longer has the burning sensation, and discomfort can be controlled with mild sedatives or tranquilizers.

The mask is left in position for 48 hours, during which time the patient is instructed to keep the face as immobile as possible and not to talk. Liquids are administered through a straw in sufficient quantity to maintain adequate hydration and nutrition. It is best to keep the patient's head elevated approximately 20 degrees. Bed rest is mandatory. Bathroom privileges are allowed, but the nursing service must be instructed that the patient should be assisted going to the bathroom, since edema of the eyelids may cause a temporary problem with the vision. There is little change in the edema during the second 24 hours. However, the skin begins to weep beneath the mask, and the patient experiences a sensation of having fluid running under the mask and should be warned to expect this.

REMOVAL OF THE MASK

After the mask has been in position for 48 hours, the patient is given additional tranquilizers by mouth. In some individuals a narcotic is necessary since the removal of the mask can be painful. On one occasion we had to give the patient a brief general anesthetic in the operating room in order to remove the mask. The removal is quite simple and is usually initiated by grasping the edge of the mask with forceps and gently pushing away the underlying skin with a sterile cotton-tipped applicator. Beneath the mask is an edematous, weeping surface resembling a second-degree burn. The mask is carefully and slowly teased away from the face and discarded. One can see the epithelium adherent to the undersurface of the mask, and the epithelium that does not stick to the mask can be seen lying gently on the face (Fig. 19-3D). It is not necessary to remove the remainder of the epidermis; it has already been exfoliated and will spontaneously separate in a short time.

APPLICATION OF THYMOL IODIDE POWDER

Once the mask has been completely removed, the treated area is coated with thymol iodide U.S.P. powder. This coating can be done in a number of ways, but our preference is to use a cotton-tipped applicator and carefully roll the powder onto the weeping surface. The powder adheres quickly and forms a golden brown crust. Reapplication of the powder is carried out 2 or 3 times during the day until a heavy crust is formed. Thymol iodide is a bacteriostatic agent.

SEPARATION OF THE CRUST FROM THE FACE

The following day—that is, 24 hours following the application of the thymol iodide powder (and 72 hours from the beginning of the treatment)—a softening ointment is applied to the crust, which hastens the spontaneous separation from the face. This ointment is used daily as necessary until the crust is separated. A and D ointment has proved to be quite satisfactory, but topical antibiotic agents can be used also. It has been our experience that the antibacterial agents cause a high degree of skin sensitivity and the treating physician should be alerted to this factor and change the ointment if a problem occurs. On the fourth or fifth day following the initiation of the treatment, cool tap-water soaks are utilized on the face. Gently putting the face into a cool shower or irrigating nozzle helps to wash away the debris and make the patient more comfortable. Most of the crust will have separated by the sixth or seventh day, and the face then appears to be quite red and edematous.

EARLY POSTTREATMENT CARE

Approximately 1 week after the treatment has begun, it is necessary only to wash the face once or twice a day and keep an emollient on the skin in order to keep the face comfortable. Refrigerated hydrogenated vegetable oil, such as Crisco, is well known to most patients, is readily acceptable, and works well. Itching can be a problem during the early phase of treatment and is more prevalent during the night because of venous congestion. We advise the patients to get out of bed and apply ice packs directly to the treated surface. Antihistamines by mouth can be of benefit, and occasionally topical steroids are utilized to help control the itching and skin irritation. The use of adequate sleeping medication during the first few nights of treatment is recommended. The length of time required in a hospital or a clinic varies according to the intelligence, stability, and cooperation of the subject, as well as the home situation. Most patients are able to leave the hospital or clinic on the fourth or fifth posttreatment day. From the seventh to the twenty-first day of treatment, the skin takes on a granular appearance and milia may form. No specific treatment is indicated except to keep the face well lubricated and clean. The extreme red color persists from 2 to 3 weeks and the reddish appearance for another 6 to 12 weeks, gradually fading away to a pinkish hue, which is usually not too objectionable. By the fourteenth to the twenty-first day, most patients are able to wear cosmetics and are encouraged to do so for short periods of time. There are several products on the market that will cover or camouflage the reddish appearance of the skin, and a great many of these contain sunscreens, which are advisable. Lipstick may be used much earlier, since it is not applied to any of the treated areas. After the skin begins to retain its normal appearance, the patient is advised to return to routine skin care and is encouraged to use a moisturizing lotion or cream at night. Most patients question the physician regarding recommendations about specific cosmetics, and it is better psychologically to make these specific recommendations than to give mere generalizations. Patients can best be encouraged to maintain skin care and they will give more attention to the proper use of cosmetics and their overall appearance.

LATE CARE

It has been histologically demonstrated that a significant number of the melanin-producing cells of the basal layer of the epidermis are removed by the peeling process (Fig. 19-4). Therefore, the treatment lightens or diminishes the skin color, reducing the natural protection of the skin from the sun [14, 15]. Patients who have undergone chemical face peeling should be advised to avoid direct or even reflected sunlight for extended periods of time in the 3 to 6 months following the treatment. Adequate sunscreens should be recommended, and it is best to suggest a specific product rather than make generalizations. With reference to sun exposure, the advice should include the following:

1. Stay out of direct or indirect sunlight for 3 to 6 months, especially during the middle of the day. Wear a wide-brimmed hat.
2. As a routine, utilize an effective sun protector daily for 3 to 6 months.
3. Avoid reflected sunlight, which is particularly a problem in riding in an automobile for extended periods of time.

We have seen cases in which patients developed irregular pigmentation on the side of the face that was chronically exposed to the sun while driving. There have been no problems with blotchy facial pigmentation following the chemical peel in individuals who have rigidly followed the instructions on avoiding sunlight.

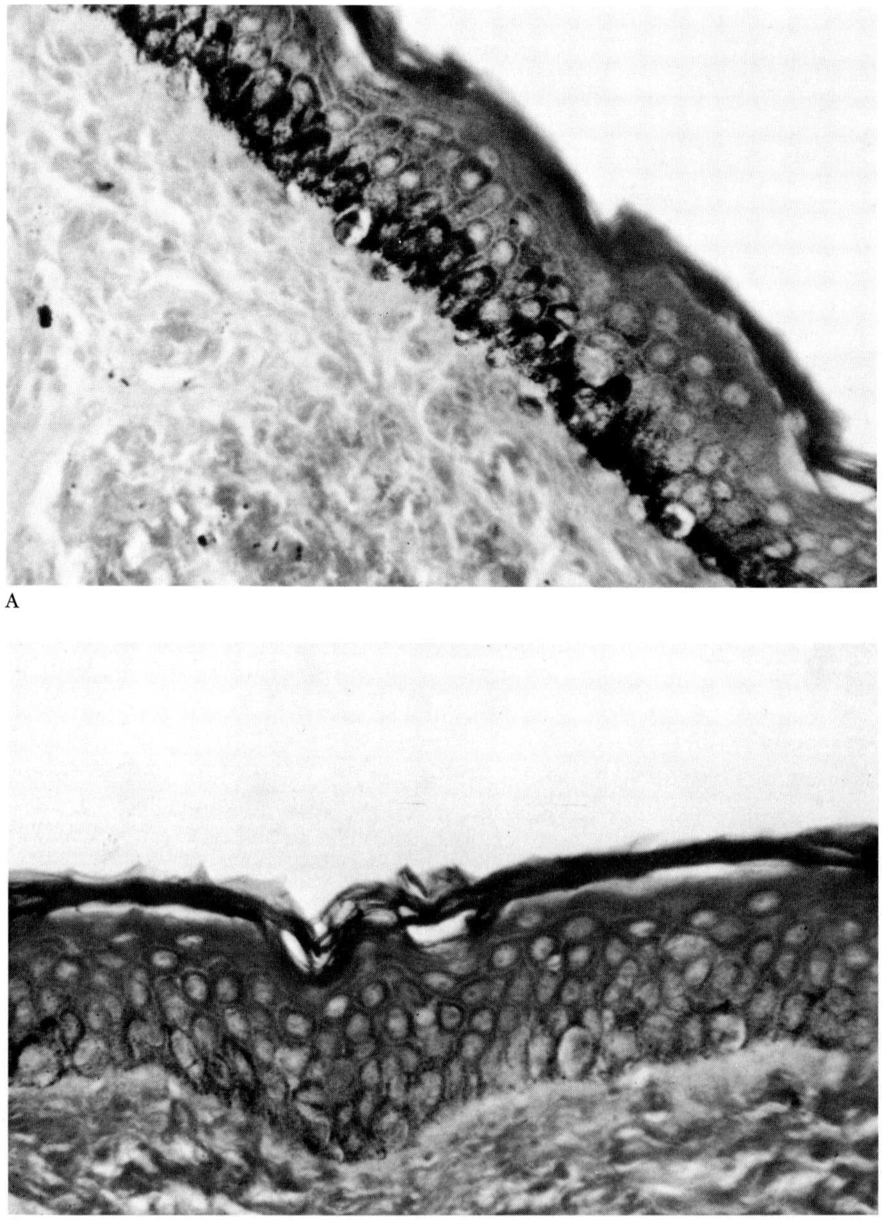

A

B

Figure 19-4
A. Note the melanin-producing cells in the basal layer of the epidermis in the pretreated skin.
B. Note the marked reduction of the melanin-producing cells in the basal layer of the epidermis. This finding is consistent and accounts for the decrease in the gross appearance of the skin as far as the amount of pigment is concerned.

COMBINED CHEMICAL PEEL AND RHYTIDECTOMY

When the aging face is critically analyzed, it can be seen to have two basic problems:

1. A generalized sagging of the facial tissues as a result of the body's losing its battle with gravity
2. Intrinsic changes in the skin, exhibited by fine wrinkling over the face along with deep lines around the forehead, mouth, and eyes

As stated previously, chemical face peeling will put a smooth skin on a sagging face. However, if the patient is in need of a rhytidectomy, this should be done in combination with the chemical peel, but *not at the same time.*

For patients who have both problems, it is wise to discuss the overall anticipated procedures with them, outlining the basic need for a rhytidectomy to alter the effects of gravity and for a chemical peel to alter the changes that are occurring intrinsically. The patients are advised that they might subsequently need to undergo a rhytidectomy following the chemical peel or, conversely, have the rhytidectomy first and the chemical face peel at a later date. If both procedures are to be done, an interval of at least 3 to 4 months should separate the two procedures. Personal preference is to do the rhytidectomy first and face peeling later [4, 6, 7, 32].

REGIONAL CHEMICAL PEELING

There are instances in which only an isolated area of the face needs to be treated—most commonly the upper lip (Fig. 19-5). Patients requesting rhytidectomy are often very concerned about the radiating lines around the mouth, particularly the upper lip, where lipstick bleeds into these wrinkles. This area responds very well to regional chemical face peeling [8, 13]. The skin of the "mustache area" is frequently a different color from that of the rest of the face prior to treatment. Since it will be lighter following the treatment, it does not offer a significant problem for most patients. The "mustache area" is a circumscribed unit of the face, bordered by the nose, upper lip, and nasolabial folds. The identical formula, as advocated above, is utilized in regional peeling. The mixture should be applied just onto the vermilion border, and the entire upper lip, including the nasolabial folds, extending 2 to 3 mm beyond the nasolabial line, should be included. If the peel stops at the nasolabial fold, it accentuates the line rather than tending partially to eliminate it. The application of the tape, thymol iodide, and other postpeel treatment is the same as outlined above. Regional peeling is usually done on an outpatient basis in the office as an isolated procedure. If a rhytidectomy is done, the upper lip and perioral area can be treated at the same time with complete safety.

On rare occasions, the glabellar area or periorbital area is treated as an isolated section of the face for peeling, either with or without adhesive tape. When adhesive tape is not applied to the skin, the effect of the phenol is less profound.

Chemical face peeling must never be done in an area of skin that has been undermined.

PEELING IN ASSOCIATED SKIN CONDITIONS

Abnormal Pigmentation Problems

Some cases of abnormal pigmentation respond dramatically to chemical face peeling. It seems to be effective in reducing the blotchy pigmentation in most instances, regardless of the etiology [14]. Cholasma, pigmentation due to drug reactions, the brown spots of aging, and freckles all respond to the treatment. The technique is exactly the same as described earlier. The results apparently are permanent or nearly so. Abnormal pigmentation often creates a greater social and psychologic problem than the presence of wrinkles. We have seen patients with severe alterations in pigmentation so affected psychologically that

Figure 19-5

A. This patient had significant radiating lines extending from the vermilion border of the upper lip and complained that her lipstick ran into this area. There were also some smaller lines radiating from her lower lip and around the corners of the mouth.

B. The patient had a perioral chemical peel, which was quite effective in removing the lines from around the mouth. (She also underwent an upper and lower lid blepharoplasty as well as a rhytidectomy.)

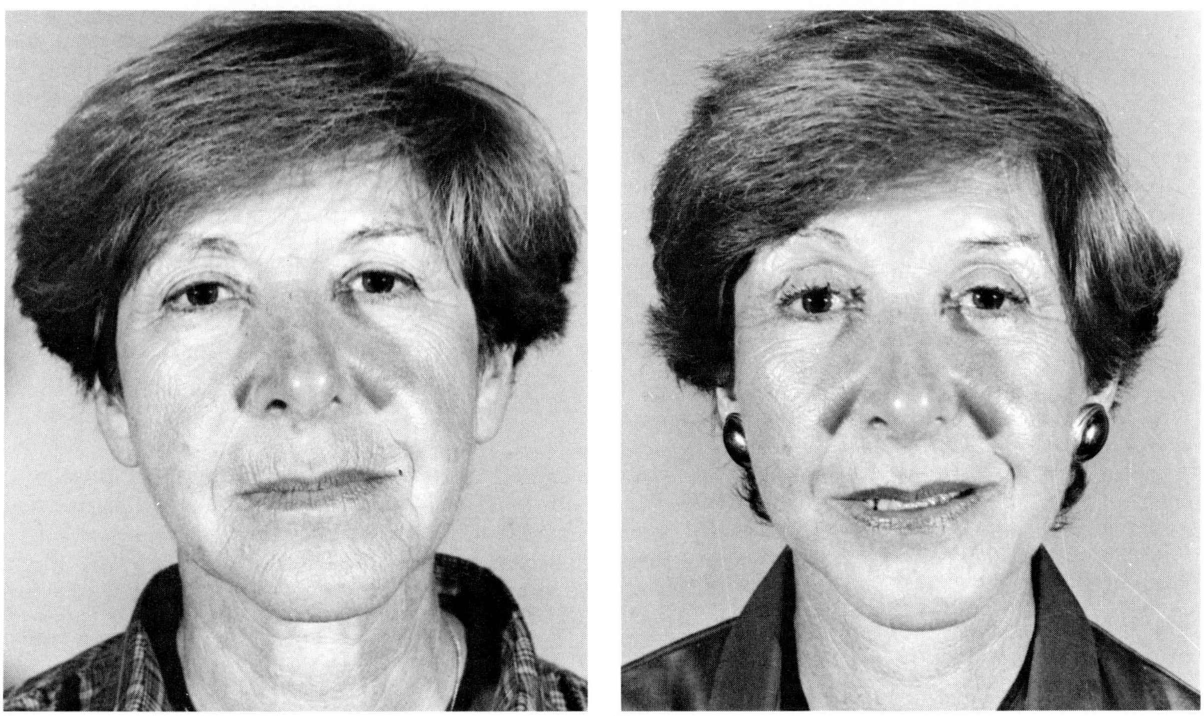

A B

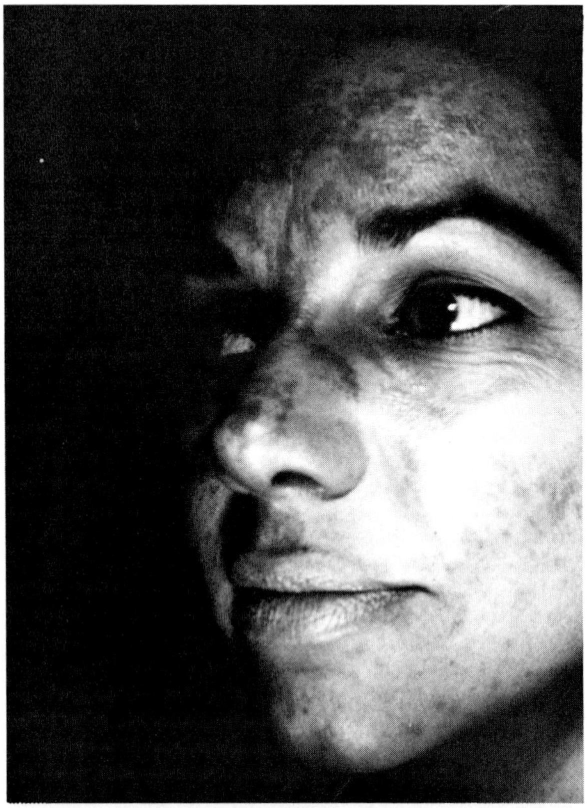

A

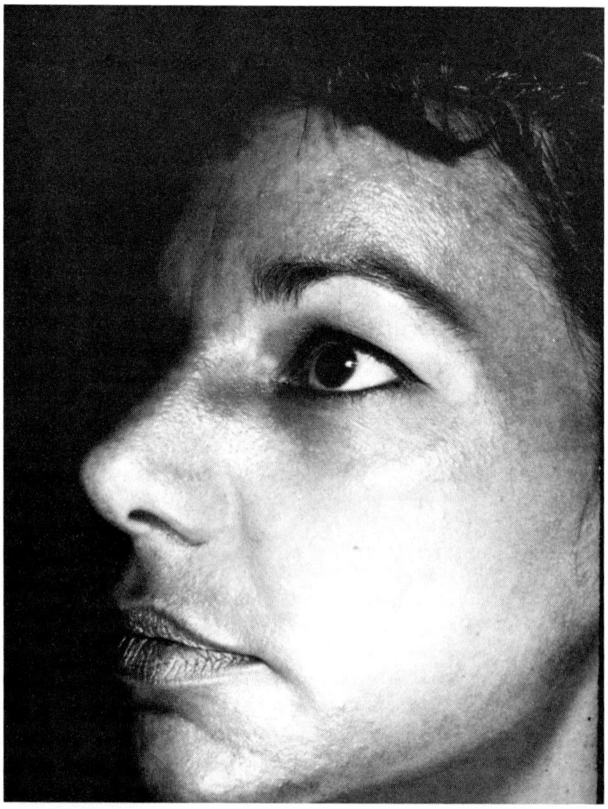

B

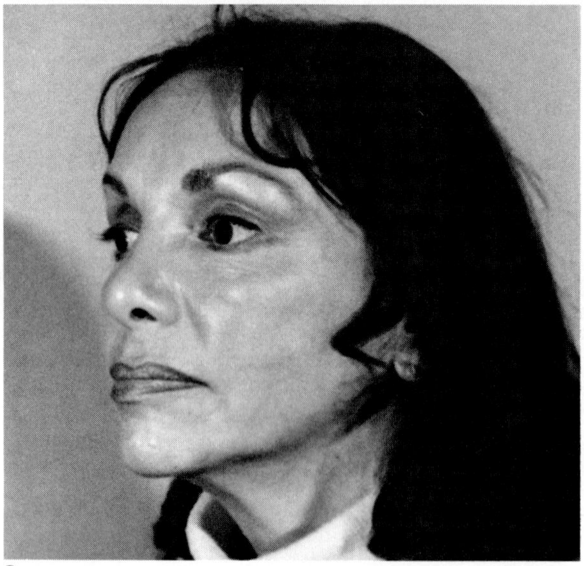

C

Figure 19-6
A. Severe hyperpigmentation of the face and blotchy appearance due to cholasma.
B. One year following chemical peeling for cholasma.
C. Fifteen years following chemical peel for cholasma. The skin remains smooth, and there is no evidence of a return of the blotchy condition.

they would not venture from their homes and became socially withdrawn. In most circumstances, the abnormal pigmentation is due to hyperpigmentation rather than a loss of pigmentation. If the individual can secure a uniform color, whether it be dark or light, this is preferable to a blotchy condition. Peeling results in bleaching of the entire area, and the hyperpigmented areas usually bleach to the same degree as the remainder of the skin that is not hyperpigmented (Fig. 19-6). This gives a homogeneous appearance to the entire skin of the face. In mild pigmentation problems, it is probably best to encourage the patient to utilize cosmetics rather than undergo a complete chemical face peel, particularly in mild cases of cholasma.

Occasionally there will be severe hyperpigmentation in the periorbital areas, which can sometimes be removed or reduced by topical application of phenol mixture in these specific areas. Again, the patient should be warned about the line of demarcation, especially since this is a limited regional application around the periorbital area. It is more likely to be noticed than the line of demarcation that would occur along the upper portion of the neck following a total chemical face peel. Most patients find the line of demarcation more acceptable than the dark circles around the eyes.

Chronic Changes Due to X-Radiation

Treatment of dermal radiation changes with the modality of dermabrasion has been disappointing. The damages experienced by individuals who have received x-ray therapy for acne scarring are not as frequent as in former years. However, some persons are still seen who suffered late gross and histologic changes in the skin due to radiation received years ago. The response to chemical treatment appears to be much the same as with dermabrasion. But long-term effectiveness seems to be greater with chemical peeling. For physicians experienced in treating this type of condition with dermabrasion, the same criteria for patient selection are utilized with chemical peeling. Most of the patients received x-radiation for the treatment of juvenile acne 15 to 30 years ago. It is usually difficult or impossible to determine the amount of radiation the patient has received, since often the treatment took place several years ago and the clinical records are unavailable. The x-ray dosage does not appear significantly to influence the response to chemical peel. Clinically, the response of the skin to the chemical face peel in this series has been the same as in patients who did not receive radiation.

Freckles

Although face peeling does remove freckles permanently, it has not been used by the author for the sole purpose of removing freckles. By coincidence, when a patient with freckles was treated for other reasons, they were removed at the same time. The freckles do not recur (Fig. 19-7).

Telangiectasia

Litton [26], in his original article, stated that chemical face peeling was of considerable benefit in the treatment of telangiectasia. However, he has subsequently said that he does not believe this to be the case, and we concur [28]. An occasional patient shows some improvement in small telangiectatic spots of the face, but for the most part these are not significantly altered and peeling is not recommended for the alteration of telangiectatic areas.

Port-Wine Stains

A number of patients have requested treatment with chemical peeling for port-wine stains. However, this has proved to have no effect in their condition. Clinical tests have also been carried out with reference to hemangiomas, and no significant benefit is seen. Chemical peeling, therefore, is not recommended.

Acne Scarring

Patients with mild superficial acne scarring, especially scarring associated with hyperpigmentation, have shown some encouraging results. Chemical face peeling is less effective in reducing the irregularities of the surface of the skin than dermabrasion. Peeling has no significant benefit in the more advanced forms of acne (Fig. 19-8).

Hypertrophied Scars and Burns

Chemical peeling has been tried for treatment of hypertrophied burn scars. On some occasions the pigmentation will be altered, making the area more homogeneous with reference to the surrounding skin. It does not, however, significantly alter the appearance of the scar and is therefore not recommended in this situation.

Hair

Chemical face peeling does not affect the growth of facial or scalp hair. Routine face peeling involves the use of the chemical mixture into the hairline, into the eyebrows, and on the fine hair of the face, and in no case has there been any alteration of hair pattern. Some individuals have the mistaken notion that chemical peeling removes hair from the upper lip. Hair follicles are not damaged by the treatment, at least not to the extent that the growth of the hair is altered.

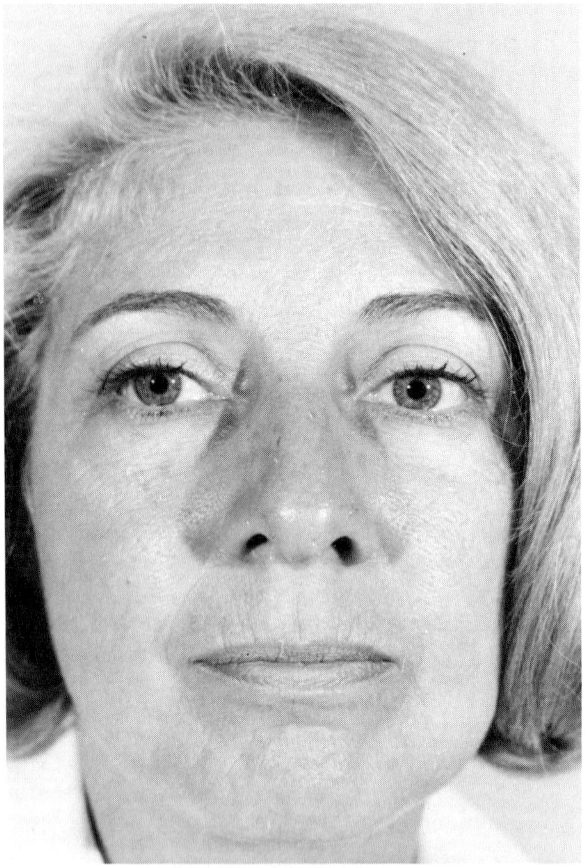

A

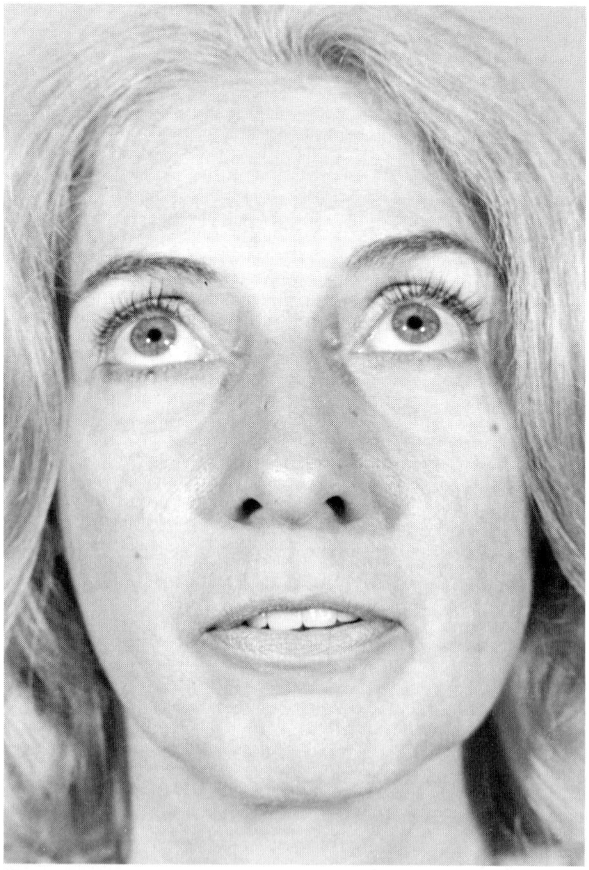

B

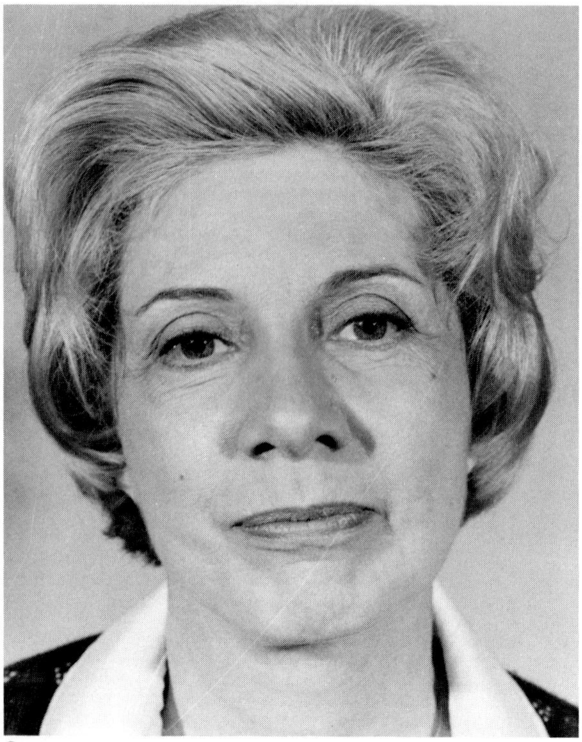

C

Figure 19-7

A. Chemical peel in this instance will remove the freckles as well as the fine lines in the skin, especially those radiating from the upper lip.

B. Ten months following complete chemical peel. Notice that the fine lines are gone from the upper lip, as well as the freckles.

C. Five and one-half years following treatment. The skin changes are very similar to those seen in Figure 19-7B. Note that the nevi of the right cheek and left malar area exhibit a darkening in color following the chemical peel.

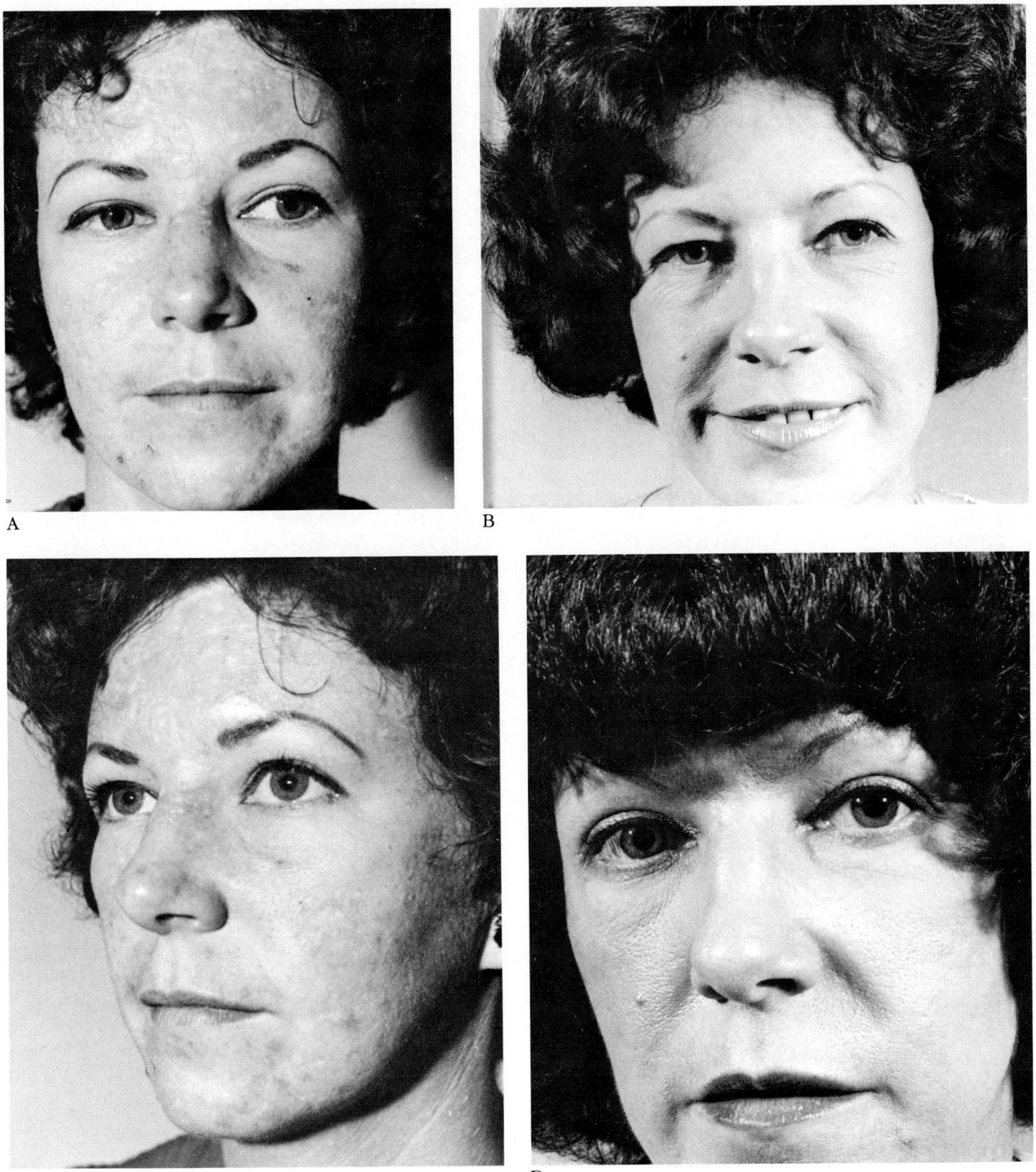

A B C D

Figure 19-8

A. Prepeel appearance of a patient with mild acne scarring and hyperpigmentation.
B. Ten years following chemical peel.
C. Lateral view of patient with superficial acne scarring and severe pigmentation problem.
D. Ten years following chemical peel. There has been no recurrence of the acne scarring or of the pigmentation problem.

SYSTEMIC TOXICITY

The use of phenol in chemical peeling involves the question as to whether systemic toxicity is produced through skin absorption. Numerous studies of this question indicate that such an effect is unlikely [22–24, 26]. A recent report by Truppman and Ellenby [39] indicates that electrocardiographic changes can occur in patients who absorb large amounts of phenol through the skin. They reached the conclusion that if the time period for application of the mixture is extended over 1 to 2 hours, the amount of phenol absorbed is probably of no serious consequence. In our own series of cases, utilizing the technique described herein, we have not noted any electrocardiographic changes in patients undergoing chemical face peeling.

A recent nationwide survey by Litton [29] failed to reveal a single case of a death being reported by a board-certified plastic surgeon.

Pure phenol is a colorless solution having an aromatic odor and a burning taste. It is obtained from coal tar or can be synthetically produced from monochlorobenzene. Pure phenol is a protoplasmic poison that affects the central nervous system. It is well known that it is absorbed through unbroken skin as well as through the mucous membranes of the body [23].

An oral dose of phenol ranging from 5 to 15 gm can result in death within 24 hours. Systemic toxic manifestations from large doses of the ingested phenol begin within a few minutes. Symptoms include faintness, muscular weakness, convulsions, weak and irregular pulse, depressed respiration, constricted pupils, coma, and even death. Detoxification and excretion of phenol that was orally administered was studied by Deichmann [22]. He reported that phenol is removed from the body by three processes: excretion, oxidation, and conjugation. In his experience, within 24 hours the experimental animal will excrete 27 percent of a toxic (half-lethal) dose in the urine. Only traces are excreted in the feces at this time. At the end of 24 hours, approximately 3 percent of the absorbed phenol may still be found in the body.

Litton reported a series of phenol blood studies in 50 patients. He examined blood samples drawn at 1-, 3-, and 5-hour intervals, and analyzed them in a spectrophotometer [26]. Utilizing approximately 3 ml of a 50% solution of phenol applied to the entire area of the face, he noted that the blood phenol levels rose to 0.68 mg/100 ml maximum within 1 hour after the application. After 2 hours had elapsed, maximum level was 0.19 mg/dl. After 4 hours, less than 0.1 mg/liter remained. This study indicates that in volumes being used for most chemical face peeling the blood phenol level is rapidly reduced in a matter of 4 hours.

There has been reported in the literature [23] a human who ingested a sufficient quantity of phenol to produce a blood level of 23 mg/dl of blood phenol. The patient survived. Obviously, there is a large margin of safety between the 0.68 mg/dl in the series reported by Litton and the 23 mg/dl level demonstrated after a human ingested oral phenol.

Our own personal experience concludes that no evidence of serious systemic toxicity is exhibited either by routine laboratory analyses or by clinical observation if the technique is carried out as described. We have used topical phenol on portions or total areas of the face in more than 2000 patients over the last 20 years. The conclusion is that the formula as utilized in this technique does not lead to significant systemic toxicity. Both Ayers [1] and Brown et al. [20] report that liquid phenol can be used with relative safety when it is applied to limited areas of the skin in restricted quantities and at proper intervals. MacKee and Kapp [30] noted that when phenol was applied to the face in one single sitting, no systemic effects were demonstrable by clinical or laboratory tests.

COMPLICATIONS

The untoward effects and complications encountered in chemical face peeling include the following:

1. Reduction in pigmentation of the skin (bleaching effect) (Fig. 19-9)
2. Increased sensitivity of the skin to sunlight
3. Milia
4. Hypertrophied scars
5. Scar contracture
6. Alteration of existing skin conditions
   a. Darkening of existing nevi (see Fig. 19-7C)
   b. Telangiectasia
   c. Increase in size of skin pores
7. Prolonged redness of the skin

Reduction in Pigmentation of the Skin (Bleaching Effect)

Dark-complexioned individuals show more bleaching effect than those with light complexions. Most problems associated with a marked line of demarcation can be avoided by proper patient selection. The ideal patient is one who has fair skin and a minimal amount of freckles or brown aging spots who has not been subjected to excessive sun exposure. Many prospective patients are not good candidates for chemical peeling, and the consulting physician should not hesitate to refuse treatment. Since the bleaching effect following a chemical peel often causes a notable line of demarcation between treated and untreated areas along the neck, an attempt is made to minimize this at the time of treatment by extending the application of the mixture to approximately ½ in. beyond the margin of the mask. Said in another way, after the mixture has been applied, the mask is brought to within ½ in. of the treated margin. It is a fact that tape on a treated area causes a more profound peeling effect [37], and therefore bringing the tape just short of the edge of the treated area tends to make the line of demarcation less conspicuous. The usual level for the cessation of treatment on the neck is just beneath the mandibular margin. This is an ideal line to limit the application of the mixture. If one elects to continue to peel down to the midportion of the neck, the

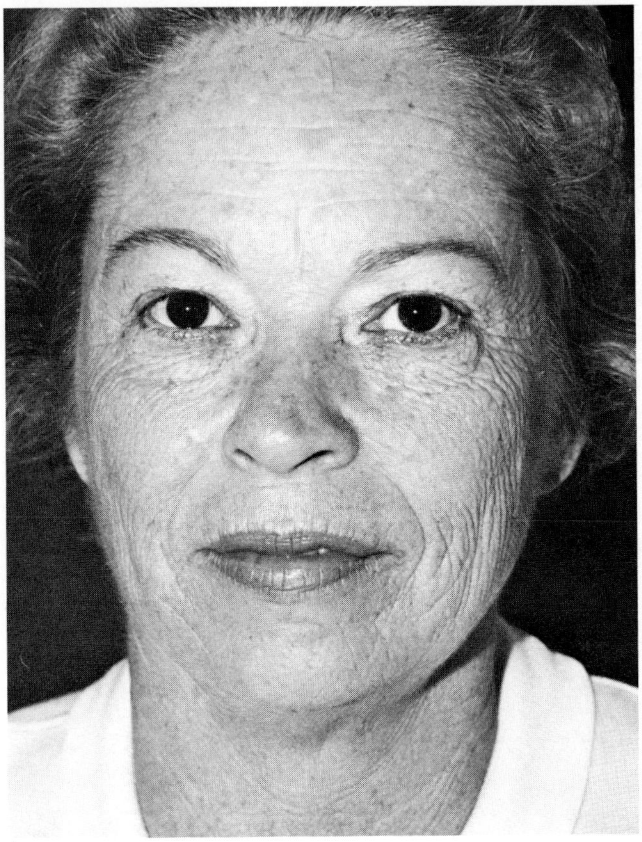

A

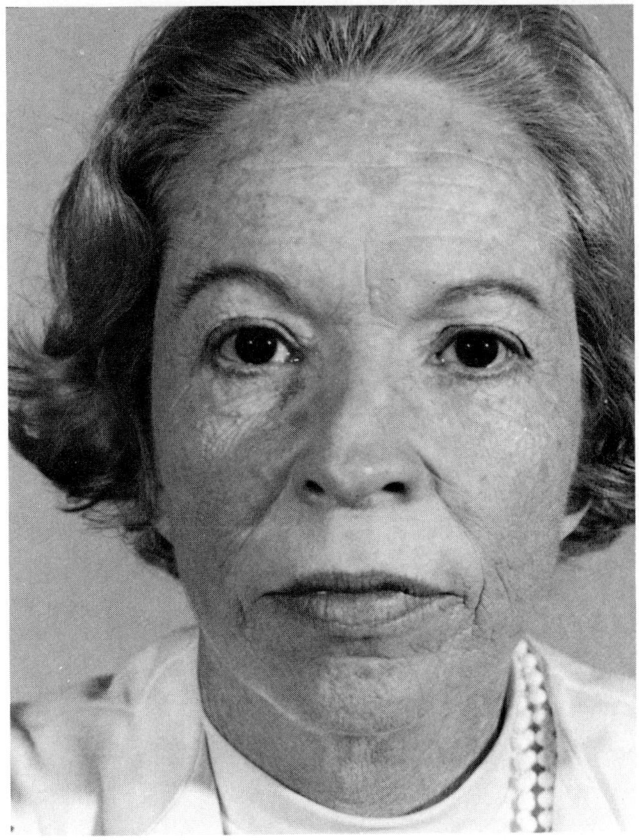

B

Figure 19-9
A. Patient who requested a chemical peel of the upper lip and was willing to accept the line of demarcation that would probably exist.
B. Seven years following chemical peel of the upper lip. Note the decreased pigmentation in this area; however, the lines have not recurred. Many patients prefer the bleached area to the lines.

treatment boundary will be much more noticeable than if one stops immediately inferior to the mandibular border. Following chemosurgery, blotchy pigmentation of the face can occur (Fig. 19-10). But if sunlight is assiduously avoided, blotchiness is rare. If blotchiness does occur, the hyperpigmented areas will have to be repeeled. Normally, 3 to 4 months should elapse before secondary peel is attempted. The blotchy areas are repeeled by means of the original formula, and usually no tape is necessary in these small areas.

Increased Sensitivity of the Skin to Sunlight

Since chemical peeling reduces the melanin-producing cells in the basal layer of the epidermis, the skin does not respond normally to sunlight and tanning does not occur. None of the patients who have received a chemical face peeling have been able to develop a suntan. Therefore, it must be stressed that these patients should use a sun protector on the skin at all times and avoid sunlight whenever possible. No cases of sunburn have been observed following chemical peeling.

Milia

Milia are rarely seen following chemosurgery, but they can occur. Following dermabrasion, milia are common. This condition will usually regress spontaneously, but if it does not after 3 to 4 months, the patient should be advised to use a soft complexion brush on the skin several times daily. If there are resistant milia that do not disappear, they may necessitate surgical intervention, with a fine scalpel blade. In no instances have milia been found to be permanent.

Hypertrophied Scars

Fortunately, hypertrophied scars are seldom encountered. We have seen a number of cases in which severe scar contracture of the face and neck occurred in patients being treated by "lay operators." Six individuals, however, developed small transverse hypertrophied scars in the midportion of the upper lip between 2 and 3 months following treatment. In each instance the patient had undergone a chemical peel of the upper lip at the same time as rhytidectomy. No cases of hypertrophy of the scar of the upper lip have been seen when the upper lip was done as an isolated procedure, or when the lip was treated not in

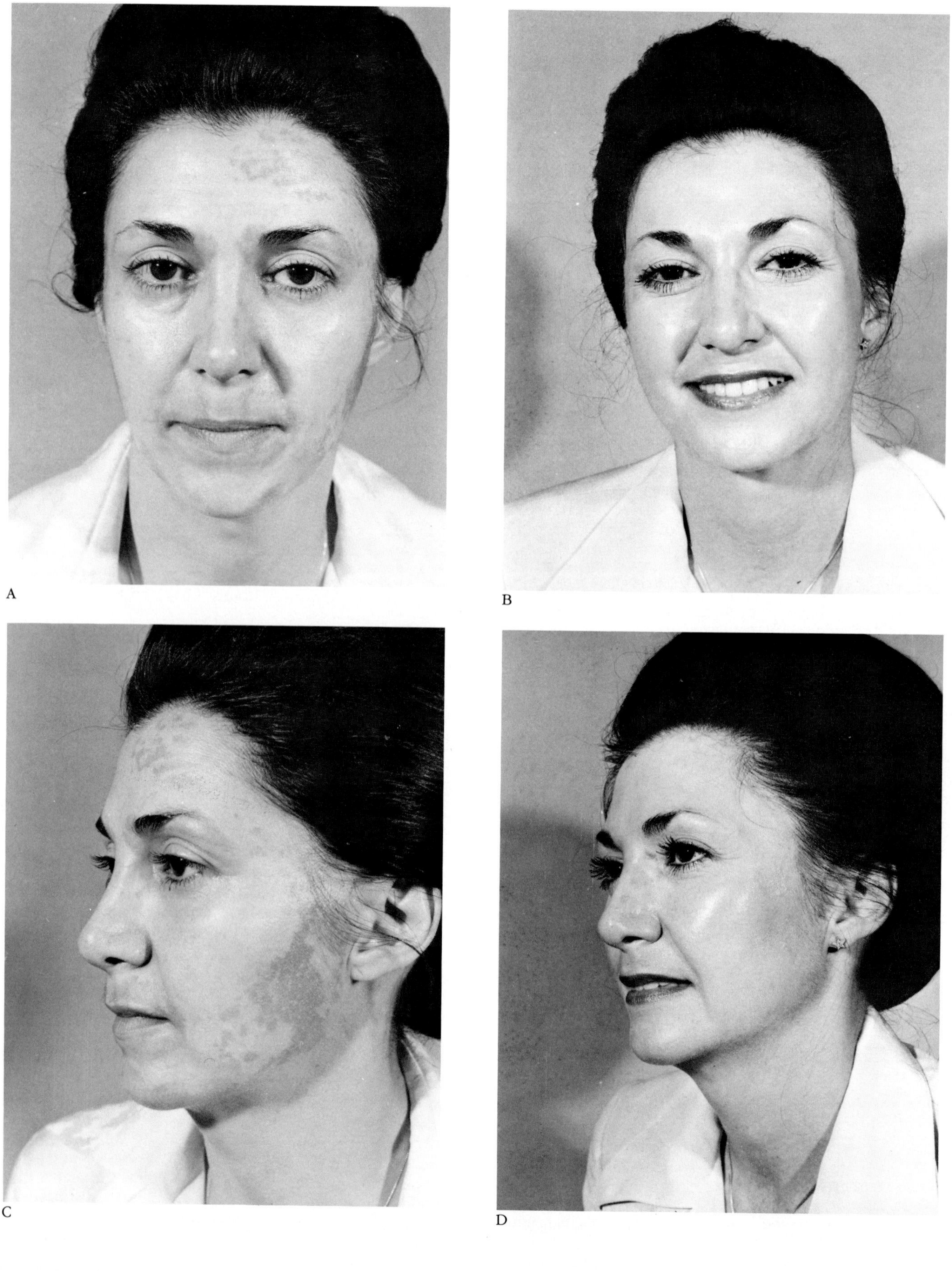

A B C D

association with any other surgical procedure. The conclusion is that scar hypertrophy is probably due to the excessive edema present from a rhytidectomy. A better technique is to treat the entire upper lip (if a rhytidectomy is being done at the same time) by applying a tape strip only along the skin just above the vermilion border and not to tape the entire lip. Since we have been utilizing this technique, no scar hypertrophy of the upper lip has occurred in the past several years. Although hypertrophied scarring has been reported following chemical peeling, it is very rare (less than 1%). Nevertheless, for medicolegal reasons, it is best to explain to the patient that it is a possibility. A consent form for chemical peeling should be utilized. The authors have had no medicolegal problems in their 22 years of experience.

Alteration of Existing Skin Conditions

DARKENING OF EXISTING NEVI

Patients have noted that "moles" appeared on their faces following therapy. When the preoperative photographs are reviewed, usually a pale nevus can be seen in the area prior to the chemosurgery. Hyperpigmentation of the nevi does occur following chemosurgery, and the patient should be forewarned. No instances of melanoma or other malignancies have been noted in the skin of patients who have undergone chemical peeling.

TELANGIECTASIA

In patients who have "thin skin," telangiectatic areas are occasionally noticeable following a chemical peel. In most cases, the telangiectatic spots were present prior to therapy. If a patient has telangiectasia before the peel, this condition should be pointed out to the patient and carefully discussed before the treatment is carried out.

INCREASE IN SIZE OF SKIN PORES

It is well known that, following dermabrasion, pores appear larger in many areas of the face. The same is true in patients undergoing chemical peeling. There is no clinical problem associated with the enlarged pores, but it is important that the patient be aware of this possibility. Some individuals request chemical peeling for the treatment of enlarged pores and have the mistaken idea that chemical peeling will reduce their size. The reverse is true.

Figure 19-10

A. Several blotchy areas remain from a previous chemical peel. This patient probably had early exposure to the sun without effective screening.

B. Six months following secondary chemical peel in the blotchy areas only. There has been no evidence of recurrence of the pigmentation.

C. The blotchy area of the left cheek was more pronounced because of exposure through passenger side car window. There was probably early exposure to the sun without adequate sunscreen.

D. The blotchy areas were peeled secondarily and there has been no evidence of recurrence of the blotchy pigmentation.

Prolonged Redness of the Skin

In some persons the skin remains reddish or pink for several weeks following the treatment. An occasional patient has had redness for 12 to 18 weeks. No one has been observed who had redness remaining as a permanent condition. The clinical impression is that the patients who maintain the redness for the longest period of time subsequently have the best clinical result. When redness persists for more than 6 to 8 weeks, topical steroids are applied daily to help diminish the erythema. Again, the patient should be forewarned that prolonged redness can occur and its possibility discussed to avoid disappointment and misunderstanding.

HISTOLOGIC CHANGE IN THE SKIN

Biopsies have been secured from the skin of patients who have undergone chemical peel at intervals ranging from 3 months to 17 years [14, 15]. The biopsy material was taken from the neck of patients undergoing rhytidectomy in which a specimen could be removed containing both treated and untreated skin, including the junctional area. This allowed us to make observations of an area in which the normal control skin was immediately contiguous with the treated skin. There have been three constant findings in patients in the posttreatment phase, in both the short-term and long-term follow-up period.

1. Homogenization of the dermal collagen architecture (Fig. 19-11)
2. A marked diminution of the quantity of melanin granules present in the basal layer of the epidermis (see Fig. 19-4)
3. An increase in the amount of elastic staining tissue in the dermis as demonstrated by special elastic stains

The bleaching effect on the chemically treated skin is explained by the permanent reduction of the melanin-producing cells in the basal layer of the epidermis. The increase in elastic staining tissue in the dermis probably represents a reaction to injury, since similar histologic changes are noted in solar degeneration of exposed skin. It is speculated in a teleologic way that the occurrence of elastotic material in the superficial dermis is the body's response to injury, protecting the underlying structures from further injury, whether it be from ultraviolet penetration or chemical penetration.

There have been no findings of skin malignancies in any patients who have undergone a chemical face peel in our series. While we do not mean to imply that chemical face peeling prevents such things as basal cell carcinoma, one can speculate that peeling might conceivably reduce the incidence of sun-induced malignant degeneration. These patients usually change their life-style following the chemical peel and either are receiving less sun exposure or are protecting their skin adequately with sunscreens.

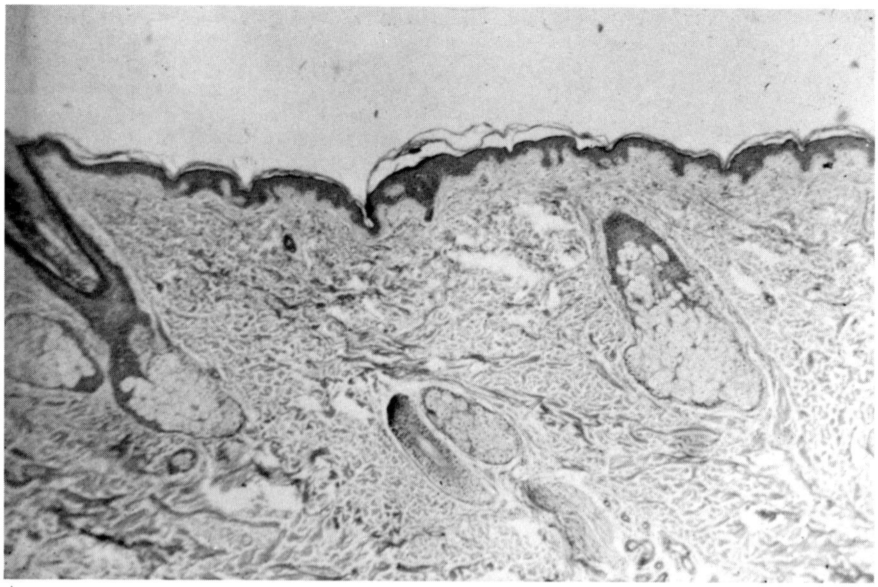

A

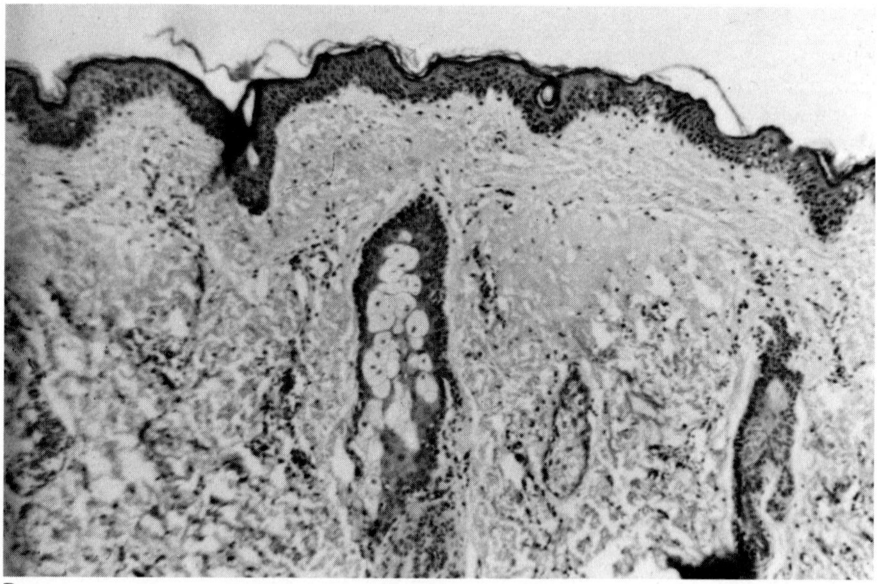

B

Figure 19-11
A. Hematoxylin-eosin stain of normal skin.
B. Hematoxylin-eosin stain in patient who has undergone a chemical peel. Note the homogenization of the collagenous layer of the dermis.

SUMMARY

Chemical face peeling has earned a place in the armamentarium of physicians who are treating aging skin as well as certain pigmentation changes that occur for a variety of reasons. Twenty-two years of experience have led the authors to conclude that chemical face peeling produces gross and microscopic changes in the skin that are permanent and predictable. Gross changes are the elimination of wrinkles, a lighter color of the skin, and a change in the texture. On occasion, the pores appear larger following a peel, as they do in skin after dermabrasion. The response of skin to chemical face peeling varies widely according to skin type, color, and texture. Utilizing proper patient selection, which has become increasingly precise in recent years, one can achieve a higher degree of success. The delicate, thin-skinned, fair-complexioned woman who has only fine wrinkles and minimal gross sagging is an ideal candidate. The poor candidate is the patient with thick, oily skin and an olive complexion who has spent too much time in the sun. Skin that has been tanned and thickened by chronic exposure to the sun will have pronounced lines of demarcation between treated and untreated areas and a tendency toward lack of color homogeneity (Fig. 19-12) after peeling. The texture and color of the skin are of greater concern in the selection of patients than is age.

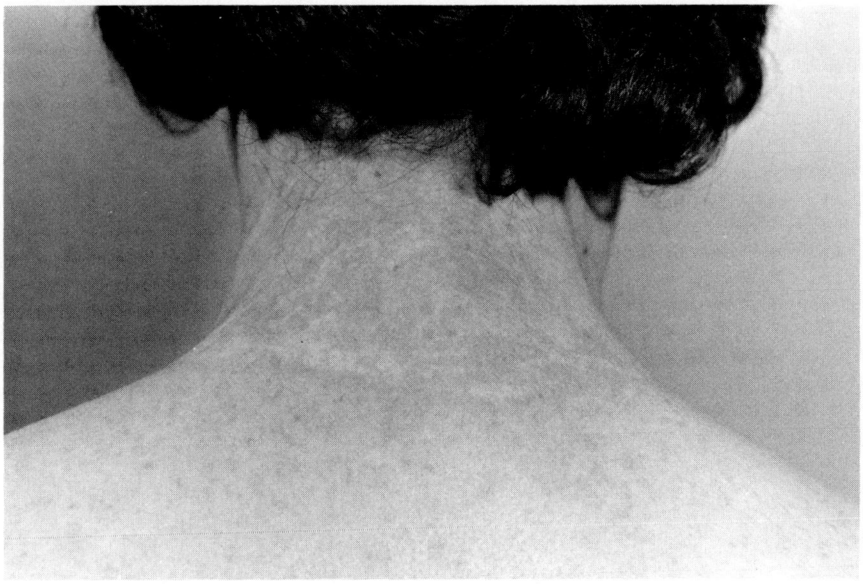

Figure 19-12. This patient had a peel of her neck and exhibited a rather frequent response on the posterior area, in that there was blotchy pigmentation. If the line of demarcation is at this juncture, it creates a problem in wearing clothing that exposes the posterior aspect of the neck.

Chemical face peeling is a safe and accepted form of treatment with proper patient selection and careful attention to the details of the technique.

REFERENCES

1. Ayers S., III. Dermal changes following application of chemical cauterants to aging skin. *Arch. Dermatol.* 82:578, 1960.
2. Ayers, S., III. Superficial chemosurgery in treating aging skin. *Arch. Dermatol.* 85:385, 1962.
3. Baker, T. J. The ablation of rhitides by chemical means: A preliminary report. *J. Fla. Med. Assoc.* 48:451, 1961.
4. Baker, T. J. Chemical face peeling and rhytidectomy. *Plast. Reconstr. Surg.* 29:199, 1962.
5. Baker, T. J., and Gordon, H. L. Chemosurgery of the face: Some warnings and misconceptions. *J. Fla. Med. Assoc.* 49:218, 1962.
6. Baker, T. J., and Gordon, H. L. Chemical face peeling: An adjunct to surgical face lifting. *South. Med. J.* 56:412, 1963.
7. Baker, T. J., and Gordon, H. L. Current approaches to facial rejuvenation. *South. Med. J.* 58:1077, 1965.
8. Baker, T. J., and Gordon, H. L. Chemical face peeling and dermabrasion. *Surg. Clin. North Am.* 51:387, 1971.
9. Baker, T. J., and Gordon, H. L. The Chemical Face Peel: Indications, Technique, and Complications. In F. W. Masters and J. R. Lewis, Jr. (eds.), *Symposium on Aesthetic Surgery of the Face, Eyelid, and Breast.* St. Louis: Mosby, 1972. P. 65.
10. Baker, T. J., and Gordon, H. L. Chemical Face Peeling. In R. M. Goldwyn (ed.), *The Unfavorable Result in Plastic Surgery: Avoidance and Treatment.* Boston: Little, Brown, 1972.
11. Baker, T. J., and Gordon, H. L. Chemical Peel with Phenol. In E. Epstein and E. Epstein, Jr. (eds.), *Skin Surgery* (4th ed.). Springfield, Ill.: Thomas, 1977. P. 613.
12. Baker, T. J., and Gordon, H. L. Chemical Peel. In E. H. Courtiss (ed.), *Aesthetic Surgery: Trouble—How to Avoid It and How to Treat It.* St. Louis: Mosby, 1978. P. 145.
13. Baker, T. J., and Gordon, H. L. Chemical peeling as a practical method for removing rhytides of the upper lip. *Ann. Plast. Surg.* 2:209, 1979.
14. Baker, T. J., and Gordon, H. L. Effects of the Chemical Peel. In R. M. Goldwyn (ed.), *Long-Term Results in Plastic and Reconstructive Surgery.* Boston: Little, Brown, 1980. P. 629.
15. Baker, T. J., Gordon, H. L., Mosienko, P., and Seckinger, D. L. Long-term histological study of skin after chemical face peeling. *Plast. Reconstr. Surg.* 53:522, 1974.
16. Baker, T. J., Gordon, H. L., and Seckinger, D. L. A second look at chemical face peeling. *Plast. Reconstr. Surg.* 37:487, 1966.
17. Bames, H. O. Truth and fallacies of face peeling and face lifting. *Med. J. Rec.* 126:86, 1927.
18. Batstone, J. H., and Millard, D. R., Jr. An endorsement of facial chemo-surgery. *Br. J. Plast. Surg.* 21:193, 1968.
19. Brown, A. M., Kaplan, L., and Brown, M. E. Cutaneous alterations induced by phenol: A histologic bio-assay. *J. Int. Coll. Surg.* 34:602, 1960.
20. Brown, A. M., Kaplan, L. M., and Brown, M. E. Phenol-induced histological skin changes: Hazards, techniques, and uses. *Br. J. Plast. Surg.* 13:158, 1961.
21. Combes, F. C., Sperber, P. A., and Reich, M. Dermal defects: Treatment by chemical agent. *N.Y. Phys. Am. Med.* 56:36, 1960.
22. Deichmann, W. B. Phenol studies: Distribution, detoxification, and excretion of phenol in mammalian body. *Arch. Biochem.* 3:345, 1944.
23. Deichmann, W., and Schafer, L. J. Phenol studies: I. Review of the literature; II. Quantitative spectrophotometric estimation of free and conjugated phenol in tissues and fluids; III. Phenol content of normal human tissues and fluids. *Am. J. Clin. Pathol.* 12:129, 1942.
24. Deichmann, W. B., and Witherup, S. Phenol studies: VI. The acute and comparative toxicity of phenol and l-, m-, and p-cresols for experimental animals. *J. Pharmacol. Exp. Ther.* 80:233, 1944.
25. Hoopes, J. E., Wolfort, F. G., and Dalton, W. E. Chemical Rhytidectomy. In F. W. Masters and J. R. Lewis, Jr. (eds.), *Symposium on Aesthetic Surgery of the Face, Eyelid, and Breast.* St. Louis: Mosby, 1972. P. 73.

26. Litton, C. Chemical face lifting. *Plast. Reconstr. Surg.* 29:371, 1962.
27. Litton, C. Observations after chemosurgery of the face. *Plast. Reconstr. Surg.* 32:554, 1963.
28. Litton, C. Follow-up study of chemosurgery. *South. Med. J.* 59:1007, 1966.
29. Litton, C., and Trinidad, G. Complications of chemical face peeling as evaluated by a questionnaire. *Plast. Reconstr. Surg.* 67:738, 1981.
30. MacKee, G. M., and Kapp, F. L. The treatment of post-acne scars with phenol. *Br. J. Dermatol.* 64:456, 1952.
31. Monash, S. The uses of diluted trichloroacetic acid in dermatology. *Urol. Cutan. Rev.* 49:119, 1945.
32. Rees, T. D. Chemobrasion with special reference to the rehabilitation of the aging face. *Geriatrics* 20:1039, 1965.
33. Roberts, H. L. The chloracetic acids: A bio-chemical study (two-part article). *Br. J. Dermatol.* 38:323, 375, 1926.
34. Sperber, P. A. Chemexfoliation—a new term in cosmetic therapy. *J. Am. Geriatr. Soc.* 11:58, 1963.
35. Sperber, P. A. Chemexfoliation for aging skin and acne scarring. *Arch. Otolaryngol.* 81:278, 1965.
36. Sperbe, P. A. *Treatment of the Aging Skin and Dermal Defects.* Springfield, Ill.: Thomas, 1965. P. 3.
37. Spira, M., et al. Chemosurgery: A histological study. *Plast. Reconstr. Surg.* 45:247, 1970.
38. Spira, M., Gerow, F. J., and Hardy, S. B. Complications of chemical face peeling. *Plast. Reconstr. Surg.* 54:397, 1974.
39. Truppman, E. S. and Ellenby, J. D. Major electrocardiographic changes during chemical face peeling. *Plast. Reconstr. Surg.* 63:44, 1979.
40. Wood-Smith, D. and Rees, T. D. Chemabrasion and Dermabrasion. In T. D. Rees and D. Wood-Smith (eds.), *Cosmetic Facial Surgery.* Philadelphia: Saunders, 1973. P. 213.

20. Ancillary Facial Procedures

Numerous patients requesting complete facial rejuvenation will also want a specific deformity corrected, e.g., lip lines, crow's-feet. If the problem is ignored in favor of the generalized rhytidectomy, the patient will often be disappointed with the result and immediately point out the original deformity. Further compounding the dilemma is which type of procedure to do—excision, dermabrasion, chemical peeling, or injection therapy.

Surgical Rejuvenation of the Lips

Rodolphe Meyer
Ulrich K. Kesselring

The perioral region is, together with the periocular, the most important site of facial expression [9]. Among the many operations recommended for correction of its imperfections or signs of aging are the following small procedures, which can be performed as isolated entities or as ancillary procedures to a rhytidectomy: (1) correction of deep nasolabial folds, (2) augmentation cheiloplasty, (3) smoothening of wrinkled upper lip, (4) height reduction of upper lip, (5) deepening of shallow philtrum, (6) reduction of fullness of the lips, (7) correction of the sagging double-contour lower lip, (8) deepening of the labiomental folds, and (9) correction of tethered lip.

CORRECTION OF DEEP NASOLABIAL FOLDS

Deep nasolabial folds may be hereditary or acquired and often project a disgusted attitude, much to the dismay of the individual. They have been one of the unanswered questions in treatment of the aging face. Complete excision seemed a radical operation in most cases; silicone and collagen injections had no or little durable effect. Undermining and subsequent dermabrasion of the whole length of the groove was not much better. Even the good results achieved by subdermal implantation of dermal grafts, which we practiced for several years, were of short duration. Only where we used a dermal flap, obtained from an excision around the alar base, instead of a graft was the effect more lasting. However, this procedure was suitable only for the correction of the upper part of the nasolabial fold. Having obtained little satisfaction with these minor procedures, we decided to use mattress sutures to evert the crease and at the same time to fix temporarily a dermafat graft, which was introduced through a short incision in the nostril crease (Fig. 20-1A).

A vermicular dermis graft is taken from the retroauricular fold or, if the procedure is done in connection with a rhytidectomy, from the preauricular skin. Sutures (5-0) of nonabsorbable material cross beneath the dermis graft in a zigzag line from one side to the other along the everted fold. It is important that the zigzag stitch be led back through the same skin hole it came out through in order to minimize scarring. We usually divide the length of the nasolabial crease in two to three suture segments, facilitating their removal (Fig. 20-1B). Temporary eversion of the crease, we feel, is an important detail of the procedure leading to results superior to those obtained by mere subcutaneous dissection and dermafat graft implantation (Fig. 20-2). A similar procedure can be used for the correction of a frontoglabellar crease.

AUGMENTATION CHEILOPLASTY

In the aging face, the upper lip gradually thins and becomes ptotic. It is the first and most evident senile stigma. Thin vertical wrinkles on the upper lip are unsightly and are poorly camouflaged with lipstick. To create or recreate the normal fullness of the lip with a harmonic Cupid's bow, we have devised and published a simple but effective method that has given us satisfaction during the last 12 years in more than 100 cases [8, 9].

With a very fine pen the vermilion border is marked (Figs. 20-3A and 20-5B). Then the desired additional lip area is designed; an initial hypercorrection must be obtained in order to compensate for the retractive forces. An incision is made along the actual and the future vermilion and the area in between is deepithelialized (Fig. 20-3B). After being undermined, the vermilion can be advanced into its new site, where it is fixed with a single 6-0 suture on either side of the philtrum ridges. The remaining wound is closed with an intradermal running nonabsorbable 5-0 suture on each half (Fig. 20-3C,D,E). In rare cases the lips not only need to be enlarged but also require additional volume, and in this event we employ free der-

Figure 20-1

A. To attenuate deep nasolabial folds a dermafat graft has to be introduced very superficially—practically intradermally—into a tunnel that has been dissected from a small incision in the alar crease.

B. Zigzag sutures evert the nasolabial fold and keep the graft in place for 3 to 4 days.

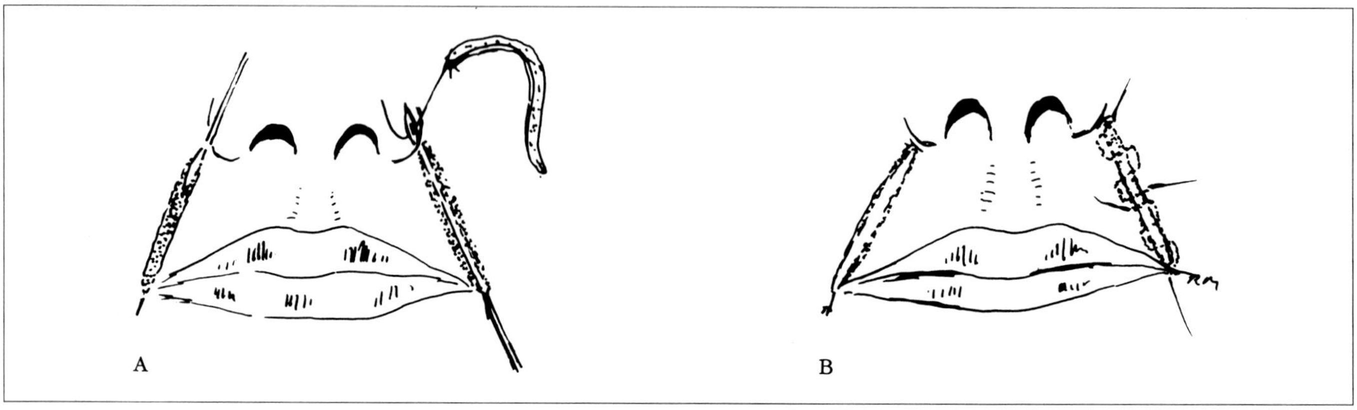

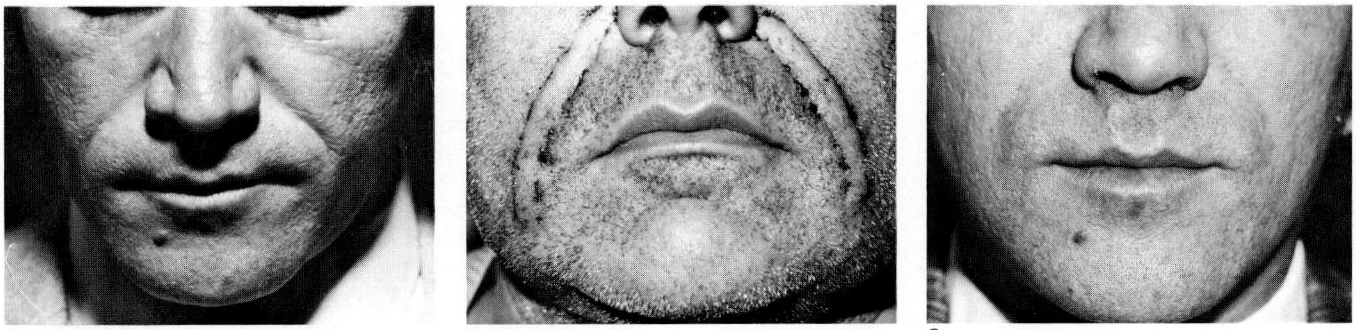

A B C

Figure 20-2. Nasolabial fold correction.
A. Preoperative view.
B. Three days after operation.
C. Result after 5 months.

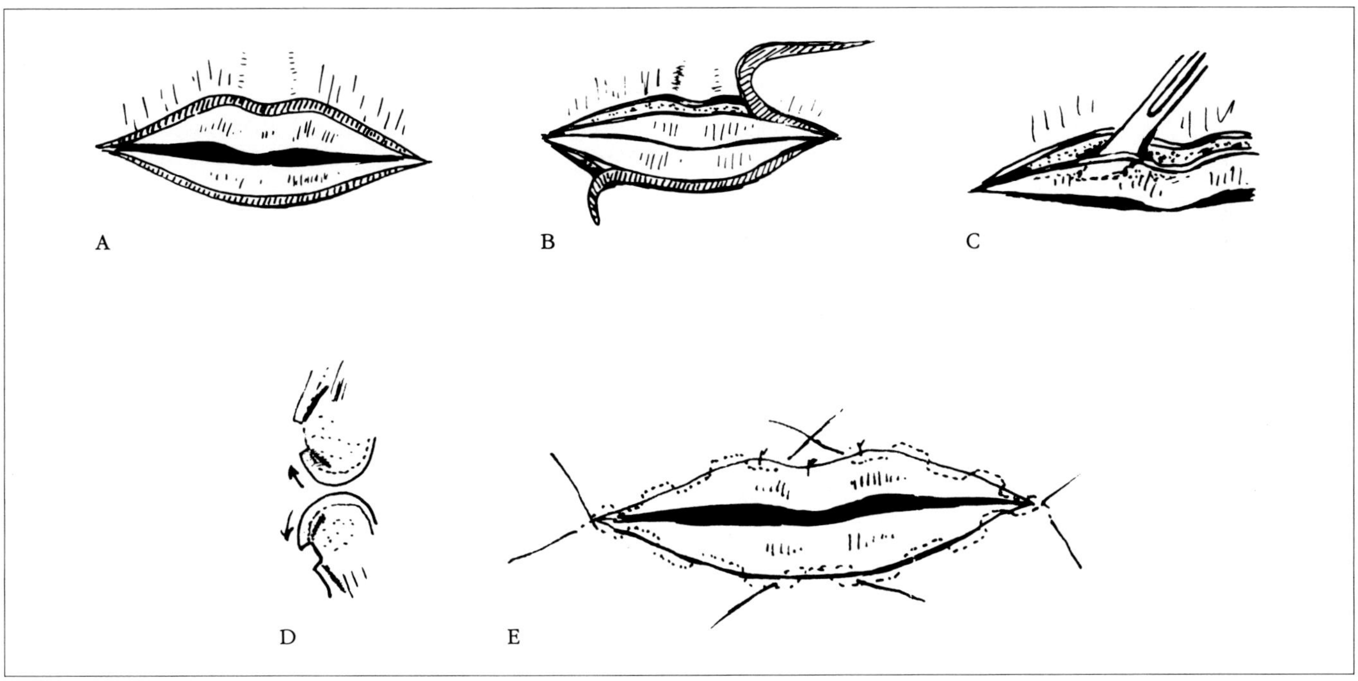

Figure 20-3
A, B. The skin delimited by the incisions along the old and the newly designed vermilion border has to be resected very superficially.
C. The vermilion itself is dissected 5 mm wide in a horizontal plane.
D, E. The vermilion "flap" can then be advanced into its newly created bed.

mal grafts introduced through small incisions in a subcutaneous pocket beneath the lip. Some years ago a method was described by Delerm and Elbaz [2] for this kind of augmentation, which consists of a V-Y advancement, a mucosa-plasty, and a muscle-plasty. We believe, however, that the same result can be achieved by our simple procedure.

Occasionally, increased fullness of the upper or lower lip can be accomplished with sliding flaps of mucosa or underlying submucosal tissue. A translabial mattress suture can occasionally help to keep the vermilion border advanced. If the deficiency is located essentially in the center of the lip, especially in the upper lip, a V-Y advancement of the central portion of the mucosa is indicated for creating a balanced contour with a forward and downward projection of the central margin.

SMOOTHENING OF WRINKLED UPPER LIP

Many methods to remove the wrinkles of the upper lip have been tried. Hinderer [4] suggested the temporary implantation of a silicone sheet, which, by formation of a connective tissue membrane, might prevent a new fixation of the cutaneous and muscular layers. For many years we have been using intradermal silicone injections and dermabrasion as well as chemical peeling. In our hands the combination of skin undermining followed by a dermabrasion 3 days later as advocated by Schmid [14] has given the best results. Since in most cases of senile lip wrinkling, the upper vermilion has become sunken and thin, we like to combine vermilion advancement with this technique, taking advantage of this approach for undermining (Figs. 20-4 and 20-5).

Figure 20-4. Undermining of the wrinkled labial skin.

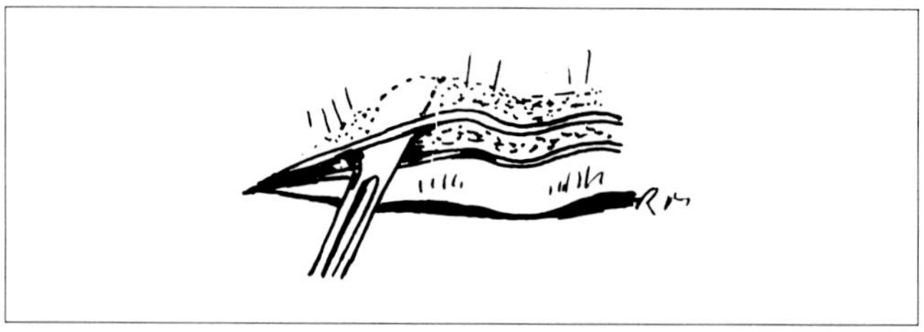

HEIGHT REDUCTION OF UPPER LIP

A long upper lip is emphasized by Cupid's bow displacement and an unpleasantly pointed nasolabial angle. A buffalo horn–shaped excision along the nasolabial junction solves both problems and leaves an inconspicuous scar (Fig. 20-6A). The excision can sometimes be reduced to a V-shaped one at the columellar base and at the alar bases (Fig. 20-6B).

DEEPENING OF SHALLOW PHILTRUM

Quite often it is not only the lip border that needs reshaping but also the philtrum, which is too shallow. The delicate philtrum, whose normal anatomy has been rather neglected until recently, gives the face a youthful and tender expression. We approach it by a short incision along the vermilion border. The dimple of the philtrum is deepened by dissecting the subcutaneous tissue (Fig. 20-7A,B) and shaping two inferiorly based flaps, which subsequently are pulled into two narrow tunnels running beneath the philtrum ridges (Fig. 20-6C). This technique

Figure 20-5. Patient before and after correction of wrinkled upper and lower lip.
A. Preoperative view.
B. Outline of resection.
C. Result after 1 year.

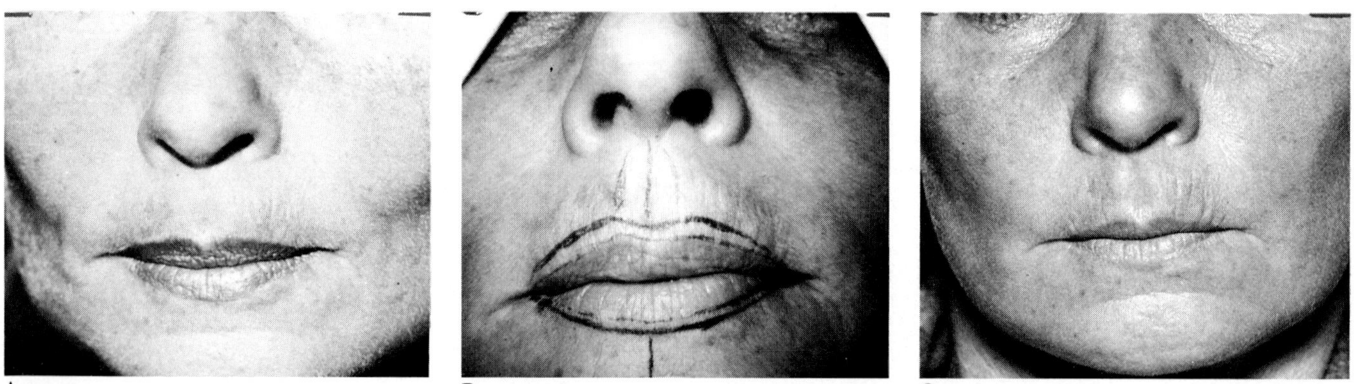

A B C

Figure 20-6
A. A buffalo horn–shaped excision along the nasolabial junction shortens a too long upper lip.
B. Another possibility is to shorten the lip by three isolated V-shaped resections at both alar bases and at the columellar base.

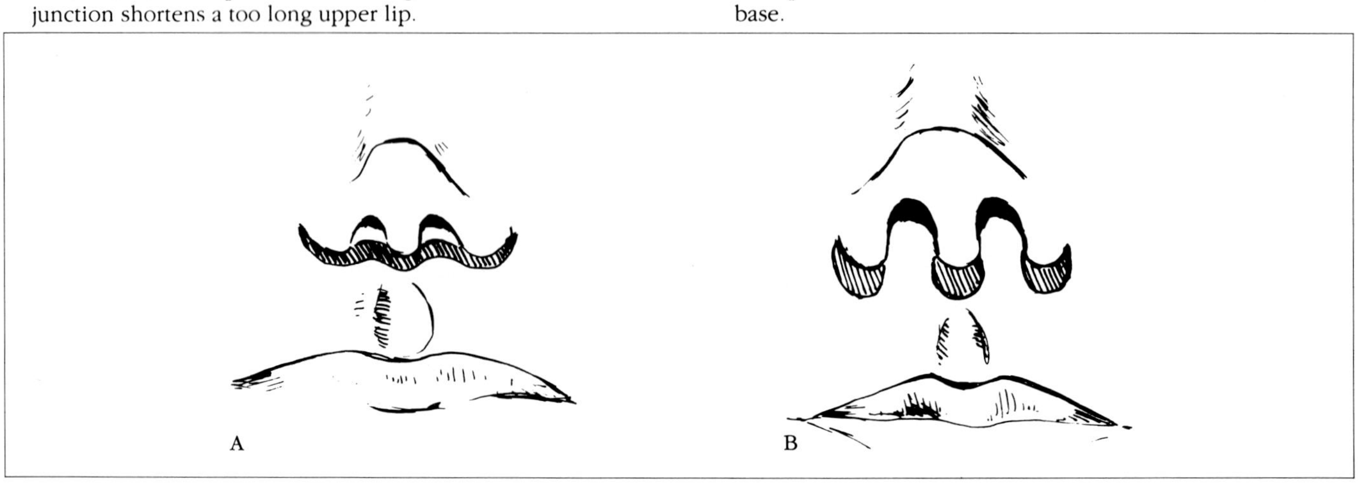

is somewhat similar to the one described by O'Connor and McGregor [10]. Mattress sutures tied over a small oval plastic sheet prevent hematoma and help maintain the desired concavity and depth during the healing process (Fig. 20-6D). In very selected cases we introduce a shell-shaped graft of auricular cartilage as reinforcement according to the method of Schmid [13].

REDUCTION OF FULLNESS OF THE LIPS

The aged upper lip is occasionally oversized and protruding, thereby causing a disproportion in the face elements. The enlarged lip can be corrected by excision of a wedge of soft tissue on the mucosal side going beyond the commissure and into the buccal mucosa on both sides. An underlying wedge of submucosa and some orbicularis muscle fibers are often included in the wedge (Fig. 20-8). For closure we use an over-and-over running suture. When an asymmetry or an irregularity of the free border of the lip results, we can still trim the edge and approximate with fine interrupted sutures. Care must be taken to avoid small dog-ears at both ends of the resection and not to interfere with the commissure. Often dog-ear resection is necessary in the mucosa. When we trim the free edge of the lip, the resulting scar has to hide inside the lip contact line when the lip is closed.

CORRECTION OF THE SAGGING DOUBLE-CONTOUR LOWER LIP

This deformity, frequently found in Mediterranean and Near Eastern populations, can be corrected by simple excision of the redundant tissue. Usually there is a ptosis of the inferior edge of the lower lip at the insertion of the ptotic quadratus labii inferioris muscle (Fig. 20-9).

DEEPENING OF THE LABIOMENTAL FOLDS

A straight lip-chin line makes an otherwise well-proportioned chin look ungracefully heavy. Gaining access through an incision at the vermilion border, we can dissect an adipodermal flap on an inferior pedicle. This flap is then turned over and pulled by means of transcutaneous sutures into a pocket dissected at the peak of the chin (Fig. 20-10). The too straight profile line is corrected in two ways: (1) by the depression halfway between lower lip and chin due to creation of the flap and (2) by the additional horizontal chin projection from the transposed flap volume.

CORRECTION OF THE TETHERED LIP

The too short tethered upper lip, usually encountered in young patients, can occasionally be a problem to be solved

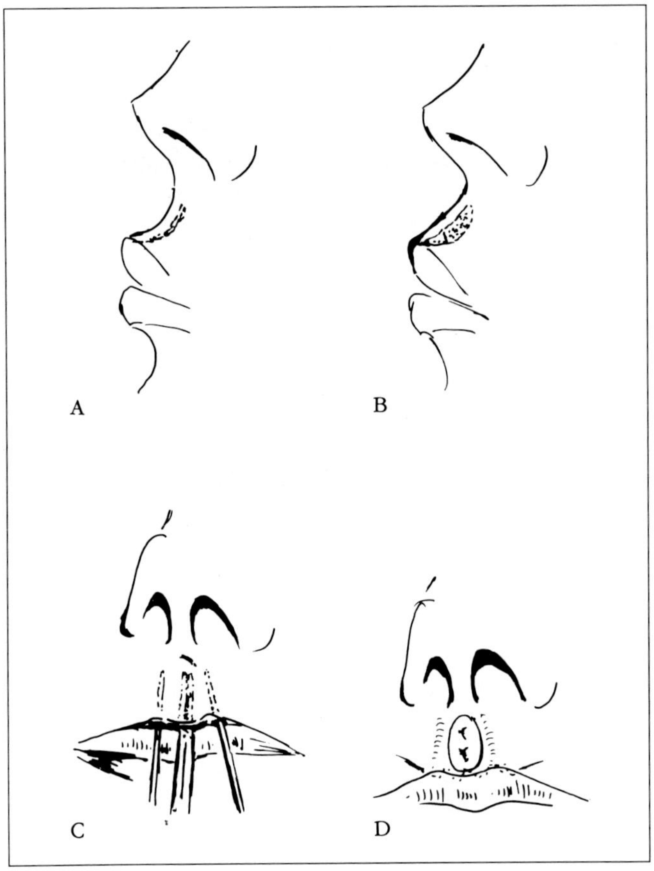

Figure 20-7
A, B, C, D. A shallow philtrum is on the one hand deepened by resection and on the other hand accentuated by the insertion of small thin dermis flaps into the philtral ridges that have been tunneled beforehand. A plastic sheet cut exactly to the form of the philtrum and mattress sutures serve as a stent dressing.

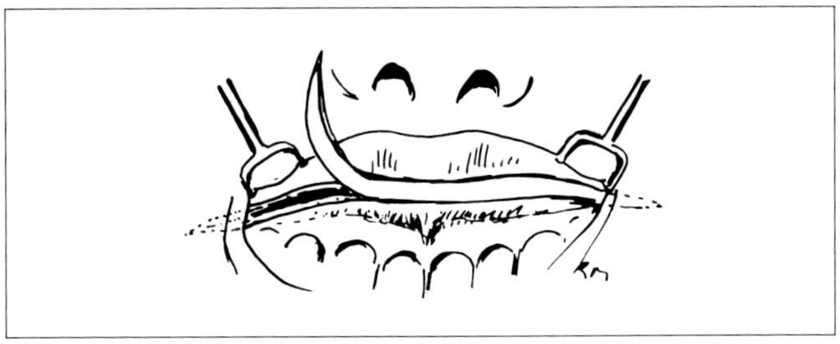

Figure 20-8. If a too voluminous lip has to be reduced, a wedge resection can be performed. Care has to be taken that the resection is done on the inner side of the lips where the vermilion blends into the mucosa.

in aging individuals, in whom the typical "Bugs Bunny" look may be even more obvious and unpleasant than in younger people [12].

This deformity is often associated with a narrow hump nose and with an increased projection of the anterior nasal spine. The upper lip is fixed to the maxilla at too high a level. We can push down the insertion of the whole lip by reducing the spine, dissecting the gingiva from the lower

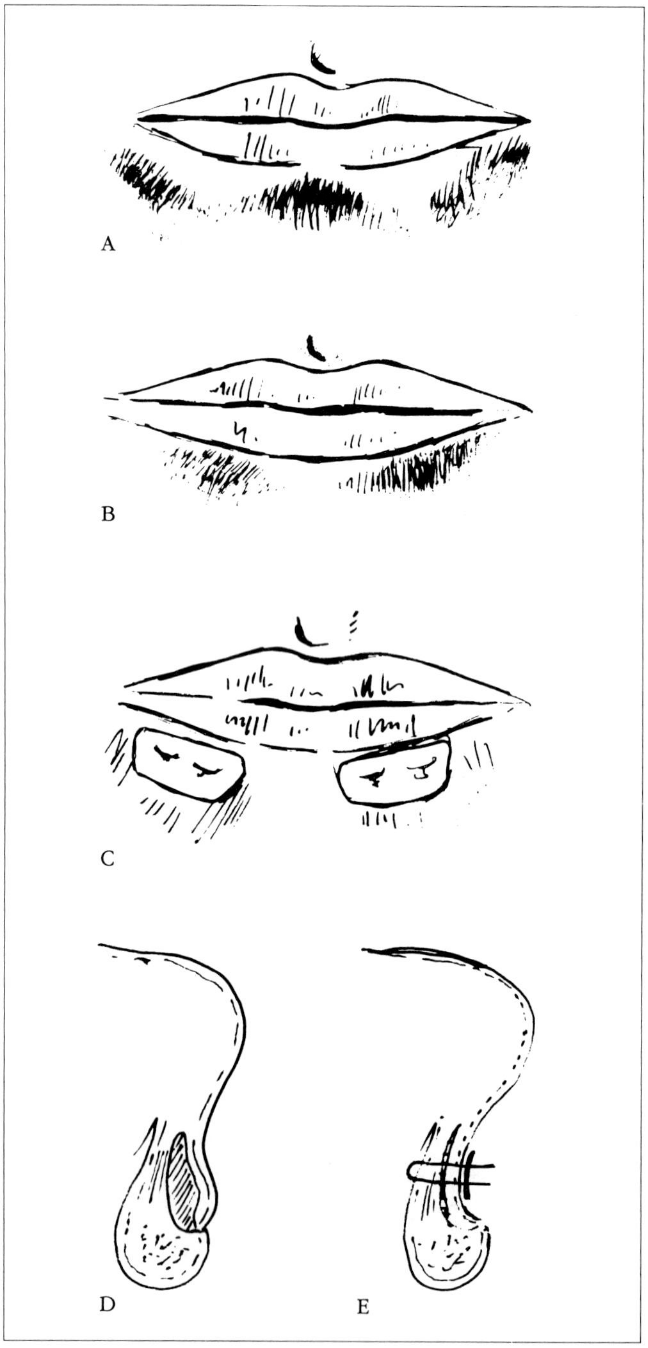

Figure 20-9
A, B, D. The sagging double-contour lower lip is resected by simple excision of the redundant tissue.
C, E. Translabial mattress sutures are kept in place for 4 to 5 days to prevent hematoma.

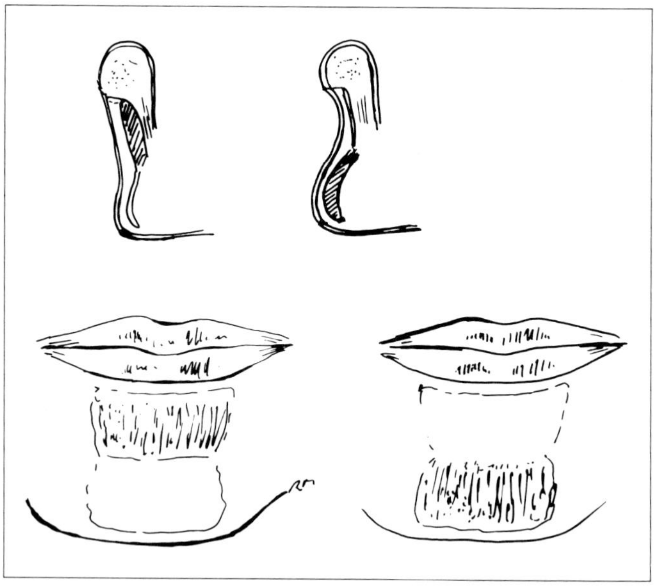

Figure 20-10. A straight lip-chin line can be resculptured by shifting dissected tissue from below the lower lip as a pedicle flap into the chin.

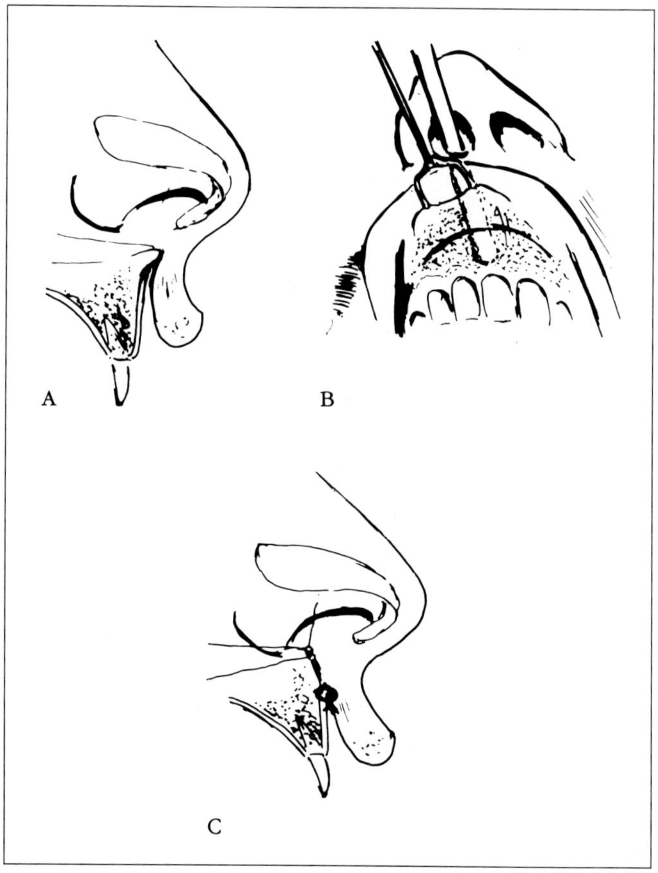

Figure 20-11
A. Tethered upper lip not covering the upper teeth.
B. Correction by dissection of the gingiva. Access is through the floor of the nasal vestibule.
C. Fixation of the soft tissue to the alveolar periosteum in a lower position.

rim of the piriform aperture nearly to the free border at the teeth in order to relax the labial soft tissue (Fig. 20-11). The depressor septi nasi muscle has to be severed beneath the spine, and sometimes sutures are necessary to fix the soft tissues in the now lower position to the alveolar periosteum. Reduction rhinoplasty can in addition be helpful by lowering the columellar base.

Collagen: A Complement to the Surgeon

Hale Tolleth

Need has long existed for a safe, effective material with which to replace lost or damaged dermal tissue. Autogenous tissue has been considered the ideal implant material, but the possibility of resorption, donor site morbidity, and late alteration of contour, and the necessary complexity of the surgery create limitations. As an alternative, various alloplastic materials, mainly of polymeric chemicals, have been successfully implanted [3]. However, these have yielded, at best, mixed results.

In 1977 Knapp et al. [6] published the results of a study in which highly purified bovine dermal collagen was injected into certain dermal contour defects. They postulated that the material would be integrated into the skin and vascularized, and contour improvement would occur [7]. The work has continued, and widely varying clinical conditions have been treated, at this point in approximately 20,000 patients [1].

Production of injectable collagen includes the selective enzymatic hydrolysis of the telopeptide end regions of the collagen molecule, these nonhelical portions being the site of most intraspecies and chemical variability and therefore of most antigenicity [11]. The solubilized collagen is dispersed in physiologic saline and 0.3% lidocaine to allow it to be injected through a fine-gauge needle. When this dispersion of collagen is injected and warmed to body temperature, the saline is absorbed and a form implant of collagen fibrils is created. The implant generally elicits neither foreign body response nor immunologic rejection. Moreover, unlike alloplastic materials, it is assimilated into the tissue and therefore is not subject to migration from the implant site. Later supplemental injections may be required to maintain correction as the bovine collagen is subject to the same stresses and enzymatic processes as human collagen.

INDICATIONS

Collagen has been used to enhance contour by elevating depressed lesions to the level of surrounding skin. The stigmata of aging, scars resulting from acne, infection, disease, surgery, and trauma have been treated [5, 15]. The tissue loss from linear scleroderma, Romberg's disease, lipodystrophy, and steroid injection has been augmented. Collagen has been used both before and after surgery to enhance results, the best indications being small-volume architectural and textural defects. It is not indicated for sagging or redundant skin. It does not replace surgical procedures such as rhytidectomy, dermabrasion, or chemical peeling; however, it has been of value in "fine tuning" the surgical results. Certain complications of cosmetic surgery have been improved.

PATIENT SELECTION

Prior to treatment, a medical history is taken to determine whether the patient has a significant history of allergy or autoimmune disease. Thus far, there is no evidence that collagen injections might exacerbate such a disease, but it seems prudent to avoid challenging the patient so afflicted with another potential antigen.

A screening skin test is given in the forearm, using a 0.1-ml dose, intradermally. Signs of sensitivity include local erythema, tenderness, swelling, and induration persisting more than 6 hours or occurring 24 hours after injection. In order to exclude patients having a delayed response, treatment is deferred for 28 days following skin testing. Positive skin tests have been noted in approximately 3 percent of patients.

TREATMENT PRINCIPLES

The outcome of treatment depends both on the choice of the lesion to be treated and on the technique used. Unknowns that might affect the final result include the configuration of the lesion, induration, skin thickness, area, tension, presence of scar, vascularity, motion, aging process, and disease processes.

There are three guiding principles of great importance: Treat supple shallow lesions, inject intradermally, and overcorrect when possible. Although collagen can be injected subcutaneously, the padding effect of fat obscures its presence unless large volumes are required.

LESION SELECTION

Injectable collagen affords the best correction in soft, distensible lesions, without significant induration. It has been observed that firm scarred areas, as in acne, sometimes seem to soften after injection. Certain lesions, such as the "ice pick" acne scars and viral pox scars, have been difficult if not impossible to improve.

Since the condensed implant represents only about 30 percent of the injected volume, multiple treatments are required at a minimum of 2-week intervals. Overcorrection at the time of each injection enhances the possibility of the smallest number of treatment sessions. The patient is usually told that at least three, and possibly more, treatment sessions will be needed since only about 30 percent of the volume placed represents collagen.

METHOD

Prior to injection, makeup is removed and the area is cleansed. The lesion is marked with a surgical marking pen, with the patient in the sitting position since contour change will occur with the patient supine. Usually the patient is asked to check the marking to make certain the area of concern will be treated.

A 27- or 30-gauge needle is gently inserted very superficially, intradermally, with the bevel down, giving a firm, blanched appearance to the skin as the collagen is injected. Injection intradermally as the needle is withdrawn, or by multiple insertions, is acceptable technique, although the latter may give a more superficial application and therefore be more effective. Some practice is required, and inadequacy of results in the earliest cases done by a physician can often be traced to lack of experience.

TREATMENT PROBLEMS

Acne

Injectable collagen works best in well-resolved, soft, distensible, saucer-shaped scars. Immature, indurated, sharply marginated, or ice pick lesions are difficult to inject. Experience has shown that injection of collagen into these indurated areas may be followed by some degree of softening. Areas of atrophy due to steroid injection may be effectively treated.

Scars

Soft, atrophic, and distensible scars can often be improved. Linear contracted scars are more likely to be amenable to Z-plasty or similar methods. Injectable collagen is not indicated for hypertrophic or keloidal scarring. Depressed scars, and the depression associated with skin grafts, may show improvement although, as previously noted, marginated viral pox scars, e.g., chickenpox scars, have been disappointingly resistant.

Atrophy

Experience with lipodystrophy, scleroderma, and hemifacial atrophy has been good when the defect is not too extensive. Surgical methods, as with dermal fat grafts, may be indicated, to be followed by "feathering" of the edges or "touch-up" with collagen.

AESTHETIC SURGERY

Not all of the patients who request collagen therapy are good candidates for its use. Careful assessment and judgment based on experience will allow the plastic surgeon to advise whether surgery, collagen injections, or both should be used (Fig. 20-12). Rarely, the alternatives are of equal value, and a choice will require considerations of expense, morbidity, and complications.

Deepening of the nasolabial folds, glabellar creasing, and perioral wrinkles have been most commonly and effectively treated (Fig. 20-13). In each of these areas, some sophistication of judgment is required since the alternative surgical method such as forehead and facial rhytidectomy, dermabrasion, or phenol peel may be more appropriate.

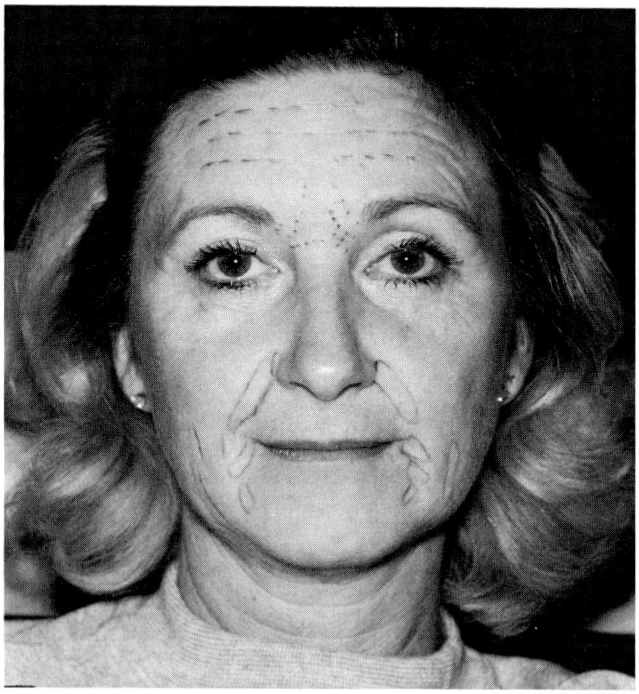

Figure 20-12. Pretreatment markings for contour irregularities due to aging process. Patient was treated with a total of 22.7 ml in six treatment sessions.

The improvement of transverse creases of the forehead and neck has been uneven—sometimes excellent and sometimes not. The best results are obtained with multiple, very superficial injections, as opposed to injection as the needle is withdrawn. When this procedure is successful, the improvement is arguably superior to that achieved with surgical methods.

The periorbital wrinkles should be approached with a certain amount of caution, in terms of both what one is trying to accomplish and the amount to be injected. Since the periorbital and lid skin is very thin, the collagen may be visible for prolonged periods as small, whitish prominences. For the same reason, overcorrection should be avoided. Injection must be very superficial, particularly when one is modifying an excessively prominent nasoorbital furrow at the junction of the nose skin and lid.

Vertical cheek furrows are rather like nasolabial folds in response to the treatment. Results have been gratifying. Less gratifying is the effect of the injection on fine, numerous parallel lines caused by too much sun. One might be better advised to consider alternatives.

There are often multiple fine oblique wrinkles about the commissure of the mouth that do not qualify as the usual perioral wrinkles. These can be successfully treated. The "commissural shadowing" or hollowness just inferior and lateral to the commissures can often be improved, a worthwhile project since it may be present after an excellent rhytidectomy.

Other contour deformities following rhytidectomy are occasionally seen, including excessively hollow cheeks, depressions along the mandible, and alterations of contour caused by defatting of the neck (Fig. 20-14). Treatment of these problems with injectable collagen offers a superior alternative to the surgical possibilities.

The small parallel depressions occasionally seen on the dorsum of the nose after rhinoplasty have been treated by injection with good results (Fig. 20-15). Recontouring the pinched tip, symmetrizing the tip, and expanding a hidden columella have been essentially unsuccessful. Injection has brought reasonable results with minor degrees of saddlenose. Tissue tension may thwart one's best efforts.

LONG-TERM EFFICACY

The major concern with the use of this modality is the length of time that correction will be maintained. It should be used with the understanding that in at least one-half of the patients additional injections at 12- to 24-month intervals may be required. These supplemental "touch-ups" vary from 20 to 40 percent of the original volume used. The many possible factors contributing to resorption have not been delineated although the degree of cross-linking in the material may be important and amenable to adjustment in the future. Since certain patients seem not to sustain correction for any appreciable period, patient consultations should be conservative.

PROBLEMS AND CONCERNS

Problems associated with the injection of collagen have been relatively few. Skin tests were reported as positive in 3 percent of patients and included swelling, pinkness, tenderness, and induration at the skin test site; 0.6 percent of patients skin-tested reported both local complaints and systemic complaints of myalgia or arthralgia.

At the treatment site, adverse responses were similar, occurring in 1.3 percent of patients (40 percent of whom had unreported positive skin tests). Sensitization occurred in 0.6 percent of patients, usually within 2 weeks of the sensitizing dose. Treatment with antihistamines and steroids has brought temporary improvement, and all reactions have subsided with time, usually 3 or 4 months.

Immunologic testing has shown that in subjects in whom antibodies could be measured they were found only in those with adverse skin responses, and they were targeted to the implant, not to the type I and III collagen of the human skin.

SUMMARY

Injectable collagen is a useful adjunct in the treatment of contour and textural deformities seen in certain diseases, trauma, scarring, and aging. Complications and problems are local and few in number. Persistence of correction in any individual is uncertain, and supplemental injections will often be required.

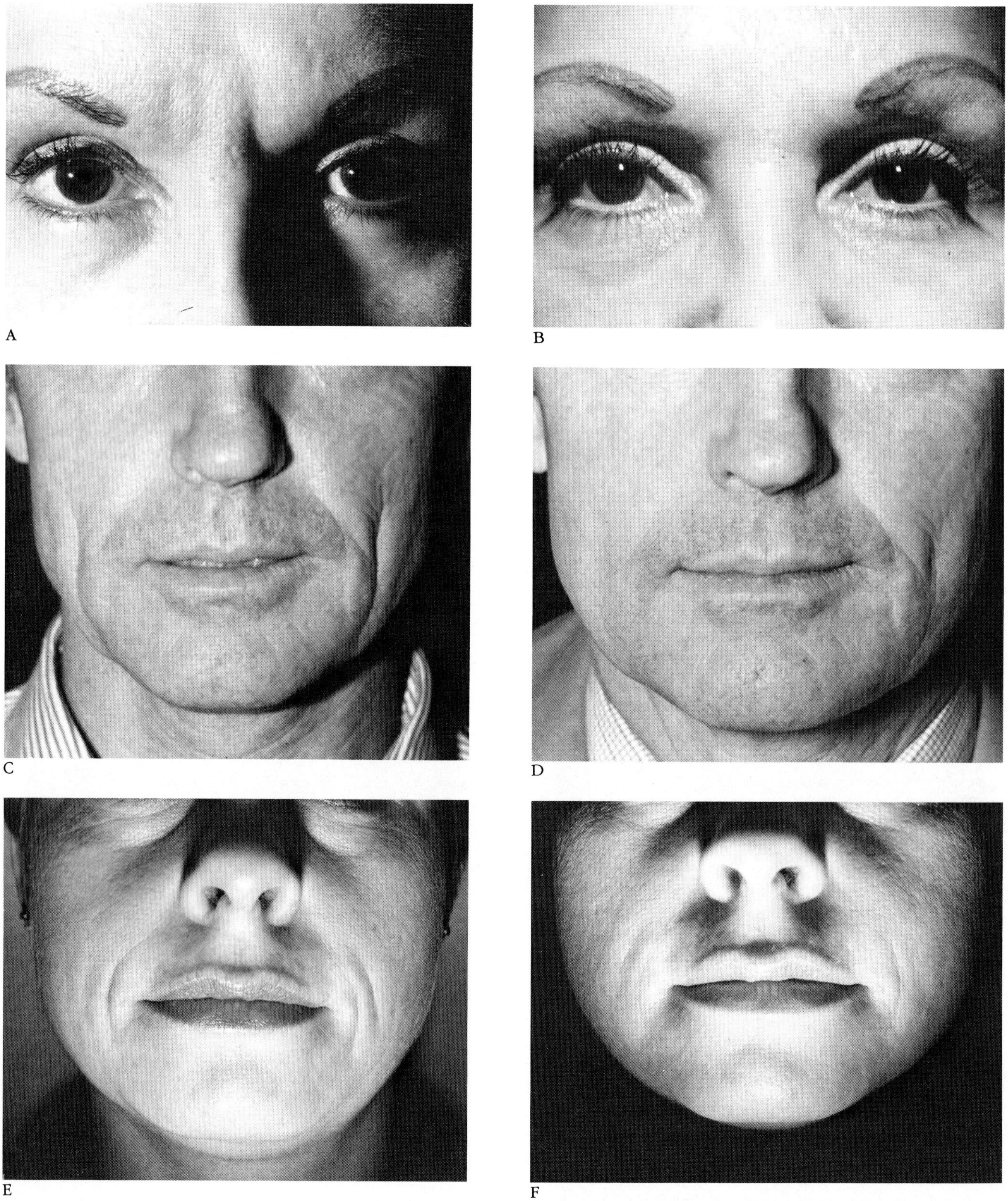

Figure 20-13. Pretreatment condition and posttreatment result following collagen injection.

A, B. Deep glabellar creases treated over a period of 18 months with average injection volume of 0.6 ml; 15 months after treatment.

C, D. Deep parallel cheek creases treated with 2.7 ml in six treatment sessions; 1½ months after treatment.

E, F. Nasolabial creasing treated with 6 ml over a 3-month period; on completion.

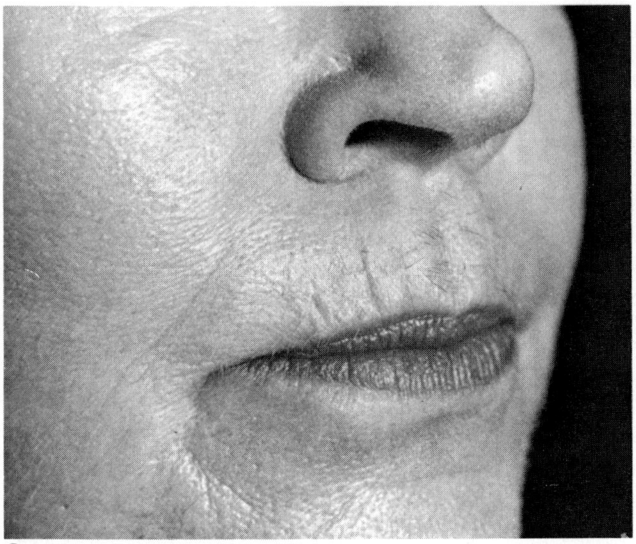

G

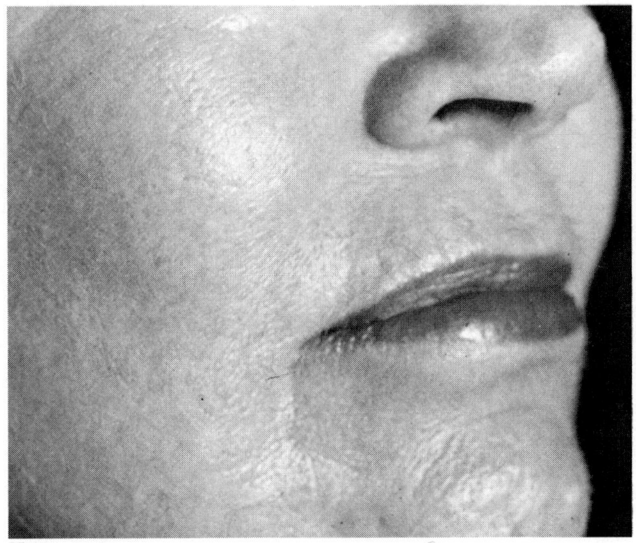

H

Figure 20-13 (continued)
G, H. Perioral wrinkles treated with 1.7 ml in two treatment sessions; 2 months after last treatment.

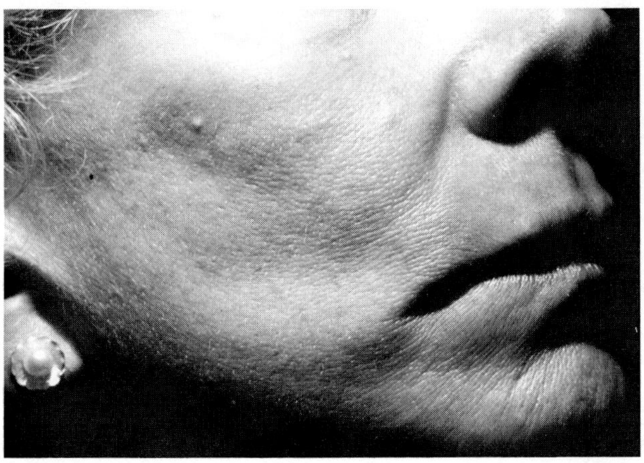

A

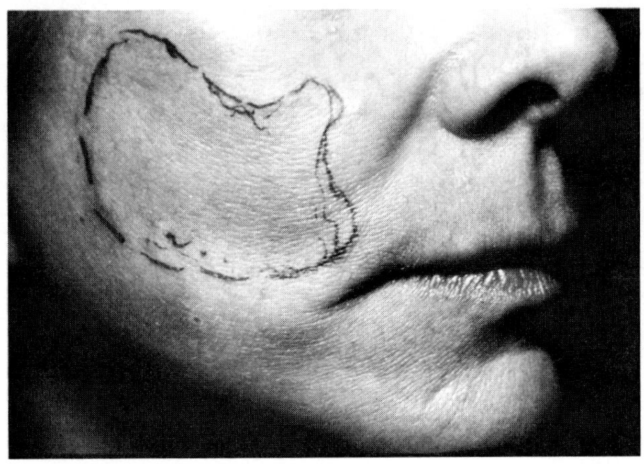

B

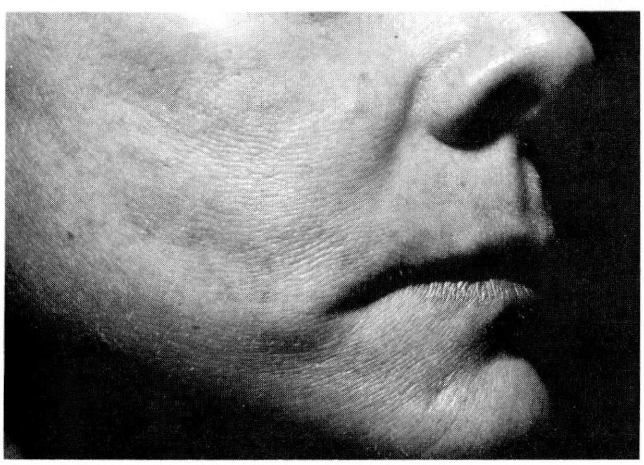

C

Figure 20-14
A, B. Hollowness of cheeks following rhytidectomy.
C. Treated with 9 ml for each cheek in three sessions.

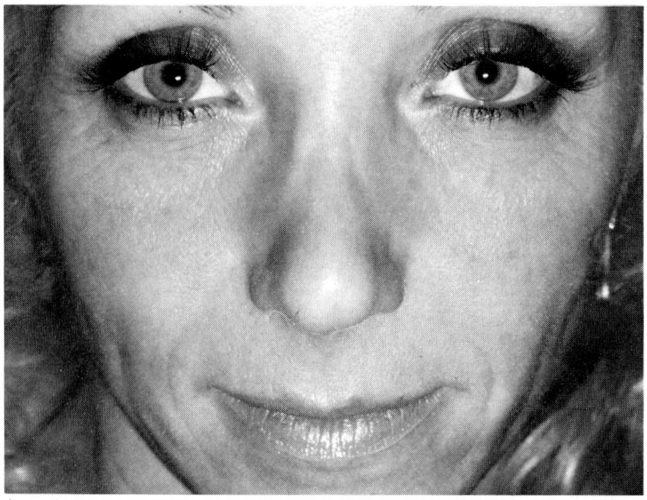

A

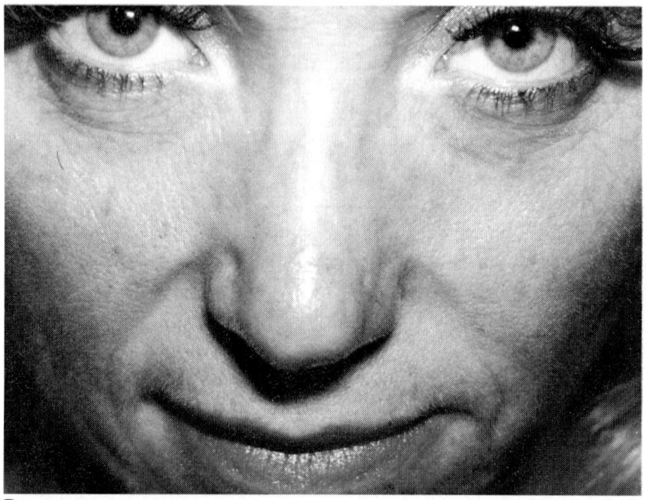

B

Figure 20-15
A. Postrhinoplasty depressions on nasal dorsum treated with 3 ml over a 3-month period.
B. One year after treatment.

Comparison of Techniques

Paule Regnault

At present there are four ways to avoid or delay signs of aging or to achieve complete facial rejuvenation: local excision, dermabrasion, chemical peeling, or injection therapy. Selection is not only objective but subjective. While patients must express their desire on the basis of the advantages and disadvantages of each technique, it is wise to consider also that the surgeon may be more skilled in one technique than the others. In this section, objective reasons are offered for using one specific procedure according to local conditions only.

DISSEMINATED FACIAL DEFECTS

Wrinkles Caused by Solar Exposure

Chronic sun exposure often produces numerous small, deep wrinkles in a dried skin with loss of elasticity. Although a face-lift can improve their appearance, it must be completed by either a dermabrasion or a chemical peel, at a separate stage. It seems that a chemical peel gives a more lasting result, but the permanent blanching and risk of peripheral pigmentation are greater, especially for those with dark complexion. Therefore, the author performs a mixed treatment in such a case: face-lift, dermabrasion 3 months later, and injection of the remaining wrinkles at 6 months.

Acne Scars

Deep and numerous pits require a mixed treatment. In young patients, dermabrasion is performed several times, usually at 3- to 6-month intervals, with gradual fading of the depressions. Local excision of deeper scars is beneficial and may be done in conjunction with dermabrasion. Local infiltration of collagen is performed once dermabrasion is completed and gives good results in the softer, more superficial scars. A classic face-lift with skin undermining of the cheeks and suturing under tension is useful in older individuals where there is sufficient elasticity of the skin.

Actin Keratoses

Multiple skin lesions due to sun exposure or aging can be treated by dermabrasion using a scalpel held tangentially, a prep sponge, or mechanical dermabrasion with diamond cylinders or wire brushes.

Pigmentation

Darkening of the skin can follow use of estrogens, chemical peeling, or dermabrasion. It may be improved by a dermabrasion, but all sun exposure and estrogen therapy must be suppressed for 6 months. Also, a maximum protective sunscreen must be worn daily.

LOCALIZED DEFECTS

Some areas or defects benefit more than others from localized treatments: (1) glabellar and upper nasal area, (2) crow's-feet, (3) perioral wrinkles, (4) nasolabial folds, and (5) chin wrinkles. With any of these problems the following procedures are available: excision, dermabrasion, chemical peeling, or injection therapy. It is often very difficult to decide objectively which one is the best. In cases of uncertainty, or when all four techniques have grounds for hesitation, the situation should be explained to the patient and the choice left to the individual who must accept the sequelae. If the patient cannot decide, the surgeon's skill and preference is the next consideration. However, the author has developed certain guidelines based on observation of results obtained over the past 20 years.

Glabellar Wrinkles

Previously, the author used direct excisions, but the final scar was unpredictable — often very good but occasionally terrible and of great concern to the patient. Therefore, direct excision is *not* now advocated. Instead, a forehead-lift with subcutaneous muscular resection is preferred. When the forehead-lift is refused, my second choice is injection therapy using collagen. From previous experience with liquid silicone, the results of injection therapy in this region are excellent. Dermabrasion is the third choice.

Crow's-Feet

These wrinkles are part not only of the palpebral complex but also of the temporal region, marking the junction between face and forehead. Usually they are treated as part of a face-lift or blepharoplasty. Occasionally they are corrected as an isolated entity several years after another procedure. When the lines are *not* deep and have recently appeared, collagen injection is sufficient and is tried first. If injections do not give satisfactory results, dermabrasion or chemical peeling may be used. When the lines are *deep* and permanent, a temporal rhytidectomy with direct traction on the orbicularis oculi muscle is the best treatment. The favored technique is a curved incision inside the temporal hair or at the hairline (according to the patient's and surgeon's preference) with undermining over the total temporal region down to the canthal area. The orbicularis oculi muscle is left attached, but its lateral edge is spread and sutured to the deep fascia at several points. More skin may be removed when the scar is located in front of the hairline. A direct excision of a large part of the wrinkled area may be undertaken at the same time, in the shape of a triangle, as is done in the upward face-lifting.

Perioral Lines

Lip lines, especially on the upper lip, are often associated with some degree of atrophy; i.e., the lip is thin and the vermilion is reduced. In the younger patient, with few and superficial wrinkles, injection therapy is the best treatment. When the lip volume is satisfactory but the wrinkles are more numerous, chemical peeling or dermabrasion offers excellent results. When wrinkles are numerous and deep, surgery is the best solution. In women, the removal of a 2-mm strip of epidermis at the upper limit of the vermilion, on the skin side, as described by Meyer gives good improvement. In men, it is better to remove a 2- to 3-mm strip of full skin at the upper limit of the lip with undermining of the wrinkled skin down to the vermilion. Surgery of the upper lip brings some swelling for 1 to 2 months. Scars are rarely visible, but occasionally it may be necessary to do a secondary dermabrasion of the scar.

Nasolabial Folds

These folds sometimes require specific treatment apart from rhytidectomy. In certain patients, deep folds may appear in the twenties, because of local features and muscle anatomy. In these cases injection therapy may help to diminish the depth of the folds but will never eradicate them. Peeling or dermabrasion has a very temporary effect, while a classic face-lift with defatting offers a better result. In older individuals, when a face-lift has been done recently or is contraindicated, direct excision of the fold remains the only way to eliminate the excess skin. The fold itself is replaced by a fine scar, which is less visible than the previous skin pleat.

Chin Wrinkles

Chin skin is very thick and often sebaceous; wrinkles may be deep. Although few people complain about them, some patients may be very concerned. Surgery is not indicated in this area except for a change of volume. The best way to remove chin lines is chemical peel or dermabrasion. Only when lines are recent is injection therapy of benefit. When they are deep, injections offer little improvement on account of skin thickness and fibrosis.

REFERENCES

1. Collagen Corporation, collected patient data, 1982.
2. Delerm, A., and Elbaz, J. S. Cheiloplastie des lèvres minces: Proposition d'une technique. *Ann. Chir. Plast.* 20:243, 1975.
3. Helseth, D. L., Lechner, J. H., and Veis, A. Role of the amino-terminal extra-helical region of Type-1 collagen in directing the 4D overlap in fibrogenesis. *Biopolymers* 18:305, 1979.
4. Hinderer, U., and Meise, T. Treatment of the deep wrinkles of the upper lip by means of temporary subdermal implantation of silicone sheets. *Rev. Esp. Cir. Plast.* 3:265, 1970.
5. Kaplan, E. N., Falces, E., and Tolleth, H. Clinical utilization of injectable collagen. *Ann. Plast. Surg.* In press.
6. Knapp, T. R., Kaplan, E. N., and Daniels, J. R. Injectable collagen for soft tissue augmentation. *Plast. Reconstr. Surg.* 60:398, 1977.
7. Knapp, T. R., Luck, E., and Daniels, J. R. Behavior of solubilized collagen as a bioimplant. *J. Surg. Res.* 23:96, 1977.
8. Meyer, R. Dauerhaftigkeit, Gefahren und Misserfolge kosmetischer Eingriffe im Gesichtsbereich. *Aesthet. Med.* (Berlin) 13:273, 1964.
9. Meyer, R., and Kesselring, U. K. Aesthetic surgery in the perioral region. *Aesthetic Plast. Surg.* 1:61, 1976.
10. O'Connor, G. B., and McGregor, M. W. Surgical formation of the philtrum and the cutaneous upsweep. *Am. J. Surg.* 95:227, 1958.
11. Piez, K. A. Primary Structure. In G. N. Ramachandran and A. H. Reddi (eds.), *Biochemistry of Collagen.* New York: Plenum, 1976. Pp. 1–44.
12. Rees, T., and Wood-Smith, D. *Cosmetic Facial Surgery.* Philadelphia: Saunders, 1974.
13. Schmid, E. The Use of Auricular Cartilage and Composite Grafts in Reconstruction of the Upper Lip with Special Reference to Construction of the Philtrum. In *Transactions of the Third International Congress of Plastic Surgery.* Amsterdam: Excerpta Medica, 1964. P. 306.
14. Schmid, E. Surgical method for removing wrinkles, *Chir. Plast.* 2:239, 1974.
15. Stegman, S. J., and Tromovitch, T. A. Implantation of collagen for depressed scars. *J. Dermatol. Surg. Oncol.* 6:450, 1980.

V. Breast Surgery

21. Breast Reduction

Paule Regnault
Rollin K. Daniel

Reduction mammaplasty reduces breast size by glandular resection and improves shape by tightening the skin brassiere. In the past decade, patients' expectations have expanded to include a more aesthetically shaped breast with acceptable scars rather than just a size reduction. Surgical techniques can be divided into two basic methods: the preplanned pattern with a parenchymal paddle versus a "cut as you go" lateral wedge resection. The square breast characteristic of previous eras is being replaced by a more projecting conical breast with an acceptable complication rate.

HISTORY

Reduction mammaplasty began in antiquity for treatment of massive virginal hypertrophy and later for reduction of large breasts. The divergent methods of nipple-areola complex (NAC) transposition versus NAC graft were gradually resolved in favor of a one-stage transposition, with free grafts reserved for massive hypertrophy or medical indications [94]. Numerous historical reviews are available to the interested reader. A recent overview by Letterman and Schurter [41] is particularly rewarding.

It is our preference to view the evolution of reduction mammaplasty as related to its three basic components: (1) transposition of the NAC, (2) glandular resection, and (3) skin excision. In the early 1900s Morestin and Guinard reported their experience with discontinuous resections of up to 1400 gm performed via an inframammary incision [41]. Following World War I, Aubert, Passot, and Axhausen extended these procedures to include NAC transposition via a periareolar incision, lateral wedge resection of glandular tissue, and excision of excess skin [41]. However, it was Biesenberger [8] who devised a reproducible, reliable operation, as detailed in his classic text *Deformitaten und kosmetische Operationen der weiblichen Brust.* His operation consists of a preliminary periareolar skin resection followed by extensive skin undermining, lateral gland resection, circular rotation of the remaining breast tissue, and skin closure in an inverted-T configuration. Until the 1960s, this technique, as modified by Gillies and McIndoe [3, 30], was the principal method of reduction mammaplasty [95].

After World War II, plastic surgery centers were established throughout the world, and large reduction mammaplasties became commonplace. The Biesenberger operation was found to have a high complication rate, due to its extensive skin undermining, which resulted in skin sloughs and compromise of the NAC. Strombeck [87–91] introduced a horizontal bipedicled flap method that was based on the Schwarzmann [78] concept of dermal vascularization of the NAC and the Wise pattern of skin incisions. His procedure was quickly accepted as complications were few and the technique easily mastered [59]. Pitanguy [54–56] stressed that incisions should be modified for each breast and that contour resection should be done, followed by plication to improve aesthetic contour. Skoog [80, 81] introduced a pedicled modification whereas McKissock [45–48] dramatically advanced the operation by transposing the NAC on a vertical bipedicle. Currently, the vertical bipedicle has been split into a superior pedicle by Weiner et al. [96, 97] and an inferior pedicle by Courtiss and Goldwyn [14, 15]. However, the latter technique denotes a distinct shift from thin circumferentially isolated pedicles toward broad parenchymal paddles that retain their attachment to the chest wall. These techniques retain the basic inverted-T incision, a parenchymal blood supply to the NAC, and resection of glandular tissue both medially and laterally.

In contrast, the lateralizing procedures introduced by Dufourmentel and Mouly [17–19] consist of a lateral wedge resection of breast tissue plus upward transposition of the NAC [49, 76]. The problem of lateral extension into the axilla was eliminated by Regnault [64–67] with introduction of the B-technique. The advantages of this method include minimal risk to the NAC as it is not isolated on a pedicle, en bloc resection of the glandular tissue, elimination of a medial scar, and an aesthetic shape that improves with time. Currently, breast reduction is a safe operation with an acceptable complication rate [51].

PATHOPHYSIOLOGY AND CLASSIFICATION

Anatomically, the breast is an ectodermal organ derived from skin whose glands penetrate the underlying mesoderm and become surrounded by fat. At puberty, breast growth is manifested by both glandular development (ductal, lobulareolar, stromal) and fat deposition. The relative amounts of glandular tissue versus fat, as manifested by firmness of the breast, are a critical factor for determining the method of breast reduction. The patient with breast hypertrophy most commonly consults a plastic surgeon at three different life stages, each with distinct pathology and surgical limitations.

Developmental Hypertrophy

Breast development is stimulated by the action of estradiol, progesterone, and prolactin on receptors within the breast tissue. It is theorized that breast growth ceases once the limited number of receptors have been stimulated. In the nongravid young (age 15–25) female, breast hypertrophy is primarily due to glandular enlargement, which results in a firm, minimally ptotic breast. In addition, it may be associated with three systemic conditions that the plastic surgeon must diagnose: moderate obesity, virginal hypertrophy, and endocrine abnormalities. Obese hypertrophy is characterized by increased fat deposition and exogenous obesity. Virginal hypertrophy is caused by an abnormal end organ response rather than elevated hormone levels. Although progesterone therapy may arrest hypertrophy, surgery is necessary to reduce the volume, but it is best delayed until age 16 if possible. Endocrine hypertrophy is due to endocrine abnormalities and is signaled by precocious puberty, thus mandating evaluation by an endocrinologist.

Pregnancy Hypertrophy and Postpartum Involution

During the third to fourth month of pregnancy, human placental lactogen causes the breasts to enlarge, resulting in hypertrophy and hyperplasia of the glandular tissue. As the breast and areola increase in size, the skin envelope is stretched and the dermis may "fracture," causing development of striae. Following cessation of lactation, the glandular-fatty ratio of the breast generally returns to its prepregnancy state provided absolute weight gain was limited. Unfortunately, rapid size increase stretches both the skin and the internal connective tissue envelope. In the postpartum patient who previously wore a C or D cup bra, the breast generally remains ptotic, with flatness superiorly and fullness inferiorly. Certain patients will become hypoplastic and remain ptotic, requiring either augmentation or mastopexy. In some cases, postgravid hypertrophy will persist and the breast will be larger than before. This lack of involution results in persistence of ductal and stromal hypertrophy as well as increased fat deposit.

Postmenopausal Involution

Following passage of the childbearing years and stabilization of marriages, many middle-aged women will seek breast reduction. The constant triad of heaviness, pain, and clothing restrictions plus increasing ptosis causes them to look for correction. In certain patients, breast growth will actually occur in the menopausal period. It is characterized by lobular atrophy with fat replacement. Thus, a detailed history of breast development and changes is essential to understand the patient's problems.

Classification of hypertrophic breasts can be made according to their shape and consistency, or on the predicted volume of excision (Figs. 21-1 and 21-2, Table 21-1). Excisional volumes are based on the difference

Table 21-1. Classification of breast hypertrophy

I. Consistency
- Hypertrophic
  - Limited ptosis, upper quadrants full
  - Predominance of glandular tissue
  - Tight skin brassiere
- Pendulous
  - Significant ptosis, upper quadrants flat
  - Predominance of fat
  - Loose, sagging skin brassiere

II. Volume in excess

0–200	minor
200–500	moderate
500–1500	major
Over 1500	gigantomastia

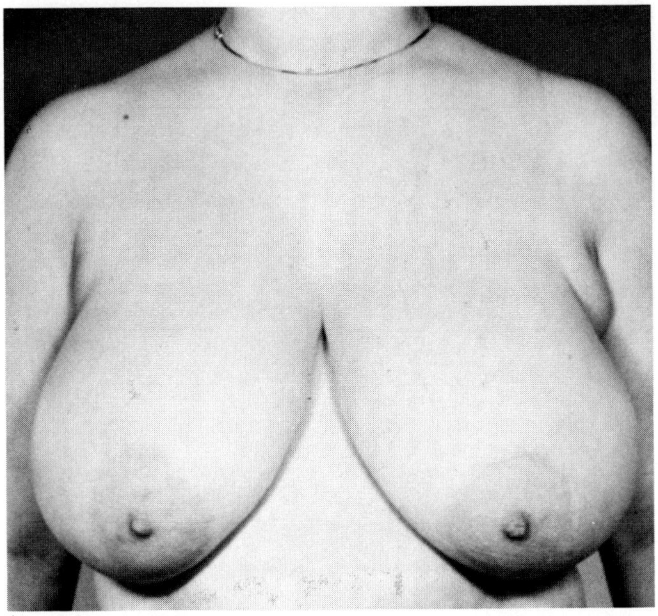

A

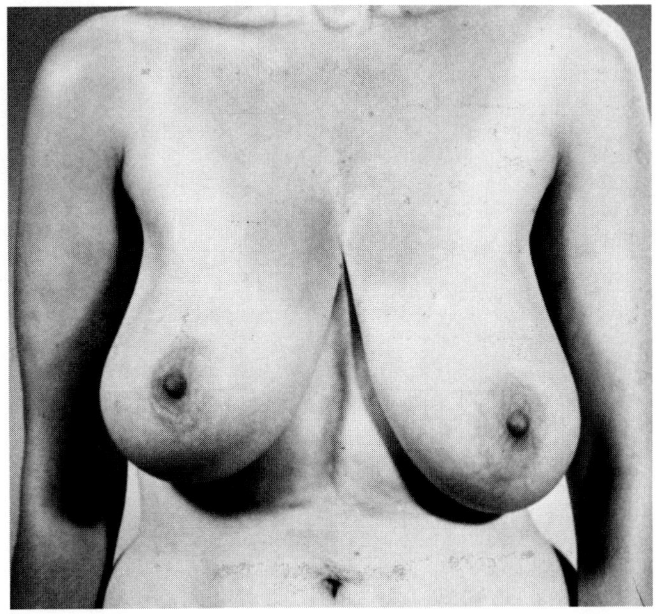

B

Figure 21-1. Classification of hypertrophy based on breast shape and consistency.
A. Firm tense breast with upper quadrant fullness and tight skin brassiere.
B. Ptotic large breasts with upper quadrant flatness and a loose sagging skin brassiere.

between preoperative and desired brassiere cup size. For patients with a 36 to 38 brassiere band size, 200 cc per cup size approximates the amount of tissue excision. Thus, a patient with a brassiere size of 38DD will require a minimum excision of 600 gm to reach a 38B. Differences in skin redundancy and glandular composition will also influence the excision.

CONSULTATION

Medical History

A medical history is taken with emphasis on the breasts. An inquiry is made as to specific complaints: breast pain, poor posture, personal hygiene, and psychologic problems. Next, breast development is reviewed: growth at puberty, influence of hormone ingestion (especially birth control pills), planned or previous pregnancies, current breast condition (pain, masses, tenderness, fibrocystic disease), brassiere size, and previous breast surgery. Increasing use of the periareolar incision for breast biopsy makes it necessary to ask specifically about biopsies. A general inquiry is made in regard to cardiopulmonary state, metabolic diseases, medications, and other factors influencing candidacy for general anesthesia.

Indications and Contraindications

The indication for a reduction mammaplasty is a combination of physical and psychologic complaints including reduction of weight for comfort, reduction in size for clothing, and aesthetic improvement. Large pendulous breasts are themselves painful and can cause significant physical deformities. Cervical arthritis with compensating kyphosis and respiratory difficulties in the older patient are documented. As reported by Pitanguy [55], the primary complaints in order of frequency for patients seeking reduction mammaplasty are premenstrual discomfort, back pain, bad posture, psychologic problems, and shoulder strap marks. Intertrigo in the submammary fold also occurs. Since ready-to-wear clothes are based on a 34B size, these patients find it hard to buy clothes, especially properly fitting brassieres. In addition, many athletic activities are either difficult or socially embarrassing. Psychologically, these patients are sensitive about the size of their breasts and constantly vulnerable to an endless series of jokes and remarks with sexual innuendos. As emphasized by Goin and Goin [31], teenagers are especially concerned about their self-image and are quite labile emotionally. In contrast to the volume reduction requested by teenagers, most women who have had children want both a volume reduction and correction of the pendulous deformity.

The operation is specifically contraindicated in the patient who is not willing to accept *significant* scars, the possible loss of nipple sensitivity, and potential inability to lactate. General constraints are those of any elective surgery.

Motivation

The patient is asked why she wishes to have the operation at this time and what her expectations are in regard to final size, shape, and scars. The majority of surgeons believe that patients will be satisfied with a reduction in bulk and any improvement in shape is a bonus. However, the study

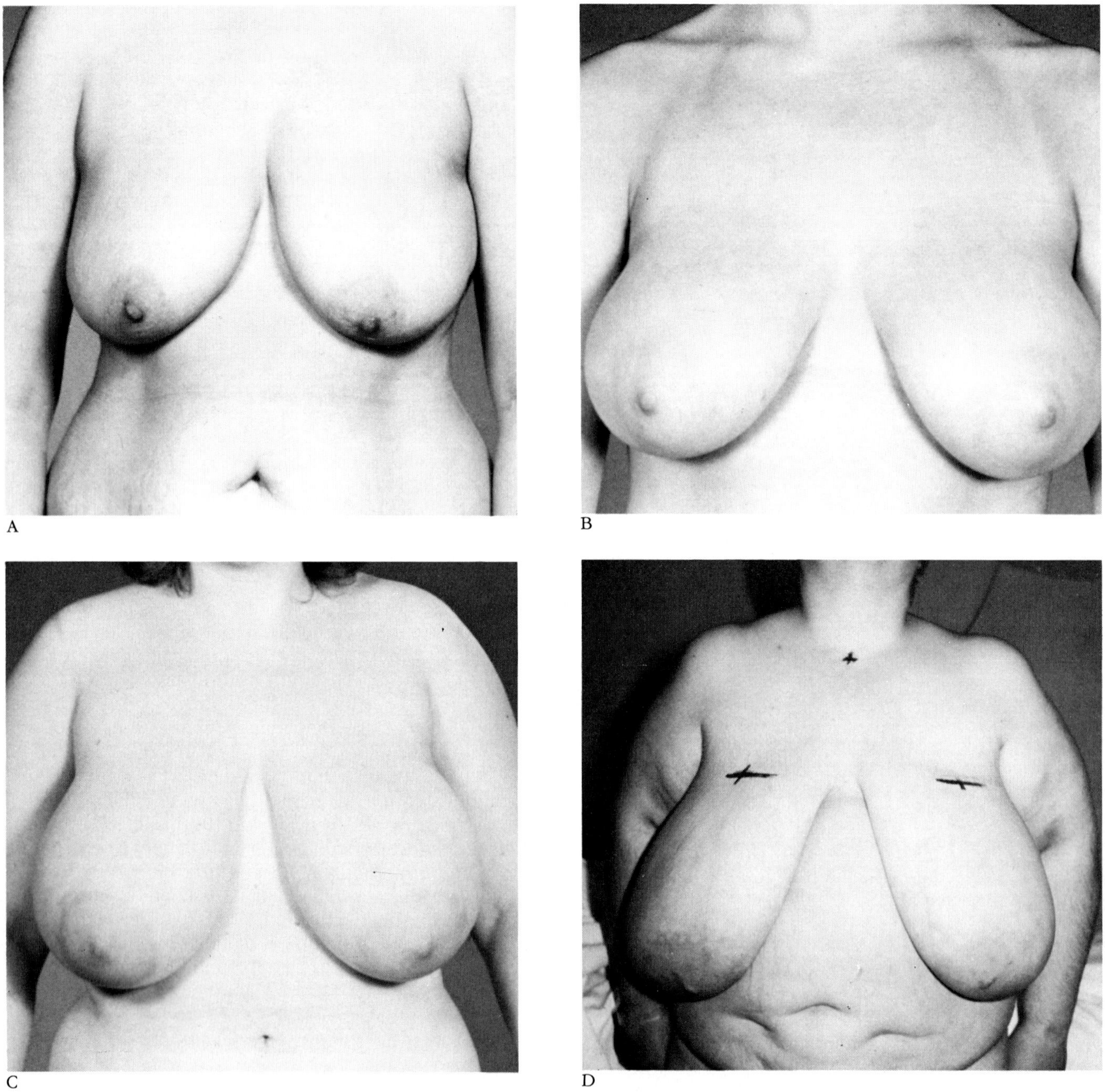

Figure 21-2. Classification of breast hypertrophy based on volume excess in *each* breast.
A. Minor (0–200 gm excess); volume excised was 175 gm.
B. Moderate (200–500 gm excess); volume excised was 350 gm.
C. Major (500–1500 gm excess); volume excised was 950 gm.
D. Gigantomastia (over 1500 gm excess); volume excised was 2900 gm.

of Goin and Goin [31] on patients undergoing breast reduction procedure indicates that all patients expect both a reconstructive component ("to feel physically better") and an aesthetic component ("to look better"). Also, the surgeon should not forget the significance of the breast or the effect surgical procedures have on the patient: "Reduction mammaplasty is an operation that, like the dreaded mastectomy, cuts, scars, bruises, desensitizes, and puts at risk a psychologically central part of the woman's body; an anatomic structure that is a nidus of her sexuality, femininity, and nurturing role as a mother" [31]. From in-depth psychiatric interviews of eight patients, it was evident that postoperative psychologic disturbances occur in a high percentage of cases (62%), ranging from body image disturbances to grief reactions to sexual disturbances [32]. In order to help the patients through this adjustment period, the surgeon should forewarn them that a period of adjustment is often required and that unusual feelings may develop. Since the female breast is the critical component determining feminine identity, it is mandatory that the aesthetic surgeon learn more about patient motivation and management [31]. The patient whose friends have had the operation are far more realistic.

Physical Examination

The patient is examined nude from the waist up in both the sitting and supine positions. A systematic breast examination is done including the axilla and supraclavicular areas. Palpation of the breasts should rule out any masses. If masses are encountered, the patient is referred to a general surgeon for investigation. With the patient sitting, the breast-to-torso relationship is evaluated, especially relative breast size and body obesity. Measurements are made bilaterally of the distance between sternal notch and nipple and sternal midline and nipple, and of the degree of ptosis. Nipple sensation is checked, especially if previous biopsies were done, and any asymmetry is shown to the patient. From palpation and measurements, one is able to classify the breast as to shape, consistency, location of hypertrophy, degree of ptosis, and required nipple elevation. The skin is examined for its turgor, elasticity, scars, striae, and dermatologic conditions. Breast volume has been measured with volumetric devices and molds [93]. In general, these techniques are time-consuming, inaccurate, and often messy. Brassiere cup sizes are a more acceptable method of generalizing breast size provided the patient is wearing a well-fitted bra. The majority of large-breasted women tend to deemphasize their breasts by wearing smaller cup sizes and larger band sizes, thus flattening the breasts (Table 21-2). Therefore, the surgeon is obligated to measure personally the patient with her brassiere on and confirm the breast size. The brassiere and cup size are determined with a tape measure (Fig. 21-3).

Although complicated formulas exist, the simplest method is to measure the patient sitting with arms by the side and *wearing a bra.* The band size is ascertained by measuring the chest circumference just under the arms. If it is an odd number like 33, the next highest even number is used, i.e., 34. Then the fullest part of the breast is measured across the nipples. If the number is 1 in. more than the band size, the cup size is A; 2 in. = B, 3 in. = C, 4 in. = D, and 5 in. = DD. For reductions, we use the following numbers to estimate excisional volumes, each cup size corresponding to the following volumes: 32 to 34 (100 gm), 36 to 38 (200 gm), 40 to 42 (300 gm), 44 to 46 (400 gm). Thus, a patient wearing a 36D brassiere would require a minimal excision of 400 gm to reach a size 36B. In cases of asymmetry, hemithorax measurements are used, and each inch difference equals half the assigned value (i.e., 32–34 [50 gm], 40–42 [150 gm]). To rule out thorax deformities, one should routinely palpate the costal cartilages and examine the patient for spinal curvatures.

Table 21-2

Brassiere relationships

32	A	B	C	D				
34		A	B	C	D			
36			A	B	C	D		
38				A	B	C	D	
40					A	B	C	D

Estimated cup volume

32–34	100 gm
36–38	200 gm
40–42	300 gm
44–46	400 gm

Figure 21-3. Brassiere size can be determined by two basic breast measurements.
A. Body circumference is measured under the arms to determine band size (34).
B. The fullest part of the breast is measured across the nipples to determine cup size (38). Each 1-in. difference equals a cup size. This patient should wear a 34D brassiere.

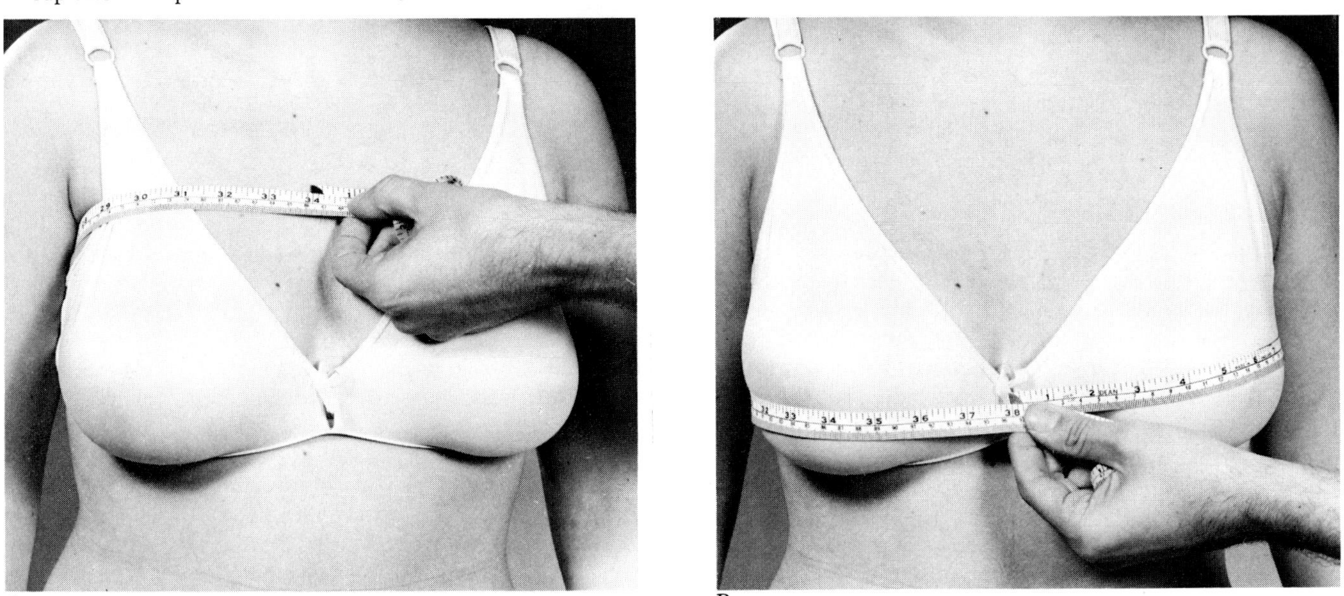

A

B

From this examination, the surgeon should have a general idea of the volumetric reduction required and thus be able to classify the deformity and select the appropriate operation. The examination is concluded with notations regarding any shoulder grooving, spinal or abdominal compensatory deformities, and respiratory or neurologic deficits.

Aesthetic Goals

At this point the surgeon should review the patient's objectives and then recommend a specific surgical technique. This discussion is best done in the examination room, where the patient can demonstrate what she does not like and the surgeon can outline how the operation is done. The breast is elevated until the desired nipple height is achieved and infolded to give the desired shape. Then, with the patient's permission, the anticipated scars are drawn on one breast, the angle of a felt-tipped pen being altered from a 2-mm circumareolar mark to a 4-mm mark in the inframammary region. It is emphasized to the patient that the trade-off is a reduced size and an improved shape for permanent scars. The patient's desire regarding areolar size is asked, and it is pointed out that any striae in the upper quadrants will not be improved and may even be accentuated.

Informed Consent

The significance of the surgery, its complications, and the unfavorable long-term sequelae must be clearly stated. A breast reduction is major surgery with the attendant risks of general anesthesia. The early complications of hematoma and fat necrosis are explained, but emphasis is placed on the 1 to 2 percent possible loss of the nipple-areola complex. Of the late results, the patient must be told to expect the following: (1) significant scarring, (2) a diminution in sensation with a 4 to 8 percent chance of total anesthesia, (3) difficulties with lactation and nursing, which correlate with the amount resected, and (4) a shape that will be somewhat ptotic and flat. Despite these admonitions, the majority of gravid patients and those with virginal hypertrophy will proceed while the younger patient whose primary complaint is ptosis will wisely reconsider, usually returning at a later date.

Instructions to Patient

The patient is required to have photographs and a mammogram [74]. Any aspirin-containing medication and birth control pills are discontinued 2 weeks prior to surgery. Although it is desirable to avoid the week of maximum breast engorgement that commences 3 days prior to menses, scheduling difficulties often preclude this possibility. In cases of breast reduction expected to exceed 1000 gm per breast, it is wise to anticipate significant blood loss and prepare for autotransfusion. The patient gives a unit of blood within 3 weeks of surgery and is started on daily iron supplements. The obese patient who is determined to lose weight should do so prior to surgery and is encouraged to see a dietitian.

ANATOMY

The breast consists of 15 to 25 separate glands, each composed of lobules of secreting acini interconnected by a ductal system. The terminal lactiferous ducts each end on the nipple. The secreting lobules are separated by a heavy stroma, which lies within the subcutaneous fat. It is the relative changes in composition that alter the density of the breast (fat: soft; glandular: firm).

In young females, the nipple overlies the fourth intercostal space. The breast extends vertically from the second to the sixth intercostal space and transversely from the parasternal to the anterior axillary line. It is contained entirely within the anterior and posterior lamellas of superficial fascia, which is continuous above with the superficial cervical fascia and below with Cooper's abdominal fascia. Cooper's ligaments are suspensory ligaments that arise from the anterior lamellas and attach the breast to the nipple and overlying skin. It must be emphasized that Cooper's ligaments are only 5 to 6 mm in length and run from the anterior lamellas through the subcutaneous fat to the dermis. The actual fascial network in which the breast is suspended consists of the anterior and posterior lamellas plus interlamellar connective tissue. Breast ptosis is due to stretching not of the suspending ligaments but rather of the deeper interconnecting bands within the stroma. Posteriorly, the breast is separated from the pectoralis major muscle by the retromammary space areolar tissue. As evidenced in retromammary augmentations, this space is traversed by a few musculocutaneous arteries arising from intercostal arteries and loose connective tissue bands. Two-thirds of the breast rests on the pectoralis major muscle. The lateral one-third overlies the serratus anterior muscle and continues upward as the axillary extension. The pectoralis major muscle is fan shaped, with a clavicular and sternal head plus an attachment to the external oblique aponeurosis in front of the rectus muscle. Its anterior fascia continues onto that of the serratus anterior, while the posterior fascia often connects with that of the pectoralis minor muscle. The latter interconnecting band as well as the fascial origin arising from the external oblique muscle must be divided in certain types of retropectoral breast augmentations.

Blood Supply

The breast is supplied from three different arterial sources: (1) internal mammary, (2) lateral thoracic, and (3) intercostal. The anterior perforators of the internal mammary artery, which nourish the deltopectoral flap, are often interconnected by a vertical branch that descends to the nipple-areola complex. Although the major contributions are from the second and third anterior perforators, additional medial blood supply comes from the remaining perforators. The lateral mammary artery is derived from a branch of the lateral thoracic, which passes around the lateral border of the pectoralis major muscle to enter the gland. This vessel is often encountered in transaxillary breast augmentations. The vessels penetrate the gland and give small branches to the overlying skin prior to terminating as a superficial arcade beneath the areola. Although Salmon [75] was able to demonstrate lateral branches of the intercostal arteries entering the posterior surface of the gland, their contribution is questionable, especially in view of the paucity of vessels seen in developing a retromammary pocket for augmentation mammaplasty. On the basis of anatomic dissections and dynamic arteriograms by Edholm and Strombeck [20], the anterior perforators of the internal mammary arteries is the dominant source, with the lateral mammary artery playing a minor role and the intercostal arteries contributing minimally. However, it must be remembered that skin flaps survive on less than 20 percent of their normal blood flow, and many of the reduction mammaplasty procedures create well-vascularized flaps with a wide base and short length.

Of even greater concern is the blood supply to the nipple-areola complex. Recent proponents of reduction mammaplasty employing an inferior pedicle (Ribeiro [70], Robbins [71, 72], Ariyan [2], Courtiss and Goldwyn [14]), have demonstrated that the nipple can easily survive on a purely glandular flap without any dermis. As advised by Climo [11], it appears prudent to preserve a circular dermal ring.

Lymphatics

An extensive lymphatic plexus exists in the breast with drainage through four pathways: axillary, internal thoracic, posterior intercostal, and cutaneous. It is estimated that 75 percent of lymph flow passes through the axillary nodes and the rest through the internal thoracic node with minimal flow through minor pathways until obstruction occurs. In most aesthetic procedures, the internal thoracic chain is not traumatized, nor are the superior afferent lymphatics to the axilla. However, the posterior intercostal system and many of the lateral afferents to the axilla would be compromised by penetration into the subglandular space or a transaxillary approach. Clinically, edema of the breast is a relatively rare event, and a higher incidence of problems has not been reported with any particular technique.

Innervation

The innervation of the breast consists of both sensory and sympathetic fibers. Nerves enter the breast from three directions: (1) laterally—the anterior rami of the lateral cutaneous branches of the third to sixth intercostal nerves, (2) medially—anterior branches of the second to sixth intercostal nerves, and (3) superiorly—supraclavicular branches of the cervical plexus. Of particular importance for the axillary approach are the contributions of the costobrachial and the third and fourth lateral cutaneous branches to the axillary tail area. Sensory innervation of the nipple-areola complex is primarily by the anterior rami of the lateral cutaneous branch of the fourth intercostal nerve. As originally emphasized by Edwards [21] and later detailed by others, the lateral branch comes off the intercostal nerve at the axillary level, penetrates the intercostal muscles, and divides into a posterior and an anterior sensory branch [26]. The anterior ramus continues beneath the fascia of the serratus anterior muscle to the lateral border of the pectoralis major muscle. It then turns anteriorly and enters the mammary gland. Thus, the key reference point is the juncture of the fourth intercostal space with the lateral border of the pectoralis major muscle. It passes upward through the breast tissue to become superficial at the nipple-areola complex. The terminal branches consist of five fascicles, with three to the areola, one to the nipple, and one to the parenchyma above the nipple. These branches approach the areola at the 7 o'clock position on the right and the 5 o'clock position on the left. Since this nerve provides primary innervation of the nipple-areola complex, its preservation is desirable. Surgically, the nerve can be avulsed at its entrance into the breast by vigorous dissection of the lateral pocket. Its terminal branches are often severed with a 3- to 9-o'clock incision, thus perhaps explaining the 15 percent alteration in sensation seen after periareolar augmentation mammaplasty. The sympathetic fibers that control the circumareolar muscles, the lactiferous ducts, and the sweat glands are mixed within the sensory nerve branches.

Form

The size and the shape of the breast are highly variable within the population and over an individual's life span. In males and young females, breast tissue is found only beneath the nipple-areola complex. During puberty, breast development occurs in a five-stage sequence: (1) initial flat preadolescent form, (2) elevation of a mound with increase in areolar diameter, (3) general enlargement of breast and areola but with no contour separation, (4) areola and papilla forming a distinct secondary mound, and (5) mature breast with the areola part of the general contour and only nipple projection. This evolution to sexual maturity is a distinct sequence that may allow classification of certain breast deformities. The cone shape of the juvenile breast gradually gives way to the mature breast with its flattened superior and medial quadrants. In adulthood, the effects of pregnancy and gravity, compounded by breast mass, often result in ptotis.

Although the "ideal" shape changes with each civilization, the full 34B breast is currently in vogue. In addition to the standard brassiere measurements, certain prescribed distances have been defined [6].

AREOLAR DISTANCE

The normal areola-nipple complex is 3.7 cm in diameter with a range of 2.8 to 4.5 cm. In the marking of breast operations, it is critical to distinguish whether measurements for the new nipple site refer to the nipple center or the top of the areola.

DISTANCE FROM STERNAL NOTCH TO NIPPLE

This distance is generally 21 cm with a range of 18 to 24 cm. Variations are relative to the patient's height, thorax, and breast size. It should be noted that many measurements change on recumbency; i.e., the skin marking of the sternal notch may ascend by 2 to 3 cm.

DISTANCE FROM INFRAMAMMARY CREASE TO NIPPLE
In the young conical breast, this distance is 6.5 cm with a range of 5.0 to 7.5 cm based on cup size. The inframammary crease itself rises on recumbency and can be altered in certain mastopexy procedures. The level of the inframammary crease as expressed on the breast surface is now considered by many surgeons the most important reference point for new nipple site in reduction mammaplasty.

INTRANIPPLE DISTANCE
The location of the nipples represents the base of an equilateral triangle whose sides are measured from the sternal notch to the nipple line; each limb of the triangle is 20 to 24 cm long. The nipples are often actually 1 to 2 cm lateral to the midclavicular line and 11 to 13 cm lateral to the midsternal line.

It must be emphasized that breast terminology is far from precise. For example, the nipple–inframammary crease distance may vary at either end point: Is it center of nipple, top of nipple, or top of areola? Is the patient standing or lying down? Are the arms by the sides or extended? Is the natural inframammary fold to be used or a new level to be created? Variations in terminology are found throughout the literature, and precise definitions are critical for success.

SURGICAL PRINCIPLES

Any method of reduction mammaplasty must correct three basic problems: (1) excessive breast tissue, (2) an inferiorly displaced nipple, and (3) a stretched skin envelope (Fig. 21-4). Obviously, the severity of each component will vary with the individual. The younger patient may have a large hypertrophic tense breast contained in a firm skin brassiere and with minimal nipple displacement; the postmenopausal woman may have fatty ptotic breasts contained in a stretched skin brassiere and with nipples pointing downward. The surgeon should approach each patient with specific objectives and prepared for modifications in operative technique [9].

Frequently, patients seeking a breast reduction will have ptosis rather than hypertrophy as their primary problem. Any attempt to apply breast reduction techniques directly to the ptotic breast will result in disappointment for patient and surgeon. Multiple modified procedures for dealing with the ptotic breast have been devised [29, 34, 35, 38, 42, 98]. However, certain younger patients with minor to moderate hypertrophy of the breasts will regard ptosis as their primary problem. This condition is of significant concern in soft breasts with a severely stretched skin envelope causing a major ptosis with a flattened appearance. In such cases a reduction of the lower quadrants is done plus a small subpectoral augmentation (125–175 cc) to restore the desired superior fullness.

Objectives

The fundamental goals of any breast reduction operation include the following: (1) excision of glandular tissue, (2) attainment of an aesthetic symmetric shape with the nip-

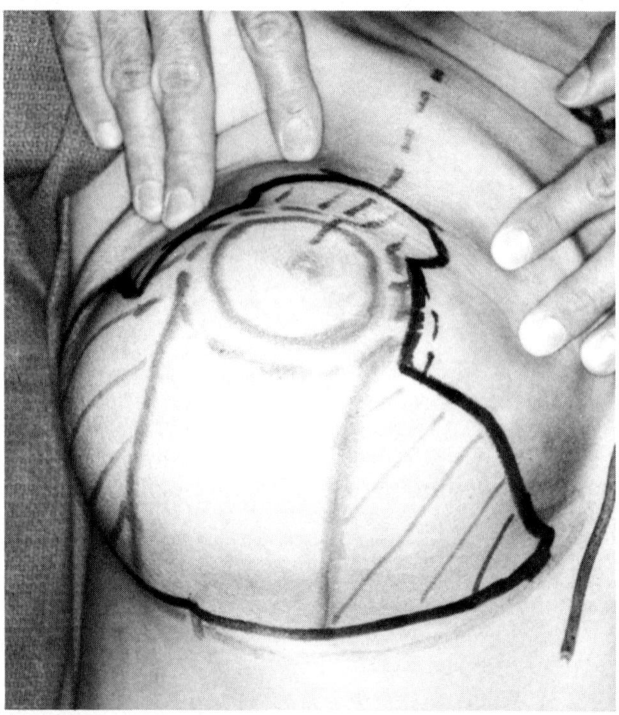
A

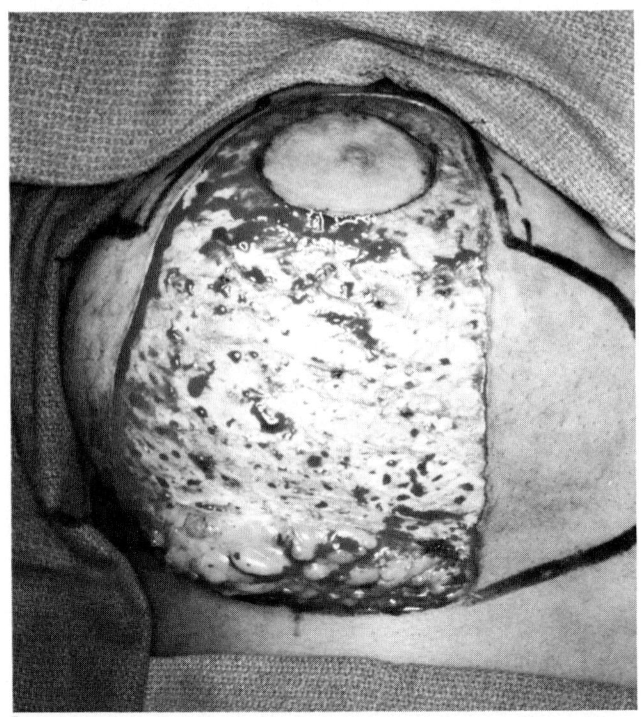
B

Figure 21-4. Principles of a breast reduction.
A. Markings for an inferior pedicle breast reduction using the technique described by Goldwyn and Courtiss.
B. Deepithelialization of an 8-cm-wide inferior pedicle.

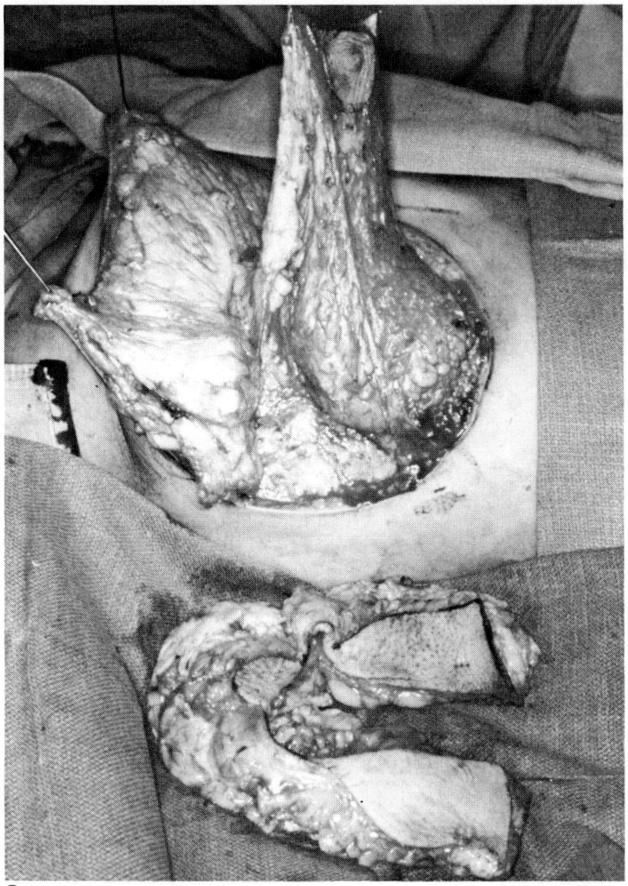

C

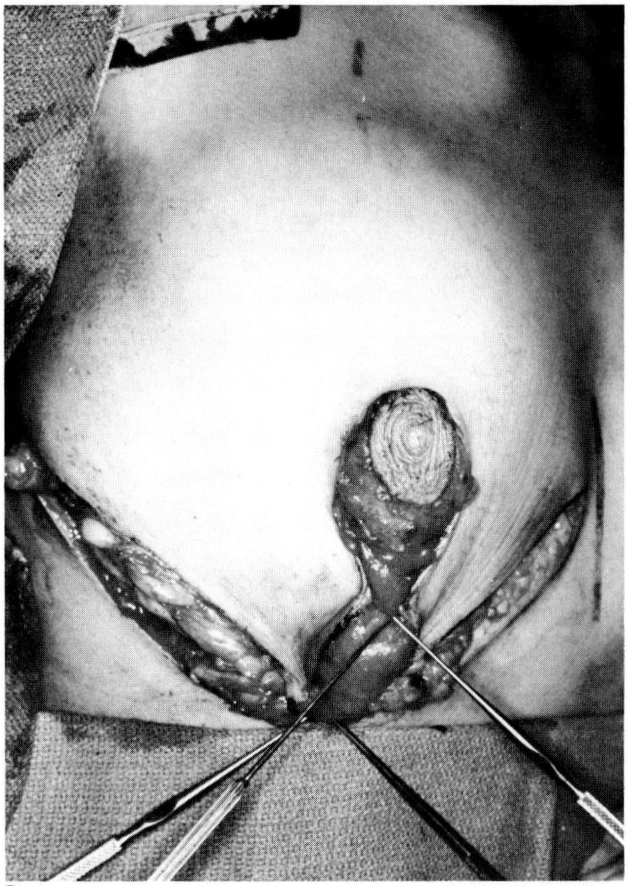

D

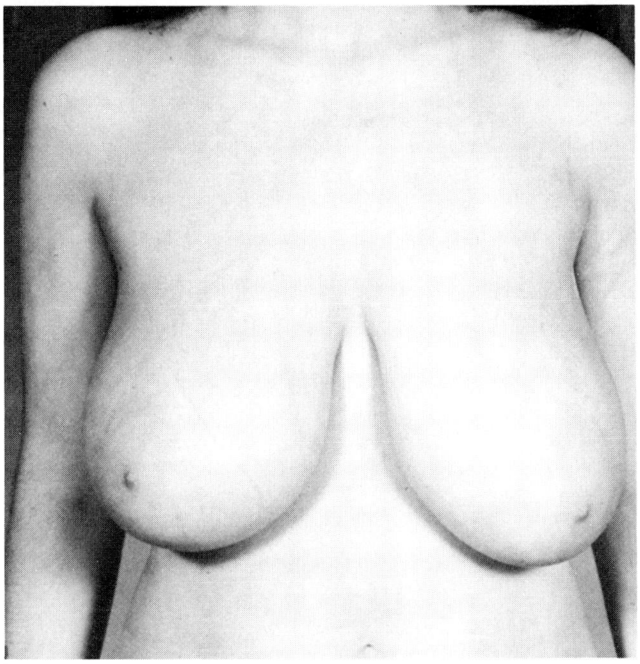

E

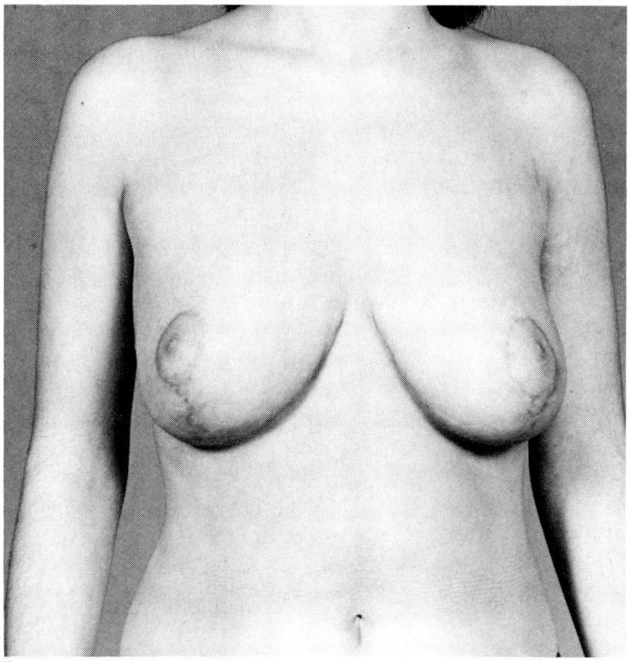

F

Figure 21-4 (continued)
C. Following removal of 680 gm, the tapered parenchymal pedicle is clearly evident.
D. Traction in a central direction precludes dog-ears.
E. Preoperative condition.
F. Postoperative result.

ple at its vertex, (3) minimal-length scars placed in nonvisible locations, (4) a safe, simple, and short operative procedure, (5) maintenance of sensation, (6) potential for lactation, and (7) permanence [33].

Marking

Currently, the surgeon must decide whether to adhere rigidly to a preplanned pattern or to sculpt a breast according to individual breast tissue and skin laxity [84]. The only common points in various methods are the following: (1) The multiparous NAC averages 4.5 cm in diameter for large-breasted women; (2) the new nipple location is generally 20 ± 2 cm from the sternal notch; (3) the new NAC site should be at the level of the inframammary fold; and (4) the distance from the inframammary fold to the lower border of the areola should *not* exceed 5 cm. The extent of preoperative planning depends on whether one is merely marking the new NAC location, with all subsequent decisions made intraoperatively in the supine position, or is marking the new skin brassiere in the upright position.

Nipple Transposition

The NAC is circumscribed with a concomitant areolar reduction, isolated onto either a dermal pedicle or a dermaglandular base, and elevated to a new site [4]. Dermal pedicles are generally being abandoned in favor of parenchymal paddles as the latter do not require meticulous deepithelialization or risk compression. In addition, the possibility of future lactation and retained sensation is improved.

Glandular Resection

The volume and location of the excess breast tissue to be excised are determined preoperatively. As emphasized by Wise [99–102] and Regnault [64–68], it is possible to preplan the volume to be excised according to brassiere cup size. A full B cup size is considered ideal for the young, thin individual whereas a smallish C cup size may be more acceptable to the older, heavyset patient. Thus, the volume that must be excised can be calculated on the basis of a cup size, as previously described. In general, redundant breast tissue is located inferiorly and laterally with little excess superiorly. Thus, most glandular resection is in the inferior quadrants, with lateral tailoring a common requisite. The contributions of Pitanguy [56] and Dufourmentel and Mouly [17] in regard to the site of glandular resection in the deep surface of the breast are noteworthy. It must be emphasized that glandular resection is determined by localization of excesses and not by the configuration of a predetermined skin envelope. The need for blood transfusion has decreased markedly because of infiltration with dilute epinephrine (1:200,000), limited undermining, and use of a cutting cautery. In a series of 20 consecutive inferior pedicle breast reductions with a mean total glandular resection of 1080 gm (452–2750 gm), we found that blood transfusion was *not* required in any cases as the mean decrease in hematocrit was 7.5 percent (3–14%). Closure of the breast is usually in a vertical manner with medial rotation of lateral tissue to achieve a more conical breast. Controversy exists as to whether breast contouring by suture plication is permanent or serves merely as an immediate mold over which excess skin is draped for estimation of excision. In contrast to breast plication, it is generally accepted that most types of breast suspension are not permanent, i.e., fascial strips from breast to pectoral fascia.

Skin Brassiere

Most surgeons agree that final breast shape is determined by the skin brassiere, and thus its excision should be guided by an attempt to achieve the ideal configuration and volume capacity [53, 59]. Either of two guidelines for determining the amount of skin excision can be used: compression of the breast in the supine position with subsequent adjustment *or* preoperative pattern markings in the vertical position that are rigidly adhered to throughout the operation. The skin excision is generally from the circumareolar area and both inferior quadrants. Historically and quite recently, attempts have been made to perform breast reductions through a periareolar incision by means of a toroidal technique. The results are unacceptable as the scars are massive and difficult to revise [8]. Skin closure differs markedly between the lateralizing operations, which employ either simple approximation or interdigitating edges, and pattern operations, which require creation of true skin-gland flaps that close over an underlying pedicle or paddle. A tight skin approximation will result in a square flat breast whereas a loose closure will lead to early ptosis with an upwardly displaced NAC.

SURGICAL TECHNIQUES

During recent years an almost limitless number of new techniques for breast reduction have been presented [5, 7, 52, 58, 92]. Conversion from bipedicles to unipedicles and, lately, parenchymal paddles has led to better shape and fewer complications [23]. A common theme has been survival of the NAC on a single quadrant of breast tissue, with or without the dermis [11, 37, 39, 73, 104]. Attempts to mold the breast by plication produce impressive early results in the ptotic breast, but long-term follow-up of its use in breast reduction has been disappointing [10, 24]. As noted by Georgiade et al. [27], one cannot apply the same technique to every breast hypertrophy.

B-TECHNIQUE

Since 1959 the senior author has personally performed more than 1800 reduction mammaplasties. Until 1969 the principal methods employed were those described by Strombeck, Dufourmentel, and Pitanguy. The results were good with any technique, provided the reduction was a small one and the skin envelope favorable. Once the reductions exceeded 500 gm, most cases were disappointing at 2 years because of extensive scars, secondary glandular ptosis, upward nipple migration, and a flat pancakelike deformity of the breast. The B-technique was devised to avoid these problems.

The three principles of the B-technique are (1) nipple transposition on a dermaglandular paddle, (2) glandular resection in the inferior quadrants, and (3) a Z-plasty type of closure composed of interlocking lateral and medial flaps but without skin undermining. In contrast to most methods, this procedure creates a final shape that improves with time and results in a short hidden scar without any medial extension. The name is derived from the skin markings, which resemble the letter *B*.

Marking

To simplify the breast markings, one can conceive of the B-technique as a periareolar skin excision and an inferior glandular resection with interdigitating flap closure. With the patient *sitting* and arms at the sides, a line is drawn from the sternal notch to the nipple (Fig. 21-5). At a point 15 to 22 cm from the sternal notch, a long transverse line is drawn perpendicular to the sternum. This represents the maximum skin resection and will become on closure the upper areolar point (UAP). The exact point varies with the amount of anticipated resection and firmness of the breasts, but generally it is no more than 4 cm above the existing inframammary fold.

It must be emphasized that this point is made on the sternal notch–nipple line, not the midclavicular-nipple line, which is used in most pattern techniques. The areola is marked in the usual manner as a 4.5-cm circle plus quadrant lines to ensure correct expansion of the areola. After induction of anesthesia, skin preparation, and draping, the rest of the markings are made in the *supine* position with the arms at right angles. The medial excision line is placed parallel 9 to 11 cm from the midsternal line. The distance from the nipple to the medial line is measured and replicated symmetrically on the lateral side of the nipple. Next, the inferior excision area is determined. The breast is pushed downward, and the old inframammary fold is marked. A new fold is traced 1 cm above as a wide curve parallel to the natural fold. From this new fold, one measures 4 cm upward to locate the lower border of the periareolar skin excision. Medially, the juncture consists of a small 1-cm angular flap located at the lower limit of the areola. Laterally, a gentle S-shaped curve is designed to run inferiorly and terminate at the inframammary fold. This line is determined by compressing the breast and estimating the amount of excision. The overall markings resemble the letter *B*. Although difficult to diagram, the markings are quite simple, usually done in 1 to 2 minutes and individualized for each patient.

Technique

MINOR AND MODERATE REDUCTION

With resections less than 500 gm, the basic technique varies primarily as to the amount of glandular and skin resection. Technically, the operation consists of only three steps: periareolar deepithelialization, excision of breast tissue, and closure. Once the technique is mastered, most bilateral reductions can be done by a single surgeon in less than 1½ hours (Fig. 21-6).

As with any procedure, attention to detail is critical for success. The areola is circumscribed and the periareolar skin area in the upper portion of the *B* is deepithelialized. A 1-cm margin of dermis is left below the new areola. Then the lateral breast flap is created by a deep incision across the deepithelialized infraareolar margin and medial lower border and in the inframammary fold. Following the incision, the inferior edge of the breast is reflected off the pectoral fascia and brought upward to allow elevation of the inframammary fold. Parenchymal resection is accentuated medially and brought transversely to create a true lateral breast flap. The flap is pulled medially and the predicted amount of excision evaluated, thus avoiding excessive resection especially in the firm breast. The areola is brought upward and anchored with a 4-0 Vicryl suture. Then the triangular medial flap is brought across and sutured to the corresponding lateral indentation. If the approximation is tight or areolar movement restricted, the deepithelialized dermis is incised vertically on either side. The areola is sutured at all four quadrants. The breast tissue is plicated with three heavy 0 Vicryl sutures and the flaps are approximated at several key points. If the final incision is too lateral, additional skin is excised medially, whereas periareolar skin can be excised to ensure a circular areolar shape. In most cases, a split silicone drain is inserted. The skin is sutured with a continuous running subcuticular 4-0 Vicryl suture taking short superficial bites on the lateral flap and larger broader bites on the convex medial edge. The redundant medial fold or inferior flatness tends to resolve within several weeks of surgery. A comparable purse-string type of suture is continued around the areola with long broad bites of the surrounding skin. The dressing consists of wide strips of paper tape, gauzes over the drain, and a firm elastic wrap. In small reductions, the results are generally excellent, with a natural contour and short scars (Fig. 21-7).

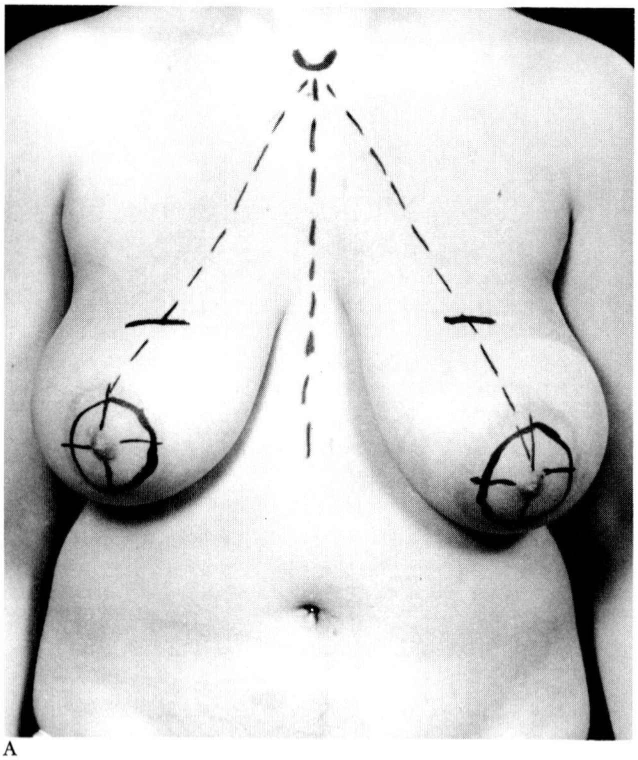

A

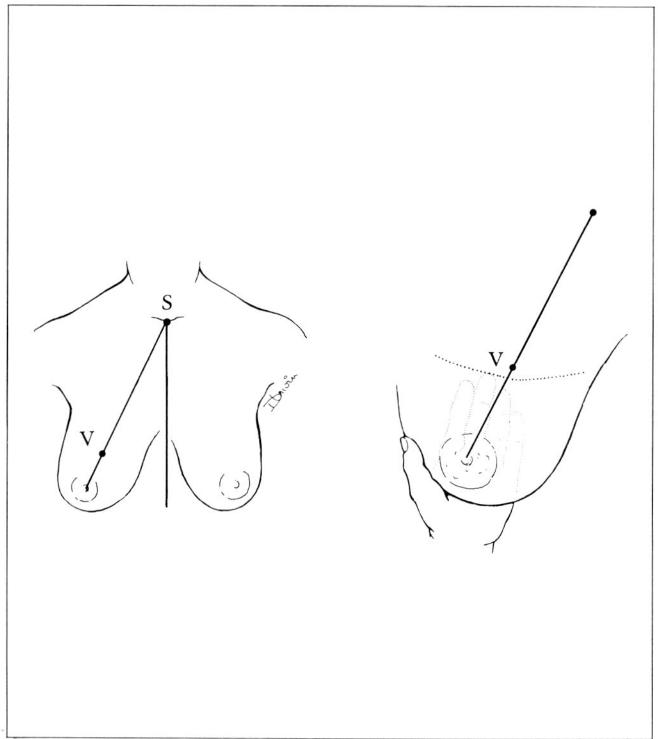

B

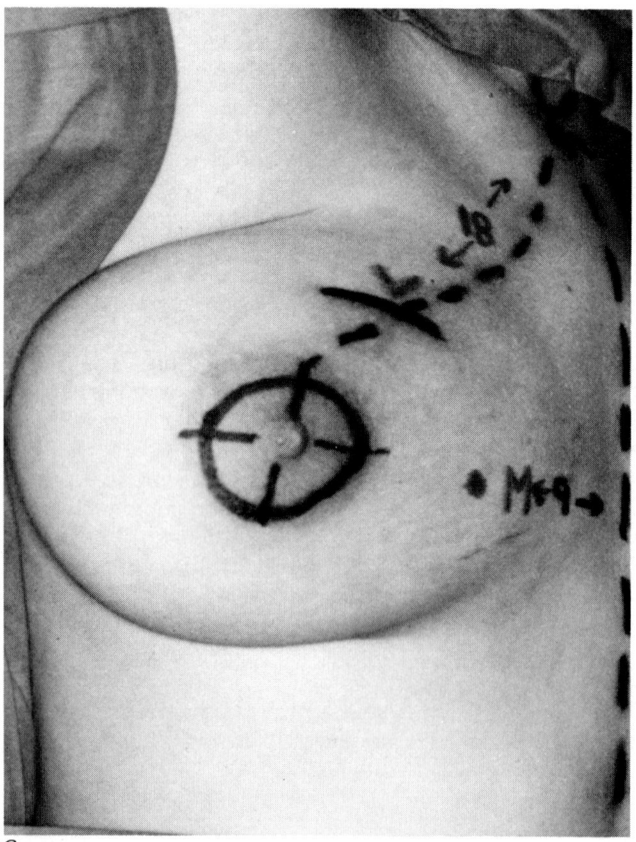

C

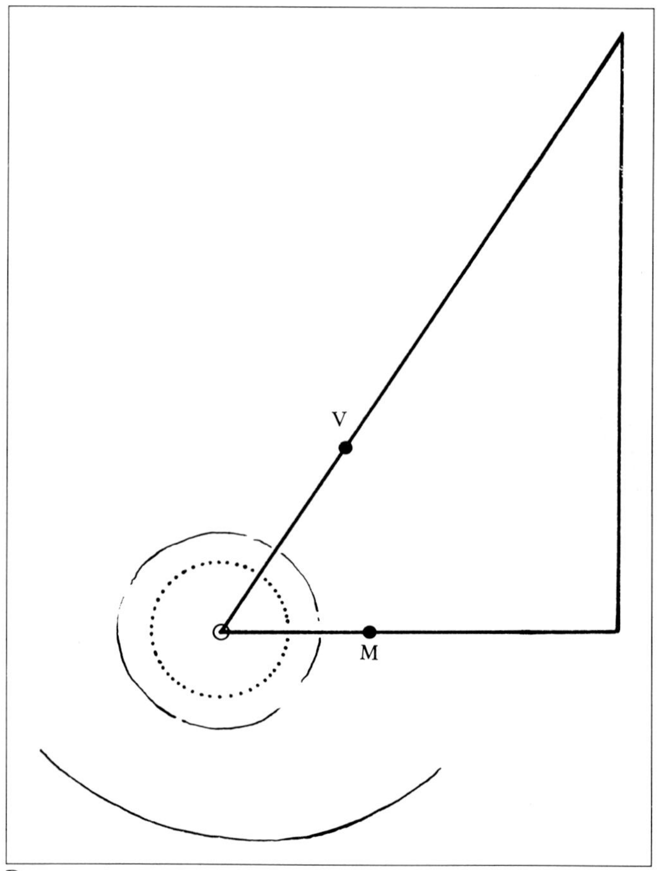

D

Figure 21-5. Sequential steps of a B-technique breast reduction.

A, B. With the patient *standing,* a line is drawn from the sternal notch to the nipple. Point V is located on the anterior surface 1 cm above the transposed inframammary fold. It is usually between 16 and 24 cm from the sternal notch. The new areola is drawn as well as quadrant lines.

C, D. With the patient *recumbent,* point M is located 8 to 12 cm from the midline. A rule of thumb is that M is half the distance of VS. The new areola averages 4.5 cm.

E, F. Next, the incision line (FF′) is marked 1 cm above the inframammary fold. Line LM is perpendicular to and bisected by VS.

G, H. An ellipse is drawn connecting LVM.

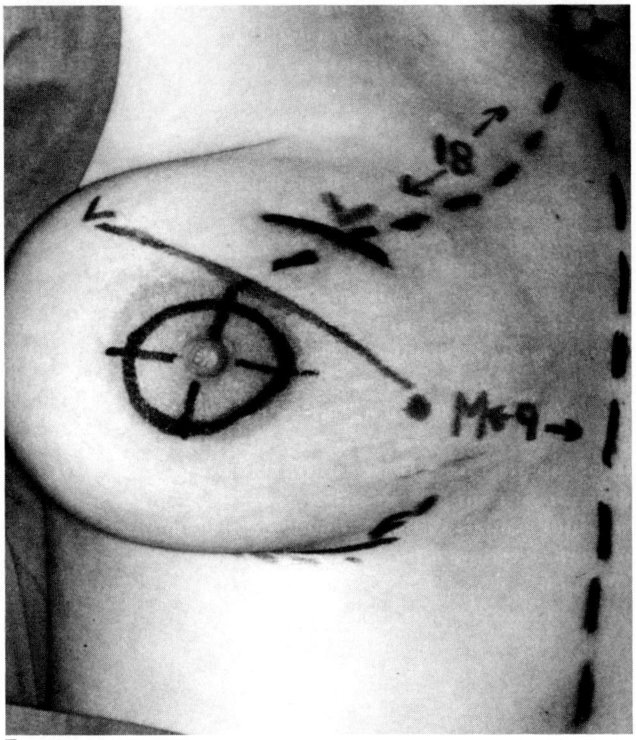

E

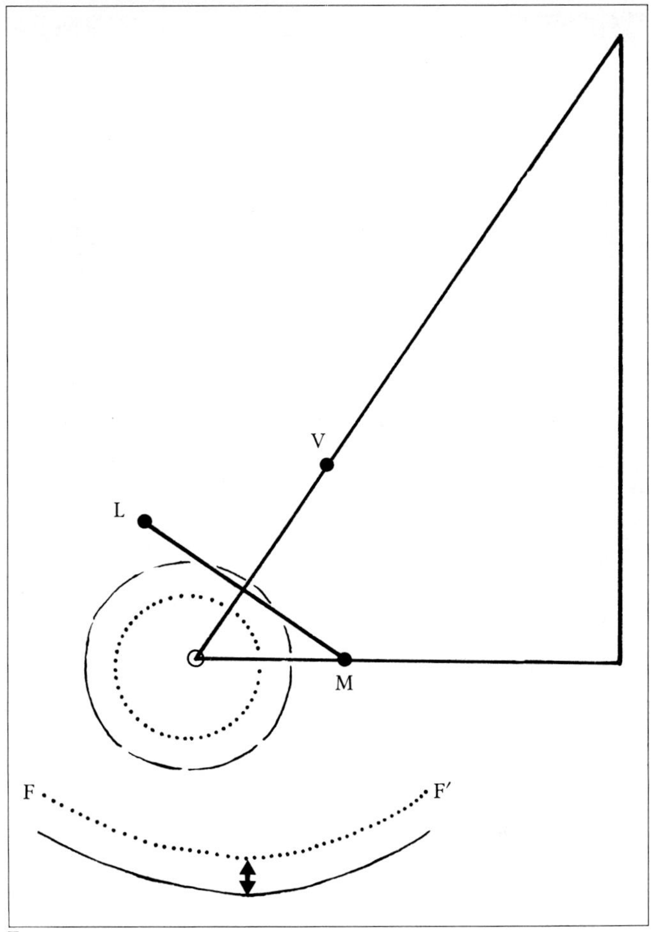

F

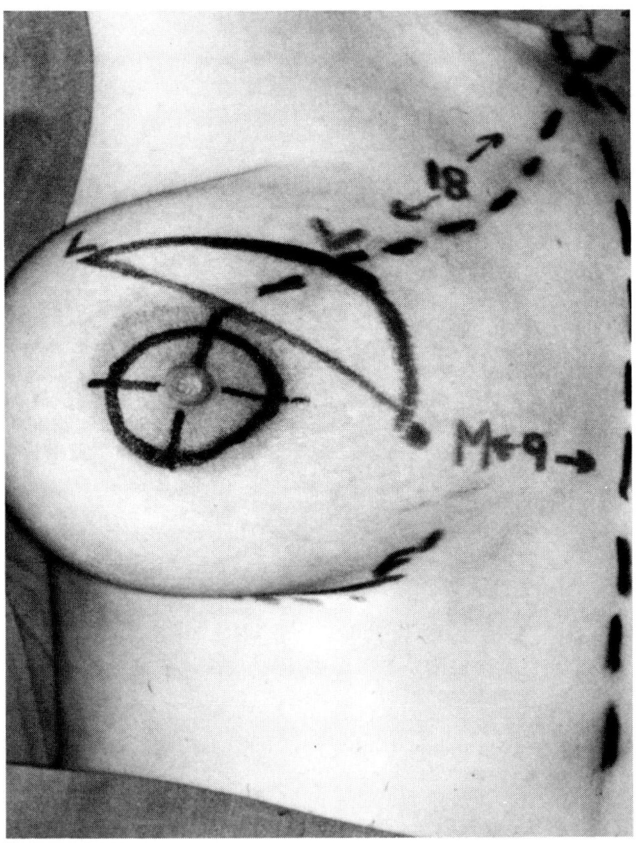

G

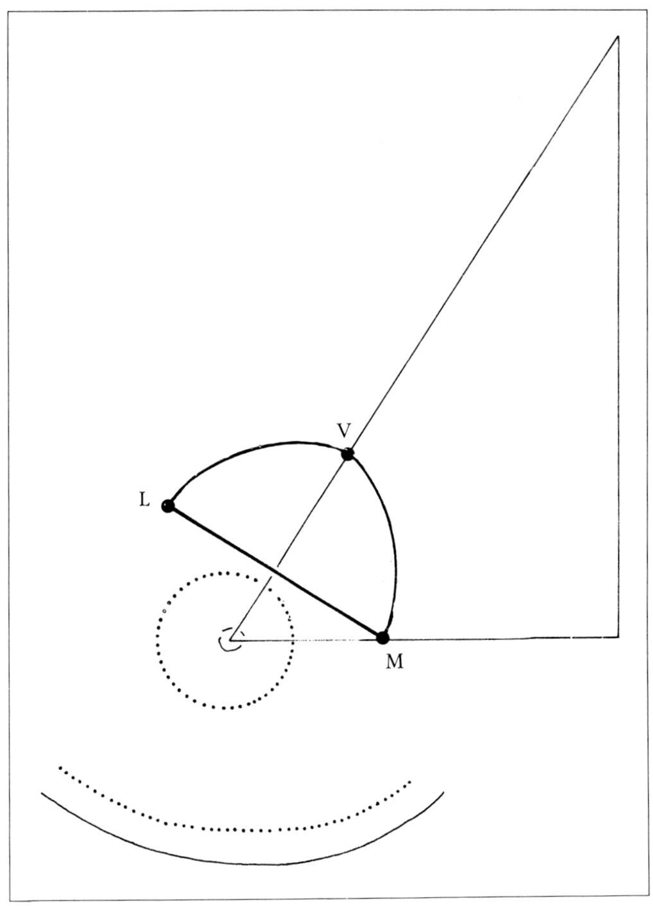

H

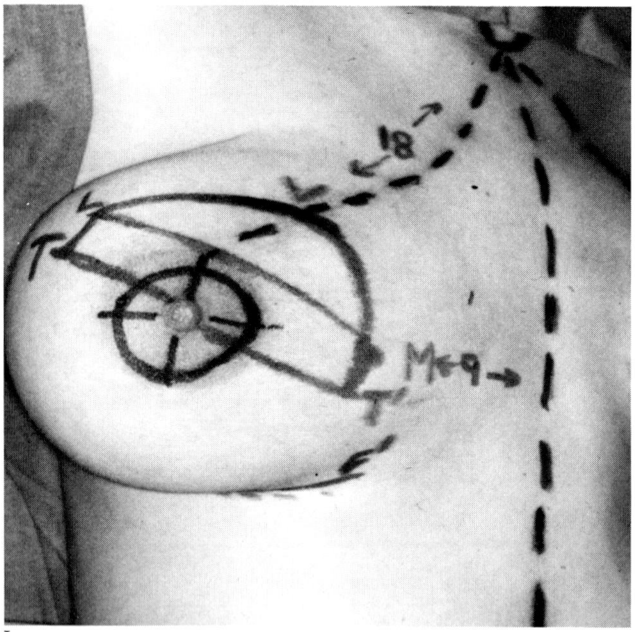

I

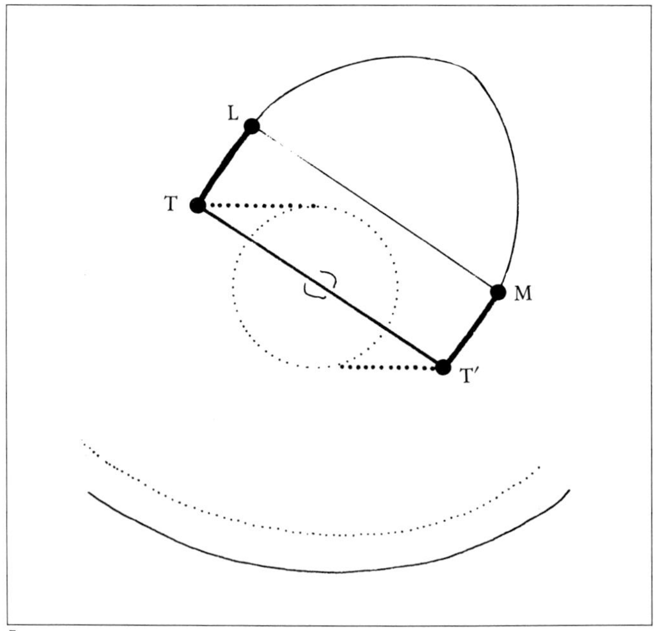

J

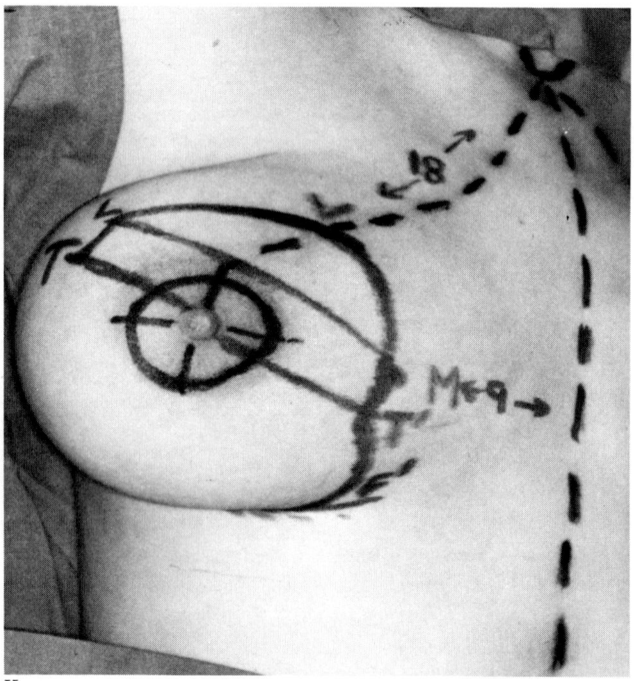

K

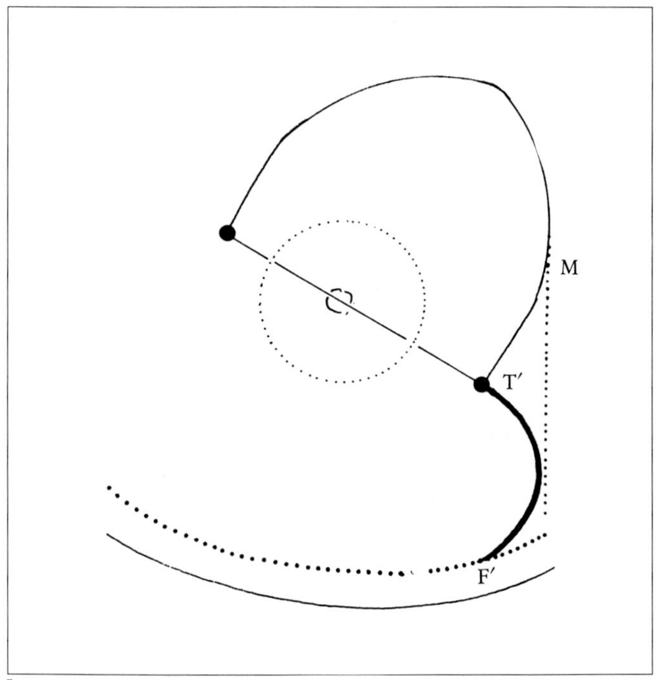

L

Figure 21-5 (continued)

I, J. Points T and T′ are drawn parallel to the top and bottom of the new areola respectively and are added to the ellipse as a parallelogram.

K, L. A vertical line is dropped from M, and then a curved line is drawn from T′ to F′. It averages 6 cm.

M, N. The breast tissue is pinched to determine the approximate amount of tissue that can be removed. The maximum skin width is marked CC′.

O, P. Curve TCF is marked parallel to T′C′F′. Line TT′ curves just below (5–10 mm) the new areola. The cross-hatched area will be deepithelialized, whereas the inferior portion will be excised. At time of closure, T will be sutured to T′, C sutured to C′.

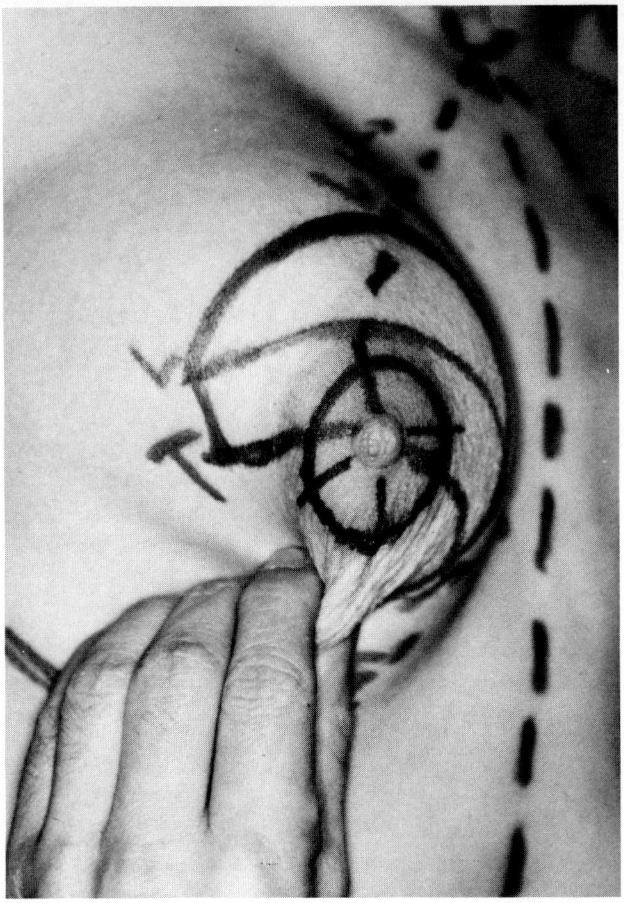

M

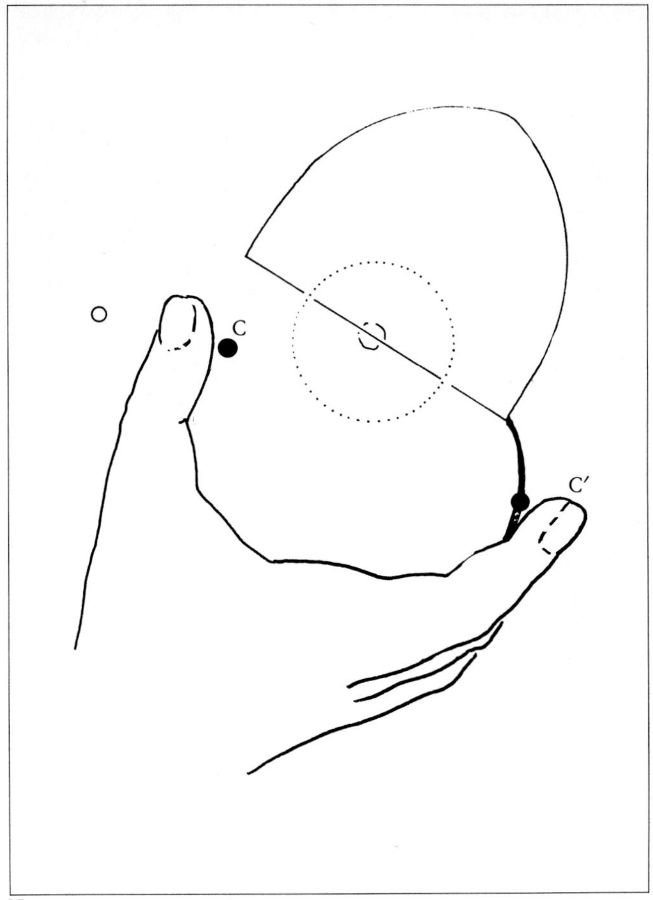

N

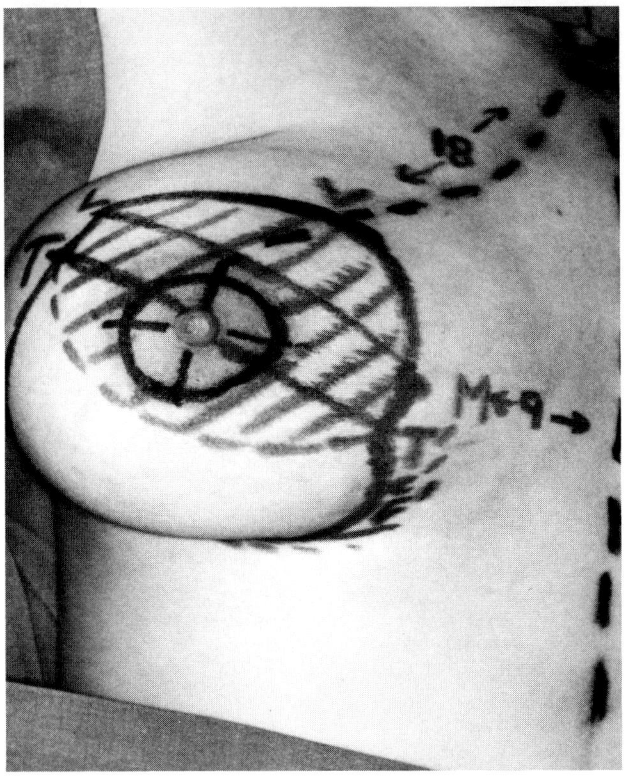

O

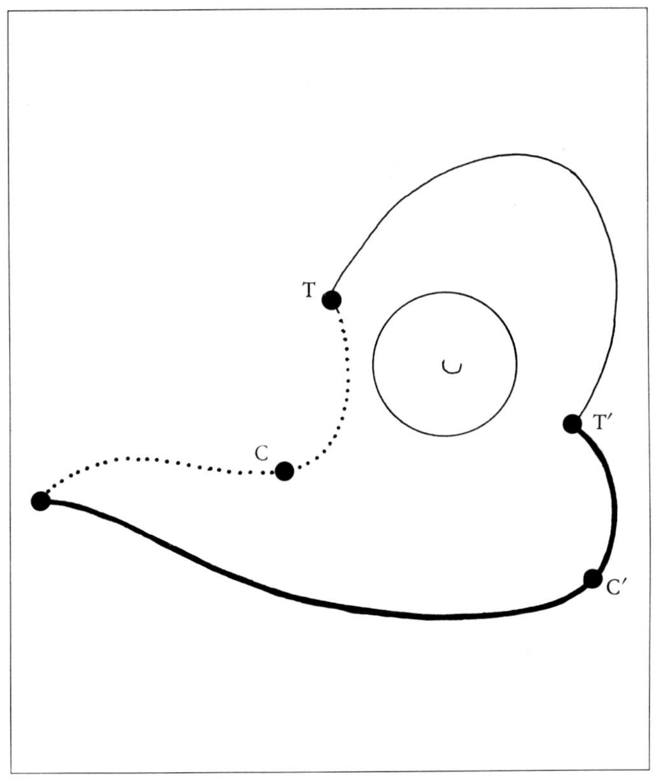

P

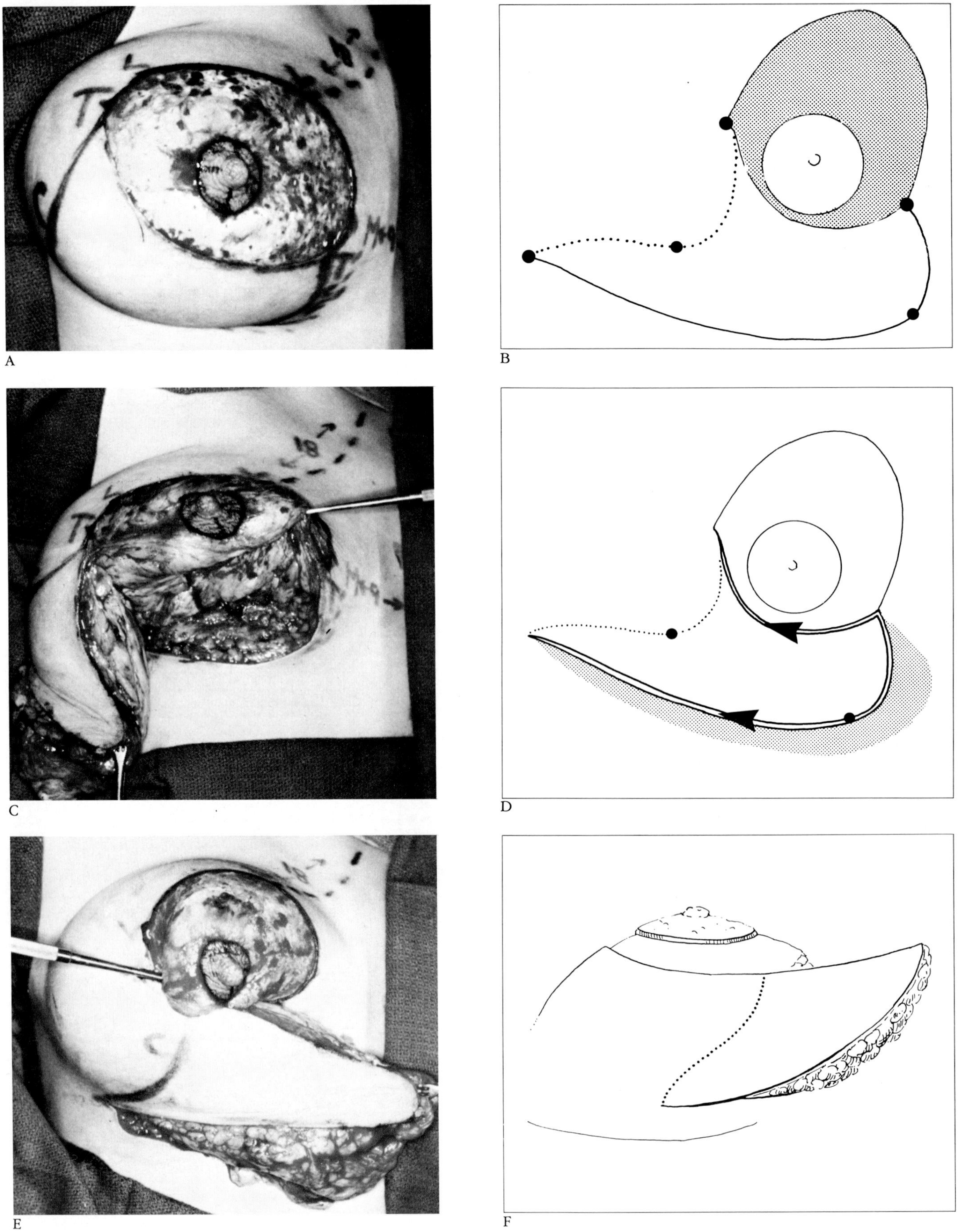

Figure 21-6

A, B. The operation begins with deepithelialization of the shaded periareolar area.

C, D. Next, a breast flap is created along TT′ and FF′ incorporating the lower poles and as much breast tissue as required to effect the reduction (see Fig. 21-8). Note that the shaded area is undermined at the time of incision.

E, F. With traction on the flap, the excision line is checked and the excess removed.

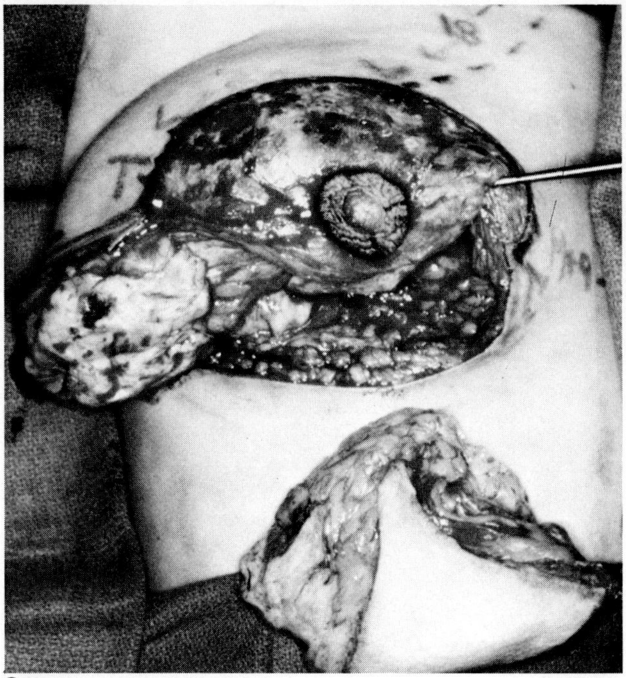

G

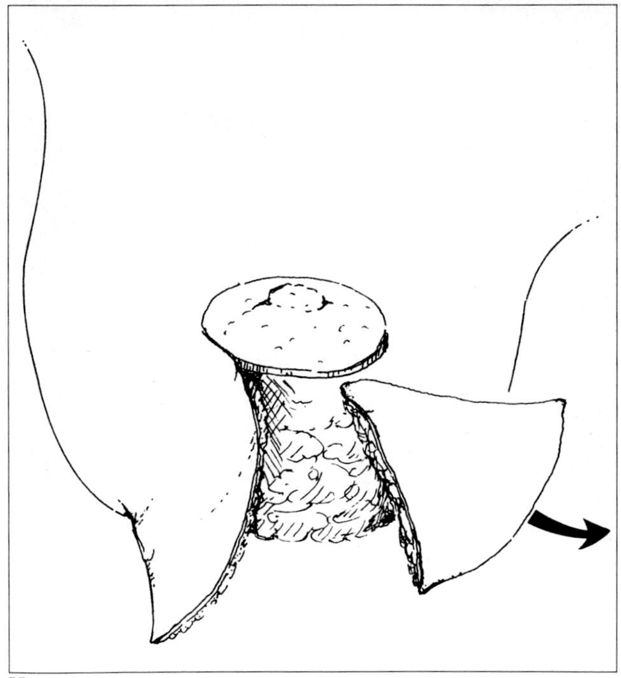

H

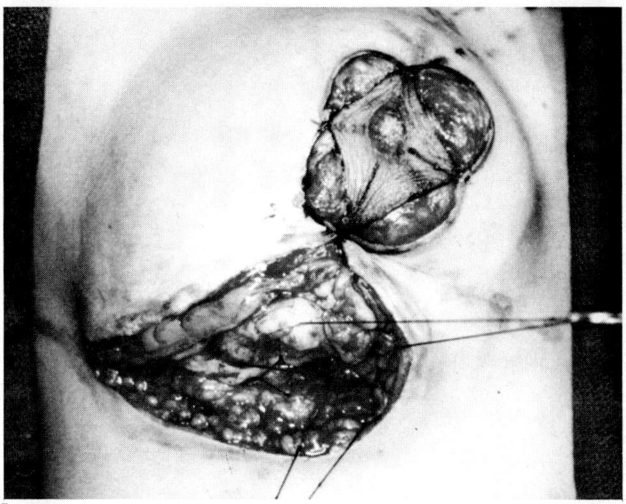

I

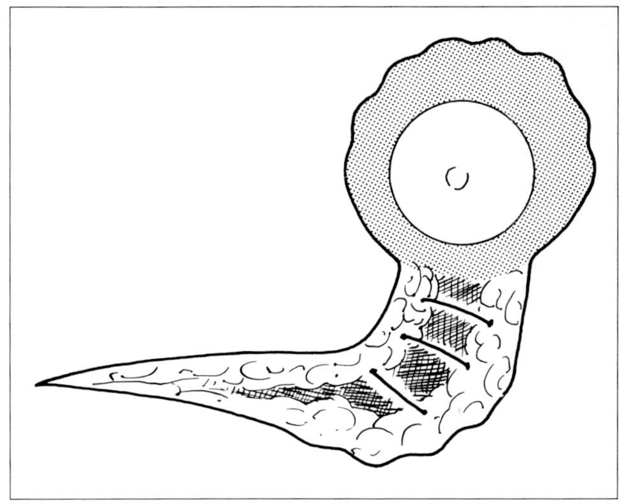

J

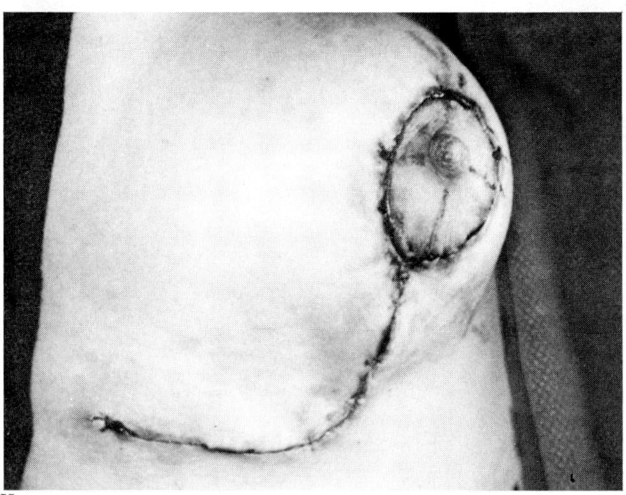

K

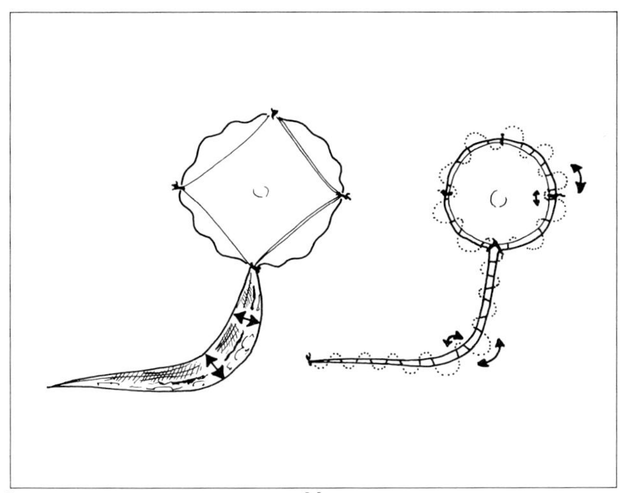

L M

G, H. Breast tissue has been excised from both lower quadrants and beneath the areola.

I, J. The direction of closure is from T to T′ and C to C′. The closure begins with deep plication of the breast tissue using 0 Vicryl. Next, the breast flaps are approximated with 4-0 Vicryl.

K, L, M. Skin closure is done with a continuous 4-0 Vicryl suture. Medial redundancy is lessened by taking short straight bites on the lateral flap and long curved plicating bites on the medial flap. Closure creates marked breast projection and upper quadrant fullness.

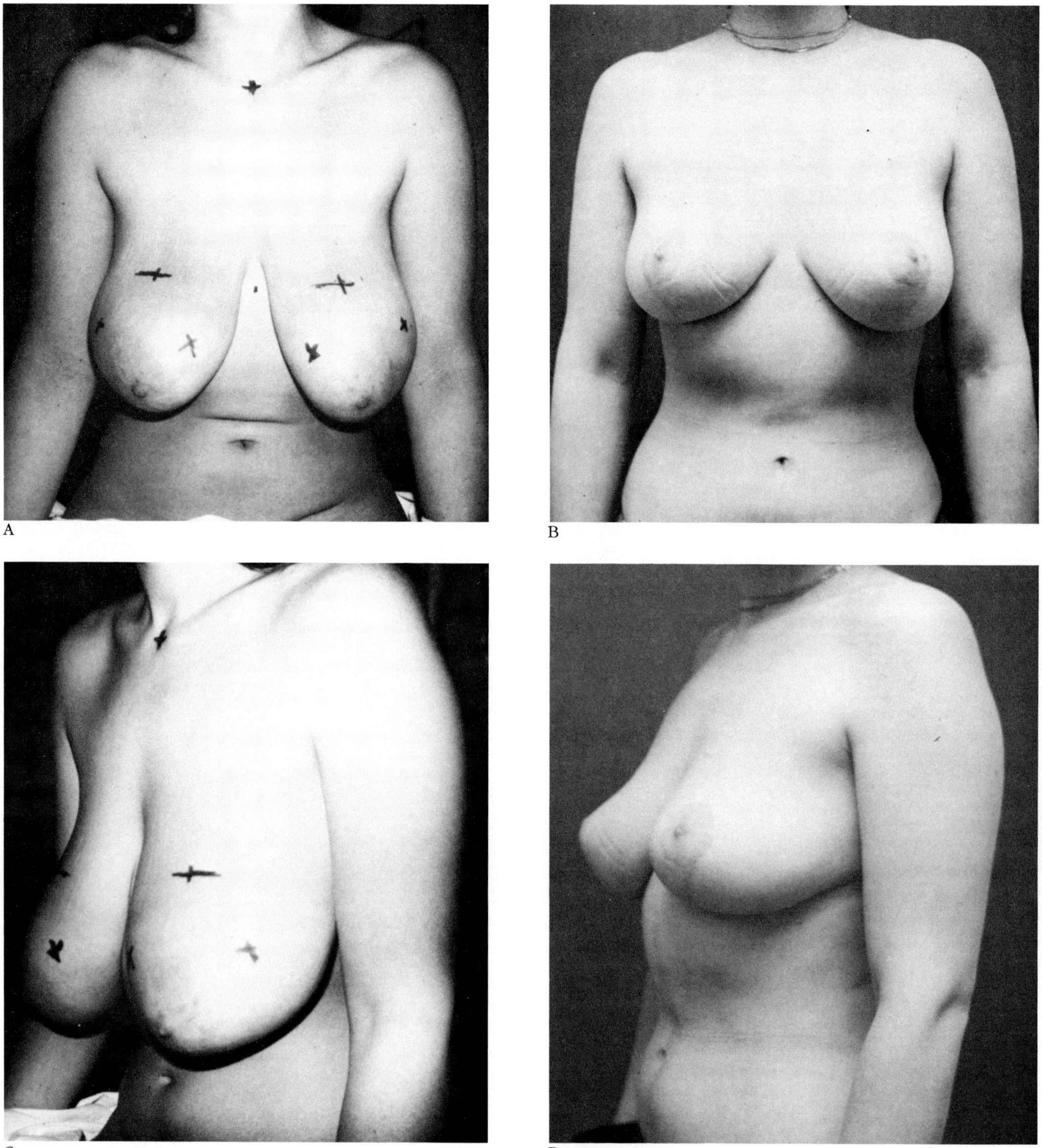

A B C D

Figure 21-7
A, C. Moderate breast hypertrophy in a 25-year-old female.
B, D. Result at 2 years after use of B-technique with resections averaging 550 gm. Note absence of medial scar.

Table 21-3. Classification of advised treatment

Minor reduction
Breast firm: refuse
Breast soft: T or B
Moderate reduction
Breast firm: T or B
Breast soft: T or B
Major reduction
Breast firm: T or B before menopause
Breast soft: T or B before menopause, areolar graft after menopause
Gigantomastia
1500–2000: virginal, T reduction, others, areolar graft
Over 2000: always areolar graft

Since the B-technique is quite flexible, it can be applied to breast reductions ranging from minimal skin mastopexy to large 1500-gm resections (Table 21-3). The critical variations are primarily in the location of the breast tissue excised and secondarily in the width of the breast flap. For minor reductions, the periareolar deepithelialization is circular, the width of the breast flap is limited, and breast tissue is excised only from the lower quadrants (Fig. 21-8A). For moderate reductions, the periareolar deepithelialization is more vertical, the width of the breast flap is expanded in both directions, and breast tissue is excised from the lower quadrants and beneath the areola (Fig. 21-8B). For major reductions, the periareolar deepithelialization extends farther upward, the breast flap expands in both directions, and breast tissue is excised from all quadrants (Fig. 21-8C). Expansion in the width of the skin flap occurs with greater resections (Fig. 21-9).

MAJOR REDUCTION

With the patient standing, the sternal midline is marked and a line drawn from the sternal notch to the nipple. Then the upper areolar limit is marked 20 to 22 cm from the sternal notch with the breast supported. It is important that the projected new inframammary fold not be more than 1 to 2 cm above the natural inframammary fold. Following induction of anesthesia, the medial point is marked 10 to 12 cm from the midline. This distance is longer than in small reductions and the areolar diameter is 5 cm rather than 4 cm. The basic marks remain the same, with the angle between the medial curves at the level of the lower limit of the new areola and the lateral notch at the level of the upper limit of the new areola.

The operation begins with an incision around the new areola followed by deepithelialization of the upper portion of the B-design (Fig. 21-10). Glandular resection must be more extensive in all directions than in a moderate reduction. The dissection is done medially and superiorly before the laterally based flap is created. Since the lateral portion of the breast is stretched toward the midline, it is left twice as thick as the fixed medial component. Resection may require removal of the entire deep portion of the gland to its upper limits. This progression in the extent of resection is similar to the resection of Pontes (variation II) [58]. Preoperative determination of the amount of glandular resection is based on brassiere cup size while the location of resection, especially the lateral component, is readily evident. With experience, it becomes possible to predict accurately the amount of excision. In general, the best results are obtained in firm breasts where the skin envelope is not stretched (Fig. 21-11). Patients with significant ptosis and flatness that require a large skin resection and limited glandular reduction will have more medial pleating and a higher incidence of scar revision. In tense glandular breasts, moderate tension on closure is well tolerated and produces excellent contour. In ptotic fat breasts, characteristic of older patients, no tension is placed on the deep sutures as there is a tendency to develop fat necrosis or even partial flap loss due to poor vascularization. Correction of dogears may be required laterally to equalize differences between the edges.

Postoperative Management

The drain is removed at 1 to 3 days, and the only dressing thereafter is a soft brassiere. No antibiotics are given, and postoperative pain is comparable to that with other techniques. The patient is reassured that any significant medial fullness or inferior flatness will round out during the ensuing weeks. In more than 1800 cases there has not been a complete NAC loss although two partial losses were encountered in reductions greater than 1500 gm. Unaesthetic shape is usually due to insufficient skin resection and is easily corrected.

Advantages and Disadvantages

The advantages of the B-technique are numerous and significant, justifying the effort of mastering a judgmental surgical procedure. The disadvantages of this technique are primarily philosophic rather than practical.

FLEXIBILITY

The skin markings are tailored to fit the individual's breasts rather than forcing the breast into a standard design. This approach requires a certain amount of surgical judgment and concentration to detail that pattern procedures excuse. Although they may find it initially disconcerting, most plastic surgeons will welcome escape from repetitive procedures, a transformation that is comparable to switching from the numbered rigidity of the Tennison cleft lip repair to the Millard lateral advancement technique.

IMMEDIATE APPEARANCE

Although excellent upper quadrant projection is present at the end of the operation, there is often a tendency toward flatness inferiorly and along medial skin folds. However, gradual postoperative rounding out occurs and an aesthetic youthful breast remains (Fig. 21-10H).

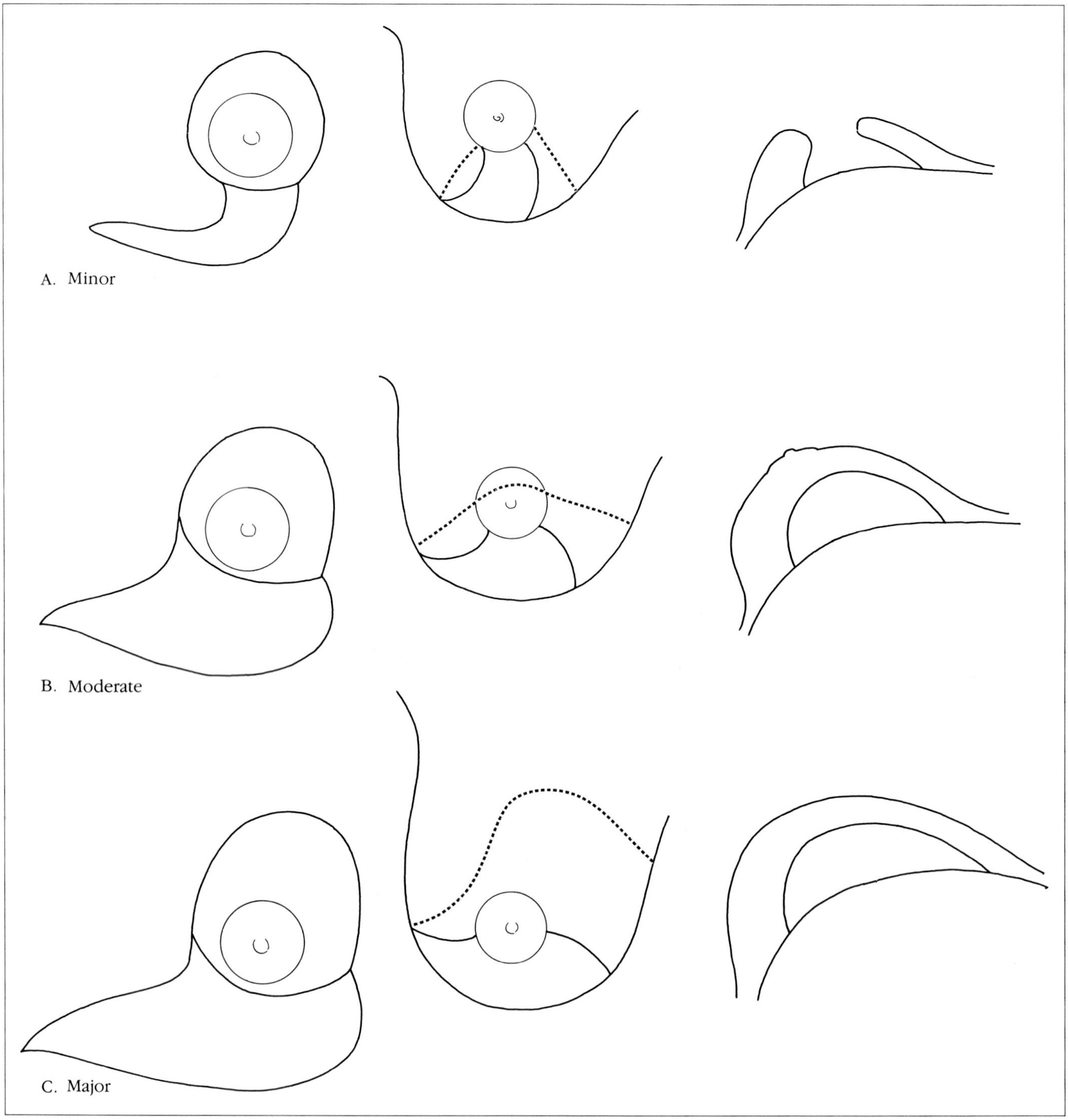

Figure 21-8. Significant changes in markings and technique occurs as glandular resection increases.

A. Minor reduction. Skin excision is limited, and resection of breast tissue is confined to the lower quadrants as seen in the anterior and inferior views.

B. Moderate reduction. The inferior skin excision is significantly greater and the periareolar deepithelialization expanded. Resection of breast tissue extends up to the areolar level as seen in the anterior and inferior views.

C. Major reduction. Skin excision is a bit larger than with a moderate reduction, but the breast resection extends throughout all quadrants as indicated by the dotted line.

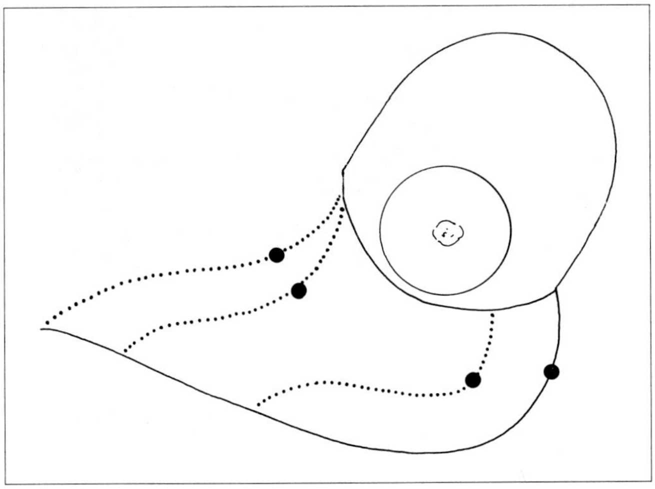

Figure 21-9. Variations in the size of the breast flap for minor, moderate, and major breast reductions.

SAFETY
The NAC maintains its surrounding dermal and underlying parenchymal circulation, thus minimizing vascular compromise. Equally important, the skin is *not* undermined and thus true skin flaps are not developed.

SHAPE
Since the glandular excision is primarily in the inferior quadrants and the breast is plicated medially, one is able to achieve excellent projection. The skin brassiere produces a conical configuration by utilizing the interdigitating flaps. In contrast to most techniques, the B-technique lets the shape of the breast improve with time, and glandular sagging has not been a problem.

OPERATING TIME
In essence, one has only to deepithelialize the circumareolar area, create a laterally based flap, which is then tailored, and close the resulting wound. Because of a single-component resection and short incision, it is possible for a single experienced surgeon to perform the operation *bilaterally* in less that 1½ hours with a nurse assistant.

SCARS
Since there is no medial incision, the scar is confined inferiorly to a short lateral extension within the inframammary fold without axillary extension. The scar is within the brassiere area and resists stretching by its Z-plasty closure. As emphasized by others, medial scars are most prone to hypertrophy and are a persistent source of sadness for many women [65].

APPLICABILITY
The B-technique is truly a universal method that gives excellent results in breast reductions, mastopexies, and asymmetries.

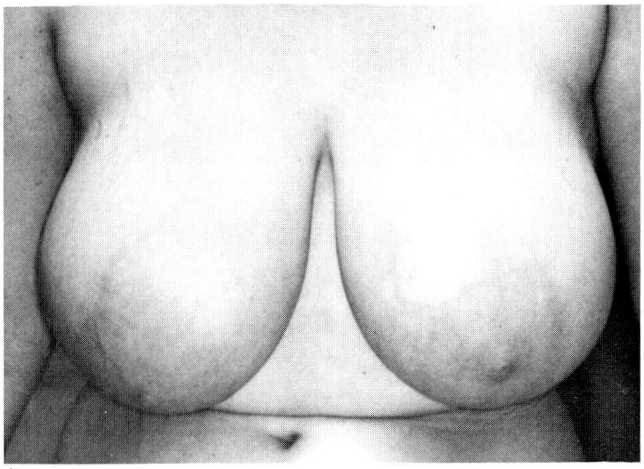
A

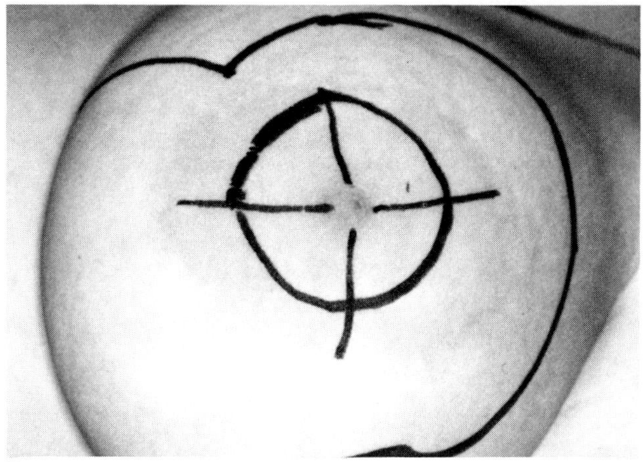
B

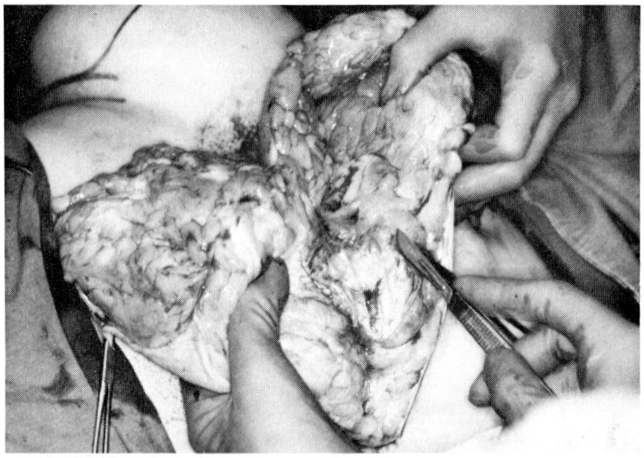
C

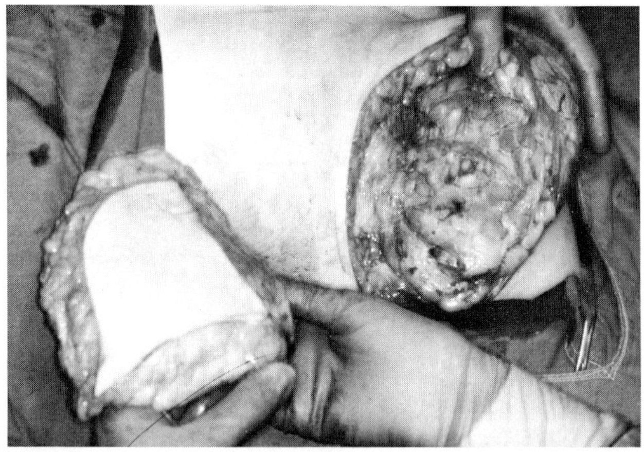
D

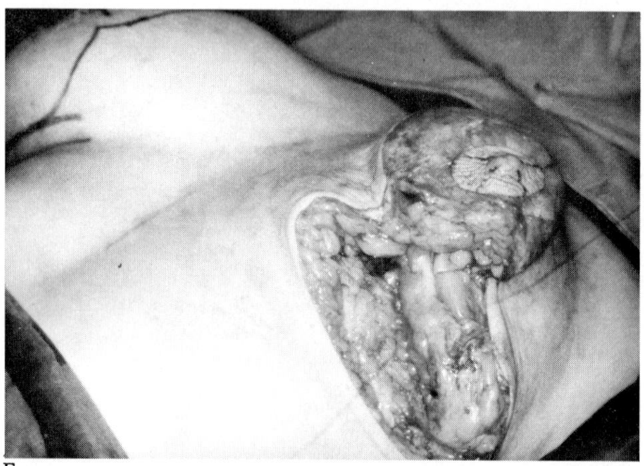
E

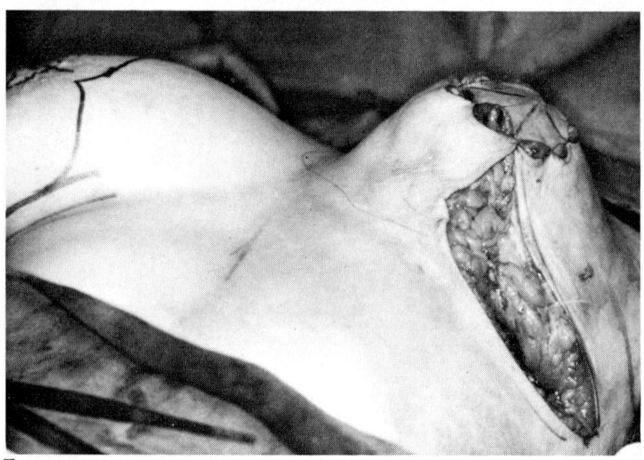
F

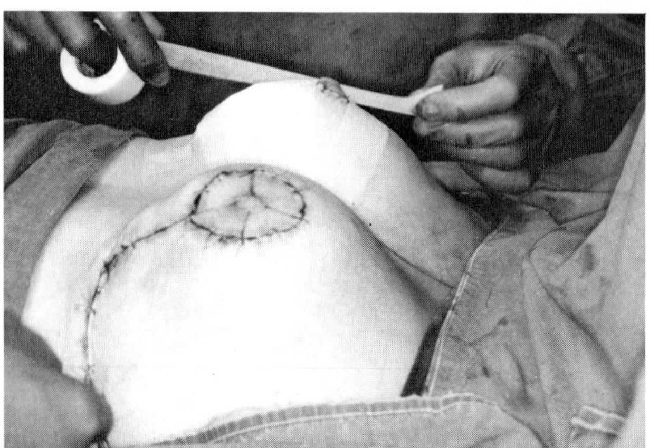
G

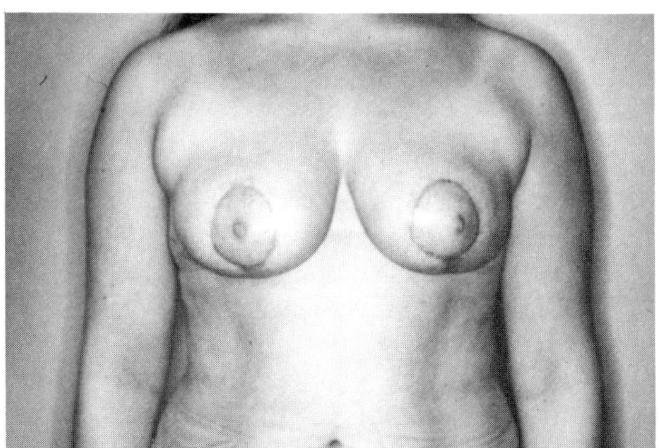
H

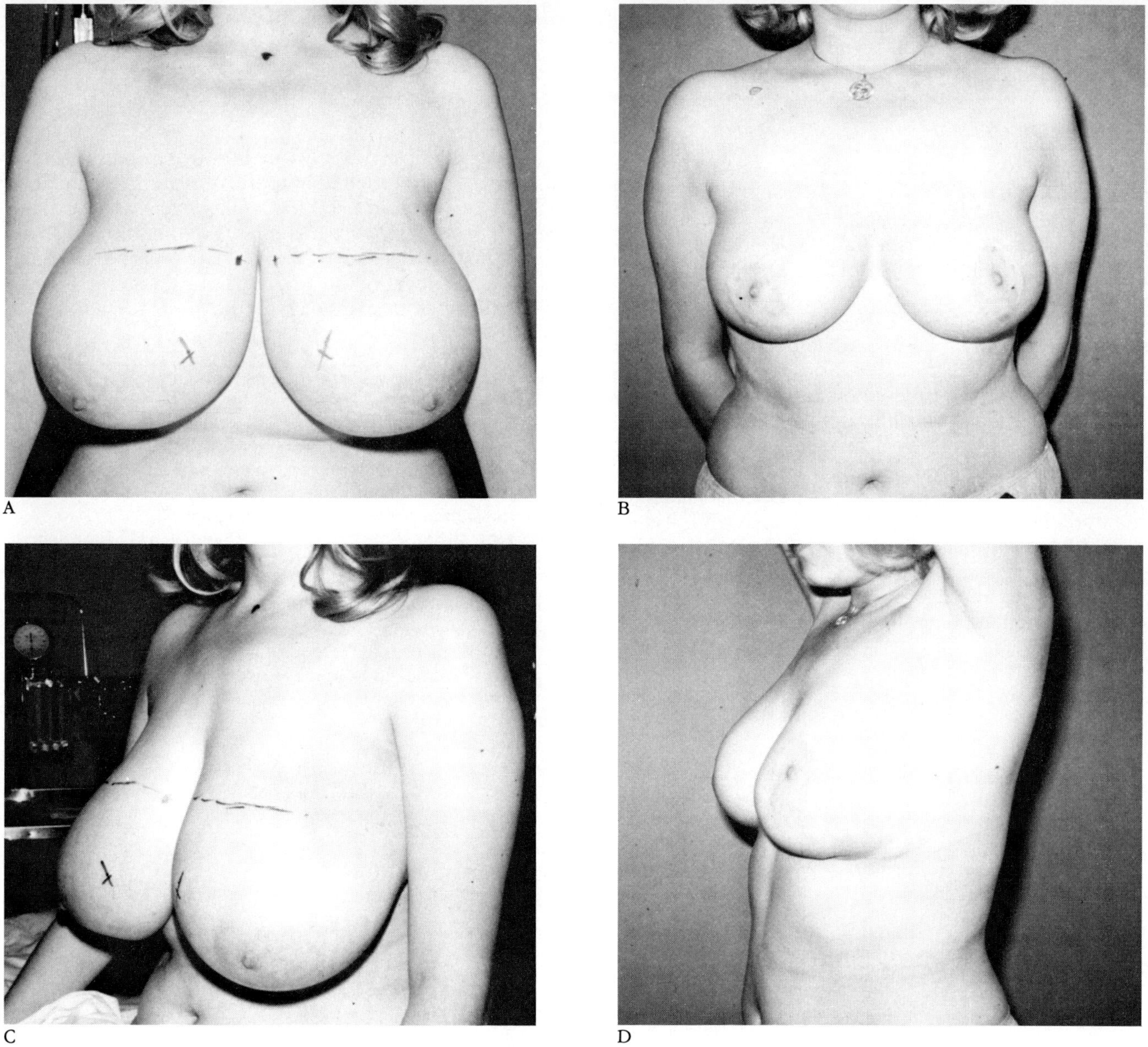

Figure 21-11
A, C. Patient with major breast hypertrophy.
B, D. Result at 1 year following 1000-gm resection per breast. Natural breast contour without upper quadrant flattening.

Figure 21-10. A 600-gm breast reduction using the B-technique.
A. Preoperative condition in an 18-year-old female with a 38D breast hypertrophy. Patient sitting.
B. Standard B-technique markings as completed with the patient recumbent.
C. Resection of breast tissue including medial and lateral lower quadrants but also extending beneath the areola and including a portion of the upper quadrants.
D. En bloc resection but with skin removal confined to the lower quadrants.
E. Following tissue excision, upper quadrant fullness remains. Note deepithelialized periareolar area.
F. Closure is begun with deep plicating breast sutures, which restores conical configuration and spreads out NAC.
G. Single subcuticular suture is used for closure followed by paper tape dressing. Note excellent breast contour.
H. Early postoperative result. In contrast to the inferior pedicle technique, breast shape improves with time (see Fig. 21-11).

Inferior Pedicle Technique

Robert M. Goldwyn
Eugene H. Courtiss

Reduction mammaplasty by the inferior pedicle technique was described by Ribeiro [70], Robbins [71], and Courtiss and Goldwyn [14, 15]. Its popularity is increasing because of the following advantages [2, 28, 69, 77, 82]: (1) It has an axial pattern blood supply [104] to the nipple, areola, and remaining breast tissue through perforators from the internal mammary artery and the external branches from the lateral thoracic artery; (2) it allows the surgeon latitude to resect breast tissue wherever needed; (3) it preserves normal or almost normal sensation to the nipple and areola because it spares the important cutaneous branches of the third, fourth, and fifth intercostal nerves; (4) it can be used for breasts that are mildly or moderately large or those that are gigantic—in the latter case without recourse to nipple and areola grafting; (5) the aesthetic results are excellent; and (6) the operation is relatively easy to learn.

MARKING

With the patient standing, a line is drawn from the middle of the clavicle through the nipple. A finger is then placed behind the breast in the inframammary fold and, with the breast *partially supported,* the level of the fold is marked across the first line drawn (Fig. 21-12A). This becomes the future upper level of the areola. Thus, the nipple is 24 to 25 cm from the sternal notch on the midclavicular line. A

Figure 21-12. Markings for the inferior pedicle technique of breast reduction.

A. With the breast partly supported, the proposed upper margin of the new areolar site is marked where the level of the inframammary crease transects the midclavicular line. The nipple is usually and ideally 24 to 25 cm from the sternal notch on the midclavicular line.

B, C. First, the keyhole and the future medial and lateral skin flaps are marked. Next, the inferior pedicle is outlined with its inferior margin 1 cm above the entire length of the inframammary fold. Alternatively, for very large reductions and greater transpositions, more of the inframammary fold may be used as the inferior margin. A split-thickness skin graft is removed from the surface of the inferior pedicle. Note the rim of dermis left superior to the areola.

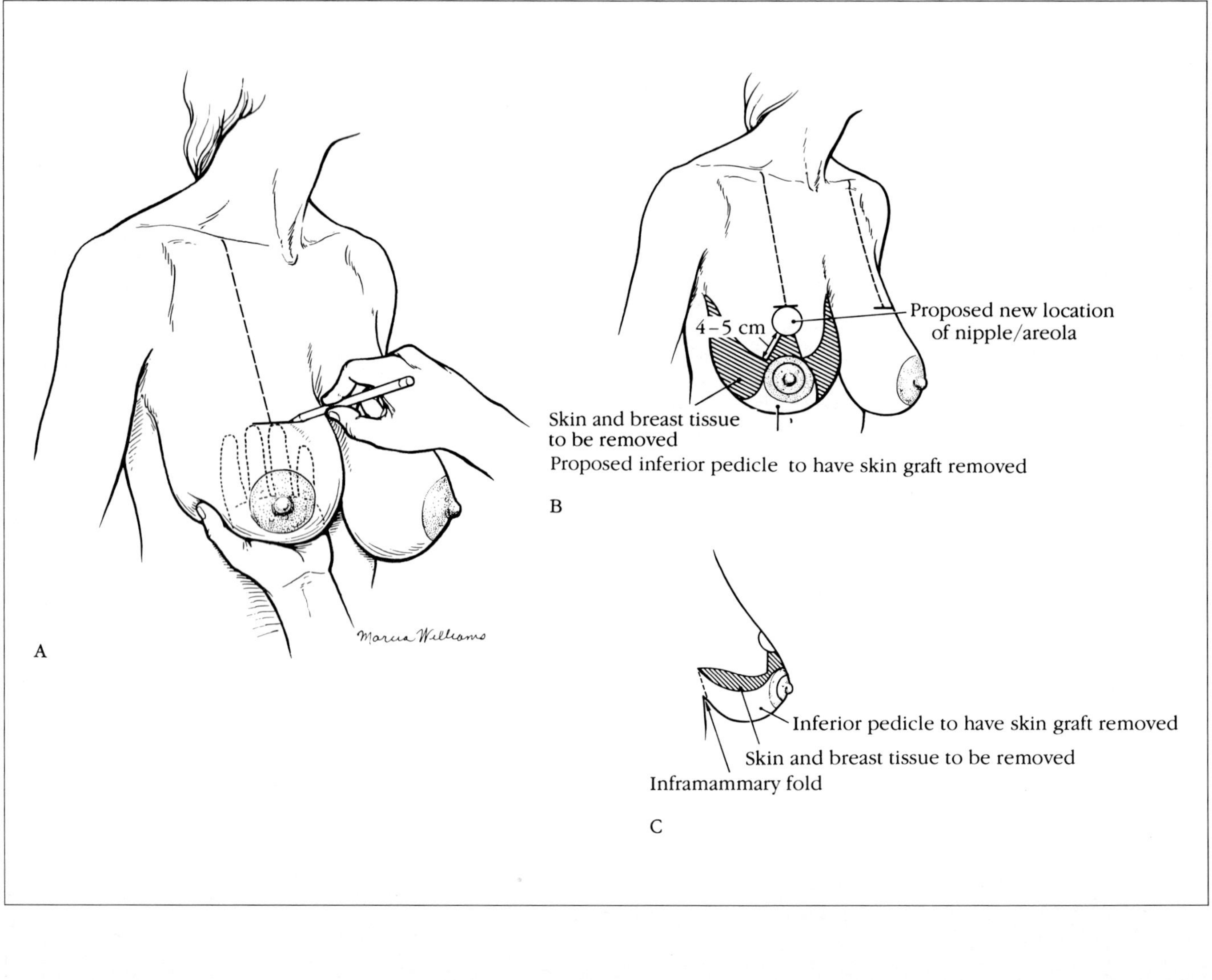

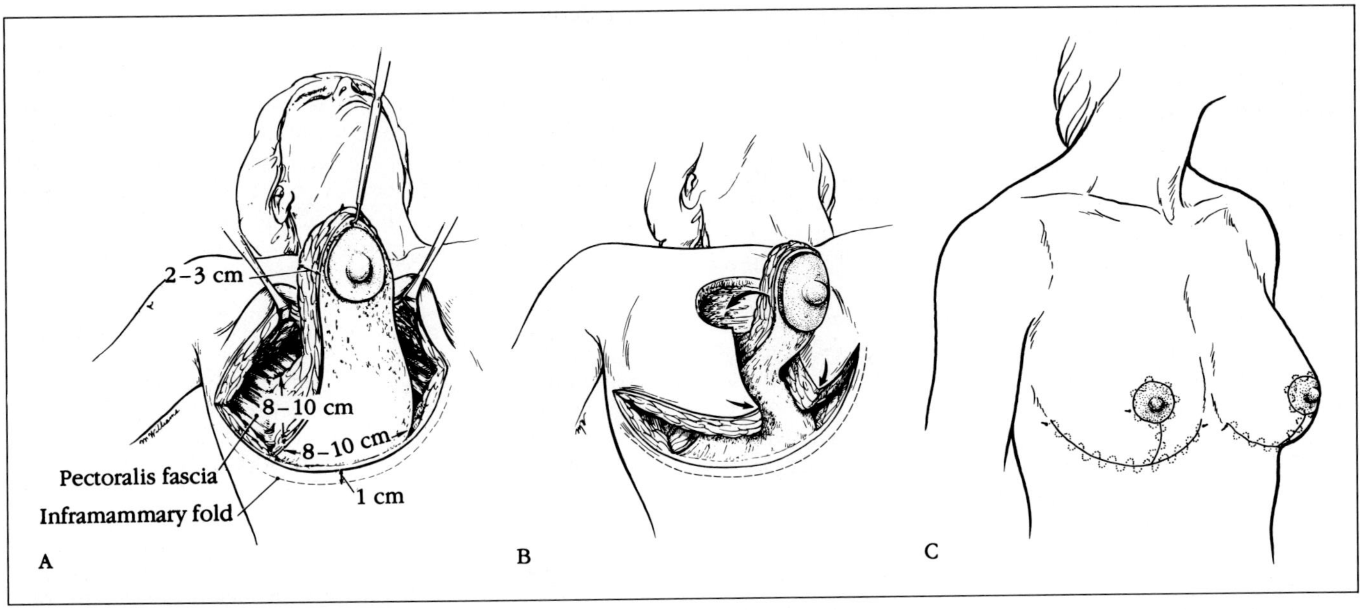

Figure 21-13. Operative technique.
A. The inferior pedicle dissected through the breast to the pectoral muscle. Care is taken to maintain a 3-cm thickness beneath the nipple-areola complex and 8 to 10 cm at the base of the pedicle. It is better to leave more tissue on the pedicle initially and to trim it later in the operation if required.
B. The nipple and areola on an inferior pedicle raised and attached to the circular part of the keyhole. The medial and lateral skin flaps are approximated beneath the areola.
C. Closure. Drains may be used depending on the surgeon's preference.

keyhole wire pattern* is placed on the breast with its top at this location so that the medial limb goes directly inferiorly and the lateral limb somewhat outward. By this means, the horizontal length of the medial and lateral flaps is equalized. The limb should not be too divergent in order to avoid an excessively tight closure. To prevent the final location of the nipple from being too high, the medial limb should be 4 to 5 cm long. The inferior borders of the lateral and medial skin flaps are defined by lazy-S extensions (Fig. 21-12B, C).

An areola marker (4.5–5.0 cm in diameter) is centered on the nipple, which is slightly tense by pressure, and the area is circumscribed. The base of the inferior dermal pedicle is marked by a line running 1 cm above the inframammary fold. Its width is usually 8 to 10 cm but should be greater in gigantomastia.

OPERATIVE TECHNIQUE

The upper border of the dermal pedicle is incised to the subcutaneous fat. A cutting electric current is used to dissect the breast pedicle, which is held forward away from the chest. If the vertical length of the inferior pedicle is less than 15 cm, the inferiorly based dermal pedicle flap can remain attached to the pectoralis muscle at the base with a thickness of 8 to 10 cm (Fig. 21-13A). The dermal pedicle is kept approximately 3 cm thick beneath the nipple-areola. Maintaining thickness avoids inversion as well as ischemia. Preserving bulk at the base ensures not only a good contour but adequate vascularity and sensation because the crucial vessels and nerves remain uninjured.

It is important not to injure the arteries and veins to the nipple and areola as one is dissecting the pedicle. Therefore, it is advisable to dissect slightly outward and laterally from the pedicle and to preserve a rim of dermis, about 1 cm in width, superior to the proposed areola.

Redundant breast tissue is resected, and final medial and lateral breast contouring is done with the patient semiupright to minimize later discrepancies because of gravity.

At the time of closure, if more projection of the areola is desired, the rim of dermis can be sutured backward to the tissue below the areola, or, alternatively, a deepithelialized dermal platform can be preserved in the keyhole area at the beginning of the operation [77].

Closure proceeds in the usual fashion (Fig. 21-13B). Georgiade and his associates [28] have suggested a Y-type closure to lessen the length of the scars both medially and laterally. A multilayered closure is performed (Fig. 21-13C) with running, everting sutures of 4-0 Prolene. A drain, either suction or Penrose, may be placed laterally, to be removed in 48 hours.

ADVANTAGES AND DISADVANTAGES

The advantages of this technique have been previously mentioned and are shown in a variety of cases (Figs. 21-14 to 21-17). However, as with every method, the surgeon does not simply cut on a dotted line but must take into account the specific problems of each patient and the three-dimensional nature of the human body. To achieve an optimal result, adjustments must be made during the

* McKissock Keyhole Pattern, Padgett Instruments, Kansas City, Mo.

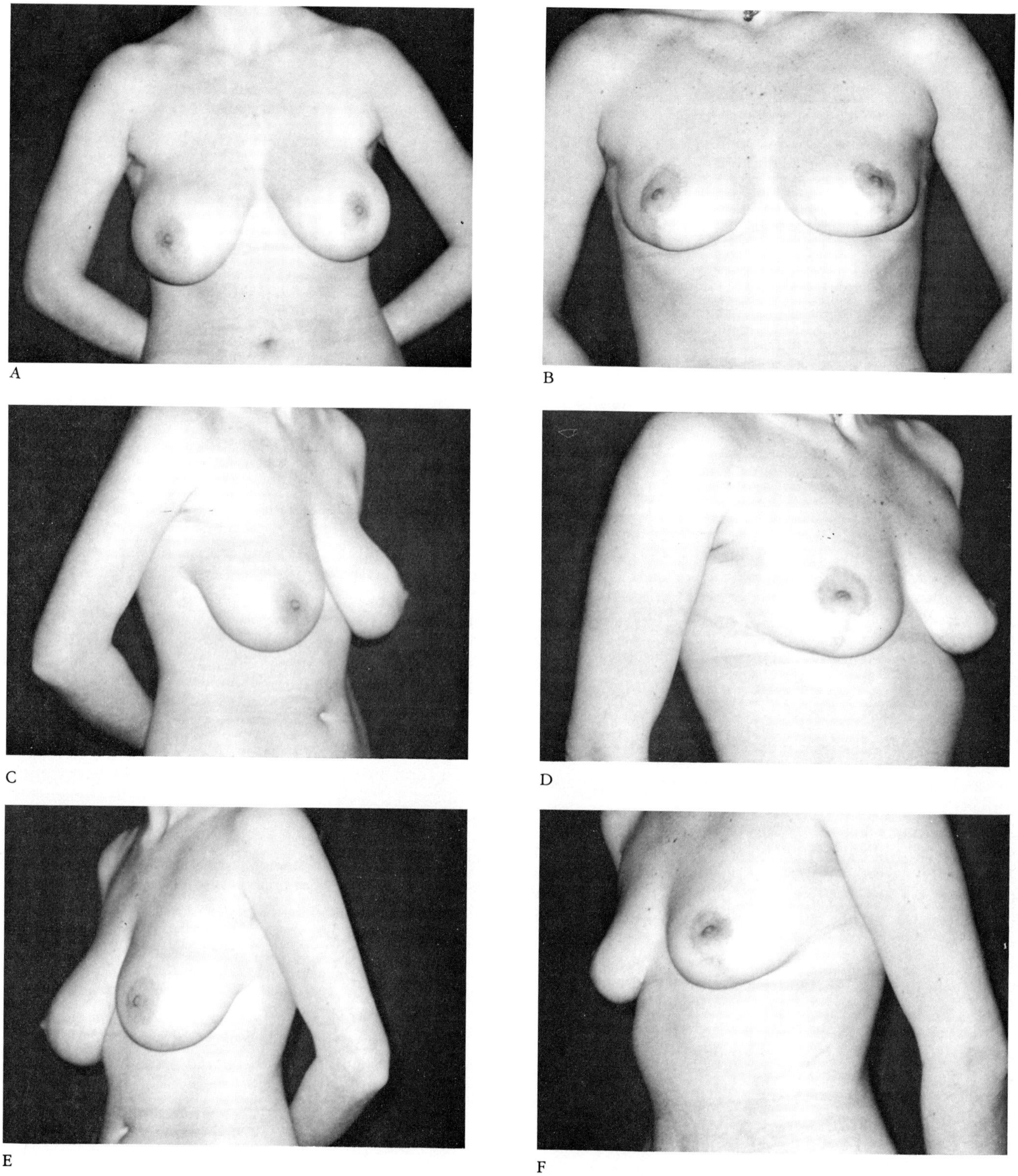

Figure 21-14
A, C, E. Preoperative views of 22-year-old female.
B, D, F. Postoperative views 12 months after an average of 368 gm was removed from each side.

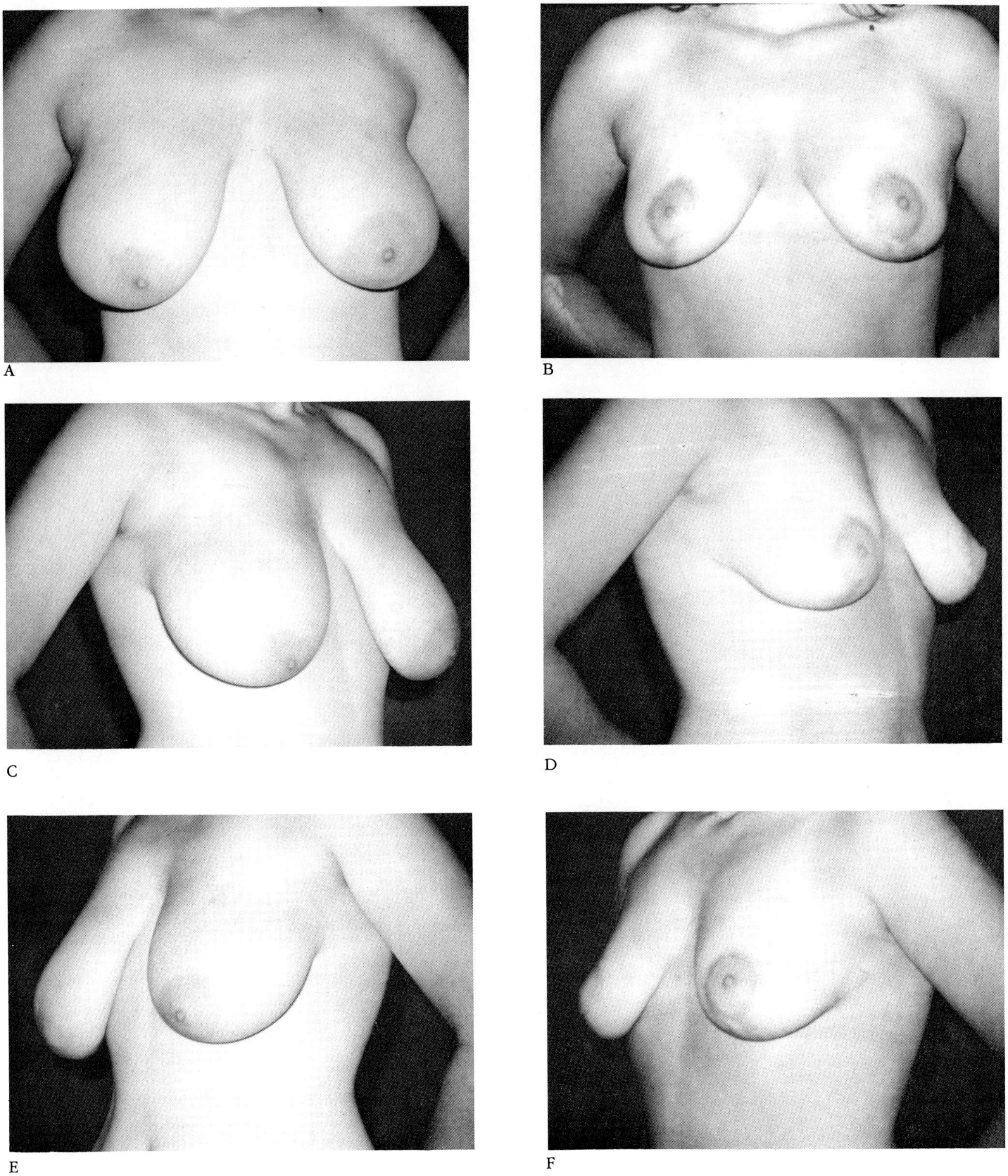

Figure 21-15
A, C, E. Preoperative views of 20-year-old female.
B, D, F. Postoperative views after 12 months with an average of 388 gm removed from each side.

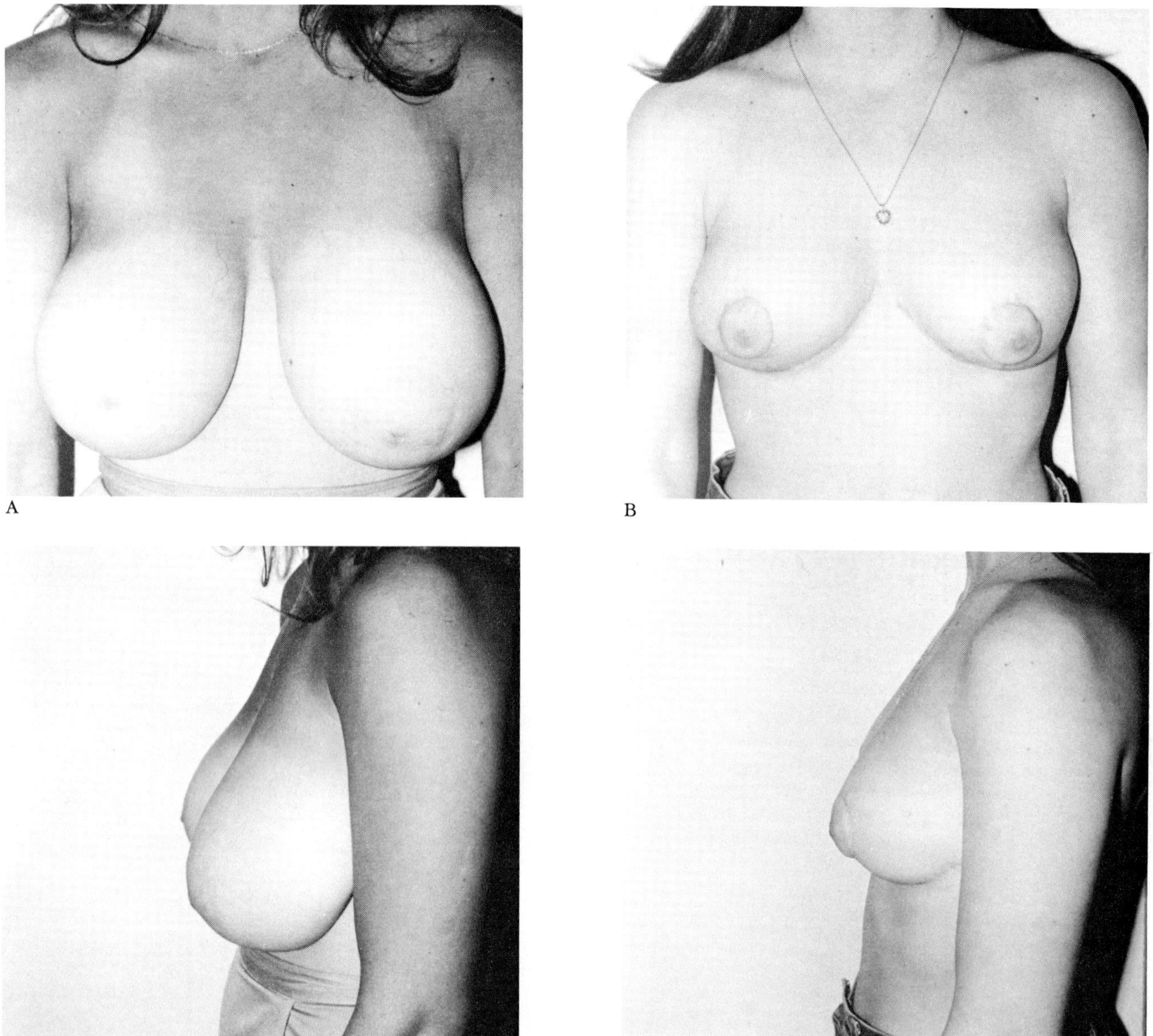

A B C D

Figure 21-16
A, C. Preoperative views of 19-year-old female.
B, D. Postoperative views after 14 months with an average of 510 gm removed from each side.

operation. The fact that the inferior pedicle technique has great safety and versatility does not mean that a prospective patient should not be informed about possible complications: death from the operation, infection, hematoma, altered sensation in the nipple and areola(s), necrosis of the nipple and areola, decreased ability to nurse, and the inevitability of scars, which may be more prominent than is desirable. The patient should understand also that the breasts will match, in all likelihood, but absolute symmetry, though ideal, is rarely achieved.

FREE NIPPLE GRAFT

Free nipple grafts are considered for patients with very large breasts where the predicted glandular resection is greater than 1500 gm in younger patients or 1200 gm in older women [36]. Some surgeons have based the indications for the procedure on the degree of ptosis and specifically the distance of nipple transposition; i.e., a nipple 45 cm from the sternal notch (normal being 22 cm) would be moved more than 20 cm. This latter indication no longer exists as the length of the inferior pedicle does not increase significantly [3]. Free nipple grafts are done because survival of the NAC as a graft is a virtual certainty, whereas long pedicles and tight closures risk complete loss. The concern for a rapid procedure with minimal blood loss remains essential in obese, middle-aged pa-

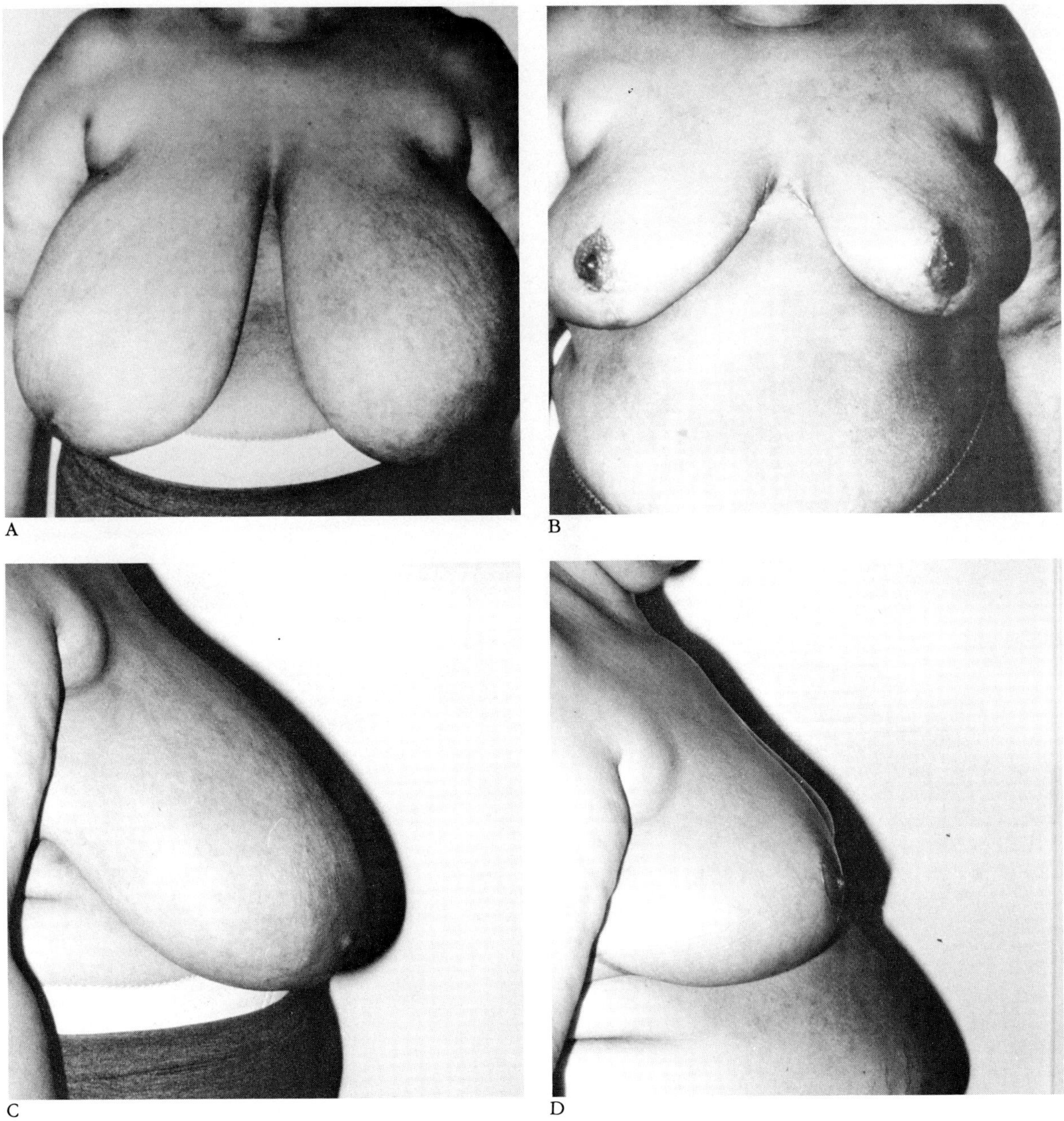

Figure 21-17
A, C. Preoperative views of 64-year-old female.
B, D. Postoperative views after 18 months with an average of 2100 gm removed from each side. Although more tissue could have easily been excised, this patient, who was older, wanted to be certain that she remained "large like my body."

tients with cardiopulmonary problems or in certain cases of virginal hypertrophy [1].

With the patient standing, the new nipple site is marked 24 to 28 cm from the sternal notch as removal of the pendulous breast will allow contraction of the skin and a more natural nipple location postoperatively (Fig. 21-18). The inframammary fold is marked in its natural crease as well as its midpoint. With the patient recumbent and the breast displaced laterally, the vertical medial line of resection is marked by joining the nipple to the submammary fold. Next, the breast is pushed medially and the vertical lateral line marked from nipple to inframammary fold. Each line is 7 cm long and the lines are joined obliquely to the inframammary fold. The final configuration is a three-wing star. As noted by Wise [100], one can use a standard pattern procedure but deepithelialize the new nipple site and split it to facilitate flap closure, rather than resecting it, as is routinely done in most reduction mammaplasties [25]. The nipple-areola is 4 cm in diameter and is excised as a full-thickness graft. The lines are then excised down to pectoral fascia, the glandular tissue removed without undermining, and the flaps brought together at the midpoint of the submammary fold. The new nipple site is deepithe-

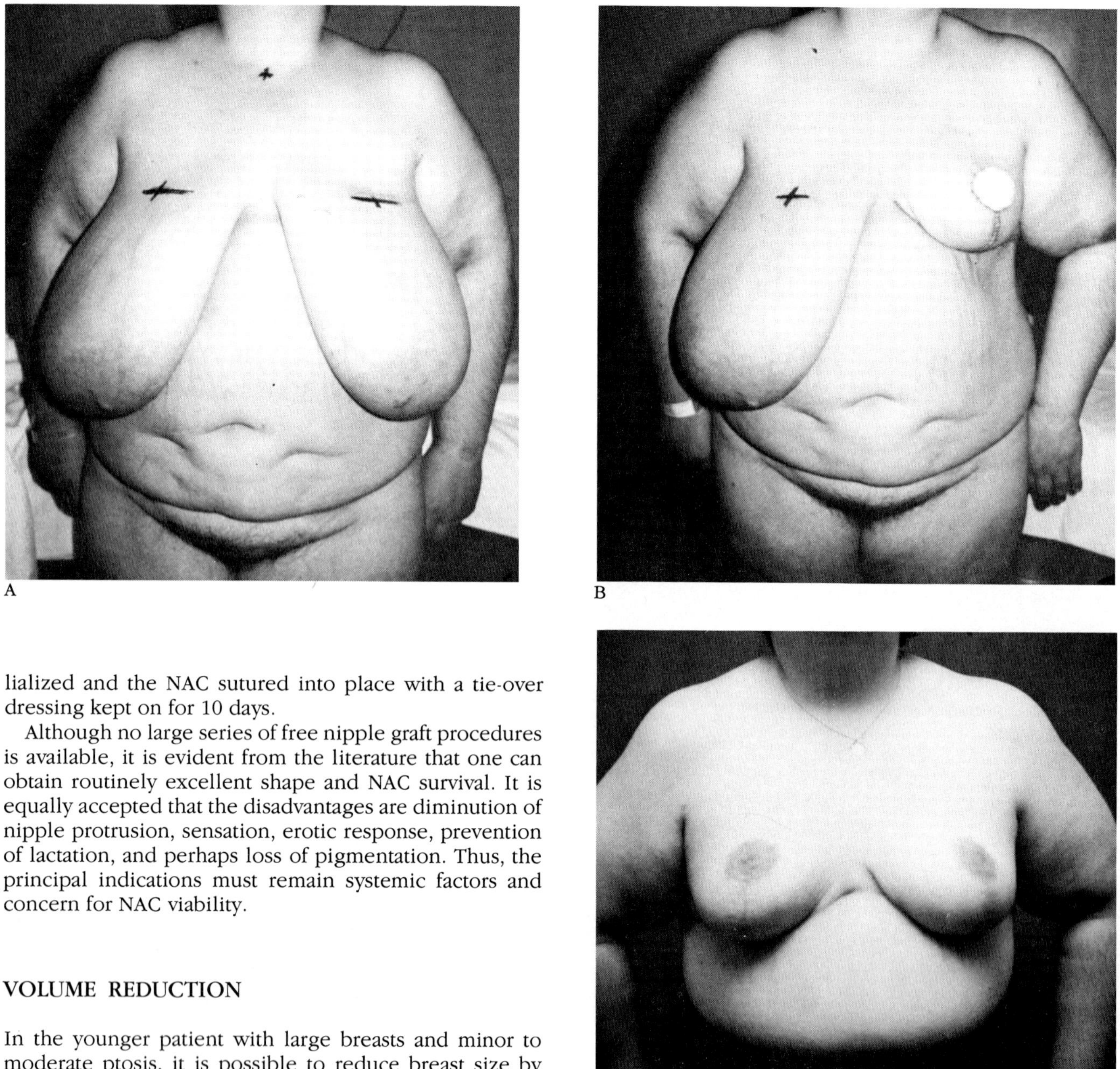

A

B

C

Figure 21-18

A. An obese patient with significant anesthetic risk due to cardiopulmonary incompetency necessitating two-stage reduction mammaplasty using a free nipple graft technique.
B. Following unilateral reduction.
C. Result after resection of 3300 gm on the right and 2500 gm on the left.

lialized and the NAC sutured into place with a tie-over dressing kept on for 10 days.

Although no large series of free nipple graft procedures is available, it is evident from the literature that one can obtain routinely excellent shape and NAC survival. It is equally accepted that the disadvantages are diminution of nipple protrusion, sensation, erotic response, prevention of lactation, and perhaps loss of pigmentation. Thus, the principal indications must remain systemic factors and concern for NAC viability.

VOLUME REDUCTION

In the younger patient with large breasts and minor to moderate ptosis, it is possible to reduce breast size by means of the volume reduction mammaplasty. As reported by Cloutier [12], one removes 200 to 400 gm of tissue from the undersurface of the breast through an inframammary incision and allows the skin envelope to contract spontaneously (Fig. 21-19). Obviously, the procedure will not make major changes in shape or improve major ptosis. Therefore, the procedure is most frequently used in the younger patient with firm breasts who wants smaller cup size. It is possible to convert a D cup to a full B cup with minimal scars. The adolescent patient is the ideal patient as their symptoms are often psychologic rather than physical.

A 6- to 10-cm-long incision is marked in the inframammary fold with the patient standing. The incision passes downward, and the entire breast is elevated off the pectoral fascia. Breast tissue is then excised leaving 4 cm beneath the areola and 3 cm under the surrounding skin. Hemostasis is obtained, a drain inserted, and the wound closed with a continuous 4-0 Vicryl suture. A pressure dressing is applied.

The operation has definite advantages in carefully selected cases: (1) Scarring is minimal and restricted to the inframammary crease; (2) the duct system is undisturbed,

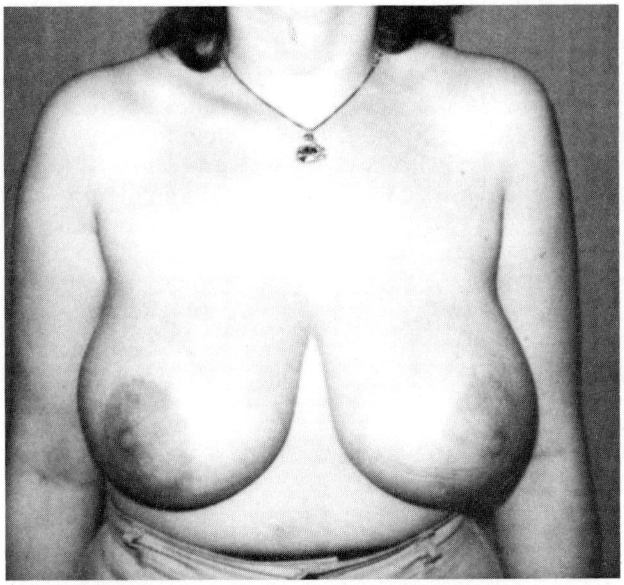

A

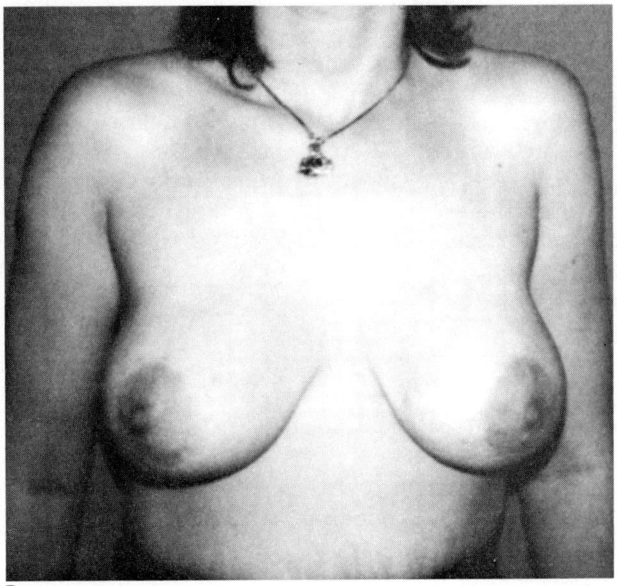

B

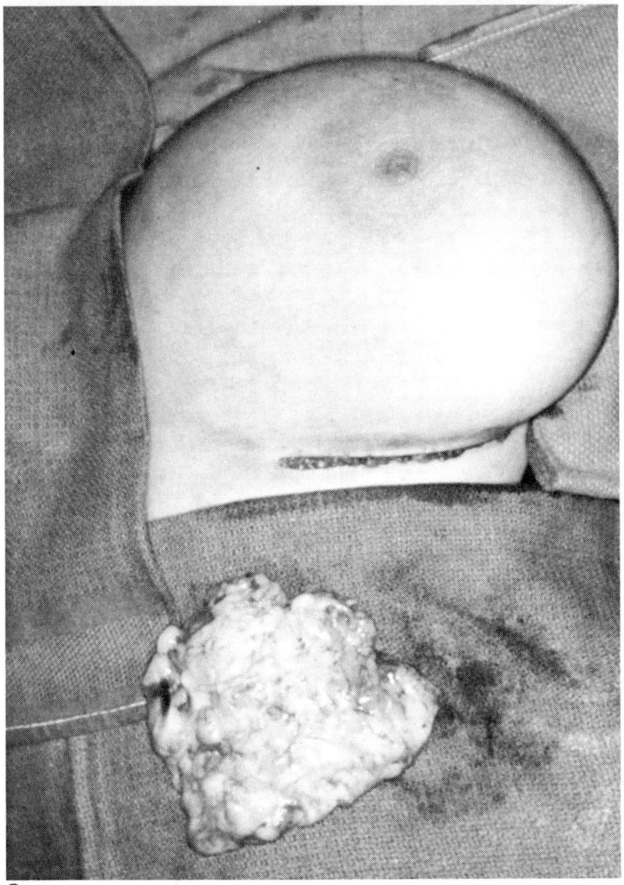

C

Figure 21-19
A. Patient with moderate breast hypertrophy.
B. Result at 1 year following removal of 350 gm of tissue through an inframammary incision only. (Case courtesy of Albert Cloutier, M.D., Montreal, Canada.)
C. Volume reduction technique for excising disk of breast tissue.

and lactation is possible; (3) the procedure is safe and simple; (4) the result has a natural appearance; and (5) subsequent revision with a pattern or B-technique is possible. The disadvantages include the following: (1) Significant degrees of ptosis are not correctable; (2) the patient must be reassured that early wrinkling of the skin and flattening will disappear with time; and (3) the breast may have a flattened, sawed-off appearance.

ANCILLARY PROCEDURES

Webbed Breasts

Extension of the breast's skin envelope across the sternal midline can produce a webbed effect. This failure to form two distinct breasts can be of great concern to the younger patient or a minor annoyance to the patient with pendulous breasts. The deformity is best treated as an extension of a reduction mammaplasty. McKissock [45–48] solved this problem by carrying the upper and lower limbs of the medial incision across the sternum, but with interjection of a superiorly based vertical V-shaped flap. Although the triangular flap minimizes hypertrophic scar formation, the patient must be aware of the risks. Since the majority of webbed breasts occur in modestly obese patients, one may attribute the defect to fat accumulation. Defatting can be done from beneath with acceptable results.

Axillary Breasts

The axillary breast is the most common type of ectopic breast and is composed of parenchyma, stroma, or NAC. Since it is essentially normal breast tissue, it will respond to both physiologic and pathologic stimuli. Patients often complain that the axillary breast drops over the hypertrophic breasts and further emphasizes their "full figure."

Although a direct incision is possible, Kaye [40] outlines the axillary breast and then draws a transverse incision above its superior border high in the axilla. With the arm abducted and the patient under local anesthesia, a curvilinear incision is made and the entire axillary breast excised with contouring into the subcutaneous tissue. The redundant skin is excised by means of a vertical split to determine the excess without tension on closure. Hemostasis must be meticulous. The wound is closed with a deep layer of 3-0 Vicryl sutures and a running subcuticular suture of 4-0 Vicryl.

COMPLICATIONS

Because of the extent of the operation, complications in reduction mammaplasty are more frequent than in other types of breast surgery (Table 21-4). The need for meticulous hemostasis and accurate wound closure cannot be overemphasized. The incidence of complications tends to vary with the size of the resection and the degree of skin undermining. Strombeck [89] reported a 16 percent complication rate in reductions greater than 1000 gm versus 1.8 percent for reductions of 250 to 500 gm. In a similar series of cases, Strombeck had an 8 percent overall complication rate compared to 14 percent by McIndoe and Rees [44] utilizing the wide undermining of the Biesenberger method [8].

Intraoperative Complications

The most common intraoperative problem is a tight skin closure, a problem that is most disconcerting when sufficient volume has already been excised. The problem is best avoided by adherence to accurate preoperative markings. If an inverted-T pattern is used, closure should begin at the outer limits and continue to the midline, with excess skin excised centrally. As emphasized by McKissock [48], deviation from a preplanned pattern often leads to disaster and must therefore be done cautiously. If difficulties arise, one can undermine the inframammary crease and incorporate the central area in the closure as a dart, thereby lessening flap tension.

Early Complications

HEMATOMA

Postoperative accumulation of blood is due primarily to severed arterial perforators entering from the chest wall. General oozing from the dermal pedicle or secondary to coagulation disorders rarely causes problems. Although most hematomas occur in the first 24 hours, McKissock [47] has noted that hematomas can occur up to 9 days following surgery and even consecutively in the same patient. Drainage of the hematoma must be immediate in order to avoid compromise of the nipple and skin flaps. Since hematomas are often associated with subsequent infection (37%, or 3 out of 8), every effort must be made to prevent them.

NIPPLE-AREOLA AND SKIN FLAP NECROSIS

Loss of a significant portion of the nipple-areola complex or of skin flaps is fortunately a rare event. In 362 reductions (average resection of 724 gm), McKissock [48] had no complete nipple losses and only five partial losses (1.4%). According to Rees [62, 63], the etiology of these complications includes (1) excessive resection with compromise of the pedicle, (2) congestion secondary to a hematoma, (3) tension, torsion, or kink of the dermal pedicle, and (4) excessive tightness of the skin brassiere with compression of the pedicle. Since frequent inspection for nipple cyanosis is a routine postoperative order, early recognition is possible. If a problem is encountered, the dressing should be completely removed and the breast palpated for possible hematomas (Fig. 21-20A). If the breast is tense and a hematoma is present, an "induced dehiscence" may be effected by removal of the sutures. Although subsequent scar revision will be necessary, the general breast contour can be retained by careful taping of the skin flaps. The critical point is that, if the cyanosis is recognized within 8 hours postoperatively, salvage by decompression of the pedicle is possible. Singer and Krant [79] have reviewed the subject and demonstrated the value of fluorescein in assessing the dusky NAC. In four cases of early exploration, compression of the pedicle was found. Wray and Luce [103] presented two cases of impending nipple necrosis managed by conversion to a free nipple graft. After bilateral reduction mammaplasty with a McKissock technique, one nipple was found to be cyanotic and

Table 21-4. Complications of breast reduction

Complication	Strombeck [91] (670 patients)	McKissock [47] (362 patients) (mean resection 724 gm)
Early		
Hematoma	2.7%	2.2% (8)
Nipple-areola slough	0.02% (3) complete	1.4% (5) partial
Skin flap loss	0.03% (5) grafting	0.4% (3) healed spontaneously
Infection		0.3% (1)
Fat necrosis	2.1%	
Wound dehiscence		1.1% (4)
Late		
Scarring		65%
Anesthetic nipple		8%

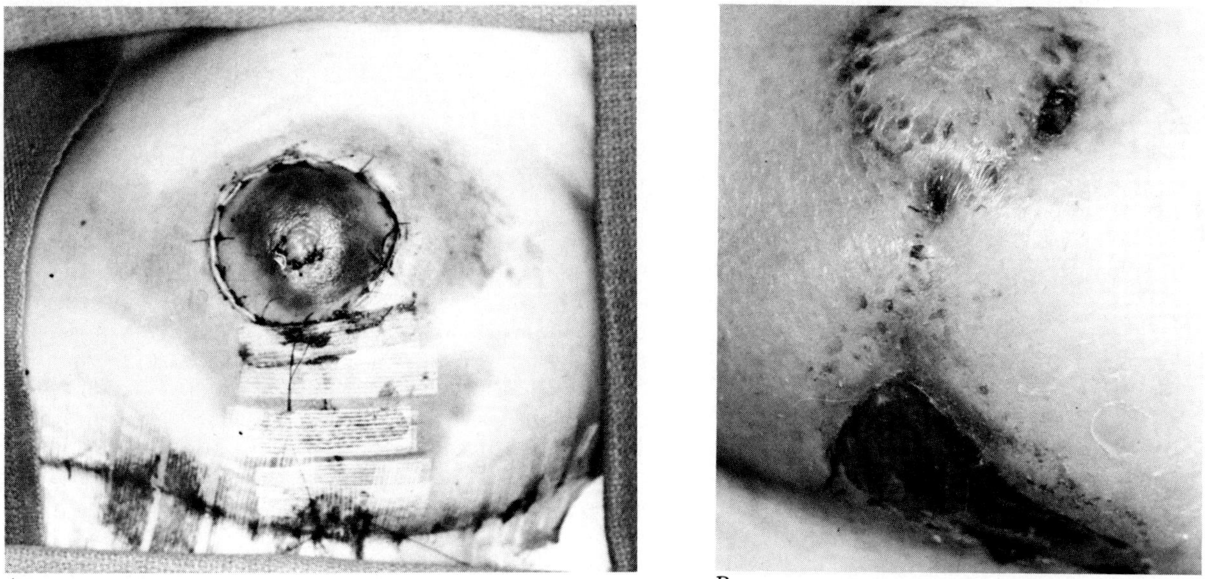

A B

Figure 21-20. Complications.
A. Cyanosis of the nipple and surrounding ecchymosis. Fluorescence was present, and the nipple survived without further surgery.
B. Skin slough at the inverted T. Healing occurred by secondary intention over 8 weeks.

without fluorescence. On reoperation, the central portion of the pedicle was found to be avascular, it was debrided, and the NAC was sutured as a free graft to the viable superior portion of the pedicle. The NAC survived completely and closely matched its pedicle counterpart in regard to color, contractibility, and projection. Although partial nipple loss may be circumferential or segmental, final eschar separation at 3 to 4 weeks is often not as severe as believed perhaps due to wound contracture.

Large skin sloughs are equally uncommon, but, in contrast, they should be treated aggressively. The demarcated area is excised, the edges are closed primarily, and the wide scar is revised secondarily. Since granulation tissue requires several weeks to develop, skin grafts are employed only as a last resort.

INFECTION

The occurrence of a primary deep infection without associated hematoma or fat necrosis is a rare event (<1%). Once an infection occurs, irrespective of its etiology, a broad-spectrum antibiotic is indicated. Although the organism may occasionally be a beta-hemolytic streptococcus, most cultures demonstrate a penicillin-resistant *Staphylococcus aureus.*

FAT NECROSIS

Necrosis of poorly vascularized fat tissue occurs as either a sterile or an infected abscess. Strombeck [91] reported a 16 percent incidence of fat necrosis in the obese patient having a resection greater than 1000 gm. It is often manifested by pain or tenderness, with a temperature elevation beginning on the third to fourth postoperative day. If aspiration is not done, a sinus tract will often develop. It is best to decompress the liquefaction through the communicating incision line as the inevitable scarring can be confined and easily revised. Although culture often discloses minor skin contaminants, immediate initiation of broad-spectrum antibiotics is indicated to prevent secondary infection. On occasion, debridement with secondary closure is necessary. In certain cases palpation of the area discloses a firm nodule that raises the patient's concerns regarding a possible cancer. Routine biopsies will show this to be necrotic fat. If the mass does not become softer over several months, biopsy is warranted.

WOUND DEHISCENCE

Significant separation of the incision occurs most frequently as a complication of long-term steroid therapy and occasionally as an intentional action to salvage a compromised NAC.

MALIGNANCY

The incidental finding of carcinoma in patients seeking breast reduction is reported to be 0.4 percent [85]. This figure is based on 19 of 5008 cases, with detection of the cancer on preoperative examination (5), intraoperative on frozen section (5), or postoperative on routine pathologic examination (9). For this reason, the resected tissue is always sent to Pathology and the patient told the result. If a carcinoma is found, the patient is referred to a general surgeon for definitive treatment [86].

Late Complications

SCARRING

The location of scarring is related to the surgical technique while the severity varies with the location and individual factors [22]. In an inverted-T incision, the vertical scar tends to spread (1 cm or wider) whereas the inframammary and periareolar scars often hypertrophy. McKis-

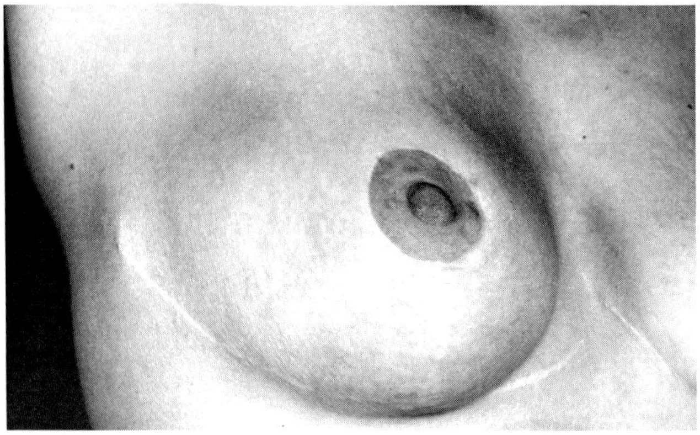

A

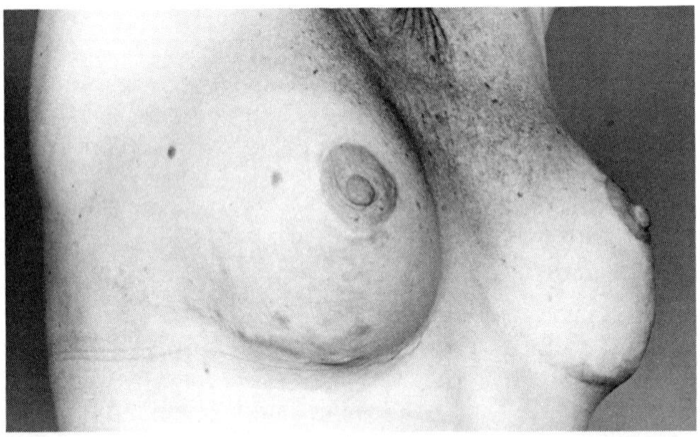

B

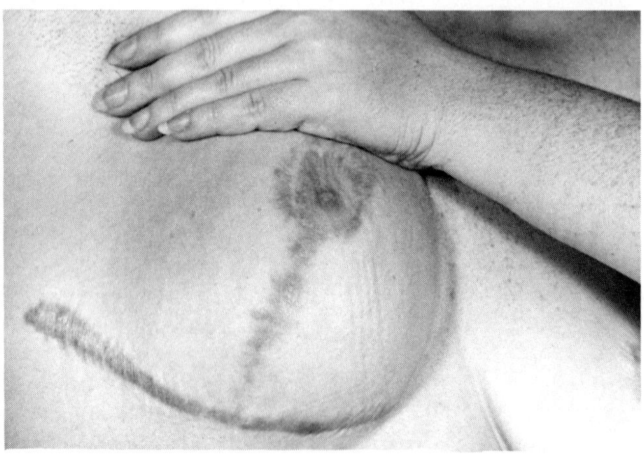

C

Figure 21-21. Degree of scarring after inverted-T reduction mammaplasty.

A. Excellent scars at 5 years postoperatively. The scars are hidden with arms by the side.
B. Average scars with some hypertrophy of the inframammary portion and spreading of the vertical component; 2 years postoperatively.
C. Poor scars with significant hypertrophy despite revision 1 year postoperatively. Subsequently, patient had steroid injection of the inframammary scar. It is now 2 years since surgical revision.

sock [48] reported that 65 percent of patients will develop a hypertrophic scar and that surgical revision is often unrewarding. At 3 to 6 months, the scars are often red and highly visible, but they tend to fade by 1 year (Fig. 21-21). After 10 years, Strombeck [91] found, patients considered their scars excellent (23%), good (30%), fair (30%), and ugly (17%).

SENSORY CHANGES

Courtiss and Goldwyn [14] objectively assessed the sensory modalities of pain, crude touch, and light pressure, before and after breast surgery. Following reduction mammaplasty performed by dermal pedicle transposition, virtually all breasts were insensitive immediately after operation and the majority remained insensitive at 6 months. At 1 year, the peripheral skin was approximately normal, but only 65 percent of the patients had nipple sensation at 2 years. Sensory changes were directly related to the *amount* of tissue resected, and not to the technique employed. A mitigating factor is the association of "sensuality," which has both a psychologic and an anatomic component, the latter being a general appreciation of firm touch rather than pain. Erectility of the nipple represents sympathetic fiber reinnervation of the areolar muscle, and it precedes return of all sensory modalities.

McKissock [48] reviewed his series of 362 breast reductions and had the following findings: (1) Immediately postoperatively, 92 percent had some loss; (2) at 6 months, 80 percent had some sensation; (3) at 2 years, 22 percent were essentially normal, 8 percent were permanently anesthetic, and 70 percent had varying amounts of reduced sensation. Of those with an alteration in nipple sensitivity, 65 percent felt the change was not significant. It is reasonable to inform the patient that she risks an 8 percent chance that the nipple will be permanently anesthetic; an incidence that may change with adoption of the inferior pedicle technique.

RECURRENT HYPERTROPHY

Numerous cases of recurrent breast enlargement have been reported, but they are usually instances of virginal hypertrophy. To avoid these problems, certain authors advocate that surgery be postponed, if possible, until the patient is 16 years old. In cases of moderate recurrence, Pitanguy [55] suggests that continued breast growth is best monitored by measuring increases in the height of the vertical scar, a 2.5-cm gain confirming the diagnosis.

INTERFERENCE WITH LACTATION

If the nipple remains in continuity with underlying glandular tissue, subsequent lactation is possible, depending on the amount of gland remaining [60, 61]. On the basis of a 10-year follow-up, Strombeck [91] has concluded that a patient has a 50 percent possibility of being able to nurse, with the highest probability in the patient having less than 500 gm resected.

NIPPLE DEFORMITIES

These problems can be divided into three groups: (1) nipple retraction, (2) nipple malposition, and (3) areolar deformity. In contrast to nipple inversions, retraction of the nipple occurring after a reduction mammaplasty implies tension on the underlying pedicle. Correction is best done at the time of operation by mobilization of the restraining pedicle or 4 months postoperatively by undercutting the nipple with division of the ducts. A secondary factor causing a flat nipple is failure of projection due to excessive resection of the underlying breast tissue. Correction of this deformity is difficult but can be attempted with a purse-string suture. It must be emphasized that approximately 50 percent of patients with postoperative nipple inversion had the condition preoperatively; thus, a detailed, recorded preoperative examination is warranted.

Nipple malposition usually occurs in the vertical axis and is further accentuated by the inevitable descent of the breast. Correction usually requires inferior transposition of the areola to a new site, with a resulting superior scar. In certain cases the skin flaps may be elevated and resected to shorten the areola–inframammary crease distance. A less frequent alternative is to perform an augmentation mammaplasty to provide additional fullness and projection.

Numerous areolar deformities are possible, including discrepancies in size (too small, too large) or shape (teardrop) and asymmetries. These problems are best avoided by precise measurements, preoperative quadrant markings of the areola, and extensive mobility of the pedicle without tethering.

BREAST DEFORMITIES

According to McKissock [47], subsequent loss of shape is a disappointing reality in 50 percent of cases by 1 year. This progression from a pleasing conical contour is characterized by a flattening of the superior breast quadrants, a descent of the inferior quadrants, and a too high location of the nipple [43]. It is believed to be caused by stretching of the inferior skin brassiere, descent of the glands, and fixation of the nipple at its original point. Prevention of this secondary ptosis is considered to be achieved by a larger resection at the primary operation. Strombeck [91] noted that patients regard the operation as excellent on cosmetic criteria in 41 percent of cases while shape was thought very good by 60 percent but ptotic by 14 percent. As stressed by McKissock [47], the greatest challenge in breast reduction now lies in artistic craftsmanship, which requires a classic breast without a squared-off appearance but with the correct amount of resection to avoid unsightly bulges.

RESULTS

Short-Term Results

The majority of patients are satisfied with the results of reduction mammaplasty. The breasts are smaller and less ptotic, and the fine incisions are rather inconspicuous. Dissatisfaction is expressed by patients with healing problems, excessive resections, or funny shapes. The initial office visits are enjoyable as the patients express their satisfaction and changes in life-style due to increased physical activity. As the scars become progressively hypertrophic, patients are more concerned with redness and visibility. Repeated reassurance will usually overcome this period of concern (3–9 months). As edema decreases and upper quadrant fullness disappears, patients will express disappointment with the flat upper quadrants. At the end of the first year, most patients remain satisfied with the results, the exceptions being younger patients who expected a more aesthetic result with minimal scarring.

Long-Term Results

Strombeck [91] reported a series of patients evaluated 10 years after reduction mammaplasty. As seen in Table 21-5, 86 percent were satisfied with the result although only 58 percent considered it very good. Significantly, 94 percent would have the procedure done again. De Castro [16] found a similar satisfaction rate. In the majority of cases, breast shape will remain unaltered after the first year provided there are no pregnancies or massive weight changes (Fig. 21-22).

Table 21-5. Results (Strombeck) [91]

1. Does result correspond to expectations?	86% yes	13% doubtful	1% no	
2. Would you have procedure again?	94% yes	5% doubtful	1% no	
3. What is your opinion of result?	58% very good	20% fair	1% bad	
4. Cosmetic result?	41% excellent	32% good	19% fair	5% bad
5. Shape of breasts?	60% very good	29% ptosis	14% too big	4% too small
6. Scars?	56% invisible	34% disturbing	10% ugly	
7. Position of nipple?	85% satisfactory	12% too high	3% too low	
8. Nipple shape?	64% round and even	8% uneven	27% inverted	
9. Nipple sensitivity?	57% unchanged	27% somewhat reduced	16% poor	
10. Back pain?	42% completely free	45% improved	13% unchanged	

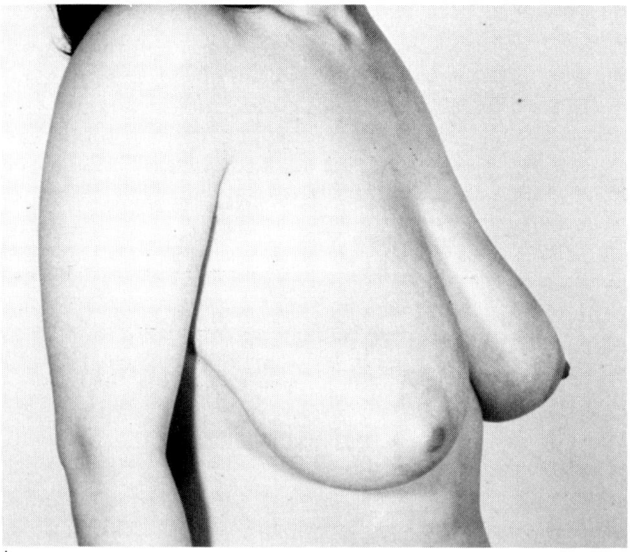

A

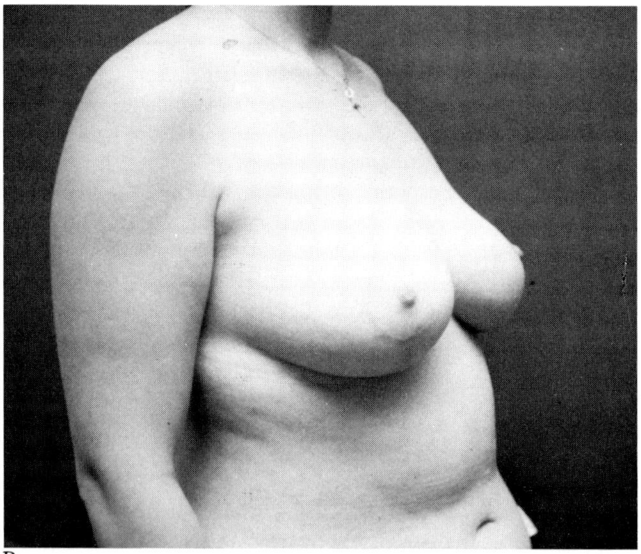

B

Figure 21-22. Long-term result following an 800-gm breast reduction using the B-technique.
A. Preoperative condition.
B. Result 9 years later.

SECONDARY SURGERY

Despite the frequency of breast problems following breast reductions, few articles have been published on secondary breast surgery. McKissock [47] has called attention to common errors resulting in unsatisfactory results. Smith and Gillen [83] described seven patients requiring secondary surgery for too high placement of the NAC. One must also expect a "learning curve" with any new procedure; its consequences can usually be minimized by careful study and implementation on minor cases of hypertrophy [82]. From our cases and those treated elsewhere, secondary surgery is a significant factor in breast reduction (Fig. 21-23). Before selecting the procedure, one must assess NAC position relative to the sternal notch, breast volume, and shape. Limited procedures are preferred whenever possible as total secondary reductions risk loss of the nipple in almost 50 percent of cases.

Scars

Scar revisions are not corrected before 1 year, and most are treated first with triamcinolone. Surgical revision is reserved for those wider than 1 cm.

Volume

With a pattern technique, the most common error is inadequate resection, especially in the lateral portion. In this event, patients will continue to complain of fullness under the arms and spilling out of their brassieres. Isolated quadrant resection can distort the breast, and one must consider a more tapered volume reduction. Occasionally, excessive resection will occur, and a secondary augmentation is required. Asymmetries are relatively rare as the skin envelope is generally constant.

Areolar Malposition

When the NAC is too low, secondary correction is relatively simple, and one utilizes the previous scars. With the NAC too high, the problem can be either absolute or relative as determined by its distance from the sternal notch [50]. If the nipple is less than 16 cm from the sternal notch, lowering of the NAC will leave a vertical scar. In severe cases it may be necessary to utilize interdigitating flaps from the lower portion of the breast. If the NAC is too high relative to the breast scars but not in relation to the sternal notch, the lower breast quadrants can be reduced and the submammary fold elevated until the nipple-to-fold distance is the desired 4.5 cm.

Glandular Ptosis

This deformity occurs when a large amount of breast tissue remains in the lower quadrants while the NAC is elevated to its ideal site. Thus, the gland is ptotic in relation to the NAC. In most cases, excess tissue is resected from the lower quadrants. However, if the breast volume is limited, an augmentation for upper quadrant fullness is required to balance the breast.

Unaesthetic Shape

Virtually any shape can be produced: too flat, squared off, too pointed, or irregular in lower contours. Unaesthetic shapes may be due to initial surgery or complications, especially fat necrosis. The flat breast, which most often occurs after an inverted-T resection, requires tightening of the skin in the lower quadrant and occasionally insertion of a breast implant. The square breast calls for reduction of lateral fullness plus mobilization of the glandular tissue

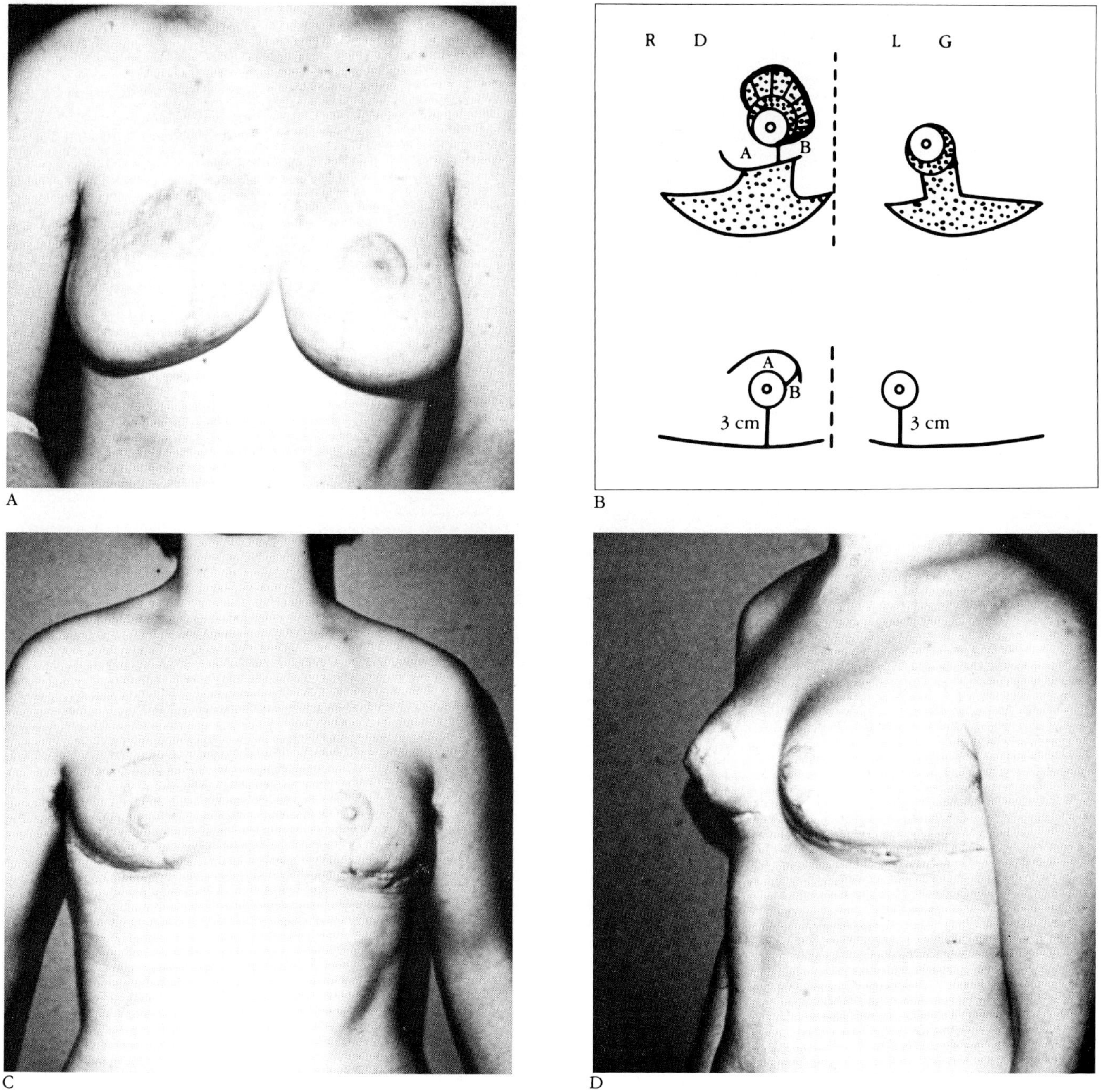

Figure 21-23. Secondary breast surgery.
A. Catastrophic result following breast reduction done elsewhere. Excessively high NAC cannot be lowered without scarring in the upper quadrants.
B. Operative plan involving transposition of the nipples, scar revision, and lower quadrant resections.
C, D. Early result following revision.

and central plication. The pointed breast may occur after lateral procedures. Conversion to a rounder shape requires periareolar skin reduction and occasionally resection of breast tissue beneath the areola.

REFERENCES

1. Adams, W. M. Free composite grafts of the nipple in mammaplasty. *South. Surg.* 13:715, 1947.
2. Ariyan, S. Reduction mammaplasty with the nipple areola carried on a single, narrow inferior pedicle. *Ann. Plast. Surg.* 5:167, 1980.
3. Arons, M. S. Reduction of very large breasts: The inferior flap technique of Robertson. *Br. J. Plast. Surg.* 29:137, 1976.
4. Arufe, H. N., Erenfryd, A., and Saubidet, M. Mammaplasty with single vertical superiorly-based pedicle to support the nipple-areola. *Plast. Reconstr. Surg.* 60:221, 1977.
5. Aston, S. J., and Rees, T. D. Breast Reduction and Mastopexy. In T. D. Rees (ed.), *Aesthetic Plastic Surgery.* Philadelphia: Saunders, 1980.
6. Aufricht, G. Mammaplasty for pendulous breasts: Empiric and geometric planning. *Plast. Reconstr. Surg.* 4:13, 1949.
7. Balch, C. R. The central mound technique for reduction mammaplasty. *Plast. Reconstr. Surg.* 67:305, 1981.
8. Biesenberger, H. *Deformitaten und kosmetische Operationen der weiblichen Brust.* Vienna: Maudrich, 1931.
9. Bostwick, J., III. *Aesthetic and Reconstructive Breast Surgery.* St. Louis: Mosby, 1983.
10. Cardona-Loya, O., Arrillaga, A., and Ryan, R. F. Toroidal breast reduction: An unsatisfactory procedure. *Plast. Reconstr. Surg.* 70:46, 1982.
11. Climo, M. Intercostothelial circulation: Nipple survival in reduction mammaplasty in the absence of a dermal pedicle. *Ann. Plast. Surg.* 4:98, 1980.
12. Cloutier, A. M. Volume reduction mammoplasty. *Ann. Plast. Surg.* 2:475, 1979.
13. Courtiss, E. H., and Goldwyn, R. M. Breast sensation before and after plastic surgery. *Plast. Reconstr. Surg.* 58:1, 1976.
14. Courtiss, E. H., and Goldwyn, R. M. Reduction mammaplasty by the inferior pedicle technique: An alternative to free nipple and areola grafting for severe macromastia or extreme ptosis. *Plast. Reconstr. Surg.* 59:500, 1977.
15. Courtiss, E. H., and Goldwyn, R. M. Update. A reduction mammaplasty by the inferior pedicle technique: An alternative to free nipple and areola grafting for severe macromastia and extreme ptosis. *Plast. Reconstr. Surg.* 66:646, 1980.
16. DeCastro, C. C. Late results after reduction mammaplasty with curved incisions. *Plast. Reconstr. Surg.* 61:862, 1978.
17. Dufourmentel, C., and Mouly, R. Plastie mammaire par la méthode oblique. *Ann. Chir. Plast.* 6:45, 1961.
18. Dufourmentel, C., and Mouly, R. Développements récents de la plastie mammaire par la méthode oblique latérale. *Ann. Chir. Plast.* 10:227, 1965.
19. Dufourmentel, C., and Mouly, R. Modification of "periwinkle shell operation" for small ptotic breast. *Plast. Reconstr. Surg.* 41:523, 1968.
20. Edholm, P., and Strombeck, J. O. Influence of Mammaplasty on the Arterial Supply to the Breast. In J. O. Strombeck, *Macromastia in Women, Acta Chir. Scand.* [Suppl.] 341:1, 1965.
21. Edwards, E. A. Surgical Anatomy of the Breasts. In R. M. Goldwyn (ed.), *Plastic and Reconstructive Surgery of the Breast.* Boston: Little, Brown, 1976. P. 37.
22. Elbaz, J. S., and Verheecke, J. La cicatrice en L dans les plasties mammaires. *Ann. Chir. Plast.* 17:283, 1972.
23. Ely, J. F. Guidelines for reduction mammoplasty. *Ann. Plast. Surg.* 6:424, 1981.
24. Erol, O. O., and Spira, M. A mastopexy technique for mild to moderate ptosis. *Plast. Reconstr. Surg.* 65:603, 1980.
25. Felix, E. R., et al. Strombeck mammaplasty with free nipple grafts. *Plast. Reconstr. Surg.* 45:47, 1970.
26. Georgiade, N. G. *Reconstructive Breast Surgery.* St. Louis: Mosby, 1976.
27. Georgiade, N. G., et al. Is there a reduction mammoplasty technique for "all seasons"? *Plast. Reconstr. Surg.* 63:765, 1979.
28. Georgiade, N. G., et al. Reduction mammaplasty utilizing an inferior pedicle nipple-areolar flap. *Ann. Plast. Surg.* 3:211, 1979.
29. Gillies, H., and Marino, H. The "periwinkle shell" principle in the treatment of the small ptotic breast. *Plast. Reconstr. Surg.* 21:1, 1958.
30. Gillies, H., and McIndoe, A. H. the technique of mammaplasty in conditions of hypertrophy of the breast. *Surg. Gynecol. Obstet.* 68:658, 1939.
31. Goin, M. K., and Goin, J. M. *Changing the Body.* Baltimore: Williams & Wilkins, 1981.
32. Goin, M. K., Goin, J. M., and Gianini, M. H. The psychic consequences of a reduction mammaplasty. *Plast. Reconstr. Surg.* 59:530, 1977.
33. Goldwyn, R. M. (ed.). *Plastic and Reconstructive Surgery of the Breast.* Boston: Little, Brown, 1976.
34. Goulian, D., Jr., and Conway, H. Correction of the moderately ptotic breast. *Plast. Reconstr. Surg.* 43:478, 1969.
35. Gruber, R. P., and Jones, H. W., Jr. The "donut" mastopexy: Indication and complications. *Plast. Reconstr. Surg.* 65:34, 1980.
36. Gsell, F. Reduction mammaplasty for extremely large breasts. *Plast. Reconstr. Surg.* 53:643, 1974.
37. Hugo, N. E., and McClellan, R. M. Reduction mammaplasty with a single superiorly-based pedicle. *Plast. Reconstr. Surg.* 63:230, 1979.
38. Kahn, S., Hoffman, S., and Simon, B. E. Correction of nonhypertrophic ptosis of the breasts. *Plast. Reconstr. Surg.* 41:244, 1968.
39. Kaplan, I. Reduction mammaplasty: Nipple-areola survival on a single breast quadrant. *Plast. Reconstr. Surg.* 61:27, 1978.
40. Kaye, B. L. Axillary breasts. *Plast. Reconstr. Surg.* 53:61, 1974.
41. Letterman, G., and Schurter, M. Facilitation of the upward advancement of the nipple-areola complex in reduction mammaplasty by Kiel resection. *Plast. Reconstr. Surg.* 67:793, 1981.
42. Marchac, D., and De Olarte, G. Reduction mammaplasty and correction of ptosis with a short inframmary scar. *Plast. Reconstr. Surg.* 69:45, 1982.
43. Mathes, S. J., Nahai, F., and Hester, T. R. Avoiding the flat breast in reduction mammaplasty. *Plast. Reconstr. Surg.* 66:63, 1980.
44. McIndoe, A. H., and Rees, T. D. Mammaplasty: Indications, technique and complications. *Br. J. Plast. Surg.* 10:307, 1958.
45. McKissock, P. K. Reduction mammaplasty with a vertical dermal flap. *Plast. Reconstr. Surg.* 49:245, 1972.
46. McKissock, P. K. Reduction mammoplasty by the vertical bipedicle flap technique: Rationale and results. *Clin. Plast. Surg.* 3:309, 1976.
47. McKissock, P. K. Reduction Mammaplasty. In E. H. Courtiss

(ed.), *Aesthetic Surgery: Trouble—How to Avoid It and How to Treat It.* St. Louis: Mosby, 1978.
48. McKissock, P. K. Reduction Mammoplasty and Correction of Ptosis of the Breast. In W. C. Grabb and J. W. Smith (eds.), *Plastic Surgery* (3rd ed.). Boston: Little, Brown, 1979. P. 737.
49. Meyer, K., and Kesselring, U. Reduction mammaplasty with an L-shaped suture line. *Plast. Reconstr. Surg.* 55:139, 1975.
50. Millard, R. D., Jr., Mullin, W. R., and Lesavoy, M. A. Secondary correction of the too-high areola and nipple after a mammaplasty. *Plast. Reconstr. Surg.* 58:568, 1976.
51. Nicolle, F., and Chir, M. Improved standards in reduction mammaplasty and mastopexy. *Plast. Reconstr. Surg.* 69:453, 1982.
52. Peixoto, G. Reduction mammaplasty: A personal technique. *Plast. Reconstr. Surg.* 65:217, 1980.
53. Penn, J. Breast Reduction, II. In *Transactions of the International Society of Plastic Surgery, Second Congress, London, 1959.* Edinburgh: Livingstone, 1960.
54. Pitanguy, I. Breast Hypertrophy. In *Transactions of the International Society of Plastic Surgery, Second Congress, London, 1959.* Edinburgh: Livingstone, 1960.
55. Pitanguy, I. Surgical treatment of breast hypertrophy. *Br. J. Plast. Surg.* 20:78, 1967.
56. Pitanguy, I. Personal Preferences for Reduction Mammaplasty. In R. M. Goldwyn (ed.), *Plastic and Reconstructive Surgery of the Breast.* Boston: Little, Brown, 1976. P. 167.
57. Planas, J., and Mosley, L. H. Improving breast shape and symmetry in reduction mammoplasty. *Ann. Plast. Surg.* 4:297, 1980.
58. Pontes, R. Reduction mammoplasty: Variations I and II. *Ann. Plast. Surg.* 6:437, 1981.
59. Poy, N. G. Is the Strombeck breast reduction viable? *Ann. Plast. Surg.* 3:47, 1979.
60. Ragnell, A. Operative correction of hypertrophy and ptosis of the female breast. *Acta Chir. Scand.* 94:113, 1946.
61. Ragnell, A. Further Experience of Preservation of Lactation Capacity and Nipple Sensitivity in Breast Reduction. In *Transactions of the International Society of Plastic Surgery, First Congress, Sweden, 1955.* Baltimore: Williams & Wilkins, 1957.
62. Rees, T. D. *Aesthetic Plastic Surgery.* Philadelphia: Saunders, 1980.
63. Rees, T. D., and Flagg, S. Untoward Results and Complications Following Breast Reduction Mammaplasty. In R. M. Goldwyn (ed.), *The Unfavorable Result in Plastic Surgery: Avoidance and Treatment.* Boston: Little, Brown, 1972.
64. Regnault, P. Reduction mammaplasty by the "B" technique. *Plast. Reconstr. Surg.* 53:19, 1974.
65. Regnault, P. Reduction Mammaplasty by the "B" Technique. In R. M. Goldwyn (ed.), *Plastic and Reconstructive Surgery of the Breast.* Boston: Little, Brown, 1976. P. 269.
66. Regnault, P. Gigantomastia by the B technique. *Aesthetic Plast. Surg.* 1:115, 1977.
67. Regnault, P. Breast Reduction. In J. Q. Owsley and R. A. Peterson (eds.), *Symposium on Aesthetic Surgery of the Breast.* St. Louis: Mosby, 1978. P. 58.
68. Regnault, P. Breast reduction: B technique. *Plast. Reconstr. Surg.* 65:840, 1980.
69. Reich, J. The advantages of a lower central breast segment in reduction mammaplasty. *Aesthetic Plast. Surg.* 3:47, 1979.
70. Ribeiro, L. A new technique for reduction mammaplasty. *Plast. Reconstr. Surg.* 55:330, 1975.
71. Robbins, T. H. A reduction mammaplasty with the areola-nipple based on an inferior dermal pedicle. *Plast. Reconstr. Surg.* 59:64, 1977.
72. Robbins, T. H. Innervation of the nipple-areola complex. (Letter to the Editor.) *Plast. Reconstr. Surg.* 68:453, 1981.
73. Robertson, D. C. The technique of inferior flap mammaplasty. *Plast. Reconstr. Surg.* 40:372, 1967.
74. Robertson, J. L. A. Changed appearance of mammograms following breast reduction. *Plast. Reconstr. Surg.* 59:347, 1977.
75. Salmon, M. Les artères de la glande mammaire. *Ann. Anat. Pathol.* (Paris) 16:477, 1939.
76. Schatten, W. E., Hartley, J. H., Jr., and Hamm, W. G. Reduction mammaplasty by the Dufourmentel-Mouly method. *Plast. Reconstr. Surg.* 48:306, 1971.
77. Schultz, R. C., and Markus, N. J. Platform for nipple projection: Modification of the inferior pedicle technique for breast reduction. *Plast. Reconstr. Surg.* 68:208, 1981.
78. Schwarzmann, E. Die Technik der Mammaplastik. *Chirurg* 2:932, 1930.
79. Singer, R., and Krant, S. M. Intravenous fluorescein for evaluating the dusky nipple-areola during reduction mammaplasty. *Plast. Reconstr. Surg.* 67:534, 1981.
80. Skoog, T. A technique of breast reduction, transposition of the nipple on a cutaneous vascular pedicle. *Acta Chir. Scand.* 126:453, 1963.
81. Skoog, T. *Plastic Surgery.* Philadelphia: Saunders, 1974.
82. Smith, G. A., and Schmidt, G. H. Experience with the Ribeiro reduction mammaplasty technique. *Ann. Plast. Surg.* 3:260, 1979.
83. Smith, J. W., and Gillen, F. J. Repairing errors of nipple-areolar placement following reduction mammoplasty. *Aesthetic Plast. Surg.* 4:179, 1980.
84. Snyder, G. B. The combined use of the Strombeck pattern and the McKissock keyhole pattern in marking macromastia. *Plast. Reconstr. Surg.* 62:122, 1978.
85. Snyderman, R. K., and Lizardo, J. G. Statistical study of malignancies found before, during or after routine breast plastic operations. *Plast. Reconstr. Surg.* 25:253, 1960.
86. Springer, H. A. Reduction mammaplasty with discovery of occult breast carcinoma in twins. Case reports. *Plast. Reconstr. Surg.* 62:122, 1978.
87. Strombeck, J. O. Mammaplasty: Report of a new technique based on the two pedicle procedure. *Br. J. Plast. Surg.* 13:79, 1960.
88. Strombeck, J. O. Reduction Mammaplasty. In T. Gibson (ed.), *Modern Trends in Plastic Surgery.* London: Butterworth, 1964. P. 237.
89. Strombeck, J. O. Reduction Mammaplasty. In W. C. Grabb and J. W. Smith (eds.), *Plastic Surgery: A Concise Guide to Clinical Practice.* Boston: Little, Brown, 1968. Pp. 821–835.
90. Strombeck, J. O. Reduction mammaplasty. *Surg. Clin. North Am.* 51:453, 1971.
91. Strombeck, J. O. Late Results After Reduction Mammaplasty. In R. M. Goldwyn (ed.), *Long-term Results in Plastic Surgery.* Boston: Little, Brown, 1980. P. 722.
92. Tanski, E. V. A new method for prophylactic mastectomy, reduction mammaplasty, and mastopexy. *Plast. Reconstr. Surg.* 65:314, 1980.
93. Tegtmeier, R. E. A quick, accurate mammometer. *Plast. Reconstr. Surg.* 23:263, 1970.
94. Thorek, M. Plastic reconstruction of the breast and free transplantation of the nipple. *J. Int. Coll. Surg.* 9:194, 1946.
95. Vilain, R. Modification of the Biesenberger Procedure. In R. M. Goldwyn (ed.), *Plastic and Reconstructive Surgery of the Breast.* Boston: Little, Brown, 1976. Pp. 155–163.
96. Weiner, D. L., et al. A single dermal pedicle for nipple transposition in subcutaneous mastectomy, reduction mammoplasty or mastopexy. *Plast. Reconstr. Surg.* 51:115, 1973.

97. Weiner, D. L., Dolich, B. H., and Miclay, M. I., Jr. Reduction mammoplasty utilizing the superior pedicle technique: A six-year retrospective. *Aesthetic Plast. Surg.* 6:7, 1982.
98. Whidden, P. G. The tailor-tack mastopexy. *Plast. Reconstr. Surg.* 62:347, 1978.
99. Wise, R. J. A preliminary report of a method of planning the mammaplasty. *Plast. Reconstr. Surg.* 17:367, 1956.
100. Wise, R. J. Surgical Management of the Hypertrophic Breast. In F. W. Masters and J. R. Lewis, Jr. (eds.), *Symposium of Aesthetic Surgery of the Face, Eyelid and Breast.* St. Louis: Mosby, 1972.
101. Wise, R. J. Treatment of breast hypertrophy. *Clin. Plast. Surg.* 3:289, 1976.
102. Wise, R. J., Gannon, J. P., and Hill, J. R. Further experience with reduction mammaplasty. *Plast. Reconstr. Surg.* 32:12, 1963.
103. Wray, R. C., and Luce, E. A. Treatment of impending nipple necrosis following reduction mammaplasty. *Plast. Reconstr. Surg.* 68:242, 1981.
104. Zelnick, J. N., Pearl, R. M., and Johnson, D. Use of an axial flap for reduction mammaplasty. *Ann. Plast. Surg.* 7:204, 1981.

22. Breast Ptosis

Paule Regnault
Rollin K. Daniel

Breast ptosis has occurred when the nipple is at the inframammary fold or below it. A mastopexy is a surgical procedure for correcting ptosis when the breast volume is satisfactory or hypoplastic. Cases with hypertrophic volume are excluded because a breast reduction procedure is required rather than a mastopexy. Management of breast ptosis calls for careful analysis of the problem and the patient's desires, as well as selection of the optimal operation.

HISTORY

The diversity of surgical procedures used to correct the ptotic breast is replicated in their evolution. Letterman and Schurter [24] divide the available operations into four groups: (1) skin resection alone; (2) mastopexy, with or without attachment of the mammary gland to the anterior chest wall; (3) plication of the glandular element into a more conical shape; and (4) augmentation. The pioneering skin excisions of Pousson [33] and Verchere [39] were expanded by Girard [13] to include suspension of the gland from the second rib by heavy catgut sutures. In 1923 Lotsch [28] defined a true skin mastopexy technique based on a vertical incision with transposition of the nipple-areola compex superiorly and removal of skin inferiorly. For the next four decades, mastopexy procedures represented modifications of reduction techniques utilizing the methods of Biesenberger [3] and Strombeck [38]. Gillies and Marino [12] attempted to produce a more conical breast by transposition of breast tissue away from the full lower quadrants to the flattened upper quadrants. Dufourmentel and Mouly [7–9] extended the concept with their lateral approach and placement of redundant tissue into the retromammary space.

Subsequent advances occurred with Regnault's [34–36] report of correcting minor ptosis by augmentation mammaplasty alone while utilizing a mastopexy plus augmentation for moderate or major ptosis. In 1971 Goulian [14–18] reported a technique of skin excision without undermining followed by upward transposition of the nipple-areola complex (NAC). This method was designed exclusively for mastopexy and was subsequently expanded by Hinderer [20–22] to include dermal fixation to the pectoralis fascia. Recently, Erol and Spira [10] and others have promoted wide periareolar skin undermining, and plication of the breast, to achieve improved appearance, especially upper fullness and projection.

PATHOPHYSIOLOGY AND CLASSIFICATION

In the young female, the breast is located between the second and sixth intercostal spaces, the nipple is in front of the fourth rib, and sufficient skin support exists so that no inframammary fold is formed. In the mature breast, the nipple lies over the fifth rib and slightly below the center of the breast. As ptosis develops, the breast turns around the inframammary fold. The distance between the nipple and the fold changes very little, while the distance between the nipple and the clavicle increases progressively.

The causes of breast ptosis are gravitational, glandular hormonal regression (postpartum or menopausal), weight loss, dermatochalasis, and postoperative following breast reduction. A detailed history will reveal that many patients were previously pregnant or experienced significant weight fluctuations (±15 pounds) with resulting change in breast volume and permanent dermatochalasis [25, 26]. Alternatively, many women undergo glandular regression following menopause. In addition, active women in their late thirties develop ptosis secondary to gravitational effects alone. Although ptosis can occur by age 16 in heavy-breasted patients (C or D cup), its presentation in small-breasted patients (A or B cup) is usually secondary to the above etiologies.

Breast ptosis is said to be present when the nipple is at the level of or lower than the inframammary fold. The severity of the ptosis may be classified by the relationship of the nipple to the inframammary fold and to the breast itself (Figs. 22-1 and 22-2).

Minor Ptosis

The nipple lies *at* the level of the inframammary fold but above the lower contour of the gland and skin brassiere.

Moderate Ptosis

The nipple lies *below* the level of the fold but remains above the lower contour of the breast and skin brassiere.

Major Ptosis

The nipple lies below the level of the fold and *at* the lower contour of the breast and skin brassiere.

Two other conditions exist that may confuse the diagnosis (Table 22-1). *Pseudoptosis* is characterized by a hypoplastic breast where the full lower quadrants appear to have descended while the nipple remains above the inframammary fold. The basic pathology is a loose skin brassiere, which is best corrected by an augmentation. *Glandular ptosis* is a much rarer entity characterized by descent of the lower breast quadrants with retention of the nipple at its normal level. It occurs most commonly following breast reduction and is corrected by resection of lower breast tissue.

Table 22-1. Ptosis: classification

Minor	Nipple at inframammary fold
Moderate	Nipple below the fold but above lower breast contour
Major	Nipple at lower breast contour
Pseudoptosis	Nipple above fold, gland ptotic, hypoplasia
Glandular	Nipple above fold, but breast has descended, usually secondary to previous reduction mammaplasty

CONSULTATION

Medical History

A general medical history is taken with emphasis on the breasts. Breast development is reviewed: growth at puberty, influence of hormone ingestion (especially birth control pills), planned or previous pregnancies, current breast condition (pain, masses, tenderness, fibrocystic disease), brassiere size, and previous breast surgery (biopsies or aesthetic procedures). It is important to determine the cause of the ptosis and whether a volume change has occurred. The patient who was always a 34A has different expectations from those of someone who was a 34C prior to multiple pregnancies and now presents with a ptotic 34B.

Indications and Contraindications

Patients seeking mastopexy have a wide range of deformities and high expectations. The primary indication is the patient with adequate volume (B cup) who wishes to have the nipple elevated and will accept the requisite scars. If inadequate volume or severe flattening of the upper quadrants exists, then an augmentation mammaplasty in addition to mastopexy must be considered. Patients requesting mastopexy will often seek the operation for the wrong reasons. Many patients need a reduction mammaplasty rather than a mastopexy [41]. Those with small hypoplastic breasts will benefit from an augmentation without extensive skin incisions. The surgeon should reject the patient who is unwilling to accept the necessary scars and who repeatedly minimizes their permanence. In contrast, many patients will refuse surgery once they are aware of what is required. Mastopexy is contraindicated in patients with severe fibrocystic disease, multiple scars, psychologic problems, and systemic medical diseases.

Motivation

The patient is asked why she wishes to have surgery at this time and what her expectations are in regard to final breast shape and scars. Most patients are 30 to 45 years of age and were always satisfied with their breasts until the nipple descended and the upper quadrants became flattened. Motivation and patient satisfaction are directly proportional to the severity of the problem. The patient with major ptosis will gladly accept the requisite scarring if the nipple is returned to its normal location. Patients with minor ptosis want to be the "same as before, but without any scars." They consider the required surgery very minor. As they pinch the inferior skin and elevate the nipple, they say, "If you could just do this, it would be perfect."

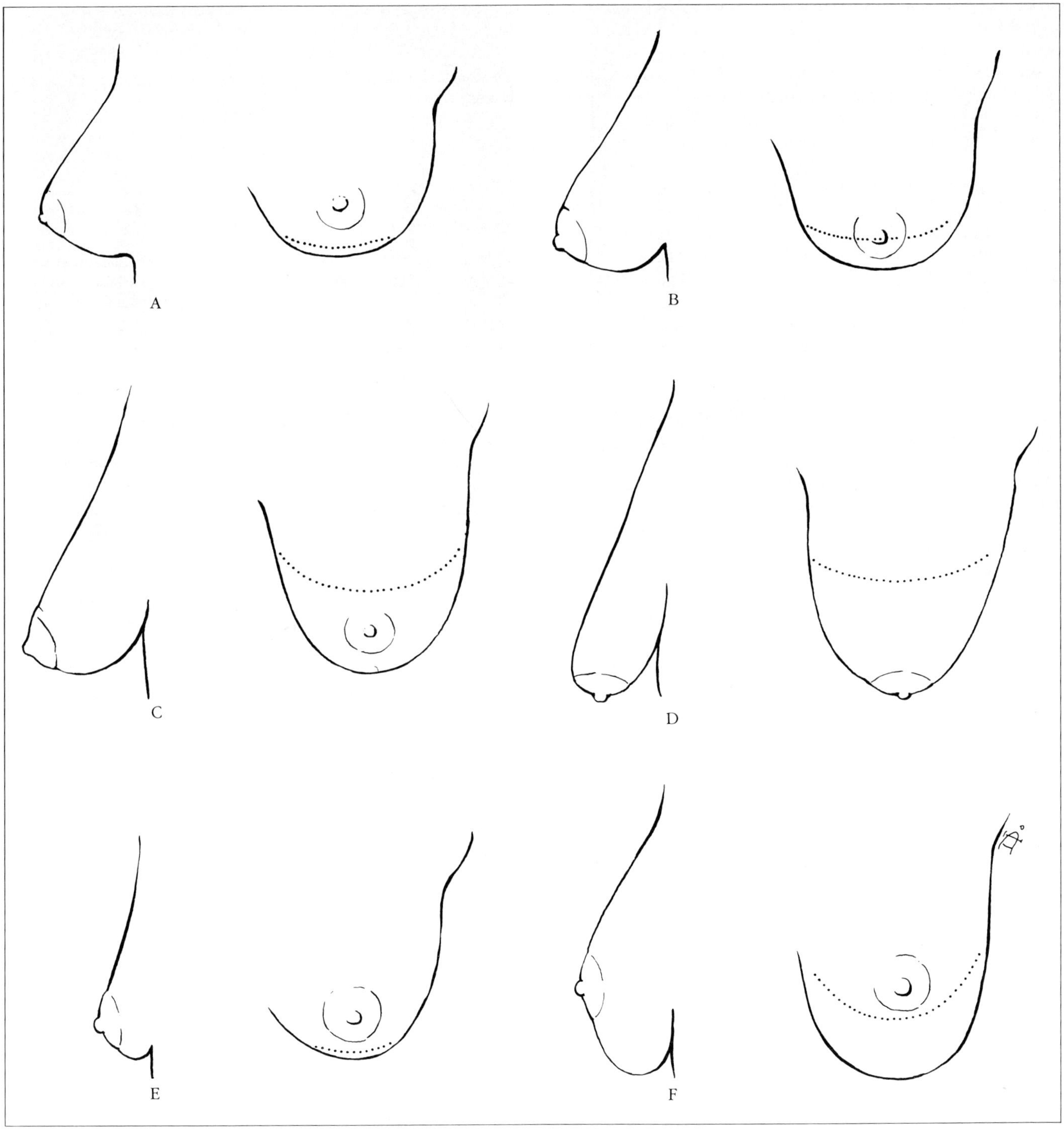

Figure 22-1. The degree of ptosis is determined by the relationship of the nipple to the inframammary fold.
A. Normal breast with nipple above the inframammary fold.
B. Minor ptosis, with nipple at the level of the fold.
C. Moderate ptosis, with nipple below the fold but above the lower breast contour.
D. Major ptosis, with nipple at the lowest point on the breast.
E. Pseudoptosis creates the impression of a ptotic breast, but the nipple remains above the inframammary fold.
F. Glandular ptosis is usually associated with a previous reduction mammaplasty. It is denoted by descent of the gland and nipple elevation.

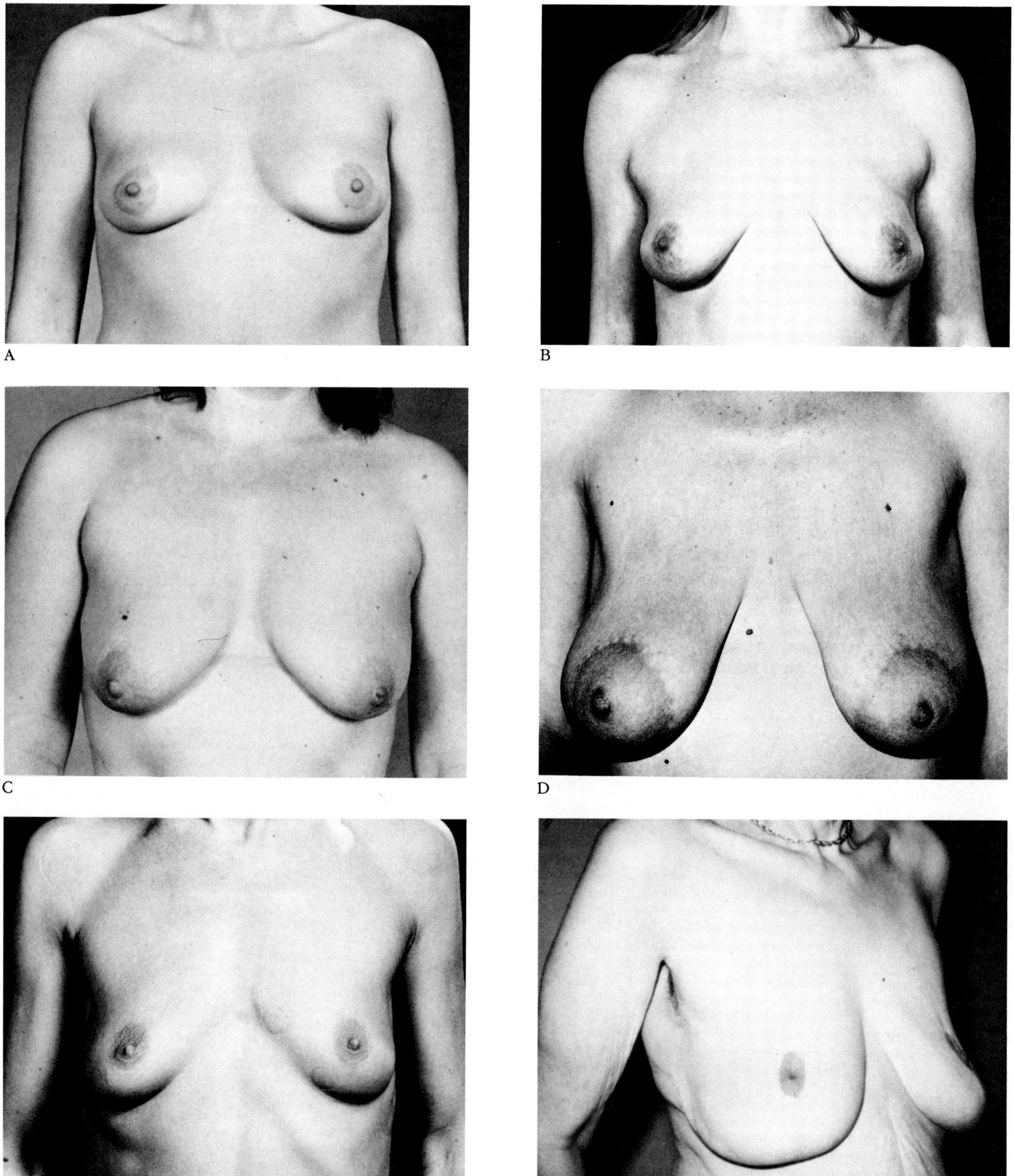

Figure 22-2. Different types of breast ptosis.
A. Normal 34B breast with nipple above the inframammary fold.
B. Minor ptosis, nipple at the fold.
C. Moderate ptosis, nipple below the fold.
D. Major ptosis, nipple lowest point on breast.
E. Pseudoptosis, as the nipple is above the inframammary fold but the breast appears ptotic.
F. Glandular ptosis following reduction mammaplasty seen on referral for secondary surgery.

Physical Examination

The surgeon should utilize part of the physical examination period to educate the patient, pointing out any abnormalities while inquiring what the patient wants, especially in regard to volume and shape. Also, the surgeon must classify the deformity in terms of ptosis and breast volume. Selection of the optimal operation requires significant patient involvement (Table 22-2). The patient is examined nude from the waist up in both the sitting and supine positions. A systematic breast examination is done including the axilla and supraclavicular areas. With the patient sitting, the breast size relative to the torso is evaluated as well as any deformities of the thorax. Next, one determines nipple position relative to the inframammary fold and the breast itself, thereby permitting classification of the deformity. From palpation, one should determine breast shape, consistency, and degree of hypoplasia. The skin is examined for its elasticity, scars, and striae. Next, the distances from the nipple to the sternal notch and sternal midline are recorded. Breast volume is determined with the patient wearing a well-fitted brassiere. One must point out any asymmetries, especially minor volumetric discrepancies or NAC location, which can be difficult to adjust in the smaller breast. The breast examination is completed with the patient recumbent.

Aesthetic Goals

At this point the surgeon should present his findings, ask the patient what she specifically wants, and then recommend an operation. The surgeon's opinion refers to the severity of the ptosis and adequacy of the breast volume, especially in the upper quadrants [11, 27]. The patient is asked whether she considers her breast volume sufficient and whether there is adequate fullness in the upper quadrants. If the volume is *sufficient,* the method of nipple elevation and resection of excessive skin brassiere is outlined. It is emphasized that the greater the severity, the longer the scar. If the volume is *insufficient* or upper quadrant fullness is desired, an augmentation mammaplasty is recommended. In minor ptosis, an augmentation alone may suffice whereas a mastopexy with augmentation is necessary for moderate and major ptosis if volume is inadequate. Despite protestations to the contrary, the mastopexy patient wants a normal, soft, conical breast without scars. It must be stressed repeatedly that the breasts can be improved over their present condition but that the prepregnancy or adolescent breast is an impossibility. With the patient's permission, the predicted scars are drawn on the breast with a felt-tipped pen. The patient is urged to think about the procedure, discuss it with others, and decide whether the trade-offs are worth it.

Table 22-2. Treatment of ptosis

Minor	
Normal volume	VOQ ± prosthesis
Inadequate volume	Prosthesis
Moderate	
Normal volume	B-mastopexy
Slight hypoplasia	B-mastopexy + 100-cc lower pole reduction
Hypoplasia	B-mastopexy + prosthesis
Major	
Always reduce lower pole by 1–200 cc	
Normal volume	B-mastopexy + augment excision volume *only*
Hypoplasia	B-mastopexy + augment excision volume *plus* desired volume
Pseudoptosis	Augment to B cup

Informed Consent

Once a mutually agreeable plan is devised, the possible complications are reviewed. Because of the diversity of procedures available and limited long-term follow-up, an informed consent must be generalized. Critical factors for discussion include the following: (1) Hematoma and wound infection are relatively rare (1–2%) but may occur; (2) despite every effort to minimize their occurrence, scars will always be visible on close inspection; (3) breast sensation will be decreased immediately postoperatively but will gradually return by 6 months, although there is a slight possibility that nipple sensation will be either completely lost or decreased permanently; (4) breast shape will be improved, but perfect symmetry is impossible; (5) the nipple will be elevated above the inframammary fold; (6) if an augmentation is done, capsular contracture will occur as part of the normal healing process and will produce a breast that is firmer than normal in approximately 20 percent of cases.

Preoperative Instructions

The patient is photographed. Any aspirin-containing medication is discontinued 2 weeks prior to surgery. A complete medical history and physical examination are done plus appropriate preoperative studies (blood profile, chest x-ray examination, electrocardiogram). Prescriptions are given for pain or sleeping, and a broad-spectrum antibiotic if an augmentation is scheduled.

The patient is told to shower with pHisoHex prior to surgery and to shave the axillae. Postoperatively, she should (1) watch for excessive swelling or pain, especially unilateral, and call the office immediately if either occurs; (2) take medication as directed; (3) return to the office for a change of dressing (if there are drains, return in 2–3 days; if no drains, return in 1 week); (4) limit arm and shoulder exercises for 1 week, and refrain from driving a car, sleeping on breast; and (5) return after 3 months to check scars or before 3 months in case of painful, itchy scars.

SURGICAL TECHNIQUES

Minor Ptosis

When the nipple is at the level of the inframammary fold, the solution is a breast augmentation with or without

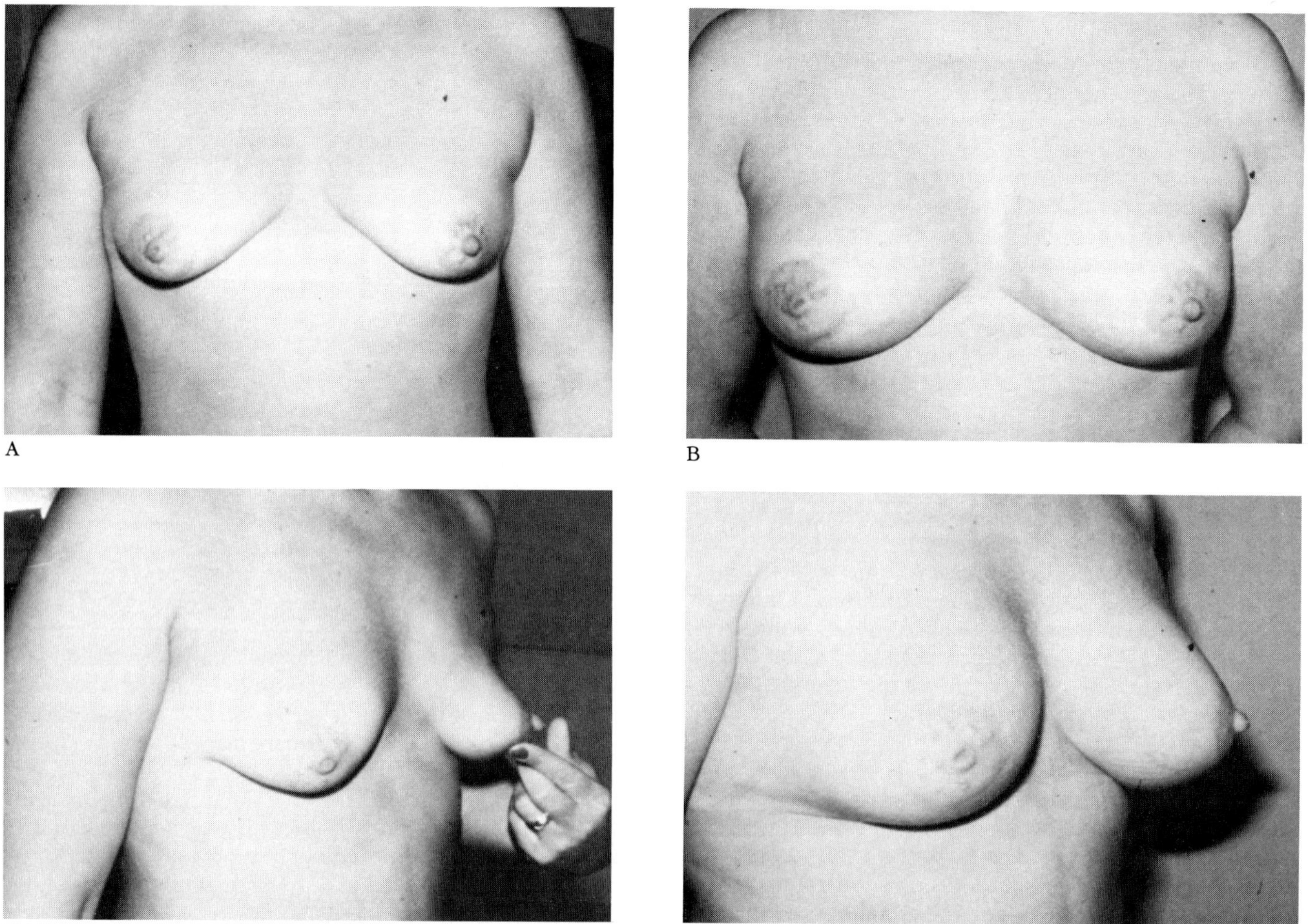

A B C D

Figure 22-3. Correction of minor ptosis by augmentation mammaplasty alone.
A, C. Preoperative condition showing nipple at the fold and the patient indicating the desired elevation.
B, D. Result at 1 year with elevation of nipple above the inframammary crease produced by a 300-cc prosthesis.

elevation of the nipple. The critical factor is the patient's impression of breast volume and acceptability of both scars and an implant. For the patient who wants increased volume and minimal scars, an implant alone is the solution (Fig. 22-3). For those who refuse an implant, a VOQ procedure will elevate the nipple and allow tightening of the skin brassiere. In an intermediate group are patients with loose skin and hypoplasia, in whom a large implant would be required. For these individuals a VOQ plus augmentation is ideal. Since few patients in our practices refuse implants, approximately 80 percent of minor ptosis is corrected with an implant alone, 15 percent by VOQ with implant, and 5 percent have a skin mastopexy only.

VOQ TECHNIQUE

The VOQ name is derived from the excision (VO) and the final scar (Q) (Fig. 22-4). Excess skin must be removed from the periareolar area (O) as well as the stretched inferior quadrants (V). Any attempt to excise only periareolar skin will result in tension in the circumareolar scar and eventual enlargement of the areola. Gruber and Friedman [19] reported 13 cases of "donut" mastopexy in which a circumareolar skin reduction was done with resulting problems of areolar spreading (13 out of 13) and hypertrophic scarring (7 out of 13). The periareolar incision allows one to transpose the NAC and to reduce areolar diameter. The vertical V excision tightens the skin brassiere and redirects tension.

If an implant is not used, the markings can be rigidly followed. With the patient sitting, a line is drawn from the sternal notch to the nipple. At a point 16 to 20 cm from the sternal notch, a transverse line is drawn perpendicular to the sternum. It represents the upper areolar point (UAP) and is generally no more than 3 cm above the transposed inframammary fold. After skin preparation and draping, the rest of the markings are made in the *supine* position with the arms at right angles. The distance from the center of the nipple to the new UAP is measured and becomes the radius of a periareolar circle. The areola itself is marked with a 4.5-cm diameter. The vertical excision should have a width equal to the circle's radius and a length extending downward toward the inframammary fold. The amount of excision can be tested by pinching the skin together to ensure its adequacy.

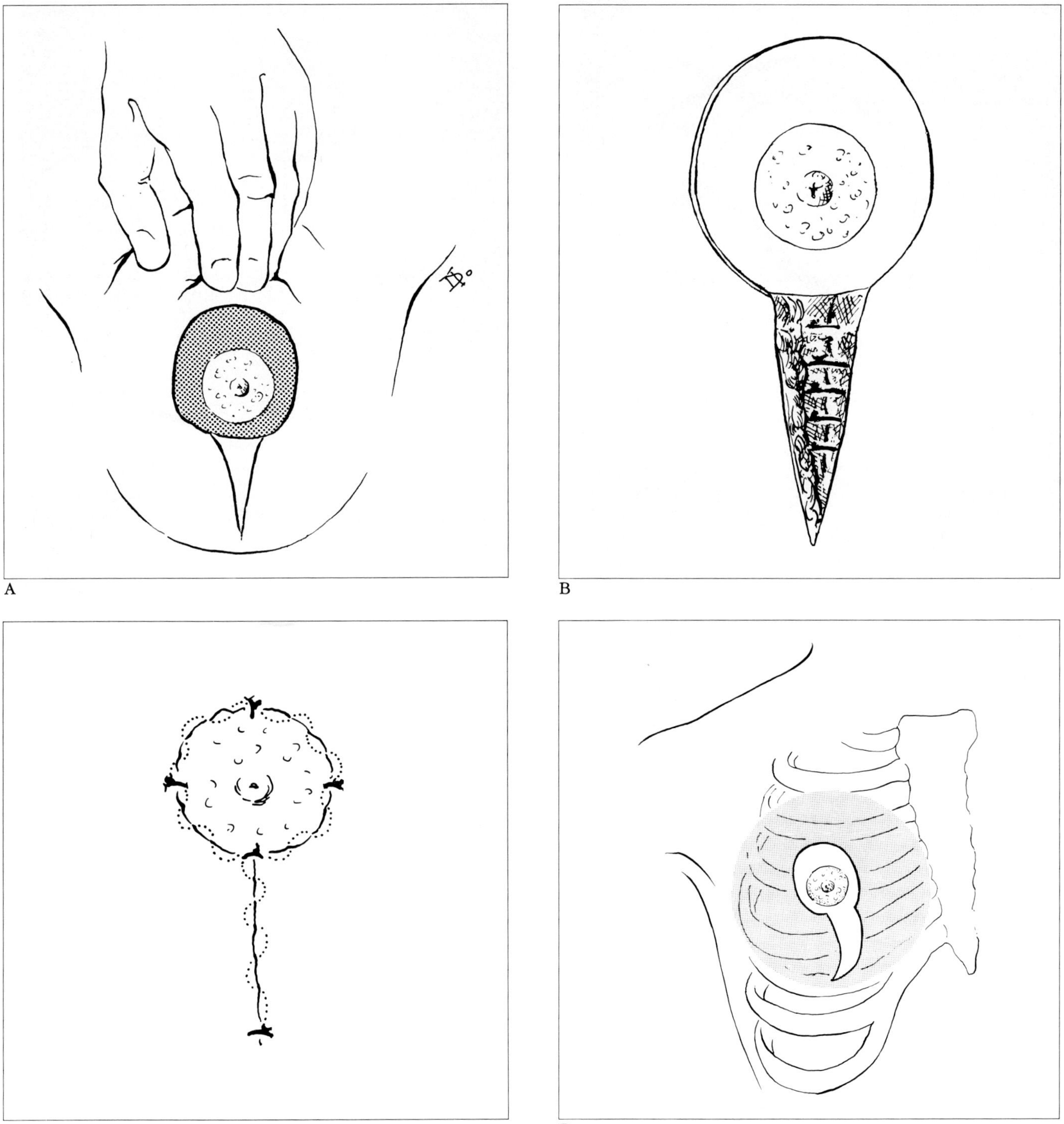

A B C D

Figure 22-4. The VOQ operation for minor ptosis.
A. The infraareolar V tightens the skin brassiere while the periareolar O allows nipple elevation; closure produces a Q.
B. The breast is plicated to produce a more conical shape.
C. Quadrant areolar sutures are inserted followed by closure with a subcuticular suture, resulting in a Q shape.
D. Most frequently the VOQ is done with a simultaneous breast augmentation.

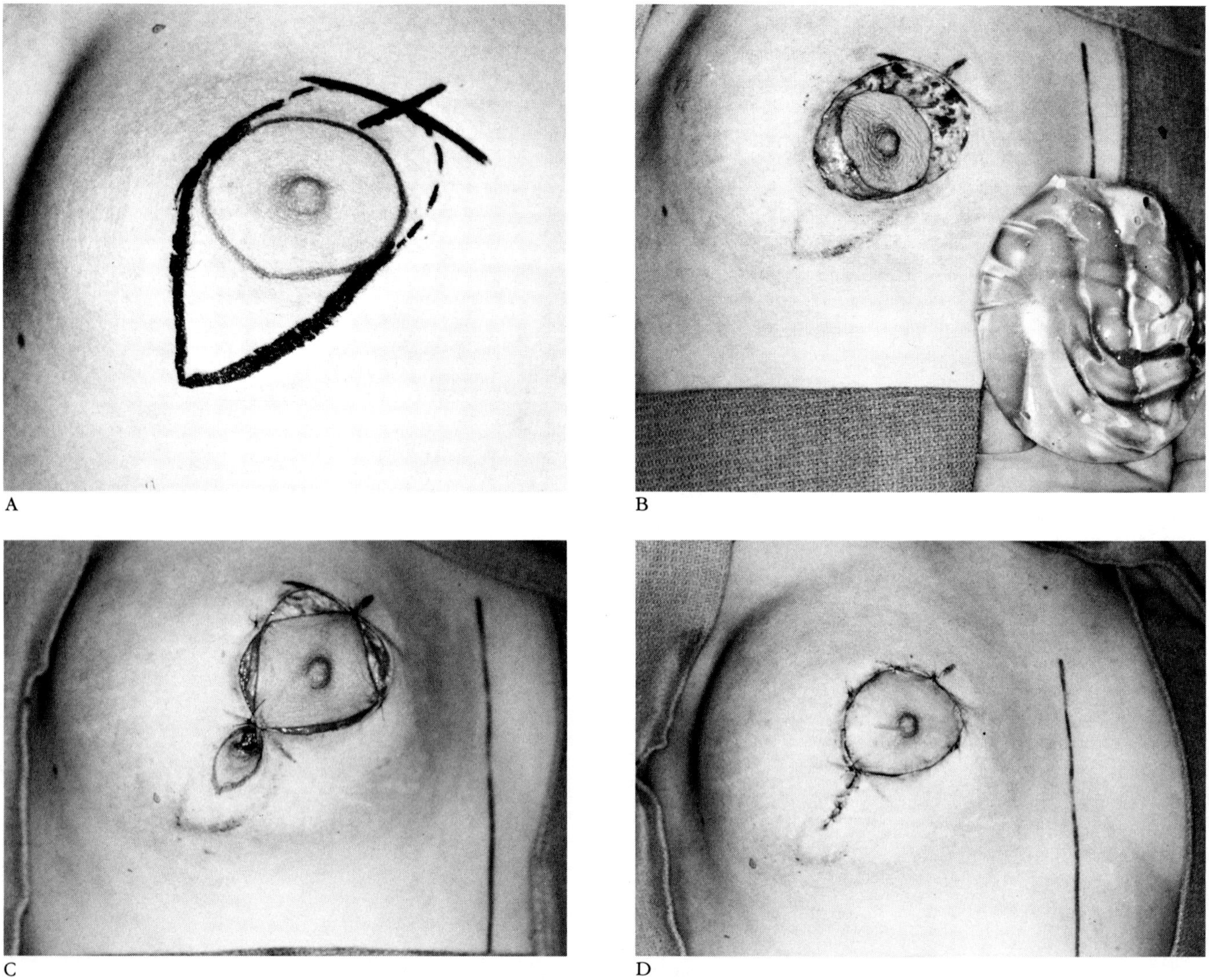

Figure 22-5. VOQ with breast augmentation for correction of minor ptosis.
A. VOQ is outlined for 2-cm elevation of NAC.
B. Periareolar deepithelialization, subcutaneous dissection, and partial division of pectoralis major muscle.
C. Elevation of nipple with limited skin excision.
D. Wound closure.

If the patient is to be under intravenous sedation and local anesthesia, an intercostal block (levels 2–6) is done bilaterally and the breast area is also injected. The incisions and areas of excision are injected with a dilute solution of 1:200,000 epinephrine and lidocaine. The areolar and periareolar markings are incised, and the intervening skin is deepithelialized. The vertical wedge is excised down to breast gland. Hemostasis is obtained with an electric cautery. The upper portion of the NAC is elevated and fixed at the UAP level with a single interrupted 4-0 Vicryl suture. The breast tissue at the edges of the V excision is plicated with 3-0 Vicryl. The nipple is sutured to the various quadrants. Then a running subcuticular suture of 4-0 Vicryl is inserted, with equal bites on the vertical component but gathering bites around the areola. Small drains are rarely required. Skin tapes are applied to the incision, and a light gauze is placed over the breasts. The patient's brassiere is used as a supporting bandage.

If an implant is required in conjuction with a VOQ procedure, the height of the skin excision is kept the same but the width is reduced (Fig. 22-5). The goal is to tighten the skin while accommodating the increase volume of the prosthesis. The width of the lower V is generally 1 to 2 cm less than a simple skin reduction. If doubt exists, one limb of the V is incised and the second removed following augmentation. Access to the subpectoral pocket is gained by elevating the breast tissue at the lower part of the vertical incision. The muscle is exposed and divided in the usual fashion for a breast augmentation.

The VOQ procedure has the following advantages: (1) elevation of the NAC to a normal level with limited scarring, (2) plication of the lower quadrants, producing a conical breast, (3) absence of a scar in the inframammary fold, and (4) easy access for breast augmentation.

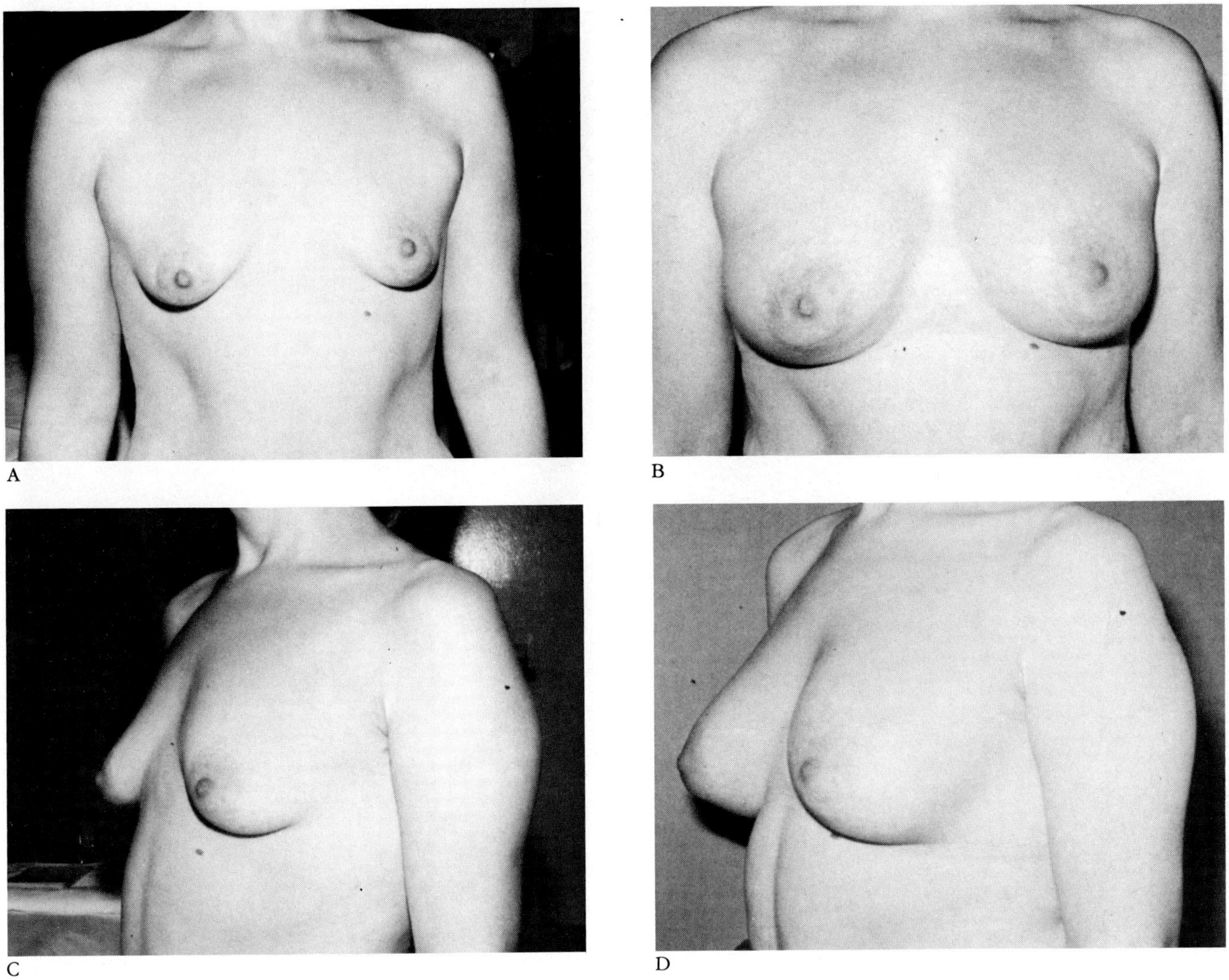

Figure 22-6
A, C. Patient with asymmetric breasts; left breast with pseudoptosis, right breast with minor ptosis.
B, D. Result following bilateral breast augmentation with 270-cc prosthesis.

Pseudoptosis

Pseudoptosis is merely hypoplasia of the breast in which the skin and gland have descended, leaving the nipple above the inframammary fold. Patients with pseudoptosis often request a mastopexy. The correct diagnosis is easily demonstrated by elevating the lower pole and marking the inframammary fold location, which is below the nipple. Once the condition is diagnosed, the optimal treatment is breast augmentation without mastopexy (Fig. 22-6). The augmentation volume is discussed with the patient, and a volume is suggested that is in relation to her body. The average case requires an increase from size A to B, with the usual implant ranging from 120 to 200 cc. A large woman may need 200 to 300 cc.

Moderate Ptosis

By definition, in moderate ptosis the nipple is below the inframammary fold but above the lower contour of the breast. Excision of redundant skin is mandatory. Although many patients desire only an augmentation, it must *not* be done, as ptosis will remain (Fig. 22-7). An occasional patient will want, for professional reasons, an extra large augmentation and accept a low breast rather than scars. Frequently one sees unhappy patients who had an augmentation without ptosis correction. Although a VOQ is possible in certain cases of moderate ptosis, a B-technique mastopexy is usually necessary to ensure adequate skin excision.

The patient has to assess her own breast volume and the adequacy of fullness in the upper quadrants. If volume and fullness are acceptable, a B-mastopexy with skin excision alone is done. If the volume is acceptable but fullness is inadequate, a B-mastopexy plus augmentation is suggested, so that prosthetic volume will equal the amount of lower pole excision. Thus, one is able to keep breast volume constant while achieving fullness in the upper

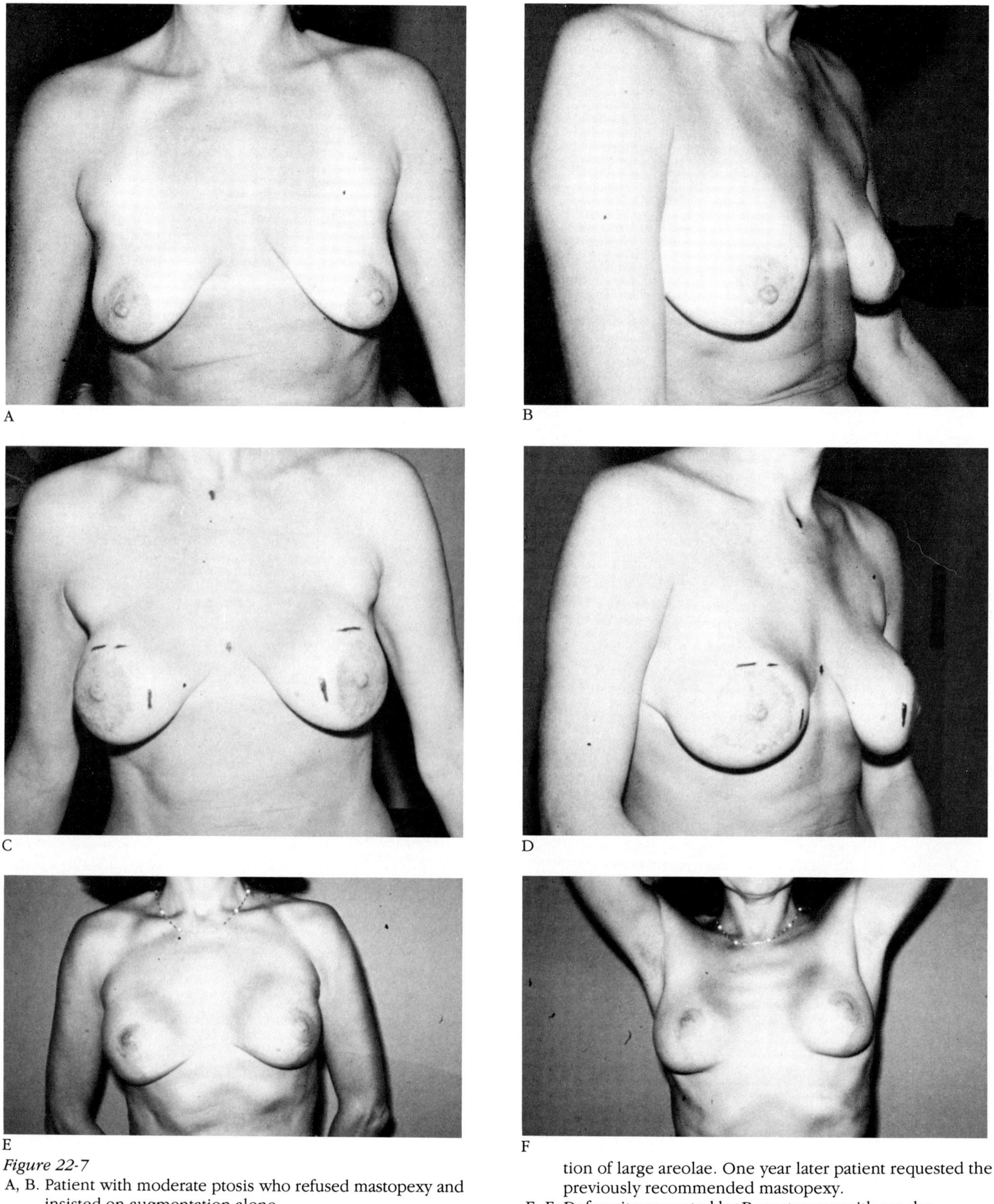

A B C D E F

Figure 22-7

A, B. Patient with moderate ptosis who refused mastopexy and insisted on augmentation alone.

C, D. The expected "rock-in-the-sock" deformity and accentuation of large areolae. One year later patient requested the previously recommended mastopexy.

E, F. Deformity corrected by B-mastopexy with areolar reduction and subpectoral placement of the prosthesis.

quadrants. If the implant is unacceptable, a smaller breast volume must be accepted as the accentuated lower quadrants must be reduced to harmonize with the flatter upper quadrants. If the volume is inadequate and the upper quadrants are flat, a B-mastopexy with augmentation is performed. The frequency of the three procedures is approximately as follows: (1) B-mastopexy, 20 percent, (2) B-mastopexy with lower pole excision, 20 percent, and (3) B-mastopexy with augmentation and lower pole excision, 60 percent. Note the term *pole* refers anatomically to the inferior quadrants of the breast or aesthetically to the most dependent part of the breast as seen on anterior view.

B-MASTOPEXY

A step-by-step description of the B breast reduction technique is presented in Chapter 21 and should be reviewed. The patient is marked in the sitting position with hands at her sides. A line is drawn from the sternal notch to the nipple. The new UAP is marked 16 to 20 cm from the notch and should be no more than 4 cm above the existing inframammary fold. A new 4.5-cm diameter areola is drawn as well as reference quadrant lines. After skin preparation and draping, the rest of the markings are made in the *supine* position with the arms at right angles (Fig. 22-8). The medial excision line is placed 9 to 11 cm from and parallel to the midsternal line. The distance from the nipple to the medial excision line is measured and replicated symmetrically on the lateral side of the nipple. The breast is then pushed downward and the existing inframammary fold is marked. A new fold is drawn as a wide curve 1 cm above and parallel to the existing fold. From the new fold, one measures upward 4 cm to locate the lower border of the periareolar excision. Medially, the juncture consists of a small 1-cm triangular flap located at the lower level of the areola. Laterally, a gentle S-shaped curve is designed to pass inferiorly and terminate at the inframammary fold. The overall excision resembles the letter *B*.

If the procedure is performed under intravenous sedation and local anesthesia, a bilateral intercostal block is done plus injection in the retroglandular space. The incision lines and excision area are injected with dilute epinephrine and lidocaine. The operation begins with deepithelialization of the periareolar skin. The lower periareolar border is then incised down to gland and the incision continued medially and inferiorly to create a skin flap. The lower border of the breast is elevated off the pectoral fascia to allow creation of a new inframammary fold. The lateral flap is then brought medially to check the resulting tension and excised. The areola is sutured to the UAP. The breast is infolded over the surgeon's finger. A single triangular suture of 0 Vicryl approximates the lower breast edges and the pectoralis fascia. Additional plication sutures are inserted to achieve a conical shape. Subcutaneous sutures are used to approximate the flaps. The medial and lateral skin tabs are brought together at the lower areolar point. The nipple is fixed at its medial and lateral quadrants. Final closure is achieved with a running 4-0 Vicryl subcuticular suture. Smaller superficial bites are taken on the short lateral side, but longer wider bites are taken on the redundant medial side. This bidirectional gathering suture is critical to achieve a purse-string closure in the periareolar area. Drains are rarely required, and a paper tape dressing is applied.

The principal advantages of the B-mastopexy technique are absence of a medial scar, excellent projection, ensured nipple viability, speed, and flexibility (Fig. 22-9). In contrast, pattern techniques that utilize an inverted-T incision produce an objectionable medial scar and tension at the critical closure point [1]. Many of the dermal pedicle techniques complicate and prolong the operation without any proved benefit [14, 21, 42]. In contrast to certain lateralizing operations, the B scar remains under the breast and is not visible in the axilla [5, 37]. The disadvantage of the B-technique is that it is a less rigid cut-as-you-go method requiring some degree of surgical finesse similar to the Millard cleft lip repair.

Major Ptosis

By definition, major ptosis occurs when the nipple is the lowest point on the breast contour. Obviously, skin reduction is essential, and frequently an augmentation is necessary to restore breast fullness [23, 29]. If the breast tissue is firm, a B-mastopexy without augmentation is possible. Patients who refuse an implant and those with breast diseases that preclude a prosthesis are also corrected by means of a B-technique with lower pole resection. A skin mastopexy with lower pole resection is done in approximately 40 percent of cases. In all cases of major ptosis, the lower pole of the breast is excised, approximately 100 to 200 gm, in order to minimize subsequent descent and to ameliorate accentuation of upper quadrant flatness. The result is a smaller breast with a more youthful shape. The ideal operation for major ptosis is a B-mastopexy with lower pole resection and augmentation; it is done in 60 percent of patients with major ptosis (Fig. 22-10). For women with normal volume, the augmentation is a small one (100–200 cc) and merely replaces the excised volume. Tightening of the skin brassiere gives a better shape while the implant provides superior quadrant fullness. Skin mastopexy alone does not correct either superior quadrant flatness or lower quadrant ptosis. When hypoplasia and major ptosis coincide, the implant must be larger to replace the resected lower quadrants (100–200 cc) and to allow an increase in cup size (100–150 cc).

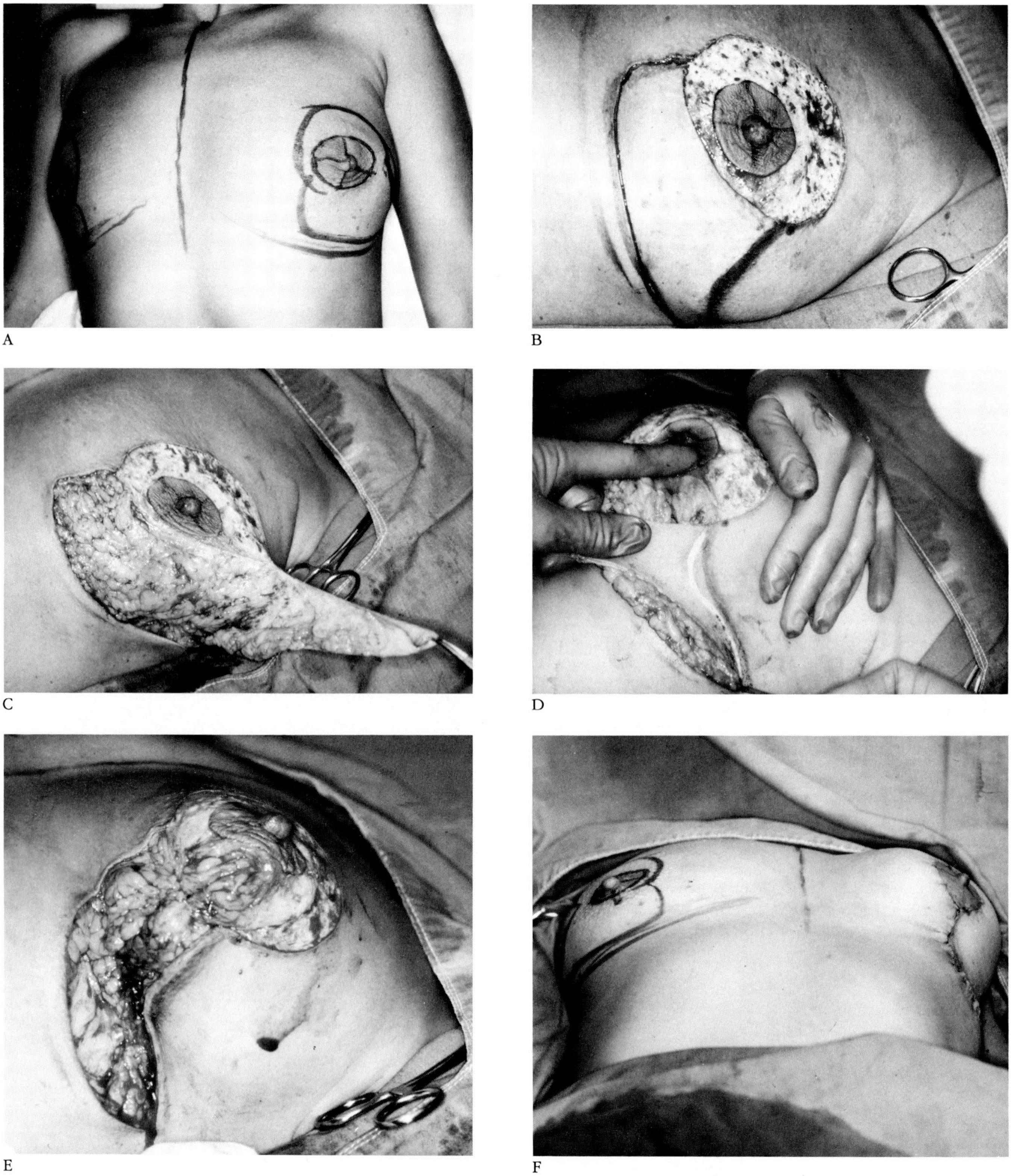

Figure 22-8. Mastopexy for moderate ptosis.

A. Markings. Note planned elevation of the inframammary fold.
B. Periareolar deepithelialization followed by incision of the breast flap.
C. The lateral flap is elevated back to the anticipated line of excision. Also, the lower breast is elevated off the pectoralis fascia, thus allowing creation of a higher inframammary fold.
D. While the breast is folded, the breast flap is brought medially to determine the desired tightening, then excised.
E. Closure begins with plication of the breast tissue.
F. Result shows dramatic improvement in breast contour and projection achieved *without* a prosthesis.

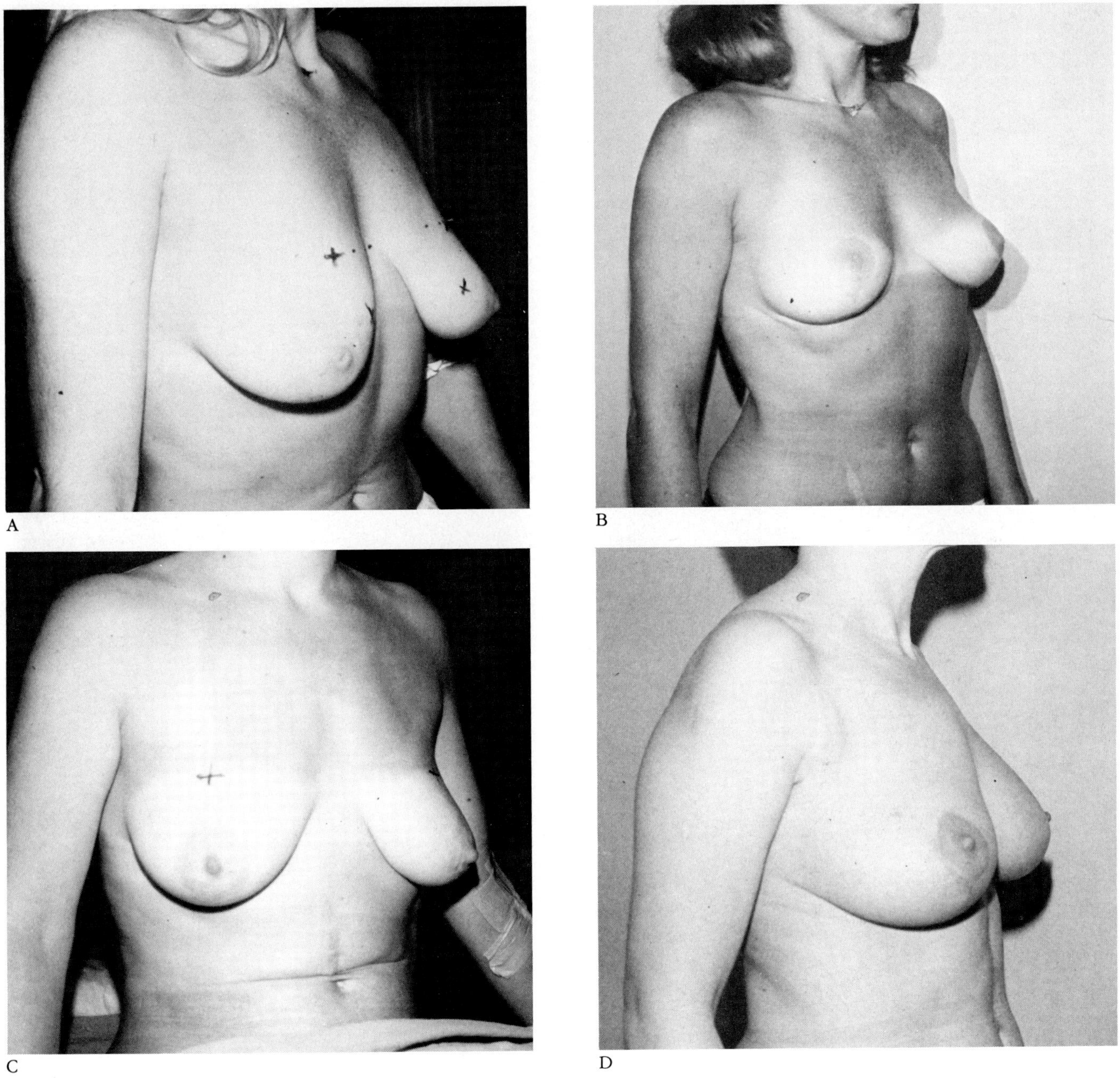

Figure 22-9. Two patients with moderate ptosis treated differently because of a significant difference in upper quadrant fullness despite a similar breast volume.

A, B. Patient with moderate ptosis. Result at 2 years following skin mastopexy alone.

C, D. Patient with moderate ptosis corrected by B-mastopexy and augmentation; superior quadrant fullness due to prosthesis. Note: An augmentation provides a marked increase in the upper quadrants. Compare upper quadrants preoperatively (A and C) versus postoperative condition (B and D).

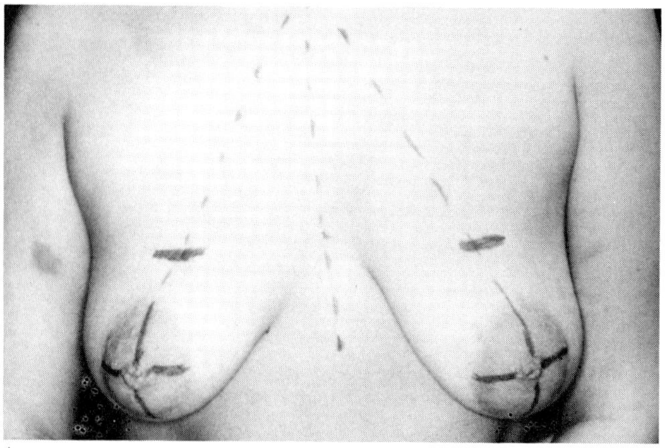

A

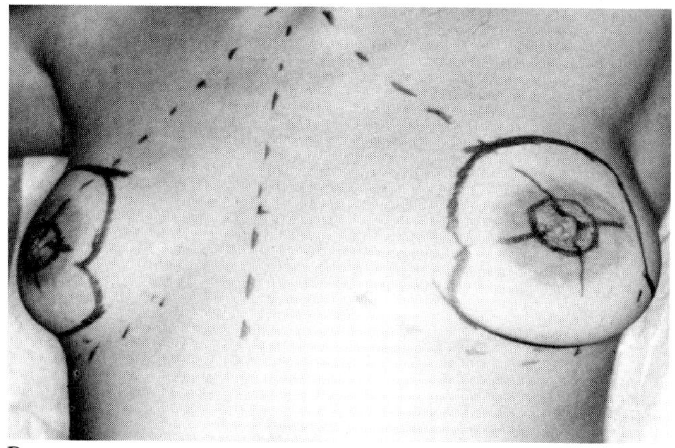

B

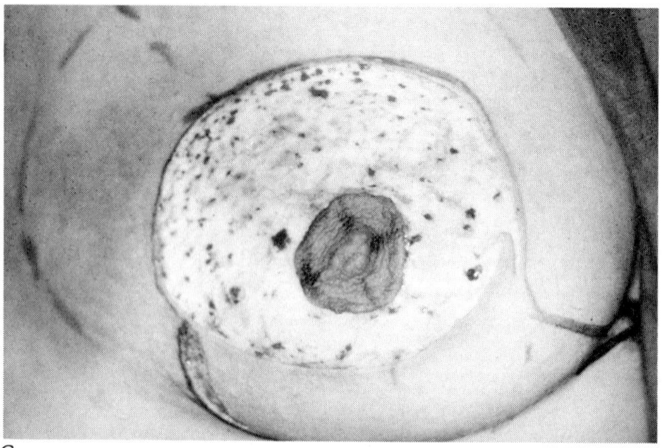

C

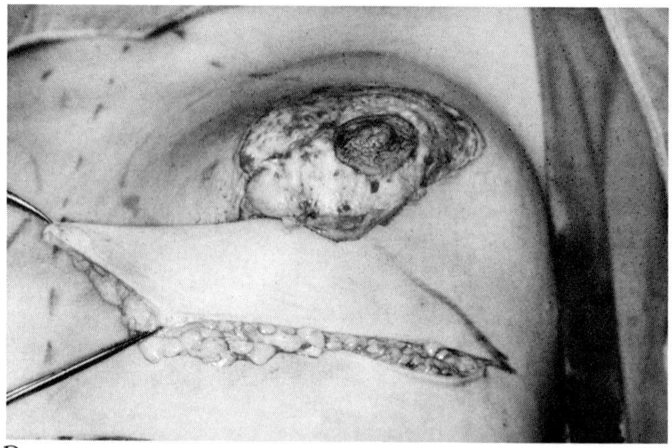

D

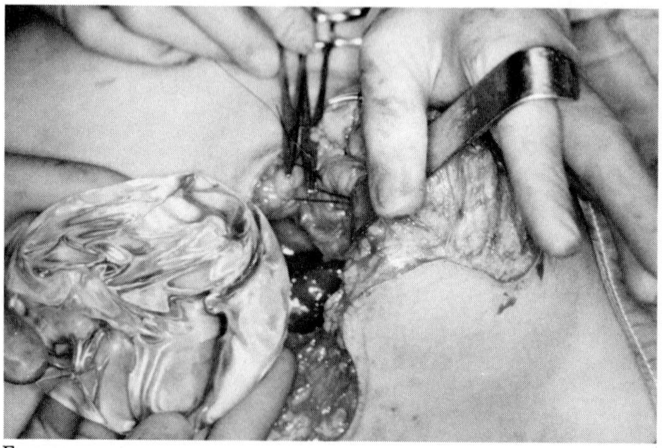

E

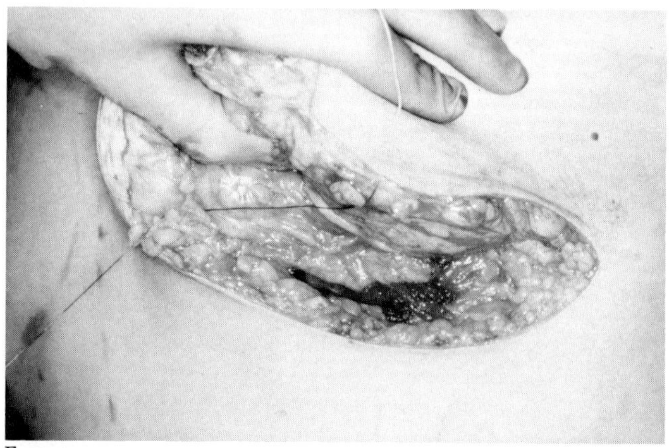

F

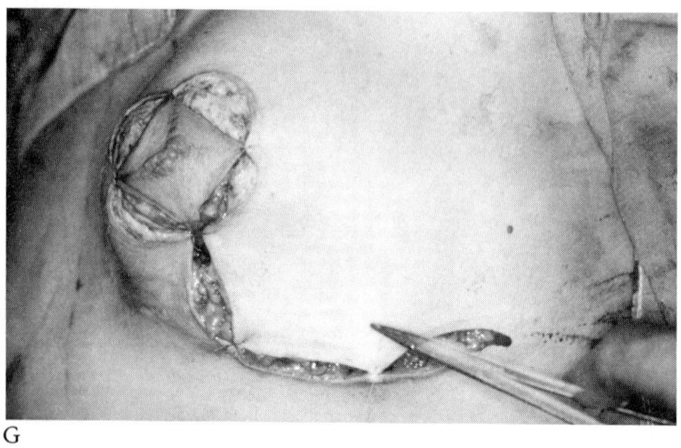

G

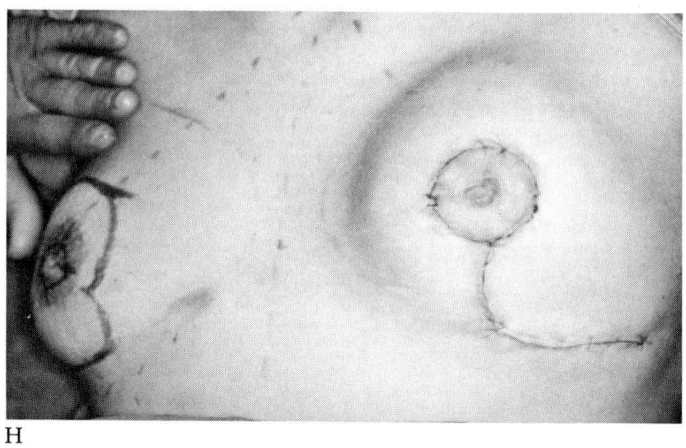

H

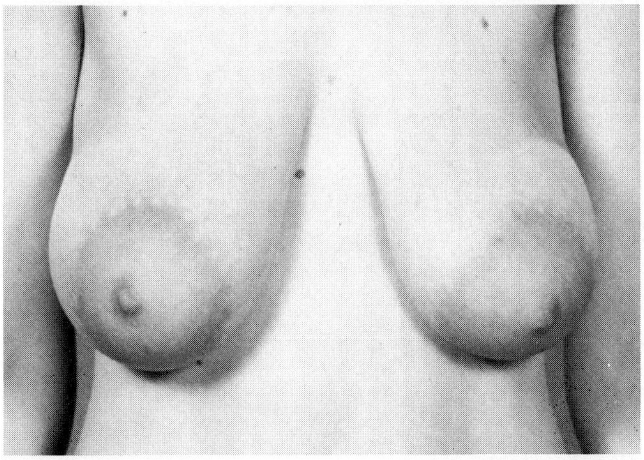

I

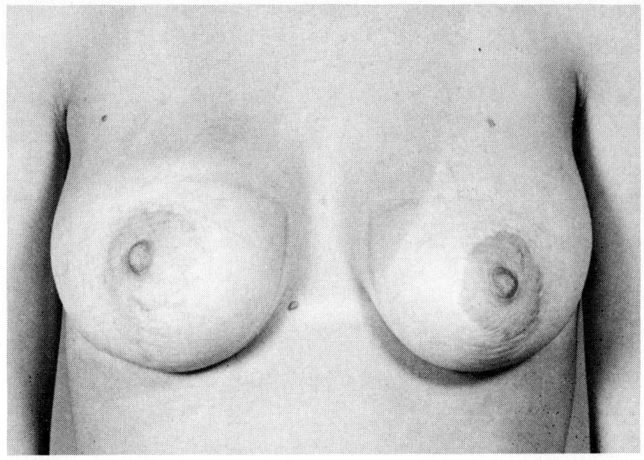

J

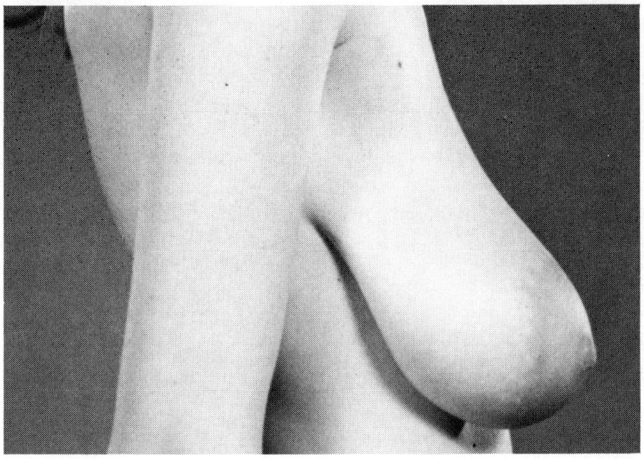

K

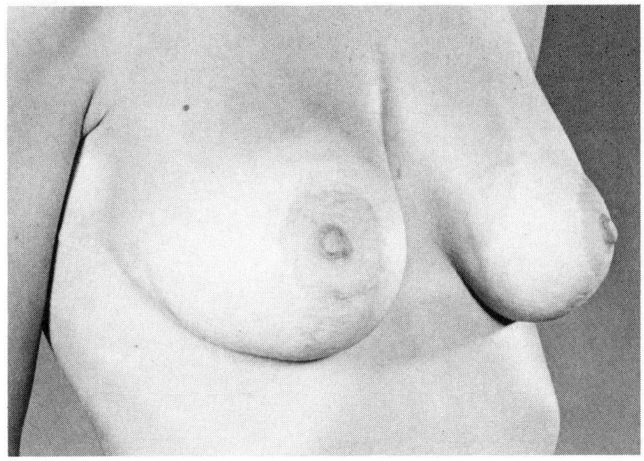

L

Figure 22-10. B-mastopexy with augmentation.

A. With the patient sitting, the reference points are marked, including midline, upper areolar point, and areolar quadrant lines.

B. The B-mastopexy excision markings are completed with the patient recumbent.

C. As seen from below, the first step is periareolar deepithelialization.

D. The breast flap is created, including the desired lower pole glandular excision.

E. Temporary plication sutures are inserted but left untied prior to the placement of the prosthesis.

F. Following determination of desired tension, the breast flap is excised and multiple plication sutures are inserted.

G, H. Closure consists of initial tacking sutures followed by a running subcuticular.

I, K. A 20-year-old patient with major ptosis and giant areola. Treated by a "minus-plus mastopexy" involving resection of the lower poles (200 gm) and an augmentation (165 gm) to fill the upper quadrants.

J, L. Result at 2 years.

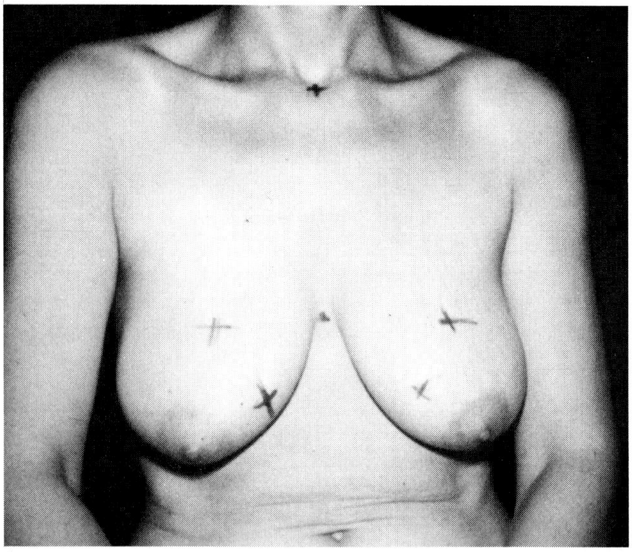
A

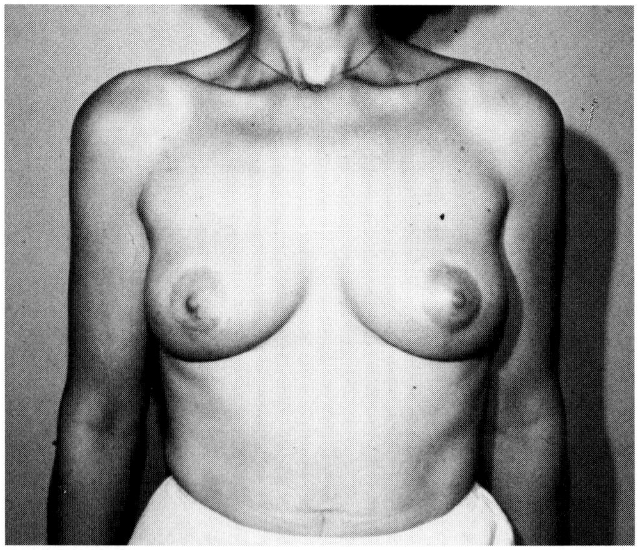
B

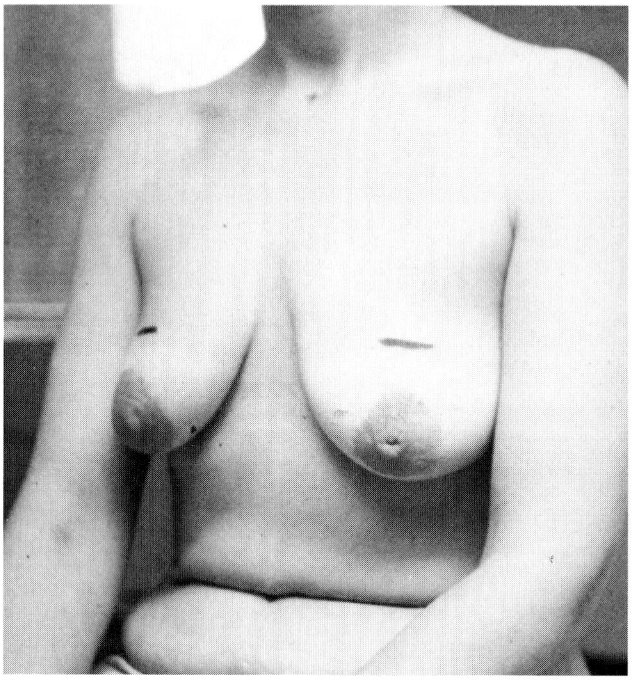
C

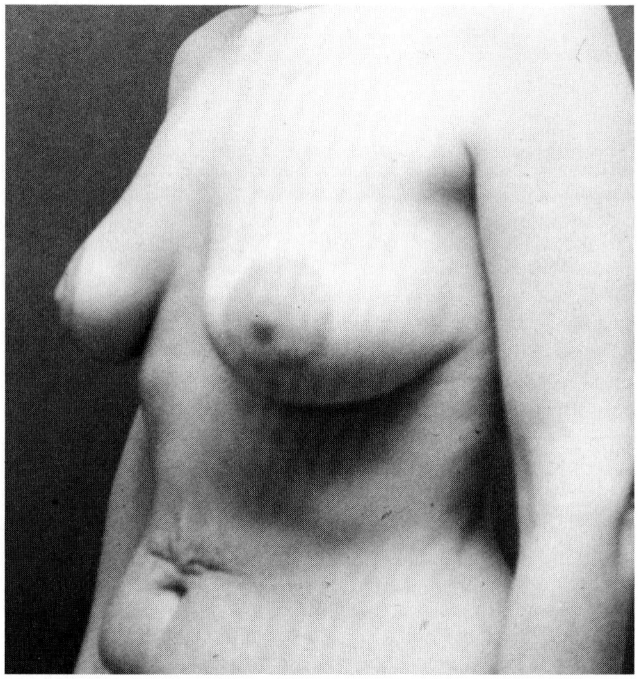
D

Figure 22-11. Two patients with major ptosis treated differently.
A, B. Patient having firm breasts and major ptosis corrected by B-mastopexy with lower pole excision. Breasts are elevated, but upper quadrant flatness remains as implant was refused.
C, D. Patient having flat, saggy breasts and major ptosis corrected by B-mastopexy with lower pole excision (150 gm) and augmentation (200 gm). Upper quadrant fullness was achieved with a prosthesis, which represented an additional volume of only 50 cc.

B-MASTOPEXY TECHNIQUE WITH AUGMENTATION

The breast markings are done in the aforementioned manner. Since one will be increasing volume, a sequential operation is performed consisting of periareolar skin excision, creation of a lateral flap, insertion of the prosthesis followed by excision of the lateral flap, and closure (Fig. 22-11). After the periareolar deepithelialization is completed, the lower pole of the gland is dissected and the pectoralis major is exposed. A retropectoral pocket is developed with division of the pectoralis major muscle from the 3- to the 9-o'clock area. The prosthesis is inserted in the partial subpectoral location. The lateral breast flap is then brought medially and with correct tension on the fold the excess skin and gland is excised. Closure is completed in the standard fashion.

Owsley and Brownstein [31] warn that excision of skin prior to insertion of the prosthesis can produce excessive tightness and limit implant size. To avoid this error, they recommend temporary skin plication sutures and assessment of breast shape with the patient in a semisitting position [30, 32]. In contrast, Baroudi and Lewis [2] complete the skin excision and vertical closure prior to insertion of the prosthesis, which merely serves to project the remodeled breast. The combination of a mastopexy, lower pole glandular resection (usually 100–200 gm), elevation of the inframammary fold (usually 1–2 cm), and augmentation provides a better shape than is possible with mastopexy alone. Whenever flatness of the upper quadrant exists, one cannot expect correction by simple skin mastopexy. The principal disadvantages of a combined procedure are nonacceptance of the implant and the risk of capsular contracture.

COMPLICATIONS

Intraoperative Complications

Viability of the flap is rarely threatened, but a difficult or tight closure can occur in combined procedures. In this event, one should use a smaller prosthesis. Obviously, prevention is achieved by delaying definitive skin excision until the prosthesis is inserted. The concept of reducing the skin envelope first and then augmenting the breast ignores the central premise that breast volume determines breast contour while risking skin necrosis.

Early Complications

The early complications of hematoma, NAC necrosis, fat necrosis, and wound infection are exceedingly rare in skin mastopexy or in minor glandular resection. However, all of the potential problems of augmentation mammaplasty are possible with an implant. Perhaps the most distressing complication is the patient who is immediately dissatisfied with the result. Such a patient requires careful management and frequent reassurance, especially that the scars will fade with time.

Late Complications

With skin mastopexies, the incidence of sensory loss and unacceptable scars is less than with virtually any other breast surgery. If a lateralizing operation is done, the only hypertrophic scar is periareolar, and simple revision is possible. Goulian [17] has reported significant scarring in dermal mastopexy. However, it has not been forthcoming in connection with the B-mastopexy technique, perhaps because of the Z-plasty closure and absence of a three-point closure characteristic of T-shaped incisions. If an augmentation is done, the occurrence of sensory loss and capsular contracture is as previously described. Although inversion of the nipple is unlikely, small breast asymmetries as well as areolar inequalities or deformities can occur. Gradual improvement may take place, but simple revision under local anesthesia is possible. Certain patients will feel that the surgery did not achieve the expected result (Fig. 22-12). In most of these cases skin-only mastopexies left flatness of the superior quadrant. The more time one spends preoperatively determining the patient's desires and expectations, the less one has to spend postoperatively justifying the result.

RESULTS

Patient satisfaction with mastopexy procedures is directly related to preoperative decisions. If preexisting breast volume was excessive, the patient will be disappointed with the rapid recurrence of the ptotic heavy breast. As shown by Goulian [17], a mastopexy is not a substitute for a breast reduction because the initial improvement will fade within 6 months. For the small breast with major ptosis, the initial superior quadrant fullness will gradually settle, producing a hypoplastic breast. If the optimal procedure is correctly done, ptosis rarely recurs and improvement can last for 15 to 20 years. As noted by Vilain and Mitz [40], the condition at 1 year will show little change over the next 10 years provided pregnancy and major weight fluctuations do not occur.

SECONDARY PTOSIS

After mastopexy, the main reason for secondary ptosis is weight loss, especially in the older age group. A loss of 5 kg will be significantly reflected in breast shape. In normal aging without weight loss, sagging occurs less often.

Classification

Three types of ptosis may develop secondarily: (1) total ptosis of breast, skin, and NAC as seen with volume changes following pregnancy, (2) total ptosis with diminution of volume, and (3) partial or glandular ptosis with the NAC located above the fold, as often seen after T-mastopexies. In these cases the degree of ptosis is usually moderate, except when a very significant weight loss has occurred. They are treated exactly like a primary ptosis except that the scars of the previous surgery are removed and thus the choice of technique is limited if one does not want to make additional incisions.

TOTAL PTOSIS

The NAC usually remains at an almost normal level because the skin in the superior quadrants is not as distended as that inferiorly. In a few cases, the entire skin envelope is redundant, as if the patient has not been operated on.

After previous inverted-T operations, the main change is elongation of the lower quadrants so that correction requires a skin reduction following the same pattern as the first operation but tightening the lower portion of the vertical scar. Relocation of the NAC follows the same rules as any mastopexy or reduction. The location of the inframammary fold should be carefully defined as it has often descended and is located below the horizontal scar. The lower pole of the gland should be elevated, thus allowing the fold and the horizontal scar to coincide.

After a B-mastopexy, secondary ptosis tends to reflect the influence of gravity much as a normal breast does. By utilizing the same scars, one can reduce the entire skin brassiere after determining the desired NAC level with the patient standing.

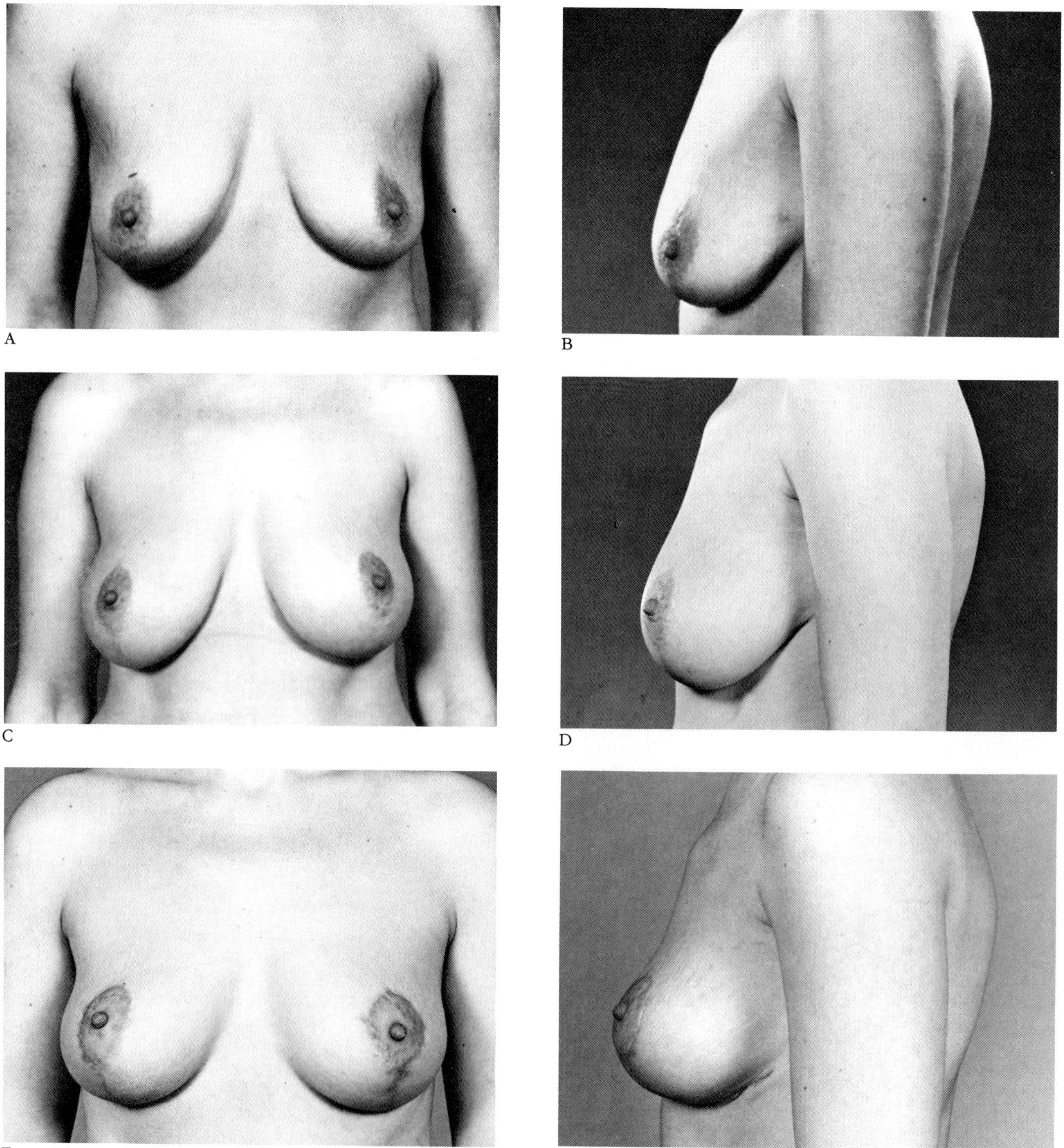

Figure 22-12

A, B. Patient requested correction of "drooping breasts" but refused a B-mastopexy.

C, D. After three consultations, VOQ mastopexy with augmentation (200 cc) was done. Postoperatively, patient considered breasts too heavy and thought that ptosis remained. Technically, the nipple had been elevated by the VOQ and ptosis did not exist. The true cause of patient dissatisfaction was the increase in breast volume (in the lower quadrants) and persistence of upper quadrant flatness, giving the breast a ptotic appearance.

E, F. One year later, the patient agreed to a B-mastopexy with removal of the prosthesis, lower pole excision, and replacement of excised volume (150 cc) as an augmentation to enhance the upper quadrants. Thus, her breast volume remains the same as at the initial consultation, but it has been transferred to the upper quadrants, giving a more pleasing and youthful appearance to the breasts.

TOTAL SECONDARY PTOSIS

This condition happens often in conjunction with a change of volume, usually weight loss. An augmentation will correct the problem. Since an implant is indicated, it is advantageous to reduce the ptotic lower poles and thus minimize another recurrence. The size of the augmentation varies according to the excised volume and the additional volume requested by the patient. Rarely will secondary ptosis occur following an augmentation of volume.

GLANDULAR PTOSIS

This condition occurs mainly after breast reduction but it may also follow mastopexy. It is usually associated with too high a location of the NAC, while the gland with its skin envelope and inframammary fold have migrated downward. The best solution is a reduction of the lower breast pole with relocation of the inframammary fold, care being taken to keep a very short vertical scar. It may be necessary to insert an implant to correct the flatness of the upper quadrants and NAC area. The desired volume is discussed with the patient.

REFERENCES

1. Aston, S. J., and Rees, T. D. Breast Reduction and Mastopexy. In T. D. Rees (ed.), *Aesthetic Plastic Surgery.* Philadelphia: Saunders, 1980. P. 903.
2. Baroudi, R., and Lewis, J. R. The augmentation-reduction mammaplasty. *Clin. Plast. Surg.* 3:301, 1976.
3. Biesenberger, H. *Deformitaten und kosmetische Operationen der weiblichen Brust.* Vienna: Maudrich, 1931.
4. Biggs, T. M. Brauer, R. C., and Wolf, L. E. Mastopexy in conjunction with subcutaneous mastectomy. *Plast. Reconstr. Surg.* 60:1, 1978.
5. DeCastro, C. C. Mammaplasty with curved incisions. *Plast. Reconstr. Surg.* 57:596, 1976.
6. Dempsey, W. C., and Lathan, W. D. Sub-pectoral implants in augmentation mammaplasty. *Plast. Reconstr. Surg.* 42:515, 1968.
7. Dufourmentel, L., and Mouly, R. Plastie mammaire par la méthode oblique. *Ann. Chir. Plast.* 6:45, 1961.
8. Dufourmentel, L., and Mouly, R. Développements récents de la plastie mammaire par la méthode oblique latérale. *Ann. Chir. Plast.* 10:227, 1965.
9. Dufourmentel, L., and Mouly, R. Modification of "periwinkle shell operation" for small ptotic breast. *Plast. Reconstr. Surg.* 41:523, 1968.
10. Erol, O. O., and Spira, M. A mastopexy technique for mild to moderate ptosis. *Plast. Reconstr. Surg.* 67:543, 1981.
11. Georgiade, N. G. Correction of the Ptotic Breast. In N. G. Georgiade (ed.), *Reconstructive Breast Surgery.* St. Louis: Mosby, 1976. P. 113.
12. Gillies, H., and Marino, H. The "periwinkle shell" principle in the treatment of the small ptotic breast. *Plast. Reconstr. Surg.* 21:1, 1958.
13. Girard, C. Uber Mastoptose und Mastopexie. *Arch. Klin. Chir.* 92:829, 1910.
14. Goulian, D., Jr. Dermal mastopexy. *Plast. Reconstr. Surg.* 47:105, 1971.
15. Goulian, D., Jr. Dermal mastopexy. *Clin. Plast. Surg.* 3:171, 1976.
16. Goulian, D., Jr. Ptosis and Its Correction. In R. M. Goldwyn (ed.), *Plastic and Reconstructive Surgery of the Breast.* Boston: Little, Brown, 1976.
17. Goulian, D., Jr. Mastopexy. In E. H. Courtiss (ed.), *Aesthetic Surgery: Trouble—How to Avoid It and How to Treat It.* St. Louis: Mosby, 1978.
18. Goulian, D., Jr., and Conway, H. Correction of the moderately ptotic breast: A warning. *Plast. Reconstr. Surg.* 43:478, 1969.
19. Gruber, R. P., and Friedman, G. D. Periareolar subpectoral augmentation mammaplasty. *Plast. Reconstr. Surg.* 65:603, 1980.
20. Hinderer, U. T. Cirugía plástica mamaria de aumento y reduccíon. *Ann. Acad. Méd. Quir. Esp.* 50:3, 1965.
21. Hinderer, U. T. The dermal brassiere mammaplasty. *Clin. Plast. Surg.* 3:349, 1976.
22. Hinderer, U. T. Mammaplasty: The dermal brassiere technique. *Aesthetic Plast. Surg.* 2:1, 1978.
23. Kahn, S., Hoffman, S., and Simon, B. E. Correction on nonhypertrophic ptosis of the breasts. *Plast. Reconstr. Surg.* 41:244, 1968.
24. Letterman, G., and Schurter, M. History of Surgical Correction of Mammary Ptosis. In J. Q. Owsley and R. A. Peterson (eds.), *Symposium on Aesthetic Surgery of the Breast.* St. Louis: Mosby, 1978. Pp. 183–189.
25. Lewis J. R., Jr. Classification and Surgical Correction of Ptosis of the Breasts. In F. W. Masters and J. R. Lewis, Jr. (eds.), *Symposium on Aesthetic Surgery of the Face, Eyelid, and Breast.* St. Louis: Mosby, 1972. P. 183.
26. Lewis, J. R., Jr. *Atlas of Aesthetic Plastic Surgery.* Boston: Little, Brown, 1973.
27. Longacre, J. J. Surgical reconstruction of the flat discoid breast. *Plast. Reconstr. Surg.* 17:358, 1956.
28. Lotsch, F. Uber Hangebrustplastik. *Zentralbl. Chir.* 50:1241, 1943.
29. Mahler, D. Rejuvenation of the atrophied breast. *Aesthetic Plast. Surg.* 5:213, 1981.
30. Owsley, J. Q. Simultaneous mastopexy and augmentation for correction of the small ptotic breast. *Ann. Plast. Surg.* 2:195, 1979.
31. Owsley, J. Q., and Brownstein, M. L. Correction of the Small Ptotic Breast with Simultaneous Augmentation and Mastopexy. In J. Q. Owsley and R. A. Peterson (eds.), *Symposium on Aesthetic Surgery of the Breast.* St. Louis: Mosby, 1978. P. 103.
32. Owsley, J. Q., and Peterson, R. A. (eds.). *Symposium on Aesthetic Surgery of the Breast.* St. Louis: Mosby, 1978. Pp. 72–82.
33. Pousson, M. De la mastopexie. *Bull. Mem. Soc. Chir. Paris* 23:507, 1897.
34. Regnault, P. The hypoplastic and ptotic breast: A combined operation with prosthetic augmentation. *Plast. Reconstr. Surg.* 37:31, 1966.
35. Regnault, P. Breast ptosis: Definition and treatment. *Clin. Plast. Surg.* 3:193, 1976.
36. Regnault, P. Ptosis, Asymetry, Tubular Breast, and Congenital Anomalies. In J. Q. Owsley and R. A. Peterson (eds.), *Symposium on Aesthetic Surgery of the Breast.* St. Louis: Mosby, 1978. P. 109.
37. Schatten, W. E., et al. Further experience with lateral wedge resection mammaplasties. *Br. J. Plast. Surg.* 28:37, 1975.
38. Strombeck, J. O. Macromastia in women and its surgical

treatment. *Acta Chir. Scand. [Suppl.]* 341 : 1, 1964.
39. Verchere, F. Mastopexie latérale contre la mastoptose hypertrophique. *Med. Mod.* (Paris) 9:540, 1898.
40. Vilain, R., and Mitz, V. The Biesenberger Technique for Mammary Ptosis and Hypertrophy. In R. M. Goldwyn (ed.), *Long-Term Results in Plastic and Reconstructive Surgery.* Boston: Little, Brown, 1980.
41. Weatherly-White, R. C. A. *Plastic Surgery of the Female Breast.* New York: Harper & Row, 1980.
42. Weiner, D. L. A single dermal pedicle for nipple transposition in subcutaneous mastectomy, reduction mammaplasty, or mastopexy. *Plast. Reconstr. Surg.* 51 : 115, 1973.

23. *Breast Augmentation*

Paule Regnault
Rollin K. Daniel

During the past two decades, breast augmentation has been performed with increasing frequency because of improvements in implant design and surgical technique. Conceptually, it is a straightforward surgical procedure, which can be done on an outpatient basis under local anesthesia. The operation is personalized to fit the patient's desires in regard to incision and size of prosthesis. However, patient selection and management of breast firmness secondary to fibrous capsular contracture remain a significant challenge for the surgeon.

HISTORY

The modern era of breast augmentation began in the 1940s with utilization of dermal fat grafts by Bames [13, 14] and Maliniac [89]. These grafts were placed in the retromammary space to ensure rapid revascularization. The high incidence of absorption and infection forced abandonment of the procedure [16]. Subsequently, Longacre [87] rotated a deepithelialized abdominal flap beneath the breast. In the 1950s, prosthetic materials were introduced; initially Ivalon sponges and later Etheron. The simplicity and good early results made the procedure quite popular, but the late results were disappointing. Fibrous tissue ingrowth resulted in a rock-hard breast with contractural deformity [105].

In the 1960s, the silicone bag prosthesis, filled with either silicone gel or saline, revolutionized breast augmentation and led to its widespread popularity [32–34, 38, 45, 84]. The incidence and severity of capsule contracture, which was virtually 100 percent with sponges, dropped to 40 percent. The initial design had posterior Dacron patches to ensure fixation to the chest wall. However, breast distortion occurred because of fixation of the prosthesis and inferior displacement of the breast mass, leading to subsequent removal of the Dacron patches. Attempts to reduce the incidence of capsular contracture brought the inflatable prosthesis, the ultrathin silicone bag, the double lumen, and now the multilayered silicone bag [64]. The operative technique has been continually modified as to incision (inframammary, periareolar, axillary), placement (retromammary, retropectoral), and postoperative management [3, 58, 77, 101, 108, 143]. Although late results are not known, the high percentage of good results at 10 years justifies continuation of the procedure. The use of liquid silicone for direct injection into the breast is fraught with serious complications and is mentioned only to be condemned [19, 26, 79, 99, 102].

PATHOPHYSIOLOGY AND CLASSIFICATION

Inadequate breast volume and contour can be caused by any of the following: (1) developmental micromastia, (2) postpartum involution, (3) drastic weight reduction, (4) postsurgical deformities, (5) breast asymmetry, and (6) gender changes. The majority of young women seeking breast augmentation have breasts that are qualitatively normal but quantitatively and proportionally small. Another group consists of thin, ectomorphic patients whose body habitus is quite lean and masculine. Patients with postpartum involution generally have more redundant skin, larger areolae, and slight ptosis in contrast to those with developmental micromastia. On account of the popularity of weight reduction programs and gastroplasties, numerous women are now requesting large-volume augmentations to restore breasts proportional to their inherent endomorphic configuration. This deformity is often associated with major ptosis and severe striae and requires a more extensive procedure than augmentation alone. Occasionally, patients present with localized deformities secondary to previous biopsies and need only a small augmentation. Significant breast asymmetry requires detailed analysis of both breasts, but smaller asymmetries can be improved by slight adjustment with inflatable prostheses [35, 75]. Patients presenting with normal size breasts (B cup) may request larger breasts either because of psychologic maladjustment (feelings of inadequacy or inferiority), for economic reasons (exotic dancers), or following gender changes. Each of these groups requires careful preoperative assessment and occasionally psychiatric evaluation (Fig. 23-1).

From this analysis, it is possible to classify most patients' motives for augmentation mammaplasty into the following subdivisions: (1) hypoplasia: small breast, nipple-areola complex (NAC) at normal location; (2) aplasia: masculine type; (3) hypoplasia with ptosis (classify as to severity of ptosis); (4) asymmetry (location, severity); (5) associated deformities (muscle); and (6) males (postgender change) (Table 23-1).

Table 23-1. Classification of breast aplasias and hypoplasias

Hypoplasia, nipple-areola complex (NAC) in normal location
Complete hypoplasia (masculine type)
Asymmetry
Unequal hypoplasia
One side only hypoplastic
Hypoplasia with ptosis
Minor, NAC at level inframammary fold
Moderate, NAC lower than fold
Major, NAC at lower contour
Association with most usual breast deformities and NAC deformities
Association with thoracic deformity
Males (transvestites, gender changes)

CONSULTATION

The initial consultation and physical examination are of critical importance if the patient is to achieve the desired result and the surgeon is to select the optimal technique.

Medical History

A general medical history is taken with particular emphasis on breast pathology. Specific questions are asked related to breast development, previous pregnancies, breast feeding, and breast pathology including surgery and family history of breast cancer. In addition, all medications are detailed including aspirin and hormones or birth control pills, as are height, current weight, and weight variations. Review of the patient's personal and work situations should also be included.

Indications and Contraindications

Augmentation mammaplasty is indicated when the patient requests an increase in breast volume that will result in better-proportioned and aesthetic breasts. The majority of patients who wish this operation are concerned more about their appearance in clothes than in seminude (bathing suit) or nude situations. Thus, the desire for a normal appearance without recourse to padded brassieres coupled with an obvious deformity justifies the operation and does not necessitate a psychiatric examination. However, the psychologic motivation and expected result must be carefully elucidated at time of consultation.

Contraindications can be classified as general, specific, and psychologic. This procedure is especially contraindicated in patients with bleeding disorders, anticoagulation, or steroid therapy. Local conditions, including recent and recurrent fibrocystic breast disease with mastodynia or undiagnosed breast mass, are contraindications. Occasionally, a woman presents for augmentation who has beautiful breasts in proportion to her body. She is pleased to be informed that she already has the best and that surgery is not warranted. More frequently, patients present with pendulous breasts requesting correction by augmentation mammaplasty alone. In these cases, a mastopexy must be done as only minor ptosis can be corrected by augmentation alone [59]. A reasonable lower age limit is 18, but there is no older limit, as long as the operation is viewed with realistic expectations [124].

Figure 23-1. Range of patients seeking breast augmentation.
A. Developmental hypoplasia.
B. Complete hypoplasia, masculine type.
C. Involutional hypoplasia.
D. Hypoplasia with ptosis.
E. Mild asymmetry. Patient requested augmentation of left breast.
F. Patient requested upper quadrant fullness. Intraoperatively, marked deformity of left cartilaginous rib cage and 13-degree scoliosis became apparent.

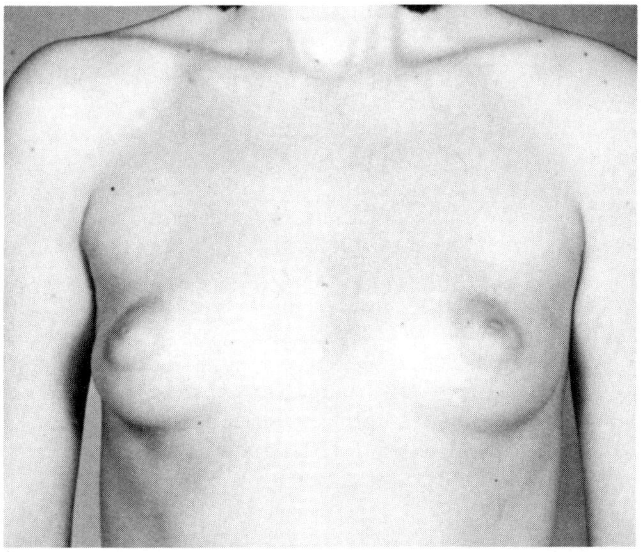
A

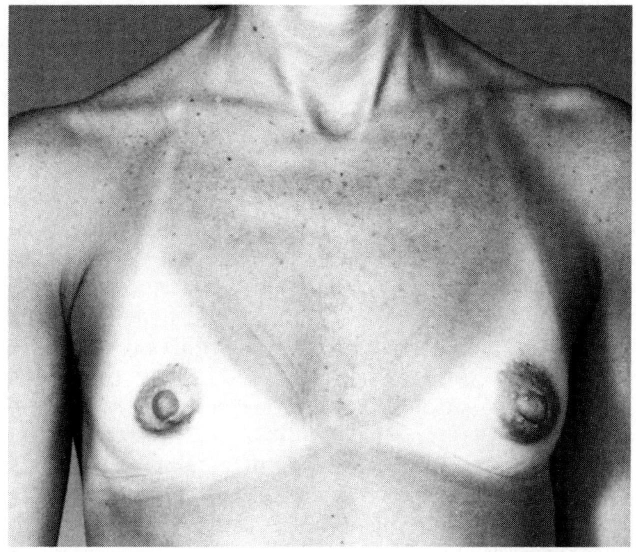
B

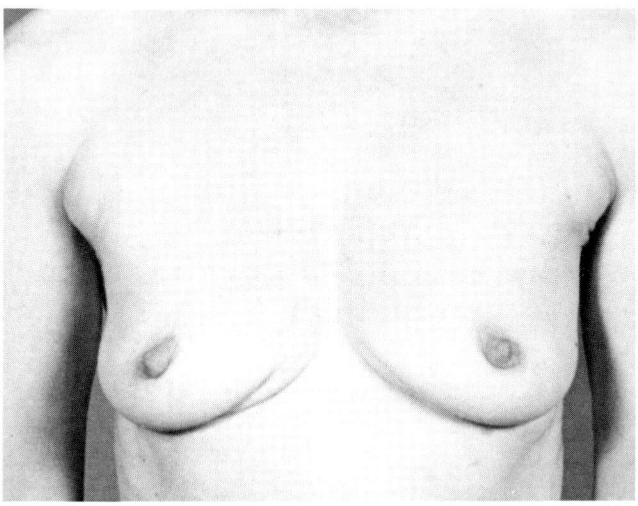
C

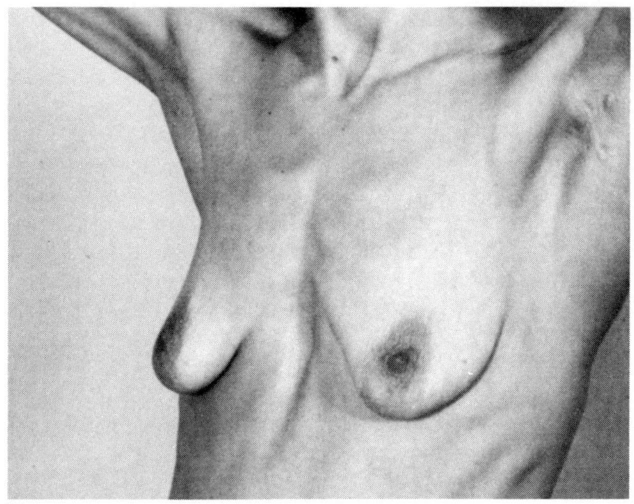
D

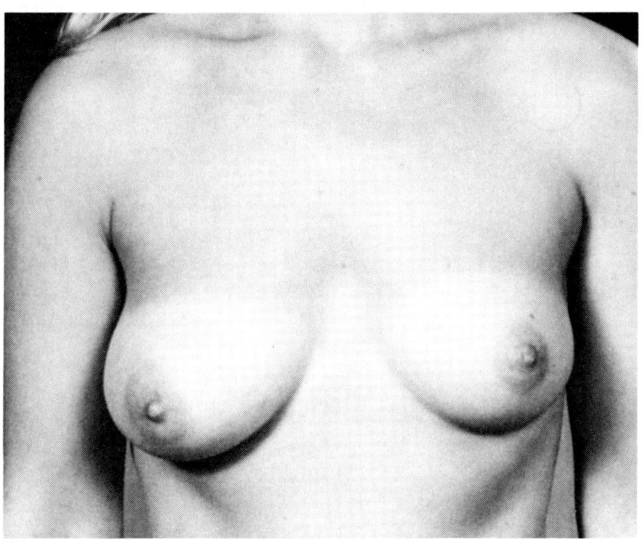
E

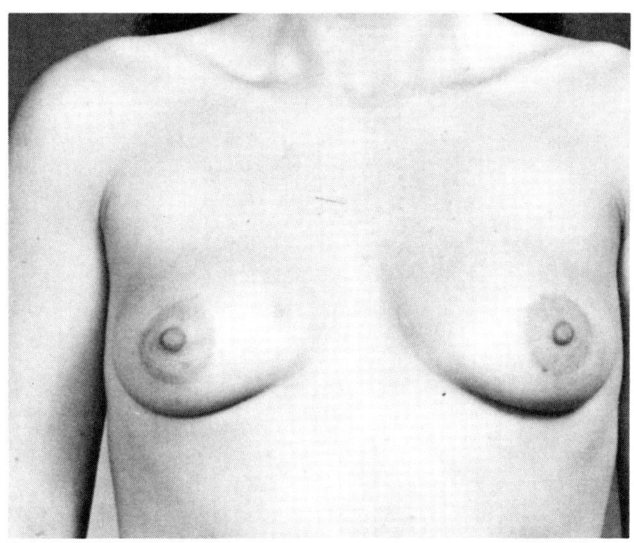
F

Motivation

If postoperative disappointment is to be avoided, the surgeon must determine the patient's motivation. Ideally, she feels somewhat inadequate about her small size and wants to look better in clothes. If the motivation is derived from marital or social pressure, the patient is best sent for counseling first. It is important to be aware of any psychiatric history in patients seeking augmentation mammaplasty. In contrast to the narcissistic compulsive personality of pioneering patients in the 1950s and the nonaesthetic patient of Scandinavia, the majority of patients in North America seek the operation out of feelings of inadequacy and low self-esteem [45]. This situation is manifested in social situations (shopping, summertime activities, sports) and sexual relations (insecurity, decreased interest) [126, 127]. It should be noted that 5 to 15 percent of patients have significant psychiatric problems (depressive reactions, neuroses) related to concern about their breast size [54]. One should inquire into the patient's expectations regarding volume, shape, scars, and softness of the breasts following augmentation mammaplasty. Since most patients are in their twenties, are married, and have at least one child, inquiry concerning satisfaction with breast size during pregnancy is often revealing. Also, 88 percent of patients wear padded brassieres preoperatively and so have increased feelings of inadequacy. Goin and Goin [57] recognize three subgroups of patients seeking augmentation mammaplasty: (1) those with small breasts who are unsure of their femininity, (2) those with postpartum hypoplasia who seek restoration of normalcy, and (3) those with psychologic instability during sexual relations.

Physical Examination

The entire body is examined for comparison and evaluation of existing breast volume in relation to hips, shoulders, and waistline as well as height and silhouette. The entire torso front and back is examined for general configuration, any bony curvatures of either the vertebral column or the thorax, and contrasts in muscle mass, especially the pectoralis major. A general observation of the torso and breast is followed by a specific breast examination. The brassiere band and cup size are determined with a tape measure. The body circumference is measured with the patient sitting and arms by the sides. The brassiere band size equals the chest circumference measured at the level of the axillary fold. Next, the fullest part of the breast is measured; in the hypoplastic breast this is at the nipple level. In contrast to the patient seeking breast reduction, it is not essential for the hypoplastic patient to be wearing a brassiere. The difference between the two circumferences yields the cup size, with a one-letter increase in cup size for each 1-in. increment; i.e., 34-in. breast, 34-in. chest = 34AA; 35-in. breast, 34-in. chest = 34A; 36-in. breast, 34-in. chest = 34B. In asymmetries, the hemithorax circumference is measured and differences are recorded. These values are mentioned to the patient, and any discrepancy from her usual brassiere size may be due to style selection, monthly variation, or weight changes. The waist circumference is also recorded.

The breast deformity is assessed according to the following criteria: (1) breast size either small or complete aplasia; (2) breast ptosis absent or present, minor, moderate, or major; (3) asymmetry; (4) presence of scars and elasticity of soft tissue; and (5) nipple-areola complex (NAC). Each of these factors is important in allowing classification of the deformity and selection of the optimal operative technique (Table 23-2). A complete breast examination is done with the patient in a recumbent position. Even small breasts vary greatly in volume, shape, and tissue elasticity. Soft, distensible breasts seem to expand and project more readily than aplastic breasts. In patients with total aplasia and a lean torso, retropectoral placement of the prosthesis is considered mandatory. Small discrepancies can often be corrected by a 20-cc difference in implants while major asymmetries call for a 50-cc increase for each inch of difference in hemithorax circumference. Since most augmentation patients have a 32 to 34 brassiere band size, 1 in. on the hemithorax equals one-half the cup size volume of 100 cc. Abnormal, protruding

Table 23-2. Classification of deformities with selection of optimal surgical technique

Hypoplasia	Small breast, normal NAC, most frequent Inframammary fold incision, partial retropectoral placement Regular prosthesis for small thorax or requested projection Low-profile prosthesis for normal thorax or limited projection If athletic, retroglandular with small prosthesis
Complete hypoplasia (masculine type)	Inframammary fold incision, partial retropectoral placement Regular implant
Asymmetry	Almost invisible, 20 cc less on larger side Easily visible, measure breasts, 1 inch = 50 cc Unilateral, measure breasts, 1 inch = 100 cc
Hypoplasia with ptosis	Minor: retropectoral, low profile, 180 cc minimum Moderate: mastopexy plus augmentation preferred; otherwise very large prosthesis, 280 cc minimum Major: resection of lower pole plus augmentation
Nipple-areola deformities	Tubular breast: correct skin envelope by circular excision or B-technique; inframammary, retropectoral, low profile Protruding NAC: reduce areola by ring excision, use same incision for augmentation with low profile Nipple invagination or hypertrophy: treat concurrently with augmentation
Males and transsexuals	Periareolar or axillary incisions Retroglandular placement, retropectoral only if lean Regular implants, size as for complete hypoplasia

areolae, tubular breasts, or nipple deformities are discussed as well as any previous scars. Following examination, the surgeon is able to determine the feasibility of the procedure and the presence of any associated deformities that must be corrected to ensure a good result. The required volume of the prosthesis can be determined from experience or discussion with the patient of the desired size.

Aesthetic Goals

Following examination, the surgeon can reconcile the patient's desires with inherent anatomic limitations. Since the vast majority of patients have always had small breasts, it is natural that they will want a significant increase. It is generally accepted that the most aesthetic cup size is the B cup, regardless of torso circumference, and it is the basis for clothes design. In addition, most surgeons feel that the incidence of capsular contracture and palpation of the prosthesis increases with prosthetic volume. If limited differences occur, the surgeon should yield to the patient's desire as it is she who will have to live with the implants for life. If a major difference occurs, a second visit or consultation with a colleague is recommended. Next, the degree of projection is discussed. A regular prosthesis is used when universal projection is requested and a round prosthesis when limited projection is desired. In general, the surgeon offers a proposed technique that is compatible with existing breast size and associated deformities. The patient is then told that alternatives exist as to the incision and prosthesis placement and is given an explanation of why the surgeon recommends a specific technique. Also, the type of implant is mentioned; inflatables are recommended when asymmetry exists [129]. Again, a mutually agreeable plan is devised and recorded in the patient's chart [52].

The question of size selection is generally based on the surgeon's experience and standard tables. Recently, Brody [21] has emphasized the value of having the patient participate directly in the selection process. As noted by Pacik [100], the patient is encouraged to purchase a brassiere of the desired size and then at the consultation try various prostheses (120–350 cc). Most patients select a size from 175 to 225 cc with an additional allowance for retropectoral placement (Fig. 23-2). With this approach, patient satisfaction was higher and revisional surgery less [130].

Informed Consent

The operative technique is reviewed and possible complications are explained. First, hematoma and infection occur in 1 to 2 percent of cases and may require removal of the prosthesis for a 3-month period prior to reinsertion. Second, capsular contracture is part of the normal healing response but will result in a breast that is firmer than normal in approximately 25 percent of cases. Although it can be treated effectively by closed compression, an open capsulotomy may be needed in about 5 percent of cases. Third, despite every effort to minimize scarring, a scar will

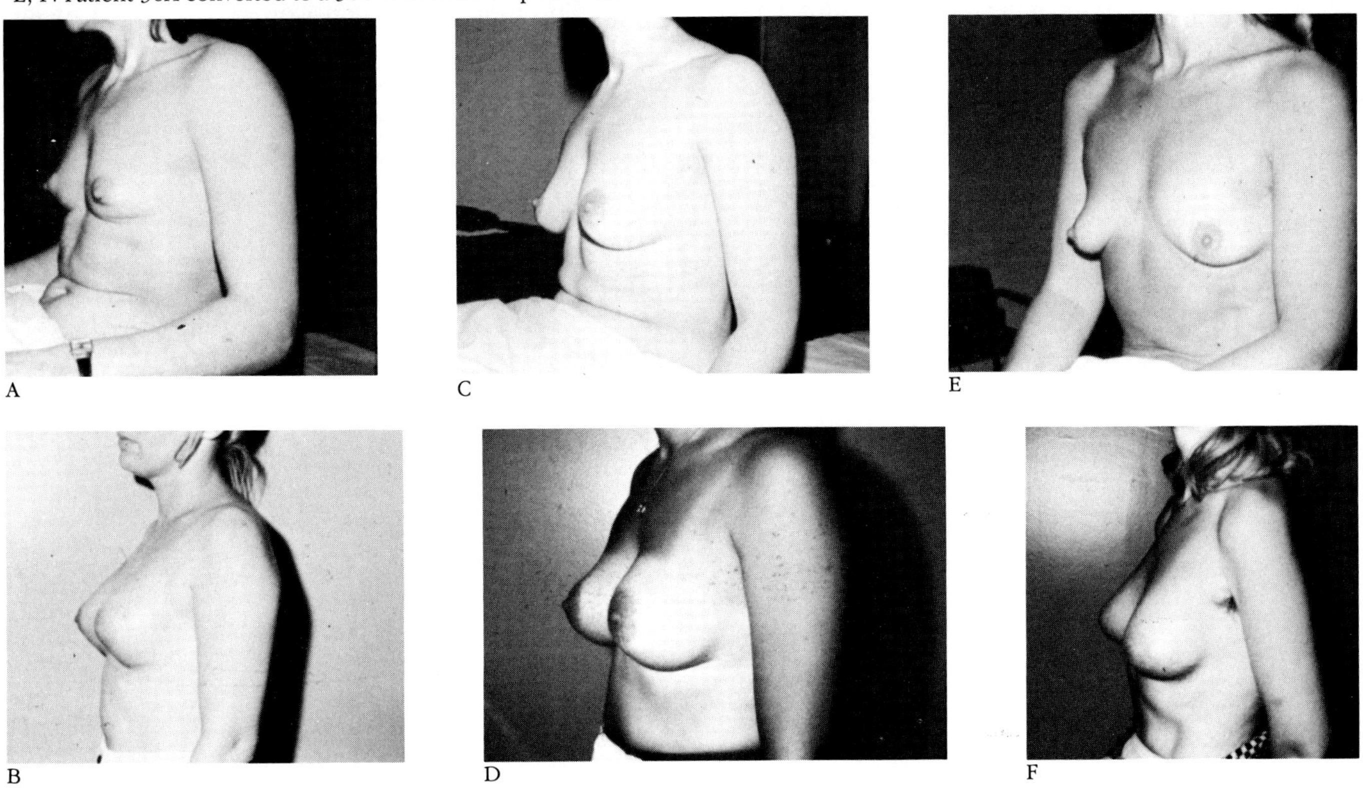

Figure 23-2. Most patients can achieve the desired B cup with an implant between 175 and 225 cc.
A, B. Patient 32A increased to 32B with a 180-cc prosthesis.
C, D. Patient 34A achieved a 34B with a 200-cc prosthesis.
E, F. Patient 36A converted to a 36B with a 220-cc prosthesis.

always be visible on close inspection. Fourth, sensation in the breast will be decreased immediately postoperatively, with a gradual return by 6 months. Rarely, nipple sensation can be either lost permanently or decreased, and the patient must consider this aspect carefully.

Preoperative Preparations

If the patient decides to proceed with surgery, photographs are taken of the torso, from navel to neck, including anterolateral, and oblique. The patient is given a prescription for (1) a broad-spectrum antibiotic, (2) pain medication (postoperative), and (3) sleeping medication. If the transaxillary technique, as described by Peterson, is used, the patient is instructed to bring a front-fastening brassiere of the desired cup size with underwire support on the day of surgery.

SURGICAL TECHNIQUES

Despite its conceptual simplicity, numerous techniques exist for augmentation mammaplasty, varying in approach, prosthetic placement, and required associated procedures (Fig. 23-3). Terminology is nonspecific, and the reader is referred to Table 23-3. One should have experience with each of the major approaches and placements to permit selection of the optimal operative technique.

Inframammary Approach and Partial Retropectoral Placement

The inframammary fold incision with partial retropectoral placement is used for many augmentation mammaplasties. Its selection is based on personal experience of the senior author with more than 2000 cases over a 20-year period employing virtually every incision, type of prosthesis, and possible placement [114–117]. The advantages and disadvantages of the evolved procedure are detailed here. However, patient preferences and circumstances mandate that the surgeon be capable of using all methods. Currently, the transaxillary approach as described by Peterson is being employed more frequently as a greater number of patients are requesting it.

The principal advantage of the inframammary incision is that it offers an acceptable scar that is located in a natural fold under the breast and excellent exposure for dissection. The incision is virtually invisible in this position and easily hidden by a small brassiere. It is worth remembering that *all* scars from augmentation mammaplasty are visible and risk hypertrophic development. The inframammary incision facilitates direct exposure of the entire area and hemostasis. It is also the best approach for evacuation of hematomas and capsulotomy.

Partial retropectoral placement of the prosthesis ensures coverage of the prosthesis superiorly while preventing the upward displacement of the prosthesis characteristic of the complete retropectoral location (Fig. 23-4). This upper padding is important in lean individuals (Fig. 23-5). Since the superior portion of the pocket is a natural cleavage plane, dissection is rapid and minimal bleeding is encountered [41, 60]. Both hemostasis and postoperative pain are less than with retroglandular undermining. Of particular importance is a lower rate of fibrous capsule contracture—approximately 15 percent for retropectoral versus 40 percent for retroglandular. The explanation is probably a result of constant natural massaging and excellent vascularization.

The disadvantages of the inframammary incision are principally its visibility, social implication, and possible hypertrophy. The partial retropectoral placement may cause distortion due to adhesion of the pocket to the upper part of the muscle, thereby resulting in lifting of the implant on contraction of the pectoralis muscle. This condition may be temporary or permanent; in the latter event enlargement of the upper pocket is required. Inferior displacement of the prosthesis may also occur and is easily corrected by resuturing the aponeurotic layer with permanent sutures. Long-term extrusion of the implant may occur following prolonged exercise, i.e., competitive sports or ceiling painting. This can be corrected by reinserting the prosthesis and prohibiting arm extension for 1 month.

Table 23-3. Surgical techniques

Approaches and incisions	Markings made on standing
Inframammary fold	Distance measured from center of nipple
	Incision in crease
Areolar	Incision subareolar, at juncture of areola and skin
	Periareolar, 1–2 mm within the areola
	Transareolar, incising through areola
	Undermining subcutaneous or transgranular
Axillary	Transverse incision
Abdominal	Via abdominoplasty
Previous scar	Via scar
Prosthetic placement	
Retroglandular	
Retropectoral	Muscle splitting, complete coverage
	Muscle detachment, partial coverage

Figure 23-3. The three most frequently used incisions for breast augmentation as shown at 1 year postoperatively. All implants placed retropectorally with detachment of the muscle.
A, B. Postpartum breast hypoplasia improved by breast augmentation (180-cc prosthesis) placed through a 4-cm inframammary incision.
C, D. Masculine hypoplasia treated by breast augmentation (200-cc prosthesis) inserted through a periareolar incision.
E, F. Developmental hypoplasia corrected by breast augmentation (200-cc prosthesis) through an axillary incision.
Note: Incisional scars are always visible and the patient must accept this fact, but the axillary is least.

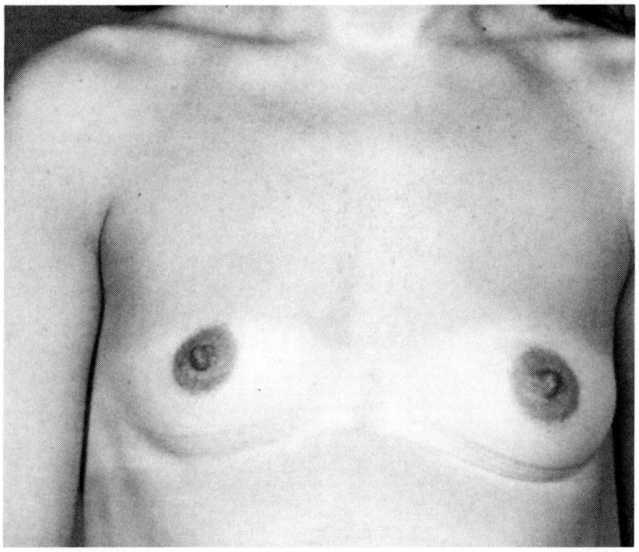

A

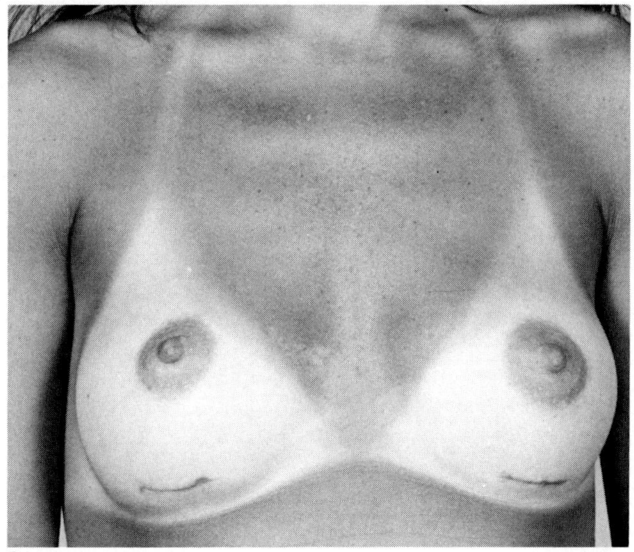

B

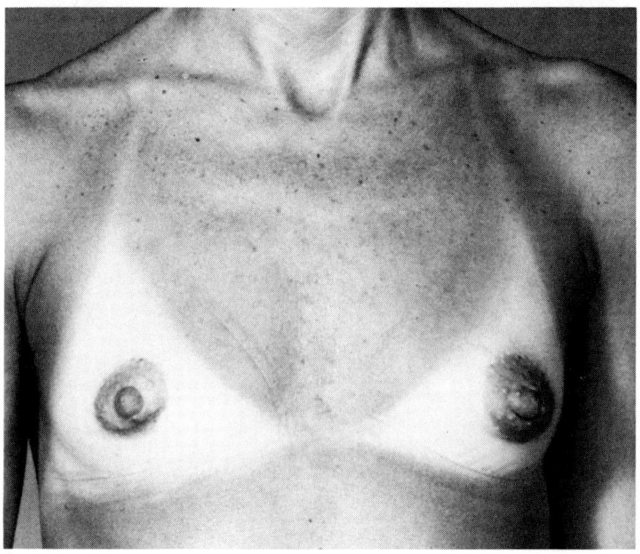

C

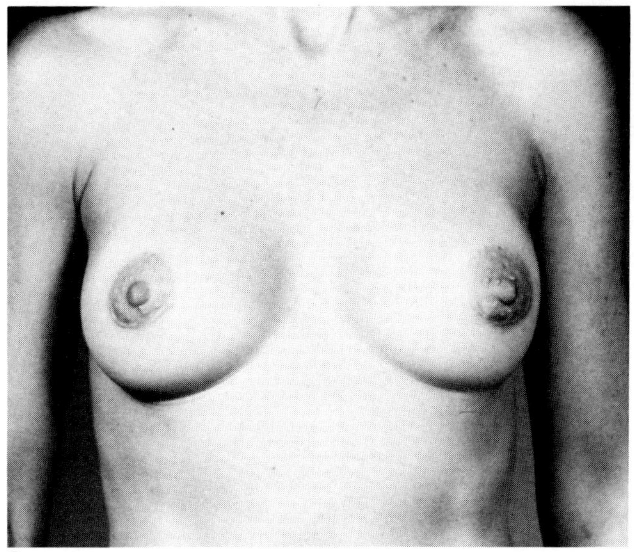

D

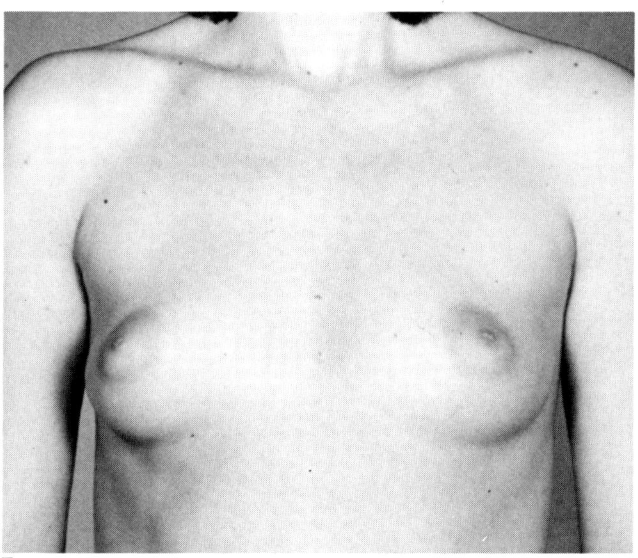

E

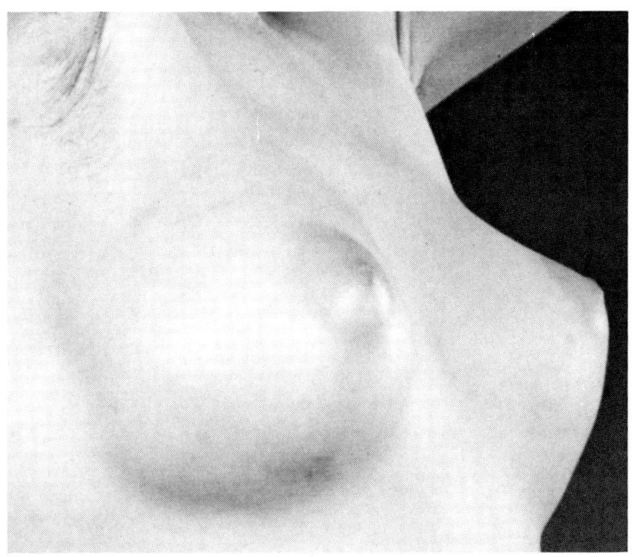

F

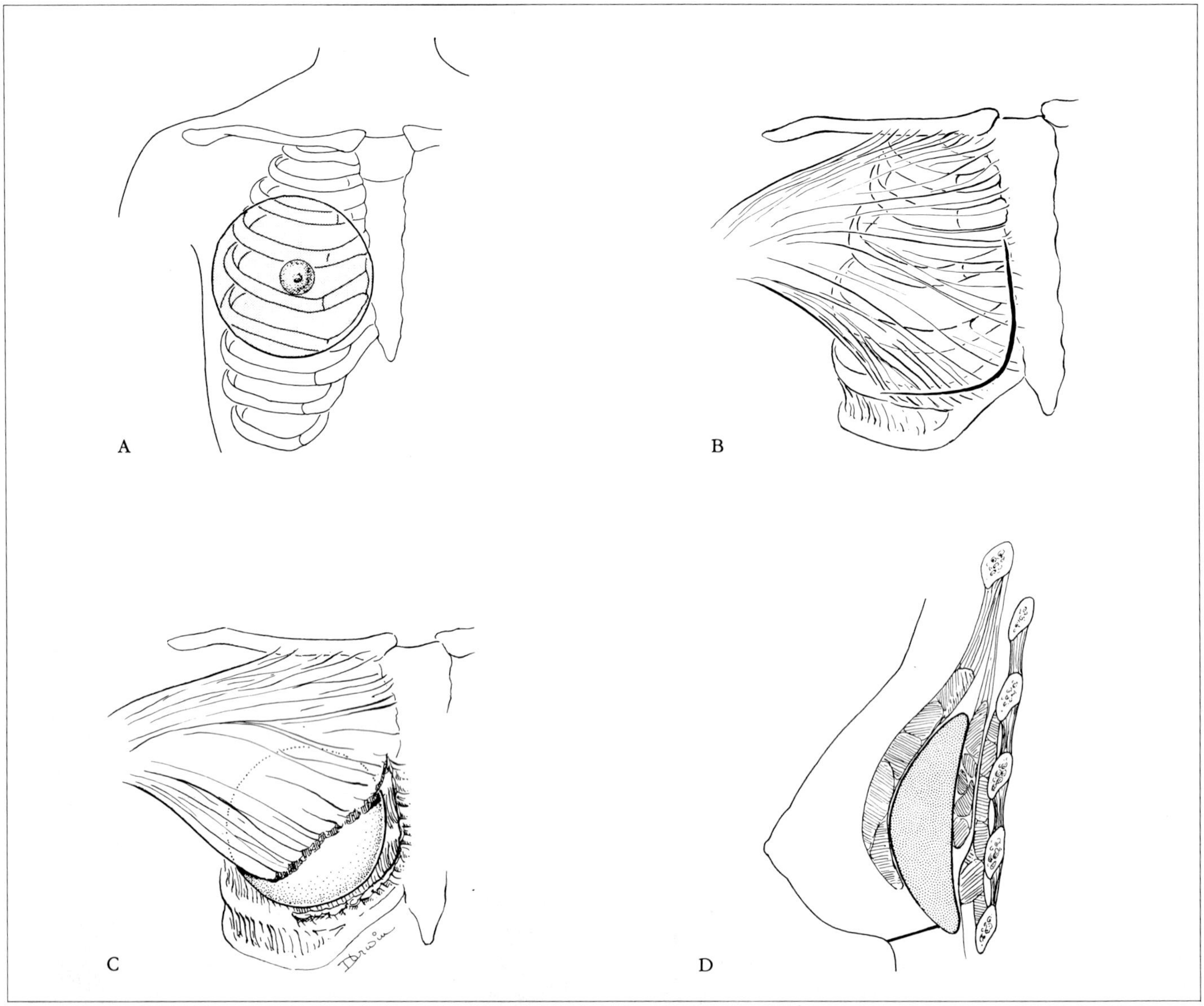

Figure 23-4. Breast augmentation with partial retropectoral placement.
A. Location of prosthesis relative to the nipple.
B. Detachment of the pectoralis major muscle completely from the rectus sheath and from its sternal origin up to the third interspace. A critical maneuver.
C. Partial coverage of the prosthesis.
D. Partial coverage of the prosthesis as seen on sectional view.

Present-day implants are a soft silicone elastomer shell filled with either silicone gel or saline. The silicone bag is composed of polymers with a moderate to high molecular weight, which has been reinforced with silica filler and additional cross-linkage. In contrast, the silicone gel has a moderate molecular weight and no fillers. The physical properties of silicone are worth remembering: It is (1) heat and time stable, (2) minimally tissue reactive and adherent, (3) nondecomposable, and (4) noncarcinogenic [51, 76]. Implants vary as to shape (round, oval, teardrop, custom-made), projection (regular, low profile), and filling (prefilled gel, inflatable) [5, 6, 83]. In general, the round gel-filled implant is used with either a low profile or regular profile according to the breast, thorax, and projection desired. Because of a significant 6 percent deflation rate, the inflatable prosthesis is reserved for difficult asymmetric deformities [111–113, 121]. Detailed studies have not confirmed a lower incidence of capsular contracture with inflatable prostheses.

Preoperative Planning

Prior to surgery, the patient is examined in the sitting position to remind the surgeon of the general breast contour. The patient is then placed in a supine position with elbows semiflexed, hands under hips. Following disinfection and draping, the midline is marked. The area of undermining is drawn vertically from the second to the sixth interspace and transversely from 2 cm lateral to the sternal border to the midaxillary line. With a hand on its superior part, the breast is pushed inferiorly and the sub-

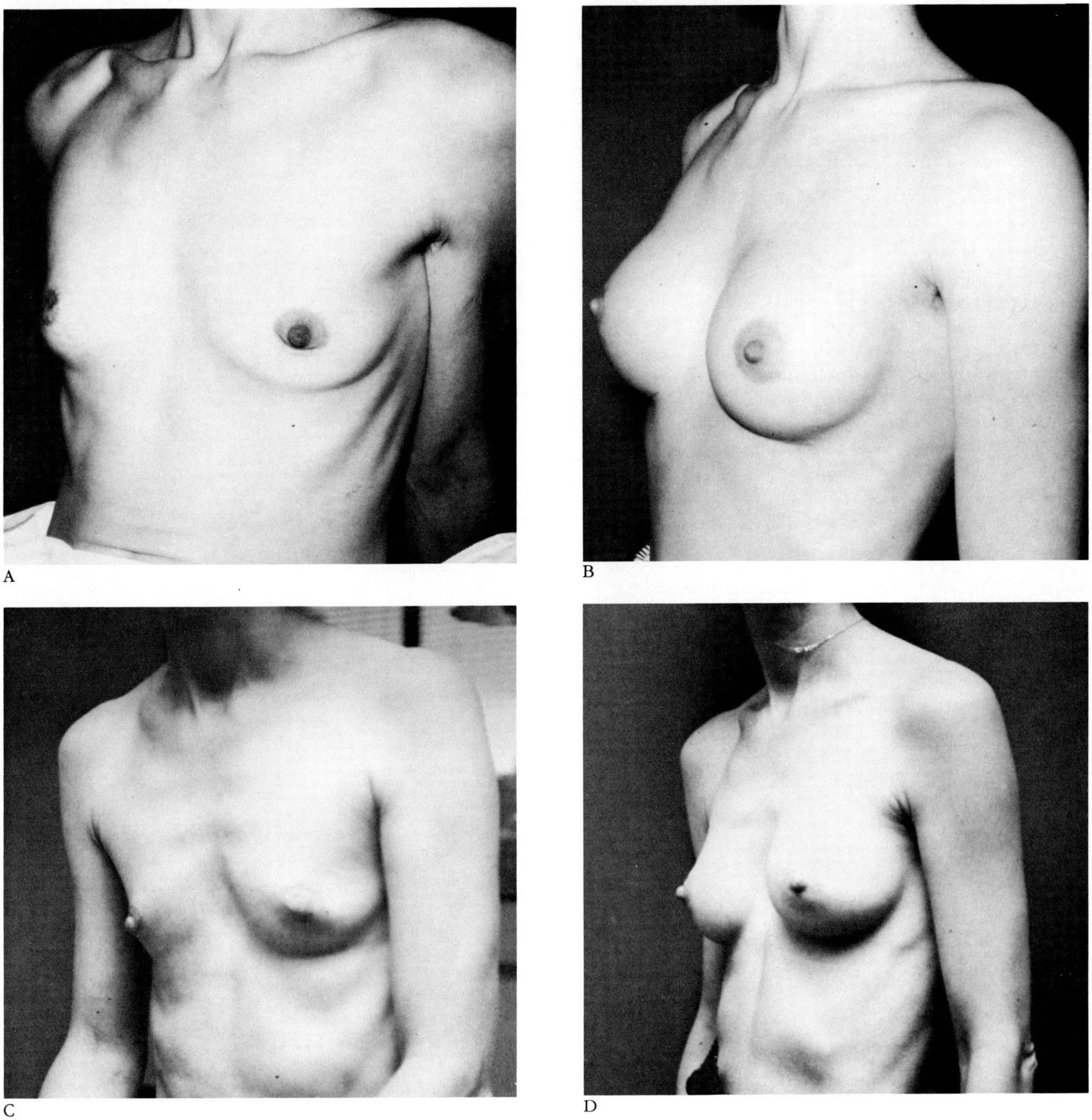

Figure 23-5. Two patients requesting augmentation.

A, B. Developmental hypoplasia corrected by partial retropectoral coverage of the breast implant inserted through an inframammary incision.

C, D. Lean individual with involutional hypoplasia. Significant contour improvement achieved by retropectoral placement. If a retroglandular pocket had been used, the prosthesis would probably have been visible in the upper quadrants.

mammary fold identified. It is important to measure the distance from the inframammary incision to the nipple center on both sides to ensure symmetry. The average distance is 6 to 8 cm depending on thorax configuration and volume of augmentation required. The incision is marked directly under the areola and the length varies from 3 to 6 cm according to implant size.

Anesthesia

Selection of the anesthesia technique is based on patient preference and economic consideration. In the anxious patient, general anesthesia is better. Otherwise, preoperative sedation (diazepam, 10–30 mg, intravenously) is followed by intercostal blocks (third to sixth nerves), and direct infiltration of the lower portion of the field is done with 0.5% lidocaine and epinephrine (1:200,000) [4, 73, 88, 92]. The total amount required is 50 cc per side. Local infiltration of the lower quadrants is done even with general anesthesia to assist hemostasis.

Surgical Technique

A 3-cm incision is made at the previously marked inframammary fold and continued down to the underlying pectoralis major muscle. It is worth remembering that the fan-shaped pectoralis major muscle varies as to its rib insertions, thickness, and tonicity. The overlying pectoralis fascia blends with the rectus abdominis inferiorly and the serratus anterior laterally. The breast itself rests almost entirely on the pectoralis, with lateral overlap of the serratus anterior. The muscle is identified in the upper medial portion of the incision, often somewhat higher than expected. It is then clamped over a 2-cm distance and severed, and the cut edge is meticulously cauterized. A finger is introduced into the retropectoral space with the pectoralis major above and the pectoralis minor below. The ribs are readily palpable. The upper portion of the dissection is done with a blunt finger while the lower portion is done by sharp dissection under direct vision. The attachment of the pectoralis major to the underlying ribs, the inferior rectus fascia, and the sternum up to the level of the third rib are sequentially clamped, transected, and cauterized. Repeated inspection and cauterization is done to ensure a dry field. The pocket should be significantly larger than the implant.

A smooth deep retractor is inserted to raise the breast, and the moistened implant is squeezed into the pocket. Once inserted, the prosthesis should be barely visible, and if bulging is seen, the pocket is enlarged by blunt dissection especially at the lateral periphery, or by relaxing the anterior muscle flap. Secondary hemostasis is then obtained if necessary, but drains are rarely required. Closure is accomplished by layers with multiple interrupted fascial sutures of 3-0 Vicryl. The pectoralis muscle is *not* sutured, ensuring that the lower third of the implant is covered only by breast tissue and subcutaneous tissue. The skin is approximated with a running subcuticular suture of 4-0 Vicryl. Paper adhesive strips are placed over the incision. Unless a drain is necessary, no other dressing is applied.

Postoperative Instructions

Mild sedatives and analgesics are prescribed although many patients will not require them. The patient is instructed to restrict pectoralis major contractions for 7 days. Thus, lifting of the arms and driving are forbidden, and vigorous sports activities are not permitted for 1 month. The patient is seen 1 week later. The breasts are usually a little swollen, and the patient is warned that they will be slightly smaller in a month. She is instructed to begin massaging the implants over the rib cage in all directions for a few minutes twice daily. Brassieres are not allowed for 3 months to allow free movement of the breasts and implants. This type of constant massage prevents unnatural localization of the implants, which often results from tight brassiere straps. Later, only a very soft brassiere is permitted, and metallic supports are contraindicated.

Periareolar Approach

James W. Smith
John E. Sherman

Although the majority of augmentation mammaplasties are performed through an inframammary approach, the periareolar approach affords an adequate surgical exposure and at the same time can provide a more aesthetic and less conspicuous scar. The limitation of this approach is that, with a very small areola, the incision may not be long enough to afford adequate exposure for creating the surgical pocket. Also, if a very large implant is needed, it may be difficult to insert the prosthesis through an incision of such limited size.

ANESTHESIA

A satisfactory scope of anesthetic techniques is currently available ranging from general anesthesia to local infiltration supplemented by intravenous sedation and including intercostal block anesthesia.

Premedication consisting of a combination of a narcotic (morphine, 5–10 mg), a phenothiazine (Compazine, 5–10 mg), and a barbiturate (Nembutal, 50–100 mg) is administered intramuscularly 1 hour preoperatively after a previous intramuscular injection of a barbiturate (Nembutal, 50–100 mg) at least 2 hours preoperatively. Intravenous sedation is obtained with morphine and diazepam (in 2.5-mg increments) after an initial intravenous dose (2–4 mg) of lorazepam (Ativan). After a satisfactory level of sedation has been achieved, the field is prepped and draped and the incision is marked. Local infiltration is obtained using lidocaine 0.5% in a solution containing a 1:200,000 dilution of epinephrine. A 25-gauge needle is employed for the initial infiltration, and a 20-gauge spindle needle is used to infiltrate in the fascial plane between the breast tissue and the pectoralis muscle.

TECHNIQUE

The breast and the chest wall are marked with the patient in the sitting position. The incision and the extent of the pocket are marked, as are the inframammary creases, the midline from the suprasternal notch to the umbilicus, and the breast meridian from the midclavicular line through the nipple.

The patient is then placed on the operating table in the supine position and prepped and draped (Fig. 23-6). Local infiltration is obtained after adequate sedation. An incision extending from the 3-o'clock to the 9-o'clock position at the junction of the hyperpigmented skin of the areola and the surrounding breast skin is made and deepened through the subcutaneous tissue to the level of the breast tissue.

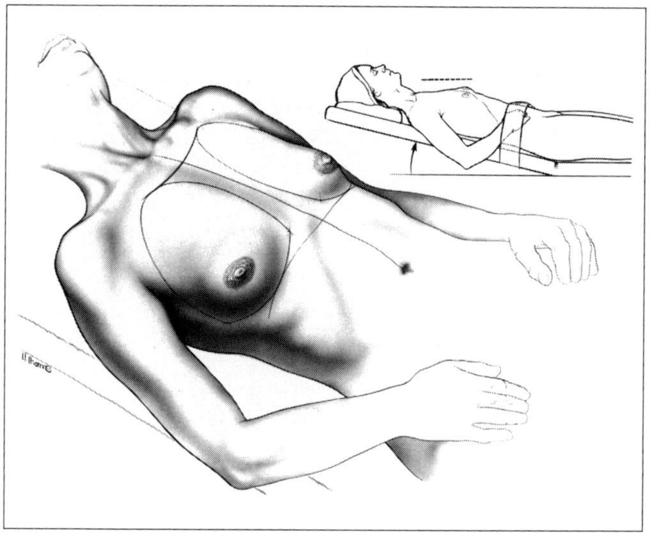

Figure 23-6. Breast forms are placed symmetrically on the chest wall and the skin is marked, to guide in the making of symmetric pockets. At the time of surgery the patient is placed in the supine position on the operating table with the head and thorax elevated approximately 30 degrees.

There are two approaches to the retromammary pocket (Fig. 23-7). One may incise directly through the gland until the juncture of the posterior breast capsule and the pectoral fascia has been reached. Or one may create a subcutaneous tunnel along the inferior aspect of the gland until the inframammary crease is reached, at which point the dissection extends cephalad at the level of juncture between the posterior breast capsule and the pectoral fascia.

The retromammary pocket is dissected from the level of the second rib superiorly to the inframammary fold inferiorly. The medial boundary is the lateral border of the sternum, and laterally the pocket extends to the midaxillary line.

A useful technique to avoid penetration of the pectoralis fascia and muscle is to place two hand retractors in the wound and elevate the breast from the chest wall. This maneuver permits a more expeditious dissection of the proper plane between the posterior breast capsule and the pectoralis fascia. A sponge forceps is an excellent adjunct for blunt dissection of this cavity. Adequate illumination of the breast pocket with either a headlamp or a fiberoptic retractor is essential for meticulous hemostasis, which is achieved with the use of electrocoagulation.

Irrigating catheters are placed at the superomedial aspect of each breast pocket (Fig. 23-8). A gel-filled round prosthesis is placed within the cavity. Wound closure is obtained with an inverting 4-0 Vicryl suture at the deep dermal-subcutaneous level and 5-0 nylon as a running subcutaneous suture. Steri-Strips are applied across the skin edges. The irrigating catheters are flushed with lidocaine with epinephrine. Then a steroid solution (20 mg Depo-Medrol) and an antibiotic solution (25,000 units bacitracin) are injected through the irrigating catheters.

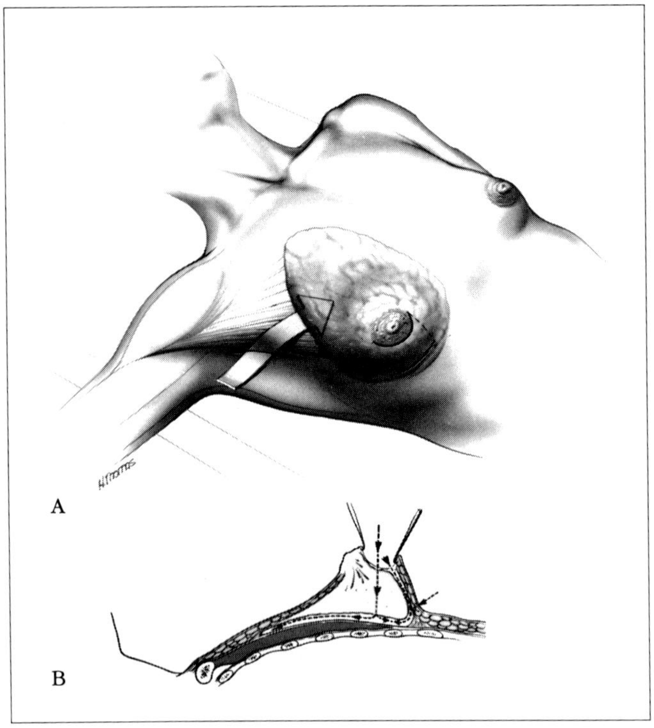

Figure 23-7

A. Most breast augmentations are carried out through one of three incisions: axillary, periareolar, or inframammary.

B. The retroglandular pocket can be approached directly through the inframammary incision, or, if the periareolar incision is chosen, dissection can be carried anterior to the breast fascia and then posteriorly along the plane of the prepectoral fascia. Most surgeons using the periareolar incision prefer to approach the retroglandular pocket by dissecting directly through the breast tissue. This choice carries with it the danger of contamination with *Staphylococcus epidermidis* or other bacteria located within the ductal system of the breast.

They are flushed with 10 ml of lidocaine with epinephrine before being removed.

The patient is placed in a support brassiere for 24 hours. The brassiere is removed and breast massage is begun on the first postoperative day. If capsular contracture occurs, attempts at closed compression are made (Fig. 23-9). If open capsulotomy is necessary, the safest way for incising the capsule surrounding the prosthesis is with an electrocautery unit. It cuts the capsule without puncturing or damaging the implant (Fig. 23-10).

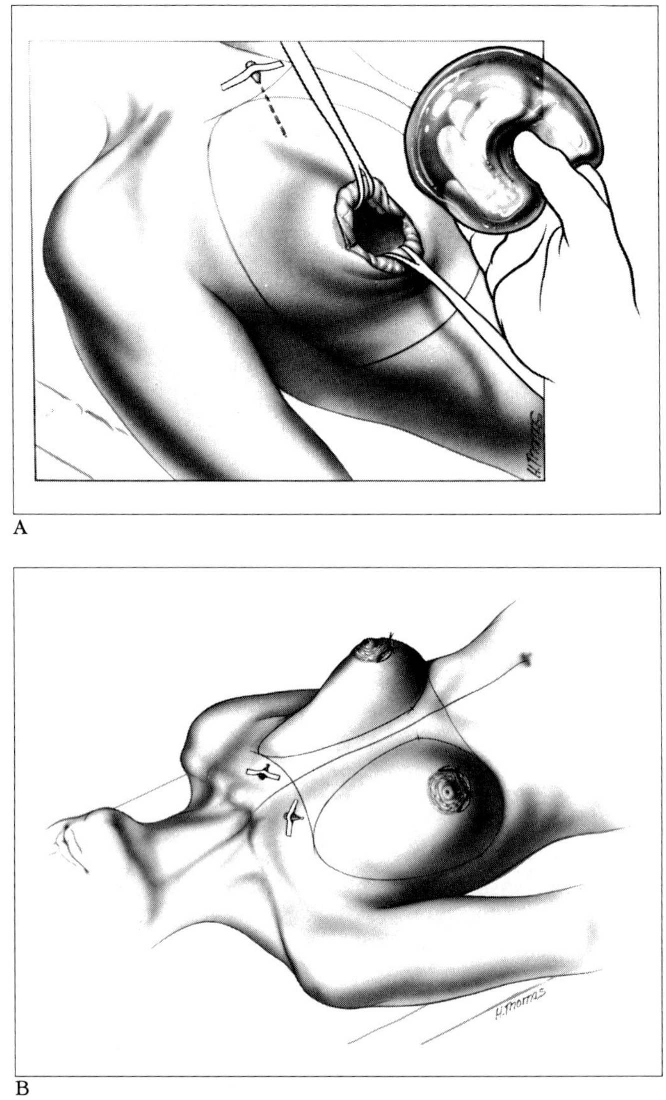

Figure 23-8

A. Once the cavities have been created and found to be symmetric, a 2-in. No. 18 intracath is placed at the level of the second intercostal space from the skin into the pocket and then taped in place.

B. This drawing demonstrates the importance of being sure that the dissection of the cavity is completed inferiorly so that with closure the nipples point forward and a good breast contour has been achieved. Sometimes it is worthwhile to raise the patient to a sitting position to be certain that the pocket is dissected enough inferiorly to create the proper contour. Once the closure has been completed, 10 ml of lidocaine containing epinephrine is instilled through the intercath to further add to the hemostasis within the cavity. Then 20 mg of Depo-Medrol is instilled into each pocket and followed by a bacitracin solution (20,000 units in 10 ml). Finally, 10 ml of lidocaine is added to be certain that the other substances have been flushed well into the cavity before the catheter is withdrawn.

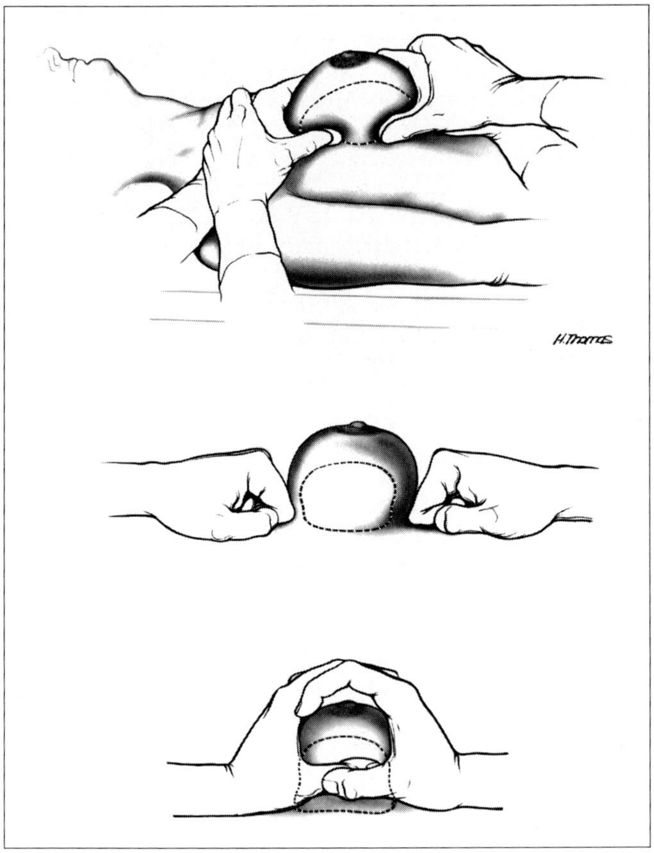

Figure 23-9. We have found the several techniques illustrated to be the most effective ways of performing a closed capsulotomy.

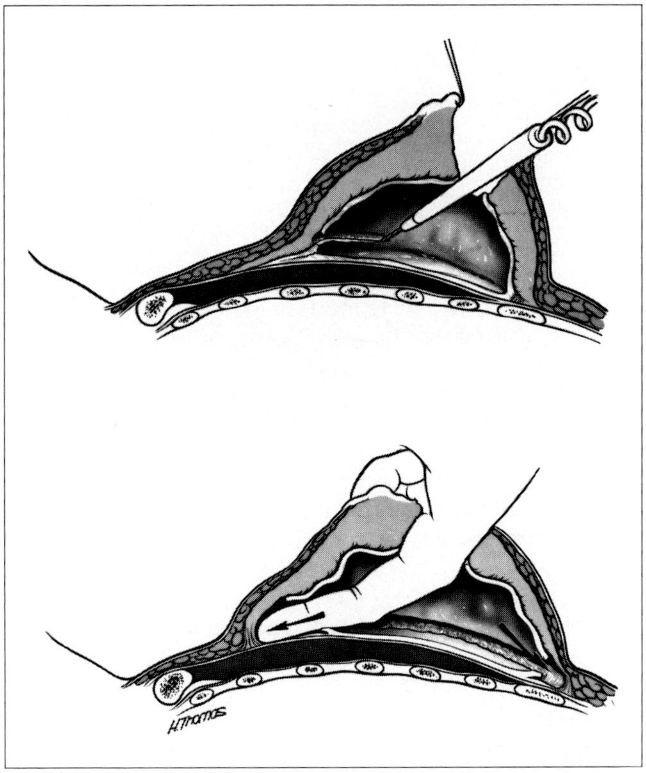

Figure 23-10. During an open capsulotomy, it is important either to separate the capsule into two components or to divide it circumferentially; an adequate capsulotomy usually will have been achieved by this technique.

Axillary Approach

Rex Peterson

In 1968 Dempsey and Latham [41] reported the retropectoral placement of mammary prostheses for breast augmentation. The transaxillary incision and approach to prepectoral mammary augmentation was described by Eiseman [46] (1974) and by Hoehler [70] (1973). In 1978 Robles et al. [120] described an enlarged retropectoral pocket for overcoming one of the disadvantages then prevalent in retropectoral implantation—the tendency of the implants to remain too superior, producing convex supraareolar breast contours. Robles split the pectoralis major muscle in line with its fibers for access to the retropectoral plane, enlarged the space by blunt dissection in all directions, then cut the origins of the pectoralis major to the fourth, fifth, and sixth ribs and dissected below the sixth rib to provide an adequate inferior retropectoral recipient area.

In following the Robles method, it occurred to this author that the retropectoral plane could quite easily be entered via the axilla, under the prominent edge of the pectoralis major muscle, and that the fourth, fifth, and sixth rib origins of the muscle might instrumentally be disrupted with the use of a urethral sound. The first case (October 15, 1978) approached by the transaxillary subpectoral mammary augmentation (TASPMA) route was incredibly easy. The dissection was facile and rapidly accomplished; there was no bleeding. The encouraging ease of the surgical method and the superior aesthetic breast contours obtained led the author to utilize TASPMA for patients with many types of breast problems that might well be benefited by mammary augmentation.

The following deformities have been corrected: (1) true hypomastia, (2) small, normal breasts requiring enlargement, (3) mild mammary ptosis, (4) breast deformities associated with scoliotic and thoracic deformities, (5) severe fibrous spherical contracture, sometimes with calcification, and (6) persistent encapsulation after several surgeries, or prior infection and prosthetic extrusion and explantation after repeated operations.

After embarking on the TASPMA procedure, the author learned from a conversation with McGraw [91] that he also was augmenting breasts by a similar approach, with considerable enthusiasm for its values. I believe that others came upon the concept at about the same time in 1978. As of this writing, I have gained sufficient continuous experience (160 cases) to understand the pitfalls, frequency of complications, distinct advantages, and good aesthetic results of TASPMA. It is now my method of choice after more than 20 years of augmentation mammaplasty experience.

Whether periareolar, submammary, or axillary, incisions are usually 5 cm in length. The areolar periphery is a very good location for a breast incision, passing, when psychologically necessary, as a biopsy scar. However, the surgical gymnastics required in a periareolar approach to dissect through the breast tissue, cut the pectoralis muscle, dissect a retropectoral plane in all directions, enlarging it surgically below the sixth rib, are hardly justifiable. The axillary incision is a direct, essentially bloodless pathway for retropectoral implantation of a breast prosthesis. If the incision is properly designed, the scar is obscure in almost all positions except that with outstretched and upraised arms, a seldom-held motion. The breast, subject of the aesthetic augmentation, is therefore left unscarred, unless some later secondary surgical procedure is recommended, as may infrequently be necessary.

The incisional placement in a natural skin crease, posterior to the pectoralis major muscle in the hair-bearing area of the thoracic portion of the axillary skin, is the most hidden of all augmentation mammaplasty scars. In twentieth century cultures, the axilla is not specially regarded as a place of erotic beauty and is not usually a focus of visual attention.

The entire operative dissection can often be achieved bloodlessly in a very few minutes. The essential steps of the dissection are as follows:

1. Axillary incision
2. Transaxillary dissection
3. Incision in the posterior edge of the pectoralis major muscle fascia
4. Digital dissection of upper two-thirds of the retropectoral space
5. Completion of the prosthesis recipient area by blunt instrumental dissection

RETROPECTORAL PLACEMENT

The retropectoral implantation is favored because the silicone prosthesis is not located within or in contact with the breast tissues. There is no relationship to or hindrance of breast function, including nursing. Manual, radiographic, or xerographic examinations of the breasts are not affected. Since the implantation does not in any way contact the breast glandular tissue, there can be no question of any relationship to any medical condition of the breast, including fibrocystic disease or cancer.

The natural submuscular plane makes for mobility of the implant and of the breast tissue, per se. Neither is bound to the other, so the breast flows over the chest wall in a normal fashion, making for more natural contours in all postures, but particularly recumbency. The TASPMA is capable of producing the most aesthetically pleasing natural breast contours of any currently used method of augmentation mammaplasty, with beautiful retroussé supraareolar contours and full convex roundness below the nipples. The breasts can assume natural lateral sessile positions when a patient is supine. This situation is preferable to the restricted mobility of the conical upright mounds of retroglandular breast implants. Also, in the author's experience, the incidence of firm or hard fibrous capsular contracture is less when the prosthesis is placed retropectorally.

SURGICAL PROCEDURE

TASPMA, in the author's practice, is an outpatient procedure, always done with intravenous sedation, intercostal blocks, and local infiltration anesthesia. A plastic cannula is inserted in a large antecubital vein for the administration of appropriate medications. Having a long and successful experience with a combination of pentobarbital (Nembutal), meperidine (Demerol), and diazepam (Valium), I use these medications exclusively unless the patient has a history of an allergic reaction to their previous use.

First, 100 mg of pentobarbital is given intravenously; 3 minutes later, 50 mg of meperidine; and 3 minutes later, another 50 mg of meperidine. The 3-minute time intervals between medications permit safety to observe the vital signs of the patient. The blood pressure and pulse rate are continuously monitored. At this time, the second to sixth intercostal nerves are blocked bilaterally with 1 to 2 ml of 1% lidocaine with 1 : 100,000 ephinephrine at each rib in the midaxillary line.

While the nurse prepares the patient's skin in the operative area, the surgeon scrubs. After sterile draping, 5 mg of diazepam is administered intravenously, and a precise local infiltration of almost 50 ml of 0.5% lidocaine with 1 : 200,000 epinephrine is placed in each breast and axilla. This requires infiltration *exactly* on the fourth, fifth, and sixth ribs (under the muscles) medially, anteriorly, and laterally. The external surfaces of the second and third ribs are injected medially adjacent to the sternum. The axillae, the zones between the latissimus dorsi muscle and the pectoralis major muscle, and the axillary portion of the pectoralis major muscle within are injected thoroughly (not subcutaneously, but deep within the musculature). This local anesthesia method suffices for any surgery of the breast. Additional 5-mg increments of intravenous diazepam are administered at safe intervals, as necessary for adequate sedation.

With the patient recumbent and the arms at right angles to the torso, the important anatomic reference points for the retropectoral prosthesis recipient area are marked (Fig. 23-11). The second, third, and fourth ribs and intercostal spaces are marked at the sternal borders. The inferior margin of the sixth rib is defined anteriorly and laterally. Anteriorly, this is usually 2.5 cm below the breast sulcus (fifth rib) or the brassiere imprint on the skin. To achieve normal breast contours at the proper level, the retropectoral prosthesis space must always extend below the sixth rib, and both dissections should be the same so that the breast sulci will be symmetric. Laterally the marking follows the edge of the breast tissue in the recumbent position, which is usually at the midaxillary vertical line.

A 5-cm incision is placed in an oblique direction on the thoracic aspect of the axilla, posterior to the pectoralis muscle margin and high enough in the axillary hair-bearing skin to be invisible in most postural positions. Preoperatively the incisional location may be marked with the patient standing, to be sure that the scars will be at the same level and hidden from view. The scars usually bear

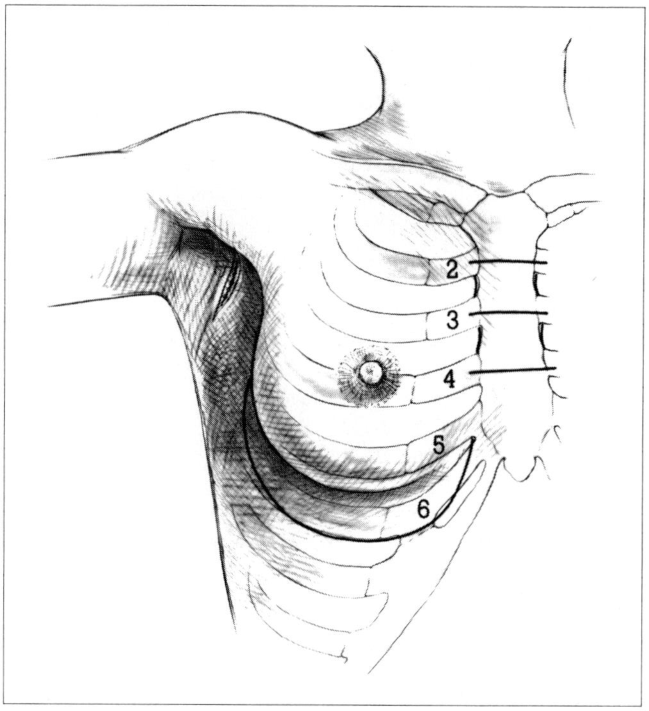

Figure 23-11. The prominent junction of the second ribs with the sternum provides an anatomic key to marking the third and fourth ribs at the sternum. The breast sulcus is at the fifth rib, so the sixth rib is about 2.5 cm inferior to the sulcus. The recipient area for the retropectoral mammary prosthesis extends superiorly to the subclavicular area, medially to the sternal margin, inferiorly to the intercostal space between the sixth and seventh ribs, and laterally to the midaxillary line over the fifth and sixth ribs. A smaller space will cause the breast to be convex in the superior half because the implanted prosthesis will reside too far superiorly. The axillary scar will be inconspicuous if the 5-cm transaxillary incision is placed in the hair-bearing axilla, posterior to the lateral margin of the pectoralis major muscle.

only slight pigmentation and only rarely are obtrusive. The breast itself is not defiled by scar.

With the skin edges retracted, the incision is deepened through the axillary fascia to identify the deep margin of the pectoralis major muscle. The lateral thoracic vein is always encountered, one or two branches being in the operative field. One of these parallels the margin of the pectoralis, and at the caudal end of the axilla one venous branch courses perpendicular to the pectoralis, sending branches into, under, and superficial to the muscle. The lateral thoracic vein and artery can almost always be safely retracted, but if injured they must be promptly controlled as the cut ends retract either into the axilla or under the muscle. The only bleeding the author has ever encountered in more than 160 patients having TASPMA has occurred in the adipose tissue of the caudal axilla.

The costobrachial nerve arises between the second and third ribs in the axilla and courses through the axilla to the medial aspect of the arm. This nerve is rarely seen, but the

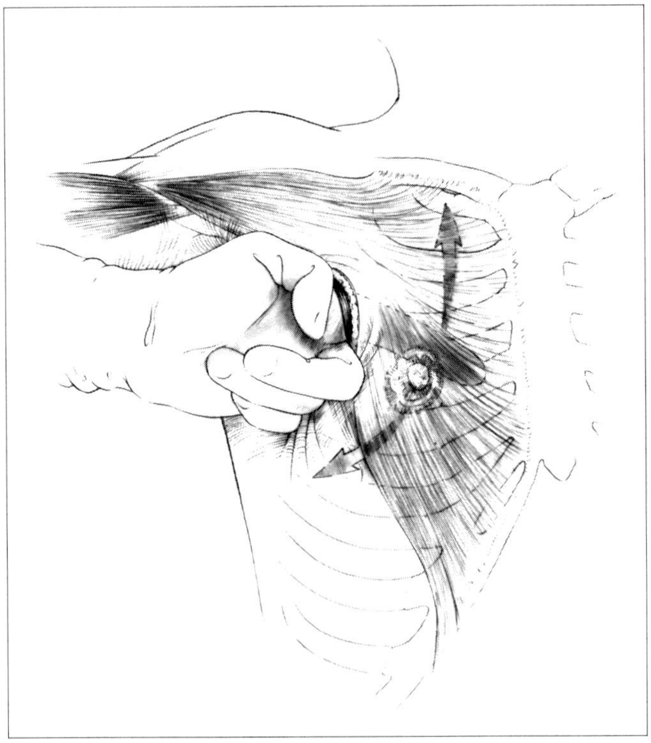

Figure 23-12. The entrance to the retropectoral plane (between the pectoralis major and minor muscles) is achieved by incising the pectoralis major fascia along the deep margin of the muscle, within the axillary incision. The branches of the lateral thoracic vessels, which course in varying positions both parallel to and perpendicular to the pectoralis major lateral margin, should be located and safeguarded as the muscle is approached by blunt scissors dissection. The subpectoral plane should be dissected digitally as far as possible superiorly, medially, inferiorly, and laterally. No fine linear strands should be disrupted, as these are either blood vessels or nerves.

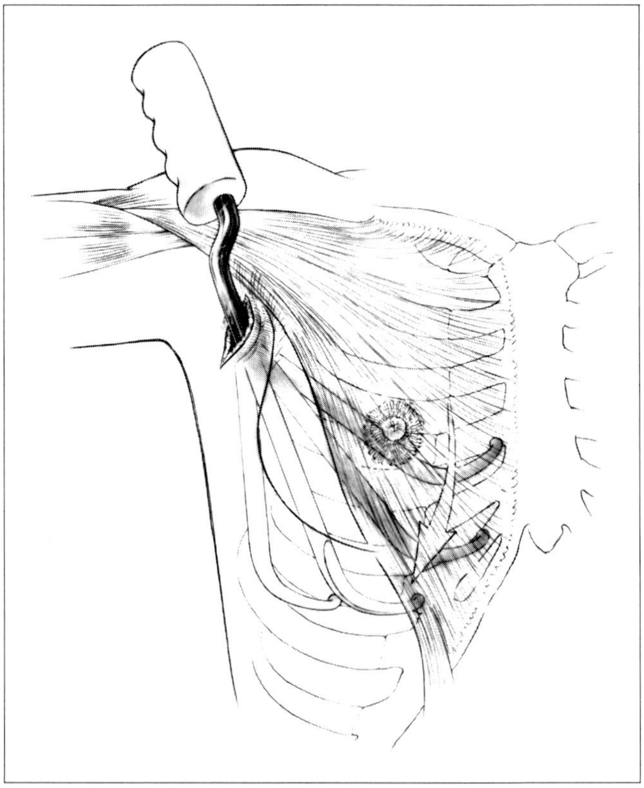

Figure 23-13. The Agris-Dingman Axillary Breast Dissector is the ideal instrument to complete the dissection because its bayonet handle, molded manual grip, and curved "working end" (modified from the design of a urethral sound) provide the leveraged force to displace the origins of the pectoralis major muscle from the fourth, fifth, and sixth costal cartilages and ribs. One uses a series of stretching, pushing, sweeping motions from the junction of the fourth costal cartilage with the sternum inferiorly and laterally to below the sixth rib margin. At times, considerable force is required; at others, the maneuvers may be quite easy.

surgeon must be aware of its location and avoid injury or there will be a resultant sensory disturbance in its distribution. The fascia over the deep axillary margin of the pectoralis major muscle is incised by scissors or scalpel, or sometimes merely penetrated by the surgeon's index finger (Fig. 23-12). The retropectoral plane must be developed between the pectoralis major and minor to ensure a rapid, bloodless digital dissection. If the pectoralis minor muscle is inadvertently raised, the plane will be ragged and the dissection difficult.

Once the proper retropectoral plane is entered, the pectoralis major is dissected with incredible facility as far superiorly, medially, and laterally as the index finger can reach: well up toward the clavicle, to the sternal border of the second, third, and fourth ribs, and laterally along the fourth rib over the anterior thorax. The dissection is free of bleeding.

For the TASPMA, the ideal instrumental dissector is the Agris-Dingman Axillary Breast Dissector.* It has sufficient length, a bayonet offset in the shaft, an enlarged or molded handle, and a terminal curve on the dissector shaft modified from a urethral sound. The design provides adequate leverage to avulse or disrupt the origins of the pectoralis major from the fourth, fifth, and sixth costal cartilages. The dissector is inserted with the end of the curved shaft toward the sternum and the bayonet-angled handle above the axilla. The instrumental dissection begins medially at the junction of the third rib and the sternum with a caudal push paralleling the sternum, to avulse the pectoralis major's musculotendinous attachment from the fourth costal cartilage (Fig. 23-13). First stretching the muscle away from the thorax, then pushing caudally, then sweeping laterally causes the origin to give way. The same maneuver is repeated over the fifth and sixth costal margins—anteriorly, then laterally (Fig. 23-14). The strength of both hands is often required. Sometimes these maneuvers are quite easy, sometimes quite strenuous. The instrument is swept medially to laterally to ensure a uniformly curved periphery to the retropectoral recipient area. As the dissector is withdrawn, a small amount of blood may flow briefly from the incision.

* Now manufactured and sold by Padgett Instruments, Kansas City, Mo.

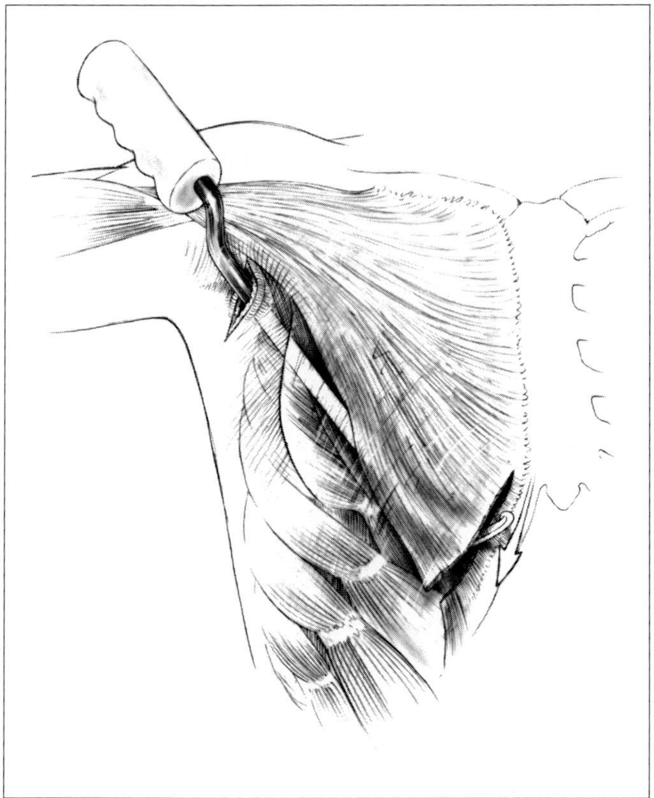

Figure 23-14. Disruption of the fourth, fifth, and sixth rib origins of the pectoralis major. Inferiorly and laterally the fasciae superficial to the muscle remain in continuity, thus preventing "escape" of the prosthesis from under the muscle and the visible deformities sometimes observed when the pectoralis is activated.

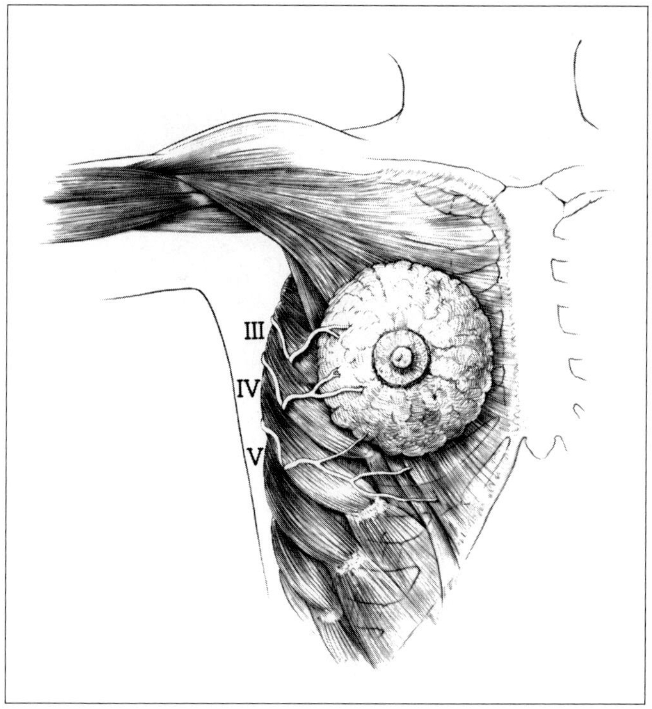

Figure 23-15. On two occasions (in more than 160 patients with TASPMA), unilateral periareolar anesthesia has occurred from disruption or stretching of the fourth intercostal-cutaneous nerve. The zones of anesthesia were approximately 5 cm in diameter and involved the nipples and most of the areolae. There was a gradual diminution of the anesthetic zone over an interval of 1 year, but sensory perception did not become completely normal. To avoid this problem, the final dissection inferolaterally is completed digitally, with careful preservation of any palpable linear structures.

The surgeon again inserts the index finger into the retropectoral plane to check the size and smoothness of the recipient space. There should be no muscle bundles attached to the ribs. If present, they are digitally disrupted, but fine linear tissue strands laterally *are not* disrupted as these may be the lateral cutaneous branches of the intercostal nerves and vessels. Their avulsion may lead to operative bleeding and later sensory deficits in the areolar skin (Fig. 23-15). For this reason, the final tailoring laterally is simply accomplished by digital stretching of the tissues.

A large Robinson catheter, with side fenestrations, is inserted into the most inferior area of the retropectoral space for saline irrigation. This is continued until the irrigant flowing from the wound is clear, a matter of a minute or so. An appropriate mammary prosthesis is inserted as the pectoralis is retracted with a right-angled retractor such as a 5-cm-wide Sims Vaginal Retractor. When breast prostheses are placed retropectorally, the volume of the implant should be 50 to 60 cc larger than retroglandular placement to attain the same degree of breast projection (Fig. 23-16).

High-profile implants offer no aesthetic advantage in TASPMA. Logically, they would tend to be more susceptible to spherical fibrous capsular contracture as they are more spherical in design than the desired lower-profile prostheses. Experience has shown that beautiful aesthetic breast contours result from the use of retropectorally implanted low-profile silicone gel–filled prostheses* (Figs. 23-17 to 23-21).

Posture, body weight, stature, breast volume, nipple position, elasticity of the tissues, and asymmetry of the thorax or breast volume are factors that determine selection of implant size. In most patients, the 250- to 275-cc implant provides an ideal aesthetic breast contour, when placed retropectorally. Less frequently the 225 cc is used and only infrequently is a 300 cc necessary.

The axillary wound is repaired in layers with two or three 3-0 Dexon sutures to the pectoralis major margins and the subadjacent fascia, a few sutures to the axillary fascia, and a few to the subdermal fascia. The final layer is a 4-0 monofilament nylon continuous dermal pullout suture. The wound edges are supported externally by 1-in. longitudinally placed Steri-Strips, and a small gauze dressing is applied over these.

The same procedures are then accomplished on the other breast. During the procedure, 1 gm of cephalosporin is administered intravenously; postoperatively, it is

* The author prefers Heyer-Schulte round low-profile silicone gel prostheses because of the durable shells 0.1 to 0.25 mm in thickness.

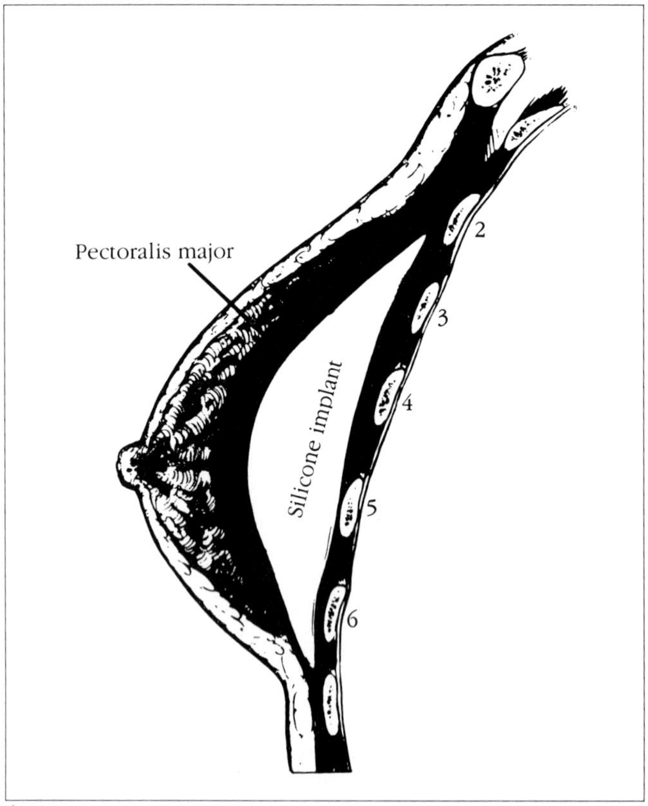

A

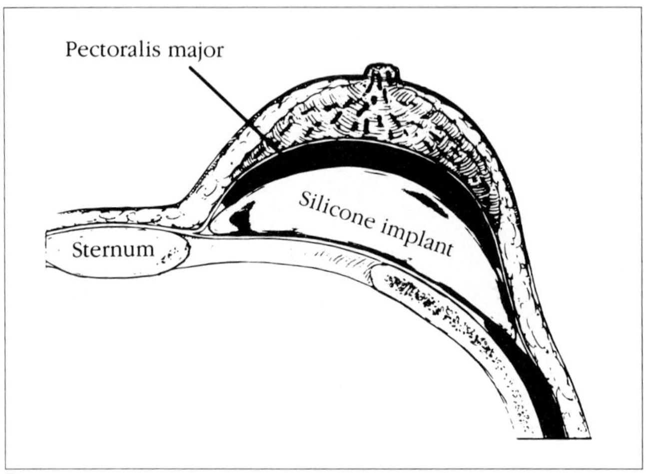

B

Figure 23-16. The prosthesis extends inferiorly to the interspace between the sixth and seventh ribs. Note the schematic interpretation of the pectoralis fasciae remaining intact inferiorly, medially, and laterally. If the recipient space is not large enough, the prosthesis will be less mobile and more susceptible to periprosthetic capsular contracture. Invariably, if capsular contracture does occur, the prosthesis moves above the breast sulcus superiorly, the superior half of the breast will be convex, or rounded, and the sulcus will be at a more superior level than the unaffected breast.

taken orally for 7 days. The patient is then elevated to a sitting position and the breast symmetry surveyed, particularly as pertains to the submammary folds and the desired concavity of the supraareolar contours. If all contours are perfect, the only dressing applied is a front-fastening underwire stretch-fabric brassiere, one size in the cup and 2 in. larger in the band than previously worn. If she wore a 32A preoperatively, the new brassiere should be a 34B. If she wore a 34B, the new bra will be a 36C.

The underwire has the function of applying pressure to the exact level of the new inframammary fold, assisting in equalizing any *minor* asymmetry of the prosthesis pockets by causing adherence of the tissues at the desired areas. This is very significant in the aftercare. Formation of the inframammary sulcus is important, but equally important is the early manipulation and upward, inward, and lateral mobilization of the breast prostheses. The recipient area is a natural sliding plane, and the postoperative cicatricial closure of the space should be limited *only* by the formation of the inferior periphery at the proper level. The author recommends that the patient move each implant at least 25 times twice a day for 6 months, at which time the frequency of capsular contracture declines markedly.

Postoperatively, there is no restriction whatsoever of any motion of the arms or any activity. The anatomy and repair of the axillary retropectoral portal is such that direct pressure on the breast cannot produce an explantation via the transaxillary incision. Furthermore, pectoral muscle motion contributes to the mobility of the periprosthetic collagenous tissues as they form and therefore serves to reduce the incidence of fibrous contracture. Thus, early arm motion is not only encouraged but required of TASPMA patients.

The TASPMA has an intrinsic advantage over other retropectoral mammary augmentation approaches in that the contiguous fasciae remain in continuity with the pectoralis major muscle and also maintain their attachments to the subdermis. Such continuity of tissues allows natural breast contours, and the pectoralis is restrained from retraction by this fascial integrity.

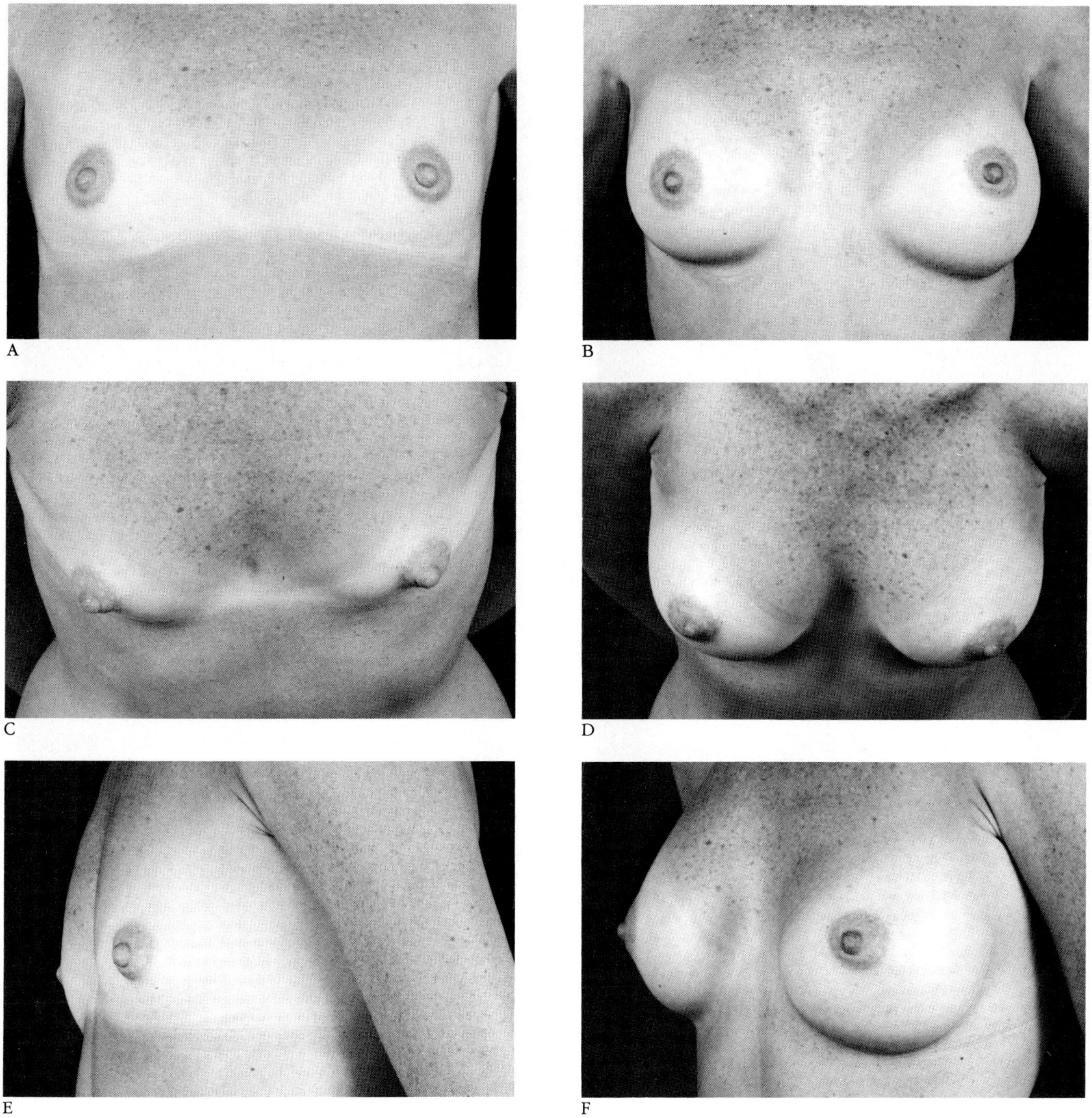

Figure 23-17. A 29-year-old married female. Hypomastia. TASPMA with 250-cc Dow Corning low-profile round silicone gel mammary prostheses; 14-month follow-up. Note sulcus of right breast slightly higher, but not unacceptably so. The slightly higher right prosthesis is also revealed by the slight convexity of the contour superiorly.

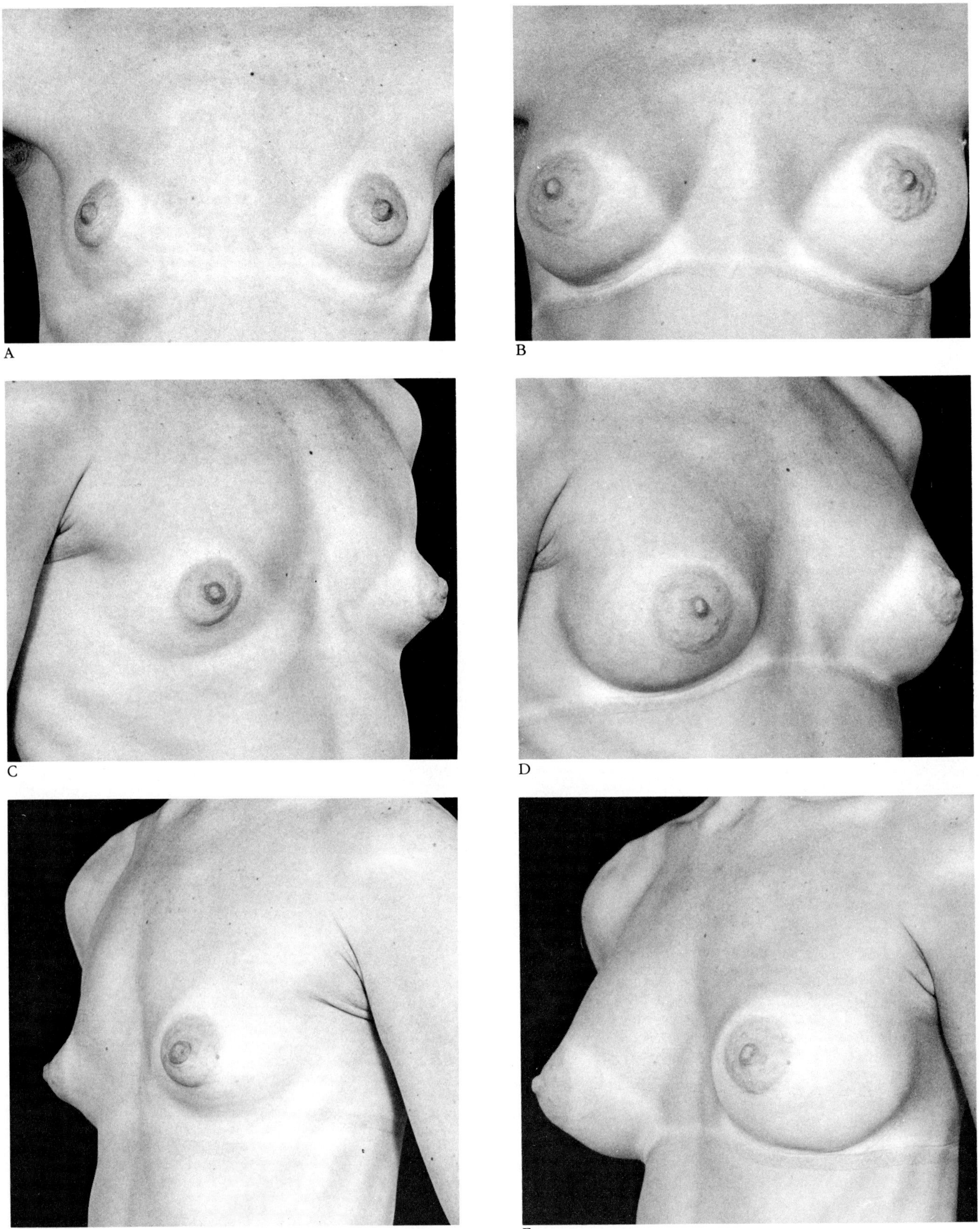

A B C D E F

Figure 23-18. Asymmetry of the breasts is often accompanied by scoliosis and rotation of the hemithorax posteriorly on the side having a small breast. The surgeon must check the patient in the erect position before finishing the surgery as it is more important to achieve symmetry for upright posture than for supine.

A 32-year-old married female. Scoliosis. The right hemithorax is rotated posteriorly so that the right breast appears smaller. TASPMA with 260-cc McGhan low-profile round silicone gel prosthesis on the right and 200 cc on the left. In the 6-month postoperative photographs (B, D, F), the right breast still appears smaller in the anterior view, but symmetric with the left in the oblique and lateral views. Ideally the author would prefer both breast implants to be smaller by 25 to 40 cc.

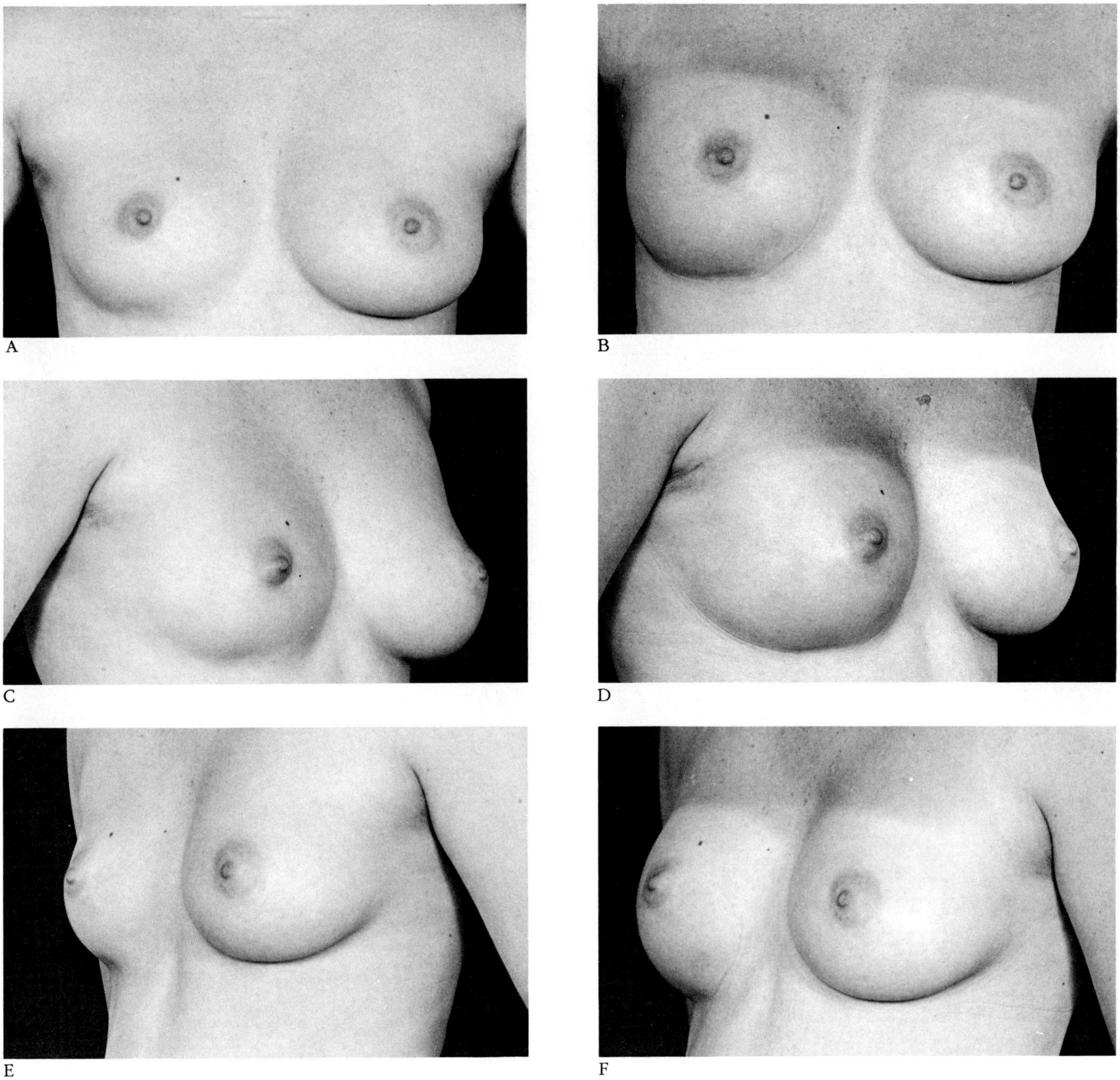

Figure 23-19. A 23-year-old married female. Mammary asymmetry with relative right hypomastia. Right TASPMA with 225-cc Heyer-Schulte low-profile round silicone gel prosthesis. A 250-cc prosthesis was implanted first but appeared too wide at surgery.

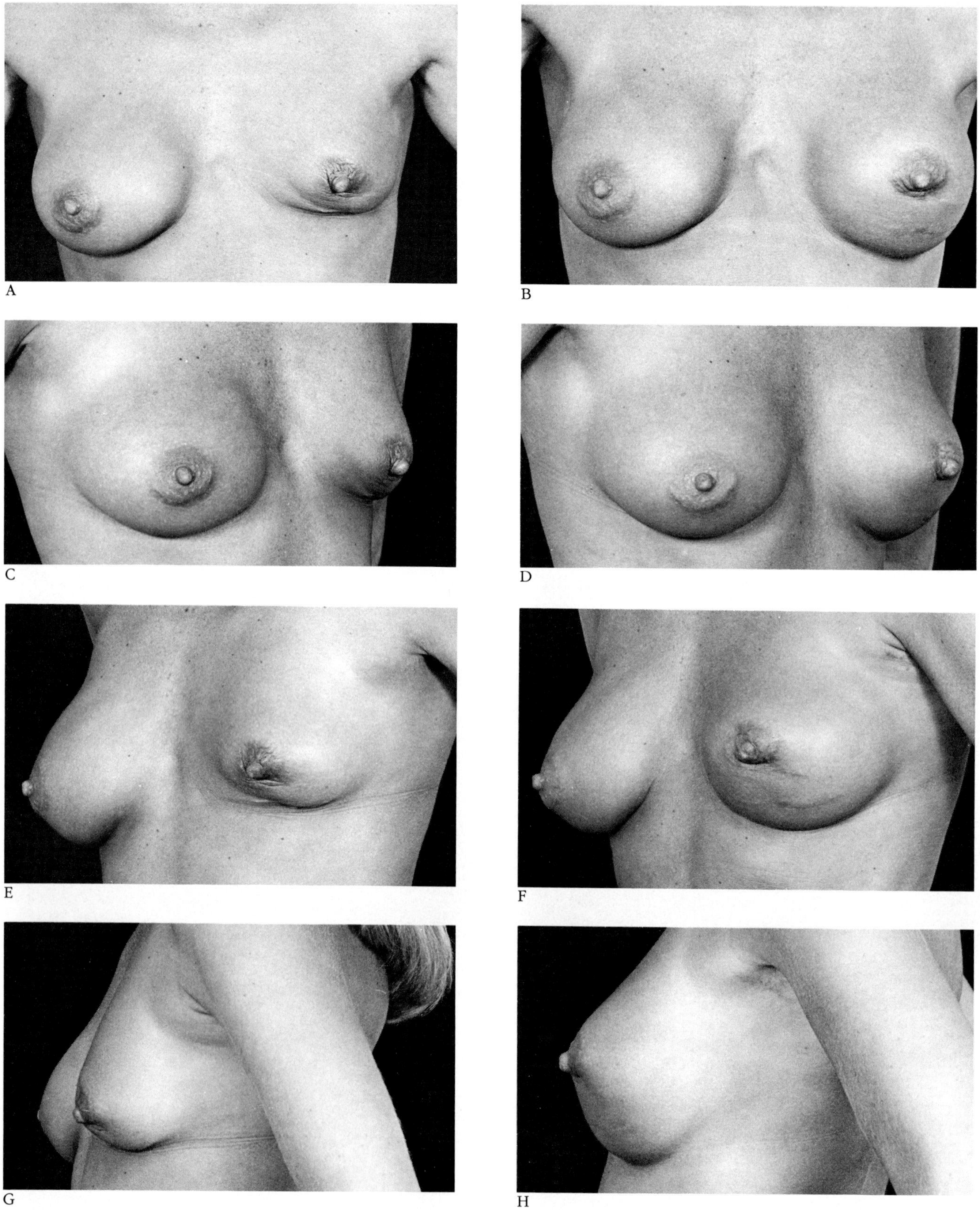

Figure 23-20. A 31-year-old married female with five previous augmentation mammaplasty procedures on the left breast, including extrusion of prosthesis through the skin following surgery via periareolar incisions. TASPMA, left breast, with 195-cc Heyer-Schulte low-profile round saline-inflatable prosthesis, did not disturb the location of the previous scars or revise the scars in any way. For 2 months postoperatively the prosthesis was rather firm, with a tendency to periprosthetic fibrous contracture. Self-administered manual movements of the retropectoral prosthesis, arm exercises, and vigorous swimming resulted in softening of the capsular scar. Photographs B, D, F, H were taken 13 months after surgery. No further problems had arisen 4 years postoperatively. TASPMA is an excellent corrective surgery for patients with recalcitrant capsular scar contracture about prepectoral prostheses.

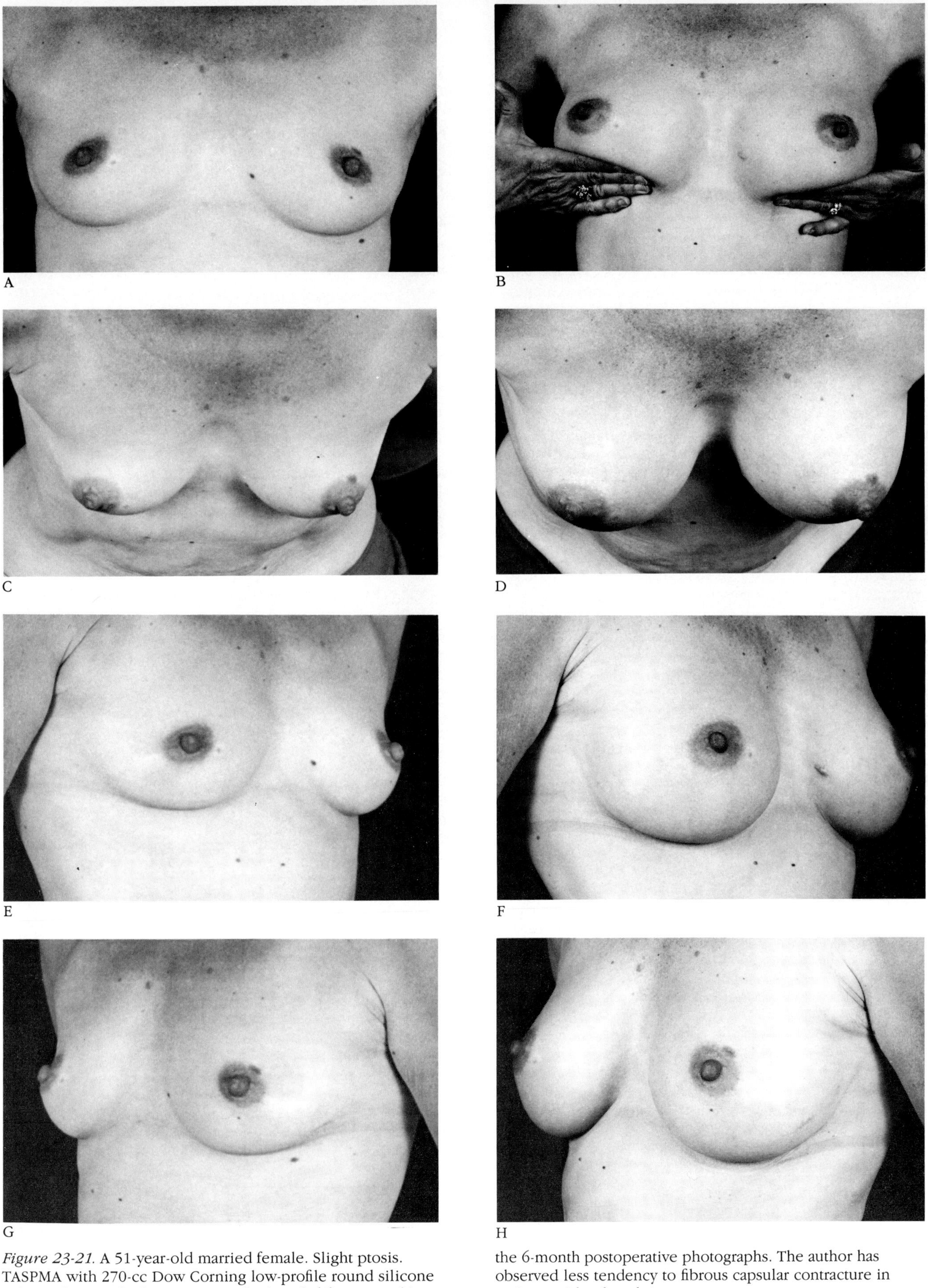

Figure 23-21. A 51-year-old married female. Slight ptosis. TASPMA with 270-cc Dow Corning low-profile round silicone gel prostheses. The breasts are perfectly soft (F), as noted in the 6-month postoperative photographs. The author has observed less tendency to fibrous capsular contracture in patients with relaxed tissues.

POSTOPERATIVE PROBLEMS

There are three complications common to all surgery: bleeding, infection, and scar. They may occur in TASPMA.

The scar process around the prostheses is natural to implantation but, if severe enough, may cause distortion of the breast contours, with the implant firmly fixed at a more superior level than is desirable. Approximately 10 percent of TASPMA patients develop a firm fibrous scar capsule about the implant. Of those who develop "capsules" of scar about the breast prosthesis, approximately one-half or 5 percent of the total patients operated on require a second corrective operation. Sometimes, in the corrective surgery, an incision is made under the breast (in the fold) to enlarge breast implant space by cutting the scar to release it. This is a disadvantage of the procedure.

Bleeding or postoperative hematoma requiring reoperation occurs in less than 1 percent of patients.

Infection requiring reoperation occurs in less than 1 percent of patients.

Disturbances of sensation of the nipple are also rare. In 2 of more than 160 patients, there was a unilateral loss of sensation of an areola, which gradually improved over a year's interval.

Asymmetry of the level of the breast sulci may result from a scar "capsule" formation about the implant, or it may occur to a lesser degree without "capsular scar." When the retropectoral dissection has been asymmetric, early treatment involves prolonged use of an underwire brassiere. If asymmetry persists, a second operation might be necessary to equalize the levels.

COMPLICATIONS

Postoperative complications of augmentation mammaplasty, regardless of the technique used, are both general (hematoma, infection, scar) and specific (sensory alteration, capsular formation). They present either early or late (Table 23-4). Any attempt to assign an absolute incidence for each complication is limited by variables inherent in each report, including patient selection, operative technique, surgical experience, and methods of assessment [40, 79, 120, 128]. However, the vast majority of postoperative problems, with the exception of capsular contracture, can be minimized by meticulous surgical technique [145].

Table 23-4. Complications of augmentations (1282 augmentations)

Capsular contracture	27%
Alteration in nipple sensation	15%
Leakage of inflatable prosthesis	6%
Hematoma formation	2%
Wound separation	1.5%
Ptosis of prosthesis	1%
Mondor's disease	1%
Infection	0
Implant erosion	0

Source: J. L. Baker, Jr., Augmentation Mammoplasty. In J. Q. Owsley, Jr., and R. A. Peterson (eds.), *Symposium on Aesthetic Surgery of the Breast.* St. Louis: Mosby, 1978.

Early Complications

BLEEDING

Intraoperative bleeding is best controlled by direct visualization under fiberoptic illumination, temporary packing with sponges, and repeated cauterization. If persistent oozing is encountered, a closed-system drain is inserted and brought out through a separate stab wound laterally.

HEMATOMA

The majority of hematomas occur within the first 24 hours following operation and are manifested by pain, swelling, and skin discoloration. Immediate evacuation of the hematoma is mandatory. The prosthesis is removed, the bleeding site cauterized, the pocket irrigated with an antibiotic solution, the prosthesis reinserted, and a pressure dressing applied. Any reluctance to reoperate should be dismissed because small hematomas often become larger or infected, necessitating removal of the prosthesis rather than the hematoma (Fig. 23-22). Bleeding can be minimized preoperatively by obtaining a detailed history to identify patients with bleeding dyscrasias and potentiating medication, and intraoperatively by utilizing fiberoptic retractors and long cautery forceps.

Figure 23-22. Patient seen for second opinion at 3 months following breast augmentation with the following history. After removal of dressing on the fifth postoperative day, a hematoma was evident on the right side and was treated "conservatively." Subsequently, the implant was removed at 3 weeks. Plan is to wait another 3 months before reinserting the prosthesis. Moral: Hematomas should be treated definitively and immediately in the operating room. A temporizing course often leads to infection and an unhappy, litigious patient.

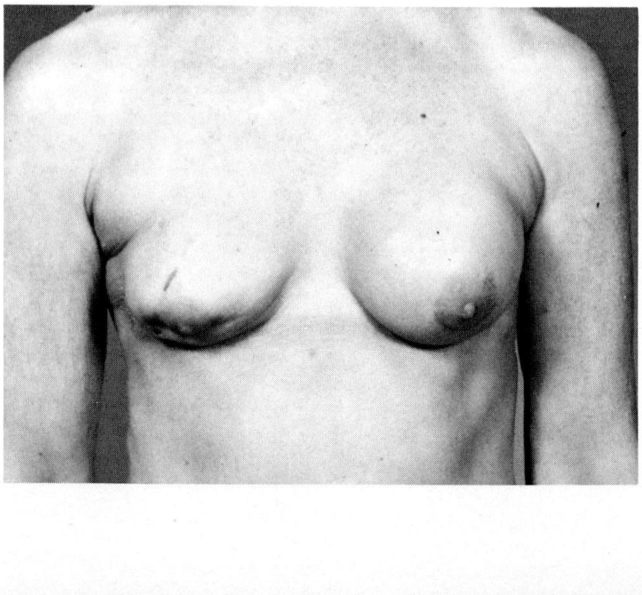

INFECTION

A review by Courtiss et al. [37] indicates that infection occurs in approximately 2 percent of augmentations, within 10 days (range 6–42 days) of surgery. The presenting symptoms vary from mild to severe inflammation, the predominant organism being *Staphylococcus aureus*. Since the basic problem is infection in tissue adjacent to the implant, it may be localized to the incisional area, allowing drainage with retention of the prosthesis, or generalized, requiring removal of the prosthesis. The initial course of action is limited to opening of the incision, culture of purulent material, and initiation of oral antibiotics for 10 days (dicloxacillin). With this regimen, approximately 50 percent of prostheses can be retained although a high incidence of capsular contracture is inevitable. If the infection persists, the prosthesis is removed, to be reinserted 3 to 6 months later [90]. Courtiss et al. [37] reported a 28 percent (2 out of 7) repeat infection rate on reinsertion, which was eventually corrected by changing from an inframammary to an areolar incision. Prophylactic antibiotics were considered *not* to be of value. The only causative factor identified is previous hematoma formation, which occurred in 25 percent or more of infections. Hipps et al. [69] reported a 1 percent (4 out of 453) incidence of infection following augmentation mammaplasty. *Staphylococcus aureus* was found on all cultures. Recently, Toranto and Malow [133] reported three cases of atypical mycobacterial periprosthetic infection. In these cases presentation is different from that with the usual breast infection: (1) later onset (14–56 days), (2) slow development characterized by pain, (3) minimal systemic and local signs of infection, and (4) massive effusion. Successful management requires a high index of suspicion for atypical mycobacteria and a somewhat complicated antibiotic regimen, detailed elsewhere [133]. An interesting observation of uncertain significance is reported by Truppman et al. [135], who identified fungi in and around implants after augmentation mammaplasty. Late infection of the implant is a rare event [66].

PHLEBITIS

Inflammation of the subcutaneous veins overlying the breast was first described by Mondor. It presents as a painful phlebitis of limited duration (5–10 days), which responds to warm compresses and analgesia. In contrast to its more superior location following reduction mammaplasties, it tends to present after augmentation mammaplasty as a tender band in the inframammary crease.

LACTATION

Spontaneous onset of lactation through the incision can occur following augmentation. Although exceedingly rare, it may necessitate removal of the prosthesis. As noted by Goldwyn [58], pregnancy following breast augmentation can result in painful breasts and preclude nursing.

Late Complications

SENSATION

Courtiss and Goldwyn [36] assessed breast sensation before and after surgery. Preoperatively, normal breast sensation has the following parameters: (1) The areola was the most sensitive part of the breast while the nipple was the least sensitive; (2) sensation was not uniform throughout the breast; (3) smaller breasts were more sensitive than large ones; and (4) sensation appeared to decrease after pregnancy. Following augmentation mammaplasty, sensation was almost always decreased, with some return by 2 months. Paresthesias generally ameliorated by 3 months, and sensation was virtually normal by 6 months. At 2 years, 15 percent of patients had decreased sensation in the nipple-areola complex. Of importance, there was no difference in sensation based on type of incision (inframammary versus periareolar), location on the areola (lower, upper, medial, or lateral half), or type of implant (gel-bag or inflatable). Thus, one is obligated to inform the patient that sensation in the nipple-areola complex and surrounding skin will be decreased immediately postoperatively, will probably improve by 2 months, and generally will return to near normal by 6 months. However, sensory loss can be permanent in about 1 percent of cases. Hetter [68] found changes of sensation to be bothersome in 9 percent of patients and a cause of severe dissatisfaction in 2 percent (3 out of 165).

MIGRATION OF PROSTHESIS

With any incision and any subcutaneous dissection to the retromammary space, it is possible for the prosthesis to be displaced if the inferior breast margin is not sutured to the pectoral fascia. Displacement of the prosthesis may occur in a very loose capsule. However, it can be corrected by fixation of the subcutaneous tissue to the pectoral fascia with nonabsorbable sutures. Displacement of the nipple below the prosthesis will occur with aging or if Dacron patches are used, which allow fixation of the prosthesis.

SHAPE

Although the vast majority of shape deformities are due to capsular contracture, a small percentage of patients will be dissatisfied with superior fullness or overall size. These problems are often due to inadequate preoperative discussion. Minor deformities of the areola and nipple may also occur. The patient must be aware that excessively large prostheses will manifest certain deformities; nevertheless, the surgeon must respect the patient's wishes (Fig. 23-23). Broadbent and Woolf [20] have noted that significant asymmetry of breasts and chest is often overlooked preoperatively and is accentuated postoperatively. "It becomes painfully evident with experience that unsatisfactory results are at times unavoidable, but when they occur *unexpectedly,* one must ask if it is the breast or the chest that is at fault. If a thorough examination, including side views, is not done, mild scoliosis and chest wall deformities (pectus excavatum or carinatum, barrel chest) can be missed only to become exaggerated postoperatively" [20].

SCARS

Problems with scars fall into three general categories: (1) placement, (2) size, and (3) pigmentation. Any inframammary incision that is placed above the crease is highly visible and difficult to correct. A breast augmentation can

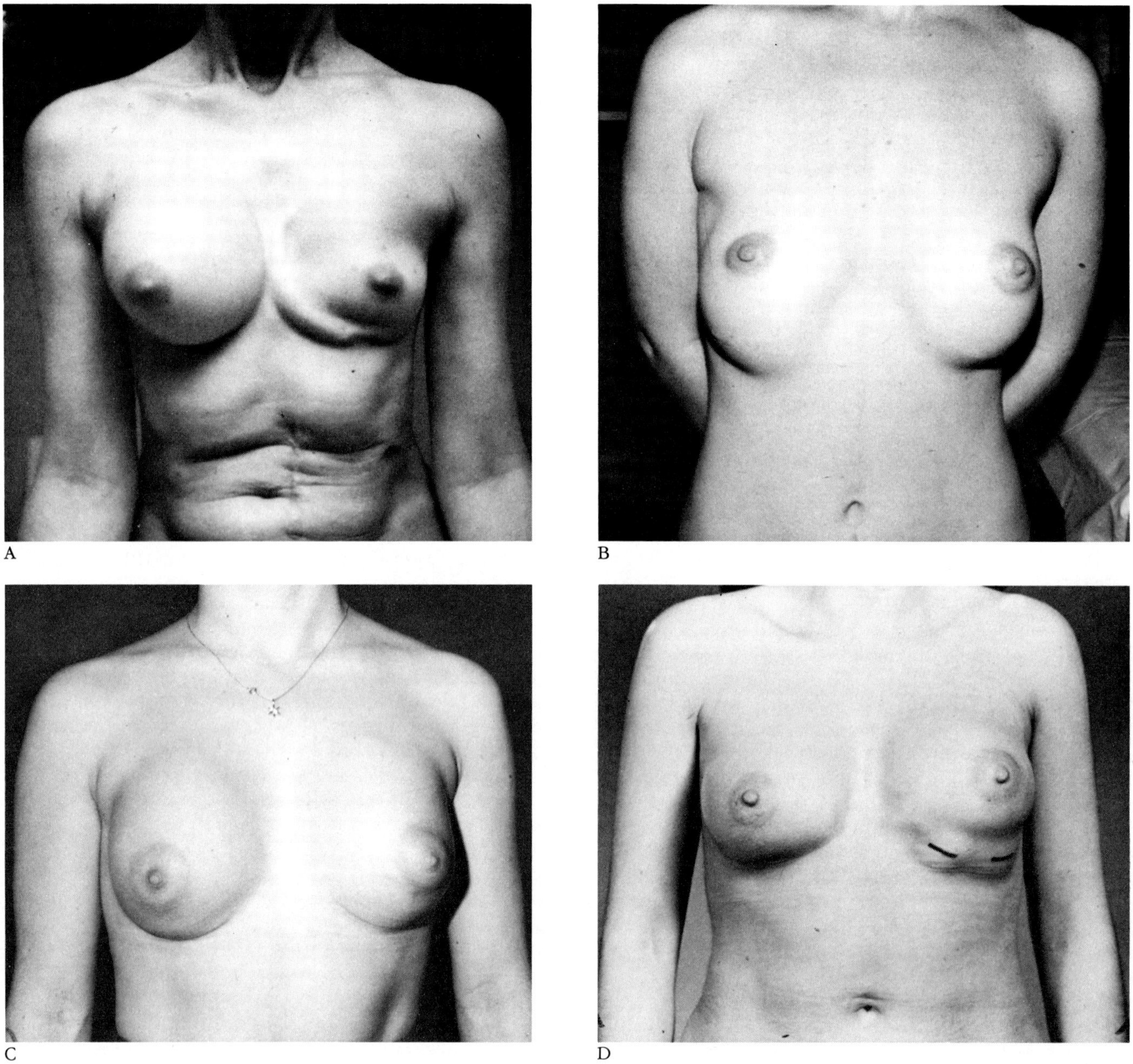

Figure 23-23. Complications.
A. Deflation of an inflatable prosthesis.
B. Migration of the implants.
C. Too big an implant with too high a placement resulting in visualization of the implant's upper border.
D. Marked asymmetry resulting from postoperative, rather than preoperative, detection of a scoliosis.

be performed easily through a 3-cm incision, and one need not resort to the commonly employed 6-cm length. Unfortunately, a small percentage of areolar incisions will undergo depigmentation. In large surveys, 90 percent of patients consider their scars unobtrusive [68].

LEAKAGE

Inflatable prostheses were developed to allow selective filling in cases of asymmetry and to minimize capsule formation. The valve mechanism is their weak point and generally results in a 2 to 8 percent deflation rate. Williams [142] reported a 76 percent (25 out of 34) deflation rate, and Grossman [61] had 7 of 8 deflate. Many surgeons feel that virtually all inflatable prostheses will deflate given sufficient time. This hypothesis is supported by Worton et al. [146], who presented six cases of spontaneous deflation between 6 and 7 years after augmentation. Although the capsular contracture rate may be slightly decreased (10%) for inflatable prostheses as compared to gel prostheses, the significant need for eventual replacement limits their value.

Recent attempts at development of an ultrathin silicone bag have resulted in "bleeding" of silicone onto the surface of the prosthesis, incorporation into the surrounding capsule, and even migration to regional lymph nodes. Baker et al. [12] determined silicone concentrations in capsular tissue and found that silicone was present and appeared to be a high-molecular-weight polymer that had diffused through the implant envelope. As a result, the pendulum is now swinging back to sturdier gel-filled prostheses. Undeniably, silicone can be found outside the implant, but whether it is a mere curiosity or a pathologic concern must await further clarification [15, 123, 136]. Silicone can be ejected beyond the capsule following high-velocity injuries or closed compression with implant rupture [23, 56, 72, 97].

EROSION

Erosion of the overlying skin with exposure of the implant is rare. It may be due to infection, direct trauma from a rigid wire-lined brassiere cup, or instillation of steroids. The previous treatment of capsular contracture by injection of Kenalog (40–60 mg triamcinolone) into surrounding scar tissue resulted in atrophy of the breast tissue and erosion. As noted by Cohen and Carrico [29, 30], placement of steroids either in the dissected pocket or in the implant will result in thinning of breast tissue, implant ptosis, and a blue discoloration that heralds extrusion [48, 80, 81, 103, 104, 107]. These events were dose related, being 60 percent for doses greater than 20 mg of Solu-medrol* and 8 percent for doses less than 20 mg although the latter percentage would probably increase with longer follow-up [25]. One must distinguish between the type of steroid (non-water-soluble triamcinolone acetonide [Kenalog]† or water-soluble methylprednisolone hemisuccinate), concentration (pure versus diluted), location (implant versus pocket), actual delivery (instillation in pocket versus injection into tissue), and timing (primary versus secondary) [139]. Oneal and Argenta [98] reported that 74 percent (17 out of 23) of inflatable prostheses containing 62 mg of Solu-Medrol had to be removed within 4 years of insertion. Also, 13 percent of these high-dose steroid-containing implants were associated with a primary capsular contracture, thus casting doubt on the value of steroids to prevent breast firmness [109]. From current evidence, steroids are not used in breast augmentation except in extenuating circumstances.

CAPSULAR CONTRACTURE

Development of a capsule around a breast prosthesis is the natural end-product of wound healing and consists of normal fibrosis consequent to inflammation induced by a foreign body [28, 55, 71, 85, 96, 138]. From numerous biopsies, Cronin and Greenberg [39] showed that the inner wound layer progresses from a capillary-rich granulation tissue to well-organized collagen fibers. The thickness of the outer layer consists of perpendicular collagen fibers [42, 53]. Treatment of the capsule is necessary only when the capsule contracture results in an excessively firm breast or distortion of the shape [137, 140]. The

* Upjohn Company, Kalamazoo, Mich.

† E. R. Squibb & Sons, Princeton, N.J.

Table 23-5. Baker classification of effects of capsular contracture

Grade I	The augmented breast feels as soft as an unoperated one.
Grade II	The breast is less soft; the implant can be palpated easily but is not visible.
Grade III	The breast is more firm; the implant can be palpated easily, and it (or distortion from it) can be seen.
Grade IV	The breast is hard, tender, painful, and cold; distortion is often marked.

reported incidence of capsule contracture varies from 1 to 80 percent depending on the surgeon's criteria, the mean being 25 percent. Despite attempts to design an accurate tensiometer, the authors use a graded clinical classification comparable to the following: grade I, breast remains as soft as preoperatively; grade II, implants palpable but like soft cysts; grade III, contour of implant is visible and firm like nasal cartilage; grade IV, rock hard with marked distortion. Baker [9] found the following distribution in 1282 augmentations: grade I (73%), grade II (10%), grade III (12%), grade IV (5%) (Table 23-5). The onset of contracture is usually within the first 6 months (62%) and in the vast majority of cases takes place by the end of 1 year (92%). Bilateral and unilateral contractures occur with approximately equal frequency.

Initial treatment of established capsular contracture is by a nonsurgical "squeeze" capsulotomy [10]. With the patient supine, the surgeon interlocks the fingers and compresses the breast between the palms—the "nutcracker" procedure [63]. Forces of up to 650 mm Hg can be generated with this technique [63]. As compared to the "finger-squeeze" or "fist-squeeze" techniques, the nutcracker procedure has the lowest level of injury to the surgeon. One should make every effort to know the brand, type, and composition of the implant, as a closed compression is not without morbidity (Table 23-6). Once a tear in the capsule is evident, audibly or palpably, the procedure is repeated but with the hands shifted 90 degrees. If the capsule is resistant or tears partially, resulting in a distorted configuration, an open capsulotomy is recommended. Baker [9] has reported a 30 percent recurrence rate following the squeeze technique, which is repeated as frequently as necessary. An in-depth review of the problem by Nelson [94, 95] disclosed several important findings: (1) Displacement of the implant occurred in 6 percent of closed compressions, (2) hematoma in 1 percent, and (3) ruptured implant in 1 percent and gel migration in 1 percent [1]. Therefore, the patient should be informed that closed compression is often a beneficial but not a benign procedure [82, 86]. Of equal concern was the discovery of ruptured implants in 16 percent of cases handled by open capsulotomy, of which 57 percent had a history of closed compression. After five closed compressions, an open capsulotomy is done. A surgical capsulotomy is done through the periareolar or inframammary incision. The following factors have been altered to minimize capsule thickening and contracture.

Table 23-6. Closed versus open capsulotomy

Complication	Percent occurrence in closed compression (30,000 cases)	Percent occurrence in open capsulotomy (5579 cases)
Hematoma	1.00	2.58
Ruptured implant	0.93	0 (found in 15.9 of breasts)
Silicone gel migration into soft tissue after implant rupture	1.14	0 (found in 4 of breasts)
Incomplete rupture of capsule with displacement of implant	4.06	0
Complete rupture of capsule with displacement of implant	2.49	2.28
Infection	0.02	0.79
Exposure of implant	0.08	0.59
Other	0.25	0
Total	9.97%	6.24%

Source: G. D. Nelson, Complications of closed compression after augmentation mammaplasty. *Plast. Reconstr. Surg.* 66 : 71, 1980.

Prosthesis Composition

In the 1960s, introduction of soft-gel prostheses resulted in a dramatic decrease of contractures, from 61 percent to 27 percent [43]. Elimination of Dacron patches minimized the occurrence of secondary ptosis and reduced the incidence of contractures. The use of saline-filled prostheses was reported by their advocates to reduce the incidence of capsules. However, their inflatable valve proved to be a weak point, and now double-lumen prostheses are offered [121, 122]. Instillation of drugs (steroids, antibiotics) within inflatable prostheses created problems far beyond any benefit, i.e., erosion or drug reaction. The report of Ellenberg and Braun [49] on instilling Solu-Medrol, 20 mg, within a double-lumen implant is worth consideration. Recent introduction of polyurethane-covered gel-filled mammary prostheses represents yet another search for the ideal prosthesis [24].

Surgical Techniques

Since hematoma formation and adherent foreign bodies (starch granules, paper drape fibers) are accepted etiologic factors, their presence must be prevented. Patients are instructed not to take aspirin and related drugs for several weeks prior to surgery. Retropectoral placement of the prosthesis is reported to have a significantly lower rate (5%) of capsule formation. Also, the current trend is to develop a larger pocket extending upward to the second rib and laterally to the anterior or midaxillary line [120]. Meticulous surgical technique and fanatical hemostasis are considered essential to avoid minute subclinical hematomas, which are considered by some surgeons to be the cause of capsular contracture [141]. The average prosthesis in most series is 220 cc; excessively large prostheses are discouraged.

Perioperative Management

Antibiotics are used routinely by most surgeons to avoid major infections and also contamination by *Staphylococcus epidermidis,* which may contribute to capsular formation [13]. The current trend is away from heavy circular dressings to light bras or simple skin tape. Long periods of immobilization are no longer recommended. Massaging of the breast is begun as early as the second postoperative day. In the final analysis, capsule formation is a normal event, but its progression to rigidity and contracture can hopefully be minimized by the modifications listed above.

RESULTS

Short-Term Results

Virtually no other aesthetic procedure provides the immediate patient satisfaction and delight that a breast augmentation does. As noted by Baker [9] and Hetter [68], patient happiness is largely influenced by continuation of a soft natural feel. If capsular contracture occurs, dissatisfaction inevitably follows, with complaints about scarring, changes in sensation, etc. Hetter [68] found that *all* patients who were dissatisfied with the procedure had capsular contracture. Answers to three questions revealed the following:

1. Did the operation meet your expectations? 96% yes
2. Were you satisfied with the results? 88% yes
3. Would you have the operation again? 96% yes

Obviously, the response to any self-administered questionnaire is relatively unscientific. In 1978 Hipps et al. [69] provided a detailed 1-year follow-up of 453 patients who had had retroglandular augmentation mammaplasty. The incidence of grades III and IV contractures was 23 percent (107 out of 453), and the need for open capsulotomy was cut in half by the use of closed-compression capsulotomy. Thus, the early result is dependent on the appearance of capsular contracture. Frequent patient visits must therefore continue through the first year, with closed compression done at the first suggestion of breast firmness.

Long-Term Results

Most of the reported long-term studies present data on the original Ivalon sponges or the thick-wall Dacron-patch breast prostheses of the early 1960s. All were inserted by the retroglandular approach, and physical activities were limited for 6 weeks. Pickering et al. [107] observed that (1) 81 percent (35 of 43) had unacceptable firmness, (2) 14 percent had subjective decrease in sensation, and (3) 58 percent (15 of 43) felt that the breast mass had drooped considerably over the intervening 10 years. Obviously, surgeons do not expect comparable problems with newer prostheses, retropectoral placement, early massage, and frequent closed compression. In a very provocative paper, Biggs et al. [18] reviewed their experience with 1567 augmentations performed over an 18-year period. It is interesting how they divide this time frame: the "primitive period" (1962–1974), the altering period (1974–1976), the developing period (1976–1977), and the modern period (1977 to present). Even at the present time, data at 1-year follow-up revealed that 2 percent of patients had a prosthesis removed because of infection, 5 percent required evacuation of a hematoma in the operating room, and 10 percent had an open capsulotomy. As a surgical technique, augmentation mammaplasty will continue to undergo refinements until a minimal incidence of breast firmness is achieved. Close follow-up over several years is essential following augmentation mammaplasty for both the patient's and the surgeon's benefit [134].

SECONDARY SURGERY

As noted previously, approximately 5 percent of patients will require a second surgical procedure to correct capsular contracture. In addition, patients will seek secondary procedures for deformities that may occur many years following a primary augmentation. The latter group requires careful preoperative evaluation and counseling.

Capsular Contracture

Surgical treatment of capsular contracture requires either a capsulotomy or a capsulectomy; the former is done routinely while the latter is reserved for thick, calcified capsules [16, 110]. If the prostheses are retromammary, they are switched to a retropectoral location with minimal treatment of the capsule unless calcific hardness mandates excision. In a detailed review of 243 cases, Baker et al. [10] performed an open capsulotomy on 18 patients (7%), of whom 37 percent (6 of 18) had a recurrence. Hetter [68] found that persistent soft breasts were achieved in 20 percent of open capsulotomies. It is because of this failure that a change in implant position is so strongly advocated, rather than a simple capsulotomy or capsulectomy [131]. Since 1977 the senior author has corrected several hundred firm breasts by changing the prosthesis from retromammary to retropectoral (Fig. 23-24). Immediate improvement occurs, and the breasts remain soft in more than 80 percent of cases. If the prostheses are retropectoral, with superior displacement, the capsule is open only in its lower circumference. Kenalog (10 mg/cc) may be injected directly into the scar tissue, deep to the subcutaneous tissue, to soften the capsule. Capsulectomy is required in less than 10 percent of cases.

Deformities

In certain cases, patients will present with ptosis of the breast over a fixed breast prosthesis (Fig. 23-25). Treatment requires correction of both breast ptosis and capsular contracture. Often, the prosthesis will have ruptured or will have fixation patches. A mammogram is done to determine the condition of the implant (intact or ruptured) and tissue reaction [31, 118, 145]. General anesthesia is often advisable where "resection" of the prosthesis is necessary. Usually, the vertical reference point for a B-mastopexy is marked, the prosthesis is removed through an inframammary incision, a new prosthesis is placed retropectorally, and a skin mastopexy is done. Occasionally, significant bleeding will occur. All specimens are sent for pathologic examination.

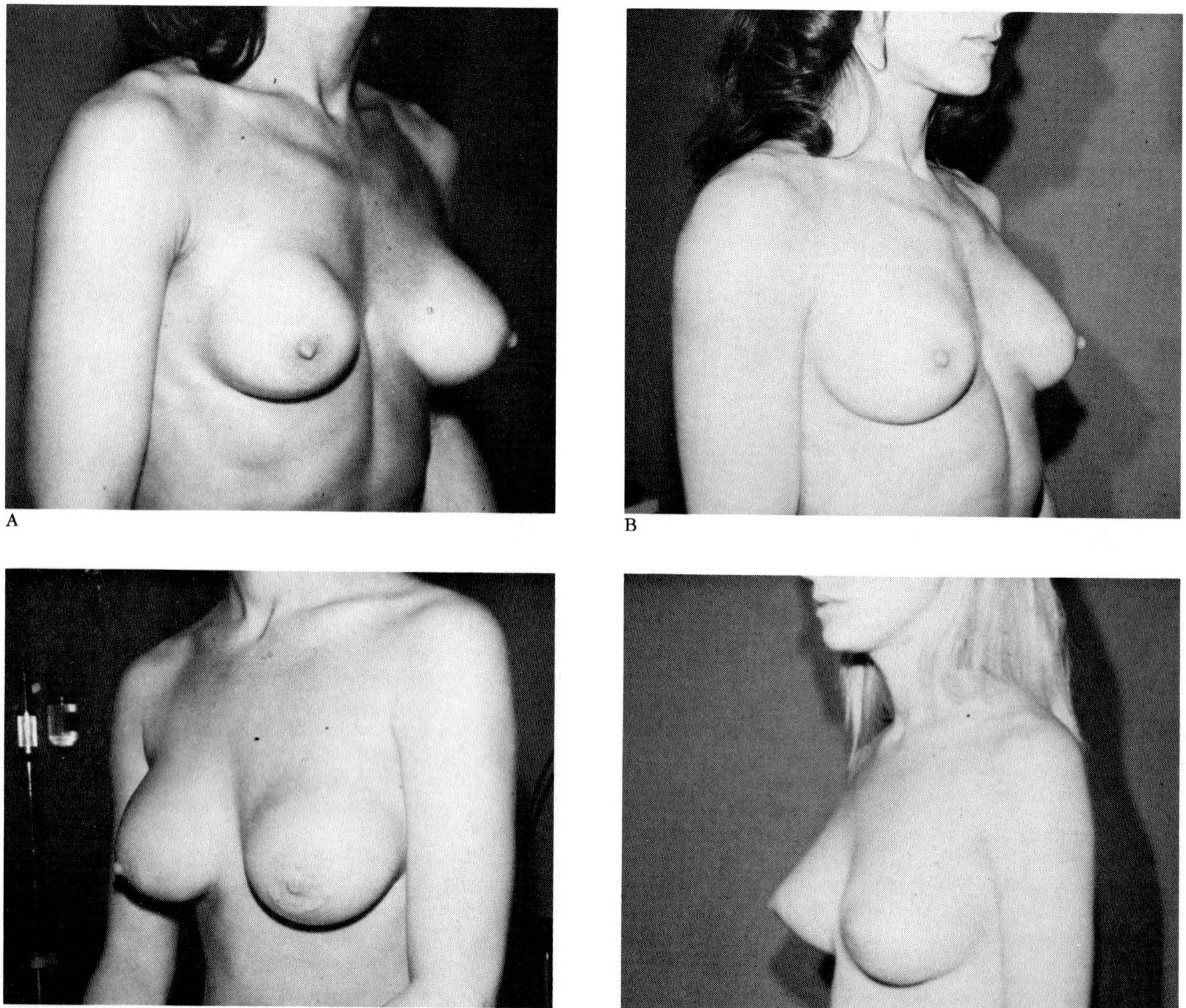

A B C D

Figure 23-24. Two patients with capsular contraction.

A. Severe capsular contracture following retroglandular augmentation with a 255-cc prosthesis.

B. Result at 1 year, subsequent to retropectoral placement of a 180-cc prosthesis.

C. Relatively lean patient with capsular contracture and downward tilt of the NAC following insertion of inflatable prostheses through a visible periareolar incision.

D. Result at 1 year, subsequent to retropectoral placement of the same-sized 260-cc gel implant.

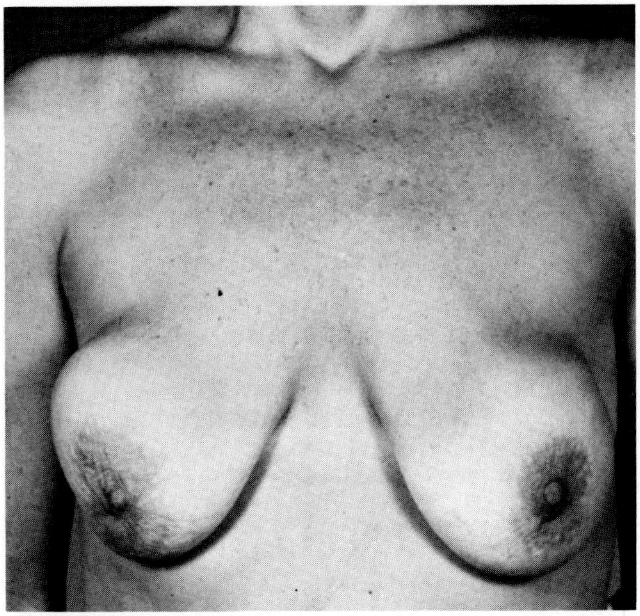

A

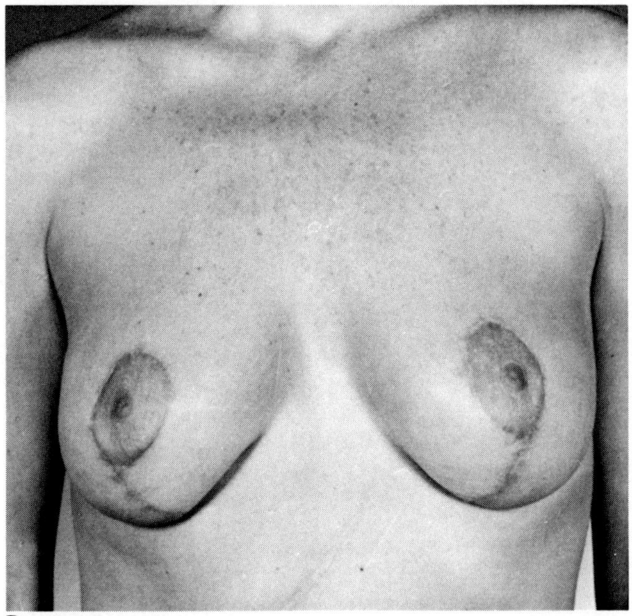

B

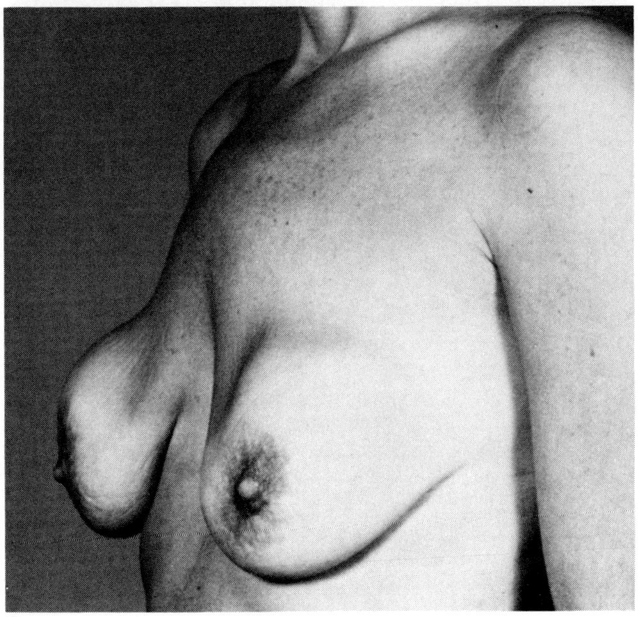

C

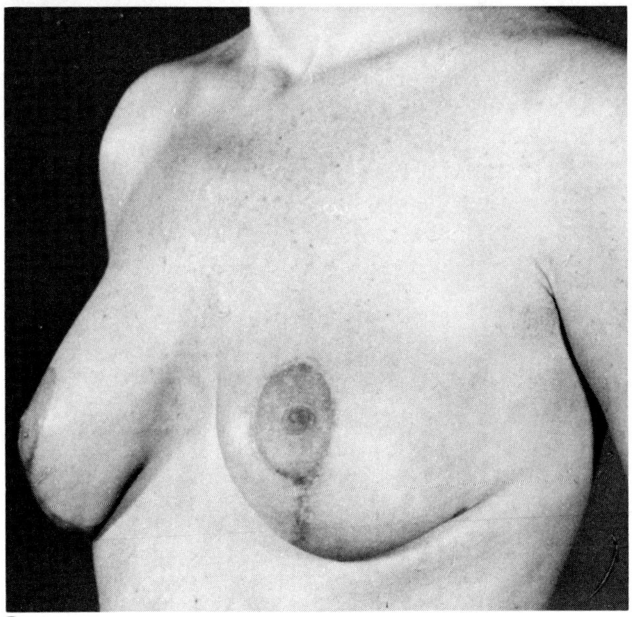

D

Figure 23-25

A, C. Patient with augmentation done 8 years previously. Capsular contracture around the implant, ptosis of the breast, and large areolae complicate the problem.

B, D. Early result following B-mastopexy and retropectoral placement of the same-sized implant.

REFERENCES

1. Addington, D. B., and Mallin, R. E. Closed capsulotomy causing fractures of the scar capsule and the silicone bag of a breast implant. *Plast. Reconstr. Surg.* 62:300, 1978.
2. Agris, J., Dingman, R. O., and Wilensky, R. J. A dissector for the transaxillary approach in augmentation mammaplasty. *Plast. Reconstr. Surg.* 57:10, 1976.
3. Arion, H. G. Présentation d'une prosthèse retromammaire. *C. R. Soc. Franc. Gynecol.* 35:427, 1965.
4. Ashbell, T. S. Commentary on outpatient breast surgery under intercostal block anesthesia by T. T. Huang, D. H. Parks, and S. R. Lewis. *Plast. Reconstr. Surg.* 65:239, 1980.
5. Ashley, F. L. A new type of breast prosthesis. *Plast. Reconstr. Surg.* 45:421, 1970.
6. Ashley, F. L. Further studies on the natural-Y breast prosthesis. *Plast. Reconstr. Surg.* 49:414, 1972.
7. Aston, S. J., and Rees, T. D. Mammary Augmentation, Correction of Asymmetry and Gynecomastia. In T. D. Rees (ed.), *Aesthetic Plastic Surgery.* Philadelphia: Saunders, 1980.
8. Baker, J. L., Jr. Augmentation Mammoplasty. In J. Q. Owsley, Jr., and R. A. Peterson (eds.), *Symposium on Aesthetic Surgery of the Breast.* St. Louis: Mosby, 1978.
9. Baker, J. L., Jr. Augmentation Mammoplasty. In W. C. Grabb and J. W. Smith (eds.), *Plastic Surgery* (3rd ed.). Boston: Little, Brown, 1979.
10. Baker, J. L., Jr., Bartels, R. J., and Douglas, W. M. Closed compression technique for rupturing a contracted capsule around a breast implant. *Plast. Reconstr. Surg.* 58:137, 1976.
11. Baker, J. L., Jr., Chandler, M. L., and LeViers, R. R. Occurrence and activity of myofibroblasts in human capsular tissue surrounding mammary implants. *Plast. Reconstr. Surg.* 68:905, 1981.
12. Baker, J. L., Jr., LeViers, R. R., and Spielvogel, D. E. Positive identification of silicone in human mammary capsular tissue. *Plast. Reconstr. Surg.* 1:69, 1982.
13. Bames, H. O. Breast malformations and a new approach to the problem of small breasts. *Plast. Reconstr. Surg.* 5:499, 1950.
14. Bames, H. O. Augmentation mammaplasty by lipo transplant. *Plast. Reconstr. Surg.* 11:404, 1953.
15. Barker, D. E., Retsky, M. I., and Schultz, S. "Bleeding" of silicone from bag-gel breast implants, and its clinical relation to fibrous capsule reaction. *Plast. Reconstr. Surg.* 61:836, 1978.
16. Benjamin, J. L., and Guy, C. Calcification of implant capsules following augmentation mammaplasty. *Plast. Reconstr. Surg.* 59:432, 1977.
17. Berson, M. Dermal-fat transplants used in building up the breasts. *Surgery* 15:451, 1945.
18. Biggs, T. M., Cukier, J., and Worthing, L. F. Augmentation mammaplasty: A review of 18 years. *Plast. Reconstr. Surg.* 69:445, 1982.
19. Boo-Chai, K. The complications of augmentation mammaplasty by silicone injection. *Br. J. Plast. Surg.* 22:281, 1969.
20. Broadbent, T. R., and Woolf, R. M. Unsatisfactory results in augmentation mammoplasty: Chest and breast asymmetry. *Aesthetic Plast. Surg.* 2:251, 1978.
21. Brody, G. S. Breast implant, size selection and patient satisfaction. *Plast. Reconstr. Surg.* 68:611, 1981.
22. Burkhardt, B. R., et al. Objective clinical assessment of fibrous capsular contracture. *Plast. Reconstr. Surg.* 69:794, 1982.
23. Capozzi, A., Du Bou, R., and Pennisi, V. R. Distant migration of silicone gel from a ruptured breast implant. *Plast. Reconstr. Surg.* 62:302, 1979.
24. Capozzi, A., and Pennisi, V. R. Clinical experience with polyurethane-covered gel-filled mammary prostheses. *Plast. Reconstr. Surg.* 68:519, 1981.
25. Carrico, T. J., and Cohen, I. K. Capsular contracture and steroid-related complications after augmentation mammaplasty. *Plast. Reconstr. Surg.* 64:377, 1979.
26. Chaplin, C. H. Loss of both breasts from injection of silicone (with additive). *Plast. Reconstr. Surg.* 44:447, 1969.
27. Christie, A. J. Silicone lymphadenopathy and synovitis (complication of silicone elastomer finger joint prostheses). *J.A.M.A.* 237:1463, 1977.
28. Cocke, W. M., Leathers, H. K., and Lynch, J. B. Foreign body reaction to polyurethane covers of some breast prostheses. *Plast. Reconstr. Surg.* 56:527, 1973.
29. Cohen, I. K. On the use of soluble steroid within inflatable breast prostheses. (Letter to the Editor.) *Plast. Reconstr. Surg.* 62:105, 1978.
30. Cohen, I. K., and Carrico, T. J. Capsular contracture and steroid related complications in augmentation mammaplasty. *Aesthetic Plast. Surg.* 4:267, 1980.
31. Cohen, I. K., Goodman, H., and Theogaraj, S. D. Xeromammography: A reason for using saline-filled breast prostheses. *Plast. Reconstr. Surg.* 60:886, 1977.
32. Conway, H. Mammaplasty: Analysis of 110 consecutive cases with end results. *Plast. Reconstr. Surg.* 10:303, 1952.
33. Conway, H., and Dietz, G. H. Augmentation mammaplasty. *Surg. Gynecol. Obstet.* 114:573, 1962.
34. Conway, H., and Smith, J. Breast plastic surgery: Reduction mammaplasty, mastopexy, augmentation mammaplasty and mammary construction. *Plast. Reconstr. Surg.* 21:8, 1958.
35. Corso, P. F. Plastic surgery for the unilateral hypoplastic breast. A report of eight cases. *Plast. Reconstr. Surg.* 50:134, 1972.
36. Courtiss, E. H., and Goldwyn, R. M. Breast sensation before and after plastic surgery. *Plast. Reconstr. Surg.* 58:1, 1976.
37. Courtiss, E. H., Goldwyn, R. M., and Anastasi, G. W. The fate of breast implants with infections around them. *Plast. Reconstr. Surg.* 63:812, 1979.
38. Cronin, T. D., and Gerow, F. Augmentation Mammaplasty: A New "Natural Feel" Prosthesis. In *Transactions of the Third International Congress of Plastic Surgery.* Amsterdam: Excerpta Medica, 1964. Pp. 41–49.
39. Cronin, T. D., and Greenberg, R. L. Our experiences with the silastic gel breast prosthesis. *Plast. Reconstr. Surg.* 46:1, 1970.
40. DeCholnoky, T. Augmentation mammaplasty: Survey of complications of 10,941 patients by 265 surgeons. *Plast. Reconstr. Surg.* 45:573, 1970.
41. Dempsey, W. C., and Latham, W. D. Subpectoral implants in augmentation mammaplasty: Preliminary report. *Plast. Reconstr. Surg.* 42:515, 1968.
42. Domanskis, E. J., and Owsley, J. Q., Jr. Histological investigation of the etiology of capsule contracture following augmentation mammaplasty. *Plast. Reconstr. Surg.* 58:689, 1976.
43. Dukes, C. E., and Mitchley, M. I. Polyvinyl sponge implants: Experimental and clinical observations. *Br. J. Plast. Surg.* 15:225, 1962.
44. Edgerton, M. T., and McClary, A. R. Augmentation mammaplasty. *Plast. Reconstr. Surg.* 21:279, 1958.
45. Edgerton, M. T., Meyer, E., and Jacobson, W. E. Augmentation mammaplasty: II. Further surgical and psychiatric evaluation. *Plast. Reconstr. Surg.* 27:279, 1961.
46. Eiseman, G. Augmentation mammaplasty by the trans-axillary approach. *Plast. Reconstr. Surg.* 54:229, 1974.

47. Eisenberg, H. V., and Bartels, R. J. Rupture of a silicone bag-gel breast implant by closed compression capsulotomy: Case report. *Plast. Reconstr. Surg.* 59:849, 1977.
48. Ellenberg, A. H. Marked thinning of the breast skin flaps after the insertion of implants containing triamcinolone. *Plast. Reconstr. Surg.* 60:755, 1977.
49. Ellenberg, A. H., and Braun, H. A 3½-year experience with double-lumen implants in breast surgery. *Plast. Reconstr. Surg.* 65:307, 1980.
50. Feleberti, M. C., Arrillaga, A., and Colon, G. A. Rupture of inflated breast implants in closed compression capsulotomy: Case report. *Plast. Reconstr. Surg.* 59:848, 1977.
51. Frantz, P., and Herbst, C. A. Augmentation mammaplasty, irradiation and breast cancer. *Cancer* 36:1147, 1975.
52. Fredricks, S. Management of Mammary Hypoplasia. In R. M. Goldwyn (ed.), *Plastic and Reconstructive Surgery of the Breast.* Boston: Little, Brown, 1976.
53. Gayou, R. M. A histological comparison of contracted and non-contracted capsules around silicone breast implants. *Plast. Reconstr. Surg.* 63:700, 1979.
54. Gifford, S. Emotional Attitudes Towards Cosmetic Breast Surgery: Loss and Restitution of the "Ideal Self." In R. M. Goldwyn (ed.), *Plastic and Reconstructive Surgery of the Breast.* Boston: Little, Brown, 1976.
55. Ginsbach, G., Busch, L. C., and Kuhnel, W. The nature of the collagenous capsules around breast implants. *Plast. Reconstr. Surg.* 64:456, 1979.
56. Goin, J. M. High-pressure injection of silicone gel into an axilla—a complication of closed compression capsulotomy of the breast: Case report. *Plast. Reconstr. Surg.* 62:891, 1978.
57. Goin, M. K., and Goin, J. M. *Changing the Body.* Baltimore: Williams & Wilkins, 1981.
58. Goldwyn, R. M. (ed.) *Plastic and Reconstructive Surgery of the Breast.* Boston: Little, Brown, 1976.
59. Goulian, D., Jr., and Conway, H. Correction of the moderately ptotic breast: A warning. *Plast. Reconstr. Surg.* 43:478, 1969.
60. Griffiths, C. O., Jr. The Submuscular Implant in Augmentation Mammoplasty. In G. Sanvenero-Rosselli (ed.), *Transactions of the Fourth International Congress of Plastic Surgery.* Amsterdam: Excerpta Medica, 1969. Pp. 1009–1015.
61. Grossman, A. R. The current status of augmentation mammaplasty. *Plast. Reconstr. Surg.* 52:1, 1973.
62. Gruber, R. P., and Friedman, G. D. Periareolar subpectoral augmentation mammaplasty. *Plast. Reconstr. Surg.* 67:453, 1981.
63. Gruber, R. P., and Friedman, G. D. The pressures generated by closed capsulotomies of augmented breasts. *Plast. Reconstr. Surg.* 62:379, 1982.
64. Hartley, J. H., Jr. Specific applications of the double lumen prosthesis. *Clin. Plast. Surg.* 3:247, 1976.
65. Hausner, R. J., Schoen, F. J., and Pierson, K. K. Foreign-body reaction to silicone gel in axillary lymph nodes after an augmentation mammaplasty. *Plast. Reconstr. Surg.* 62:381, 1978.
66. Hayes, H. Breast implant and possible late hematogenous infection. (Letter to the Editor.) *Plast. Reconstr. Surg.* 60:104, 1977.
67. Hayes, H., Jr., and McLeod, P. Indentation tonometry of breasts. *Plast. Reconstr. Surg.* 63:13, 1979.
68. Hetter, G. P. Satisfactions and dissatisfactions of patients with augmentation mammaplasty. *Plast. Reconstr. Surg.* 64:151, 1979.
69. Hipps, C. J., Raju, D. R., and Straith, R. E. Influence of some operative and postoperative factors on capsular contracture around breast prostheses. *Plast. Reconstr. Surg.* 61:384, 1978.
70. Hoehler, H. Breast augmentation: The axillary approach. *Br. J. Plast. Surg.* 26:373, 1973.
71. Hoffman, S. The dilemma of capsular contracture. (Letter to the Editor.) *Plast. Reconstr. Surg.* 66:477, 1980.
72. Huang, T. T., Blackwell, S. J., and Lewis, S. R. Migration of silicone gel after the "squeeze technique" to rupture a contracted breast capsule: Case report. *Plast. Reconstr. Surg.* 61:277, 1978.
73. Huang, T. T., Parks, D. H., and Lewis, S. R. Outpatient breast surgery under intercostal block anesthesia. *Plast. Reconstr. Surg.* 63:299, 1979.
74. Hueston, J. Unilateral Agenesis and Hypoplasia: Difficulties and Suggestions. In R. M. Goldwyn (ed.), *Plastic and Reconstructive Surgery of the Breast.* Boston: Little, Brown, 1975.
75. Hughes, E. S. R. The development of the mammary gland. *Ann. R. Coll. Surg. Engl.* 6:99, 1950.
76. Johnson, M., and Lloyd, H. E. D. Bilateral breast cancer 10 years after an augmentation mammaplasty: Case report. *Plast. Reconstr. Surg.* 53:88, 1974.
77. Jones, F. R., and Taurus, A. P. A periareolar incision for augmentation mammaplasty. *Plast. Reconstr. Surg.* 51:641, 1973.
78. Kelley, A. P., et al. Complications of the Cronin Silastic mammary prosthesis. *Plast. Reconstr. Surg.* 37:438, 1966.
79. Kopf, E. H., et al. Complications of silicone injections. *Rocky Mt. Med. J.* 73:77, 1976.
80. Ksander, G. A. Effects of diffused soluble steroid on capsules around experimental breast prostheses in rats. *Plast. Reconstr. Surg.* 63:708, 1979.
81. Ksander, G. A., Vistnes, L. M., and Fogarty, D. C. Experimental effects on surrounding fibrous capsule formation from placing steroid in a silicone bag-gel prosthesis before implantation. *Plast. Reconstr. Surg.* 62:873, 1978.
82. Laughlin, R. A., Raynor, A. C., and Habal, M. B. Complications of closed capsulotomies after augmentation mammaplasty. *Plast. Reconstr. Surg.* 60:362, 1977.
83. Lavey, E., et al. Customized silicone implants of the breast and chest. *Plast. Reconstr. Surg.* 69:646, 1982.
84. Lewis, J. R., Jr. The augmentation mammaplasty with special reference to alloplastic materials. *Plast. Reconstr. Surg.* 35:51, 1965.
85. Lilla, J. A., and Vistnes, L. M. Long-term study of reactions to various silicone breast implants in rabbits. *Plast. Reconstr. Surg.* 57:637, 1976.
86. Little, G., and Baker, J. L., Jr. Results of closed compression capsulotomy for treatment of contracted breast implant capsules. *Plast. Reconstr. Surg.* 65:30, 1980.
87. Longacre, J. J. The use of the local pedicle flaps for reconstruction of the breasts after sub-total extirpation of the mammary gland and for the correction of distortion and atrophy of the breast due to excessive scar. *Plast. Reconstr. Surg.* 11:380, 1953.
88. Mahler, D. Improved method of injecting local anesthetic solutions for breast operations. *Plast. Reconstr. Surg.* 64:566, 1980.
89. Maliniac, J. W. *Breast Deformities and Their Repair.* New York: Grune & Stratton, 1950.
90. Marsh, J. L., et al. Reinsertability after breast prosthesis pocket infection: An experimental study. *Plast. Reconstr. Surg.* 69:234, 1982.
91. McGraw, J. B., Jr. Personal communication, 1978.
92. Moore, D. C., and Briedenbach, L. D. Intercostal nerve block

in 4333 patients: Indications, technique and complications. *Ann. Anesth. Analg.* 41:1, 1962.
93. Moore, J. R. Applanation tonometry of breasts. *Plast. Reconstr. Surg.* 63:9, 1979.
94. Nelson, G. D. Complications of closed compression after augmentation mammaplasty. *Plast. Reconstr. Surg.* 66:71, 1980.
95. Nelson, G. D. Update. Complications from the treatment of fibrous capsular contracture of the breast. *Plast. Reconstr. Surg.* 68:969, 1981.
96. Nosnachuk, J. S. Injected dimethylpolysiloxane fluid: A study of the antibody and histologic response. *Plast. Reconstr. Surg.* 42:562, 1968.
97. Oneal, R. M. High-pressure injection of silicone gel into an axilla: A complication of closed compression capsulotomy of the breast. (Letter to the Editor.) *Plast. Reconstr. Surg.* 64:700, 1979.
98. Oneal, R. M., and Argenta, L. C. Late side effects related to inflatable breast prostheses containing soluble steroids. *Plast. Reconstr. Surg.* 69:641, 1982.
99. Ortiz-Monasterio, F., and Trigos, I. Management of patients with complications from injections of foreign material into the breasts. *Plast. Reconstr. Surg.* 50:42, 1972.
100. Pacik, P. T. Patients determining breast implant size. *Plast. Reconstr. Surg.* 69:1028, 1982.
101. Papillon, J. Pros and cons of subpectoral implantation. *Clin. Plast. Surg.* 3:321, 1976.
102. Parsons, R. W., and Thering, H. R. Management of the silicone-injected breast. *Plast. Reconstr. Surg.* 60:534, 1977.
103. Perrin, E. R. The use of soluble steroids within inflatable breast prostheses. *Plast. Reconstr. Surg.* 57:163, 1976.
104. Persoff, M. M. Problems with the use of soluble steroids within inflatable breast prostheses. (Letter to the Editor.) *Plast. Reconstr. Surg.* 62:106, 755, 1977.
105. Peters, W. J., and Smith, D. C. Ivalon breast prostheses: Evaluation 19 years after implantation. Case report. *Plast. Reconstr. Surg.* 67:514, 1981.
106. Peterson, H. D., and Burt, G. B. The role of steroids in prevention of circumferential capsular scarring in augmentation mammaplasty. *Plast. Reconstr. Surg.* 54:28, 1974.
107. Pickering, P. P., Williams, J. E., and Vecchione, T. R. Augmentation Mammoplasty. In R. M. Goldwyn (ed.), *Long-Term Results in Plastic and Reconstructive Surgery*. Boston: Little, Brown, 1980. P. 696.
108. Pickrell, K. L., Puckett, C. L., and Given, K. S. Subpectoral augmentation mammaplasty. *Plast. Reconstr. Surg.* 60:325, 1977.
109. Price, R. I. M. Failure of steroid instillation to prevent capsular contracture after augmentation mammaplasty. (Letter to the Editor.) *Plast. Reconstr. Surg.* 57:371, 1976.
110. Redfern, A. B., Ryan, J. J., and Su, C. T. Calcification of the fibrous capsule about mammary implants. *Plast. Reconstr. Surg.* 59:249, 1977.
111. Rees, T. D., and Aston, S. J. The tuberous breast. *Clin. Plast. Surg.* 3:339, 1976.
112. Rees, T. D., and Dupuis, C. C. Unilateral mammary hypoplasia. *Plast. Reconstr. Surg.* 41:307, 1968.
113. Rees, T. D., Guy, C. L., and Coburn, R. J. The use of inflatable breast implants. *Plast. Reconstr. Surg.* 52:609, 1973.
114. Regnault, P. One hundred cases of retromammary implantation of Etheron followed up for 30 months. In *Transactions of the Third International Congress of Plastic Surgery*. Amsterdam: Excerpta Medica, 1964. P. 74.
115. Regnault, P. The hypoplastic and ptotic breast: A combined operation with prosthetic augmentation. *Plast. Reconstr. Surg.* 37:31, 1966.
116. Regnault, P. Indications for breast augmentation. *Plast. Reconstr. Surg.* 40:524, 1967.
117. Regnault, P. Partial submuscular breast augmentation. *Plast. Reconstr. Surg.* 59:72, 1977.
118. Rintala, A. E., and Svinhufvud, U. M. Effect of augmentation mammaplasty on mammography and thermography. *Plast. Reconstr. Surg.* 54:390, 1974.
119. Robertson, J. L. A. A complication of a transareolar augmentation mammaplasty. Case report. *Plast. Reconstr. Surg.* 63:263, 1979.
120. Robles, J. M., Zimman, O. A., and Lee, J. C. A larger subpectoral pocket for breast implants. *Plast. Reconstr. Surg.* 62:78, 1978.
121. Rubin, L. R. The deflating saline implant: Facing up to complications. (Editorial.) *Plast. Reconstr. Surg.* 65:665, 1980.
122. Rubin, L. R., and Speace, G. One preventable cause of spontaneous deflation of inflatable mammary prostheses. *Plast. Reconstr. Surg.* 64:313, 1979.
123. Rudolph, R., et al. Myofibroblasts and free silicon around breast implants. *Plast. Reconstr. Surg.* 62:185, 1978.
124. Schonfeld, W. A. Body-image disturbances in adolescents with inappropriate sexual development. *Am. J. Orthopsychiatry* 34:493, 1964.
125. Shah, Z., Lehman, A., Jr., and Tan, J. Does infection play a role in breast capsular contracture? *Plast. Reconstr. Surg.* 68:34, 1981.
126. Shipley, R. H., O'Donnell, J. M., and Bader, K. F. Personality characteristics of women seeking breast augmentation: Comparison to small-busted and average-busted controls. *Plast. Reconstr. Surg.* 60:369, 1977.
127. Shipley, R. H., O'Donnell, J. M., and Bader, K. F. Psychological effects of cosmetic augmentation mammaplasty. *Aesthetic Plast. Surg.* 2:429, 1978.
128. Silver, H. L. Treating the complication of augmentation mammaplasty. *Plast. Reconstr. Surg.* 49:637, 1972.
129. Simon, B. E., Hoffman, S., and Kahn, S. Treatment of asymmetry of the breasts: A report of 30 cases of development origin. *Clin. Plast. Surg.* 2:375, 1975.
130. Souther, S. G., and Lucid, M. L. Breast implant size selection. (Letter to the Editor.) *Plast. Reconstr. Surg.* 69:1025, 1982.
131. Thompson, H. G. The fate of pseudosheath pocket around silicone implants. *Plast. Reconstr. Surg.* 51:667, 1973.
132. Tolhurst, D. E. "Nutcracker" technique for compression rupture of capsules around breast implants. *Plast. Reconstr. Surg.* 61:795, 1978.
133. Toranto, I. R., and Malow, J. B. Atypical mycobacteria periprosthetic infections: Diagnosis and treatment. *Plast. Reconstr. Surg.* 66:226, 1980.
134. Truppman, E. S., and Ellenby, J. D. A 13 Year Evaluation of Subpectoral Augmentation Mammoplasty. In J. Q. Owsley and R. A. Peterson (eds.), *Symposium on Aesthetic Surgery of the Breast*. St. Louis: Mosby, 1978. P. 344.
135. Truppman, E. S., Ellenby, J. D., and Schwartz, B. M. Fungi in and around implants after augmentation mammaplasty. *Plast. Reconstr. Surg.* 64:804, 1979.
136. Vargas, A. Shedding of silicone particles from inflated breast implants. (Letter to the Editor.) *Plast. Reconstr. Surg.* 64:252, 1979.
137. Vinnick, C. A. Spherical contracture of fibrous capsules around breast implants. *Plast. Reconstr. Surg.* 58:555, 1976.
138. Vistnes, L. M., Bentley, J. W., and Fogarty, D. C. Experimental study of tissue response to ruptured gel-filled mammary prostheses. *Plast. Reconstr. Surg.* 59:31, 1977.
139. Vistnes, L. M., Ksander, G. A., and Kosek, J. Effects of local instillation of triamcinolone on the capsules around silicone

bag-gel prostheses in animals. *Plast. Reconstr. Surg.* 62:739, 1978.

140. Wilflingseder, P., Propst, A., and Mikuz, G. Constrictive fibrosis following silicone implants in mammary augmentation. *Ann. Chir. Plast.* 2:215, 1974.
141. Williams, C., Aston, S., and Rees, T. D. The effect of hematoma on the thickness of pseudosheaths around silicone implants. *Plast. Reconstr. Surg.* 56:194, 1975.
142. Williams, J. E. Experience with a large series of Silastic breast implants. *Plast. Reconstr. Surg.* 49:253, 1972.
143. Williams, J. E. Augmentation Mammaplasty, Inframammary Approach. In N. G. Georgiade (ed.), *Reconstructive Breast Surgery.* St. Louis: Mosby, 1976. Pp. 50–67.
144. Williams, J. E. Augmentation Mammaplasty. In E. H. Courtiss (ed.), *Aesthetic Surgery: Trouble—How to Avoid It and How to Treat It.* St. Louis: Mosby, 1978.
145. Wolfe, J. N. On mammography in the presence of breast implants. (Letter to the Editor.) *Plast. Reconstr. Surg.* 62:286, 1978.
146. Worton, E. W., Seifert, L. N., and Sherwood, R. Late leakage of inflatable silicone breast prostheses. *Plast. Reconstr. Surg.* 65:302, 1980.

24. Breast Asymmetry and Deformities

Paule Regnault
Rollin K. Daniel

Breast Asymmetry

Slight degrees of breast asymmetry are virtually universal, especially in patients requiring reduction mammaplasty. However, significant discrepancies that are disturbing to the patient and obvious to the examiner are relatively unusual, occurring in 3 to 5 percent of patients seeking consultation for breast surgery [15]. Attainment of breasts that are similar in size, shape, and position is difficult. Patient satisfaction with the final result will depend on the severity of the initial discrepancy and the surgeon's ability to achieve the patient's desires or to modify them into attainable goals.

HISTORY

Since antiquity, breast asymmetry has been a medical curiosity [21]. All of the pioneering breast surgeons dealt with problems of asymmetry, usually by reducing the hypertrophic breast [9, 22]. Following introduction of breast implants, numerous surgeons reported correction of asymmetric deformities involving hypoplastic breasts. The series reported by Simon et al. [40], Rees [33], Hueston [15], and Elliott et al. [7] stressed the diversity of presentation and the difficulty of achieving perfection, especially in regard to contour. Recently, new procedures have been devised for correction of the most severe deformities (Poland syndrome) including custom-made prostheses and latissimus dorsi muscle transfers [13]. The principles derived from postmastectomy breast reconstruction are now being applied to the more devastating asymmetries.

PATHOPHYSIOLOGY AND CLASSIFICATION

In the 6- to 20-mm embryo, the nipple develops as an ectodermal thickening along the mammary line stretching from the axilla to the groin [16]. At 5 months, the mammary ducts begin to evolve and continue development until term. Between birth and puberty very few changes occur until a rise in hormone levels stimulates breast enlargement.

Aplasia is the complete absence of breast formation whereas the common term *hypoplasia* is a quantitative decrease in the number of cells in the primordium [24, 46, 49]. Breast enlargement is due either to an increased unit size (hypertrophy) or to an increase of cellular number (hyperplasia). Chest wall deformities consist of variations in Poland syndrome as well as isolated skeletal deformi-

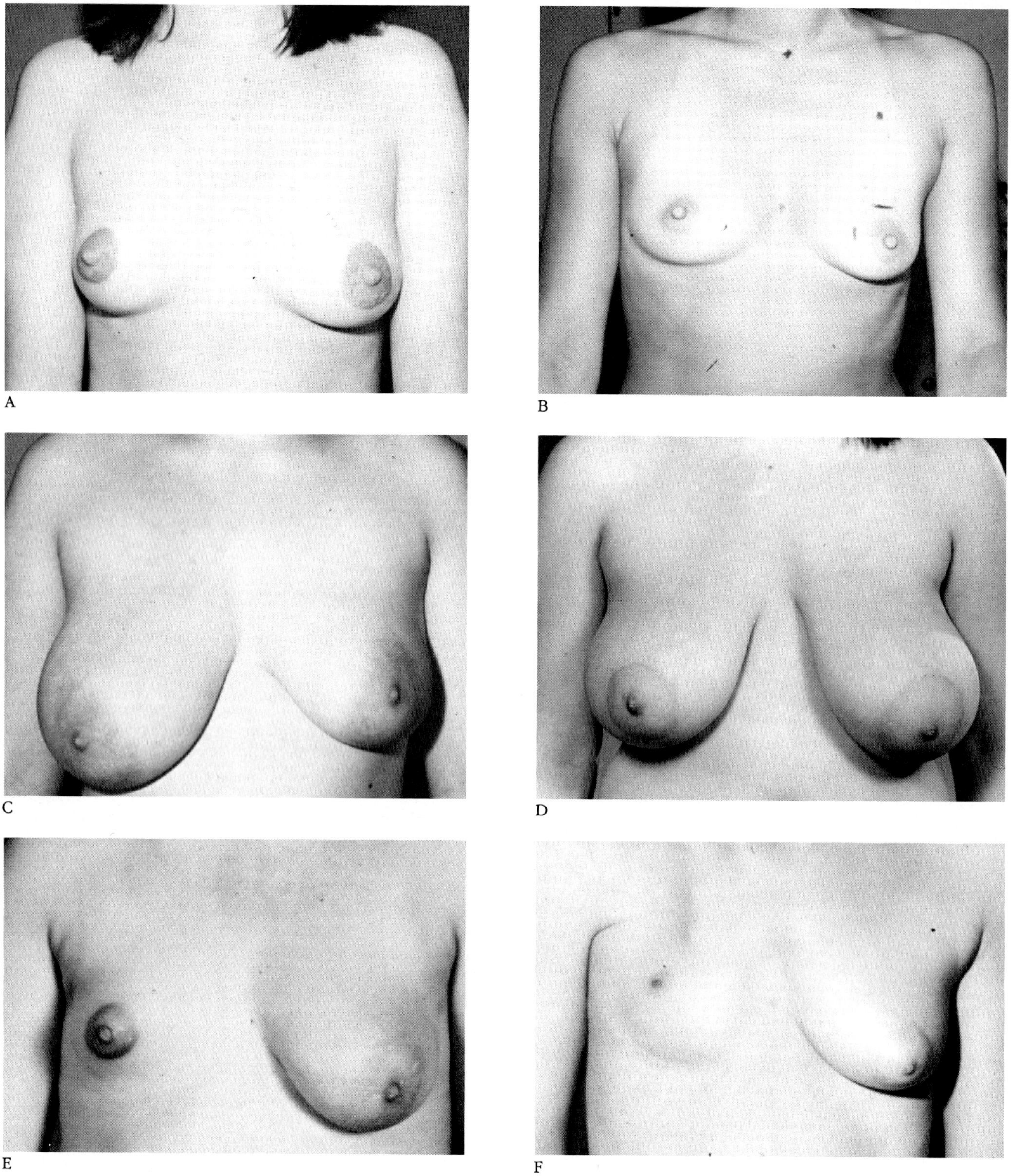

Figure 24-1. Classification of breast asymmetries.
A. Hypoplasia and normal.
B. Hypoplasia and hypoplasia.
C. Hyperplasia and normal.
D. Hyperplasia and hyperplasia.
E. Hypoplasia and hyperplasia.
F. Poland's syndrome.
Note in the latter two conditions marked differences in breast position, shape, inframammary crease, and areolar characteristics.

ties of the ribs, sternum, scapula, or vertebral column [32]. Isolated absence of parts of the pectoralis major muscle is surprisingly common, with the costosternal portion the most frequently absent. Complete expression of Poland syndrome may include numerous deficiencies: (1) amastia, (2) absence of cartilage and the anterior portion of the third to fifth ribs, (3) absence of the costosternal portion of the pectoralis major, and (4) absence of the pectoralis minor, intercostal muscles, and portions of the serratus anterior. Broadbent and Woolf [2] have emphasized the frequency of rib, vertebral column (scoliosis, kyphosis), and sternal (pectus excavatum and carinatum) deformities. One must decide whether these deformities can be camouflaged or whether a more extensive reconstruction will be necessary.

Breast asymmetries can be divided into developmental and acquired, the latter being caused by trauma, surgery, inflammation, or neoplasm. Since this latter group often falls within the realm of breast reconstruction, it will not be included in the present discussion. The classification of Simon et al. [40] of developmental breast asymmetries based on relative discrepancies can be modified to include the influence of ptosis (Fig. 24-1).

1. One breast hypoplastic, the other normal, with or without ptosis
2. Both breasts hypoplastic, but unequal in size
3. One breast hypertrophic, the other normal; either or both may be ptotic
4. Both breasts hypertrophic and unequal in size; either or both may be ptotic
5. One breast hypoplastic, the other hypertrophic
6. Hypoplasia of thorax, pectoral muscle, or breast, unilateral

In general, we consider category 6 to be a thorax deformity rather than a quantitative asymmetry [28]. Clinically, the various combinations are virtually limitless, and consummate surgical skill is required to achieve the desired symmetry [10].

CONSULTATION

Medical History

A detailed history of breast development is required. Were any breast or systemic deformities present at birth? Is there a family history of birth defects? At what age did breast development begin, and when was the asymmetry apparent? What was the age of onset for menarche, and what is the onset, duration, and regularity of the menses? Is there significant premenstrual breast enlargement? Has the patient ever taken any hormones including birth control pills, and if yes what effect did they have on breast size? Has she ever seen an endocrinologist or been evaluated by a physician for this problem? If the patient has been pregnant, what effect did pregnancy have on breast size and did lactation occur from both breasts? In most aplastic breasts, pregnancy does not increase size or cause lactation. Throughout the consultation, it is imperative that the surgeon *not* project his or her interpretation of the problem onto the patient. As emphasized by Corso [3], one should ask, "Which breast do you feel is unacceptable and which would you like corrected?" In a surprising number of cases, the patient will want changes contrary to those the surgeon would recommend. Also, this approach gives the patient an opportunity to express her feelings and concerns about body image.

Indications and Contraindications

Deformities requiring surgical correction are those that cause psychologic damage or cannot be concealed in normal clothing. Corso [3] reported that all eight patients in his series had suffered psychologically from their deformity. Primarily, they had feelings of inadequacy and inferiority in regard to femininity. Bilateral quantitative deformities, either bilateral hypoplasia or hypertrophy, did not cause serious problems. In contrast, the patient with a severe unilateral hypoplasia experienced a severe body image defect expressed as a "freak" or as a "half woman, half man" appearance. In other patients, the difficulty of camouflaging the deformity and buying clothes (brassieres, bathing suits, revealing dresses) prompted surgical intervention.

Contraindications to surgery are often psychologic and occasionally medical. Since symmetry is a fundamental objective, it is often necessary to operate on both breasts. The more severe the deformity, the more likely the patient will be to accept surgical intervention and be pleased with the result. One of the most difficult questions is the candidate's age. Should a 13-year-old girl with significant psychologic problems due to an asymmetric hypertrophic breast (36D) and a contralateral hypoplastic breast (36A) wait until physical maturity is attained? In most cases, we recommend psychiatric and medical consultation, basing our decision on the recommendations derived from that, including counsel on sexual maturity.

Surgery is contraindicated in the patient with severe fibrocystic disease, multiple scars, and medical problems precluding anesthesia.

Motivation

The principal aim is correction of body image and achievement of symmetry. The psychologic impact of breast asymmetry can be enormous but is usually overcome by surgery without permanent sequelae.

Patients with less severe asymmetries are prone to be dissatisfied unless it is clearly emphasized that perfection is rarely achieved and bilateral surgery is often necessary. In these cases it may be best for the patient to consider a delay until all pregnancies are completed, and then a definitive contouring and equalization can be justified. It is important to ask the patient how much of a problem it is to buy clothes, especially brassieres. How difficult is it to cover the deformity in street clothes and bathing suits? How self-conscious about the deformity is she? Does she permit herself to be seen nude?

Equally important, what does she expect from the surgery? Will she accept the requisite scarring and procedures on the normal breast? The more restrictive and perfectionistic the patient, the more a second visit is recommended. Since most of these patients have had the deformity for several years, why are they seeking surgery at this time?

Physical Examination

A detailed examination of the breasts and thorax is mandatory. The patient is examined nude from the waist up in the sitting position and the appearance contrasted with the clothed appearance. The breasts are evaluated bilaterally with reference to approximate size, shape, location, skin envelope, and nipple-areola complex (NAC). Hemithorax measurements are made, and the distance from sternal notch to NAC is determined. The degree of ptosis is recorded.

Testing of the pectoralis major muscle is done with palpation of the various segments. Any abnormalities in the sternum, ribs, or costal cartilages are rated and discrepancies in posture or shoulder height recorded. The patient is asked to turn, and any deformities of the vertebral column or scapula are detailed. A thorough breast examination including the axilla is completed with the patient supine.

Aesthetic Goals

At this point the surgeon should review the problem as originally stated by the patient and then present the findings made, with a recommendation for treatment. In certain cases the asymmetry will be minor, and surgery is not necessary. The patient should be reassured that she falls within the "normal" range and that mirror image breasts are virtually nonexistent. In other instances the problem will be in the musculoskeletal system or a specific breast deformity, e.g., tuberous breast. A more detailed explanation of the deformity and type of surgery is then required. For the vast majority, the problem is a disproportion, and the objective is a comparative balance of the two breasts. It must be emphasized that volumetric equality can be achieved but symmetric contour is virtually impossible unless the "normal" breast is "made to match." Although initially hesitant to have surgery on the normal breast, most patients will agree once the problem is explained in depth. A two-stage approach is often used for the adolescent or undecided patient. An augmentation is done on the hypoplastic side and volumetric equality obtained. Although appearance is normal in brassiere and bathing suit, discrepancies in shape and position compel the patient to seek a second operation on the normal breast. A minority will be pleased with volumetric approximation. The appropriate operation is proposed to the patient, possible complications are explained, and preoperative instructions are given. Informed consent and preoperative preparations vary with the selected procedures as presented in preceding chapters.

SURGICAL TECHNIQUES

Because of the diversity of presentation, the entire gamut of breast surgery may be necessary even in a small series of asymmetries. The primary challenge should be selection of the optimal procedure, with its successful execution a foregone conclusion.

Principles

The final result is usually best in bilateral similar deformities where residual volume, consistency, and scars will be comparable (Fig. 24-2). Reduction of unilateral hypertrophy will often give an acceptable result, but there can be marked contrast with the normal breast because of tight skin envelope, malposition, and NAC deformities. In general, the location and size of the hypoplastic breast's NAC are taken as reference points for contralateral procedures. Bilateral implants are often preferred to ensure symmetric contour and consistency despite a contralateral breast that is normal or hypertrophic. Since the augmented breast can rarely match the natural ptosis of the unaugmented breast, the asymmetry is preserved. The majority of implants are inflatable, with custom-made implants used for masking musculoskeletal deformities. If significant muscle loss is present, a modified latissimus dorsi muscle transfer is considered.

Despite proponents of sequential procedures that correct the most deformed breast initially, we generally prefer a one-stage operation, with a second operation reserved for finishing touches.

Hypoplasia and Normal Breast

Augmentation of the hypoplastic breast is the obvious solution, but it will rarely produce symmetry (Fig. 24-3). The augmented breast has greater superior quadrant fullness and often a different consistency. The normal breast will have some degree of ptosis except in the patient with small breasts [14, 35]. Thus, attainment of symmetry frequently requires bilateral implants with a minimum volume on the normal side.

For example, a patient presenting with a nonptotic asymmetry consisting of 34A and 34B measurements would be advised to have a 200-cc implant on the hypoplastic side and a 100-cc implant on the normal side, both placed subpectorally. If the patient refuses bilateral surgery, the inherent limitations of unilateral surgery would be reemphasized and a second visit scheduled.

The value of showing photos from previous cases should be considered. If the patient remains adamant, a unilateral subpectoral augmentation is done.

Hypoplasia and Hypoplasia

Bilateral augmentation is the obvious treatment, and volumetric equality is usually achieved (Fig. 24-4). Volumetric increases are based on the premise that each inch of difference in hemithorax measurement equals 100 cc of prosthesis [17, 37]. A more graded approximation can be

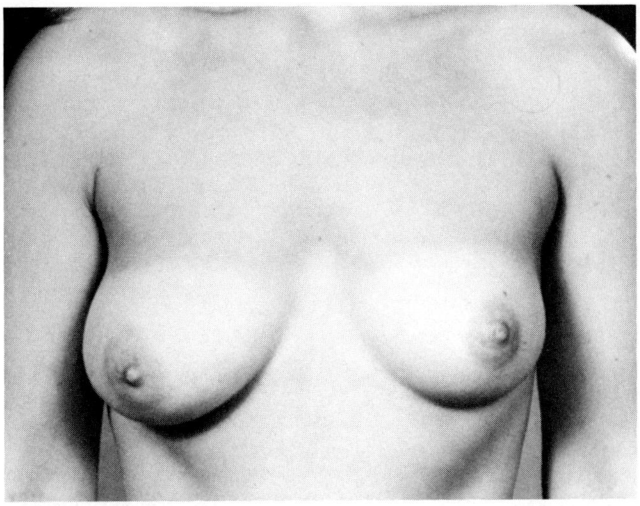

A

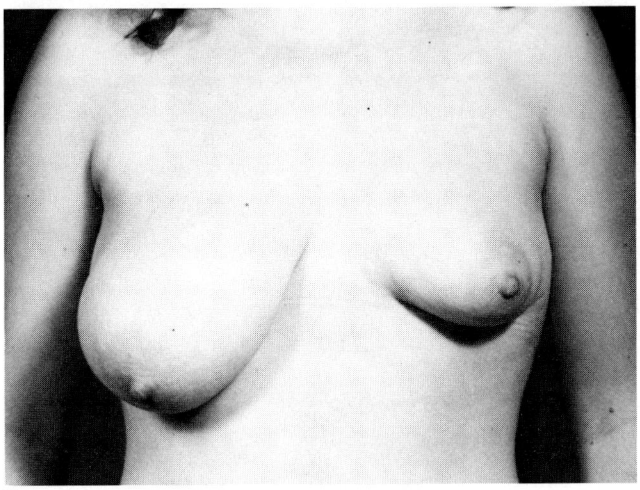

B

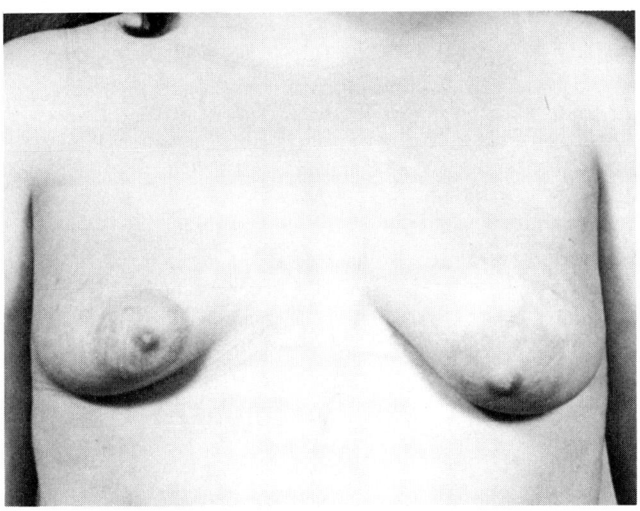

C

Figure 24-2. Ranges in degree of difficulty of average asymmetries influence the expected result.
A. Slight quantitative and NAC location asymmetry.
B. Marked quantitative asymmetry, but balance possible.
C. Deformed breasts with abnormal contour, result limited.

achieved with an inflatable prosthesis, obtaining overfill and then gradual reduction to ideal size. In general, the smaller breast is augmented to the desired size as determined by the skin envelope, and then the larger breast is increased to the same size. Contour discrepancies may require prostheses of varied shapes (low or high profile) and occasionally custom-made ones. Preoperative discrepancies in NAC position and size may persist. This problem can be minimized by a circumareolar incision with elevation of the lower NAC and circumareolar reduction of the larger areola when indicated. For example, the patient with an asymmetric 34A and 34AA configuration complicated by a higher (15-cm) and smaller (2.5-cm) areola on the more hypoplastic side would require a different procedure on each breast. On the more hypoplastic breast, a 200-cc implant would be inserted subpectorally through a periareolar incision while on the contralateral side an areolar reduction with subpectoral placement would be done. The amount of areola to be excised is determined from a pattern of the smaller breast following insertion of both implants.

Hypertrophy and Normal Breast

Unilateral hypertrophy represents the one category in which bilateral surgery is rarely necessary (Fig. 24-5). In this case, a B-technique is used, with all reference measurements taken from the "normal" breast. Thus, it is possible to achieve excellent symmetry of volume, consistency, and NAC position. However, contour similarity will depend on the condition of the normal breast [11]. The superior fullness of the adolescent breast cannot be restored to a flattened ptotic breast.

For example, the patient with an asymmetric 34D and 34B configuration would be advised to have a reduction on the hypertrophic side. It would be emphasized that approximately 400 cc of breast tissue would be excised. Also, the NAC size and location would approximate the normal side. However, fullness of the superior quadrants could not be achieved. If ptosis were present in the normal side, a skin-only B-mastopexy would be recommended, which would provide better symmetry and comparable scarring. As reported by Shulman and Westreich [39], it is possible to perform a modified volumetric reduction on the larger breast through a circumareolar incision and achieve symmetry when the discrepancy is less than 200 gm and ptosis is limited.

Hypertrophy and Hypertrophy

Bilateral hypertrophy of unequal degrees with variable ptosis allows attainment of truly symmetric breasts with similar volume, contour, NAC, and scars (Fig. 24-6). A standard B-technique reduction mammaplasty is done bilaterally with a greater resection on the larger side. Attainment of similar breasts should be the rule rather than the exception [47]. Since the majority of breast reductions have some degree of asymmetry, this category represents a variation of the typical case.

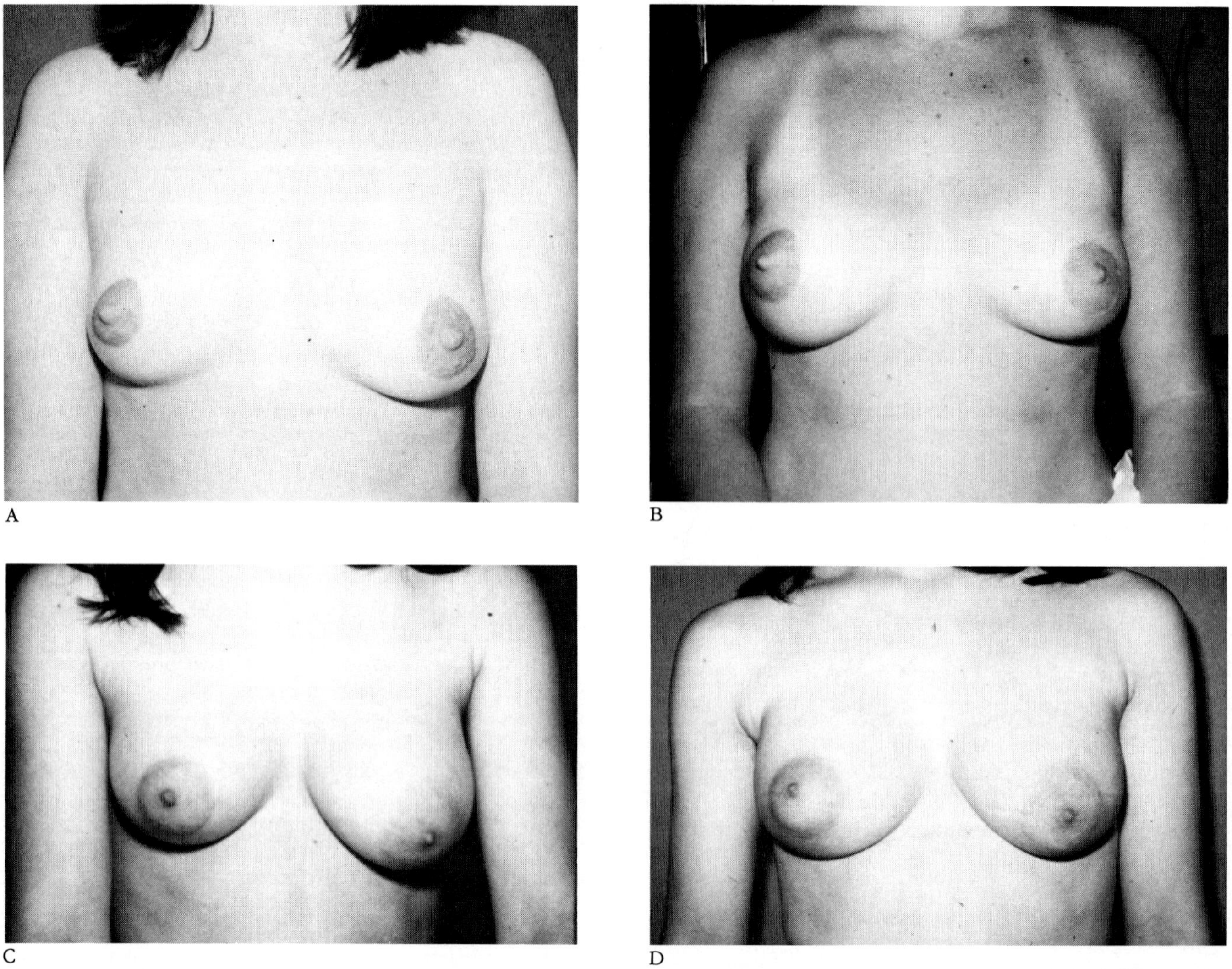

A B C D

Figure 24-3. Two patients with *hypoplasia–normal* breast deformity.

A, B. Patient with normal breast and hypoplasia corrected by 130-cc prosthesis on right. Symmetry of shape achieved.

C, D. Patient with right hypoplasia and normal left ptotic breast. Consent given for augmentation only on right side with 175-cc prosthesis. Ptosis of the normal breast remains.

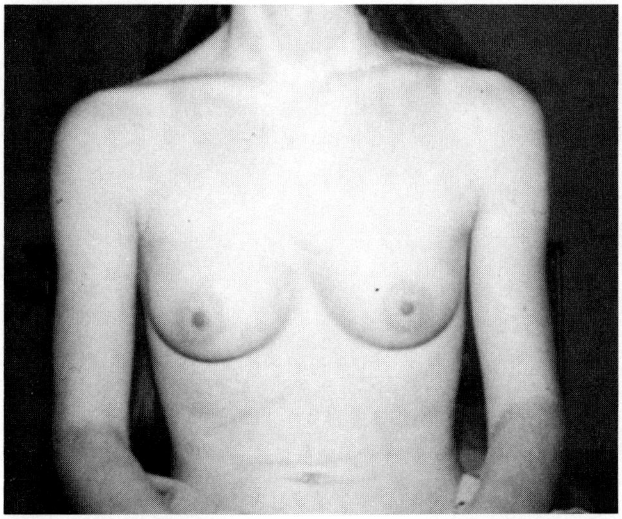

A

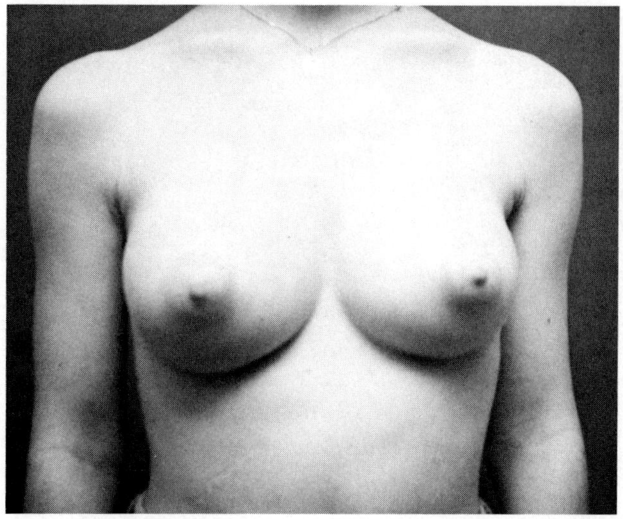

B

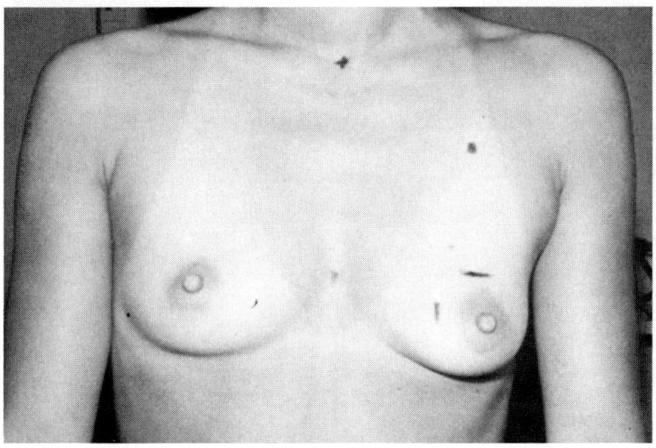

C

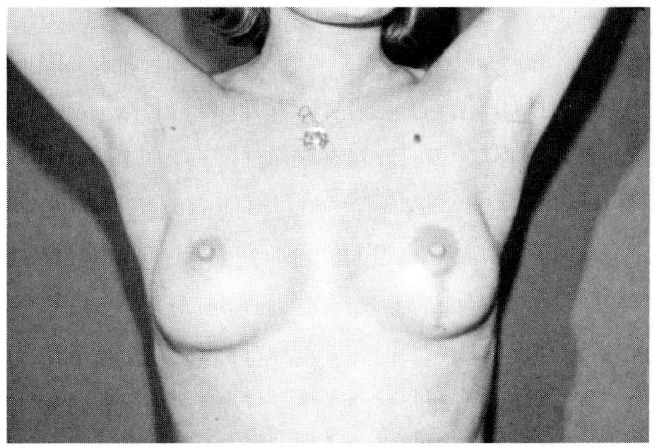

D

Figure 24-4. Two patients with ***hypoplasia-hypoplasia*** deformity.
A, B. Deformity improved with 140-cc prosthesis on right, 180-cc on left.
C, D. Bilateral hypoplasia plus asymmetric areolae and minor ptosis on left. Condition improved by bilateral augmentation (180 cc on right, 145 cc on left) plus a VOQ procedure on the left to achieve elevation of the NAC.
Note: Pure quantitative discrepancies are more easily corrected than those with areolar or glandular positional differences.

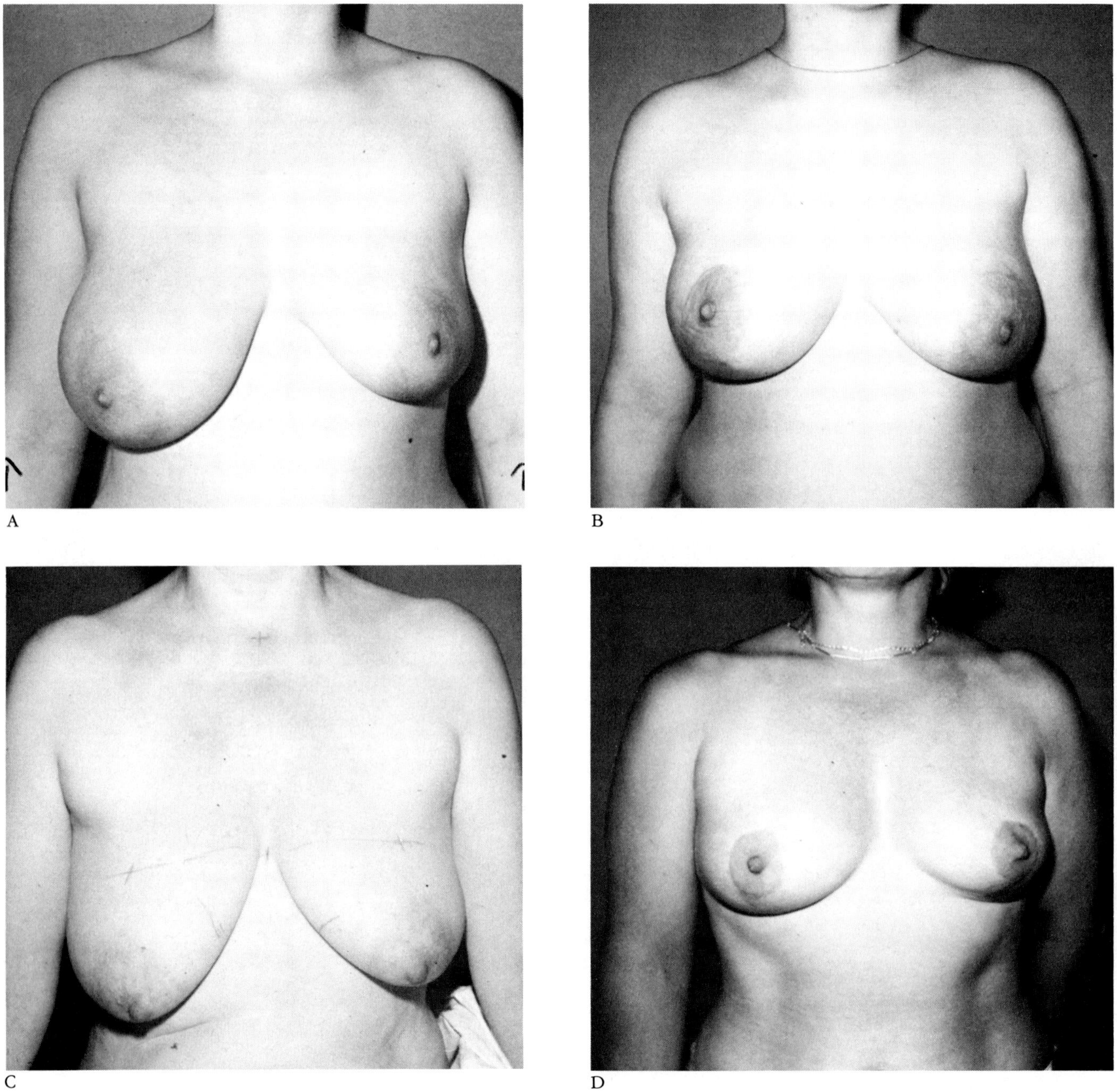

A B C D

Figure 24-5. Two patients with *hyperplasia–normal* breast deformity.

A, B. Patient with hyperplastic right breast reduced by 250 gm to match unoperated left breast.

C, D. Patient with hyperplastic right breast and ptotic left breast. Reduction of 200 gm on right and mastopexy only on left.

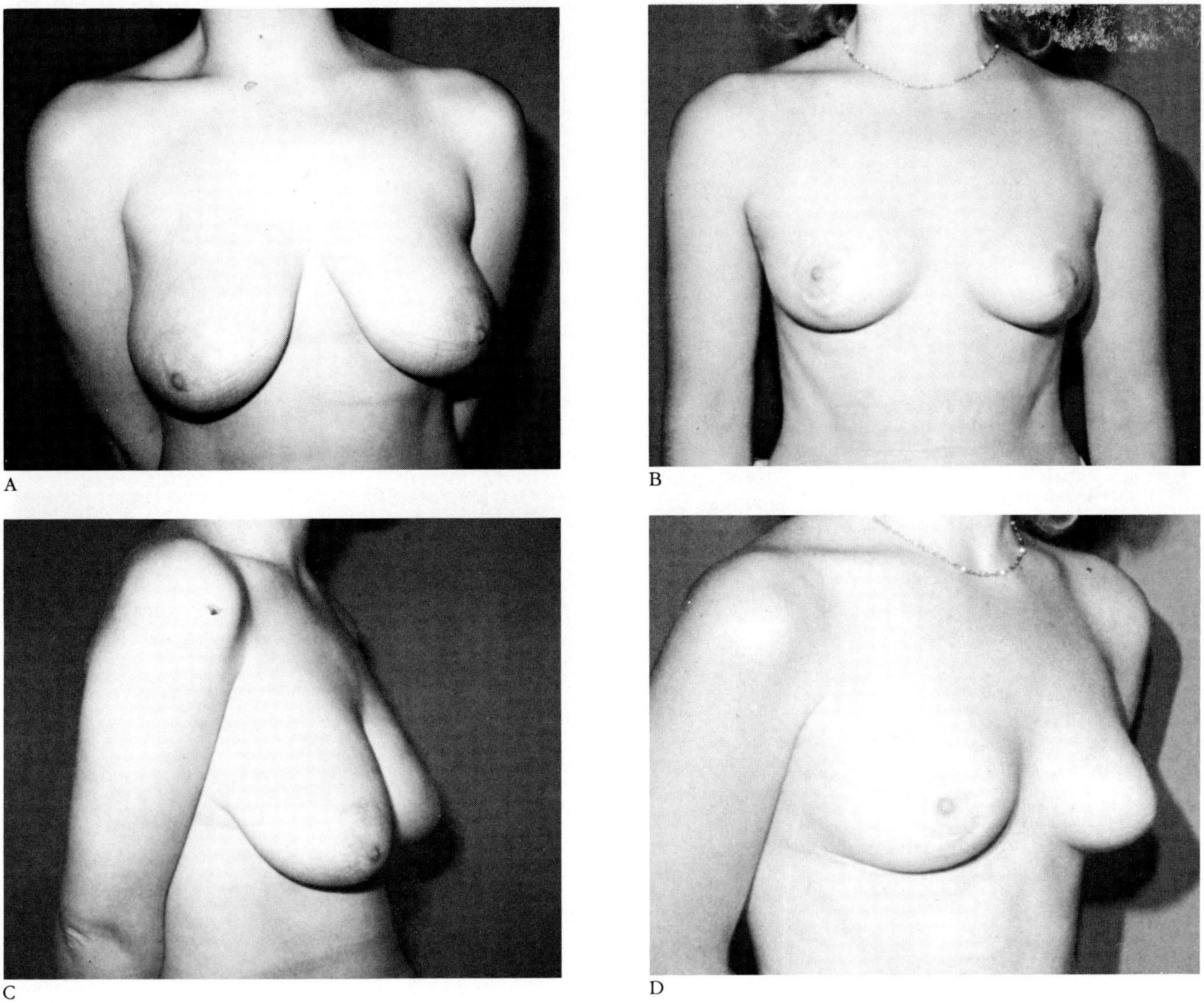

Figure 24-6. Patient with *hyperplasia-hyperplasia* deformity.
A, C. Patient with reduction 450 gm on the right and 200 gm on the left.
B, D. Result following unequal reduction.

Hypoplastic and Hypertrophic Breasts

This deformity is the most challenging of asymmetric deformities as it requires attainment of a comparative balance (Fig. 24-7). The obvious solution is an augmentation on the hypoplastic side and a reduction on the hypertrophic side [30]. Also, one must anticipate changes to be wrought by time: descent of the augmented breast or nipple elevation in the reduced breast. An implant is inserted subpectorally in the hypoplastic breast. The hypertrophic breast is reduced in accordance with measurements from the augmented breast, and a volume match is attained. Unless a small implant is simultaneously inserted in the reduced breast, contour deformities will persist.

The patient who presents with a 34A and 34D deformity would be satisfied with 34B and 34B, provided the NAC and breast contour are similar. To achieve this goal, the NAC is usually adjusted on the hypertrophic side to match the size and location on the hypoplastic side. Comparable contour can be achieved only if the patient agrees to a small augmentation behind the reduced breast.

Breast and Musculoskeletal Deformities

Correction of these problems depends on their multiplicity, their conspicuousness, and the patient's desires (Fig. 24-8). In certain cases, the patient is aware that the breasts are asymmetric but is not certain as to the causes. If the breasts can be made more equal without correction of the underlying deformity, the patient's objectives are usually achieved [5]. In other cases, simple addition of latissimus dorsi muscle will minimize pectoralis major deformities while excision of costochondral bossing will alleviate the deformity. With recent developments in breast reconstruction, the aesthetic surgeon is no longer dependent on a customized breast implant [18, 20]. Rather, one can selectively restore the individual deficiencies using latissimus muscle for pectoralis major, breast implants for breast tissue, and even areolar grafts. Previous problems of inadequate skin coverage are no longer a problem.

In 1980 Ohmori and Takada [26] reported on six patients, aged 5 to 40, who had latissimus muscle and myocutaneous flap transfers performed. Muscle was used to restore the anterior axillary border whereas a musculocutaneous flap was employed whenever an implant was necessary. Subsequently, Hester and Bostwick [13] presented eight cases: two prepubertal females, four postpubertal females, and two males. All of the female patients had insertion of an implant beneath a transferred latissimus muscle without incorporation of a skin flap. Some degree of NAC asymmetry persisted in all patients. Two postpubertal patients required procedures on the opposite breast. Thus, musculoskeletal deformities of the chest have passed from a subgroup of breast asymmetries to a type of breast reconstruction. Instead of solving the problem by augmentation alone, one employs multiple techniques.

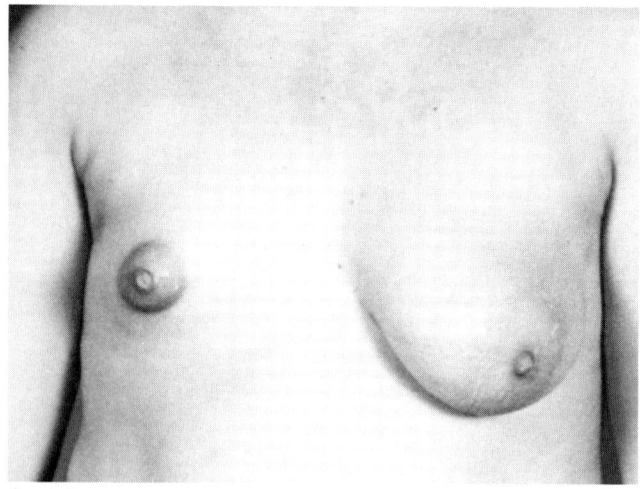

A

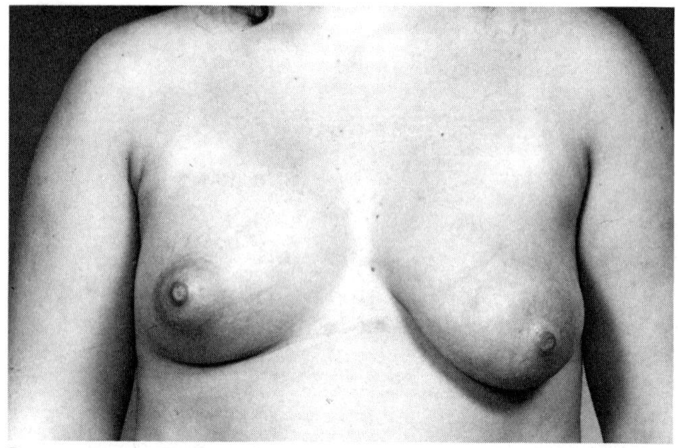

B

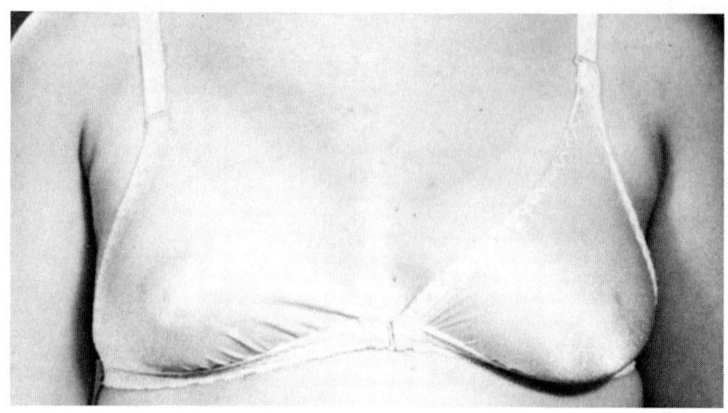

C

Figure 24-7. Patient with ***hypoplasia-hyperplasia*** deformity.
A. A 16-year-old patient with hypoplasia and hyperplasia who chose a two-stage procedure.
B. Following augmentation of right breast with a 275-cc prosthesis placed retropectorally.
C. Mastopexy with lower-pole resection (250 cc) and small upper quadrant augmentation (100-cc prosthesis) for the left breast is a future consideration. In the interim, symmetry has been improved underneath clothing.

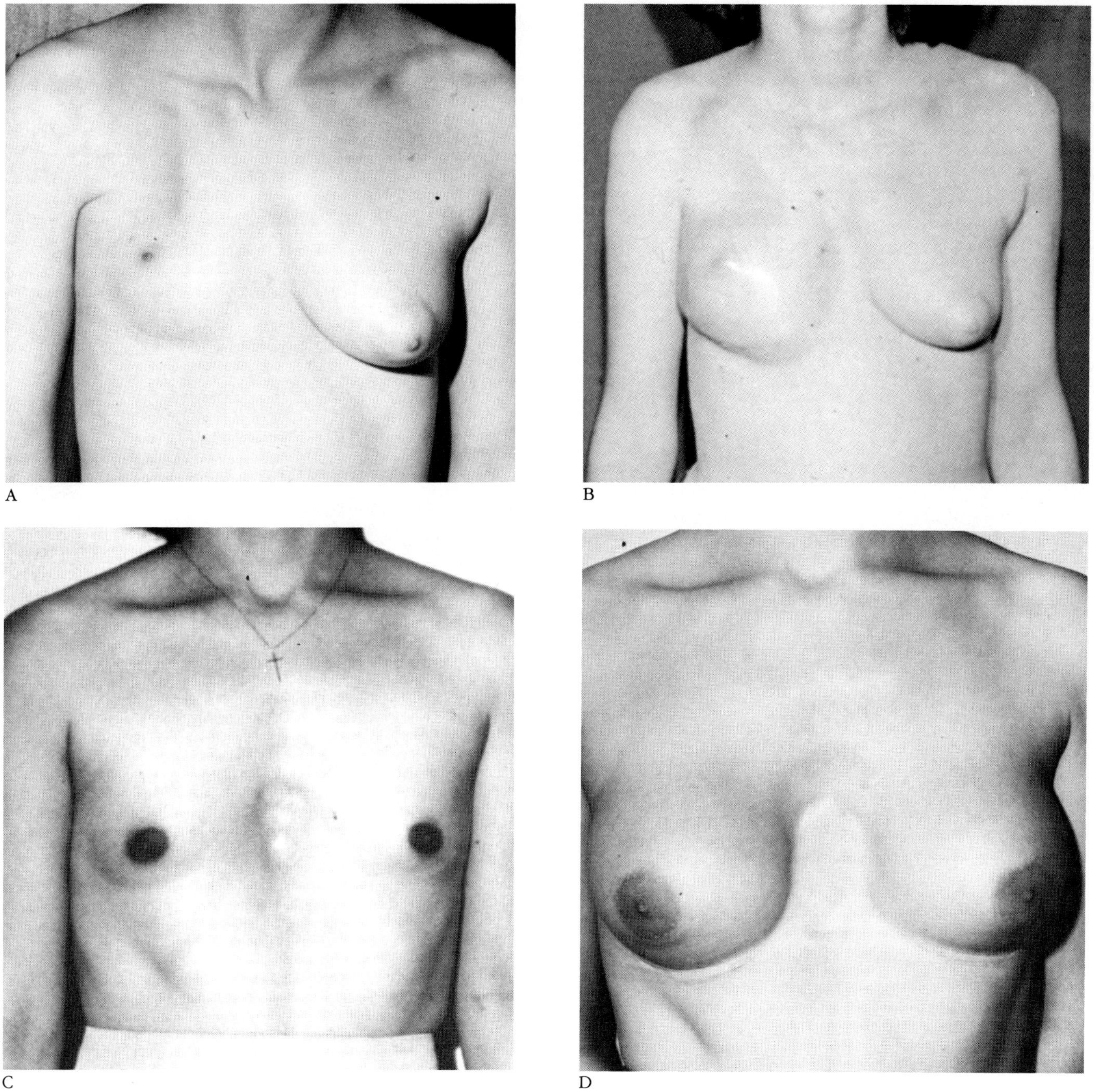

Figure 24-8. Two patients with chest wall and breast deformities.

A, B. Severe Poland's syndrome improved with unilateral custom-made implant.

C, D. Severe pectus excavatum deformity lessened with bilateral breast augmentation and custom-made sternal implant.

Pectus excavatum with breast hypoplasia is a common deformity and can be concealed by insertion of a sternal implant and bilateral augmentation mammaplasty [23]. We are opposed to a single implant incorporating all three prostheses because of the need for isolation in regard to possible occurrence of infection or capsule formation. In certain complicated problems involving breast, muscle, and bone, a custom-made breast implant can be fabricated and used to minimize the unilateral deficiency [27]. Symmetry will depend on the condition and treatment of the contralateral side.

COMPLICATIONS

The type, number, and chronologic onset of complications will be similar to those of augmentation, mastopexy, and reduction mammaplasties. However, the patient's satisfaction will be directly related to the severity of the asymmetry and inversely proportional to desire for perfection. Hueston [15] has commented that the "dissatisfied patient is more often due to lack of communication than to lack of contour." It is wise to emphasize preoperatively that one will try to minimize the difference but that perfect symmetry is impossible.

Breast Deformities

Most asymmetries represent quantitative and positional discrepancies rather than true breast deformities. Many deformities do exist that affect, singly or in combination, the nipple, areola, breast, and thorax. Discussions as to whether they represent arrested development or a true deformity tend to favor the latter [4]. Classification is virtually impossible, and most surgeons resort to a descriptive nomenclature, e.g., *tuberous breast, giant areolae.* The authors prefer to consider these problems as they affect the individual breast components plus the degree of severity.

Tuberous Breasts

The tuberous breast is characterized by a hypoplasia of the breast with a lack of fullness in the vertical and horizontal directions. Further compounding the problem may be areolar enlargement, herniation of glandular tissue into the NAC, asymmetric expression of the deformity, and ptosis. Rees and Aston [34] classify the deformity into two types: type I, a small concentric tuberous breast with herniation of breast tissue into the areola and a large areola, and type II, a flattened ptotic breast without herniation but with significant vertical dimension deficiency and a short horizontal base. Patients so afflicted consider themselves "deformed" and are generally pleased with surgical correction. A circumareolar incision is necessary to reduce areolar size and to reset the NAC into a natural position, while insertion of an implant provides shape [50].

TYPE I (TUBEROUS TYPE WITH HERNIATION)

The principal deformity is herniation of breast tissue into the areola. A standard augmentation accentuates the deformity by projecting the NAC. Correction requires a circumareolar excision with inward telescoping of the breast tissue (Fig. 24-9). For patients requesting larger breasts, the areola is reduced and telescoped while an implant is inserted through the areolar incision (Fig. 24-10). A two-stage procedure is not necessary [45]. As stressed by Williams and Hoffman [48] these cases range widely in severity, and one must be prepared to correct all three deformities: areolar herniation, volume deficiency, and ptosis.

TYPE II (TUBEROUS TYPE WITH PTOSIS)

Correction of these deformities depends on the degree of ptosis, extent of hypoplasia, and areolar size (Fig. 24-11). Since herniation of breast tissue beneath the areola is not a problem, it is possible to treat minor ptosis by augmentation alone. As noted by Rees [33], if the breast is to spread over the implant rather than project from it, the breast base must be expanded by radiating cuts from the center of the retromammary base.

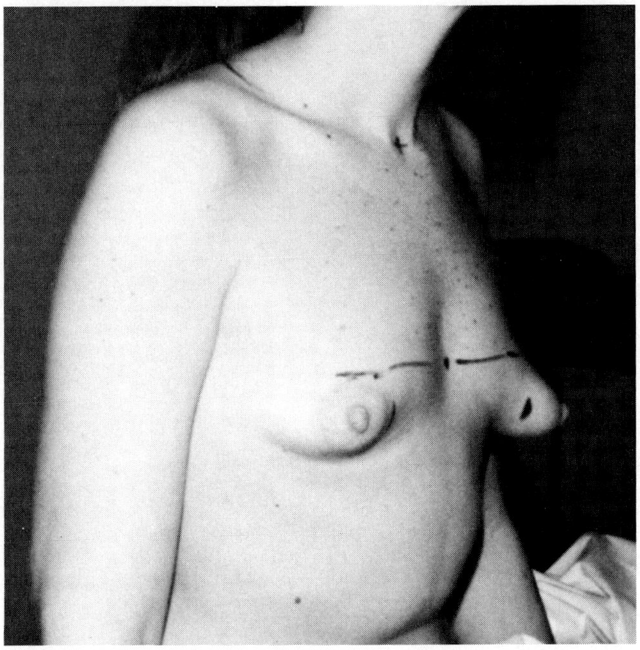

A

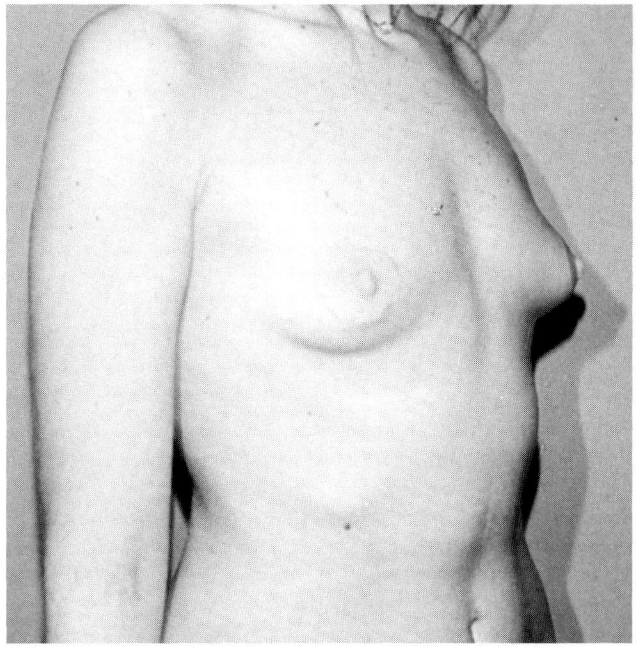

B

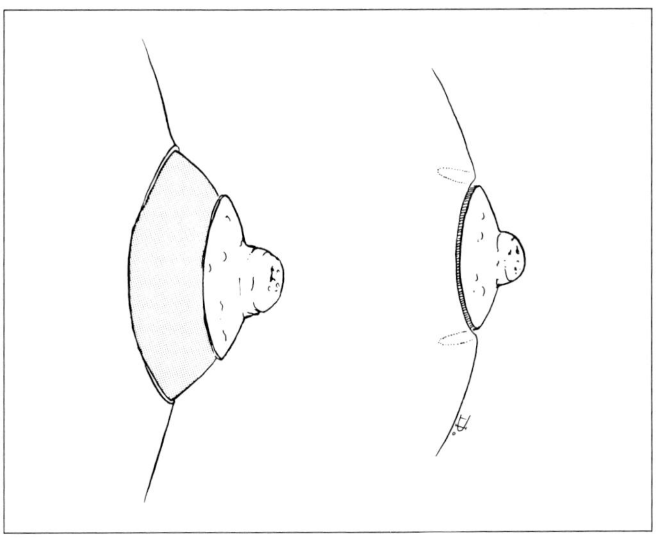

C

Figure 24-9
A. Patient with a classic tuberous breast who wished only correction of the deformity without augmentation.
B. Result following areolar strip excision and inward telescoping.
C. Operative technique.

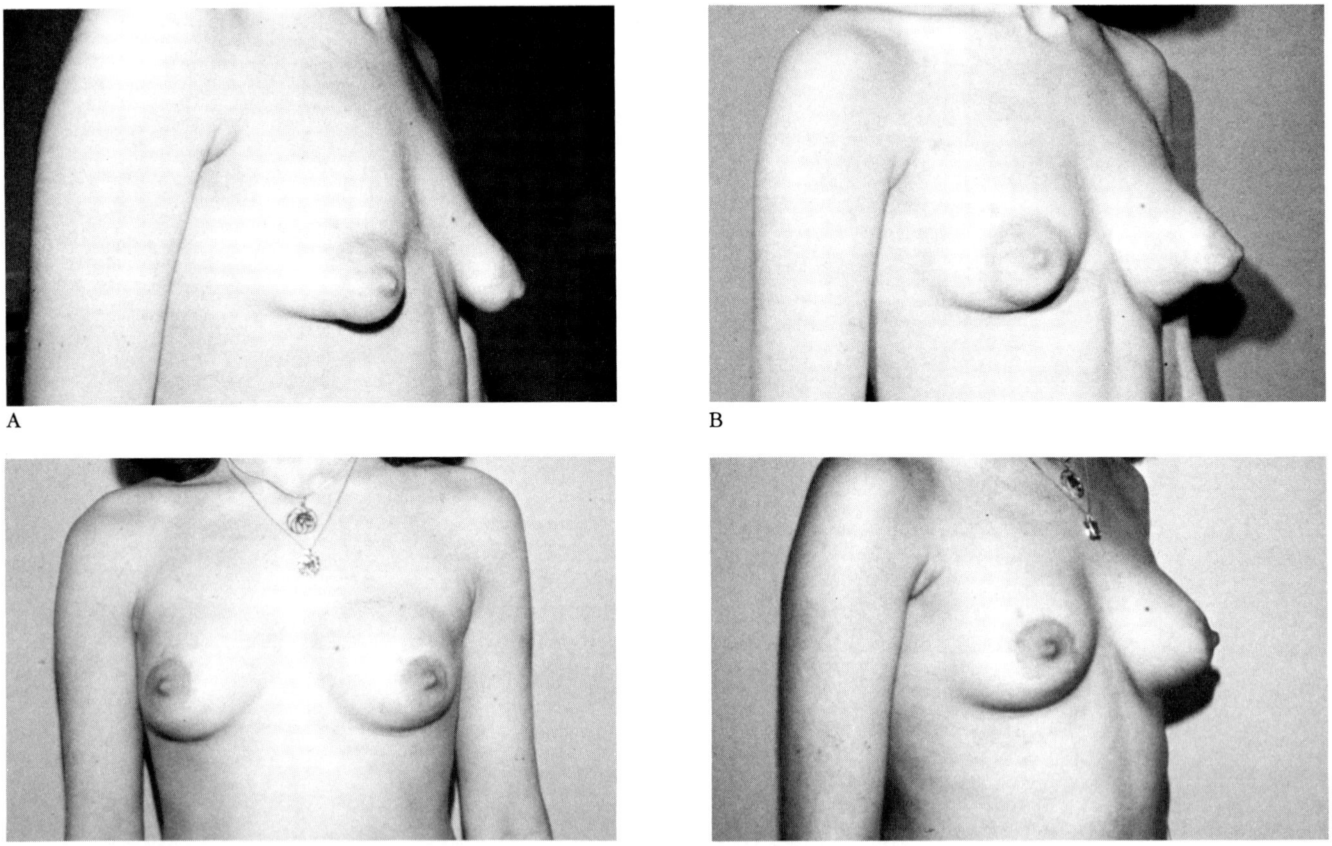

A B C D

Figure 24-10

A. Patient with tuberous breasts who insisted on augmentation and refused areolar incision.

B. The expected "Snoopy" deformity with persistent herniation of breast tissue into the areolae.

C, D. Six months later patient agreed to "telescoping" of the areolae. Neither excision of subareolar tissue nor incision of the breast was necessary; a superficial circling areolar strip excision was sufficient.

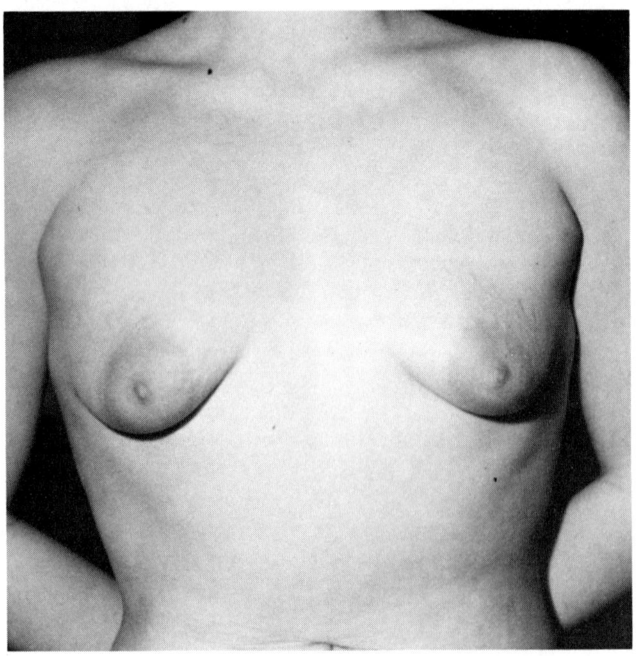

Figure 24-11. Hypoplasia with large areolae which some surgeons would consider the more subtle type II ptotic tuberous breast short in the vertical dimension.

Deformities of the NAC

In the mature patient, the nipple is an elevated portion of the areola containing the ampullae and orifices of 15 to 20 lactiferous ducts. The areola is modified skin without hair follicles or sweat glands. Color variations, from pink to brown, reflect vascularity, endocrine influences, and race. There are numerous modified sebaceous glands (Montgomery's glands), which secrete the necessary lubrication for the areola and papilla during lactation. Beneath the areola there is a superficial, nonstriated circular muscle layer in contact with the dermis and vertical muscle bands present centrally in the nipple. These muscles are controlled by the sympathetic nervous system and cause erection of the nipple. Functionally, this contraction facilitates emptying of the lactiferous ducts secondary to physical and psychologic stimulation. The present text deals with developmental aesthetic problems and not acquired deformities that necessitate reconstruction.

Common nipple deformities include supernumerary nipples, athelia, duplication, and associated skin lesions [6, 42, 43]. However, patients most frequently request correction of nipple inversion or hypertrophy.

Nipple Inversion

This condition may be classified as either umbilication, a spontaneously correctable depression, or inversion, a fixed invagination [19]. It occurs most commonly in women with large pendulous breasts, and one is wise to note its presence prior to reduction mammaplasty [29]. Basch [1] attributed inversion to absence of the underlying circular muscle fibers (Sappey's muscle). However, Schwager's [38] studies showed a diminution in the amount of dense connective tissue beneath the inverted nipple (0.4 cm versus normal 0.8 cm), indicating that the etiology is a quantitative difference. In mastectomy specimens, eversion was possible following excision of the dense connective tissue but not after isolated ductal transection.

The classic indications for surgery are a desire to nurse following pregnancy and psychologic concern for symmetry. The myriad operations available attest to the difficulties of achieving a functional everted nipple with sensation. Skoog [41] designed a starburst operation in which a more protuberant nipple is formed from folded areolar skin. Conversion of the areola into a nipple diminishes and scars the areola without everting the underlying nipple. In the majority of our cases, the patient is more concerned about the deformity, which is often unilateral, and will sacrifice function for appearance [37]. Thus, we make a short (5-mm) perinipple incision in the 9 o'clock position and, with traction on the nipple, sever the restricting connective tissue and ductal fibers until the nipple retains its eversion (Fig. 24-12). A purse-string suture is inserted around the nipple and removed in 5 days. The perinipple incision is closed with 5-0 plain sutures. In contrast to Hamilton [12], we do not insert deep sutures, nor are local flaps necessary, as suggested by Elsahy [8] and Teimoirian and Adham [44]. We also use this method for simultaneous correction of inversion associated with reduction or augmentation mammaplasty (Fig. 24-13). We have not found extensive undermining necessary. Caution is advised in the young patient who is uncertain whether she wants to nurse and who is concerned about a minimal scar or possible diminution in sensation. Ramakrishan and Rao [31] reported a series of 17 patients, of whom 3 had severance of the hypertrophied areolar muscle (Basch procedure), which failed, and 14 had release of tethering ducts (Schwager procedure), which succeeded in all cases. Of note: The deformity remained corrected at 2 years, and seven patients subsequently became pregnant and were able to nurse.

Nipple Hypertrophy

In contrast to nipple inversion, the hypertrophic or elongated nipple is rarely a presenting problem. Rather, it is often associated with hypoplasia or hypertrophy and calls for a concomitant correction. The deformity is usually bilateral and familial, with protuberance that increases after pregnancy. Nipple discharge, pain, or malignancy is rarely present. The hypertrophic nipple increases from its normal 1-cm projection and 1-cm diameter to a length of 2 cm and occasionally a diameter of 2 cm.

Surgical correction is achieved with a simple pericylindric excision (circumcision) of skin and superficial muscles (Fig. 24-14). The lower incision is made 5 mm above the areolar level and the upper incision around the nipple surface [36]. All of the intervening skin and superficial muscles are excised; no undermining is done. The nipple is then telescoped inward and the wound closed with a simple subcuticular running suture. Concurrent breast augmentation or reduction may be done (Fig. 24-15).

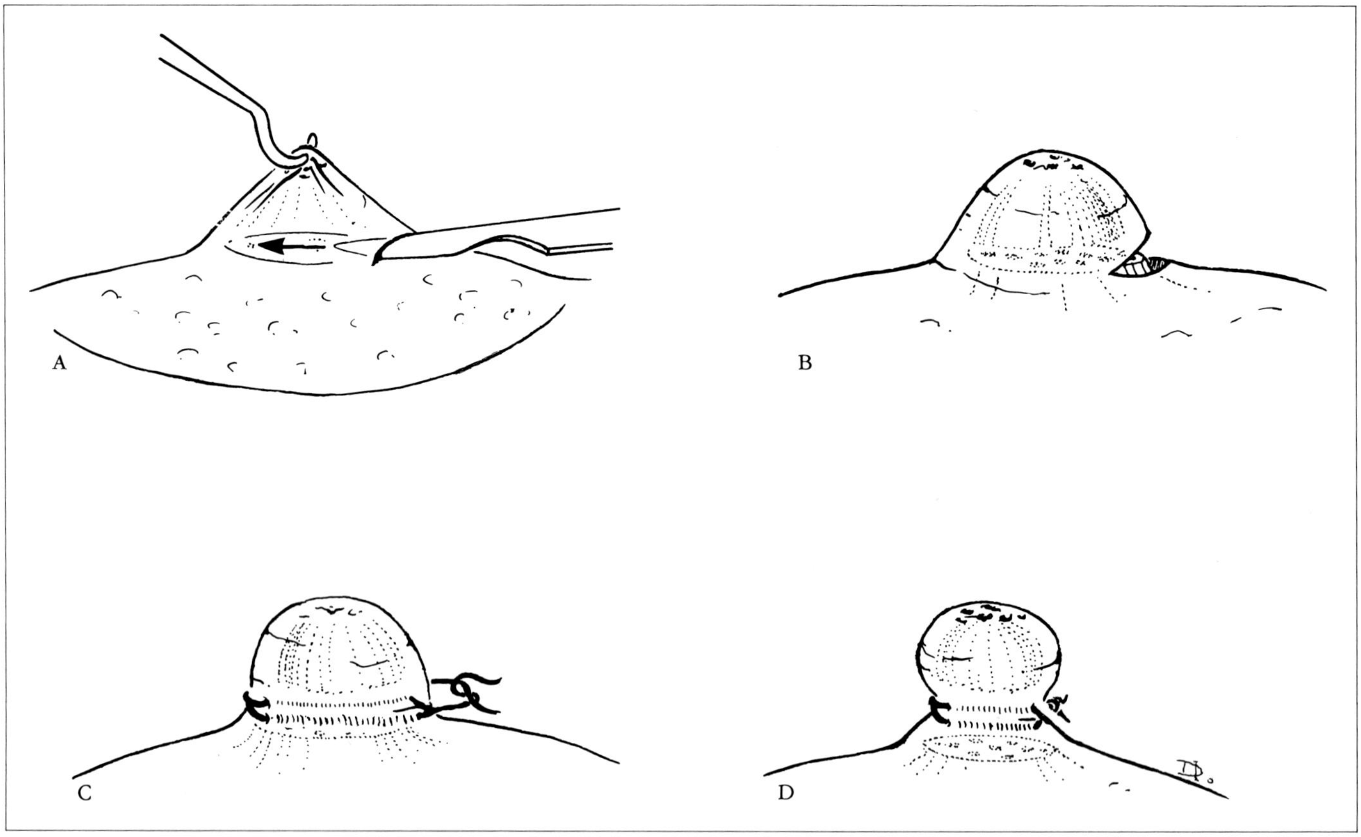

Figure 24-12. Operative technique for correcting nipple inversion.
A. Under traction, a short incision is made at the nipple base.
B. All restricting structures are cut.
C, D. Eversion is maintained with a loose purse-string suture.

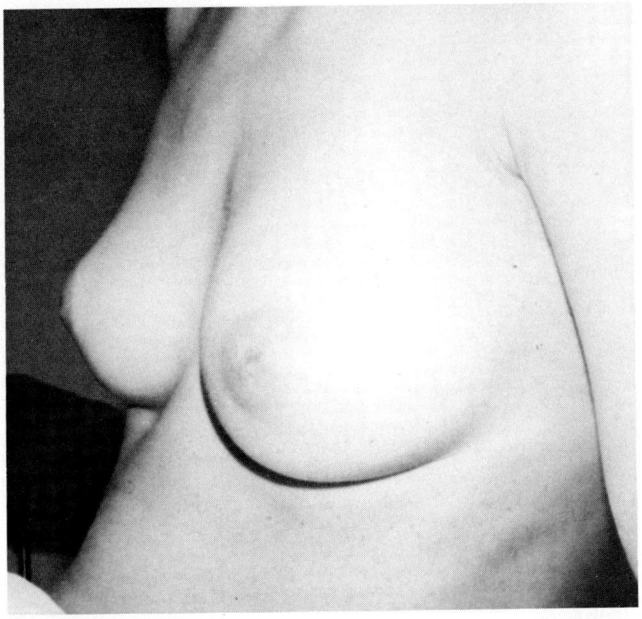

A

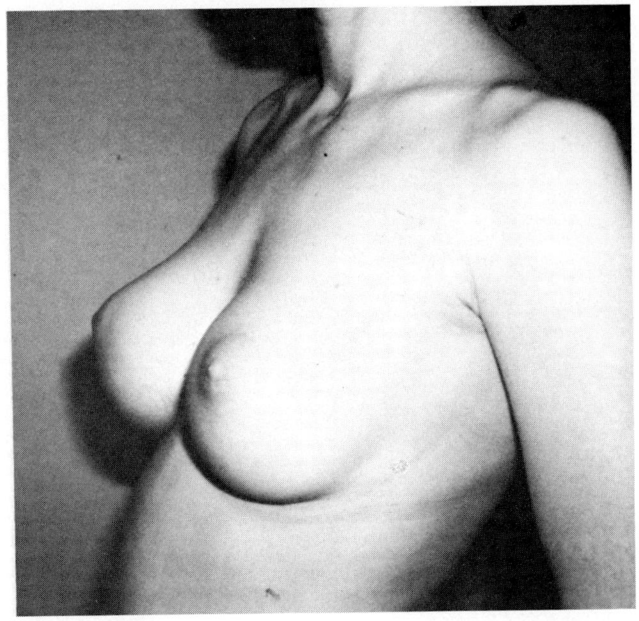

B

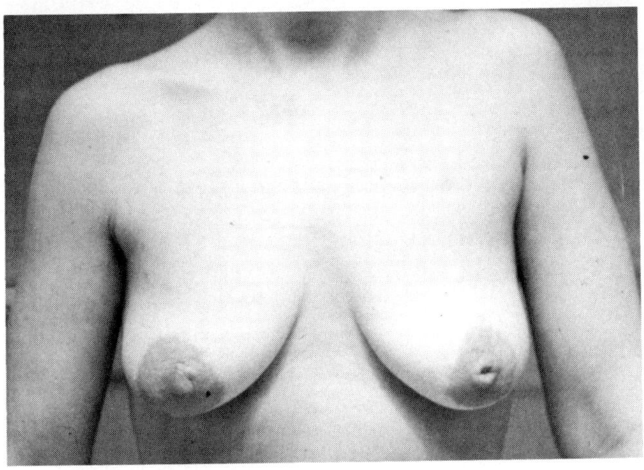

C

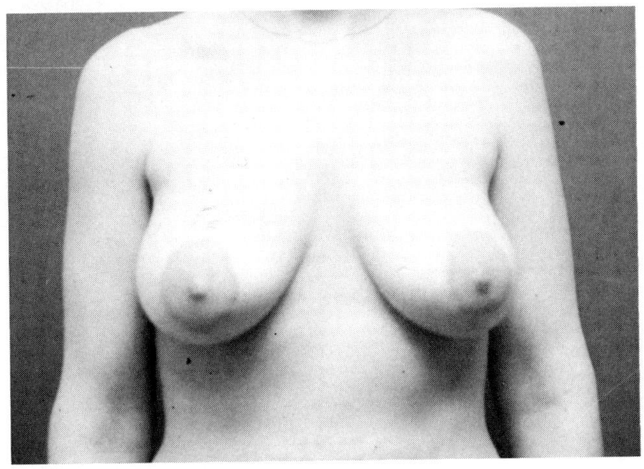

D

Figure 24-13. Two patients with nipple inversion.
A, B. Patient with nipple inversion. Result following augmentation and nipple eversion by use of the described technique.
C, D. Improvement following simultaneous breast reduction and correction of nipple inversion.

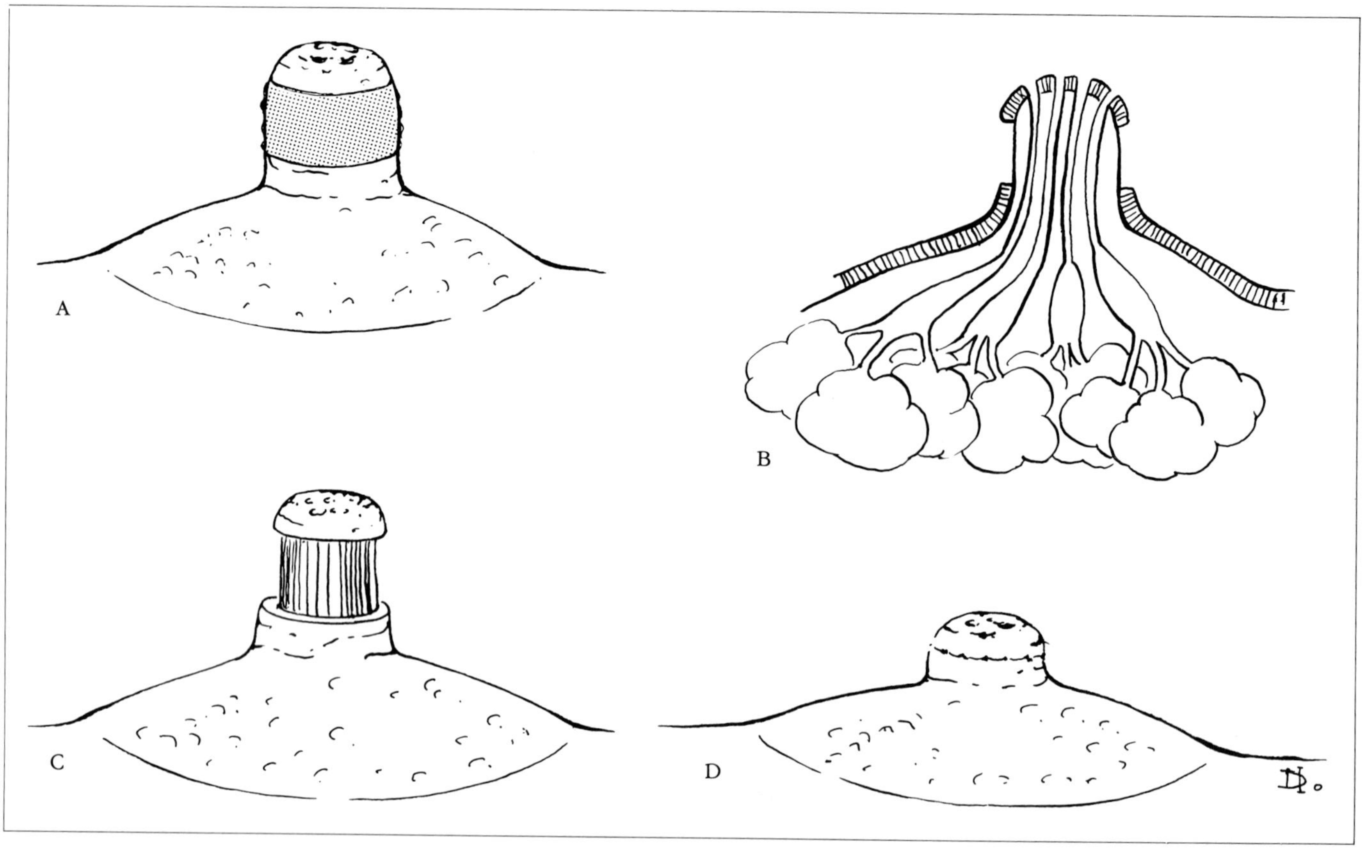

Figure 24-14. Operative technique for reduction of nipple hyperplasia.
A, B. A partial-thickness circumcision is done.
C, D. The elongated nipple is telescoped inward and sutured.

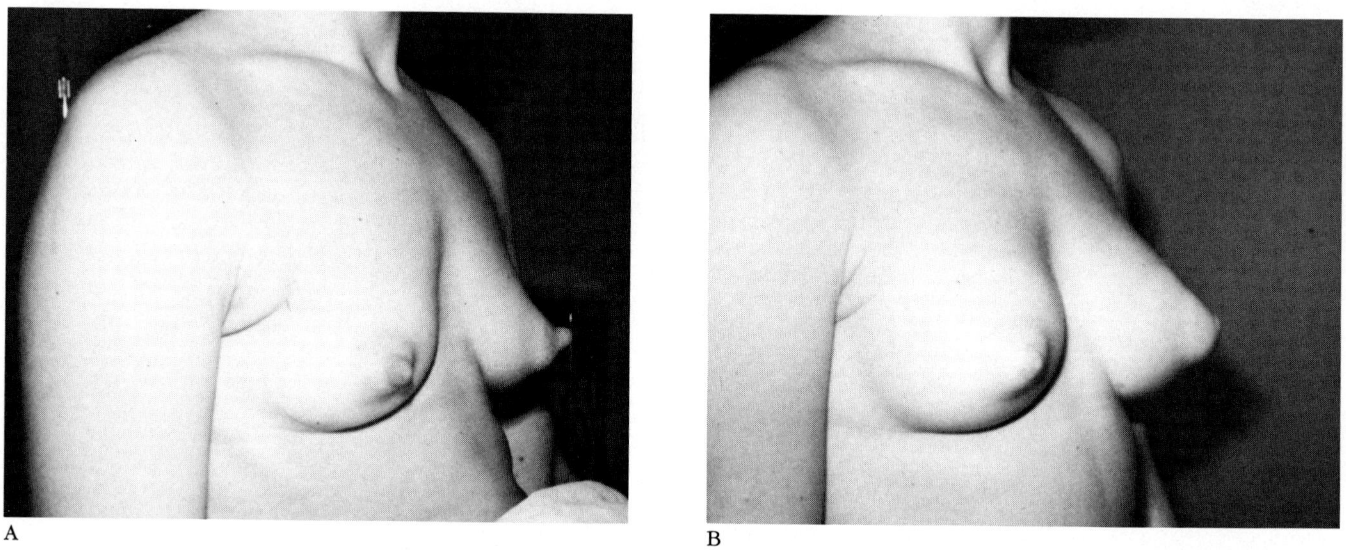

Figure 24-15. Patient with breast hypoplasia and nipple hyperplasia corrected by breast augmentation and nipple reduction.

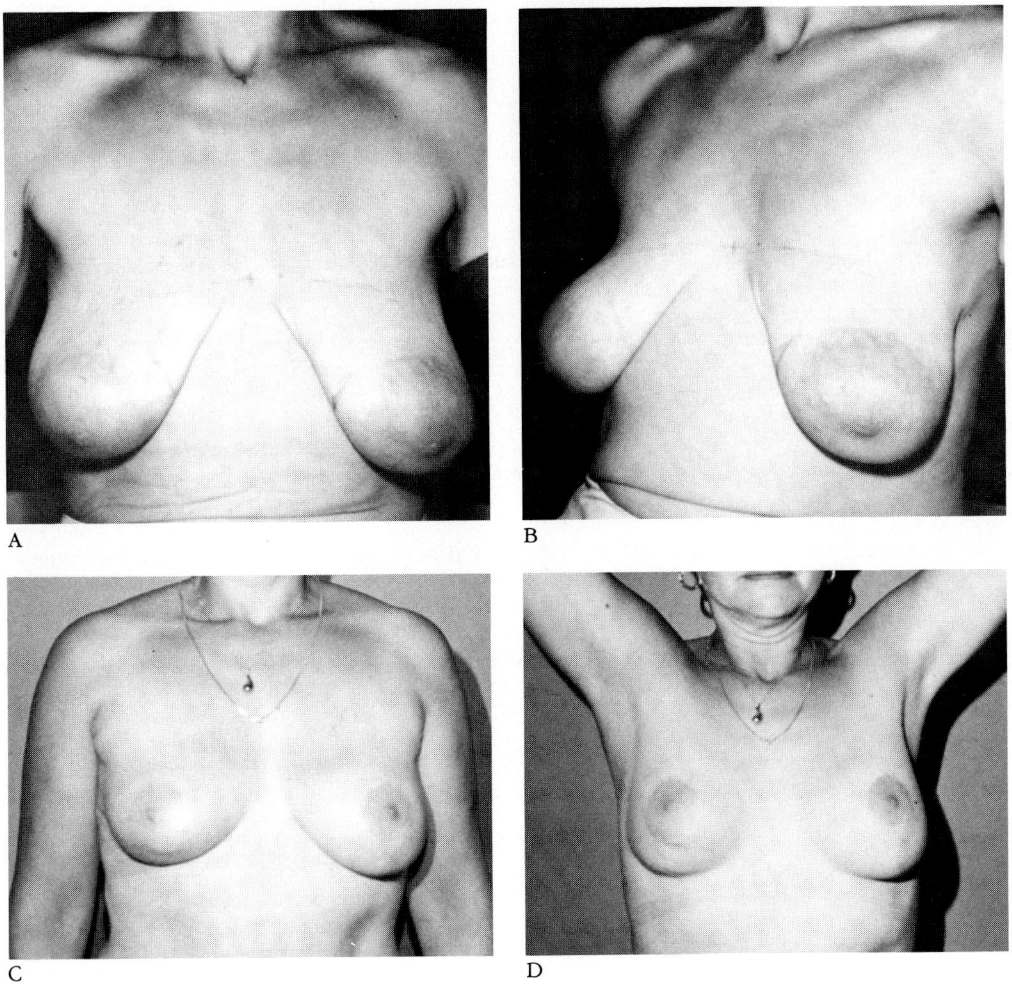

Figure 24-16
A, B. Patient with giant areolae and major breast ptosis.
C, D. Result following B-mastopexy and augmentation. Note complete excision of excess areolar tissue.

Areolar Deformities

Although a common concern of patients seeking reduction mammaplasty, areolar deformities are rarely a presenting complaint. Occasionally, patients will inquire as to the feasibility of altering a dark pigmentation and returning to a pink coloration. Equally impossible is correction of the small areola without significant scarring.

In cases of large areolae (5–10 cm) it is possible to reduce the dimension by means of a VOQ excision. Initially, one would think that a circumareolar reduction would suffice. Unfortunately, tension on the surrounding skin will stretch the areola, resulting in reestablishment of its large diameter and often an unacceptable scar. In most instances, correction of isolated areolar deformities is not worth the resulting scar. Rarely, a patient seeking a reduction mammaplasty or mastopexy will have giant areolae (>10 cm), which exceed the width of most T-pattern reductions but are easily accommodated by a B-technique that maximizes periareolar skin excision (Fig. 24-16).

It is the senior author's opinion that these areolae have a deficient muscular component that leads to excessive stretch during pregnancy but precludes constriction on involution. As noted by McKissock [25], pattern reductions used for giant areolae leave pigmentation in the lower flaps, thus necessitating a second procedure. In contrast, the B-technique with its periareolar skin resection is ideally suited for correction of giant areolae.

REFERENCES

1. Basch, K. Zur Anatomie und Physiologie dur Brustwarze. *Arch. Gynaekol.* 44:36, 1893.
2. Broadbent, T. R., and Woolf, R. M. Unsatisfactory results in augmentation mammoplasty: Chest and breast asymmetry. *Aesthetic Plast. Surg.* 2:251, 1978.
3. Corso, P. F. Plastic surgery of unilateral hypoplastic breast. *Plast. Reconstr. Surg.* 50:134, 1972.
4. Daniel, W. A., Jr. *The Adolescent Patient.* St. Louis: Mosby, 1970.
5. De Saxe, B. M. The reconstruction of unequal or absent breasts. *S. Afr. Med. J.* 51:919, 1977.
6. Elliott, R. A., and Hoehn, J. G. Asymmetrical Breasts. In N. G. Georgiade (ed.), *Reconstructive Breast Surgery.* St. Louis: Mosby, 1976. P. 89.

7. Elliott, R. A., Hoehn, J. G., and Greminger, R. F. Correction of asymmetrical breasts. *Plast. Reconstr. Surg.* 56:260, 1975.
8. Elsahy, N. J. An alternative operation for inverted nipple. *Plast. Reconstr. Surg.* 57:438, 1976.
9. Glasmer, E. *Deformities and Plastic Operations of the Female Breast.* Stuttgart: Enke, 1930.
10. Goldwyn, R. M. Problem Cases. In R. M. Goldwyn (ed.), *Plastic and Reconstructive Surgery of the Breast.* Boston: Little, Brown, 1976. P. 503.
11. Goulian, D. Mammaplasty for Asymmetric Breasts. In J. Q. Owsley and R. A. Peterson (eds.), *Symposium on Aesthetic Surgery of the Breast.* St. Louis: Mosby, 1978. P. 99.
12. Hamilton, J. M. Inverted nipples. *Plast. Reconstr. Surg.* 65:507, 1980.
13. Hester, T. R., and Bostwick, J. Poland's syndrome: Correction with latissimus muscle transposition. *Plast. Reconstr. Surg.* 69:226, 1982.
14. Horton, C. E., et al. The unilateral hypoplastic breast. *Br. J. Plast. Surg.* 23:161, 1970.
15. Hueston, J. T. Unilateral Agenesis and Hypoplasia: Difficulties and Suggestions. In R. M. Goldwyn (ed.), *Plastic and Reconstructive Surgery of the Breast.* Boston: Little, Brown, 1976.
16. Hughes, E. S. R. The development of the mammary gland. *Ann. R. Coll. Surg. Engl.* 6:99, 1950.
17. Kirianoff, T. G. Volumetric measurements of unequal breasts. *Plast. Reconstr. Surg.* 54:616, 1974.
18. Krause, J. L., Crikelair, G. F., and Cosman, B. The Cronin implant in the treatment of combined chest wall and breast deformities. *Plast. Reconstr. Surg.* 44:536, 1969.
19. Lamont, E. Congenital inversion of the nipple in identical twins. *Br. J. Plast. Surg.* 26:178, 1973.
20. Lavey, E., et al. Customized silicone implants of the breast and chest. *Plast. Reconstr. Surg.* 69:646, 1982.
21. Letterman, G., and Schurter, M. History of the Surgical Correction of Mammary Asymmetry. In J. Q. Owsley and R. A. Peterson (eds.), *Symposium in Aesthetic Surgery of the Breast.* St. Louis: Mosby, 1978.
22. Maliniac, J. W. *Breast Deformities and Their Repair.* New York: Waverly, 1950.
23. Masson, J. K., Payne, W. S., and Gonzalez, J. B. Pectus excavatum: Use of preform prostheses for correction in adults. *Plast. Reconstr. Surg.* 46:399, 1970.
24. Mathews, R. E. Bilateral absence of breasts. *N.Y. State J. Med.* 74:87, 1974.
25. McKissock, P. M. Reduction Mammaplasty. In E. H. Courtiss (ed.), *Aesthetic Surgery: Trouble—How to Avoid It and How to Treat It.* St. Louis: Mosby, 1978.
26. Ohmori, K., and Takada, H. Correction of Poland's pectoralis major abnormality with latissimus dorsi musculocutaneous flaps. *Plast. Reconstr. Surg.* 65:400, 1980.
27. Perras, C. Asymmetry of the breast and the thoracic cage. *Aesthetic Plast. Surg.* 4:117, 1980.
28. Pers, M. Aplasias of the anterior thoracic wall, the pectoral muscles, and the breast. *Scand. J. Plast. Reconstr. Surg.* 2:125, 1968.
29. Pitanguy, I. Inverted nipple. *Aesthetic Plast. Surg.* 2:53, 1978.
29a. Pontes, R. Single stage reconstruction of the missing breast. *Br. J. Plast. Surg.* 26:377, 1973.
30. Radlauer, C. B., and Bowers, D. G. Treatment of severe breast asymmetry. *Plast. Reconstr. Surg.* 47:347, 1971.
31. Ramakrishan, K. M., and Rao, D. K. Congenital inversion of the human nipple. *Aesthetic Plast. Surg.* 4:65, 1980.
32. Ravitch, M. M. Poland's syndrome: A study of an eponym. *Plast. Reconstr. Surg.* 59:508, 1977.
33. Rees, T. D. Mammary asymmetry. *Clin. Plast. Surg.* 2:371, 1975.
34. Rees, T. D., and Aston, S. J. The tuberous breast. *Clin. Plast. Surg.* 3:339, 1976.
35. Rees, T. D., and Dupuis, C. C. Unilateral mammary hypoplasia. *Plast. Reconstr. Surg.* 41:307, 1968.
36. Regnault, P. Nipple hypertrophy. *Clin. Plast. Surg.* 2:391, 1975.
37. Regnault, P. Ptosis, Asymmetry, Tubular Breast, and Congenital Anomalies. In J. Q. Owsley and R. A. Peterson (eds.), *Symposium on Aesthetic Surgery of the Breast.* St. Louis: Mosby, 1978.
38. Schwager, R. G., et al. Inversion of the human female nipple with a simple method of treatment. *Plast. Reconstr. Surg.* 54:564, 1974.
39. Shulman, Y., and Westreich, M. Treatment of mild breast asymmetry. *Plast. Reconstr. Surg.* 67:31, 1981.
40. Simon, B. E., Hoffman, S., and Kahn, S. Treatment of asymmetry of breasts. *Clin. Plast. Surg.* 2:375, 1975.
41. Skoog, T. An operation for inverted nipples. *Br. J. Plast. Surg.* 5:65, 1952.
42. Snyder, C. C., Browne, E. Z., and Pickens, J. E. Reconstructive Problems of the Nipple and Areola. In R. M. Goldwyn (ed.), *Plastic and Reconstructive Surgery of the Breast.* Boston: Little, Brown, 1976.
43. Snyder, G. B. Ptosis, Asymmetry and Tubular Breasts. In J. Q. Owsley and R. A. Peterson (eds.), *Symposium on Aesthetic Surgery of the Breast.* St. Louis: Mosby, 1978. P. 117.
44. Teimoirian, B., and Adham, M. Simple technique for correction of inverted nipple. *Plast. Reconstr. Surg.* 65:504, 1980.
45. Toranto, I. R. Two-stage correction of tuberous breasts. *Plast. Reconstr. Surg.* 67:642, 1981.
46. Trier, W. C. Complete breast absence. *Plast. Reconstr. Surg.* 36:430, 1965.
47. Weatherley-White, R. C. A. *Plastic Surgery of the Female Breast.* New York: Harper & Row, 1980.
48. Williams, G., and Hoffman, S. Mammoplasty for tubular breasts. *Aesthetic Plast. Surg.* 5:51, 1981.
49. Williams, J. E. Complete breast absence. *Plast. Reconstr. Surg.* 49:253, 1972.
50. Williams, J. E. Discussion of "two-stage correction of tuberous breasts." *Plast. Reconstr. Surg.* 67:642, 1981.

VI. Body Contouring

25. Abdominoplasty

Paule Regnault
Rollin K. Daniel

Abdominal dermolipectomies are surgical excisions of excess skin and fat in patients with obesity (abdominal lipectomies) or redundant tissue (abdominoplasties) [88]. Since the problems are quite diverse, the aesthetic surgeon must employ a variety of techniques. In addition, patients are now demanding finer aesthetic results, including a minimally visible scar and a natural-appearing umbilicus. These challenges can be met provided careful preoperative planning is combined with meticulous attention to detail.

HISTORY

In the early 1900s abdominoplasties were essentially panniculectomies, and only in the 1960s did aesthetic dermolipectomies become common. The first panniculectomy was reported by Kelly [54, 55] in 1899 and consisted of a 7450-gm resection (90 cm long, 31 cm wide, and 7 cm thick); a transverse incision was used. Subsequently, numerous procedures were devised that are best classified according to the type of incision: transverse, vertical, or mixed [49] (Fig. 25-1). Kelly's original procedure was modified by Passot [62] to include undermining and by Thorek [97, 98] to preserve the umbilicus [20, 21]. Vernon [99] introduced the concept of umbilical transposition with extensive undermining and relocation of the umbilicus.

During the 1950s dermolipectomies were done in South America by numerous surgeons including Somalo [93–95], Iturraspe, [45–47], Serson [90–92], and others [57, 87] (Fig. 25-2). However, it was Pitanguy's [63–69] publication of a series of 300 abdominal lipectomies that drew widespread interest. He used a horizontal incision with downward curvature at its extremes. In 1972 Regnault [75–82] introduced the W-technique with its incision in the upper pubic hair medially and along the inguinal fold laterally. The principle of flexing the table at the midline with tension brought onto the hips was shown for the first time. Subsequently, Baroudi [8, 9] published his experience and stressed the need for a meticulous umbilicoplasty. Grazer [35–40] modified the Pitanguy incision to a gull-wing incision, which did not encroach on the thighs, and recommended a more superior skin-line incision for the corpulent patient. The standard transverse incision was extended circumferentially by Somalo [95] and Gonzalez-Ulloa [33, 34] to achieve a "belt" lipectomy for the obese patient.

Vertical excisions were demonstrated by Babcock [5, 6] in 1916 and later championed by Fischl [26]. Mixed incisions, which have both a vertical and a transverse component, were introduced by Weinhold [104] and Galtier [28,

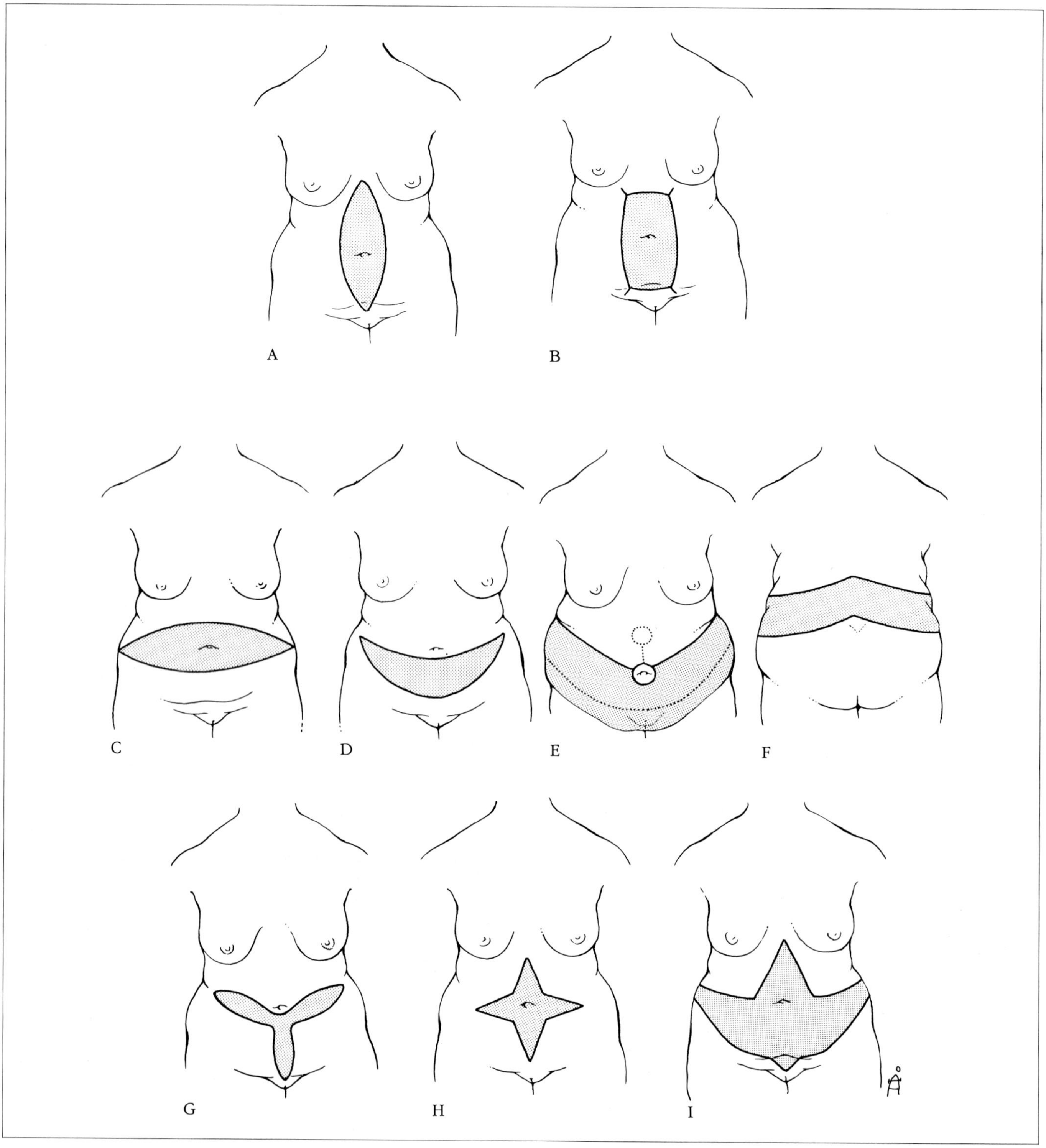

Figure 25-1. Types of incisions for abdominal lipectomy and abdominoplasty.

A, B. Vertical incisions: Babcock, Kuster.

C–F. Transverse incisions: Kelly, Thorek, and Gonzalez-Ulloa.

G–I. Combined incisions: Weinhold, Galtier, and Castanares-Goethel.

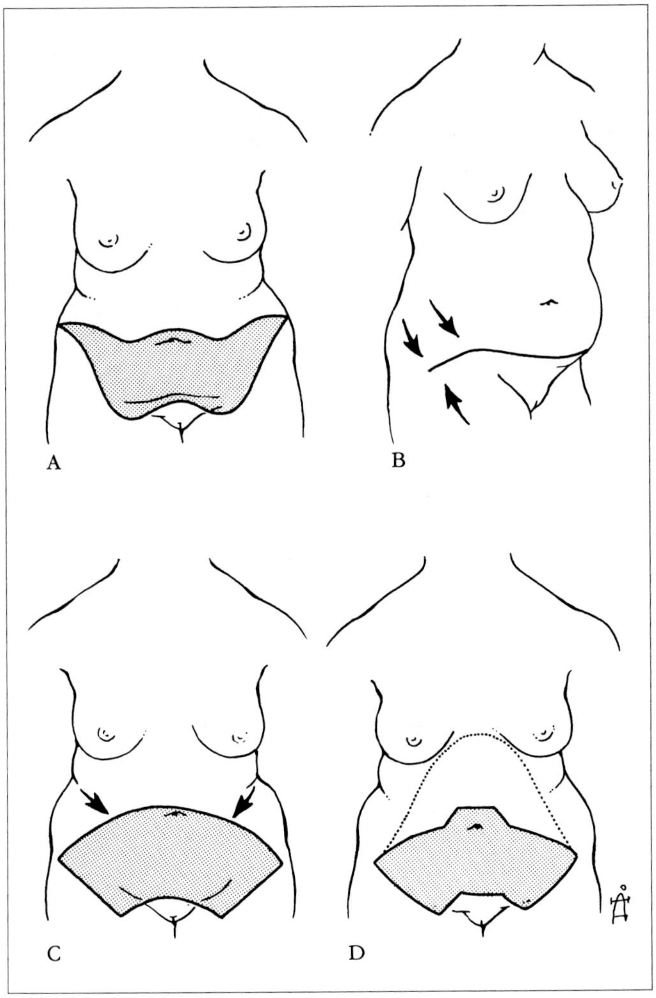

Figure 25-2. Aesthetic abdominoplasty procedures.
A. Spadafora.
B. Pitanguy.
C. Callia.
D. Serson.

29]. Later, Regnault [80] described two mixed incisions including a fleur-de-lis excision and a modified belt lipectomy for large upper abdominal adiposity.

PATHOPHYSIOLOGY AND CLASSIFICATION

The pathophysiology of abdominal wall deformities is excess fat or excess skin plus a flaccidity of the musculoaponeurotic system and scarring, either striae or surgical. Although one full-term pregnancy may cause deformities, the majority of patients seeking abdominoplasties have had multiple pregnancies. The volumetric increase of the abdominal contents during pregnancy causes laxity of the musculoaponeurotic system and diastasis of the rectus muscle plus stretching of the skin. It is generally believed that separation of the rectus muscles occurs in all pregnancies and can never be restored by exercise alone. Laxity of the skin occurs following pregnancy or dramatic weight changes. The latter etiology is discussed in Chapter 29 [53, 60]. Post partum, most patients will experience a gradual tightening of the skin over several months. If redundancy remains at 6 months, the condition is probably permanent. Most skin laxity is concentrated around and below the umbilicus while superimposed on a diastasis of the muscle fascia. The skin itself has normal physical properties except in the striae. Arem and Kischer [1] hypothesize that striae are a form of dermal scarring that follows rupture and separation of the dermal collagen with subsequent filling in of the gap.

Adipose tissue is deposited throughout the abdominal wall but is classifiable as a lower medial or upper medial obesity, with the umbilicus as a reference point [30]. The majority of patients requesting abdominoplasty fit into three major groups: (1) those with normal weight (±7.5 kg of ideal weight), (2) the mildly to moderately obese, and (3) individuals who have had massive weight loss. It is reasonable to classify the patients into those with abdominal dermatochalasis and those with abdominal obesity (lower medial or upper medial) (Fig. 25-3). Patients desiring excision of excess skin to tighten their tummies require an abdominoplasty whereas overweight individuals who want their fat excised require an abdominal lipectomy [17]. Liposuction may be of benefit in patients with moderate obesity, but it obviously cannot correct redundant skin or minimize striae or abdominal protuberance due to laxity of the musculoaponeurotic system [96]. Massive weight-loss deformities call for total torsoplasties rather than a limited anterior abdominal wall correction.

Disfiguring surgical scars, especially those from vertical cesarean section or infected appendixes and umbilical hernias, are often present in patients requesting abdominoplasty. The majority of disfiguring scars are excised within the abdominal specimen. The presence of oblique upper quadrant incisions implies severance of the superior epigastric artery and may be a contraindication to wide undermining. Umbilical hernias may appear de novo following pregnancy and require closure of the fascial defect, often in a double-layer "vest-over-pants" configuration.

CONSULTATION

Indications and Contraindications

The most frequent indications for abdominoplasty are postpartum deformities (laxity, diastasis recti, striae, flabbiness), adiposity, and surgical scars. If exercise and diet control programs have not been successful, surgery may be viewed as a last resort [10]. The moderately or severely obese patient should be reassured that surgery can ultimately be of value, but that initial consultation with a physician specializing in diet control or a surgeon specializing in intestinal bypass surgery is the first step. Contraindications are both specific and general. The presence of multiple abdominal scars above the umbilicus (cholecystectomy) are a contraindication for wide undermining as vascularity of the flap may be compromised; instead, a more localized procedure is required. Poor scars and sig-

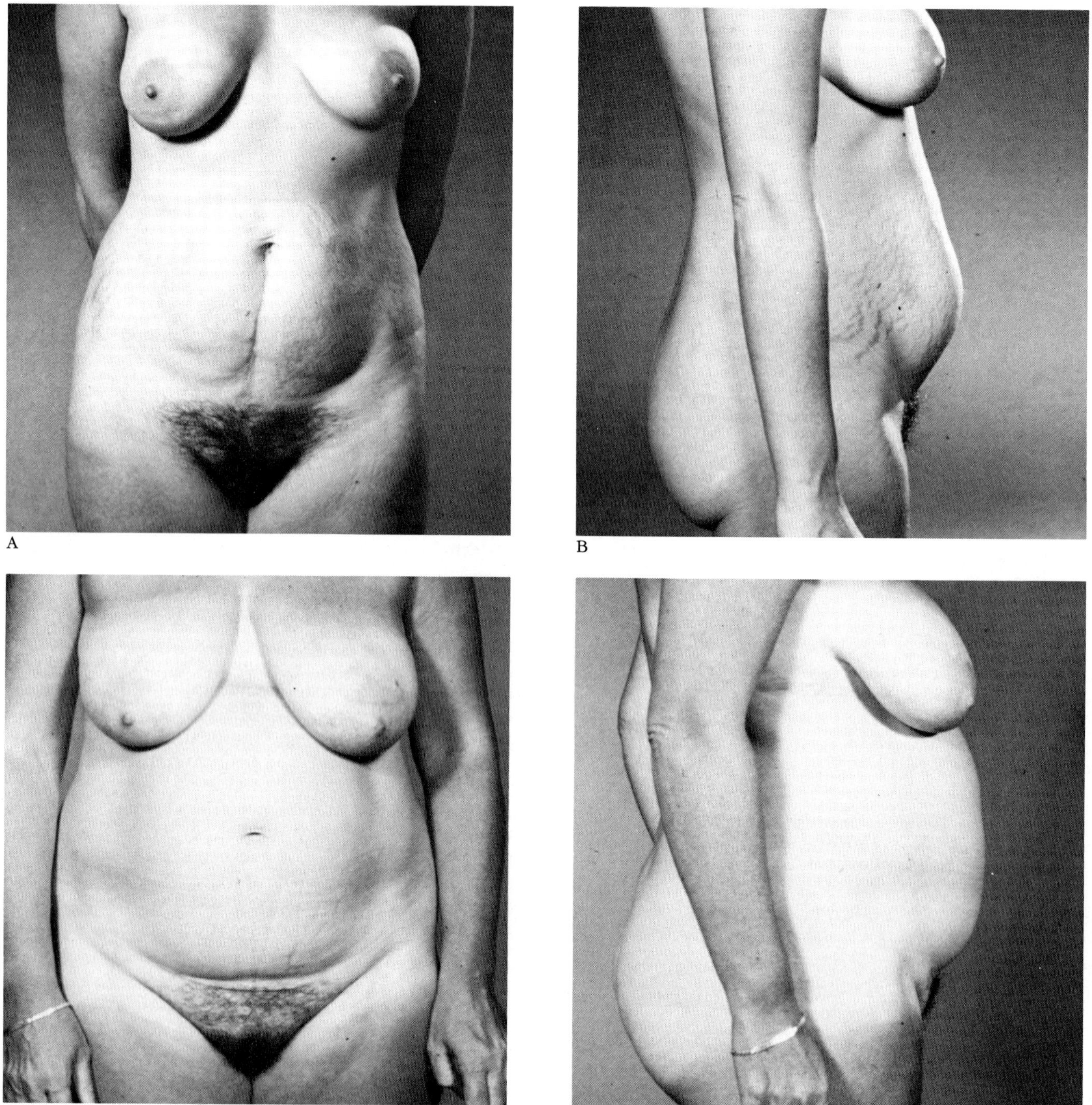

A B C D

Figure 25-3. Typical patients seeking body contour surgery.
A, B. Normal-weight individual following two pregnancies with skin laxity, abdominal protuberance, multiple striae, and cesarean scar. Abdominoplasty is indicated.
C, D. Moderately obese patient with central adiposity and abdominal laxity. Fleur-de-lis abdominal lipectomy with direct excision of fat is warranted, rather than an abdominoplasty.

nificant complications are a very real possibility, which the patient must accept. Future plans for pregnancy or unrealistic expectations are absolute contraindications. Patients with a history of thromboembolic disease require careful preoperative evaluation and a special perioperative regimen. A history of cardiopulmonary problems, diabetes, or metabolic diseases precludes elective surgery. The ideal patient is of normal height and weight with postpartum laxity and sufficient skin elasticity to ensure a transverse incision [31].

Medical History

A general medical history with emphasis on the abdomen is taken. The patient's previous pregnancies and weight ranges are reviewed. The age at initial pregnancy and the effect each pregnancy had on skin laxity, abdominal flaccidity, and striae are noted. A detailed inquiry into all surgical procedures, with any attendant complications, is made. One should determine whether the patient is satisfied with her current weight and whether future pregnancies are planned. If pregnancy is anticipated in the near future, it is best to postpone surgery. An exception is the very young woman who wants to eradicate the stigmata of a past "mistake."

Motivation

The normal-weight patient encounters difficulties either in revealing clothes that display the striae-ridden redundant skin or in tight clothing that shows the lower abdominal bulge. This deformity can be particularly debilitating during sexual relations as the patient considers it "disgusting" and "ugly."

The moderately obese patient wants the abdominal panniculus excised to improve body image and to facilitate hygiene. Every effort must be made to have the patient lose weight on a medical regimen with abdominal lipectomy reserved as a reward. Unfortunately, most patients prefer a surgical solution without dietary discipline [22]. Occasionally, a patient will have unrealistic expectations that all striae can be removed and that a fine invisible scar will be left. It is important to determine the patient's expectations in regard to both contour improvement and the resulting scar.

Physical Examination

Patients are examined nude in the standing position to allow them to demonstrate what they do not like and in the supine position to allow the surgeon to determine surgical technique. The location of scars, striae, and obesity is obvious on inspection. The degree of abdominal flaccidity and protrusion is evaluated in profile and, if uncertainty exists, with the patient on hands and knees [84]. The patient is then asked what bothers her the most. Next, the patient is examined in the supine position to evaluate diastasis of rectus muscles, skin excess, and hernias, either umbilical or incisional. The patient is asked to do a partial sit-up, which tightens the abdominal wall and allows the surgeon to palpate the muscle edges. Skin excess is determined by pinching the skin and attempting to approximate the periumbilical skin to the inguinal crease. This maneuver is particularly important, and one must decide which incision to use and at what level. Once the surgeon has selected the technique that will correct the patient's deformity, an approximation of the final scar is drawn on the patient, who is shown that the trade-off is a long scar for excision of excess skin and fat.

Aesthetic Goals

Surprisingly, the moderately obese patient has aesthetic objectives as demanding as the patient with simple dermatochalasis. One must emphasize that an improvement can be made by excising redundant skin and fat, but that the thick abdominal wall will obscure subtle body contouring. Also, the scars must be more extensive to match the greater deformity. This discussion affords another opportunity to stress that the same procedure would offer even greater rewards if the patient were able to lose 15 to 20 kg before surgery.

The patient with dermatochalasis generally wants excision of the redundant skin with as many striae as possible and tightening of the protuberant abdomen. The patient is given a realistic analysis of what improvements can be made. Next, with the patient's participation, the location of the final scar must be decided on. What types of leisure-time activities and clothing does the patient prefer? What type of bathing suit does she wear? In general, a W-incision is drawn with its lateral extension some 2 to 3 cm below and beyond the anterior superior iliac spine. The necessity for transposing the umbilicus is explained and the patient reassured that every effort will be made to replace it in a similar location.

Problems occur with the mildly overweight individual whose abdominal laxity can be corrected, but who will be disappointed with the now emphasized buttock-flank deformity. Grazer [35] notes that continued lateral extension onto the upper buttocks will allow contouring of the hips. For such a patient we prefer the extended W-plasty or liposuction of this area provided the patient is young and the skin tense.

Informed Consent

At this point the surgeon should review the problem, the patient's wishes, and the planned surgical procedure. The limitations and possible complications are emphasized, including the early problems (hematoma, seroma, marginal separation, skin slough) as well as late realities (hypertrophic scars, umbilical alterations). It is stressed that abdominoplasty is a major operation with its attendant risks (thrombophlebitis, pulmonary embolus) and those of general anesthesia. The consultation concludes with a *realistic* assessment of the result the patient can expect.

Preoperative Preparations

The patient discontinues all aspirin-containing medications and birth control pills 2 weeks prior to surgery. If blood transfusion is anticipated, as in most obese patients, the patient can donate blood in advance at 2-week intervals—as many units as required. Photographs are taken with the patient standing, nude from nipples to thighs, and include anterior, oblique, and lateral views. The patient begins bathing with pHisoHex 2 days prior to surgery. Enemas may be given the evening prior to surgery.

ANATOMY

The anterior abdominal wall is diamond shaped, bordered by the xiphoid and costal margins superiorly, the oblique muscles laterally, and the pelvic brim and inguinal ligaments inferiorly [25]. The contour varies with sex, body weight, and age, ranging from concavity in ectomorphic individuals to the slight convexity of mesomorphs to the pendulous abdomens of obese endomorphs [100–103]. The umbilicus is the most visible landmark and is located below the midpoint of the xiphoid–pubic tubercle line. Its location is relatively constant being between the waistline above and the high point of the iliac crest below. The superficial expression of the rectus muscle is the linea alba in the midline and the linea semilunaris laterally.

Skin

The skin of the abdomen is quite loose except at the bordering bony points and the midline linea alba–umbilicus. The subcutaneous tissue has a double layer of fascia interspersed with adipose tissue. The superficial fascia is Camper's fascia and the deeper layer Scarpa's fascia, which continues with the fascia lata of the thigh [61]. Under normal conditions, fat distribution extends downward from the umbilicus to the inguinal ligaments and laterally around the buttocks [23].

Muscles

The abdominal wall musculature is important in posture, locomotion, and situations requiring increased interabdominal pressure. The aponeurosis of these lateral three muscles (external oblique, internal oblique, and transversalis) have a direct correlation with the rectus abdominis muscles. The rectus abdominis originates from the pubis and inserts into the fifth, sixth, and seventh costal cartilages. The rectus muscle is enclosed by the aponeurosis of the oblique, which splits with one lamina joining that of the external oblique and the other joining the aponeurosis of the transversalis. Although this sequence varies, these aponeuroses join medially to form the linea alba. It is stretching of this musculoaponeurotic system that allows protrusion of the abdomen and requires plication.

Vascular Supply

Embryologically, the umbilicus is the dividing point for the abdomen. Thus, the vascular supply has a superior and an inferior component as represented by the superficial veins and arteries [24]. The subcutaneous veins consist of the large thoracoepigastric system, which drains into the axillary and femoral veins. The inferiorly located superficial arteries include the superficial pudendal, superficial inferior epigastric, and branches from the superficial circumflex iliac [13]. The contribution of these vessels is severed on the initial incision. Thus, the abdominal flap is totally dependent on its superior arterial blood supply including the superior epigastric perforators and numerous branches from the intercostals. Preservation of these vessels along the border of dissection is advantageous. Paired venae comitantes accompany each artery and drain into major veins in the groin or axilla.

Lymphatics

As occurs with the veins, lymphatics below the umbilicus drain to the inguinal nodes while the superior lymphatics go to the axillary nodes (Fig. 25-4A, B). Occasional edema of the abdominal flap is attributed to the need for total lymphatic drainage to progress upward into the axilla as inferior drainage is severed at operation and subsequent reestablishment blocked by the scar inferiorly [5]. This problem is most marked in the retained lateral edges, which previously drained into the inguinal nodes.

Nerves

Sensation of the abdominal wall is supplied by the lateral and anterior branches of T6 to T12 plus L1. The lateral branches pass into the subcutaneous tissue at the midaxillary line, continue circumferentially, and are retained in most abdominoplasties. The anterior branches pass upward in the middle of the rectus sheath and are severed during an abdominoplasty. Most of the skin excision comes from T10 to T12 dermatomes, and an anesthetist subsequently attempting a spinal block could be confused (Fig. 25-4C, D). The lateral femoral cutaneous nerve of the thigh penetrates the inguinal ligament 1 cm medial to the anterior superior iliac spine and runs subfascially for another 6 to 10 cm. It can be injured by cauterization or ligation. The ilioinguinal nerve emerges near the subcutaneous inguinal ring and crosses over the inguinal ligament onto the thigh.

Figure 25-4. Anterior abdominal wall anatomy.
A, B. Lymphatic drainage is directed superiorly and inferiorly from the umbilical level. Persistent postoperative edema in the area immediately above the incision may occur until new lymphatic channels develop or flow is redirected.
C, D. Conventional sensory dermatomes demonstrating area of excision. (From C. G. Carvalho, R. Baroudi, and E. M. Keppke. Anatomical and technical refinements for abdominoplasty. *Aesthetic Plast. Surg.* 1:217, 1977.)

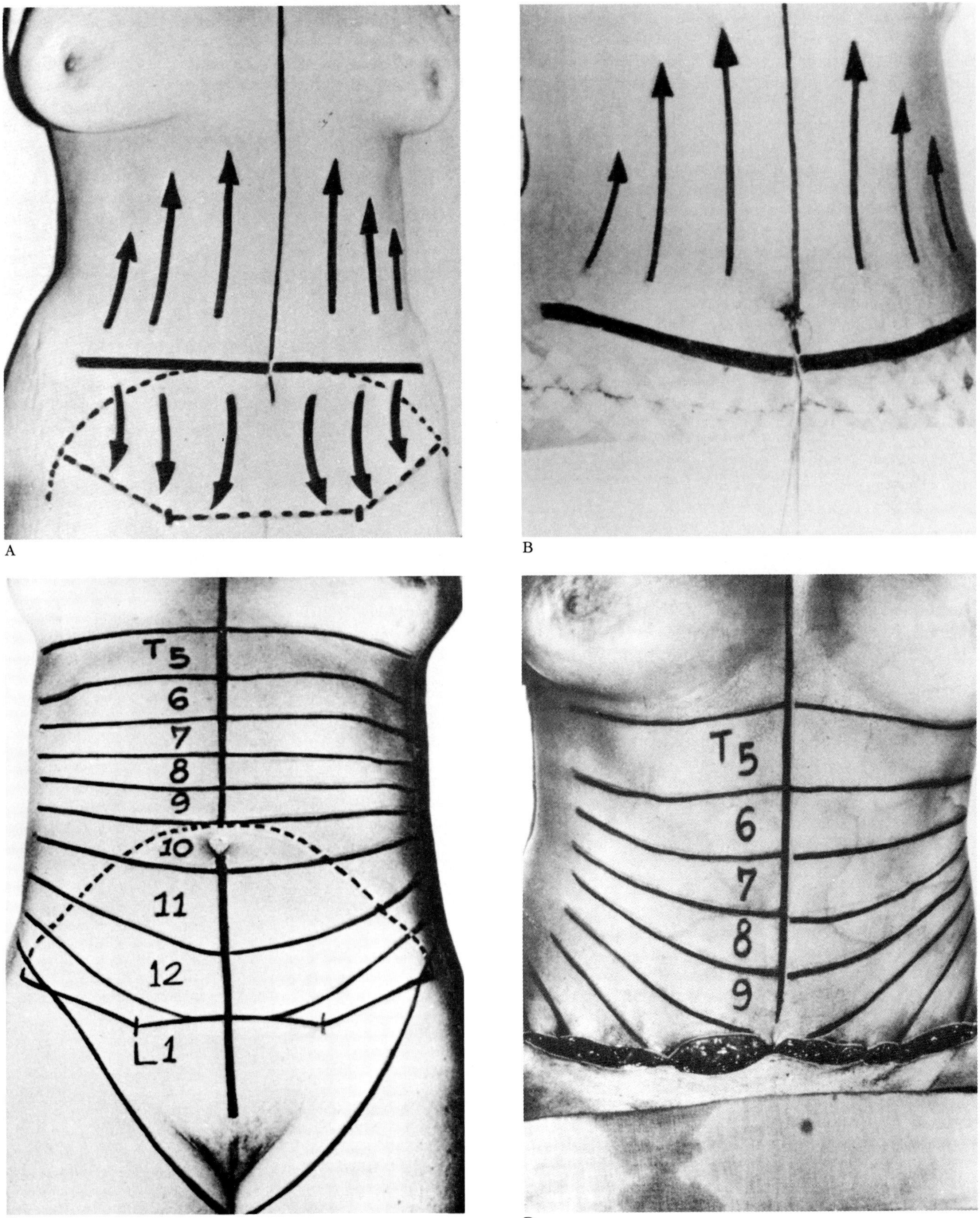

A B C D

SURGICAL PRINCIPLES

The abdominal wall has a pleasing contour with its hourglass configuration, narrow waistline, umbilical dimple, and flat profile. Selection of the optimal operation is based on the pathophysiologic deviation from this normal appearance. In contrast to abdominal lipectomy, which is basically excisional, the abdominoplasty is a more challenging aesthetic procedure. Its principles are discussed in detail and modifications for abdominolipectomy are considered later. The constraints of a well-concealed symmetric scar, a nonsurgical-appearing umbilicus, and an improved contour have forced continued refinements in surgical techniques (Fig. 25-5).

Incision

The lower incision determines the location of the final scar as modified by closure tension. Its placement is dictated by the need for concealment in swimwear plus consideration of future body sculpting procedures (thigh lipectomy). The lower border of a bikini is along the inguinal crease while the upper border parallels a line drawn on the anterior superior iliac spine. Within this area, one can move the incision superiorly in patients with minimum skin elasticity and inferiorly in those with maximum elasticity. The final scar is usually in the pubic hair and 1 to 2 cm above the inguinal folds.

What shape should the incision be? A true transverse incision has the disadvantages of extending onto the thighs, producing lateral dog-ears, and elevating the pubis in tight closures [16]. If the lines of incision and excision are of comparable length, lateral extension is reduced and dog-ears rarely occur. An incision that begins in the pubic hair and curves convexly toward the inguinal crease will minimize pubic elevation. These principles are incorporated into the W-plasty (Fig. 25-6). Medial tension on the flap obviates the need for lateral extension. Grazer [35] prefers a gull-wing incision with its lower lateral extension, which may be a necessity because of the more vertical tension on closure. Serson and Martins [91] provided geometric planning for abdominoplasty markings, but its arithmetic rigidity does not allow adaptation to a wide variety of deformities.

Although others prefer marking the incision line with the patient supine, we strongly advocate that all markings, both incision and reference points, be made with the patient standing, thereby incorporating the influence of gravity and replicating the postoperative position. Should a pattern be used, and should the contemplated lines of excision be marked preoperatively [7]? We do not use a pattern because the female body and its skin elasticity are too variable to achieve optimal results in a wide variety of patients (too little excision in the corpulent, too much in the thin athletic patient). Preoperative marking of the anticipated line of excision is important as it is often a fixed point toward which the line of incision is adjusted within the constraints of the bikini markings. This excision line passes straight from the umbilicus to the lateral limit of the incision line, tapering acutely to avoid dog-ears. The advantage of the excision line is that it ensures a symmetric resection without guesswork.

In his "vest over pants" abdominoplasty Planas [71] cuts the excision line first, to facilitate exposure and speed the operative procedure. The type and size of umbilical incision are virtually limitless: transverse, vertical, circular, and Y-shaped. We prefer a 2-cm-long transverse marquise cut, which replicates the multiparous umbilicus.

Undermining

It is generally agreed that undermining is done in the areolar plane above the muscle fascia and extends up to the xiphoid process, over the costal margins, and laterally to the anterior axillary line (Fig. 25-7A). The dissection must be symmetric, relieving any epigastric bulging, and followed by meticulous hemostasis. Guerrero-Santos et al. [41, 42] recommended additional undermining at a superficial level extending laterally toward the buttocks and inferiorly onto the thighs.

Plication

In contrast to symptomatic diastasis of the recti, laxity of the musculoaponeurotic fascia is a common occurrence following pregnancy. Thus, plication of the rectus fascia is done in 90 percent of patients undergoing abdominoplasty. It is important that this plication be symmetric, of limited width (3–10 cm), and frequent (every 2 cm) and extend from xiphoid to pubis (Fig. 25-7B, C). There is no need to open the rectus fascia, and only rarely is a slimming waistline suture of the external oblique fascia beneficial [48]. The disadvantage of plication is its suppression of the linea alba concavity and the periumbilical depression, thus accounting for the 10 percent of patients in which plication is not done. These are thin individuals with clear definition of the linea alba preoperatively who have skin laxity but minimal abdominal protuberance. These facets may be compensated for by defatting the flaps cautiously, in the midline only or around the new umbilical site or both. Birdsell et al. [11] evaluated the "staying power" of absorbable and nonabsorbable sutures used for plication in 30 women having abdominoplasty. They found that the type of suture did not matter, and that the fascial imbrication was maintained at 6 months. Thus, heavy absorbable sutures may be ideal for plication in thin patients, in whom palpation of nonabsorbable sutures can occur.

Resection

The resected tissue varies in amount and shape depending on the direction and degree of tension placed on the abdominal flap. In many techniques, the operating table is flexed and the flaps are pulled straight downward followed by straight-line excision of excess skin. However, this approach results in excessive tension, possible malplacement of the umbilicus, and increased postoperative morbidity; secondary scar revisions can approach 100 percent. Therefore, we prefer leaving the operating table flat,

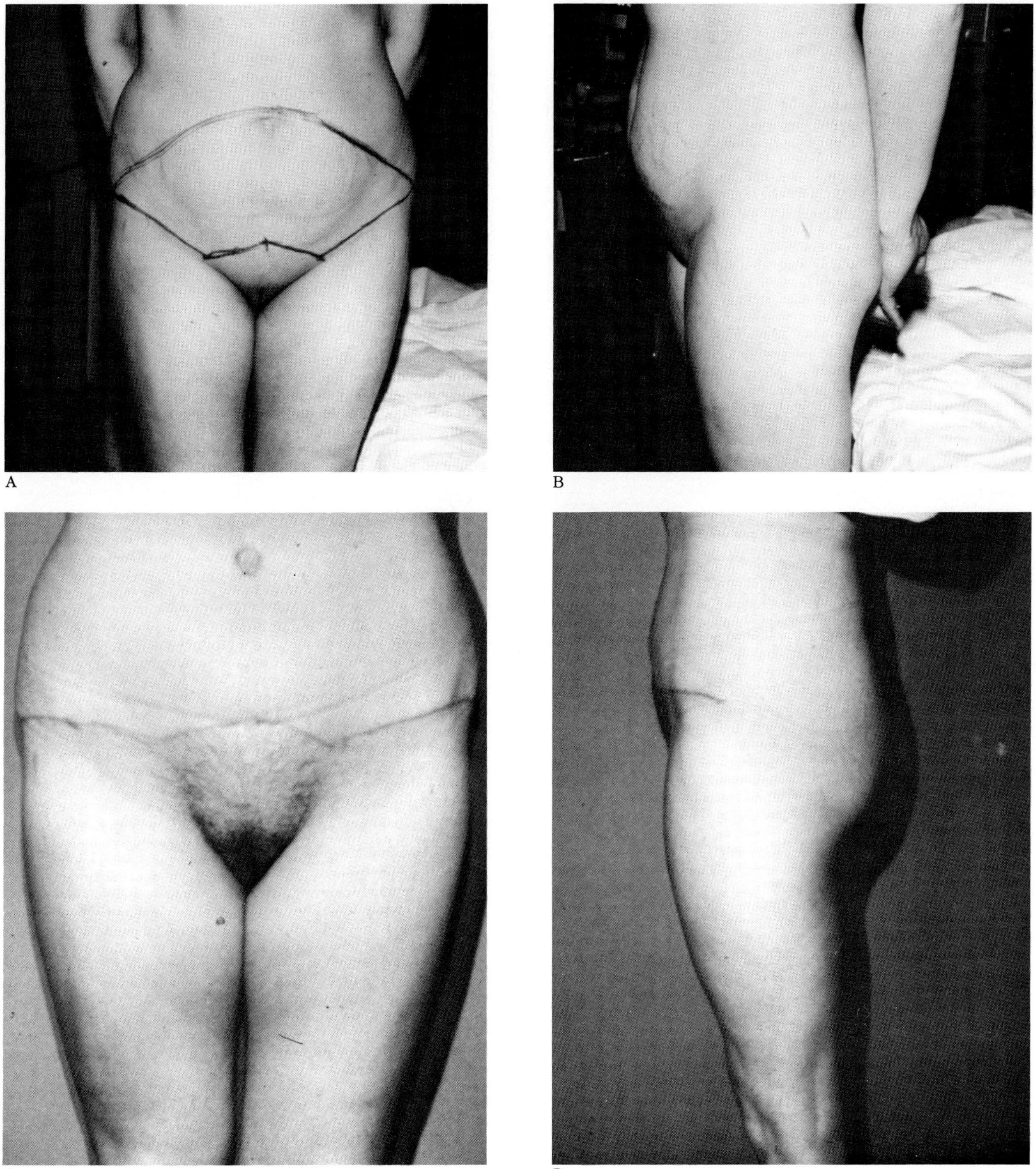

A B C D

Figure 25-5

A, B. A standard W-plasty consisting of an incision line with medial pubic and lateral inguinal components, plus the estimated excision line.

C, D. Result at 1 year with restoration of hourglass contour, flat profile, and normal umbilicus.

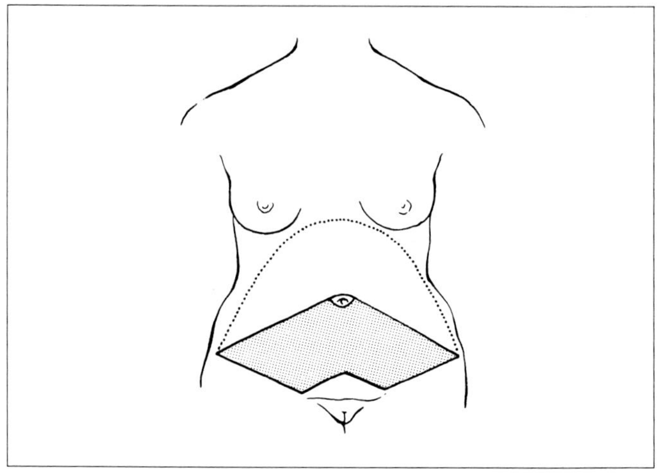

Figure 25-6. The W-abdominoplasty showing area of excision and dotted area of undermining.

Figure 25-7
A. Extent of undermining.
B. Plication is frequent and extends the entire length from xyphoid to pubis.
C. Plication brings the medial borders of the rectus fascia together.

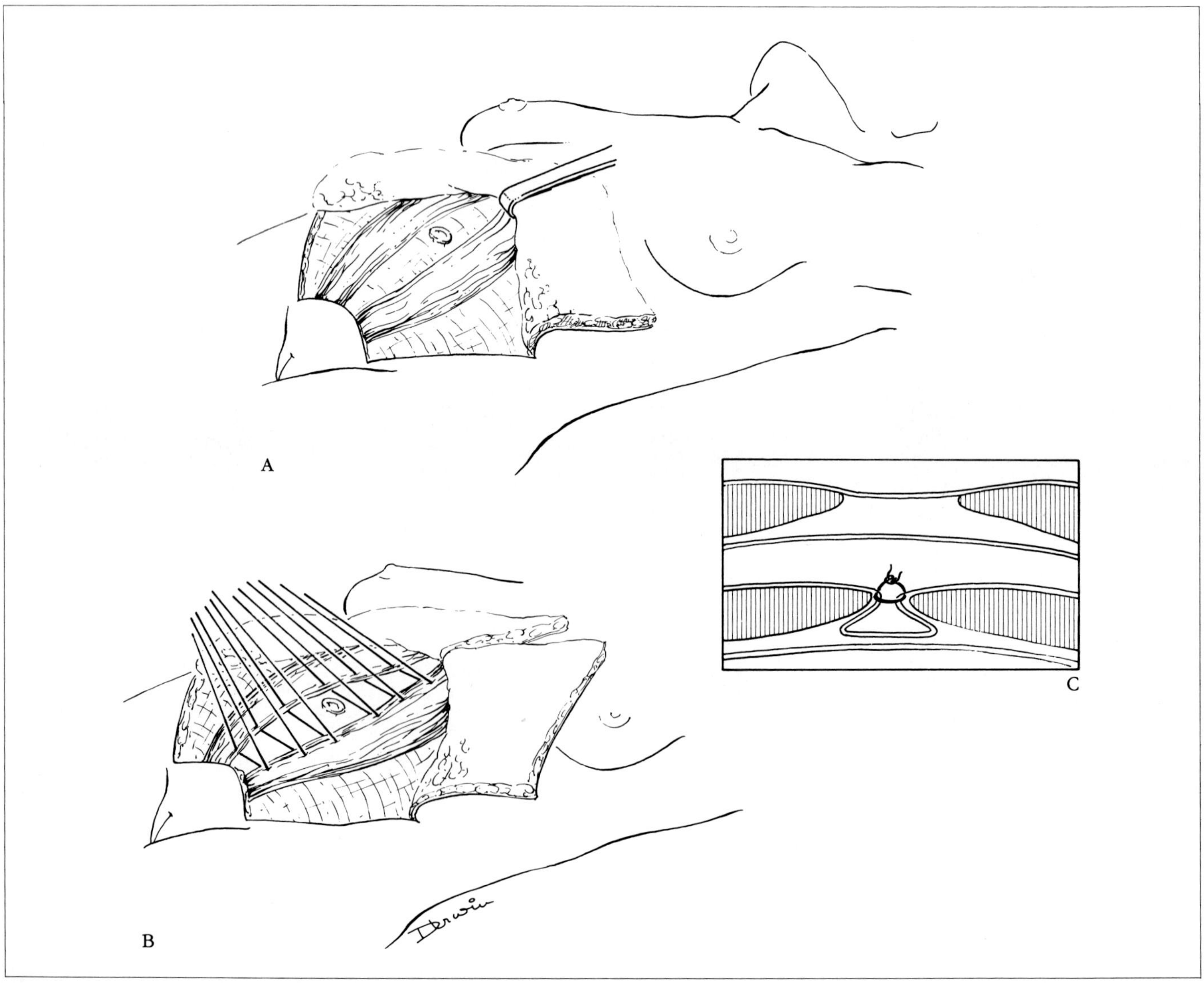

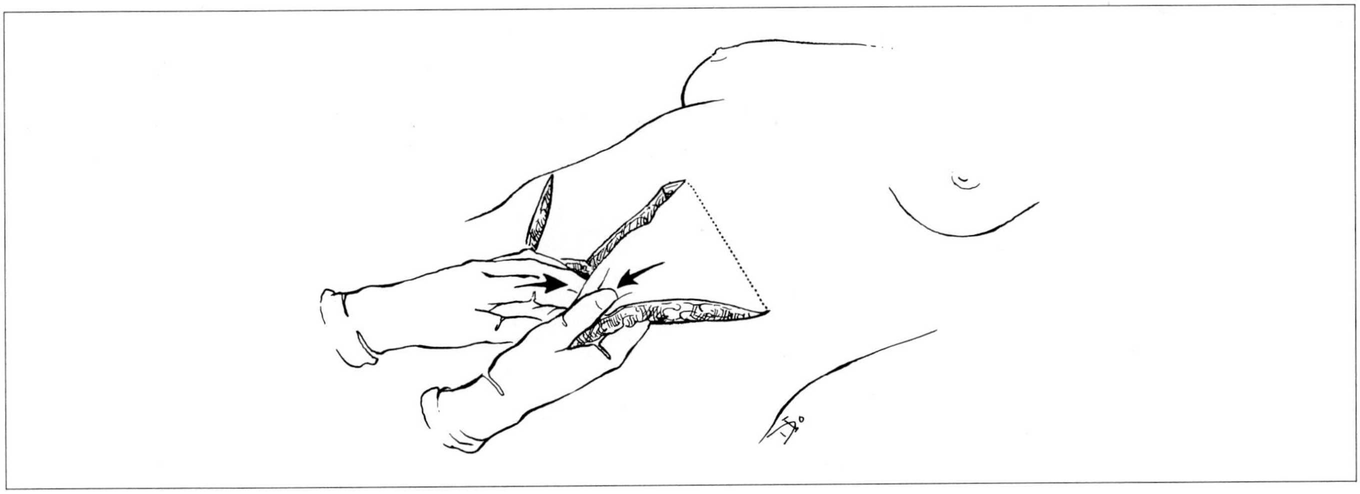

Figure 25-8. Confirmation of the excision line and determination of the site for the umbilicus are done with the table flat. The abdominal flaps are pulled downward while the pubis is pushed upward.

placing medial traction on the flaps to reduce lateral redundancy, and pushing on the pubis to determine the excess tissue (Fig. 25-8). If the anticipated resection is not possible, a line is drawn parallel to the preoperative excision line.

Umbilicoplasty

The ideal umbilicus should have the correct location, shape, and size without surgical stigmata (suture marks, scars, or distortion) (Fig. 25-9). The midline location is obvious, but the height will be approximately on a line connecting the crest of the ilium (transiliac crestline) or 3 cm above the anterior superior iliac spine or midway between xyphoid and pubis. Dubou and Ousterhout [19] measured 100 normal-weight individuals in the *supine* position, with the table flat, and found that the umbilicus coincided with the transiliac crestline in 96 percent. Deviation from the midline usually occurs from failure to mark the midline preoperatively or from lateral traction on the umbilicus due to asymmetric plication. It is generally agreed that umbilical height is determined with the operating table flat and tension on the flaps; failure to straighten out the table may result in too high an umbilical location. Umbilical shape changes with aging from the flat vertical of the nulliparous adolescent to the more hooded and transverse multiparous configuration. Baroudi [8] notes that body habitus influences umbilical shape, both preoperatively and postoperatively. Heavier patients have a deeper and wider umbilicus; thin patients have a shallow or protuberant navel. Because of the thin skin and limited fat, it may be difficult to create a deep navel in a thin individual. Since most patients are multiparous, a transverse 2-cm-long marquise cut is used to isolate the umbilicus, and a 2-cm transverse cut in the abdominal flap opens into an ellipse for insertion. Creation of a superior hood and dimpling is achieved by periumbilical defatting of the subcutaneous fat, greater in the inferior area, and fixation of the umbilicus to the abdominal fascia (Fig. 25-10). If all sutures are tied deep within the umbilicus, scarring will be minimized. Avelar [4] prefers a three-flap umbilicus incision, thereby avoiding a circular scar, whereas Freeman and Wiemer [27] use an omega-shaped flap to achieve a natural superior hood.

Closure

Tension on the closure is reduced by flexion of the operating table and maintaining this position in bed for several days (Fig. 25-11). All abdominoplasties should be drained, preferably with suction drains. Since the lower incision is beveled superiorly, a two-layer closure with staggered suture lines is possible [72, 85]. The deep sutures carry the tension, thus placing less stress on the superficial layer, which approximates the skin with less incidence of separation (Fig. 25-12).

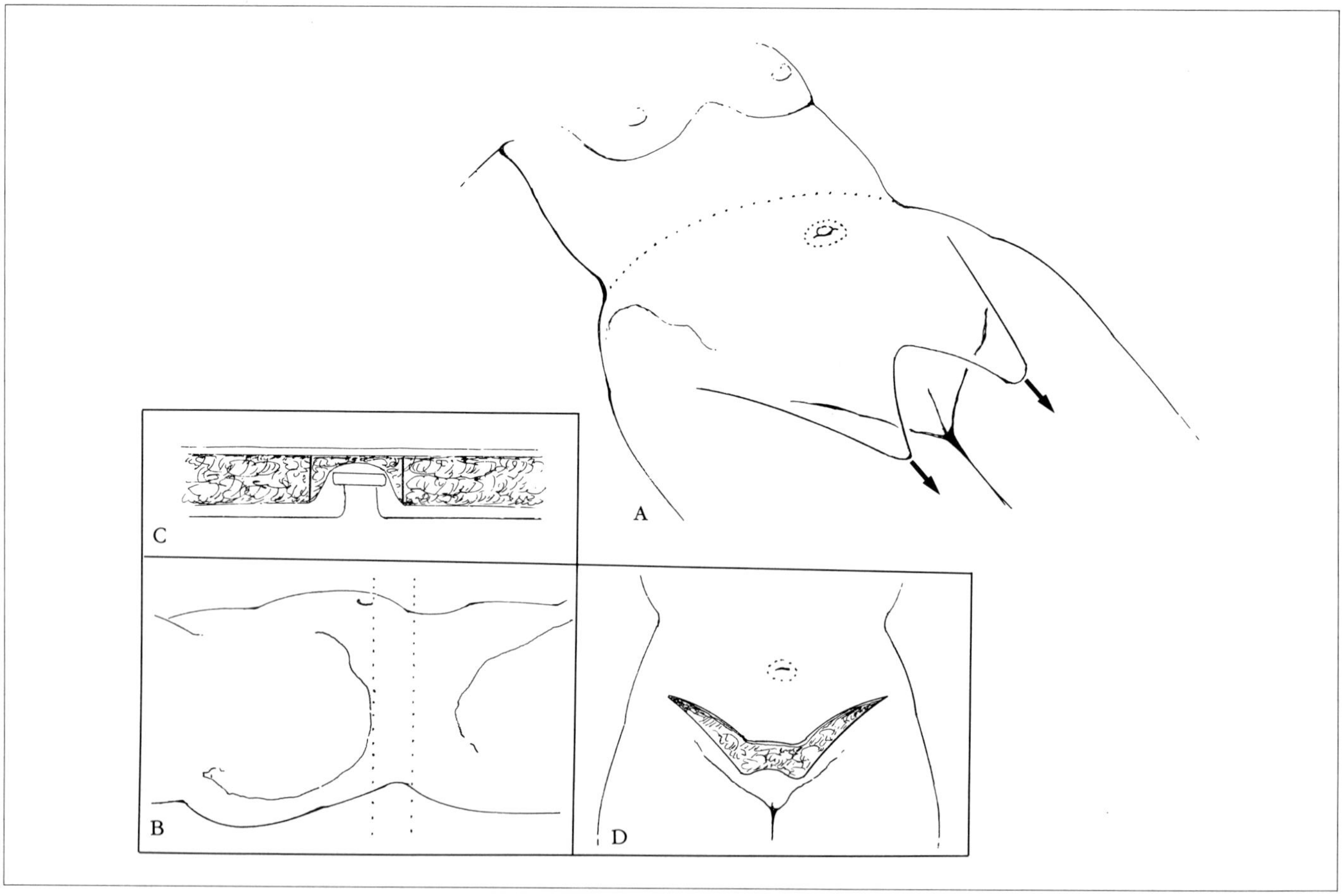

Figure 25-9. Umbilicoplasty.
A, C. With tension on the abdominal flap, the new site of the umbilicus is located on the transiliac crest line.
B. The periumbilical area is defatted, in greater amount inferiorly than superiorly.
D. Once the site is determined, the excess skin is excised.

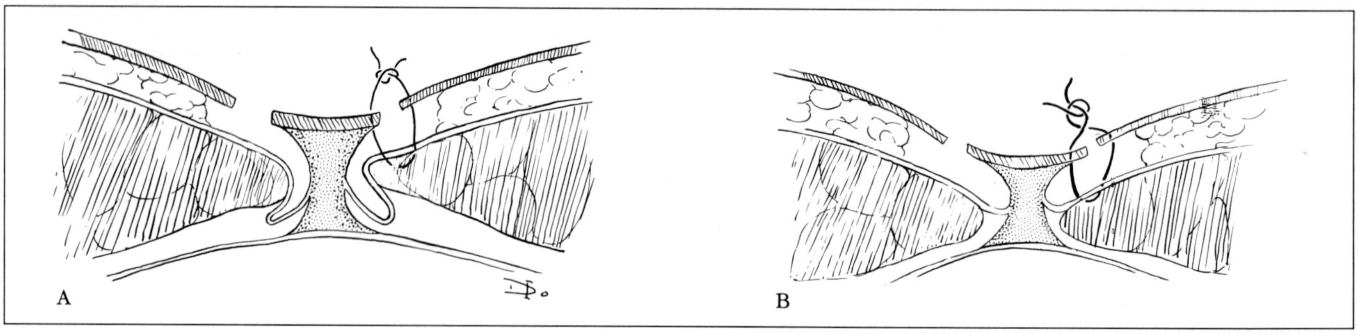

Figure 25-10. Following the periumbilical defatting, the umbilicus is sutured to the rectus fascia with quadrant sutures.
A. If plication was done, then infolding of the rectus fascia has occurred.
B. If plication was not done.

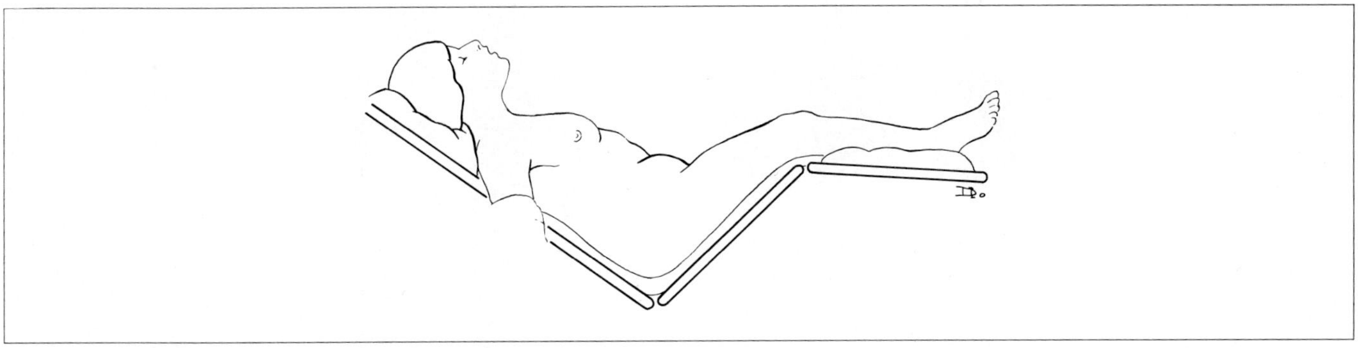

Figure 25-11. The operating table is flexed to allow closure without tension.

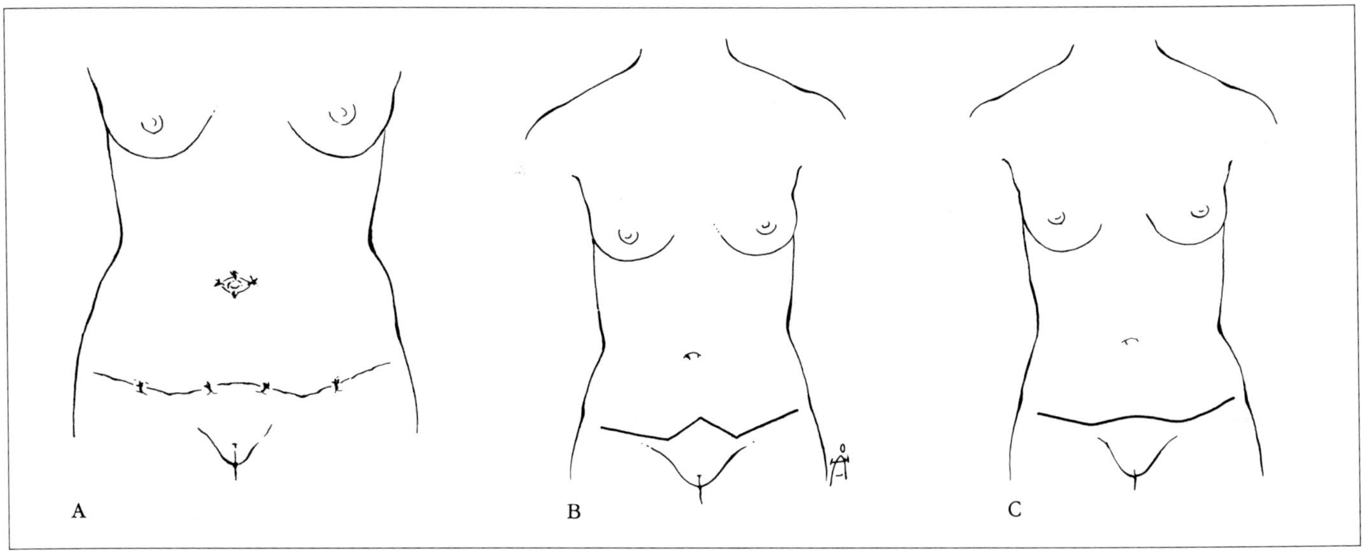

Figure 25-12
A. The incision is closed in two layers.
B. Scar will be sharply angulated in patients with great skin elasticity.
C. Scar will be straighter and higher in patients with minimal skin elasticity.

SURGICAL TECHNIQUES

Abdominoplasty

STANDARD W-PLASTY

The choice of which type of abdominoplasty (W-plasty, gull-wing, or Pitanguy) to use depends on the surgeon's preference. We prefer the W-plasty as the incision is short, in a well-concealed location, and offers maximum lateral tightening, and the technique itself is safe, easily learned, and reliable.

Marking. With the patient standing, the abdominal midline is marked from the xyphoid to the umbilicus to the pubis. The anterior superior iliac spine and lines perpendicular to the midline are drawn as reference points [3]. The incision has three components: pubic, inguinal, and excisional (Fig. 25-13). The midline point is marked 1 to 2 cm inside the pubic hair when the abdominal wall is very elastic or slightly above that point if laxity is minimal. The central pubic line extends downward to reach the inguinal fold and ascends laterally to end 3 to 5 cm below and lateral to the anterior superior iliac spine. The inguinal line is usually twice the length of the pubic line. The umbilicus is then marked as a transverse marquise cut approximately 1.5 cm in length. The excision line is a straight line from the umbilicus to the lateral end of the inguinal line. These lines can be conceived of as an arithmetic equation: $1X + 2X = 3X$. The inguinal line is twice the length of the pubic line, and the excision line is equal to or less than their sum. For patients with dermatochalasis, the lengths average: pubic (8–10 cm), inguinal (16–20 cm), and excision (24–30 cm). If dog-ears are to be avoided on closure, the excision line must never be longer than the incision lines. One can easily check the symmetry of incisions by using a fixed reference point and a plumb line.

Prior to completing the markings, it is wise to review the skin elasticity and the patient's build, which will determine the extent of excision. The greater the laxity, the easier it is to place the incisions in the pubic hair and inguinal crease. The greater the skin turgidity, the higher the incisions.

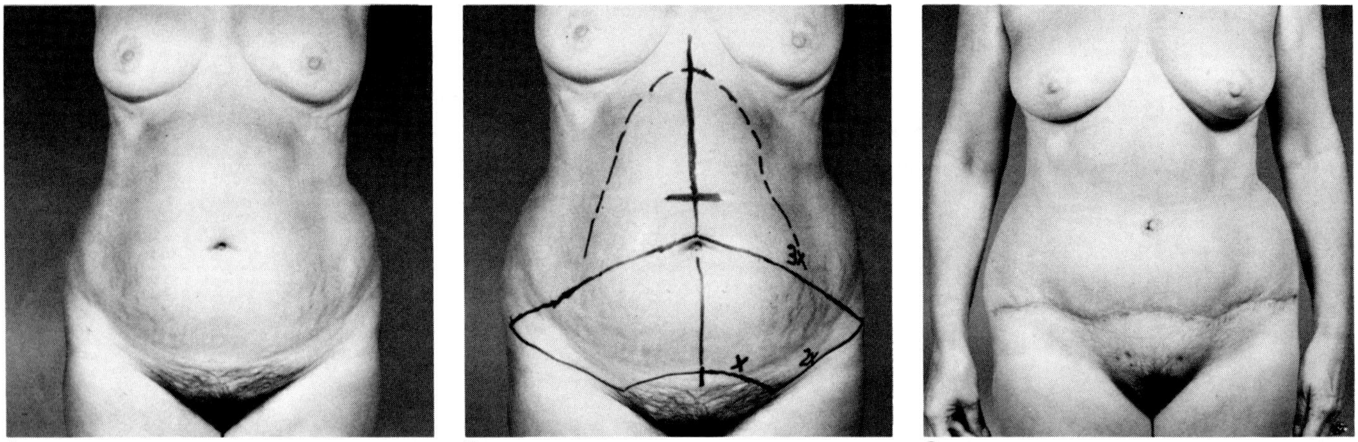

A B C

Figure 25-13
A. Middle-aged female with moderate adiposity.
B. W-plasty outlined with typical 1X + 2X = 3X configuration with actual values being 7 cm + 14 cm = 21 cm.
C. Early result.

Preparation. Abdominoplasty is major surgery and is done under general anesthesia with the patient remaining hospitalized for at least 48 hours. The patient is placed on an operating table that will allow hip flexion of 100 to 120 degrees at the time of wound closure. It must be emphasized that the operation is done with the table flat, and it is flexed only when the excision and the level of the umbilicus have been determined. Following induction of anesthesia, the upper pubic hair is shaved. Antibiotics (cephalosporin, 500 mg intravenously) are begun. The wound is prepped from inframammary fold down to the thighs and draped to permit wide exposure.

Operation. At this point the amount of tissue to be excised is reestimated by pinching the soft tissues. The lower pubic incision is made with an upward bend, which will allow sloping tangential two-layered closure. The beveled incision is carried superiorly to avoid the inguinal lymph nodes and in the center to preserve hair follicles. As noted by Guerrero-Santos, this acutely beveled incision reduces the incidence of a painful suprapubic depression and anesthesia of the lateral skin. The superficial inferior epigastric artery and vein are cross-clamped and tied on the femoral side. Once the entire incision is completed, it is carried down to fascia, where the areolar layer is preserved. Theoretically, retention of this layer aids in fluid resorption and reduces postoperative pain. Although some surgeons prefer scalpel or electrocoagulation, undermining may be done with blunt dissection and continued up to the umbilicus. Hemostasis is accomplished by cross-clamping and electrocoagulation.

Under skin hook traction, the umbilicus is circumferentially incised in a transverse direction and isolated on its stalk. The flap is then split in the midline and undermining continued upward to the xyphoid and over onto the lower ribs. With elevation complete, traction is placed on the flap and the extent of resection determined (Fig. 25-14A). If the initial lines appear correct, the redundant tissue is excised, thereby improving exposure and facilitating both hemostasis and plication of the fascia. The fascial midline is marked from xyphoid to pubis and the amount of laxity assessed by traction on either side (Fig. 25-14E). The anesthesiologist may give muscle relaxants intravenously to facilitate plication. The plication begins at the area of greatest laxity but must extend from the xyphoid to the pubis. A heavy nonabsorbable suture (2-0 Prolene) is inserted in a horizontal mattress configuration with the knots buried, and small bites are taken to prevent postoperative palpation (Fig. 25-14F). Sutures are inserted close together (1.5 cm) to prevent any postoperative bulging.

The umbilical stalk is shortened by the plication, thus helping to create a pleasing umbilical dimple. If plication is not done or the umbilical stalk remains too long relative to abdominal wall thickness, it can be further reduced by suturing it to the rectus fascia. An acceptable length is 1 cm. Location of the new umbilical site is achieved in accordance with the following guidelines: (1) It will be on the premarked midline; (2) height is at the transiliac crestline; and (3) with the table flat and traction on the flap, the umbilicus is palpated and needles are placed through the skin to indicate the desired site (Fig. 25-14B, C). With approximation of the flaps, the umbilical location is then determined, and a straight transverse 2-cm incision centered on the midline is made. The periumbilical subcutaneous tissue is excised over a distance of 4 to 5 cm in a sloping fashion with a greater amount inferiorly (Fig. 25-14D). Four sutures are passed through the skin incision, fascia, and umbilicus. They are left long and clamped with hemostats. Once the incision is closed, final insert of the umbilicus will be completed.

Resection of the flap is then performed. *Equal traction* is placed on the two halves of the divided abdominal flap in a downward and medial direction. The pubic area is pushed upward to allow estimation of redundant skin, but excess excision must be avoided. The excision line is marked. In certain cases it may be possible to excise even more skin than previously planned while in others poor elasticity may mandate a small vertical scar in the lower midline. Each flap is split up to the line of overlapping to

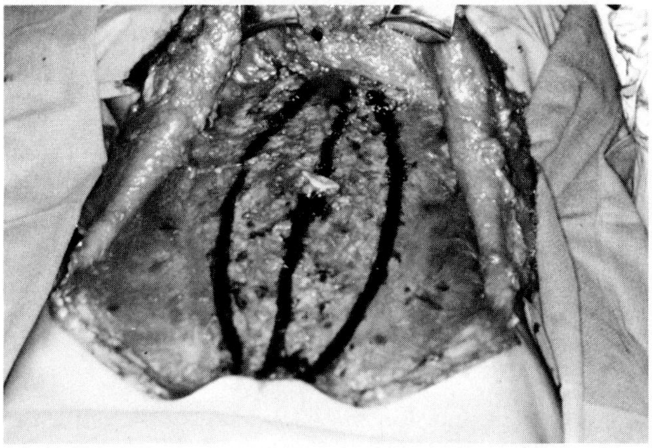

A

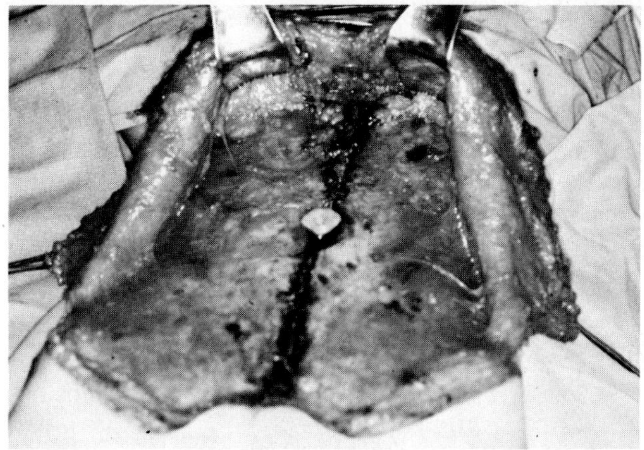

B

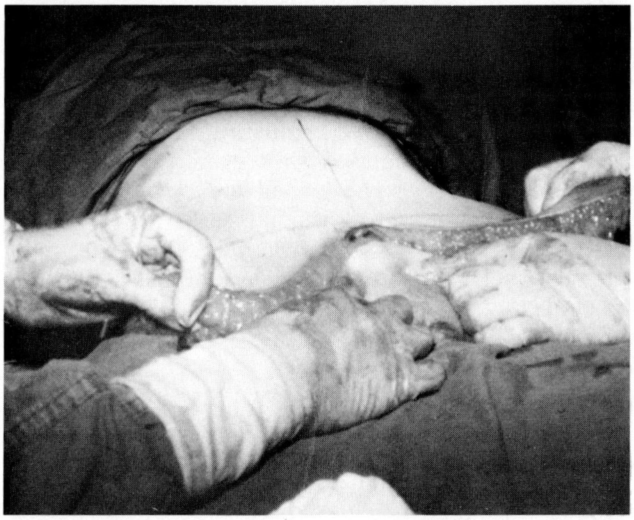

C

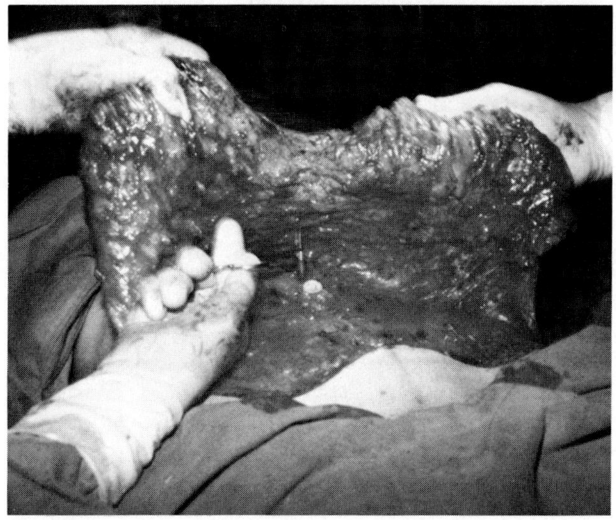

D

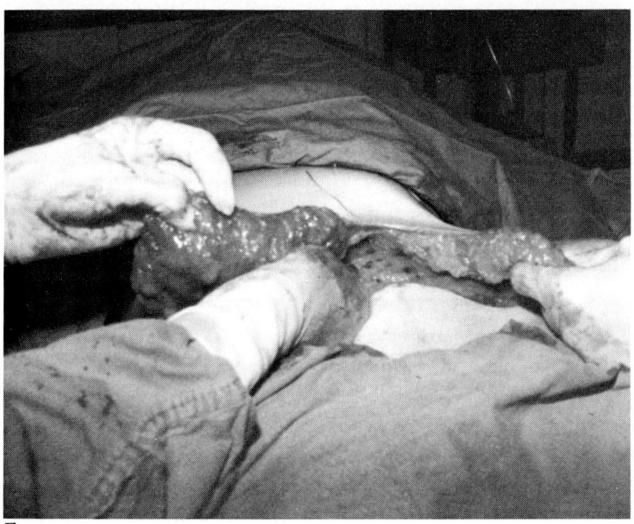

E

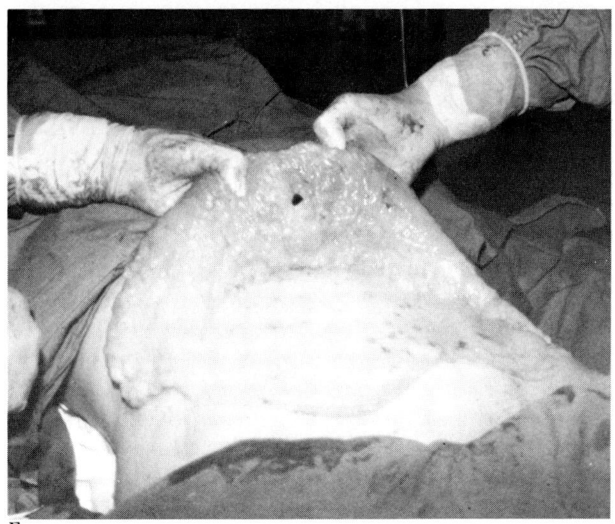

F

Figure 25-14

A. An 8-cm-wide plication tapered from xyphoid to pubis.
B. Plication completed; outer lines approximated in the midline.
C. Estimation of flap excision by pushing upward on the pubis and pulling downward on the abdominal flaps.
D. Location of the umbilicus with straight needle.
E. Umbilical placement with table flat and tension on the flap.
F. Periumbilical area defatted.

ensure correct resection. In contrast to simple transverse incisions, the W-plasty requires that the more lax lateral skin be brought medially, and thus one avoids pursuing dog-ears out onto the thigh. The subcutaneous fat on the abdominal flap is reduced by beveling with scissors to the same thickness as the inguinal skin; one removes Scarpa's fascia but not Camper's [2]. This maneuver is essential in the area overlying the anterior superior iliac spine.

The operating table is then put in a jackknife position (90–120 degrees), permitting closure without tension. Drains are placed on either side. Suturing is done in two layers: heavy absorbable (0 Dexon) interrupted sutures in the fat and fascia, and a subcuticular running suture (4-0 Dexon) in the skin. Large-bore suction drains are inserted. The lateral ends are sutured first, to avoid dog-ears. Should any skin folds be evident, they can be reduced by superficial undermining of the skin. If suturing causes elevation of the pubis, the undersurface of the pubis is sutured to the midline fascia.

The incision is covered with adhesive paper strips. A moderate pressure dressing is applied, using pads covered by elastic adhesive bandages in an X configuration. Cast and sandbags are not used, as they may compromise marginal vascularity of a flap or cause direct thermal burns. The patient is then placed in her flexed hospital bed, rather than on a stretcher, and the same position is maintained for the first 24 hours. The patient is out of bed on the first postoperative day.

EXTENDED W-PLASTY

This procedure is indicated in patients whose excess tissue extends laterally beyond the abdomen and where pulling down at the inguinal area does not reduce the lateral excess (Fig. 25-15). Very often the patients are aware of the lateral adiposity and ask for concomitant reduction. If a standard abdominoplasty is done, the lateral fullness is further accentuated and the patient is disappointed with the results.

The lower incision is similar to a standard W-abdominoplasty in the central area, but the lateral limbs are continued farther in the same upward direction (Fig. 25-16). Instead of being twice as long as the central limb, they may be three times longer, continuing onto the back. The upper line of excision is drawn from above the umbilicus to the ends of the lower one. Thus the excision line is almost horizontal rather than downward.

The technique of incision and dissection is similar to the standard procedure. The extended lateral portions do not require significant undermining when the tissues are supple enough. The procedure begins with the patient prone and the posterior portion is excised first. Suturing and taping are completed and the patient is turned to the supine position for the abdominoplasty.

MALE ABDOMINOPLASTY

Since the skin is thicker and less elastic in males, smaller amounts of soft tissues can be excised, except in the massive-weight-loss patient (Fig. 25-17). Also, the pubic hair is less well defined, and thus it is not an anatomic landmark that can be followed. The final scar is located higher, but always several centimeters below the umbilicus. Hemostasis is more difficult and takes more time. Drains are always used, even when hemostasis seems perfect. Hematomas and seromas are more frequent, even after adequate hemostasis and drainage. Scars are often hypertrophic and need protection and care. Tight belts are not worn over the scars for 6 months, and tapes are kept on incisions for a greater period of time.

Technique. The incision line is marked on the standing patient in a lazy W, above the pubis and going down but remaining approximately 2 to 5 cm above the inguinal folds. The lines then parallel the inguinal folds and continue to the back at the upper part of the buttocks, stopping approximately 10 cm from midspine. This posterior continuation is necessary, as there is less skin flaccidity, and significant improvement requires greater direct resection. The presumed line of excision starts at an acute angle in the back and follows a horizontal line toward the umbilicus, which is the termination point.

The patient is placed in the prone position, prepped, and draped. The operation begins on the back with incision of the lower line of the posterior triangle on one side. The incision is deep, with very little fat and areolar tissue left on the lumbar muscles. The flaps are elevated and resected under traction along the preplanned excision lines. The resection is carried to the lateral limit of the operating field. Defatting of the upper or lower edges is sometimes done when it could improve the final contour. However, this increases the chances of complications. Defatting beyond the terminal angle is always done to avoid redundancy. Closure is accomplished with a few deep stitches (2-0 Dexon) to approximate the deeper portion and to avoid dead spaces. The skin is closed with a subcuticular running suture of 4-0 Dexon, and drains are used routinely. A sterile drape covers the field, and the patient is turned supine. The abdomen is prepped and draped. The incision is in continuity with the lower lateral incisions and follows the preoperative markings. The dissection is done down to the areolar plane and continued upward exactly like the classic W-plasty. The undermining extends very high above the ribs up to the submammary area. Diastasis recti is rare in men, especially young males requiring this type of surgery. If separation of the linea alba is present, plication is done in the usual manner. Resection of the flap is carried in continuity with the lateral resections, before the operating table is flexed.

Location of the umbilicus in the flap is determined, on the midline at the optimum level, not higher than the iliac crest (in females it is between iliac crest and waistline). Defatting of the umbilical site over a 3-cm diameter is done, and occasionally of the upper midline. Separate sutures attach the umbilicus to the skin and rectus fascia. It should be noted that there are no specific sexual characteristics of the umbilicus, with the exception of hairiness along the upper border in the male [19]. One should attempt to reduplicate the type of preoperative umbilicus, i.e., vertical, transverse, or round. Routine closure is done.

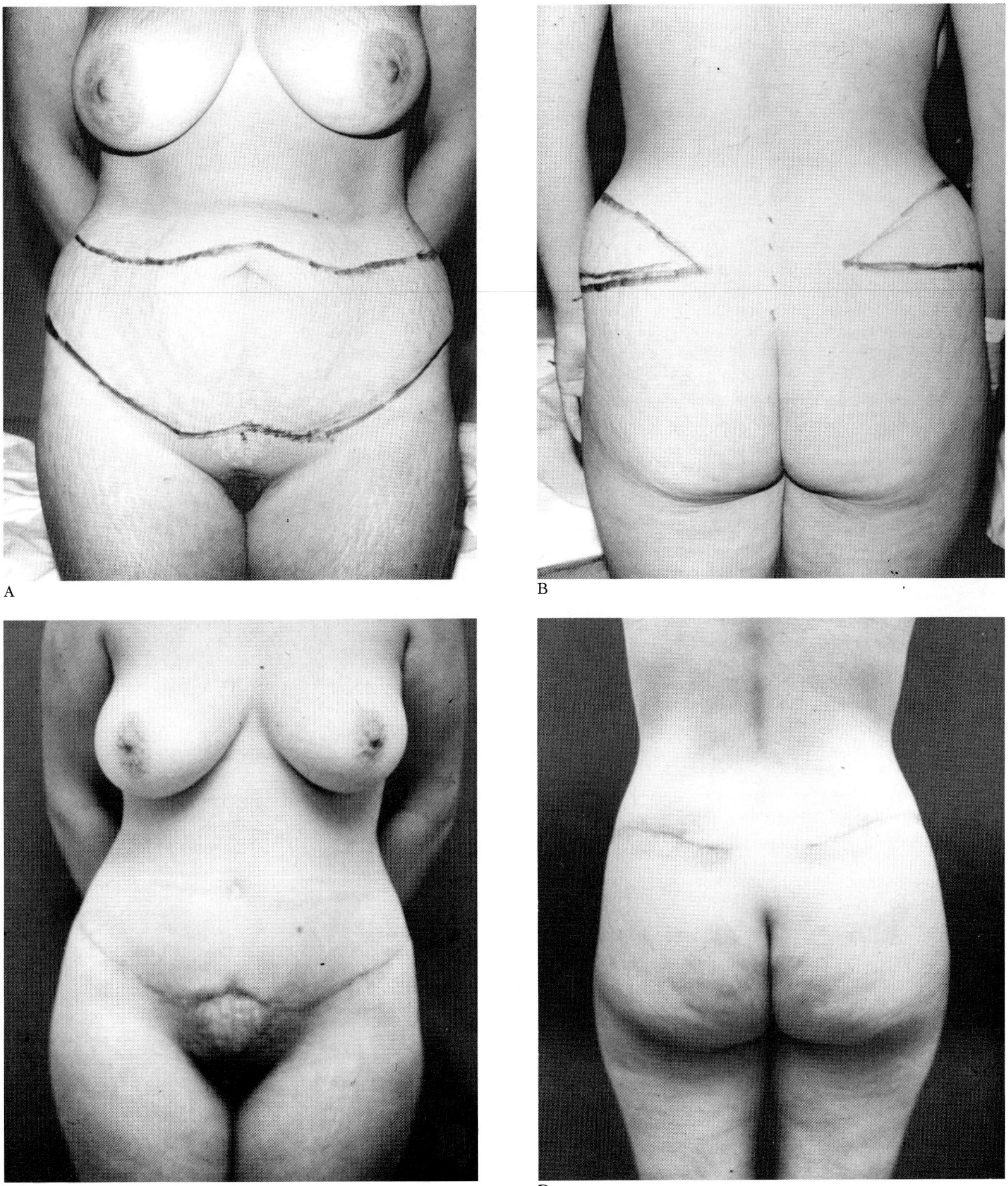

A B C D

Figure 25-15

A, B. Preoperative markings for an extended W-plasty to correct lateral fullness.

C, D. Postoperatively, the silhouette has been dramatically improved. Note 8-cm inferior movement of periumbilical mole.

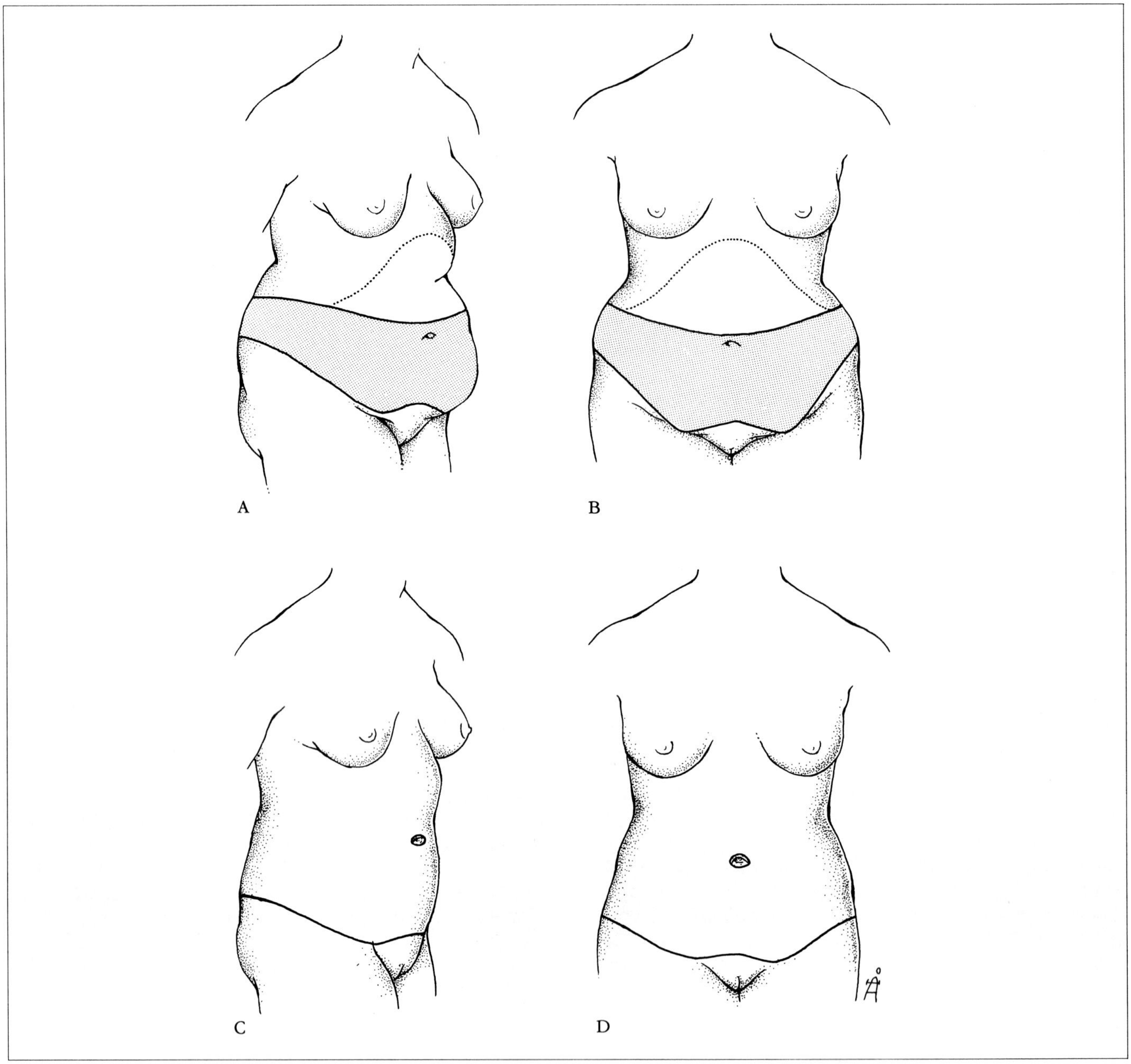

Figure 25-16
A–D. Operative plan for an extended W-plasty.

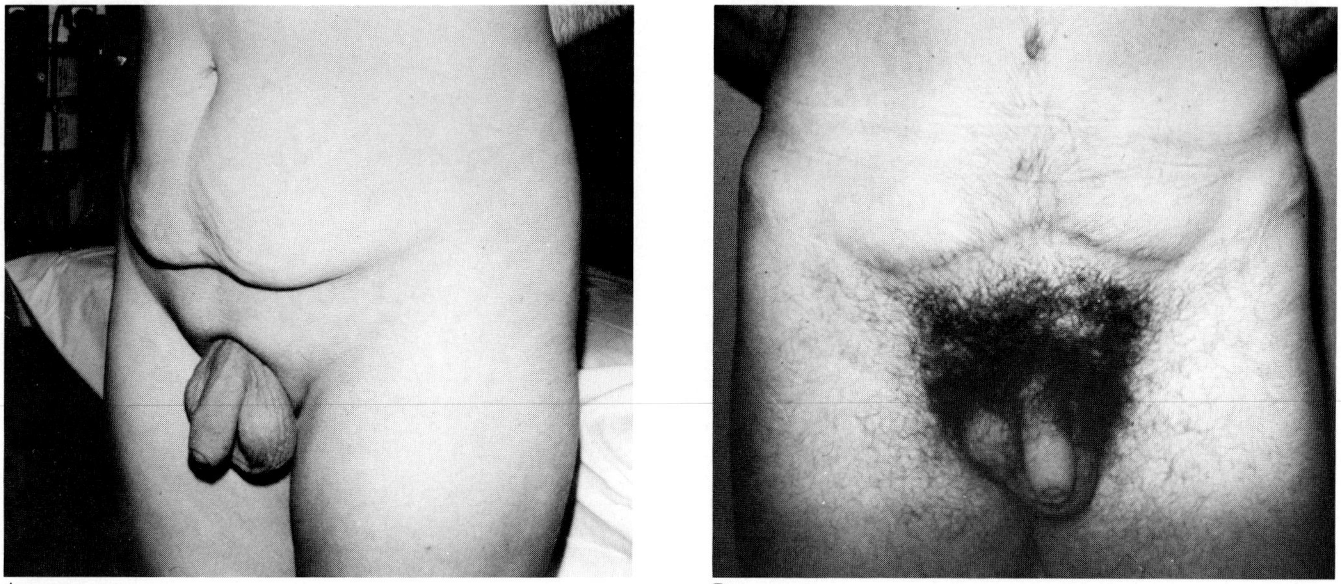

A B

Figure 25-17
A. Abdominal redundancy in a male.
B. Result following abdominoplasty.

COMBINED PROCEDURES
A wide variety of plastic, gynecologic, and general surgical procedures can be combined with abdominoplasty. The most frequent are breast surgery and vaginal hysterectomy. We discourage most general procedures (cholecystectomy), as their complications can be catastrophic, and accept gynecologic procedures (abdominal hysterectomies) only if the cost of hospitalization will be lessened, for the benefit of the patient.

Augmentation Mammaplasty. As originally proposed by Hinderer [43, 44] in 1968, the advantage of simultaneous abdominoplasty–augmentation mammaplasty is avoidance of breast scars and a second separate operation. The onus is on the surgeon to achieve as excellent a result with the combined operation as he would with separate procedures without increased complications [73]. The obvious risks to the abdominal skin flap as well as displacement or infection of breast prostheses are rare [97]. Planas [70] did not have any significant complications in his initial report of 12 cases.

The inframammary fold and breast pockets are marked in addition to the standard abdominoplasty reference points (Fig. 25-18). The abdominoplasty dissection is done and continued up to the fifth rib, where the pectoralis is divided for a routine partial subpectoral placement. Once the implants are inserted, a two-layer closure of the breast pocket is done with nonabsorbable sutures. Transfixion sutures through the skin and underlying fascia are inserted to fix the lower borders and prevent displacement of the implants. Drains are not inserted in the breast pockets. The routine abdominal closure and postoperative management are followed. Recent perfection of the transaxillary approach for breast augmentation has reduced the frequency of the abdominal approach. Since the axillary scar is so inconspicuous, we feel that an axillary augmentation plus a W-plasty has less morbidity and a higher certainty of the ideal result than the abdominal route, especially in tall individuals.

Mastopexy or Breast Reduction. Despite the magnitude of each individual procedure, it is possible to combine a breast reduction or mastopexy with an abdominoplasty (Fig. 25-19). Because of the required jackknife position for abdominoplasty closure, the breast surgery is done first and then the abdominoplasty. Hinderer [44] has noted that traction on the abdomen may lower the inframammary sulcus by 1 to 3 cm, thus minimizing the ptosis and reducing the need for nipple transposition in cases of minor ptosis. Cardoso de Castro and Daher [14] reported 30 combined cases of reduction mammaplasty and abdominoplasty. Surgery averaged 3 hours, and transfusion was necessary in only one patient. Problems with hypertrophic inframammary scars were minimized by marking the inframammary sulcus higher than normal, i.e., with downward traction on the inframammary skin, thereby compensating for the tension secondary to the abdominoplasty.

MODIFICATIONS FOR SCARS
When abdominal scars exist in the *upper quadrants,* they may produce problems according to their location, length, and number. A careful review of previous operations and complications is essential as well as physical examination to rule out incisional hernias.

Each case requires special attention. If a vertical midline scar is present, a fleur-de-lis excision is used. The usual cholecystectomy scar in the right upper quadrant, either oblique or horizontal, is considered insignificant if it is less than 8 to 10 cm in length and the procedure was done more than 2 years previously. If these criteria are met, a W-plasty is done, leaving the scar as it is. Other small scars

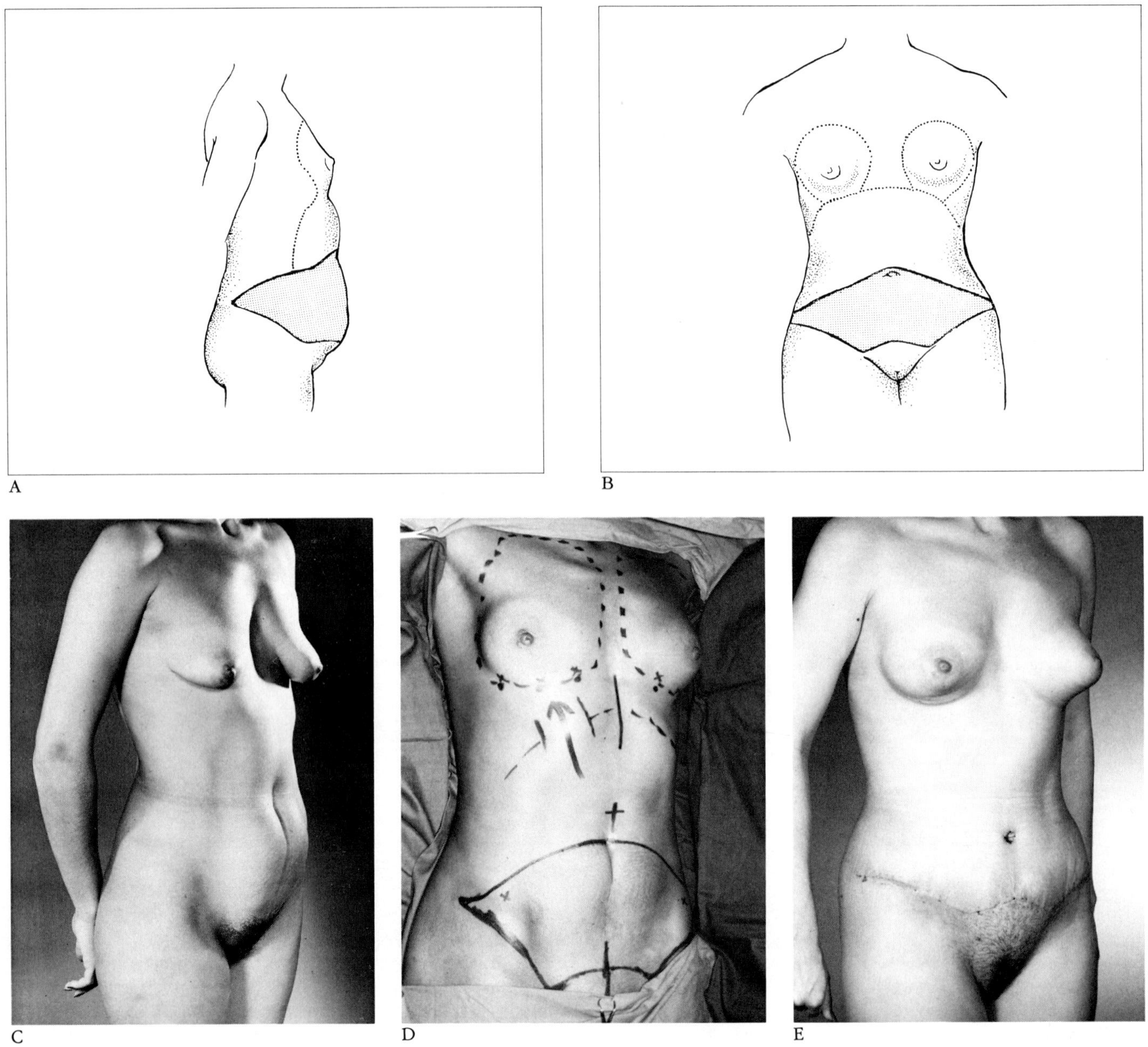

Figure 25-18. Technique for abdominoplasty with simultaneous augmentation mammaplasty.

A, B. Technique for abdominoplasty with simultaneous augmentation mammaplasty using the abdominal approach.

C. Patient with skin laxity, striae, protuberance, and cesarean scar. She requested abdominal hysterectomy, abdominoplasty, and augmentation for pseudotuberous breast deformity.

D. Preoperative markings include tunnels for subpectoral placement of the implants and anticipated descent of the inframammary crease due to abdominal tension.

E. Early postoperative result.

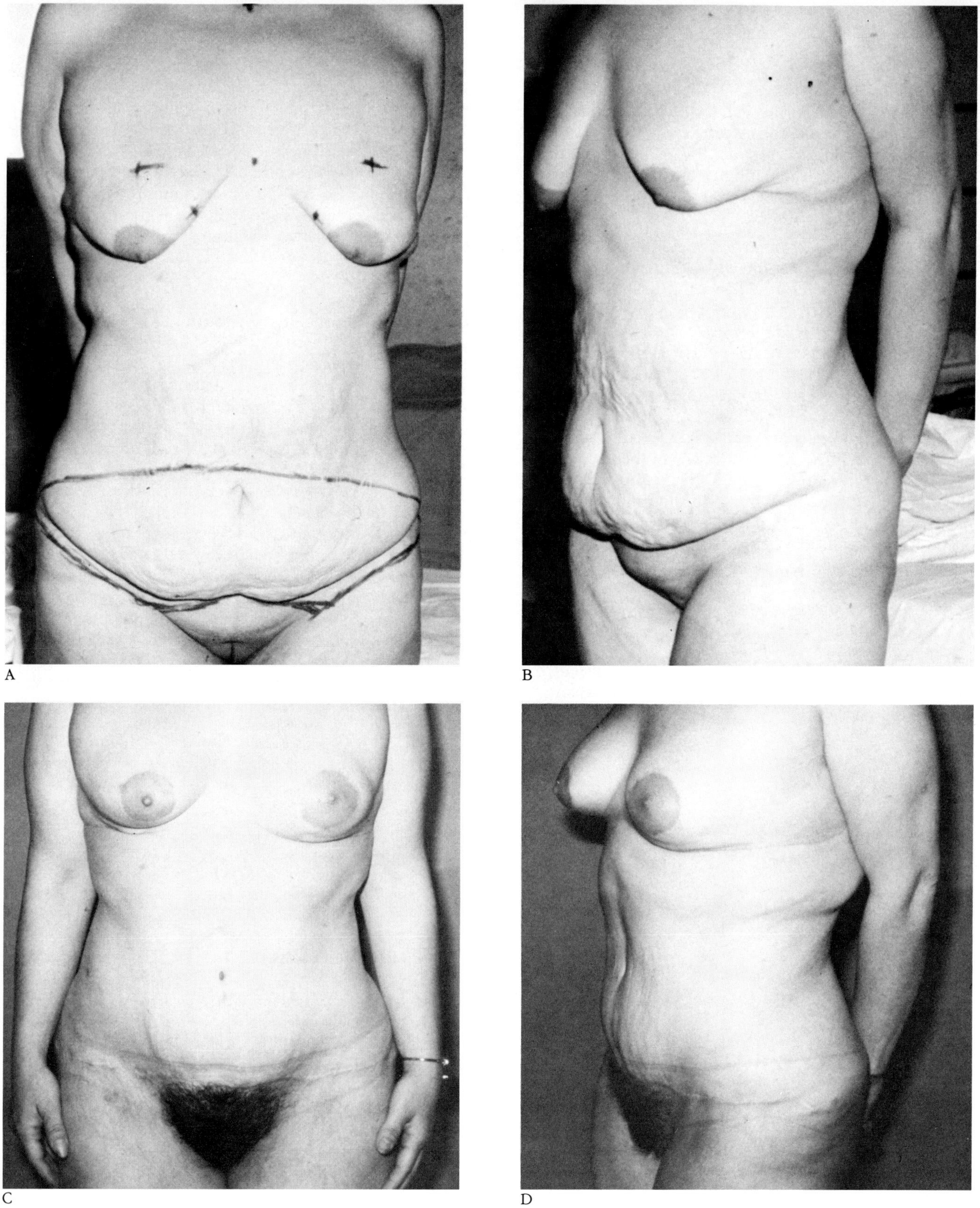

Figure 25-19

A, B. Patient requesting abdominoplasty and correction of ptotic deformed breasts.

C, D. Result following abdominoplasty and B-mastopexy with augmentation.

may also be left as they are and a W-plasty be performed. However, large or multiple scars of the upper quadrants cannot be ignored, and the requisite modification is an upper abdominoplasty. Use of a lower abdominoplasty incision may result in skin sloughs and catastrophic complications.

Marking. The markings incorporate removal of the scar plus simultaneous correction of flaccidity and adiposity. The excision is designed to leave the least visible scar while removing the largest possible fat and skin excess. Two types of designs occur as determined by the umbilical position (Fig. 25-20A, B). The umbilicus may rest within the excised area and is isolated and incorporated into the horizontal scar. Or it may remain above or below the final scar and is transposed with the flap.

The upper marking is incised and dissected downward. Traction is applied following elevation of the flap and the maximum resection determined. When the excision is rather limited, minimal or limited undermining may be sufficient. Drains are left when extensive undermining is done. Taping and moderate pressure dressing are used.

Patient acceptance of a midabdominal incision line is quite high as significant scarring already exists and often one is consolidating several scars into one (Fig. 25-20C, D). As noted by Lewis [58, 59], the midabdominoplasty scar often coincides with lines from a half-slip or panty hose. Alternatively, it may be possible to combine the inframammary incisions of a previous reduction mammaplasty with a central dart and thus perform an upper abdominoplasty, as recommended by Reich [83] and Rebello and Franco [74].

Abdominal Lipectomy

Selection of the optimal operation depends on the location of the adiposity and the patient's willingness to accept the resulting scars. The obesity may be generalized, lower medial, or upper medial. In abdominal lipectomies, the adiposity is excised where it exists without undermining or concern for the location of the final scars [89]. The patient is marked in the standing position and the amount to be excised determined by pinching the skin. Since undermining is limited and the umbilicus is rarely transposed, postoperative complications are few. The incidence of preexisting ventral or umbilical hernias is much greater in these patients, and one must be prepared to treat them definitively.

TORSO OBESITY—BELT LIPECTOMY

This circular excision is indicated for patients with adiposity of the entire torso including the back and upper buttocks (Fig. 25-21). With fingers placed above and below the umbilicus, the surgeon pinches and marks the abdominal wall. These estimates are continued around the body, producing two circles that are closer together in the back; triangles of compensation may be necessary. The usual circular adiposity does not involve the spine. Only in massive-weight-loss cases (see Chap. 29) does extreme flabbiness require a complete circular excision. The abdominal excision lines are continued in an oblique and upward direction following the natural crease lines. They terminate as two angles separated by the spine. These angles may be at the level of the waistline or slightly below.

Technique. The operation is started in the back with the patient prone. The lower incision line is made first, the surgeon dissecting along the fascia and pulling on the dissected flap to evaluate the amount of resection. Then the excess is removed as far laterally as possible. Defatting is sometimes done close to the edges and under the medial limb of the excision to avoid redundancies. Hemostasis is meticulous, and drains are inserted. A two-layer closure is done. Tapes and sterile dressing are applied, covering the operating field completely. The arms are elevated above the head and the patient is turned supine. The abdomen is prepped and draped and the lower incision line continued in front, following the preoperative markings. Dissection of the flap up to the excision line is done, the mobility checked, and the panniculus excised. Where large inequality of the edges exists, compensating triangular excisions may be required. Most often, one midline lower excision in the pubic area is required. If there is redundancy over the hips, two compensating triangles may be excised laterally.

UPPER MEDIAL OBESITY—T-EXCISION

When the adiposity is concentrated at or above the waistline, it is best treated by a T-excision or modified Weinhold technique (Fig. 25-22). With the patient standing, the excess soft tissue is pinched and marked. The superior straight circular incision line is located 4 to 5 cm above the umbilicus while the lower excision line slopes inferiorly and has a midline vertical downward component (Fig. 25-23). These incisions tighten the abdomen and allow excision of the adiposity where it exists.

The umbilicus may be located at the junction of the vertical and horizontal branches, or lower in the vertical scar, depending on where the upper line of excision is located. After the flap is lifted to the midline and separated from the umbilicus, gentle traction will show the adequate width to remove. Plication of the fascia is done. In cases of large umbilical hernia, the umbilicus is sacrificed and will be simulated by attaching the defatted wound edges at this location to the fascia. A limited defatting of the deeper fat layer can be done in the upper horizontal flap, especially in the midline (Fig. 25-23D). The deep layers are closed with 0 Vicryl and the subcutaneous tissues with 4-0 Vicryl and paper tapes. Drainage is indicated when defatting has been done.

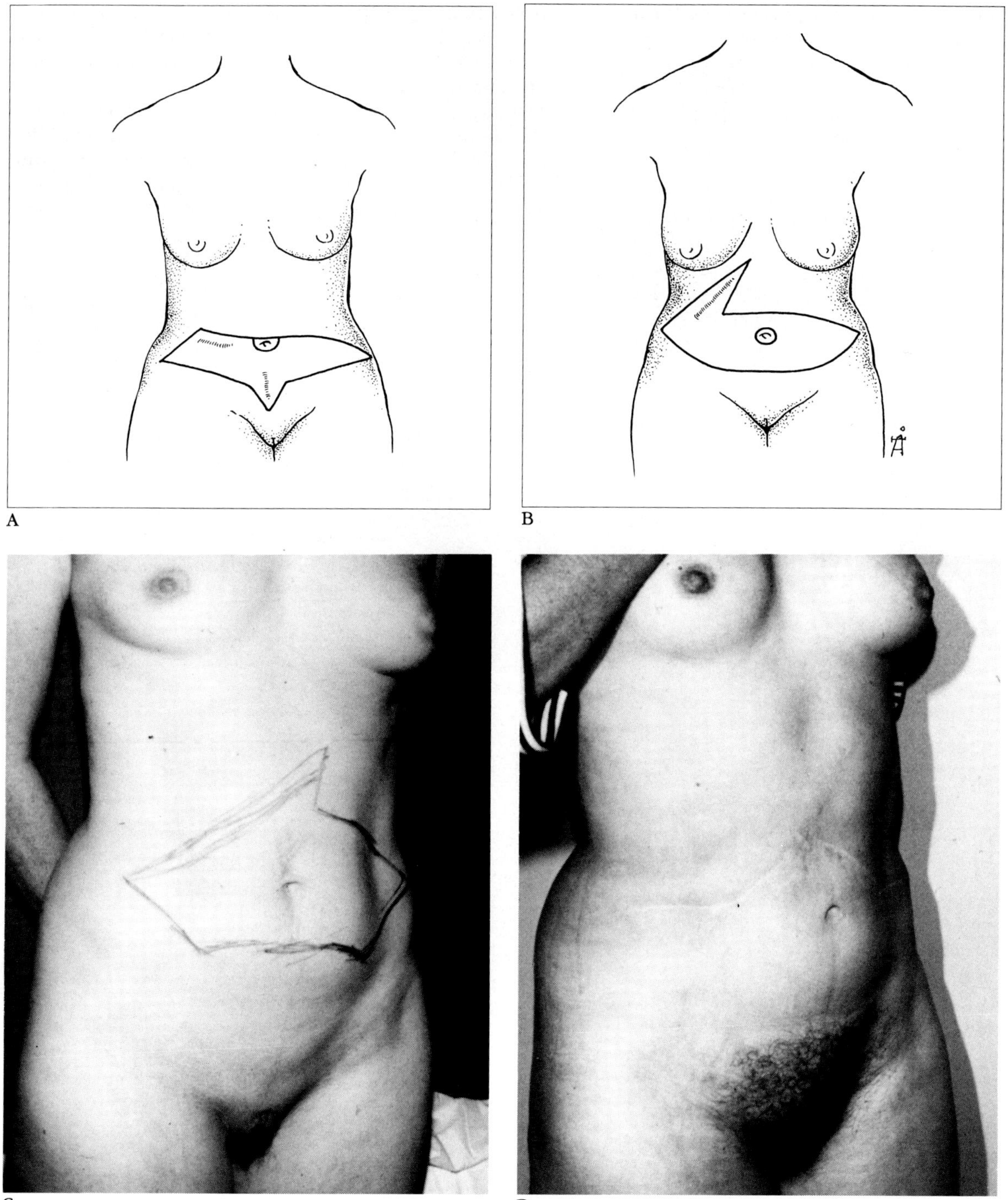

Figure 25-20. Two types of modified abdominoplasties for upper quadrant scars.

A. Periumbilical removal of tissue.
B. Incorporation of umbilicus into one limb of the excision.
C. Patient with previous cholecystectomy and midline scars.
D. Result following skin excision, plication, and creation of a natural-appearing umbilicus. Patient also had simultaneous breast augmentation through the abdominoplasty incision.

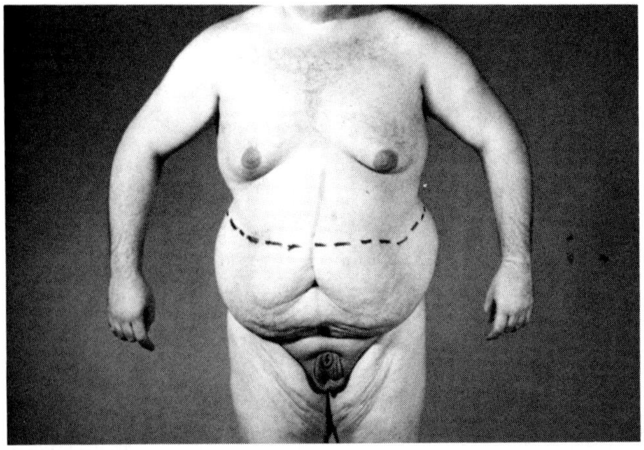

A

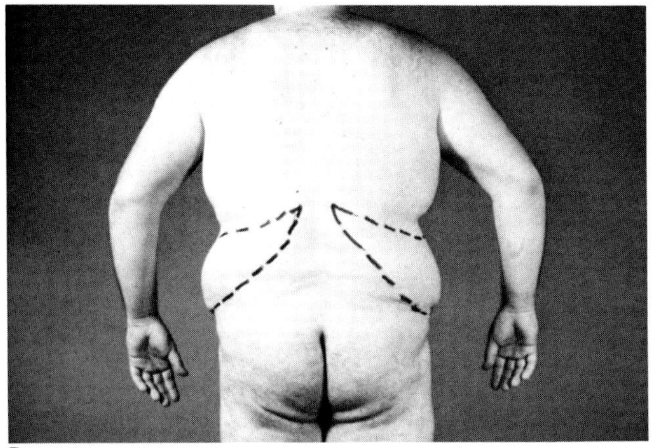

B

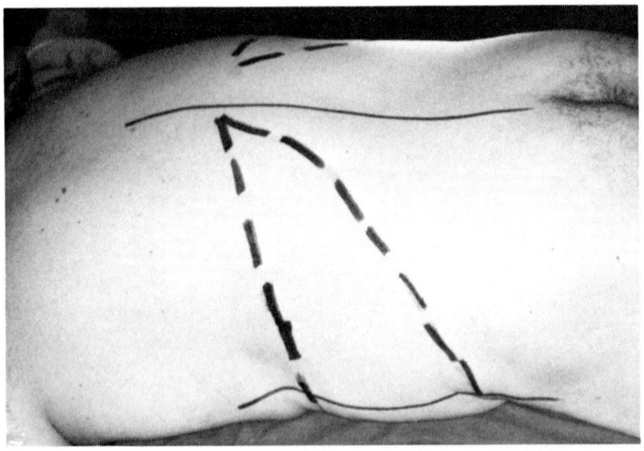

C

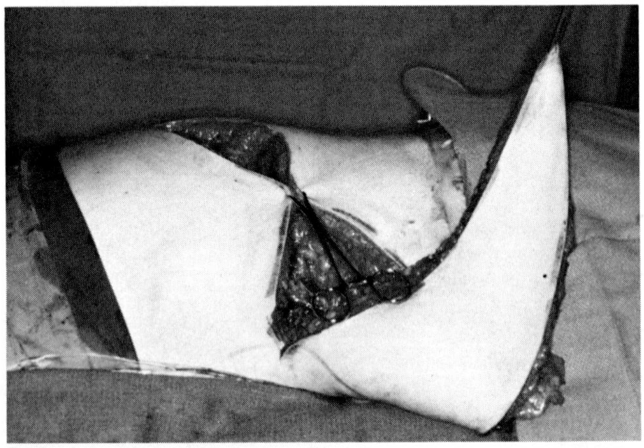

D

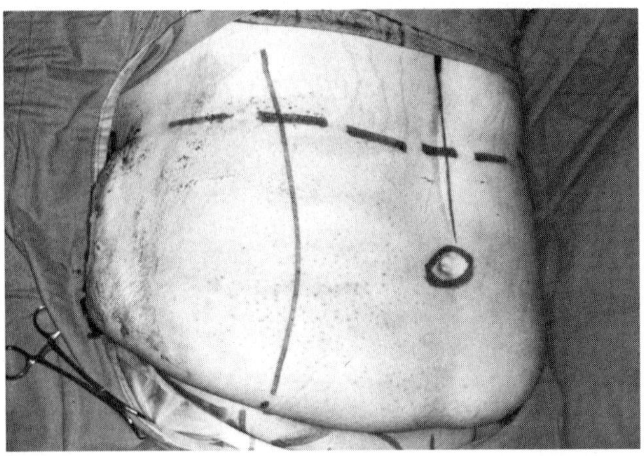

E

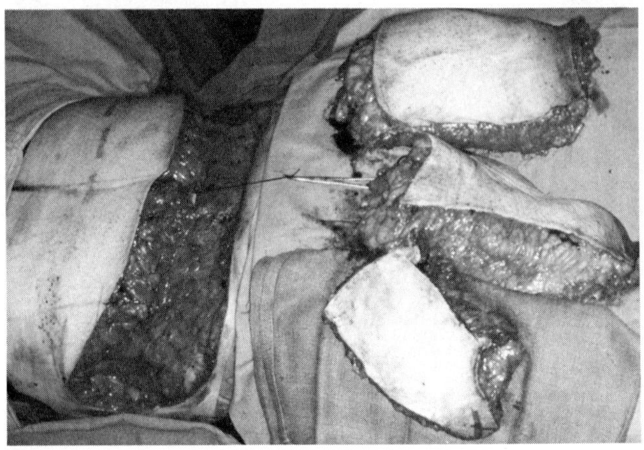

F

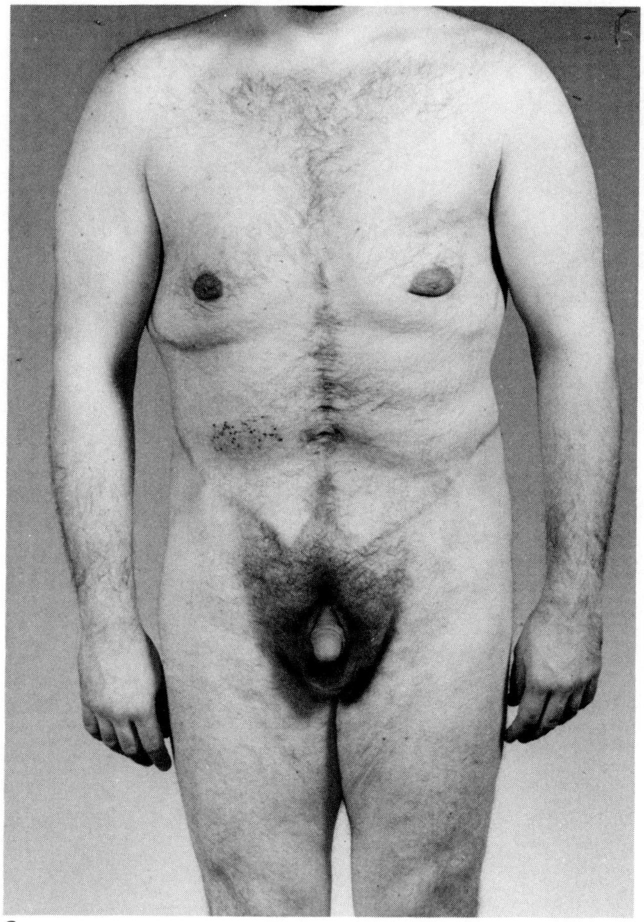

G

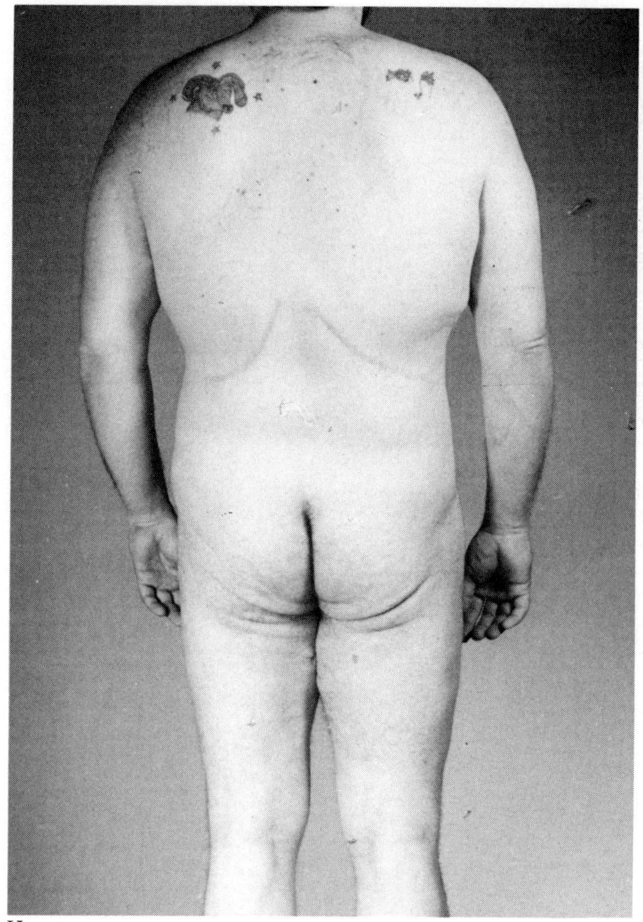

H

Figure 25-21. Modified belt lipectomy.
A, B. Preoperative markings for maximum excision of tissue redundancy.
C, D. Back excision is done first extending to the midaxillary line.
E, F. Abdominal excision is completed and the umbilicus transposed.
G, H. Postoperative result at 2 years with significant contour improvement and acceptable scarring. Patient also had a bat-wing torsoplasty with subcutaneous defatting of the breasts and a midline tightening.

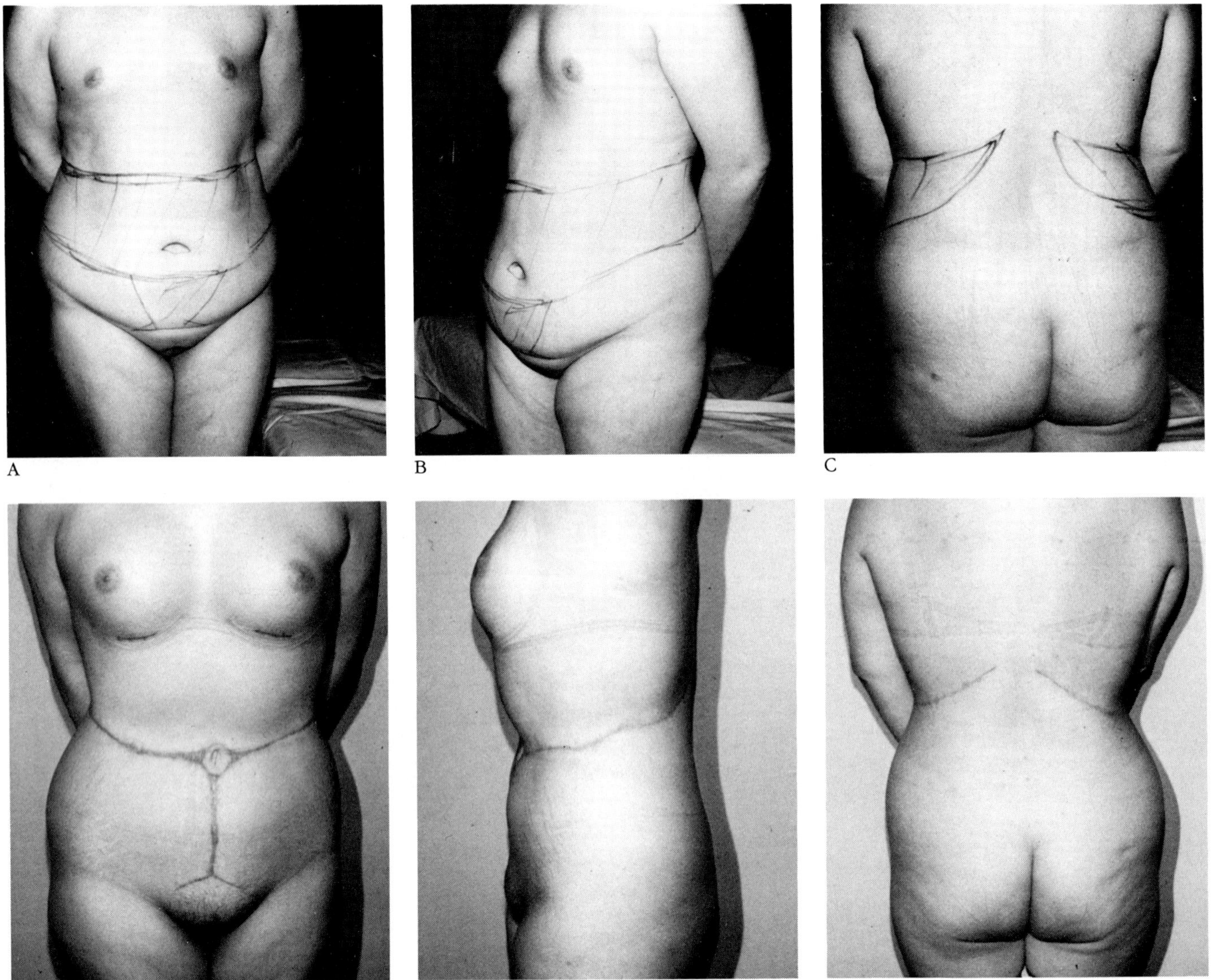

A B C D E F

Figure 25-22

A–C. Patient with significant upper medial obesity requiring a direct T-excision with no undermining; therefore, augmentation done through an inframammary incision.

D–F. Marked improvement in body contour, especially anterior and over the flanks.

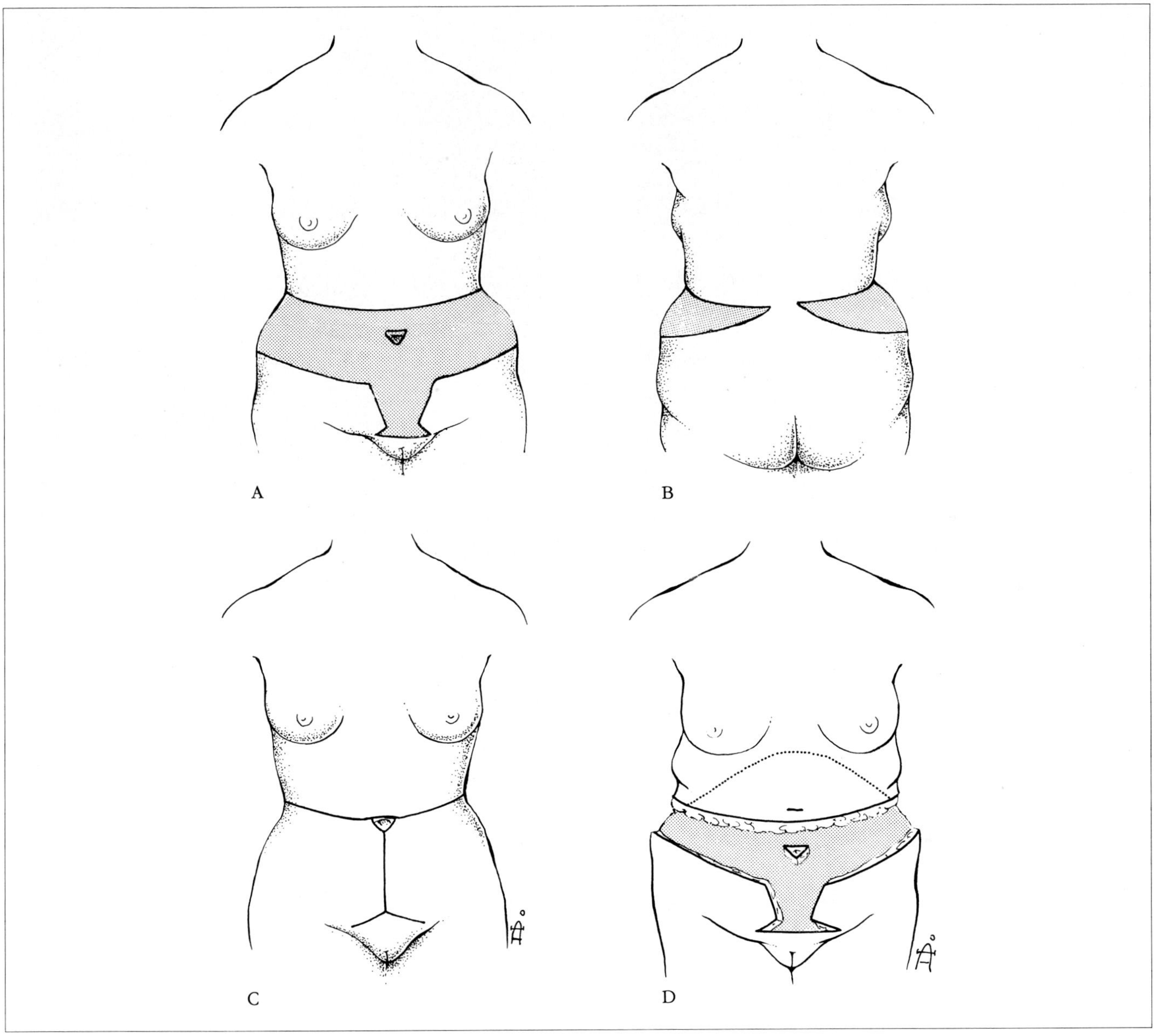

Figure 25-23
A–C. T-excision technique for upper medial obesity.
D. Extent of excision with optional defatting of the upper flap.

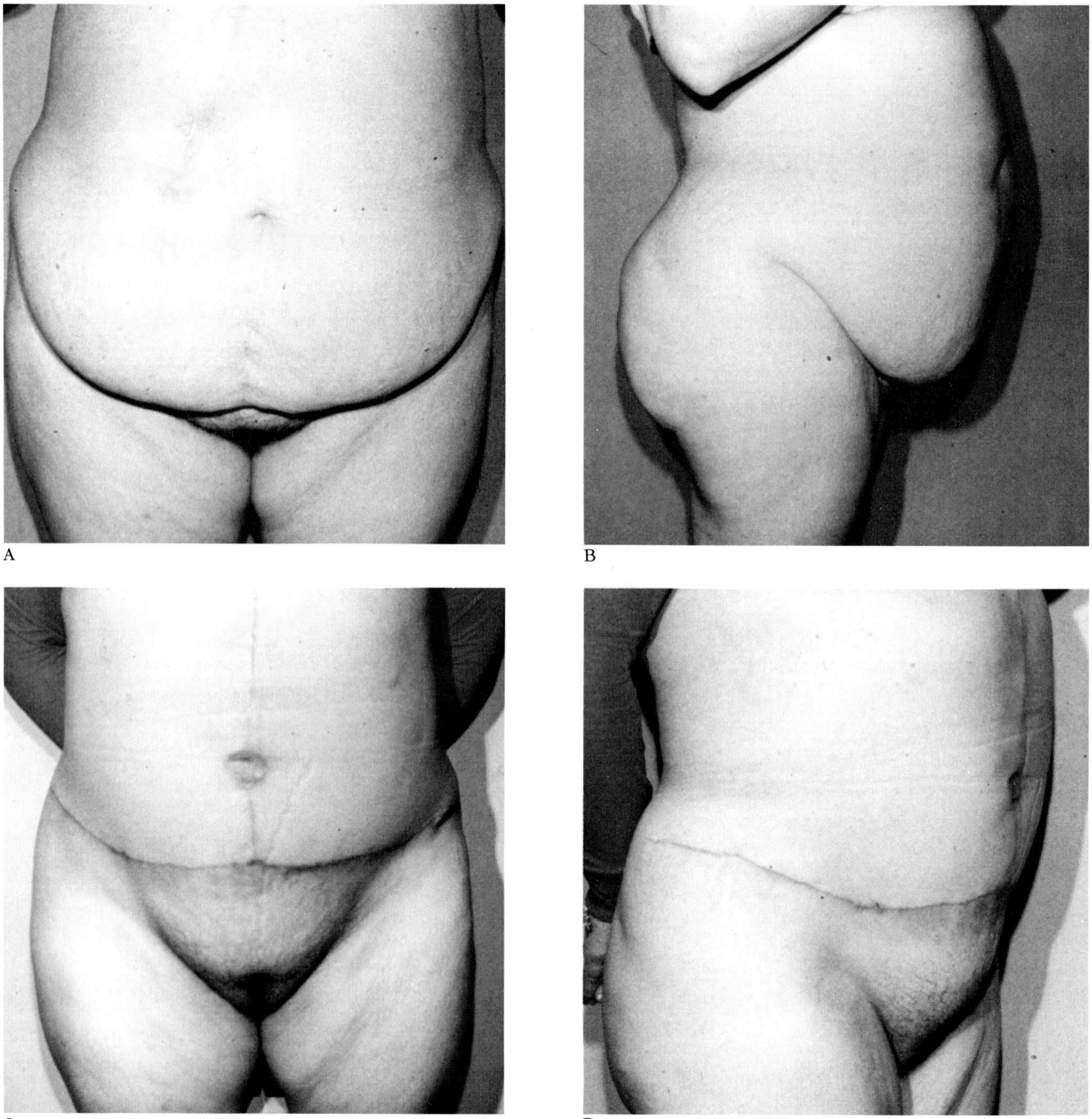

A B C D

Figure 25-24
A, B. Patients with significant obesity of the anterior abdominal wall and multiple scars.
C, D. Result following fleur-de-lis excision.

LOWER MEDIAL OBESITY—FLEUR-DE-LIS OPERATION

When the adiposity is concentrated in the lower and medial quadrants, it is best treated by the fleur-de-lis technique, a three-branched excision that not only removes excess tissue but improves the contour, especially the waistline. Frequently, patients with preexisting scars are willing to trade a scar for maximum correction (Fig. 25-24). With the patient standing, the amount of excision is estimated by pinching the soft tissues and marked with indelible ink. The lower incision follows a W design and is located 2 cm above the pubic hair and inguinal folds laterally (Fig. 25-25). The vertical and upper lateral excision lines are based on pinching the soft tissue. The umbilicus is incised in a vertical marquise cut.

The lower W-incision is continued down to the suprafascial areolar plane and continued upward until the lateral line is reached (Fig. 25-26). Each lower lateral wing is excised. Then the right side of the vertical marking is

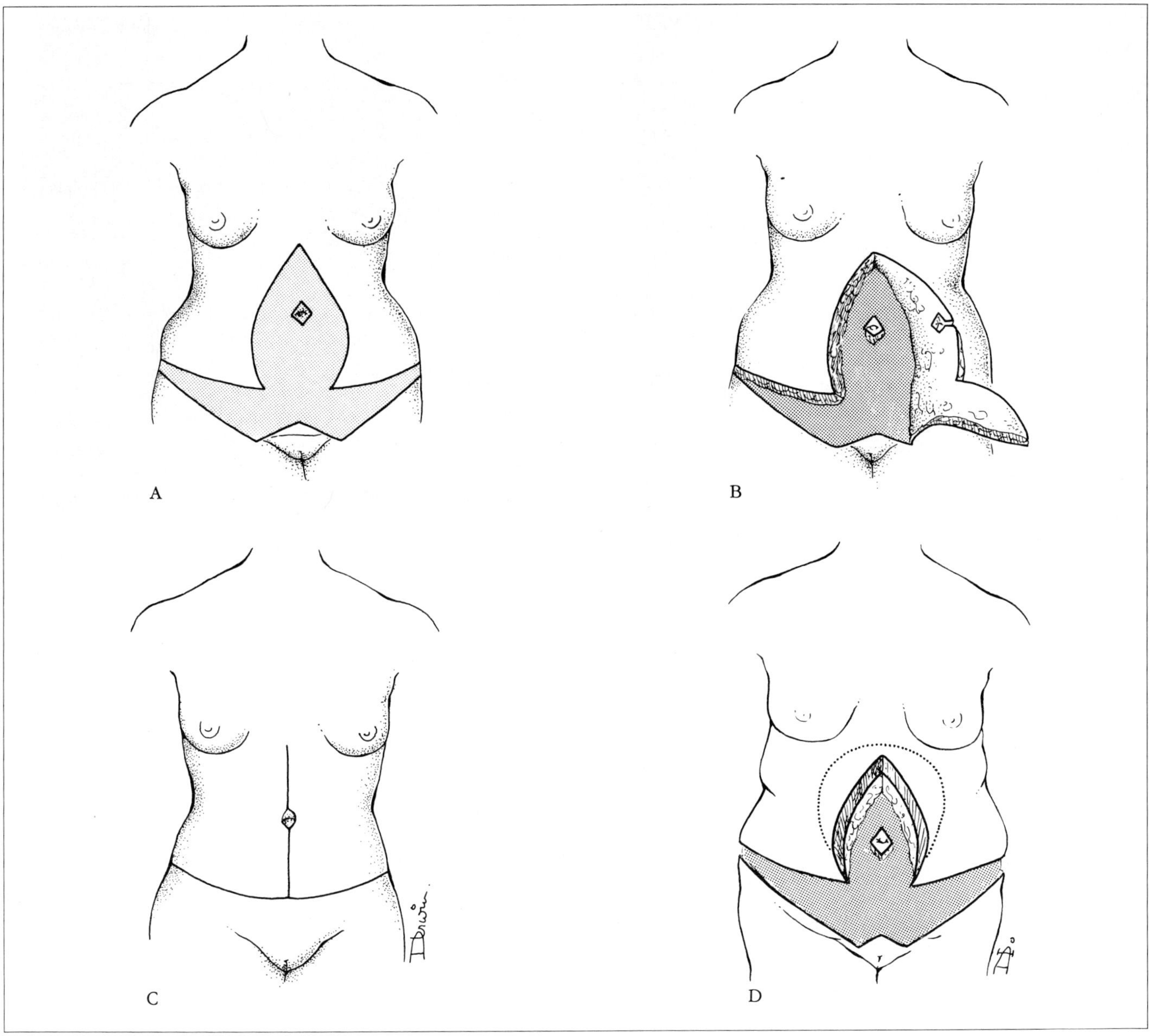

Figure 25-25
A. Standard fleur-de-lis design.
B. Incision followed by dissection to the anticipated excision line.
C. Closure resulting in an inverted-T scar.
D. In moderately obese patient, optional defatting can be done.

incised down to areolar fascia and dissected from right to left. It must be emphasized that extensive undermining is not done in abdominal lipectomies. Defatting up to Scarpa's fascia on the undersurface is done close to the edges, in the upper epigastric area, and around the umbilicus. The amount of tissue to be excised is checked to ensure that closure with *moderate* tension is possible. After complete resection, a diastasis of the recti or umbilical or ventral hernias may become apparent. Most diastases of the recti are correctable by plication with heavy nonabsorbable sutures. If a large umbilical hernia is encountered, the umbilicus is sacrificed and an umbilical hernia repair completed followed by umbiliconeoplasty at a later date. When large ventral hernias cannot be corrected by rectus fascia plication, Marlex mesh must be inserted.

A two-layer deep closure is done with heavy absorbable material in both layers and a running subcuticular suture in the skin. The vertical component is closed first, with the umbilicus located in its normal position. The repair then extends laterally, possibly requiring a flexed position for the operating table. Because of the absence of undermining, drainage is rarely required. Patient acceptance with this technique is excellent as the results are often dramatic. Waistlines are restored and dress sizes reduced markedly. Surgeon satisfaction is great as the tissue is

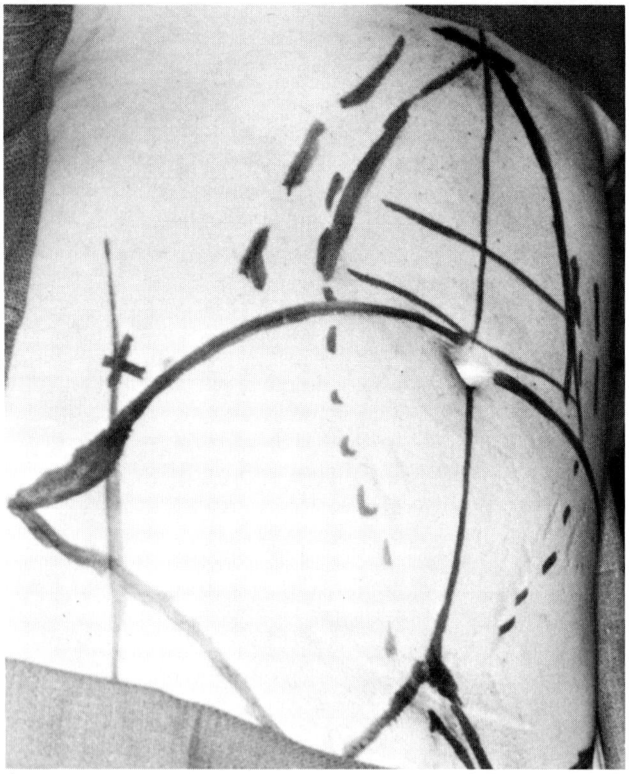
A

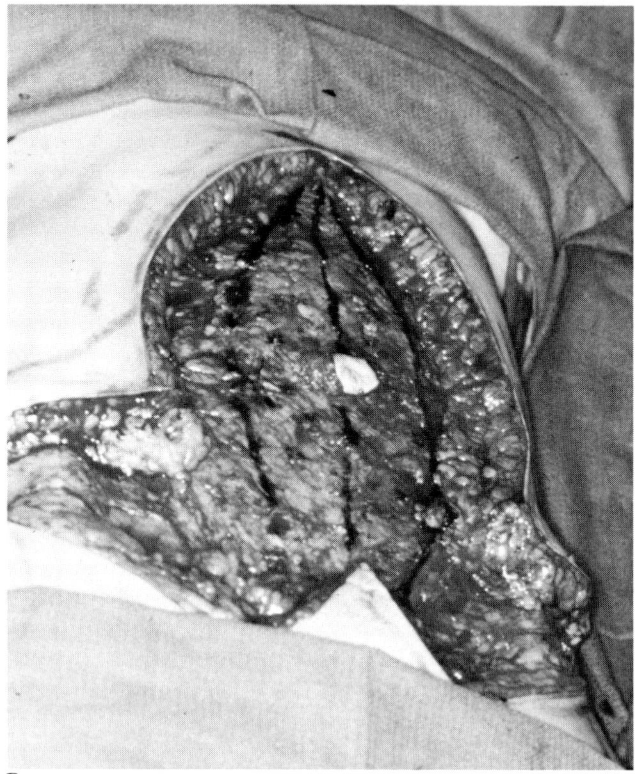
B

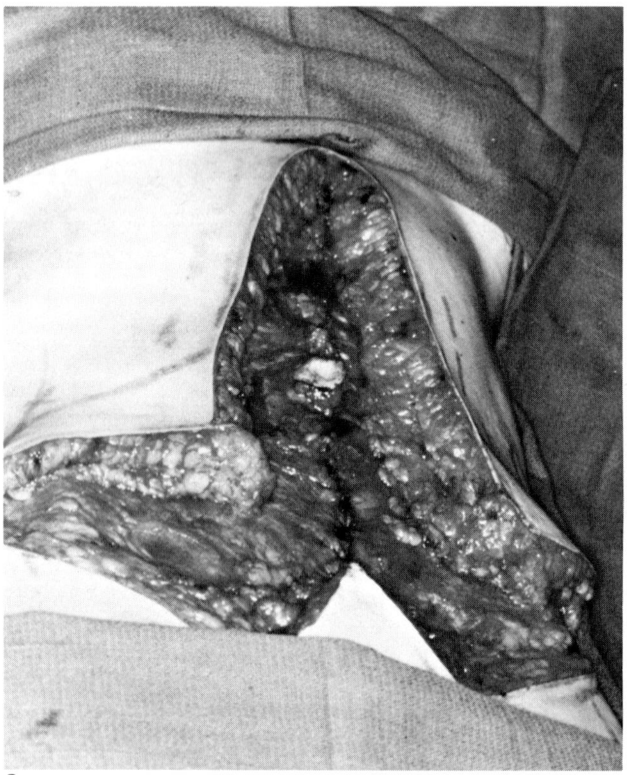
C

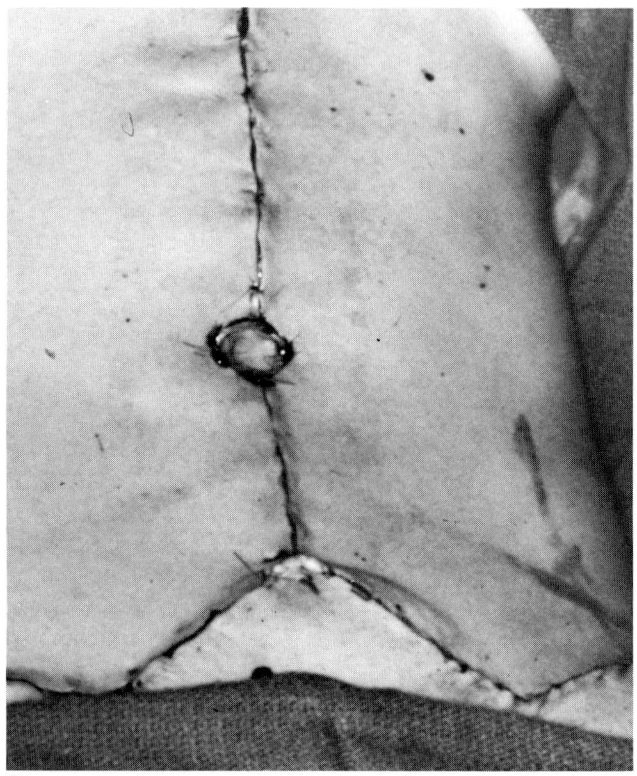
D

Figure 25-26

A. Outline for a fleur-de-lis abdominal lipectomy.
B. Following direct excision, no undermining, and proposed plication.
C. Wound edges are closer following plication of diastasis recti.
D. Subcuticular wound closure. Pubic area is usually more curved.

directly excised, undermining is minimal, there is no transposition of the umbilicus, and the procedure is quick (1–1½ hours).

COMPLICATIONS

Abdominal dermolipectomy has both frequent and potentially serious complications that must be thoroughly understood [71]. The incidence of problems approaches 10 percent (Table 25-1). Occasional deaths from pulmonary embolus occur.

Intraoperative Complications

The primary intraoperative complications are tight wound closure and lateral bulges. Since it is desirable to minimize any vertical scar, one occasionally excises more skin than is desirable. In these situations, one can extend the undermining laterally onto the upper thighs to gain increased skin mobility. In addition, the lateral flaps can be advanced and a small vertical closure performed. Every effort must be made to avoid a skin slough, which is more reprehensible than a vertical scar. If any distortion of the umbilicus occurs because of asymmetric tension on the flap or suture errors, it should be corrected immediately, with release and reapproximation of the flap.

Lateral bulges are frequently encountered, and one should minimize them at the time of closure rather than expect them to disappear postoperatively. The choices are either liposuction or extension of the incision and resection of excess tissue. Obviously, liposuction is a realistic adjunct for lipectomy and a valuable tool for reducing adjacent bulges.

Early Postoperative Complications

HEMATOMA AND SEROMA

On account of extensive undermining, hematomas and seromas are a significant problem that can be minimized by meticulous hemostasis, ligation of any severed lymph channels, suction drainage, a conforming dressing, and continued bed rest in a flexed position. Most hematomas occur within the first postoperative day and are signaled by patient discomfort and developing skin ecchymosis. Hematomas usually represent continued bleeding from one or two large vessels rather than generalized oozing. Thus, it is best to reexplore the wound in the operating room under general anesthesia with ligation of the vessels. In contrast, serous fluid accumulation occurs 3 to 5 days postoperatively and can usually be treated by aspiration through a large-bore needle. Repeated aspiration twice a week for 3 to 5 weeks may be required. Occasionally, small hematomas become visible only after the second to third week, creating small bulges, discomfort, or wound disruption. Aspiration is the treatment of choice.

Table 25-1. Complications in 539 abdominal dermolipectomies

Serosanguineous collections		5.8%
Required drainage	2.5%	
No drainage	3.3%	
Infection, dehiscence		0.3%
Skin necrosis		1.7%
Required surgery	0.3%	
No surgery	1.4%	
Suture reaction		0.9%
Hypertrophic scars		3.7%
Poor scar or body contour		0.3%
Residual adiposity (epigastrium)		0.3%
Deep vein thrombosis		NA
Total		13.0%

Source: I. Pitanguy, *Aesthetic Plastic Surgery of Head and Body.* Berlin: Springer, 1981.

INFECTION

Major infections are relatively rare but are associated with large hematomas, skin sloughs, or dehiscences. The wound should be partially opened for drainage of any abscess or loculated fluid accumulation. Following cultures, a broad-spectrum antibiotic is given and adjusted according to sensitivity studies. Wet-to-dry dressings are begun. If there is limited skin loss, the wound will usually close spontaneously.

STITCH ABSCESS AND WOUND SEPARATION

Minor stitch abscesses and wound separation occur most frequently in the obese patient. Their occurrence increases with wound tension and the use of superficial interrupted absorbable sutures. In general, these problems pass without incidence provided the patient is warned of their possible occurrence. Minor separations will close spontaneously with optimal wound management and antibiotics.

SKIN NECROSIS

Skin sloughs are a major disappointment for surgeon and patient. Skin loss usually appears in the midline and ranges from minor (2–3 cm) to major (up to the umbilicus) (Fig. 25-27). Although the obvious explanations are excessive tension, surgical trauma, and hematoma, one cannot discount variations in vascular anatomy, smoking, or previous incisions. Since compromised skin is rarely recognized before 12 hours postoperatively, meaningful intervention is usually not possible. The patient should be told that there is a problem with skin circulation and that some skin loss will occur. Fluorescence can be of value in predicting its size. Once the patient understands the problem and is reassured that she will not "fall apart," one of two treatments is proposed: either surgical debridement with application of a skin graft or gradual eschar separation with wound contracture. The former is quicker but requires a longer hospitalization and a secondary donor site; the latter requires daily dressing changes for up to 6 weeks. We prefer excision and grafting although some patients demand a conservative regimen. In both cases, a secondary scar revision is usually necessary at 6 to 9 months. During the intervening period, the patient needs and deserves the surgeon's close support and frequent reassurance that everything will be fine. Ultimately, the

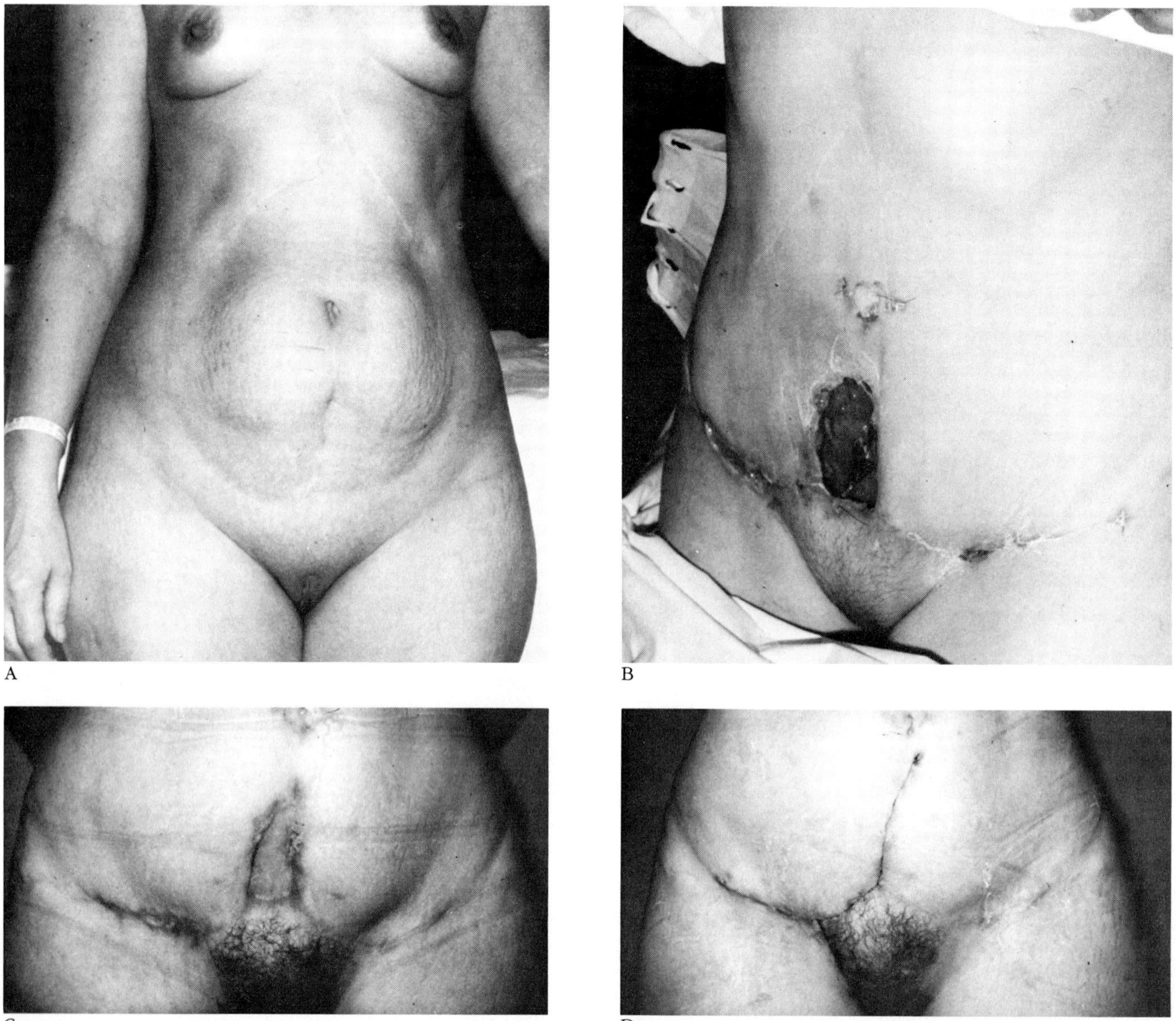

Figure 25-27
A. Patient with preexisting bilateral upper quadrant incisions who sought abdominoplasty.
B. Lower midline slough following W-abdominoplasty.
C. Defect closed with a skin graft.
D. Subsequent revision by midline flap approximation.

patient must accept the vertical scar that skin slough produces, in addition to the anticipated transverse scar.

THROMBOPHLEBITIS AND PULMONARY EMBOLUS

Thrombophlebitis with pulmonary embolus is a life-threatening complication and occasionally causes death. As detailed in the review by Grazer and Goldwyn [37], the incidence of thrombophlebitis is 1.1 percent and of pulmonary embolus 0.8 percent, with six deaths due to pulmonary embolus. Is there a specific association between abdominoplasty and pulmonary embolus or do these figures reflect the patient population? Grazer and Klingbeil [39] state that exaggerated flexion of the hips and knees does not increase venous stasis but that manipulation of the abdominal flap may result in hypercoagulability or fat emboli. Pertinent patient factors include age, obesity, previous thrombophlebitis, smoking, and birth control pills. In general, these risk factors are comparable to those of the general patient population and are not specific. In conclusion, it would appear that abdominoplasty does have a higher risk of pulmonary embolus than other body-sculpting procedures and that every effort must be made to identify the at-risk patient. The regimen recommended by Grazer and Klingbeil [39] includes (1) preoperative and postoperative fibrinogen ^{125}I scan, (2) intraoperative infusion of 1 liter of 5% alcohol–5% dextrose, and (3) minimal panniculus manipulation. The patient is mobilized on the first postoperative day and encouraged to do frequent plantar flexion. With this regimen Grazer and Klingbeil have not had a single pulmonary embolus in 200 consecutive cases. If the patient has a previous diagnosis of thrombophlebitis, a modified regimen is begun.

The junior author prefers to use subcutaneous heparin or miniheparin therapy with a dosage of 5000 units given subcutaneously 2 hours preoperatively and similar doses every 8 to 12 hours until the patient is fully mobile. The use of miniheparin for the prevention of pulmonary emboli is supported by solid scientific data [51, 52, 86]. Also, elastic stockings are applied prior to operation, and early mobilization is instituted. Since deep vein thrombosis with pulmonary embolus may occur even in young normal-weight individuals without significant risk factors, it is essential to have a high index of suspicion. Any postoperative complaint of dyspnea or pain on respiration requires an immediate workup to rule out pulmonary embolus. The onset of breathing difficulty or associated leg pain may range from 4 to 11 days. If it is detected, the patient is heparinized and given respiratory support with eventual discharge on Coumadin for 6 months.

Late Postoperative Complications

HYPERTROPHIC SCARS

The majority of hypertrophic scars are best treated by local injection of triamcinolone (10 mg/ml). Surgical revision of the scars should not be done before 1 year except in cases of previous skin separation or slough. If the patient is told preoperatively that a red raised scar occurs often because of tension on the skin, the gradual improvement with time will be better accepted.

PERSISTENT EDEMA

In a few cases edema and swelling of the abdomen may persist and are best minimized by the wearing of a soft panty girdle for several months.

ABNORMAL UMBILICAL POSITION

The umbilicus can be placed in an erroneous vertical or lateral position. Prevention is achieved by accurate preoperative markings plus careful surgical techniques. The umbilicus can be placed too high if the table is not flat when the new umbilicus site is determined and too low if proper tension does not exist on the flaps. Lateral errors are usually due to asymmetric plication, unequal flap tension, or palpation errors caused by displacement of a long umbilicus. Correction can be exceedingly difficult, requiring either a local shift with its attendant scar or redraping of the entire abdominal flap, after 1 to 2 years.

NUMBNESS AND NERVE INJURY

The majority of patients will have numbness postoperatively over the lower abdomen. Although it gradually improves with time, Grazer et al. [36] noted that 84 percent (42 of 50) of patients had persistent midline numbness on long-term follow-up. Thus, the patient should be advised preoperatively to expect some loss of sensation. The initial numbness and burning sensation slowly disappear over several weeks.

If one sutures the flaps to the deep fascia, it is possible to injure the lateral femoral cutaneous nerve.

RESULTS

Short-Term Results

If major complications do not occur, the majority of patients will be pleased with their abdominoplasty. Patient dissatisfaction is usually due to unrealistic expectations or poor preoperative counseling by the surgeon [32]. The patient must accept the fact that the defect can be corrected only partially and that the resulting long scar will hopefully fade from red to white by 1 year. Technical problems of concern to the surgeon are bulging above the incision (insufficient beveling of the abdominal flap), a surgical-looking umbilicus (myriad causes), and hypertrophic scarring.

Long-Term Results

According to Grazer et al. [40], the long-term results of abdominoplasty are excellent as a tighter, flatter abdomen without striae is achieved and justifies the long scar. An analysis of 50 patients, ranging from 1 to 10 years after abdominoplasty, revealed that 33 had no disappointments, 14 considered the scar objectionable (too long, high, or red), and 3 were unhappy with the remaining striae gravidarum. Of particular interest, the abdomen remained flat in all patients despite a 35-lb weight gain in three patients. None of the patients subsequently carried a pregnancy to term. Since the majority of patients (47 of 50) considered their deformity secondary to pregnancy rather than to significant weight change, abdominoplasty would appear to be a permanent solution provided obesity is avoided.

SECONDARY SURGERY

Revisions and Recurrences

The indications for secondary surgery include (1) bulging of the upper quadrants due to insufficient defatting or selection of the wrong operation, (2) continued lateral bulging, and (3) malposition of the scar (too high, vertical component). Recurrences are due to significant weight loss or subsequent pregnancy. In general, liposuction is a valuable modality for "touching up" any small secondary deformities, especially lateral bulges or epigastric fullness. However, it cannot correct persistent skin redundancy or umbilical deformities [96].

In a secondary abdominoplasty, the incision is placed as low as skin elasticity permits and extended laterally for removal of bulges (Fig. 25-28). As with secondary rhytidectomies, the skin excision will not be as great as in a primary procedure. The dissection is done in the previous plane, and the amount of bleeding varies. It is continued higher and farther on the sides than the initial dissection. If the problem is upper quadrant fullness, the flap above the umbilicus is extensively defatted from the undersur-

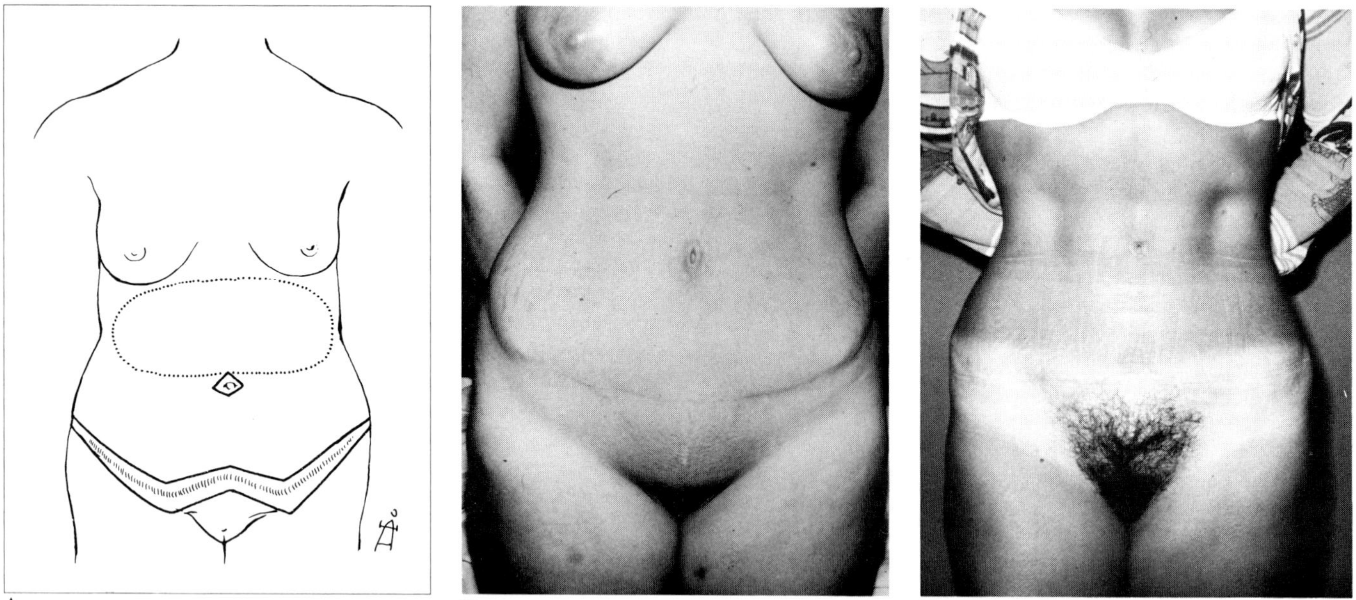

A B C

Figure 25-28
A. Secondary abdominoplasty usually requires scar revision and excision of epigastric fullness or lateral bulges.
B. Patient with previous abdominoplasty done elsewhere with retention of lateral bulges and periumbilical scar contraction.
C. Following secondary complete W-abdominoplasty, with undermining up to the xyphoid, and lateral extension, thus allowing removal of previous umbilical site. Skin resection was roughly equal to that in a primary abdominoplasty.

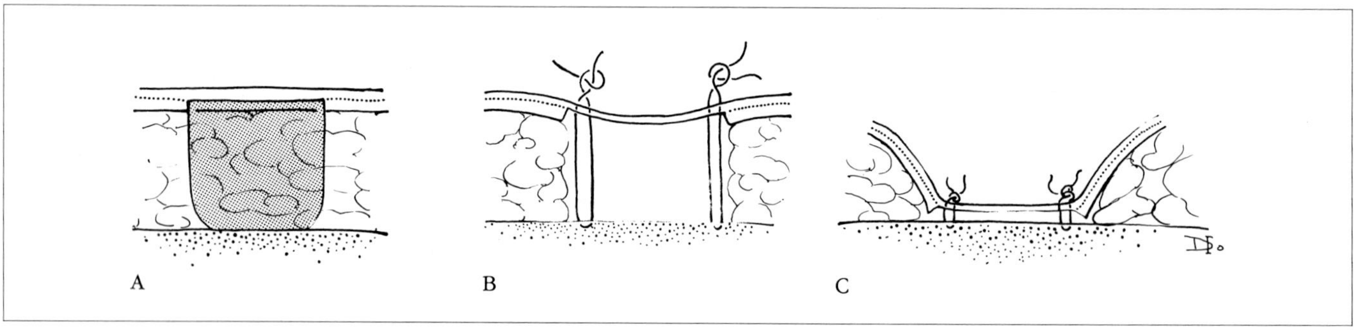

Figure 25-29. A method for creating a new umbilicus, concurrent with an abdominoplasty.
A. Fat is excised up to dermis.
B. Dermis is sutured to rectus fascia.
C. Umbilical depression is created.

face, leaving only 1 cm of adipose tissue. Lateral bulges are corrected by extension of the incision beyond the deformity, excision of the redundant tissue, and medial tension. The level of incision can be lowered by initial marking of the desired level, elevation of the flap through the previous incision, and excision of intervening tissue provided sufficient elasticity is present. Wound drainage must be excellent as defatting transects many small blood vessels.

The results of secondary abdominoplasty are generally excellent except for adhesions when secondary defatting is performed, which can be minimized by massaging.

Umbilicoplasty

The umbilicus can be a source of significant patient dissatisfaction and surgeon frustration. With the exception of hypertrophic scars, the majority of umbilical problems are due to inattention to detail. Freeman and Wiemer [27] assessed the umbilicus in 200 patients following abdominoplasties and stressed the following points: (1) Careful preoperative markings on the standing patient are essential; (2) any umbilicus greater than 1.5 cm appeared too large; and (3) hypertrophic periumbilical scars usually disappear by 18 months, thus avoiding revision.

MALPOSITION

Most often, the umbilicus is located too high because the umbilicus is inserted with the table in a flexed position. Correction can be either local or complete. In the former, a horizontal incision is made at the proper location, the umbilicus is transposed, and the resulting defect is closed, producing a transverse scar that serves as a permanent stigma of the malposition. Alternatively, one can wait 1 to 2 years until the skin's maximum elasticity is achieved and repeat the entire abdominoplasty, pulling the umbilicus into the correct position.

Lateral displacement of the umbilicus is due either to faulty localization or to asymmetric plication. The former requires simple repositioning with closure of the previous site while the latter demands a complete dissection with a secondary plication bringing the umbilicus back to the midline.

SIZE

A small umbilicus may be caused by a small initial incision, inadequate recipient site, or scar stenosis. Its dimensions can be improved by multiple Z-plasties along the periphery or a simple wedge excision at the 6 o'clock position, as recommended by Baroudi [8]. A large umbilicus is due to either a large donor or a large recipient site (>2 cm), which can be either excised or constricted with acceptable results. A protuberant umbilicus may be due to edema, lasting 3 to 6 months, or to excessive fat retained on the umbilical stump. If it persists, one can shorten the stalk or do a circumferential excision plus narrowing.

ABSENCE

The umbilicus may be absent on account of previous surgery (umbilical hernia, panniculectomy) or congenital deformity. Numerous methods for creation of a new umbilicus have been proposed [12, 15]. Creation of a new umbilicus requires tangential defatting of the periumbilical area and adherence of the skin to the rectus fascia (Fig. 25-29). If no other surgery is planned, local anesthesia is sufficient and a tristar incision with a superior flap is made, as recommended by Kirianoff [56]. If a revisional abdominoplasty is planned or the umbilicus must be sacrificed because of an umbilical hernia, subcutaneous fat is excised and the dermis of the abdominal skin sutured to the rectus fascia (Fig. 25-30).

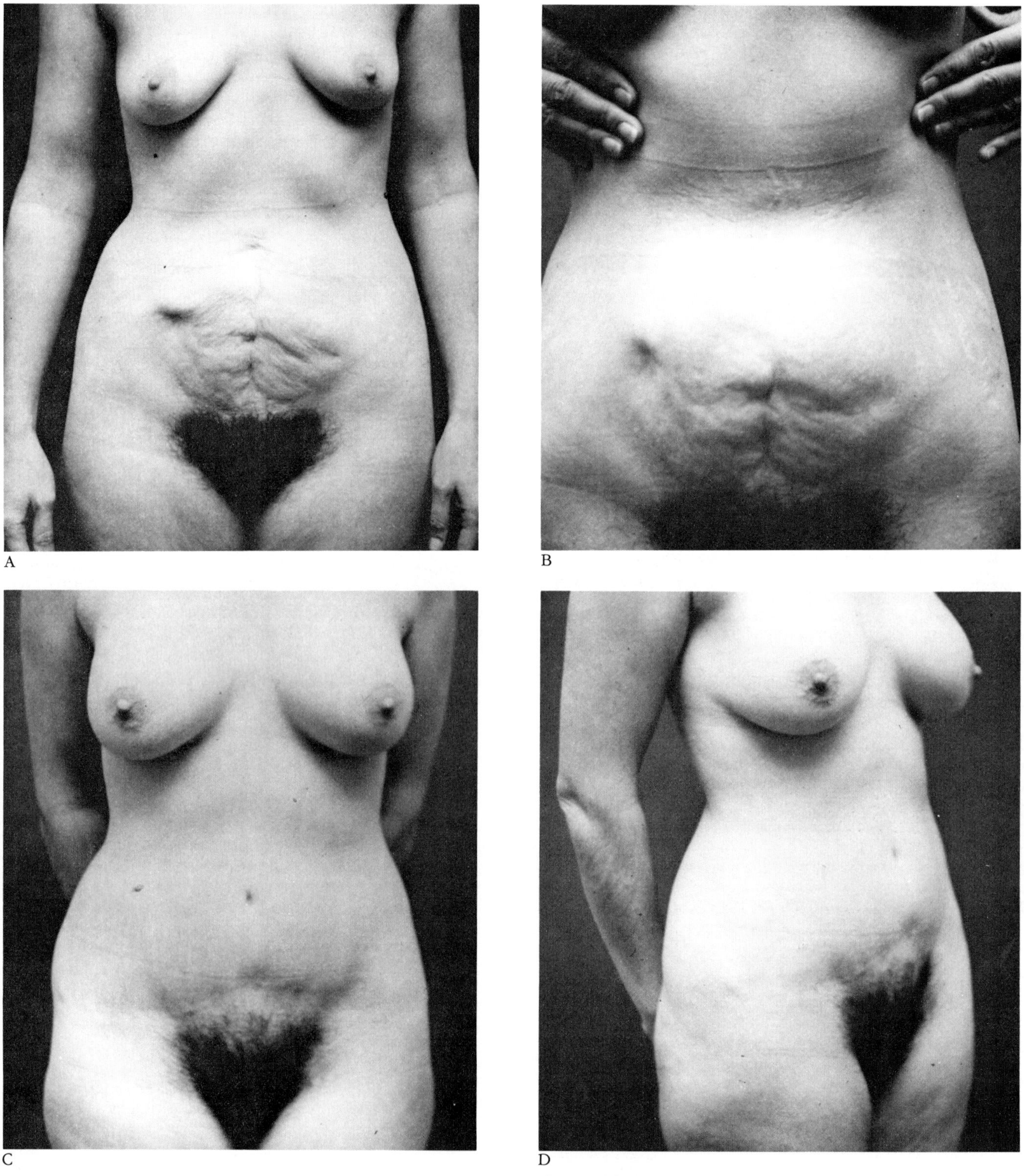

Figure 25-30
A, B. Patient with previous abdominal surgery including excision of the umbilicus.
C, D. Following a W-abdominoplasty with creation of a new umbilicus.

REFERENCES

1. Arem, A. J., and Kischer, C. W. Analysis of striae. *Plast. Reconstr. Surg.* 65:22, 1980.
2. Aston, S. J. Abdominoplasty. In T. D. Rees (ed.), *Aesthetic Plastic Surgery.* Philadelphia: Saunders, 1980. P. 1007.
3. Aston, S. J., and Pickrell, K. L. Reconstructive Surgery of the Abdominal Wall. In J. M. Converse (ed.), *Reconstructive Plastic Surgery* (2nd ed.). Philadelphia: Saunders, 1977. Vol. 7.
4. Avelar, J. Abdominoplasty: Systematization of a technique without external umbilical scar. *Aesthetic Plast. Surg.* 2:141, 1978.
5. Babcock, W. The correction of the obese and relaxed abdominal wall with especial reference to the use of buried silver chain. *Phila. Obstet. Soc.* May 4, 1916.
6. Babcock, W. On diseases of women and children. *Am. J. Obstet. Gynecol.* 74:596, 1916.
7. Baker, T. J., Gordon, H. L., and Mosienko, P. A template (pattern) method of abdominal lipectomy. *Aesthetic Plast. Surg.* 1:167, 1977.
8. Baroudi, R. Umbilicalplasty. *Clin. Plast. Surg.* 2:431, 1975.
9. Baroudi, R., Keppke, E. M., and Tozzi-Netto, F. Abdominoplasty. *Plast. Reconstr. Surg.* 54:161, 1974.
10. Bellero, V., et al. Abdominoplasty: Physiorespiratory surgery and aesthetic problems. *Plast. Reconstr. Surg.* 56:356, 1975.
11. Birdsell, D. C., et al. "Staying power": Absorbable vs. nonabsorbable. *Plast. Reconstr. Surg.* 68:742, 1981.
12. Borges, A. F. Reconstruction of the umbilicus. *Br. J. Plast. Surg.* 28:75, 1975.
13. Brown, R. G., Vasconez, L. O., and Jurkiewicz, M. J. Transverse abdominal flaps and the deep epigastric arcade. *Plast. Reconstr. Surg.* 55:416, 1975.
14. Cardoso de Castro, C., and Daher, M. Simultaneous reduction mammaplasty and abdominoplasty. *Plast. Reconstr. Surg.* 61:36, 1978.
15. Carvalho, C. G., Baroudi, R., and Keppke, E. M. Anatomical and technical refinements for abdominoplasty. *Aesthetic Plast. Surg.* 1:217, 1977.
16. Castanares, S., and Goethel, J. A. Abdominal lipectomy: A modification in technique. *Plast. Reconstr. Surg.* 40:378, 1967.
17. Clarkson, P. Lipodystrophies. *Plast. Reconstr. Surg.* 37:499, 1966.
18. Cullen, T. S. *Embryology, Anatomy and Diseases of the Umbilicus.* Philadelphia: Saunders, 1916.
19. Dubou, R., and Ousterhout, D. K. Placement of the umbilicus in an abdominoplasty. *Plast. Reconstr. Surg.* 61:291, 1978.
20. Dufourmentel, C. *Chirurgie Réparatrice et Corrective.* Paris: Masson, 1939.
21. Dufourmentel, C., and Mouly, R. *Chirurgie Plastique.* Paris: Flammarion, 1959. Pp. 381–389.
22. Edgerton, M. T., and Knorr, N. J. Motivation patterns of patients seeking cosmetic (esthetic) surgery. *Plast. Reconstr. Surg.* 48:551, 1971.
23. Elbaz, J. S. Abdominal plastic surgery: Horseshoe technique [A propos des plasties abdominales: Technique du fer à cheval]. *Ann. Chir. Plast.* 19:155, 1974.
24. Elbaz, J. S., and Dardour, J. C. Anatomy and Physiology of the Arteries and Veins of the Abdominal Wall. In *Transactions of the Sixth International Congress of Plastic and Reconstructive Surgery.* Paris: Masson, 1976.
25. Elbaz, J. S., and Flaguel, G. *Chirurgie Plastique de L'abdomen.* Paris: Masson, 1971.
26. Fischl, R. Vertical abdominoplasty. *Plast. Reconstr. Surg.* 51:139, 1973.
27. Freeman, B. S., and Wiemer, D. R. Abdominoplasty with special attention to the construction of the umbilicus: Technique and complications. *Aesthetic Plast. Surg.* 2:65, 1978.
28. Galtier, M. Surgical therapy of obesity of the abdominal wall with ptosis. *Mem. Acad. Chir.* 81:341, 1955.
29. Galtier, M. Obésité de la paroi abdominale. *Presse Med.* 70:135, 1962.
30. Georgiade, N., and Katsas, A. Topography of fat in the sacroiliac region. *Plast. Reconstr. Surg.* 49:110, 1972.
31. Glikenstein, J. Difficulties of surgical treatment of abdominal dermodystrophies. *Ann. Chir. Plast.* 20:147, 1975.
32. Goldwyn, R. M. *The Unfavorable Result in Plastic Surgery.* Boston: Little, Brown, 1972.
33. Gonzalez-Ulloa, M. Circular lipectomy with transposition of the umbilicus and aponeurolytic technique. *Cirugia* 27:394, 1959.
34. Gonzalez-Ulloa, M. Belt lipectomy. *Br. J. Plast. Surg.* 13:179, 1960.
35. Grazer, F. M. Abdominoplasty. *Plast. Reconstr. Surg.* 51:617, 1973.
36. Grazer, F. M. Plastic operation on the abdomen. *Calif. Med.* 119:64, 1973.
37. Grazer, F. M., and Goldwyn, R. M. Abdominoplasty assessed by survey with emphasis on complications. *Plast. Reconstr. Surg.* 59:513, 1977.
38. Grazer, F. M., and Klingbeil, J. R. Abdominoplasty. In E. H. Courtiss (ed.), *Aesthetic Surgery: Trouble—How to Avoid It and How to Treat It.* St. Louis: Mosby, 1978.
39. Grazer, F. M., and Klingbeil, J. R. *Body Image: A Surgical Perspective.* St. Louis: Mosby, 1980.
40. Grazer, F. M., Klingbeil, J. R., and Mattiello, M. *Long-term Results of Abdominoplasty.* Boston: Little, Brown, 1980.
41. Guerrero-Santos, J., et al. Some problems and solutions in abdominoplasty. *Aesthetic Plast. Surg.* 4:227, 1980.
42. Guerrero-Santos, J., et al. Umbilical reconstruction with secondary abdominoplasty. *Ann. Plast. Surg.* 5:139, 1980.
43. Hinderer, U. T. Problems psicologico y spiquiatrico en el paciente de cirgirgia plastica. *Rev. Esp. Piscol. Anal.* 1:31, 1968.
44. Hinderer, U. T. The dermolipectomy approach for augmentation mammaplasty. *Clin. Plast. Surg.* 2:359, 1975.
45. Iturraspe, M. C. Resultados de la dermolipectomia abdominal vertical. *Bol. Trab. Soc. Argent. Cir.* 13:648, 1952.
46. Iturraspe, M. C. Tratamiento, quirurgico de la obesidad. *Rev. Asoc. Med. Argent.* 66:340, 1952.
47. Iturraspe, M. C. Dermolipectomia vertical del abdomen. *Sem. Med.* 121:1071, 1962.
48. Jackson, I. T., and Downie, P. A. Abdominoplasty: The waistline stitch and other refinements. *Plast. Reconstr. Surg.* 61:180, 1978.
49. Jolly, R. Abdominoplasty. *Berl. Klin. Wochenschr.* 48:1317, 1911.
50. Juri, J., Juri, C., and Raiden, G. Reconstruction of the umbilicus in abdominoplasty. *Plast. Reconstr. Surg.* 63:580, 1979.
51. Kakkar, V. V., et al. Low doses of heparin in prevention of deep-vein thrombosis. *Lancet* 2:669, 1971.
52. Kakkar, V. V., et al. Efficacy of low doses of heparin in prevention of deep-vein thrombosis after major surgery. *Lancet* 2:101, 1972.
53. Kamper, M. J., Galloway, D. V., and Ashley, F. Abdominal panniculectomy after massive weight loss. *Plast. Reconstr. Surg.* 50:441, 1972.

54. Kelly, H. A. Report of gynecological cases (excessive growth of fat). *Johns Hopkins Med. J.* 10:197, 1899.
55. Kelly, H. A. Excision of fat of the abdominal wall lipectomy. *Surg. Gynecol. Obstet.* 10:229, 1910.
56. Kirianoff, T. G. Making a new umbilicus when none exists. *Plast. Reconstr. Surg.* 61:603, 1978.
57. Lagache, G., and Vandenbussche, F. Indications, contre indications et résultats de la technique de Callia dans le traitement des ptoses cutanées abdominales avec ou sans surcharge graisseuse. *Ann. Chir. Plast.* 16:37, 1971.
58. Lewis, J. R. *Atlas of Aesthetic Plastic Surgery.* Boston: Little, Brown, 1973.
59. Lewis, J. R. Midabdominoplasty. *Aesthetic Plast. Surg.* 3:195, 1979.
60. Masson, J. K. Lipectomy: The surgical removal of excess fat. *Postgrad. Med.* 32:481, 1962.
61. Mitz, V., Elbaz, J. S., and Vilde, F. Etude des fibres élastiques dermiques au cours d'opérations plastiques du tronc. *Ann. Chir. Plast.* 20:31, 1975.
62. Passot, R. *Chirurgie Esthetique Pure.* Paris: Doin, 1931. Pp. 261–267.
63. Pitanguy, I. Abdominal lipectomy: An approach to it through an analysis of 300 consecutive cases. *Plast. Reconstr. Surg.* 40:384, 1967.
64. Pitanguy, I. Abdominoplastias. *Hospital* (Rio) 71:1541, 1967.
65. Pitanguy, I. Surgical reduction of the abdomen, thighs, and buttocks. *Surg. Clin. North Am.* 51:479, 1971.
66. Pitanguy, I. Technique for Trunk and Thigh Reductions. In *Transactions of the Fifth International Congress of Plastic and Reconstructive Surgery.* Melbourne: Butterworths, 1971. Pp. 1204–1210.
67. Pitanguy, I. Thigh Lift and Abdominal Lipectomy. In R. M. Goldwyn (ed.), *The Unfavorable Result in Plastic Surgery.* Boston: Little, Brown, 1972.
68. Pitanguy, I. Abdominal lipectomy. *Clin. Plast. Surg.* 2:401, 1975.
69. Pitanguy, I. *Aesthetic Plastic Surgery of Head and Body.* Berlin: Springer, 1981.
70. Planas, J. Introduction of breast implants through the abdominal route. *Plast. Reconstr. Surg.* 57:434, 1975.
71. Planas, J. The "vest over pants abdominoplasty." *Plast. Reconstr. Surg.* 61:694, 1978.
72. Psillakis, J. M. Abdominoplasty: Some ideas to improve results. *Aesthetic Plast. Surg.* 2:205, 1978.
73. Rao-Subba, Y. V. Augmentation mammaplasty and abdominoplasty in one stage. *Plast. Reconstr. Surg.* 43:148, 1969.
74. Rebello, C., and Franco, T. Abdominoplasty through a submammary incision. *Int. Surg.* 62:462, 1977.
75. Regnault, P. Abdominal dermolipectomy. New York: International Society of Aesthetic Plastic Surgery. *Internat. Microfilm. Aesthetic Plast. Surg.* 1972.
76. Regnault, P. Abdominal lipectomy, a low "W" incision. New York: International Society of Aesthetic Plastic Surgery. *Internat. Microfilm. Aesthetic Plast. Surg.,* 1972.
77. Regnault, P. Abdominal dermolipectomies. *Clin. Plast. Surg.* 2:411, 1975.
78. Regnault, P. Abdominoplasty by the "W" technique. *Plast. Reconstr. Surg.* 55:265, 1975.
79. Regnault, P. The history of abdominal dermolipectomy. *Aesthetic Plast. Surg.* 2:113, 1978.
80. Regnault, P. Lipectomy. In W. C. Grabb and J. W. Smith (eds), *Plastic Surgery* (3rd ed.). Boston: Little, Brown, 1979. P. 838.
81. Regnault, P. Abdominal Reduction. In M. Barron (ed.), *Operative Surgery* (3rd ed.). London: Butterworth, 1981. P. 462.
82. Regnault, P., and Alfara, A. Lipodystrophie céphalothoracique de Barraquez-Simons, présentation d'un cas. *Union Med. Can.* 96:286, 1967.
83. Reich, J. The surgical improvement in appearance of the female body. *Med. J. Aust.* 2:767, 1974.
84. Ryan, R. F. Which patient needs the abdominoplasty? (Letter to the Editor.) *Plast. Reconstr. Surg.* 59:842, 1977.
85. Sanders, R. J., DiClementi, D., and Ireland, K. Principles of abdominal wound closure. *Arch. Surg.* 112:1188, 1977.
86. Sasahara, A. A., Sharma, G. V., and Parisi, A. F. New developments in the detection and prevention of venous thromboembolism. *Am. J. Cardiol.* 43:1214, 1979.
87. Schorcher, F. Kosmetische Operationen. Munich: Lehmanns, 1955.
88. Schurter, M., and Latterman, G. Abdominoplasty or abdominal dermolipectomy. *Ann. Plast. Surg.* 2:235, 1979.
89. Schwartz, A. W. A technique for excision of abdominal fat. *Br. J. Plast. Surg.* 27:44, 1974.
90. Serson, D. Planeamiento geometrico para la dermolipectomia abdominal. *Rev. Esp. Cir. Plast.* 4:37, 1971; abstracted, *Plast. Reconstr. Surg.* 48:605, 1971.
91. Serson, D., and Martins, L. C. Geometric Planning for Abdominal Dermolipectomy. In N. Owens and K. L. Stephenson (eds.), *The Year Book of Plastic and Reconstructive Surgery.* Chicago: Year Book, 1970.
92. Serson, D., and Martins, L. C. Dermolipectomia abdominal, arbordage geometrico. *Rev. Lat. Am. Cir. Plast.* 16:13, 1972.
93. Somalo, M. Dermolipectomia circular del tronco. *Sem. Med.* 1:1435, 1940.
94. Somalo, M. Dermolipectomia circular del tronco. *Cir. Plast. II, Arch. Chir. Exp.* 1:404, 1941.
95. Somalo, M. Dermolipectomia ventral cruciforme; "incision en golondrina." *Prensa Med. Argent.* 33:75, 1946.
96. Teimourian, B., et al. Suction lipectomy: A review of 200 patients over a six-year period and a study of the technique in cadavers. *Ann. Plast. Surg.* 11:93, 1983.
97. Thorek, M. *Plastic Surgery of the Breast and Abdominal Wall.* Springfield, Ill.: Thomas, 1924.
98. Thorek, M. Plastic reconstruction of the female breast and abdomen. *Am. J. Surg.* 43:268, 1939.
99. Vernon, S. Umbilical transplantation upward and abdominal contouring in lipectomy. *Am. J. Surg.* 94:490, 1957.
100. Vilain, R. Some considerations in surgical alteration of the feminine silhouette. *Clin. Plast. Surg.* 2:449, 1975.
101. Vilain, R. Surgical correction of steatomeries. *Clin. Plast. Surg.* 2:499, 1975.
102. Vilain, R., and Dubousset, J. Technique et indications de la lipectomie circulaire. 150 observations. *Ann. Chir.* 18:289, 1964.
103. Vilain, R., et al. Etude critique des complications des laparotomies. *Ann. Chir.* 21:262, 1967.
104. Weinhold, S. Bauchdeckenplastik. *Zentralbl. Gynek.* 38: 1332, 1909.

26. Lower Extremity

Paule Regnault
Rollin K. Daniel

Lower extremity dermolipectomies are surgical excisions of excess skin and fat in patients with either regionalized or generalized deformities. These procedures may be requested by persons with normal body habitus desiring an aesthetic result (thighplasty) or the moderately obese wishing a reduction in tissue (thigh lipectomy). This diversity requires selection of the optimal procedure by the surgeon. During the past decade, insight into the anatomic basis of the deformities has led to new surgical procedures that provide greater patient satisfaction. However, the magnitude of the surgery, the inconvenience of the postoperative period, and the permanent scars demand a highly motivated patient. In contrast to the high success rate of abdominoplasties, dermolipectomy of the lower extremity is often disappointing to the patient, who is left with significant scars. Recently, suction-assisted lipectomy has gained renewed interest due to its small incision, short hospitalization, lessened morbidity, and dramatic results —provided *patient selection* is carefully done. In the coming decade, a blending of lipectomy and liposuction will occur to the benefit of the patient. Throughout this chapter, we will present the classic surgical procedures, while in Chapter 27, we will deal with suction-assisted lipectomy and its relationship to surgical techniques.

HISTORY

As practiced by Kelly [16], Noël [22], and others, dermolipectomy of the lower extremities began as localized excisions of thigh fat concomitant with abdominal lipectomy. In 1957 Lewis [18] published a method of thigh-lift that established the principles of elevating the thigh by a circular incision and tightening the circumference by vertical excisions with minimal scarring and undermining. Although valuable in massive-weight-loss cases, it did not solve the problem of buttock or trochanteric adiposity. Farina et al. [11, 12] described a direct lateral incision for correcting trochanteric lipodystrophy that gave excellent silhouette improvement but produced unacceptable scars. In 1964 Pitanguy [23–25] published his semicircular excision technique, which begins at the anterior superior iliac spine, curves into the perineum, extends above the gluteal fold, and ends above the trochanter. For the first time, the incision was hidden within the bathing suit area while allowing aesthetic correction of inner thigh flabbiness, drooping buttocks, and trochanteric lipodystrophy. Subsequently, modifications of this technique have included dermal suspensory flaps and extensive undermining for excision of trochanteric fat deposits [8, 9, 29]. Vilain [36–38], Aston [2], and others have solved the problem of gluteal depression by filling it with deepithelialized tissues that previously would have been discarded. Regnault

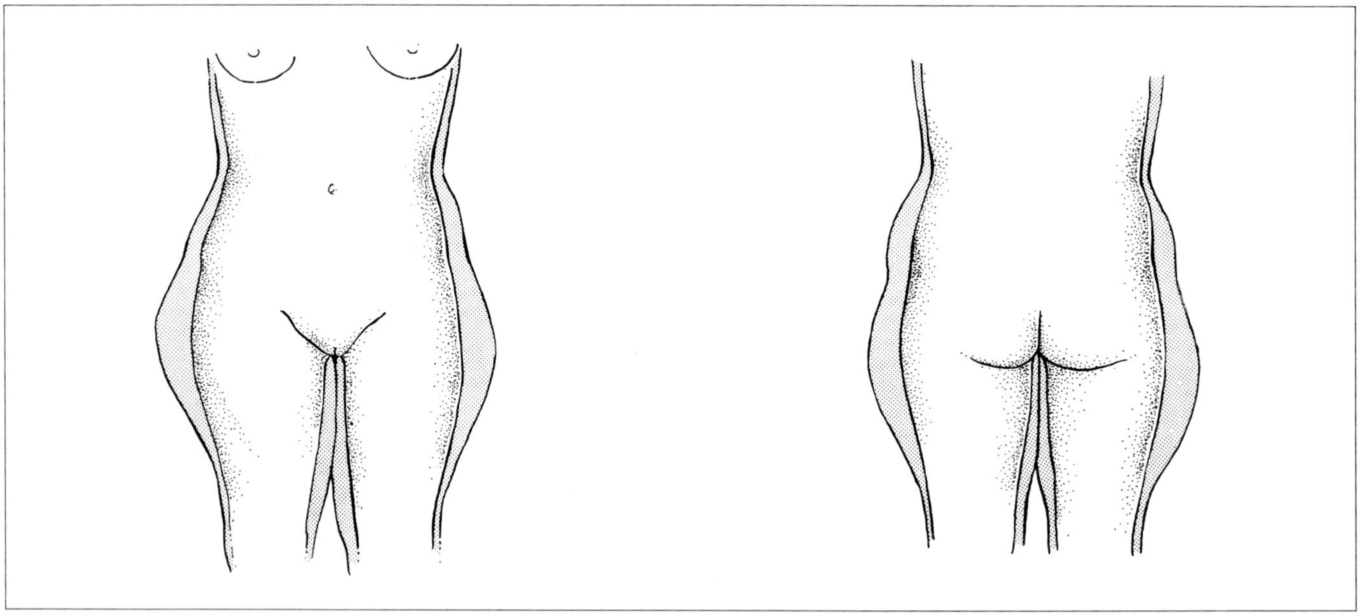

Figure 26-1. Ideal figure with silhouette of excess fat accumulation.

[30] expanded the procedure to correct entire thigh deformities by means of a circular excision plus trochanteric defatting.

PATHOPHYSIOLOGY AND CLASSIFICATION

Aesthetic deformities of the thighs are generally a result of adiposity, weight loss, or aging, with separate categories including congenital, traumatic, and massive-weight-loss etiologies. As reported by Hoffman and Simon [15], the majority of patients complain of (1) heavy thighs or general obesity, (2) trochanteric lipodystrophy, (3) medial redundancy, (4) buttock ptosis with redundancy, and (5) cellulite. It is well known that fat deposits in the normal individual are concentrated from the umbilicus down to the popliteal area (Fig. 26-1). Thus, the moderately obese patient will frequently have generalized "heavy thighs." In contrast, certain slimmer normal-weight individuals will have localized trochanteric deposits that are refractory to further weight loss or exercise. Despite claims that localized fat accumulations are in reality a regional lipodystrophy or lipomatosis, a specific pathologic entity has not been defined, nor is there a difference in fatty acid composition. Trochanteric fat deposits are a localized accumulation that may be further accentuated by a superior gluteal depression. As reported by Clarkson [6] and Regnault et al. [32], the recognized named lipodystrophy syndromes are often grotesque deformities of the entire lower extremities.

Medial redundancy and buttock ptosis are secondary to the loss of skin elasticity that occurs with aging or significant weight loss. *Cellulite* is a term frequently used in the popular press to denote the cobblestone skin appearance overlying the lateral thigh. It is attributed to an increased volume of subcutaneous fat in the superficial layer with traction on the fibrous septa that extend from muscle fascia to deep dermis. Despite advertising claims to the contrary, cellulite cannot be corrected either by massaging, exercise, or drugs. Any improvement by massaging is probably due to edema, which transiently masks the cobblestone appearance. Surgery corrects only the area that is directly excised, and the patient must understand that contour correction is possible, but not elimination of the remaining cellulite areas.

Although classification of the lower extremity deformities can be based on etiology or anatomic location, we prefer dividing them into regionalized and generalized (Fig. 26-2). Each of the three regions (medial, buttock, and trochanteric) can be corrected by a single crescent excision, or, more frequently, they can be collectively ameliorated by a semicircular approach. The more generalized deformities demand an extensive circular resection, which may include a vertical extension.

Figure 26-2. Types of patients presenting for lower limb surgery.
A. Young 26-year-old normal-weight individual with trochanteric accentuation. Candidate for suction-assisted lipectomy.
B. Patient, aged 38, with medial fullness and flaccid skin but otherwise normal lower extremity. Treatment requires limited semicircular excision with short vertical extension.
C. Classic riding breeches thigh deformity with trochanteric fat deposit, gluteal depression, and square buttocks. Treatment requires either semicircular excision with trochanteric defatting or suction-assisted lipectomy.
D. Complete thigh deformity requiring circular excision with vertical extension. Semicircular approach would leave anterior deformity, especially above the knees.

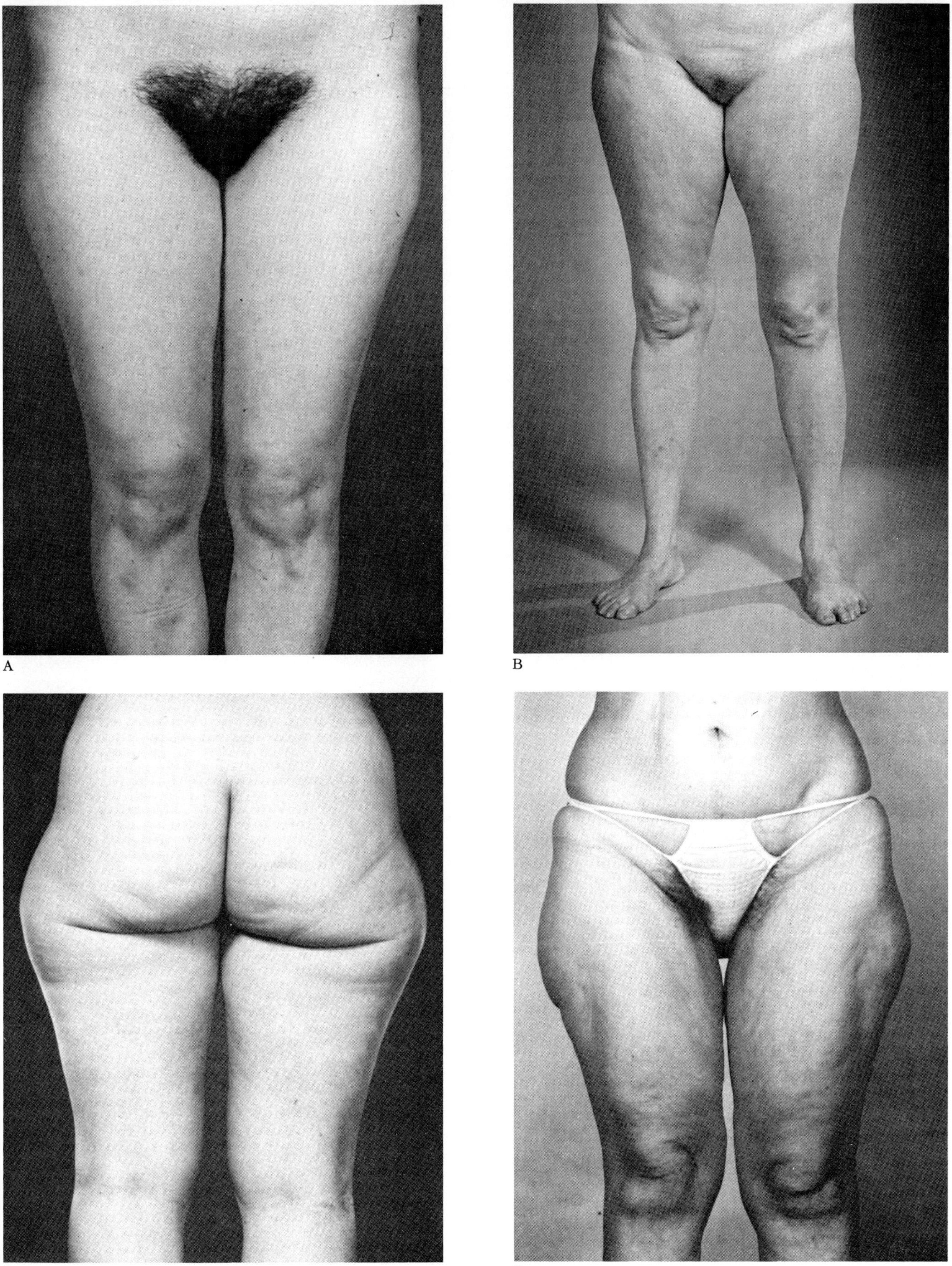

A B C D

CONSULTATION

The initial consultation for dermolipectomy of the lower limb is an opportunity for the surgeon to assess the patient's deformity and motivation. The patient is frequently surprised at the magnitude of the surgery required, the inconveniences of the postoperative period, and the permanence of the scars. A second consultation permits a more realistic patient to understand the proposed surgical procedure and helps to develop the essential patient-doctor relationship.

Indications and Contraindications

The principal indication is high motivation in a patient whose deformities are surgically correctable. In contrast to patients who request augmentation mammaplasty or rhytidectomy, thighplasty patients obtain most of their information from the popular press and do not have friends who have had the procedure. Thus, many patients will not want surgery once they are aware of the magnitude of surgery, scars, and major complications. In contrast to breast problems the more severe the lower extremity deformity, especially in cases of obesity, the less is surgical correction possible. The simple "pinch test" often indicates the degree of improvement, which is likely to be less than the patient expects. Lewis [21], the developer of the modern thighplasty, noted on review of his long-term follow-ups that "the major change in my own approach to this operation is that I now perform it only on patients needing it badly; before, I was more easily talked into doing it for less major indications." Contraindications are numerous. The patient who has unrealistic expectations and is unwilling to accept the ever-present hypertrophic scarring should not be operated upon. Equally, the patient of normal body weight but with firm adiposity over the trochanter will not obtain significant improvement except by direct excision. Patients with generalized obesity or major medical problems are not candidates.

Medical History

A detailed medical history is taken with emphasis on the cardiovascular system, peripheral vascular disease, and previous surgery of the lower limb. One must ask specifically about leg edema and any family history of lymphedema. A review of the patient's weight range and dietary habits is obtained, along with average and current weight, plus lifetime maximum and minimum. Patients who are planning to lose weight or are significantly obese are encouraged to achieve their target weight prior to surgery. Patients with significant cardiovascular disease, diabetes, or metabolic diseases are not acceptable candidates. It is wise to inquire about bleeding disorders and other coagulation problems.

Motivation

Patients are then asked what deformity they dislike, when it bothers them the most, and why they want surgery at this time. In normal-weight individuals, the majority of younger patients are concerned about trochanteric prominence while middle-aged patients dislike medial or buttock ptosis. The moderately obese patient is more concerned about heaviness and contour deformities. The patient with ptosis of the thighs is motivated by a desire to look better in leisure-time apparel, including tennis clothes and bathing suits. Patients with trochanteric lipodystrophy and heavy thighs are more concerned with bulging in pants and difficulty in buying clothes. The decision to seek a surgical solution occurs after years of failure to correct the problem by dieting and exercise.

Physical Examination

The patient is examined nude from the waist down. The general relationship of the lower extremities to the body habitus is observed and the patient is asked to point out what is disliked the most. Then the specific regions (medial, buttock, trochanteric) are examined for their adiposity, redundancy, and contour—either prominences or depressions. With the hand on the lower thigh, one can push upward to estimate the mobility of the tissues, and pinching will indicate how much excision is possible. The lower extremities are carefully examined for asymmetries, edema, and peripheral vascular problems. Significant varicose veins should be treated prior to dermolipectomy, and any edema should be evaluated by the patient's personal physician.

The surgeon should give a frank opinion as to whether the patient's deformity is correctable and whether a regional or general resection is necessary. If the patient has heavy, tense thighs, the surgeon should demonstrate their immobility and inability to pinch the tissue. Rather than rejecting the patient, the surgeon should emphasize that if a weight loss of 20 or more pounds could be achieved surgery might be possible. With the patient's permission, the location of the final scar is drawn with a 5-mm-wide felt-tipped marker, not a fine pen. The patient is encouraged to show these marks to others and to think about their permanence.

Aesthetic Goals

The majority of patients want contour correction or tightening of flabby skin, which will allow improved appearance in snug clothing and sportswear. It must be repeatedly emphasized that surgery can improve but not eradicate their problem. Cellulite will not disappear nor will fullness above the knee. An overall slimming effect can be achieved, but with significant scarring, which may be of concern to the patient and others. For those requiring a generalized resection, a description of the inconveniences of the postoperative period is warranted. The inability to sit for 2 to 3 weeks and the difficulties of toilet activities are mentioned. The problems of healing and hematoma formation are also discussed. At this point only the truly motivated patient will remain interested. Patients are encouraged to have their photographs taken and to return for a second consultation, during which the surgical procedure and potential complications are reviewed in greater detail.

Informed Consent

The patient should understand that a general improvement can be made, but the entire contour deformity cannot be eliminated. The following admonitions are particularly important. (1) The scars will be permanent and always visible. During the first year, the incision line will spread and become hypertrophic, with gradual improvement. Revision of the scar may be necessary, consisting of steroid injections or possible surgical scar revision, but not before 1 year. (2) The patient will be unable to sit for 2 to 3 weeks and will find many activities difficult. (3) The possibility of major complications is very real, including blood loss, thrombophlebitis, and pulmonary embolus. (4) Patients requiring excision of trochanteric fat must expect repeated fluid accumulation and aspirations.

Preoperative Preparations

Following completion of all laboratory tests required for general anesthesia, a decision is made whether to use autotransfusion or banked blood, the former requiring at least 6 weeks to obtain the necessary 3 units. On the day prior to surgery, the patient showers with pHisoHex and begins on a low-residue diet. Preoperative markings are made with the patient standing and using a bikini for reference.

ANATOMY

The normal body silhouette has a graceful proportional flaring of the hips that narrows down to the knees with a secondary flare at the calves. The appearance of a trochanteric projection accentuated by a gluteal depression causes great distress. The absence of a clearly defined buttock crease can be caused by either ptosis or surgery with equally distressing sequelae.

Skin

The relative proportions of skin and subcutaneous fat differ markedly as one circles the thigh from medial to lateral area. The skin in the inguinal region is quite thin, with a limited amount of subcutaneous fat. This medial area is prone to rhytidosis. Thus, correction of medial thigh deformities requires a higher placement of incisions to prevent later downward migration and resection of only the more superficial layer of subcutaneous fat. In contrast, the buttock area is characterized by a diffuse thick layer (4–8 cm) of subcutaneous fat and numerous vertical fibrous septa that create a definite gluteal fold. Vilain [36] notes that most patients requesting surgery have a straight gluteal crease resulting in a "square" buttock deformity. Temporary loss of this fold following major thigh-lifts is of concern to many patients. Over the trochanteric region, the skin may display a "cellulite" appearance due to multiple small fibrous septa and the characteristic "riding breeches deformity" secondary to a peritrochanteric fat accumulation. Although surgical correction of cellulite is impossible, one can resect the peritrochanteric fat deposit and reduce the bulging.

Muscle and Bone

The configuration of the lower extremity is dictated in part by skeletal factors, especially the flare of the ilium, the trochanteric projection, and the intervening depression. The gluteal depression is readily apparent and must not be further emphasized by excessive surgical excision (Fig. 26-3). The gluteal muscles originate within this recess. The most superficial muscle of this group is the gluteus maximus, which originates medially and passes over the trochanter to insert into the tibial tract. The free lower border of the gluteus maximum is marked by the horizontal gluteal fold separating buttock from posterior thigh.

Vascular Supply

The blood supply to the lower extremity consists of abundant musculocutaneous perforators and a few direct cutaneous arteries in the groin region. Arterial compromise is rare except in cases with extensive undermining. The major superficial veins, especially the saphenous system, should not be injured or even exposed during the medial dissection. Equally, the numerous inguinal lymph nodes and major lymphatics should not be disturbed. If injured, the lymphatics are ligated and a firm dressing is applied.

Nerves

Sensation is provided by numerous small branches that may be encountered medially (ilioinguinal and genitofemoral), or in the buttock region (L-1, 2, 3), and laterally (superior gluteal nerves and branches of the posterior femoral cutaneous nerve). Because there are numerous branches and undermining is limited, sensory loss is relatively rare.

SURGICAL PRINCIPLES

Dermolipectomies of the lower extremity are increasingly being sought for aesthetic reasons. Lipectomies originally designed for the obese patient have been refined, allowing attainment of contour correction with an acceptable, well-concealed, symmetric scar [30].

Incision

The final scar must be hidden beneath standard swimwear or leisure clothes. Thus, the initial incision is placed 1 to 2 cm above the inguinal fold and continued along the sulcus genitofemoralis into the buttock crease before crossing the buttock in the medial half. Lateral continua-

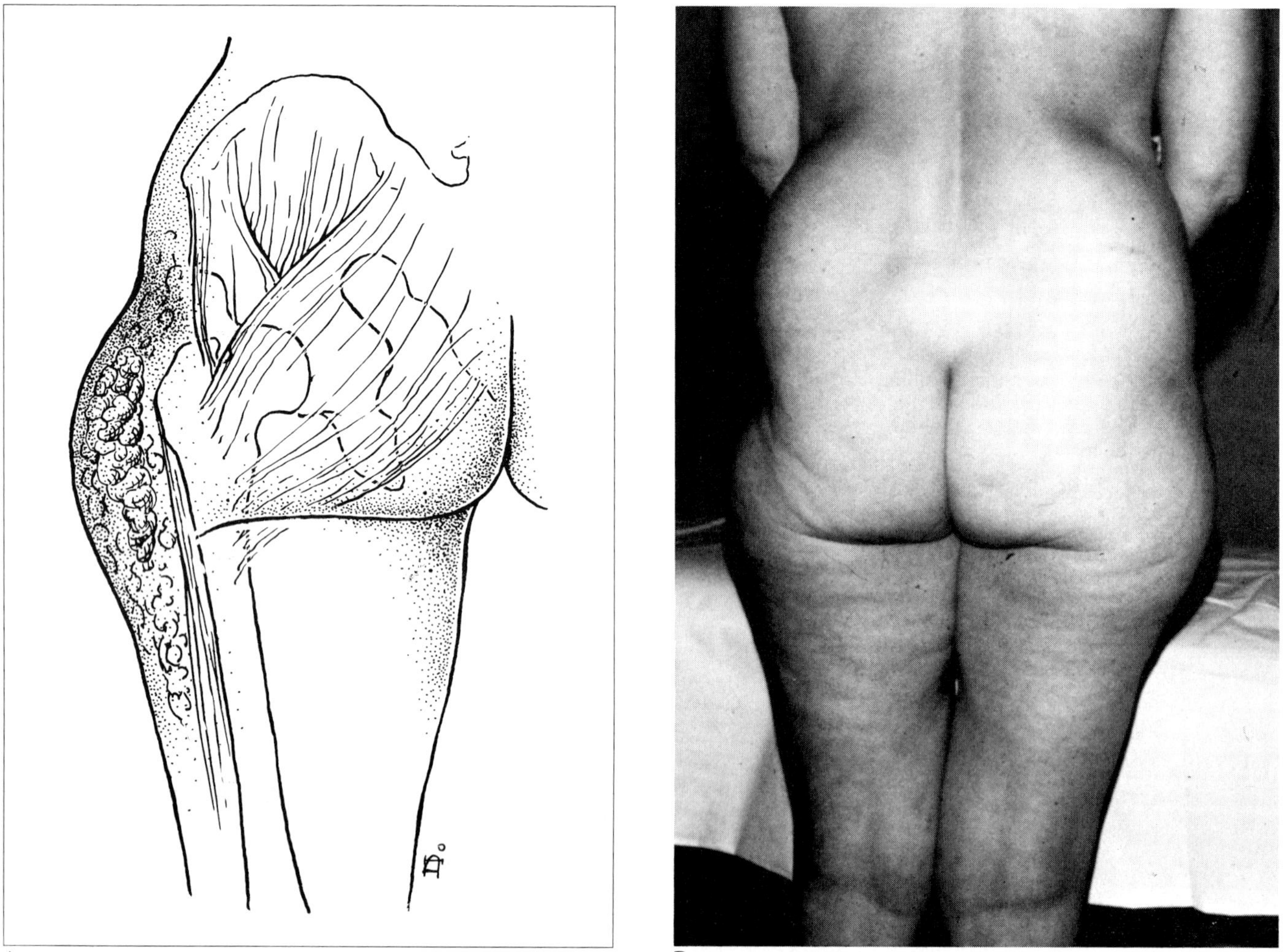

A B

Figure 26-3
A. Anatomic basis of the lower limb deformity is the gluteal depression accentuated by iliac flare and trochanteric projection with the latter further emphasized by fat deposits.
B. Clinically, the triad of gluteal depression, trochanteric bulging, and square buttocks is readily visible.

tion above the trochanter can be concealed provided the incision turns transverse before ending in a downward direction. The angle of ascent across the buttocks varies with different surgeons. We prefer a line between the lower level of Baroudi [3] and the high curve of Grazer and Klingbeil [14] (Fig. 26-4). The possible extent of resection is marked by pushing upward on the thigh tissue. Since the deformity disappears with the patient supine, all markings are made with the patient standing. If a supratrochanteric gluteal depression exists, it is marked preoperatively and the planned treatment outlined—either a limited sculptured fat excision (minor depression) or retention of a deepithelialized area (moderate depression). As recommended by Lewis [19, 20], symmetry of the incision lines can be ensured by a measuring-tape compass placed at the coccyx.

Undermining

In contrast to abdominoplasties, dermolipectomies of the lower extremity do *not* call for extensive undermining. The dissection is done above the muscle fascia with retention of some subcutaneous fat over the fascia. This principle evolved because of the prolonged hematomas and seromas that are associated with wide undermining. The one exception is direct defatting of the trochanteric fat deposits. In this operation, limited undermining of the trochanteric area is done, but a subcutaneous layer of approximately 15 mm is retained. The fat pad is directly excised and the wound drained.

Resection

The amount of redundant skin and subcutaneous fat to be excised is estimated by traction on the developed flap. The overlapping portion of the flap is split into segments to avoid excessive removal. Since tension cannot be reduced by flexion of the operating table as in an abdominoplasty, one must always err on the side of too little resection rather than too much.

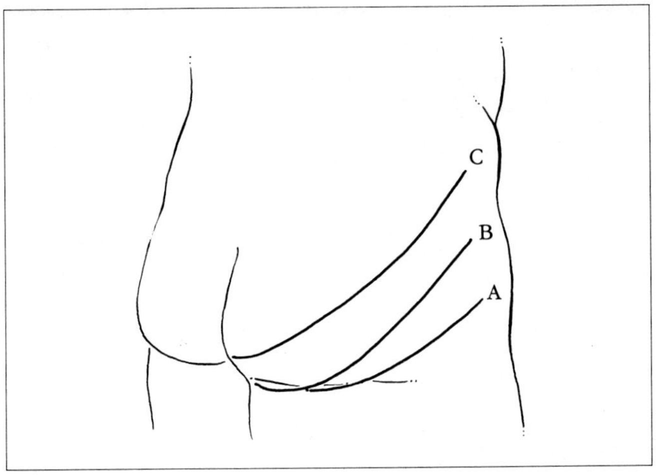

Figure 26-4. Semicircular incisions vary significantly in their posterior course: Baroudi (*A*), Regnault (*B*), and Grazer and Klingbeil (*C*).

Suspension

Agris [1] introduced the concept of reducing tension on the suture line through utilization of deepithelialized dermal flaps. Essentially, the inferiorly based suspensory flaps are fixed to fascia, thereby minimizing downward migration and hypertrophy of the scars. Unfortunately, clinical data and long-term follow-up are insufficient to confirm these objectives, and in general we do not use suspensory flaps. Vilain [37] uses a variation of this procedure with good results.

Closure

Since the goal is to tighten the thigh in a circumferential manner, cross-hatching marks are not made preoperatively. Intraoperatively, the tissues are spiraled upward to permit maximum excision and tightening; thus, final closure marks can only be made once the flaps are elevated. Anteriorly, the thigh is mobilized with medial rotation and cross-hatchings are marked. Posteriorly, the superior edge is moved laterally and the inferior edge moved medially. Skin closure is done with interrupted absorbable sutures and a subcuticular continuous absorbable suture. Sitting down is not allowed for 2 to 3 weeks to avoid tension on the suture line.

SURGICAL TECHNIQUES

Regional Deformities

Isolated deformities of the lower extremity occur in 5 to 10 percent of patients. Fortunately, the specific dislike can be corrected by a limited operation or suction-assisted lipectomy with an acceptable postoperative course. In contrast, patients having a generalized deformity require extensive surgery with significant scarring and a demanding postoperative course.

MEDIAL THIGH DEFORMITY

The usual deformity is redundancy of skin in a middle-aged normal-weight individual with a keen interest in swimming or tennis. It is important to differentiate this localized deformity from the severe ptosis extending to the knee characteristic of massive-weight-loss patients and the generalized firm adiposity characteristic of the moderately obese patient. Schultz and Feinberg [34] stress that this procedure will improve only the upper half of the thigh and will not alter the area around the knee or the lateral trochanteric region.

The patient is marked in the standing position with the knee slightly flexed and the leg rotated outward. A reference bikini line is marked and the redundant skin pinched to estimate the amount of resection possible. The excision must be conservative to prevent spreading of the scars and gaping of the labia majora. The incision line is placed 1 cm above the inguinal crease and begins just medial to the femoral triangle; it extends above the inguinal fold posteriorly to the gluteal crease. Because of tension on the suture line and the effects of gravity, the incision must be above the inguinal fold to prevent its exposure in a bathing suit while standing. The patient is placed in a supine, frog-legged position to permit exposure. The lithotomy position is not used as it places tension on the buttocks resulting in distortion of landmarks and incorrect resection. The area of planned excision is injected with 0.5% lidocaine with epinephrine (1 : 100,000). The incision is carried down to superficial fascia with preservation of the major veins and lymphatics. The flap is then undermined to the planned level of resection and split into segments, and the ease of approximation is checked. Additional undermining is not recommended nor is resection of subcutaneous fat as it causes a visible depression. Following meticulous hemostasis, a two-layer closure is done with deep interrupted absorbable sutures (3-0 Dexon) and a continuous subcuticular suture (4-0 Dexon). The edges are approximated in vertical anterior-to-posterior direction. The two edges are Steri-Stripped, and a light pressure dressing is applied. Mobilization is possible within 24 hours, and the postoperative course is usually uneventful. Firm elastic support hose are recommended for several months.

BUTTOCK DEFORMITIES

Isolated buttock deformities are relatively unusual but occur in certain minimally obese individuals or in those with aging ptotic redundance [2]. Conceptually, the redundancy lies within the buttock above the gluteal fold. Therefore, the incision is placed in the buttock crease to ensure camouflage of the scar and preservation of a distinct separation between buttock and thigh. The amount of redundancy is determined by pinching the tissue, as is its composition, skin or subcutaneous fat, or both. An elliptic area of excision extending from the medial midline to the posterolateral thigh is marked. The area is injected with local anesthetic. Excision of the skin follows, and the appropriate amount of subcutaneous fat is removed. Since excessive fat resection can cause flattening of the buttocks, careful contouring is recommended; the resection does not routinely go down to muscle fascia. In severe cases of ptosis, plication of the stretched muscle is recommended [14]. A double-layer closure is performed, and the patient should not sit for 2 weeks. Buttock augmentation, using breast prostheses, is occasionally reported along with the inevitable infection and secondary extrusion [4, 7, 10]. If the problem is one of contour in a non-weight-bearing location, temporary success may be possible. The use of prostheses to correct secondary deformities is not recommended; it is not an alternative to reoperation with preservation of deepithelialized flaps. Buttock defatting through a gluteal incision has been reported by Franco [13].

TROCHANTERIC DEFORMITIES

Accumulation of fat over the greater trochanter with obvious contour bulging is particularly disconcerting to the short normal-weight individual. Many patients expect that the fat deposit can be excised through a small incision hidden in the bikini area (Fig. 26-5). Thus, the surgeon's recommendation of long semicircular incisions with visible scars dismays the patient. Periodically, localized defattings are attempted and can produce a more noticeable depression, skin redundancy, and persistent hematomas. Excision of a large ellipse of both skin and fat extending from the medial thigh around to the anterior superior iliac spine is considered necessary to correct the total thigh deformity, which is *accentuated* by trochanteric lipodystrophy. The only exception to this rule is the secondary defatting procedure that is necessary following incomplete removal at the initial operation (see Secondary Surgery).

Generalized Deformities

The majority of patients present with generalized deformities amenable to a semicircular excision. However, certain individuals with excess throughout the upper thigh, especially anteriorly, will require a circular procedure. Following selection of the basic procedure, one must select any additional steps to correct gluteal depression, trochanteric bulging, or vertical redundancy. Preoperatively, one must decide whether the gluteal depression is merely accentuated by the adjacent bulges or is deep enough to require correction. For trochanteric bulging, one must decide whether upward traction on the thigh

Figure 26-5A, B. A 27-year-old patient who had a curettage of the trochanteric region done elsewhere. Obviously, a suction technique should have been used and a large volume (1000–1500 cc) removed. The surgical alternative would have been for the patient to lose 20 lb, followed by a semicircular thigh-lift with deepithelialization of the gluteal depression and excision of the trochanteric fat pad.

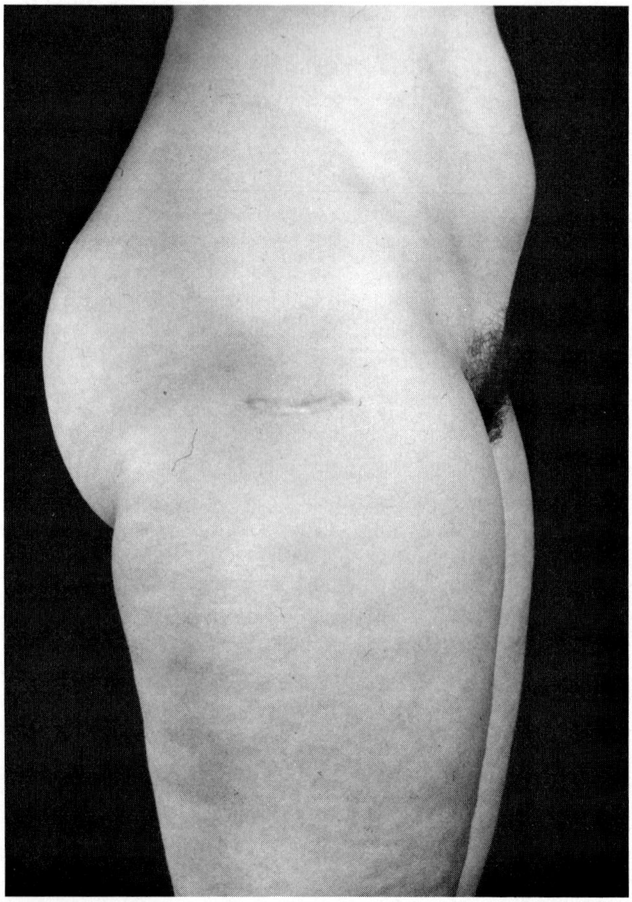

A

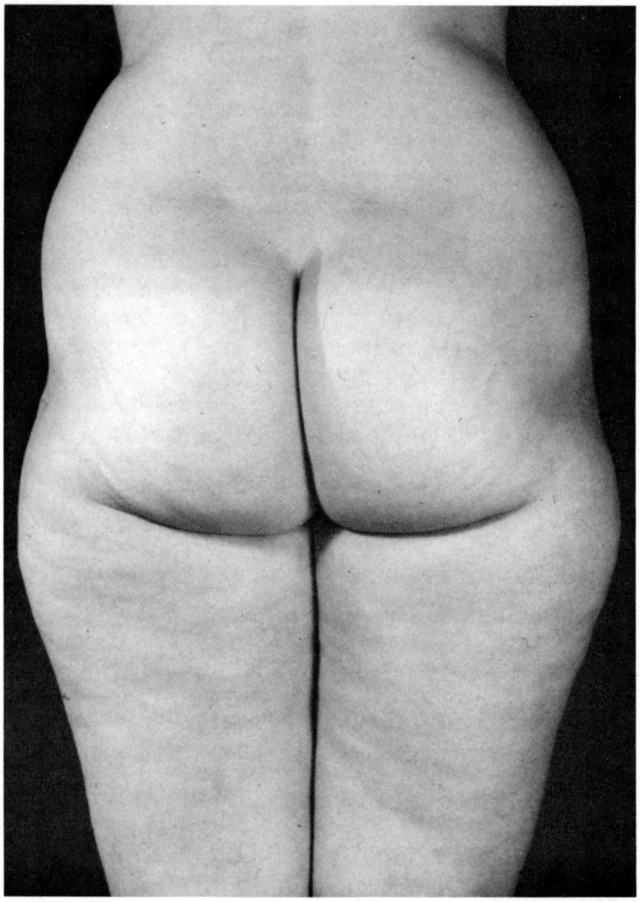

B

improves the deformity or whether defatting, surgical or suction, will be necessary. In contrast to correction of gluteal depressions, which is merely a surgical maneuver, trochanteric defatting does have a significant morbidity. It requires the patient's consent, preoperative counseling, and cooperation. If there is significant redundancy in the thigh that cannot be eliminated by upward medial traction, circumferential tightening can be accomplished by vertical excision. However, the patient must be warned that the vertical scar cannot be covered in sportswear and may be of definite concern.

SEMICIRCULAR RESECTION

A semicircular procedure permits direct excision of redundant skin and excess fat, while medial rotation on closure elevates and smooths the upper thigh (Fig. 26-6). In addition, medial thigh and buttock ptosis is improved.

Figure 26-6. Patient undergoing semicircular thigh-lift.
A–C. Use of bikini underpants for marking reference lines. Above is incision line and below is anticipated excision line.
D–F. Result showing improvement and location of scar.

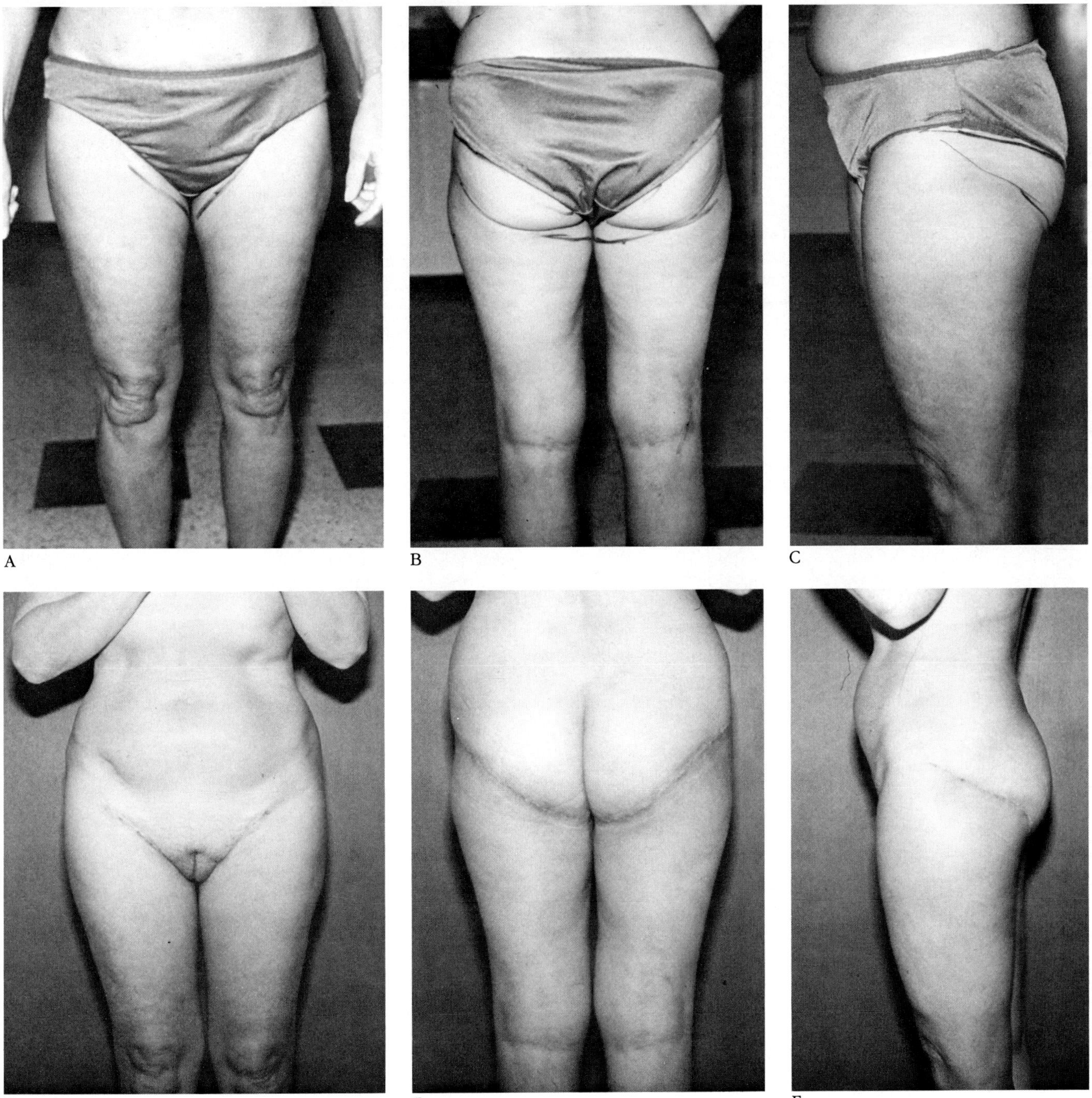

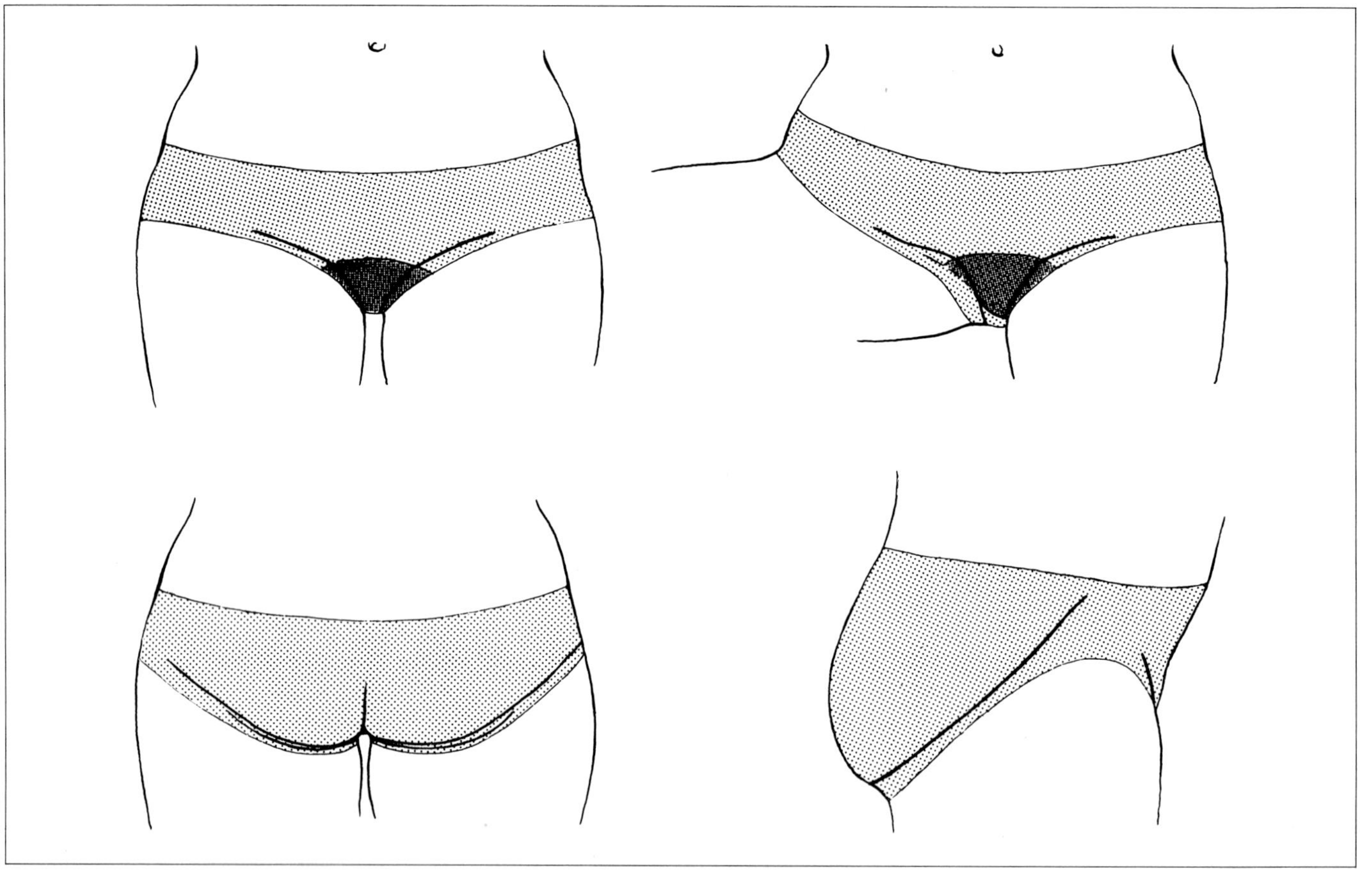

Figure 26-7. Location of incision line beneath a bikini.

Marking. With the patient standing, a reference line is marked along the lower border of the patient's bathing suit or panties (Fig. 26-7). The garment is removed and the incision line is drawn 2 to 3 cm above. It begins slightly lateral to the anterior superior iliac spine, crosses the buttock at the juncture of central and lateral third, continues 1 cm above the inguinal crease, and flares straight out at its anterior termination. It is important to note that this incision line differs substantially from standard excisions in its crescentic lateral portion, lower crossing of the buttock, and anterior flaring. The amount to be excised is determined by pushing up on the thigh and pinching the redundant tissue (Fig. 26-8). The medial and anterior estimation is comparable to a medial thigh-lift. Triangulation from a fixed sacral point ensures symmetry. One must avoid too great an excision as tension results in difficult closure, wound separation, and hypertrophic scar. At this point the degree of lateral gluteal depression is checked and marked, and a decision is made as to the best method of correction. Next, one must decide whether a specific trochanteric accumulation requires defatting. If a significant pad is present, its location and requisite area of undermining are marked.

Preparation. Lipectomy of the lower extremity is major surgery and is done under general anesthesia with the patient hospitalized for at least 4 days. The patient is placed in the supine position with the legs slightly apart. The lithotomy position is not recommended because it places deceptive tension on the tissues and makes suturing difficult. Following induction of anesthesia, the upper pubic hair is shaved and a Foley catheter inserted. Antibiotics (Kefzol, 500 mg intravenously) are begun. The wound is prepped from the umbilicus to the knee with the lower legs placed in stockinets.

Operation. The amount of expected resection is checked by pinching the soft tissues. The upper flared inguinal incision is made and continued down to superficial fascia. Since the dissection remains superficial, the major veins and nerves are not exposed nor are the inguinal lymphatics. The dissection is done bluntly by pushing with a sponge; the amount to be excised is checked and then quickly stripped as far posteromedially as possible. Undermining is not done beyond the anticipated excision line. Following hemostasis, the lower flap is rotated medially, and cross-hatches are marked. The flap is anchored to the inguinal fascia using 3-0 Dexon. A two-layer closure is done with interrupted 3-0 Dexon and a subcuticular continuous 4-0 Dexon suture. A temporary dressing is placed over the incision and then a Steridrape.

Next, the patient is turned prone by means of either a second draped operating table or the Pitanguy [27, 28] log-roll method: The arms are lifted over the head and the patient is placed at the edge of the operating table and

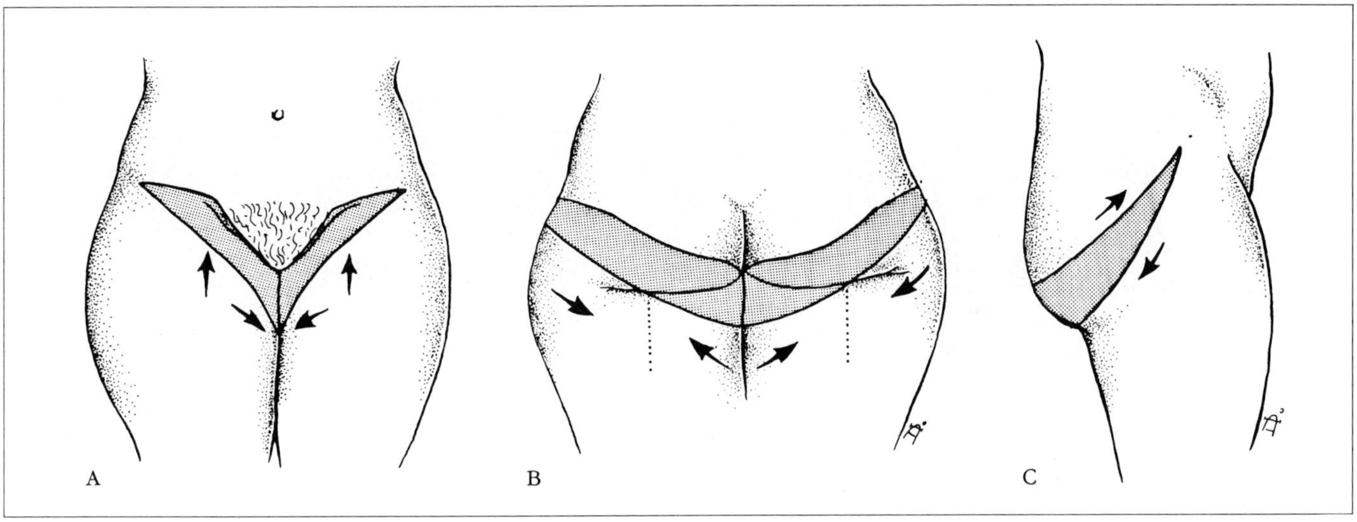

Figure 26-8. Area of excision and arrows showing direction of closure.
A. Upward flare of incision line ensures elevation while rotation on closure tightens the thigh.
B. Incision line ascends at level of rectum while excision line passes across midportion of buttock.
C. Tapered lateral extension avoids dog-ears, and countertraction lessens trochanteric prominence.

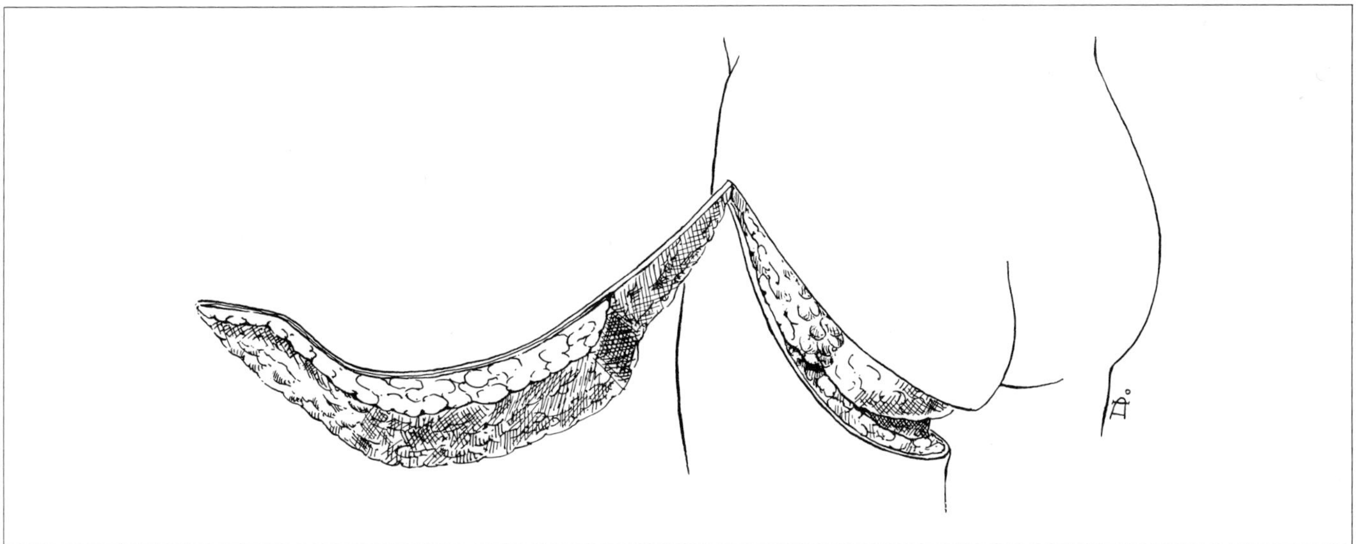

Figure 26-9. The crescentic semicircular excision with its moderate thickness medially, full thickness over the buttocks, and superficial resection in the gluteal depression.

then rolled 180 degrees. A pillow is placed under the anterior thorax, and prepped and draped [26]. The upper incision is carried down to the musculoaponeurotic plane and then dissected inferiorly with preservation of a small layer of fat on the fascia. Numerous vertical septa must be cut, and thus skin stripping is not feasible. The dissection becomes more superficial on passing from buttock to lateral thigh, thereby avoiding accentuation of the gluteal depression (Fig. 26-9). In certain cases segmental splitting of the flap and traction may be warranted to confirm preliminary markings. Special techniques may be necessary to deal with lateral gluteal depressions or trochanteric lipodystrophies. Whereas these procedures were developed for dealing with secondary deformities, they are now incorporated increasingly into the initial operation. The modifications in operative technique are the amount of tissue excised (lateral gluteal depression) and the extent of undermining (trochanteric lipodystrophy). Following meticulous hemostasis, the wound edges are approximated. The inferior edge is rotated posteriorly to minimize secondary deformities, and cross-hatchings are marked to ensure correct closure. A two-layer closure is done, and soft Penrose drains are inserted. Since there is no significant undermining, a pressure dressing is not necessary. The only dressing consists of adhesive tape strips along the incisions. The patient is allowed out of bed and encouraged to walk on the first postoperative day. Sitting is not permitted for 2 to 3 weeks.

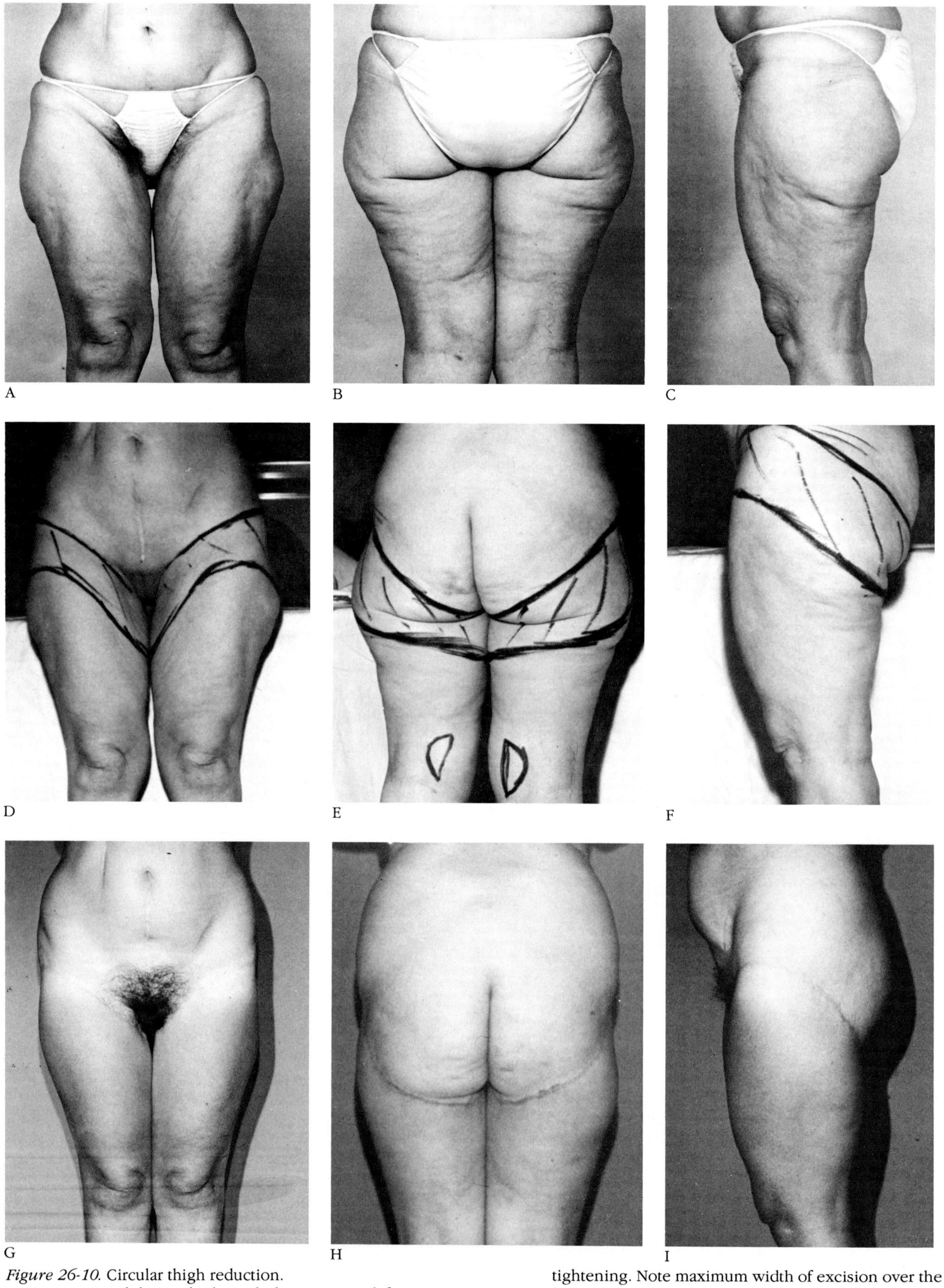

Figure 26-10. Circular thigh reduction.

A–C. Patient with heavy thighs including anterior deformity and sufficient flaccidity to warrant surgery.

D–F. Markings for a circular thigh-lift with optional popliteal tightening. Note maximum width of excision over the lateral area.

G–I. Result at 1 year shows dramatic improvement over preoperative condition.

CIRCULAR REDUCTION

In contrast to the semicircular resection, a circular reduction is designed to reduce the entire thigh at its base. The anterior extension permits direct excision of fullness on the front of the thigh, and the lateral excision is now a complete band rather than the tapered termination of a semicircular crescent (Fig. 26-10). Access to trochanteric deposits is also easier.

Marking. The reference bikini line is marked with the patient standing. A standard semicircular incision is marked and extended anteriorly above the inguinal crease but below the anterior superior iliac spine. The excision line *parallels* the incision line and is based on tissue flaccidity with the greatest spread laterally. Lateral gluteal depressions and trochanteric lipodystrophy are marked.

Operative Technique. The operation is begun anteriorly and is similar to the semicircular resection. The anterior tissue is excised first and the specimen divided as far laterally and medially as possible. The wound edges are approximated and anchored centrally. Then the medial thigh tissue is rotated medially to tighten the thigh while the lateral tissue is rotated posteriorly to minimize riding breeches deformity (Fig. 26-11). The lateral wound is extended as far as the operating table permits and closed under some tension as unexcised tissue remains posteriorly. After the standard two-layer closure, a temporary sterile dressing is placed over the incision and the patient is turned.

The amount and symmetry of the planned excision are verified. The incision is carried down to the musculoaponeurotic plane and the redundant tissue excised. The lower lateral flap is rotated inward while the lower medial flap is rotated outward. This posterior gathering of thigh tissue prevents a secondary deformity. Any associated gluteal depression or trochanteric lipodystrophy is treated in the previously discussed fashion. The suturing and dressing are similar to those in the semicircular resection.

GLUTEAL DEPRESSION

As always, the markings are done with the patient standing and they may be applied the night before with a permanent marker. The lines of a standard semicircular or circular lipectomy are drawn. Then the limits of the gluteal depression are delineated—usually spindle shaped, averaging 6 to 8 cm wide by 15 to 18 cm long and located above the trochanteric region. The depression will vary in depth from 2 to 8 cm. Minor depressions can be eliminated by preservation of the subcutaneous fat; moderate deformities require deepithelialization of the area; severe depressions are corrected by plication of the tissues (Fig. 26-12). The lipectomy is done in the standard fashion. The depressed area is kept as a deepithelialized region rather than being incorporated into the specimen. The upper and lower flaps are undermined and brought over the area. If the depressed area is of moderate proportions, the flaps are sutured with both mattress sutures on the skin and a continuous subcuticular absorbable suture (Fig. 26-13A, B). If the depression is severe and remains visible after overlapping of the flaps, the area is plicated with a heavy absorbable suture, producing an inverted tubular mound. This doubling of the area will correct virtually any depression, either primary or secondary (Fig. 26-13C, D).

TROCHANTERIC DEFATTING

Trochanteric bulging may be due to either skin laxity or firm adiposity; the former is correctable by upward traction while the latter requires direct defatting. With the patient standing, the area of undermining is carefully defined, as is the standard lipectomy excision (Fig. 26-14).

The operation is executed in a routine fashion until skin and fat excision is completed. Undermining of the trochanteric region is then done, preserving a 1-cm thickness

Figure 26-11. Area of excision and method of closure for a circular thigh reduction.

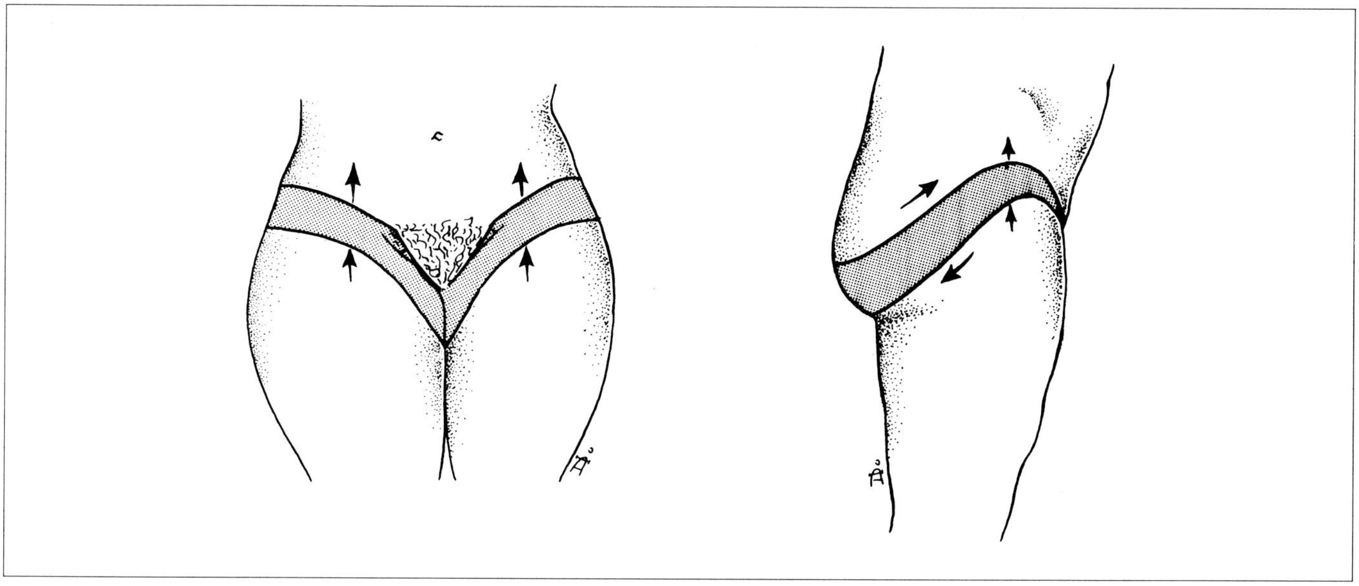

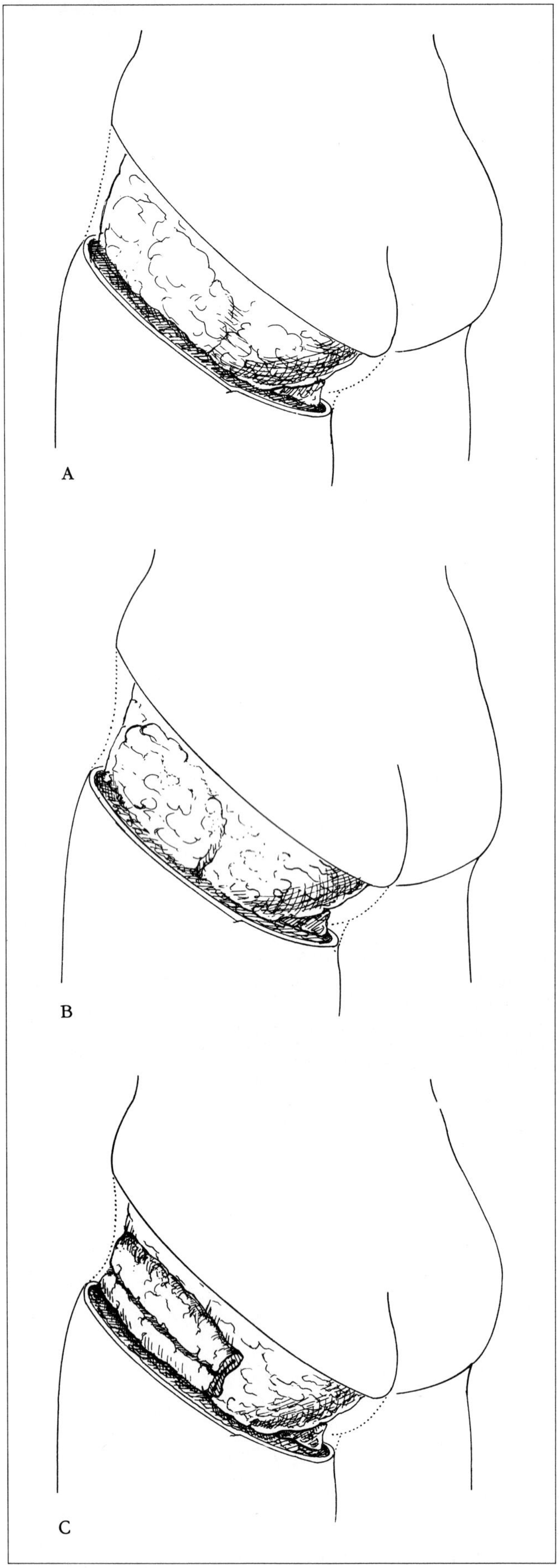

Figure 26-12. Three degrees of gluteal depression and their correction.

A. Minor depression alleviated by partial preservation of subcutaneous fat.

B. Moderate depression corrected by deepithelialization of the area.

C. Severe depression lessened by plication of the deepithelialized area.

Figure 26-13. Two patients with gluteal depression. ▶

A, B. Moderate gluteal depression corrected by deepithelialization simultaneously with a semicircular thigh-lift and no trochanteric defatting.

C, D. Severe gluteal depression on the right required plication of the deepithelialized area.

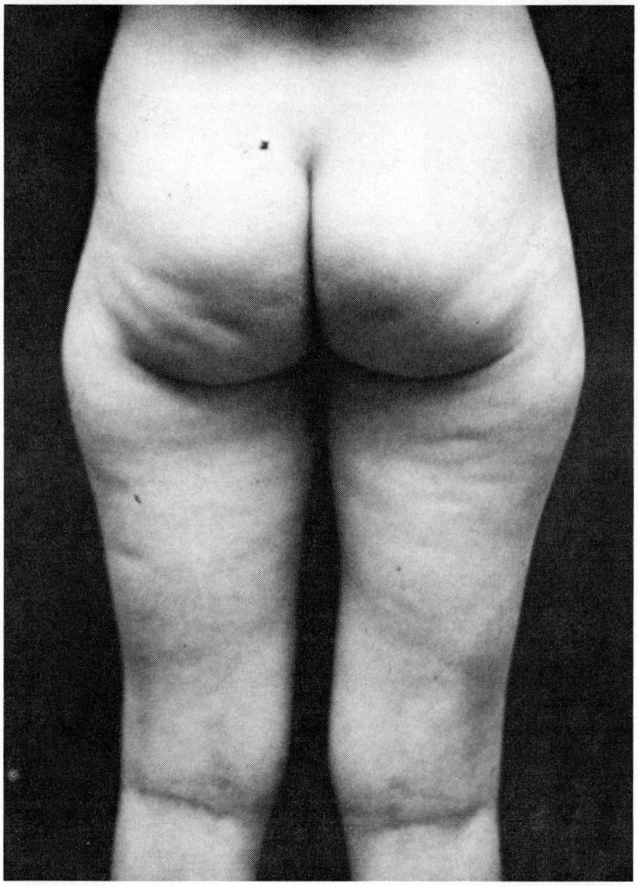

A

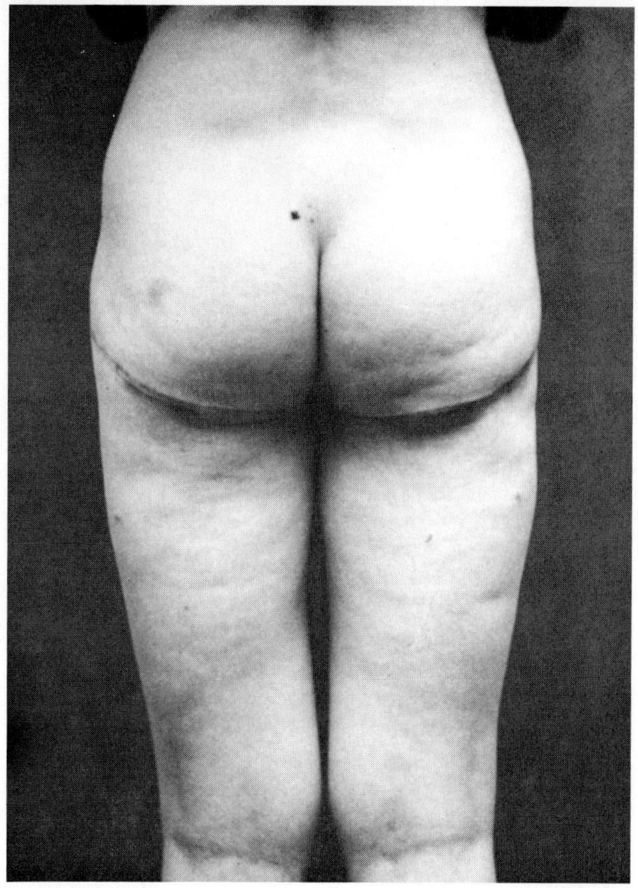

B

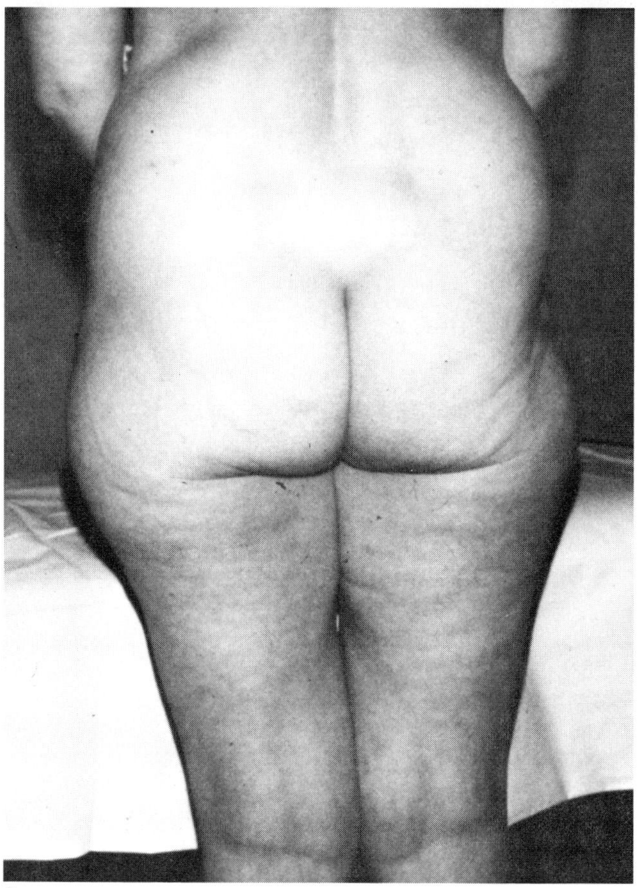

C

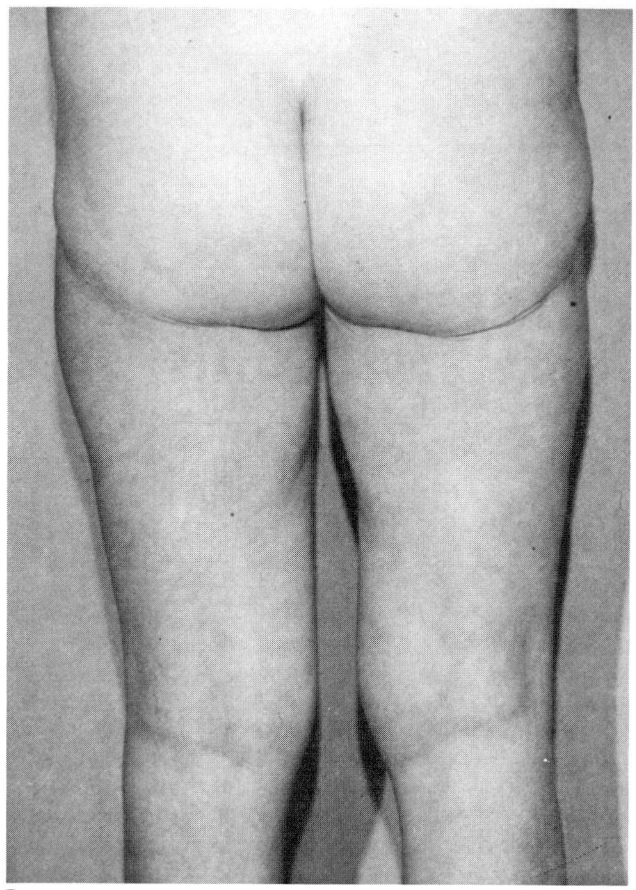

D

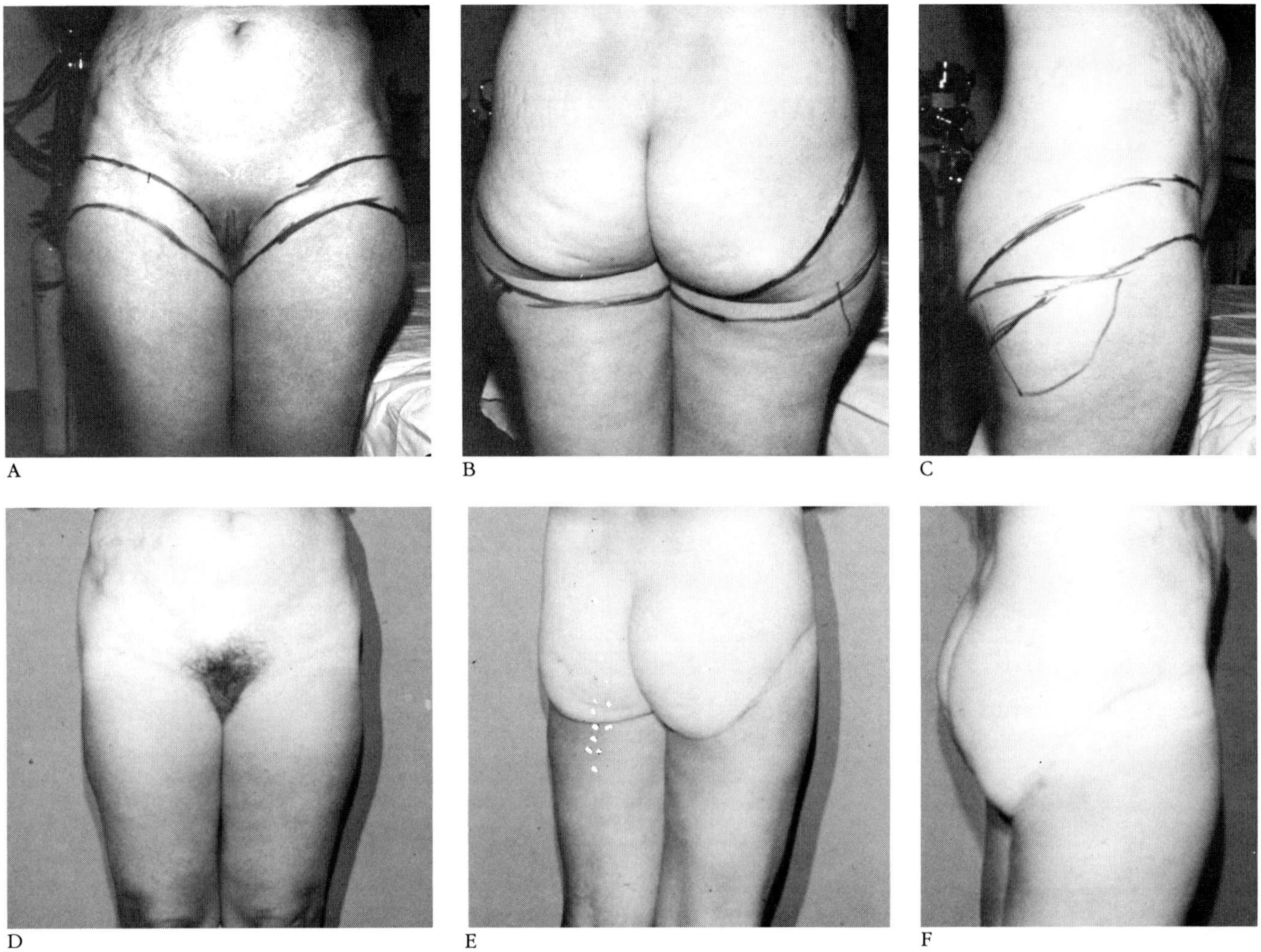

Figure 26-14
A–C. Patient requiring circular thigh-lift with trochanteric defatting.
D–F. Result at 1 year with virtually normal trochanteric contour.

of fat on the skin flap. Next, the excess fat is excised from the area, but 1 cm of fat is left over the fascia (Fig. 26-15). The latter maneuver is done to minimize chronic seroma formation. The fat excision must be carefully beveled at the periphery to avoid depressions and adjacent bulges. Profuse irrigation and suction are helpful in removing fat globules. Hemostasis must be meticulous. Two large drains are inserted in the most dependent areas and left for 24 to 48 hours. Compression taping of the area for a minimum of 10 days is very important.

VERTICAL EXTENSIONS

Isolated vertical excisions are rarely indicated except in patients with true lipodystrophies (Simons-Barraquer syndrome) [31]. Usually, they are incorporated into a semicircular or circular lipectomy (Fig. 26-16). The vertical component descends in the medial region before turning laterally above the popliteal region. The deep aponeurosis is preserved, and no undermining is done (Fig. 26-17). The lateral thigh flap is interposed between the buttock flap and the medial thigh flap to prevent a straight-line scar (Fig. 26-18). This combined procedure is used most often in massive-weight-loss cases.

Popliteal Area. Reduction of fullness above the knee can be achieved with a vertical semicircular excision done on the posteromedial aspect of the thigh (Fig. 26-19). Skin and subcutaneous fat excision is followed by a two-layer closure without undermining. This volumetric tightening reduces bulkiness while placing the scar posteriorly.

Calf. Patients request both augmentation and defatting of the calf region. Carlsen [5] has inserted custom-made silicone polymer solid implants in 37 patients desiring calf augmentation. Six patients (16%) had removal of the implants due to infection or displeasure with the appearance. The authors have seen patients in consultation following calf augmentation because of displacement, infection, or extrusion. Thus, we do not recommend prostheses in the lower extremity. With regard to reduction, lipexeresis with curets and suction curettage are the only alternatives, but the authors do not perform these procedures.

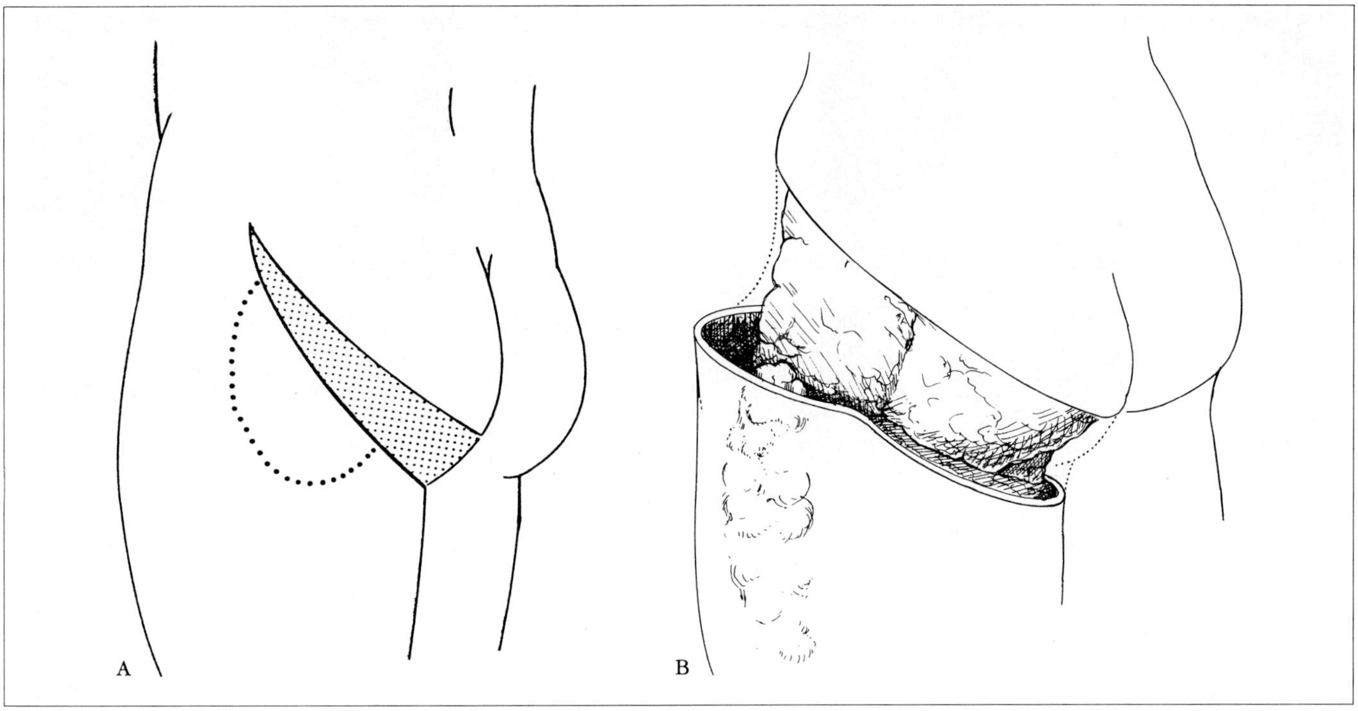

Figure 26-15
A. Area of trochanteric defatting in a semicircular thigh-lift.
B. Fat to be removed concomitant with a circular thigh reduction and moderate gluteal depression correction.

Ankle. Thickness about the ankle may be due to either fat accumulation, low origins of the various flexor muscles, or edema. Thus far, significant data are not available concerning surgery in this region.

SUCTION-ASSISTED LIPECTOMY

Many patients present with specific complaints about localized deformities over the trochanter, medial knees, ankles, and arms. They are dismayed that extensive surgery is recommended and plead for a smaller procedure. Numerous surgeons have attempted to solve this dilemma using localized resection or suction curettage. Schrudde [33] uses the term *lipexeresis* to denote localized excisions performed in the following manner: (1) The area of defatting is marked with the patient standing; (2) the skin is undermined with scissors, a 1-cm layer of fat being preserved on the skin; and (3) fat is removed from the deep surface with a curet. Four patients experienced skin loss, two healing primarily and two requiring skin grafts. However, the problem of seromas requires tight dressings for 3 weeks or insertion of an "outlet" into the most dependent part of the wound, which allows constant drainage rather than periodic aspirations.

In 1978, Kesselring [17] developed an instrument for this procedure and has extended his work to regional body areas. Teimourian and Fisher [35] reported their experience with 54 patients and noted only one hematoma. They stressed several technical points: (1) Suction curettage removes only bulging fat while preserving the arcades connecting deep fascia with skin, (2) skin contraction and adherence occurred without secondary deformity, and (3) a modified fascia lata stripper was used in addition to Kesselring instruments attached to a Bennett aspiration unit. Vogt [39, 40] cautioned against immediate acceptance of these techniques, noting that they "fell into disrepute a long time ago for body contouring, although still used by a few surgeons for localized deformities." Attempts to apply suction curettage to large deformities lead to "postoperative hemoseromas needing evacuation for several weeks, skin sloughs, and wrinkled unaesthetic looking defatted areas." Currently, suction-assisted lipectomy is receiving renewed interest and is discussed further in Chapter 27.

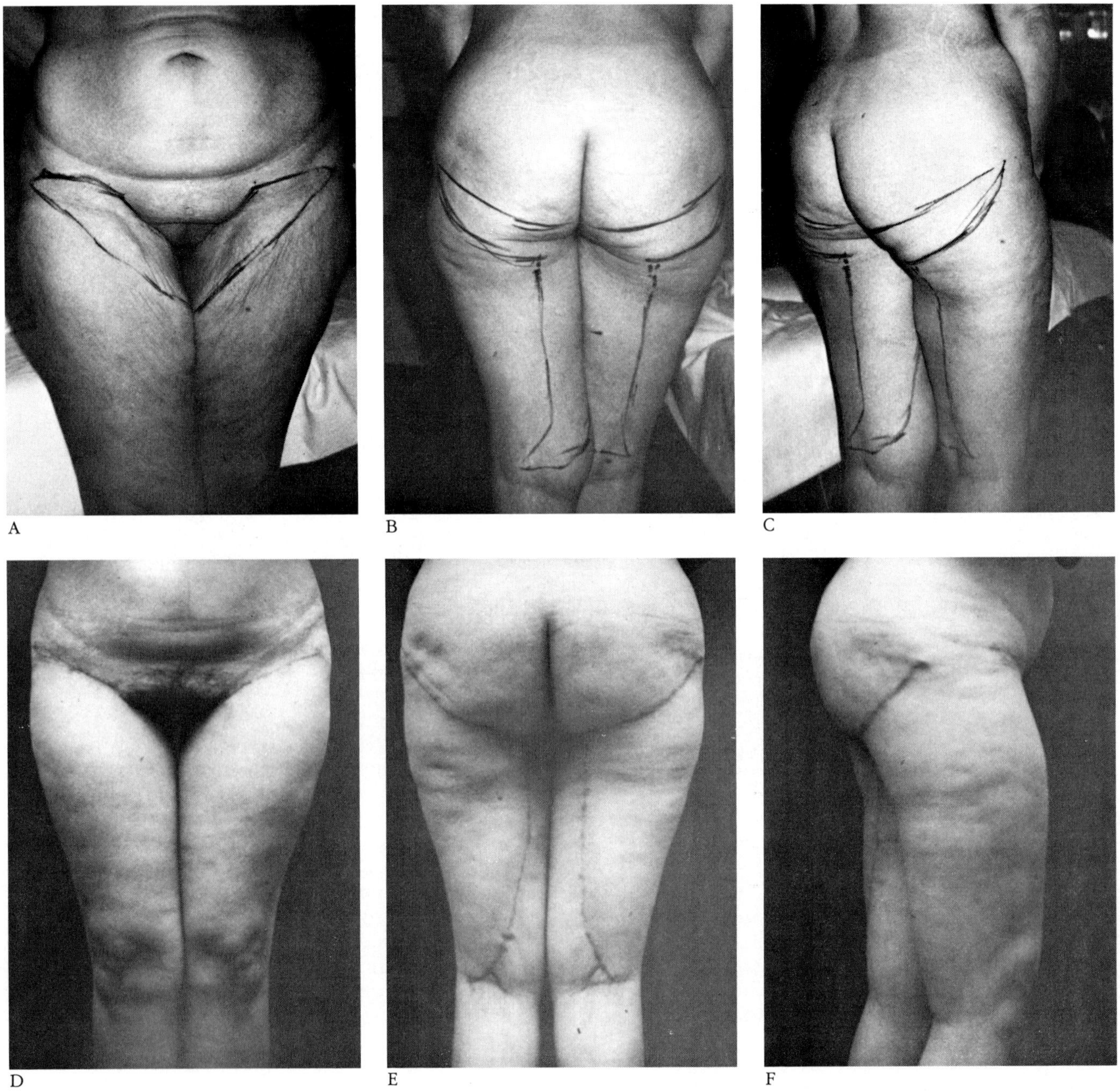

Figure 26-16
A–C. Patient with marked flaccidity requiring circumferential tightening via a vertical excision.
D–F. Result of semicircular lipectomy with vertical extension at 9 months.

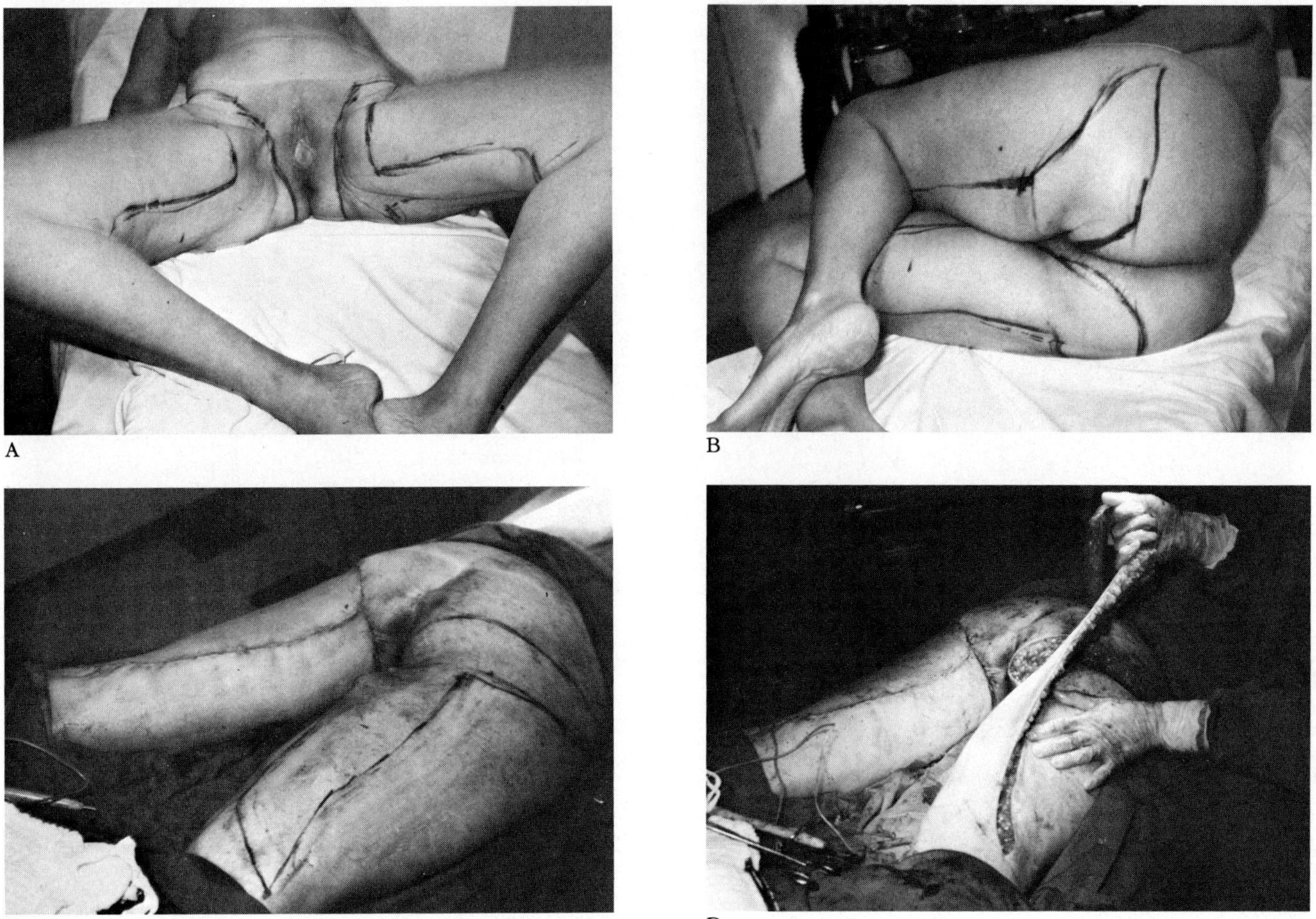

A B C D

Figure 26-17

A, B. Preoperative markings indicating wide area of excision for elevation and tightening of the thighs.

C, D. Completion of left leg demonstrates marked improvement over the right leg.

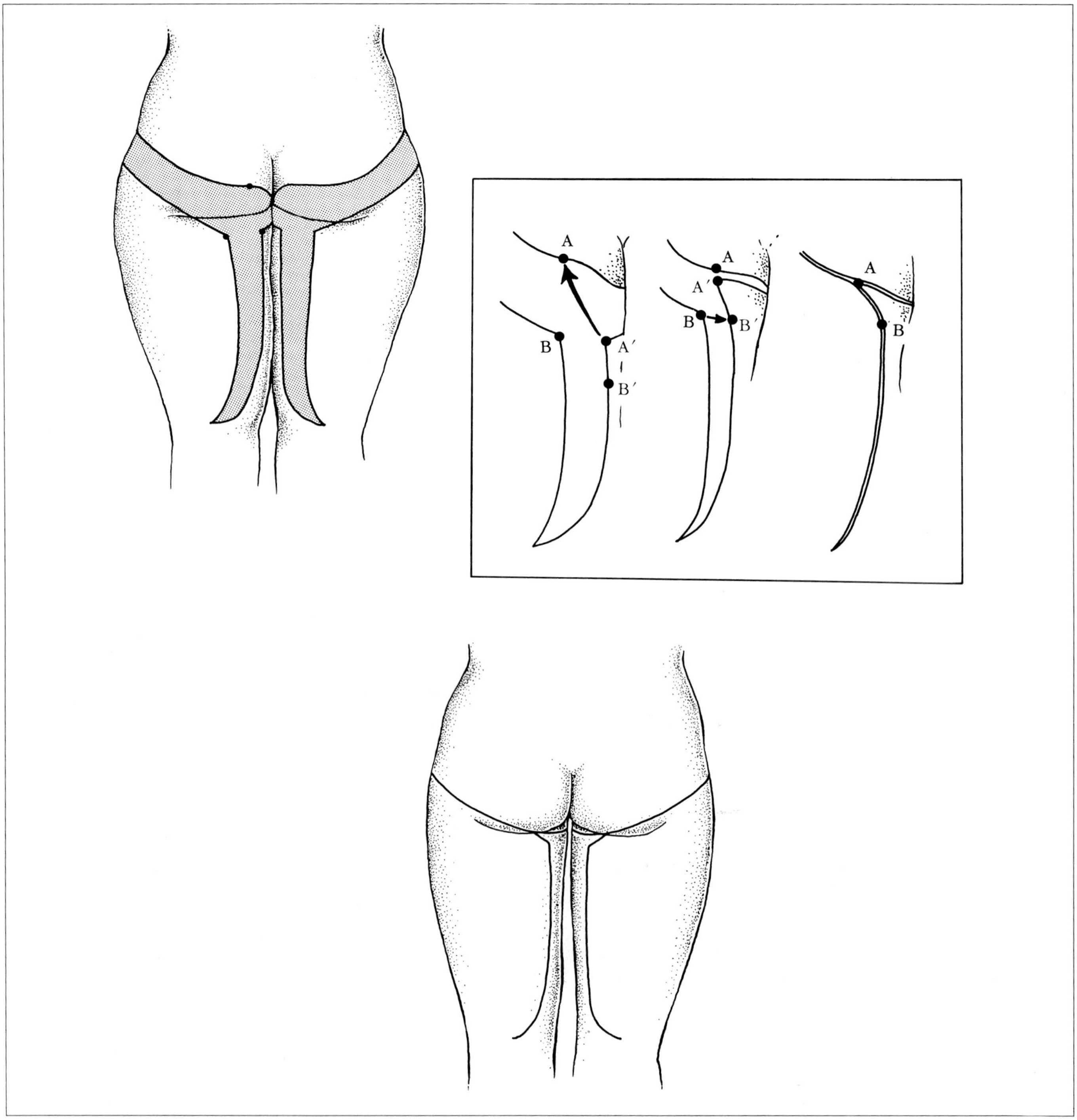

Figure 26-18. Markings and method of closure for vertical excision.

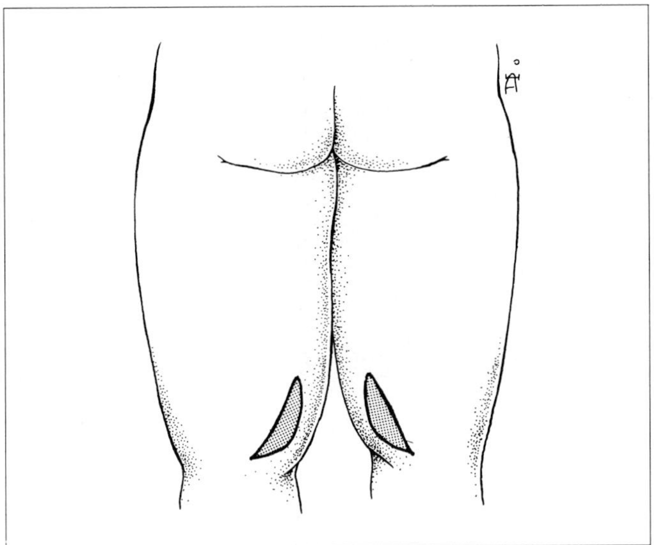

Figure 26-19. Popliteal excision for removal and tightening of fullness above the knee.

COMPLICATIONS

Surprisingly, major reviews of the incidence and types of complications following lower extremity lipectomy have not been published.

Intraoperative Complications

The major intraoperative problems are tight closure and obvious asymmetry. Overestimation of possible excision occurs infrequently and is avoided by segmental splitting of the thigh flap. Tension can be minimized by extensive undermining onto the thigh, but it increases the risk of hematoma formation. Asymmetry is best avoided but can be caused by unequal excision or unequal rotation on closure. The former is avoided by compass markings and additional resection; the latter is corrected by appropriate sutures.

EARLY HEMATOMA
The incidence of early complications tends to increase with the extent of undermining. Immediate detection and definitive treatment of fluid accumulation are necessary if one is to avoid serious wound infections and necrosis. In most lower extremity lipectomies, the incidence of hematoma is low because of limited undermining. However, hematomas are common and may approach 50 percent following trochanteric defatting procedures (Fig. 26-20). Repeated evacuations for several weeks are often necessary.

WOUND SEPARATION AND INFECTION
Minor separation of the wound edges may occur on account of patient activities and superficial infection. It is most common medially and results from maceration and friction. It is treated with local dressings, antibiotics, and separation of the thighs. Complete dehiscence of the wound is usually due to infection, which may be secondary to an infected hematoma. Large infections must be drained and allowed to heal spontaneously with subsequent scar revision.

NECROSIS
Skin sloughs are extremely rare. They are associated with infected hematomas or extensive undermining. Areas of full-thickness loss should be excised and grafted if necessary. Secondary revision is done a year later.

Late Complications

SCARS
Patient acceptance of the inevitable scarring that accompanies lower limb dermolipectomy is directly related to preoperative counseling and placement of the incision, especially in the medial area. The patient must be aware that the operative incision over the lateral area will become hypertrophic and then gradually diminish. If the scar remains objectionable at 1 year, it can be treated by injections of triamcinolone. In contrast, the inguinal scars tend to spread and descend onto the thighs, making them visible below bathing suits. This visibility is usually caused by excessive skin excision, tension on the suture line, too inferior a placement of the initial incision, or failure to rotate the thigh flap at time of closure. Secondary correction is not done before 1 year and entails excision with upward advancement. If medial depression is already present, deepithelialization of the scar followed by inferior flap advancement is recommended.

ASYMMETRY AND CONTOUR DEFORMITIES
Disproportional resections are usually due to inaccurate preoperative markings or measurements made in the prone position. All markings should be made with the patient standing and checked for symmetry by the triangulation technique. Contour deformities may be due to inadequate (bulges) or excessive (depressions) resections. Most bulges are easily corrected by undermining and curettage, whereas depressions necessitate deepithelialization and flap advancement. As always, errors of conservatism allow simple refinement whereas errors of radicalism require extensive reconstruction.

DEFORMITY OF THE VULVA AND LABIA MAJORA
Tension on the labia majora and gaping of the introitus may occur following excessive medial skin resection. This problem is best avoided by the following maneuvers: (1) an accurate limited amount of skin resection, (2) spiral rotation of the anteromedial tissues posteriorly rather than superiorly, and (3) insertion of deep suspensory sutures between the thigh flap and the inguinal fascia. Once these deformities occur, they are best treated by multiple Z-plasties and sectioning of the contracted bond.

EDEMA AND LYMPHEDEMA
If the major veins and lymphatics have been carefully preserved, edema should be of short duration. Once

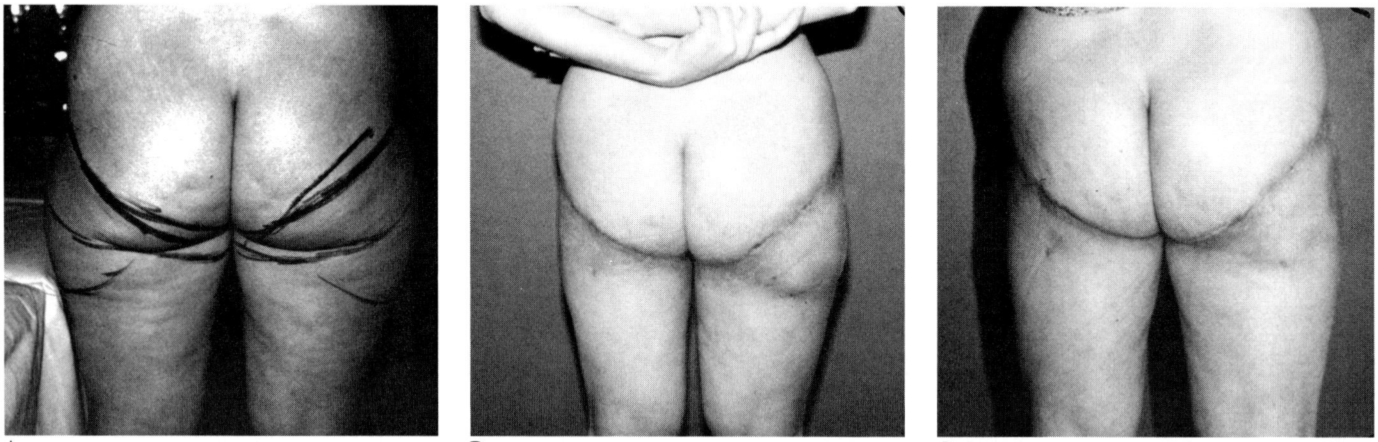

A B C

Figure 26-20
A. Patient undergoing circular thigh-lift with trochanteric defatting.
B. Presence of hematoma at 7 days.
C. Resolution at 2 months following multiple aspirations.

swelling is detected, elastic stockings should be worn for a few weeks or months. The legs should be elevated whenever possible, and exercises are recommended. Unquestionably, lymphedema is a catastrophic complication that can occur following dermolipectomy. Although only a few cases have been reported, it is most often associated with deep inguinal resections and postoperative infections. The possibility of spontaneous onset of lymphedema tarda cannot be ruled out, nor can tipping the balance between subclinical and clinical lymphedema be discounted.

RESULTS

Short-Term Results

Once the inconvenience of the postoperative period is overcome, the majority of patients are pleased with the contour improvement. A minority will be disappointed as they expected greater correction and elimination of cellulite accumulation. The first year is spent reassuring the patient that normal wound healing is progressing and that the reddening scars will become less obvious with time.

Long-Term Results

On the basis of a 20-year experience, Lewis [21] reports that the long-term benefits of thigh-lifts are generally permanent provided the patient does not undergo significant weight fluctuations. The persistent effect of gravity and aging may lead to descent of the scars. Conceptually, the medial and buttock areas are prone to the ptosis of aging whereas the lateral area will reflect increasing obesity.

SECONDARY SURGERY

Secondary surgery consists in scar revisions or correction of persistent deformities. With increasing preoperative awareness of the lateral gluteal depression and the need for direct excision of the trochanteric fat, the incidence of secondary surgery is decreasing.

Lateral Gluteal Depression

The classic thigh-lift involves resection of tissue midway between the iliac crest and the femoral trochanter. Thus, a preexisting lateral depression would be accentuated by surgical excision plus any retained trochanteric bulging (Fig. 26-21). To avoid these problems, the area of depression is marked preoperatively in the standing position. Tissue redundancy must be carefully assessed as inferior flap elevation may not be possible and treatment with a dermafat graft may be necessary. If skin redundancy permits, the depressed area is deepithelialized and an inferior flap brought over it. Extensive undermining is often necessary, and the trochanteric lipodystrophy is excised directly.

Trochanteric Lipodystrophy

If adequate skin excision was done previously, a regional trochanteric defatting may be sufficient. The prominent area is marked with the patient standing. The patient is then placed in the prone position. The incision is opened and undermining is done above the musculoaponeurotic plane, with retention of some fat. The fat pad is dissected from underneath and a 15-mm thickness of subcutaneous fat is retained. Consummate surgical skill is required to evenly sculpt the subcutaneous fat and to ensure hemostasis. A small closed drain is inserted and brought out in the most dependent part of the wound. A pressure dressing is applied and the drain left for at least 48 hours. Despite these efforts, the hematoma rate approaches 50 percent, and repeated evacuations up to 1 month are often necessary.

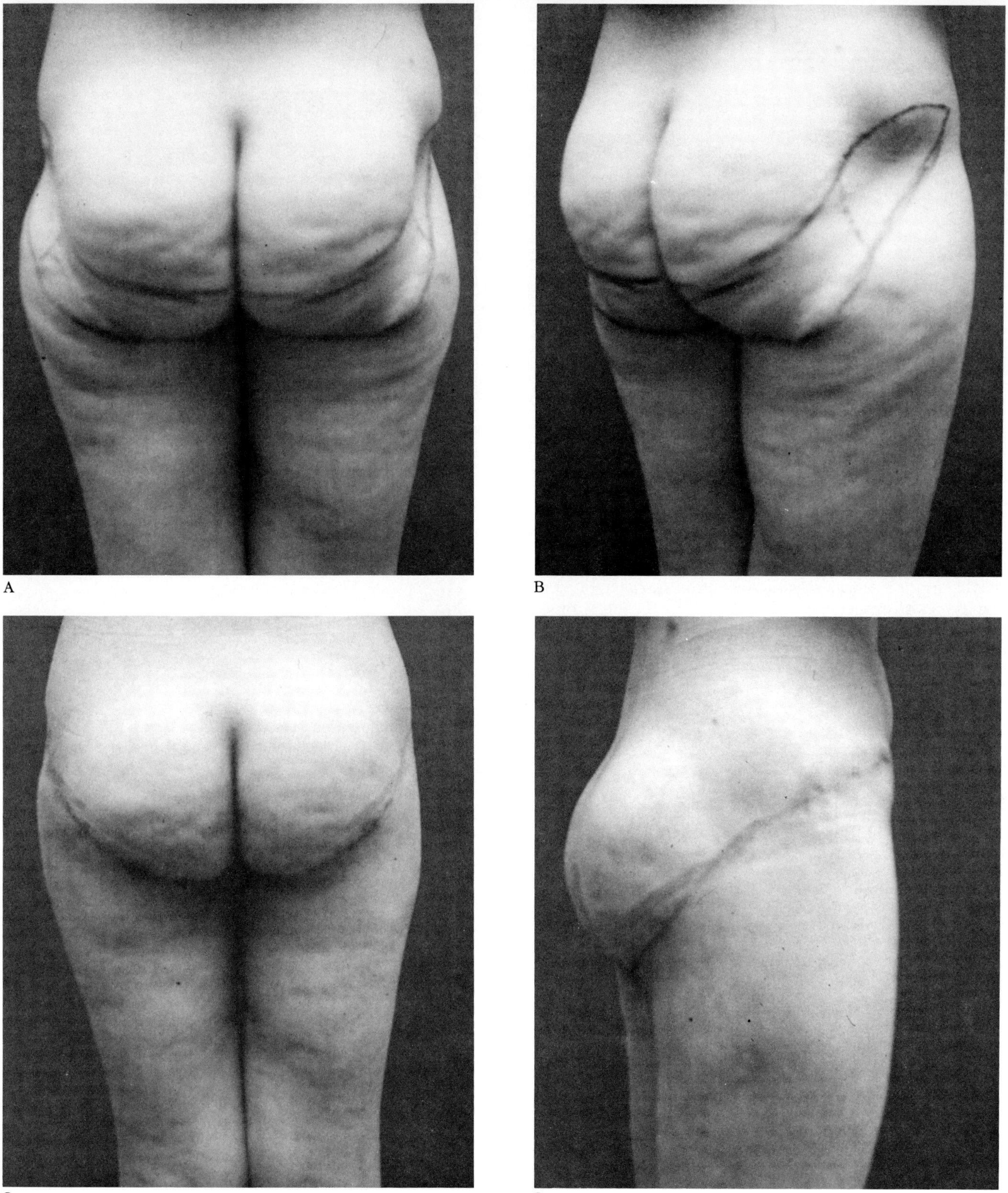

Figure 26-21. Secondary surgery.

A, B. Patient referred following semicircular thigh-lift. Obvious problems are errors of commission (resection rather than preservation of the gluteal depression) and errors of omission (failure to excise the trochanteric fat deposits).

C, D. Result following secondary surgery involving plication of the gluteal depression and excision of the trochanteric fat pad.

REFERENCES

1. Agris, J. The use of dermal-fat suspension flaps for thigh and buttock lifts. *Plast. Reconstr. Surg.* 59:817, 1977.
2. Aston, S. J. Buttocks and Thighs. In T. D. Rees (ed.), *Aesthetic Plastic Surgery.* Philadelphia: Saunders, 1980. P. 1039.
3. Baroudi, R. Thigh-Lift and Buttock-Lift. In E. H. Courtiss (ed.), *Aesthetic Surgery: Trouble—How to Avoid It and How to Treat It.* St. Louis: Mosby, 1978. P. 223.
4. Baztels, R. J., et al. An unusual use of the Cronin breast prosthesis. *Plast. Reconstr. Surg.* 44:500, 1969.
5. Carlsen, L. Calf augmentation: A preliminary report. *Ann. Plast. Surg.* 2:508, 1979.
6. Clarkson, P. Lipodystrophies. *Plast. Reconstr. Surg.* 37:499, 1966.
7. Cocke, W. M., and Ricketson, G. Gluteal augmentation. *Plast. Reconstr. Surg.* 52:1, 1973.
8. Correa, I. Tratamiento quirurgico de la obesidad. *Rev. Med. Argent.* 66:340, 1952.
9. Delerm, A., and Girotteau, Y. Plastie, Cruro "femoro" fessiere ou Circum Fessiere. *Ann. Chir. Plast.* 18:31, 1973.
10. Douglas, W. M., Baztels, R. J., and Baker, J. L. An experience in aesthetic buttocks augmentation. *Clin. Plast. Surg.* 3:471, 1975.
11. Farina, R., et al. Lipodistrofia pelvo-crurol tipo calcos de montaria (lipomatose trocanterica). *Hospital* (Rio) 57:717, 1960.
12. Farina, R., et al. Riding trousers-like type of pelvicrural lipodystrophy (trochanteric lipomatosis). *Br. J. Plast. Surg.* 13:174, 1971.
13. Franco, T. Aesthetic Surgery of Upper and Lower Limbs. In J. F. Ely (ed.), *Transactions of the Seventh International Congress of Plastic and Reconstructive Surgery.* São Paulo: Cartgraf, 1979. P. 645.
14. Grazer, F. M., and Klingbeil, J. R. *Body Image: A Surgical Perspective.* St. Louis: Mosby, 1980.
15. Hoffman, F., and Simon, B. E. Experiences with the Pitanguy method of correction of trochanteric lipodystrophy. *Plast. Reconstr. Surg.* 55:551, 1975.
16. Kelly, H. A. Excision of the fat of the abdominal wall lipectomy. *Surg. Gynecol. Obstet.* 10:229, 1910.
17. Kesselring, U. K. Regional fat aspiration for body contouring. *Plast. Reconstr. Surg.* 72:610, 1983.
18. Lewis, J. R., Jr. The thigh lift. *J. Int. Coll. Surg.* 27:330, 1957.
19. Lewis, J. R., Jr. Correction of ptosis of the thighs: The thigh lift. *Plast. Reconstr. Surg.* 37:494, 1966.
20. Lewis, J. R., Jr. *Atlas of Aesthetic Plastic Surgery.* Boston: Little, Brown, 1973.
21. Lewis, J. R., Jr. Surgery of the Hips, Buttocks, and Thighs. In R. M. Goldwyn (ed.), *Long-Term Results in Plastic and Reconstructive Surgery.* Boston: Little, Brown, 1980. P. 774.
22. Noël, A. *La Chirurgie Esthétique: Son Rôle Social.* Paris: Masson, 1926.
23. Pitanguy, I. Lipodistrofia trocanterica. *Rev. Bras. Cir.* 47:69, 1964.
24. Pitanguy, I. Surgical reduction of the abdomen, thighs, and buttocks. *Surg. Clin. North Am.* 51:280, 1964.
25. Pitanguy, I. Trochanteric lipodystrophy. *Plast. Reconstr. Surg.* 34:280, 1964.
26. Pitanguy, I. Technique for Trunk and Thigh Reduction. In *Transactions of the Fifth International Congress of Plastic and Reconstructive Surgery.* Melbourne: Butterworths, 1971. P. 1204.
27. Pitanguy, I. Aesthetic plastic surgery of the upper and lower limbs. *Aesthetic Plast. Surg.* 4:363, 1980.
28. Pitanguy, I. *Aesthetic Plastic Surgery of Head and Body.* Berlin: Springer, 1981.
29. Planas, J. The "crural meloplasty," for lifting of the thighs. *Clin. Plast. Surg.* 2:495, 1975.
30. Regnault, P. Lipectomy. In W. C. Grabb and J. W. Smith (eds.), *Plastic Surgery.* Boston: Little, Brown, 1979. P. 838.
31. Regnault, P., and Alfara, A. Lipodystrophie de platothoracique de Barraquer-Simons. Présentation d'un cas. *Union Med. Can.* 96:286, 1967.
32. Regnault, P., Baroudi, R., and Carvalho, C. G. S. Correction of lower limb lipodystrophy. *Aesthetic Plast. Surg.* 3:233, 1979.
33. Schrudde, J. Lipexeresis as a means of eliminating local adiposity. *Aesthetic Plast. Surg.* 4:215, 1980.
34. Schultz, R. C., and Feinberg, L. A. Medical thigh lift. *Ann. Plast. Surg.* 2:404, 1979.
35. Teimourian, B., and Fisher, J. B. Suction curettage to remove excess fat for body contouring. *Plast. Reconstr. Surg.* 68:50, 1981.
36. Vilain, R. Some considerations in surgical alteration of the female silhouette. *Clin. Plast. Surg.* 2:449, 1975.
37. Vilain, R. Surgical correction of steatomeries. *Clin. Plast. Surg.* 2:467, 1975.
38. Vilain, R. C., Dardour, J. C., and Bzowski, A. Use of dermalfat flaps in treating abdominal scars, in abdominoplasty, and in subtrochanteric lipectomy. *Plast. Reconstr. Surg.* 60:876, 1977.
39. Vogt, T. Combined medicosurgical torsoplasty. *Aesthetic Plast. Surg.* 4:109, 1980.
40. Vogt, T., and Dicksheet, S. Suction curettage and alternatives to remove excess fat. *Plast. Reconstr. Surg.* 69:724, 1982.

27. Suction Lipectomy

Basic Principles and Indications of Liposuction

Paule Regnault

The role of liposuction in aesthetic surgery is constantly expanding, both as to the number and types of cases performed [1]. As with any new procedure, its application will be defined and confined to specific problems. At the present time, the primary determinant of excellent results is tissue firmness. The age of the patient is not the critical factor. When the tissues are quite loose, surgical excision is indicated as it permits removal of skin and fat at the same time. The difficult cases are those with moderate flabbiness where liposuction and surgical excision are combined. Preferably, the two are done at the same time, but in certain cases a two-stage approach is preferred beginning with liposuction, doing surgical excision several months later when the swelling has completely disappeared.

INDICATIONS ACCORDING TO LOCALIZATION

After 3 decades of experience with surgical procedures for body contouring, the author was initially hesitant to embrace liposuction as a valid technique. The reasons were multiple. Were the results really good? Did it have something new to offer? Were the complications acceptable? After attending several lectures and having the opportunity to assist both Drs. Fournier and Kesselring at surgery, it became obvious that dramatic improvement was attainable without significant scars or complications in *carefully selected cases.* Therefore, liposuction has now become a part of my surgical armamentarium and the following observations appear warranted.

The choice of the technique is a matter of personal preference. Currently, the tunnelization technique described by Illouz-Fournier is more popular than the pocket technique of Kesselring. One cannot obtain a pocket without tearing vessels and superficial nerves, which brings us back to sharp defatting with less bleeding. Forming tunnels between vascular bundles while tearing only the lesser ones is an obvious advantage. Using the wet or dry techniques does not seem to change the result very much, but it appears that infiltrating the area with a diluted solution or local anesthesia (1 : 200,000) causes less bleeding and ecchymosis. It is imperative to use local infiltration in facial defatting. A tight conforming dressing is critical to success.

Lower Extremities

The primary indication for liposuction in the lower extremities is the riding breeches deformity. In firm cases, liposuction alone is indicated whereas for flabby or loose tissues excision is combined with liposuction. Total reduction of the thighs may be done by completely suctioning the periphery of the thighs in selected cases. A secondary excision may be necessary and patients are always warned about this necessity. The same applies to buttocks, whether they are defatted as an isolated entity or combined with thigh correction. The medial aspect of the thighs is an area where the skin is very thin and loose and where suction alone is rarely warranted. It is better to excise a wedge of superficial tissue following the natural upper crease with posterior extension as indicated. The calves may be defatted by liposuction as shown by several authors. It is an area where one should expect persistent edema requiring elastic stockings and massaging for a long period. When a limited area such as the ankles is done, the swelling will disappear faster than when a larger area is defatted.

Torso

The primary indication for liposuction is a very firm adipose fat layer. Thus, men are good candidates as are some women who have gained weight but have not had a previous pregnancy. In the case of flabbiness, it is imperative to *combine* liposuction and excision, preferably at the same time. This allows for smaller excisions. In selected cases, suction will permit avoidance of umbilical transposition by simply excising a W or horizontal ellipse including full-thickness skin and fat in the suprapubic area. The addition of liposuction to standard abdominoplasty techniques permits defatting of the thorax, lateral waistline, and hips, which are very often justified.

The posterior part of the trunk follows the same indications. The waistline and posterior hips can be defatted in cases where the tissues are firm enough. If the tissues are flabby, then excision plus liposuction is warranted whereas excision alone is used in most massive weight loss cases.

Upper Extremities

Liposuction is indicated in the firm, tense arm for which surgery has little to offer. A total circular liposuction of the arm may be done in one or two stages. In flabby tissues, liposuction allows for smaller excisions and thus shorter scars. For example, a total arm reduction may be reduced via a moderate excision using liposuction to correct deformities at either end. The preaxillary adipose deformity requires either a smaller skin excision, which can be placed in the axillary area (double W), or no excision at all when the adiposity is firm enough.

Breast

Alterations in the breast itself are not done with liposuction as glandular tissue cannot be removed, and emptiness of the skin brassiere would accentuate or increase ptosis. However, it is of value in men for selected cases of gynecomastia where adiposity is the primary problem rather than excess glandular tissue. Also, liposuction can be used to avoid dog ears at the end of breast reduction excisions, as well as for axillary rolls and fat accumulation in the sleeve hole area.

Face

Liposuction can improve the results of rhytidectomy as it allows fat removal from areas where sharp defatting is considered "taboo." The cheeks, especially above the nasolabial folds, the midcheek, and lower cheek can be defatted by liposuction. Thus, one can sculpture the face without the dangers of nerve damage, profuse bleeding, or hematoma fixation. The submental and cervical areas can be easily defatted with liposuction. However, great care is required in using liposuction in the neck. Smaller cannulas and careful manipulation are required. The platysma is often very thin and can easily be penetrated allowing injury to various nerve branches. One must be constantly aware of both cannula direction and location in relation to the skin and deep structures.

Body Sculpturing with Suction-Assisted Lipectomy

Ulrich K. Kesselring
Rodolphe Meyer

Subcutaneous lipectomy through a buttonhole incision has been performed by a number of physicians for more than 10 years. Among the various instruments used for this purpose are the uterine curet, the fascial stripper, power morselizing devices, and the Aspiradeps.

Although we had very satisfactory results using the uterine curet in the early seventies as recommended by Schrudde [10], we were not very happy with the purely practical aspect of the technique involved, which required squeezing and rinsing of the subcutaneous wound in order to remove the avulsed fat. After the experimental use of several prototypes, Kesselring designed a suction curet in 1976, which was presented in 1978 [8]. Currently, the instrument is manufactured in nine different forms (Fig. 27-1) by the Ulrich Company in St.-Gall, Switzerland, under the name *Aspiradeps.*

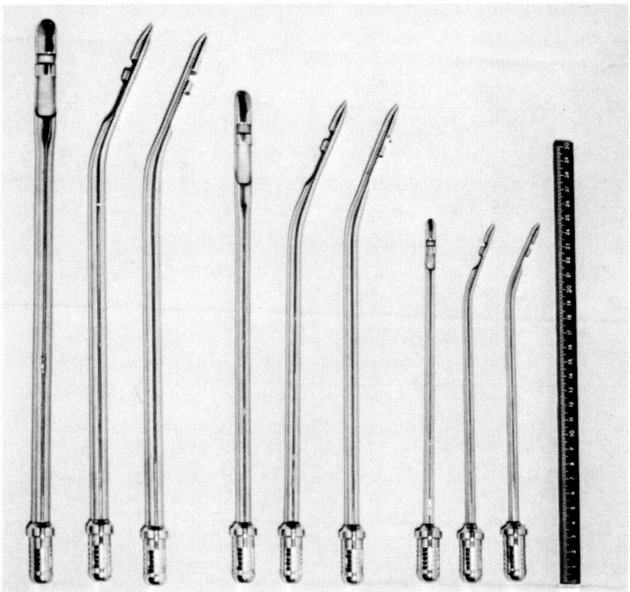

Figure 27-1. The Aspiradeps is manufactured in nine different forms and sizes.

WHY SUCTION-ASSISTED LIPECTOMY

The combined use of suction and mechanical fat resection, suction-assisted lipectomy (SAL) has the following advantages: (1) The avulsed fat globules are immediately removed from the wound, and (2) blood is simultaneously and constantly removed, so that no traumatizing manipulations like squeezing and rinsing are necessary to clean the wound. Minimal trauma favors uncomplicated healing.

The special shape of the Aspiradeps with its sharkhead tip (Fig. 27-2) is essential; it enables one to achieve a clean feathering at the transition point, thereby avoiding a depressed step area. The slightly recessed blade gives a smooth contour at the desired level as only the aspired fat is cut.

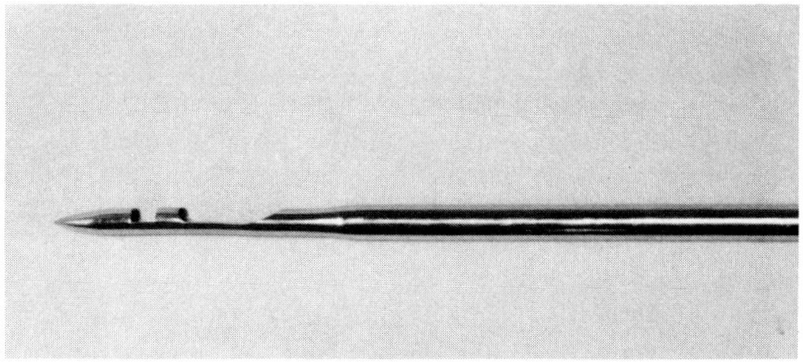

Figure 27-2. The blunt sharkhead tip is essential for achieving a feathered border at the transition from the excess fat area. The slightly recessed blade provides a clean plane without cutting anything but the aspired fat globules.

Indications

Today there is practically no site of the human body contour that has not been recommended for an SAL procedure (Fig. 27-3). Without going into detail on every possibility, as we have done elsewhere [7], we would like to insist on the very important criteria that have to be observed before undertaking an SAL procedure:

1. Is an operation really necessary; i.e., does the patient have really persistent localized adipose tissue excess, or would a diet plus exercise solve the problem?
2. Has the patient a good skin tone and enough skin elasticity to permit a smooth readherence to the new body contour? Already existing laxness or skin sagging is a contraindication.
3. Can this blind procedure be performed in the desired region without being a hazard to important vessels or nerves? We practically never perform this kind of operation in patients who are over 35.

One must always bear in mind that the two critical factors in this type of surgery are the uniformity and smoothness of the operated area and the readhesion of the skin to the new contour. To remove any amount of excessive subcutaneous fat is easy; to make the skin retract is quite another matter—particularly in regions like the upper arms, the inner thighs, and the abdomen in individuals nearing their thirties.

By far the most frequent and in our hands the most satisfactory indication is the local fat excess in the peritrochanteric region in the young woman. This typical feminine fat accumulation can often be observed in otherwise slender girls who despite diet and regular and frequent body exercise do not seem to be able to get rid of the undesired fat.

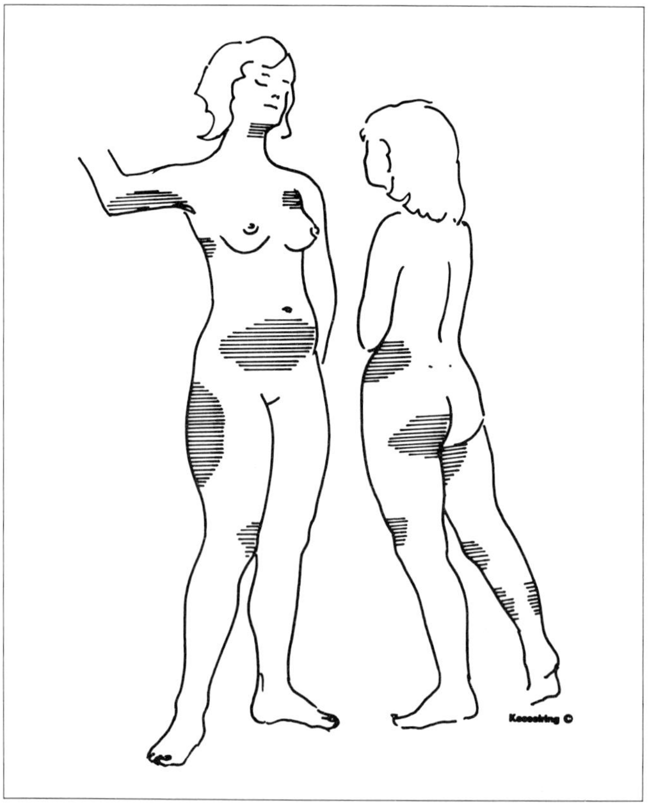

Figure 27-3. The different sites recommended by various authors for an SAL procedure are the submental area, preaxillary region, upper arms, lateral thoracomammary region, abdomen, hips, outer and inner thigh, buttocks, knee region, and calf-ankle region.

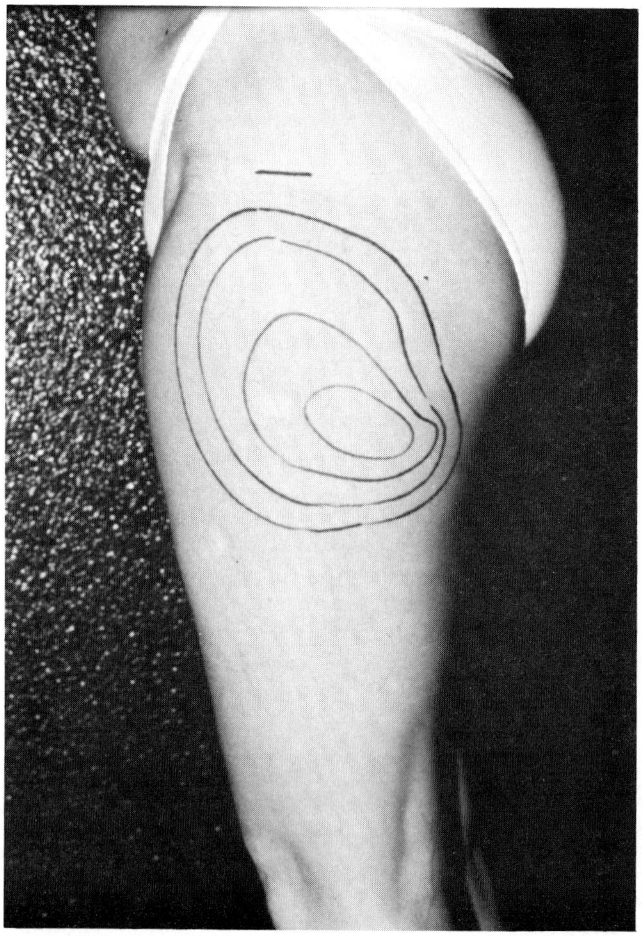

Figure 27-4. The access through a 2-cm incision in the bikini area of the hip is very convenient. The equidistant curves help to localize the maximum amount of fat once the patient is in a horizontal position.

TECHNIQUE

The patient is examined in a standing position and the excessive fat area is marked. We have found it to be most helpful during the operation if the prominence is marked with equidistant curves in order to indicate irregularities and maximum elevation as in a geographic map (Fig. 27-4).

The surgical access can be chosen either in the bikini area of the hip (Fig. 27-4) or in the infragluteal fold (Fig. 27-5). The latter is indicated especially where the fold has to be remodeled or where it is nonexistent.

From the 2-cm incision, we pass the Aspiradeps vertically down to the fascia, without the suction turned on, and create bluntly a plane beneath the marked area. Any other long blunt instrument can be used. Since the plane is relatively avascular, bleeding is minimal (Fig. 27-6).

At this point the aspiration is turned on, the negative pressure being between 0.3 and 0.9 atmospheres, and the whole marked area is planed from the fascia toward the skin, the palm of the left hand being used to control the action as the instrument proceeds. A residual panniculus

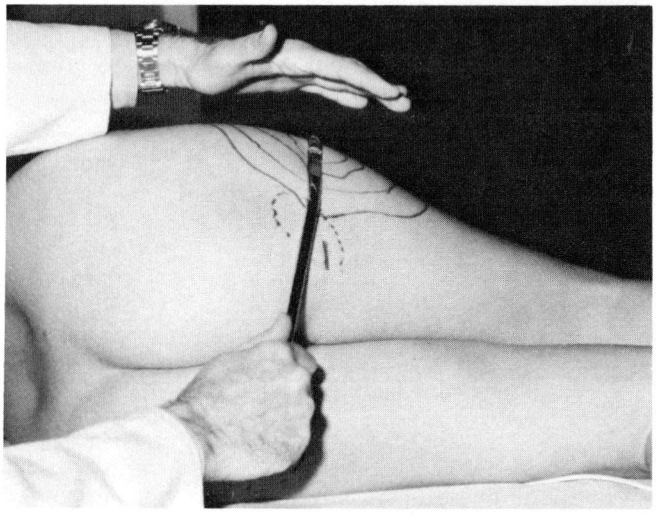

Figure 27-5. For the infragluteal access we use the angulated suction cannula. If the infragluteal crease is to be remodeled, the planing must come right up to the skin.

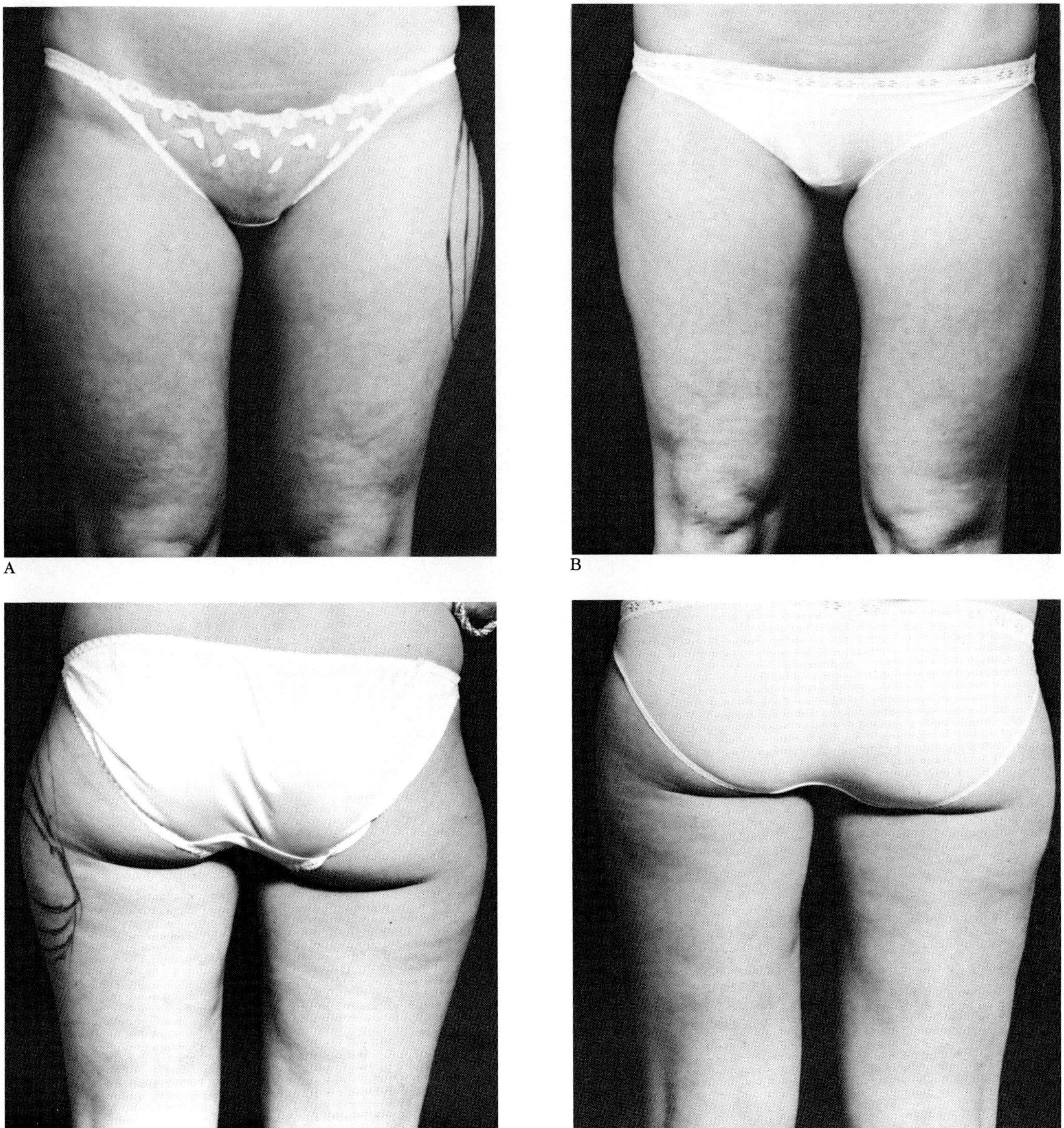

Figure 27-6. Standard hip approach, and result after 3 months.
A, C. Preoperative view.
B, D. Postoperative view.

of 1 cm has to be left beneath the skin. To control the evenness of the procedure we stretch the skin across the outmost circle for 2 cm all around the resection area.

A 5-mm Penrose drain is pulled through a small stab incision at the most caudal point of the cavity, the access incision is closed in two layers, and the thigh is bandaged.

If we choose the infragluteal approach, the maneuvers remain basically the same with two exceptions (Fig. 27-7). If the infragluteal crease has to be remodeled or accentuated, we plane right up to the skin along a previously marked line, leaving no residual panniculus. The Penrose drain is pulled out through the incision.

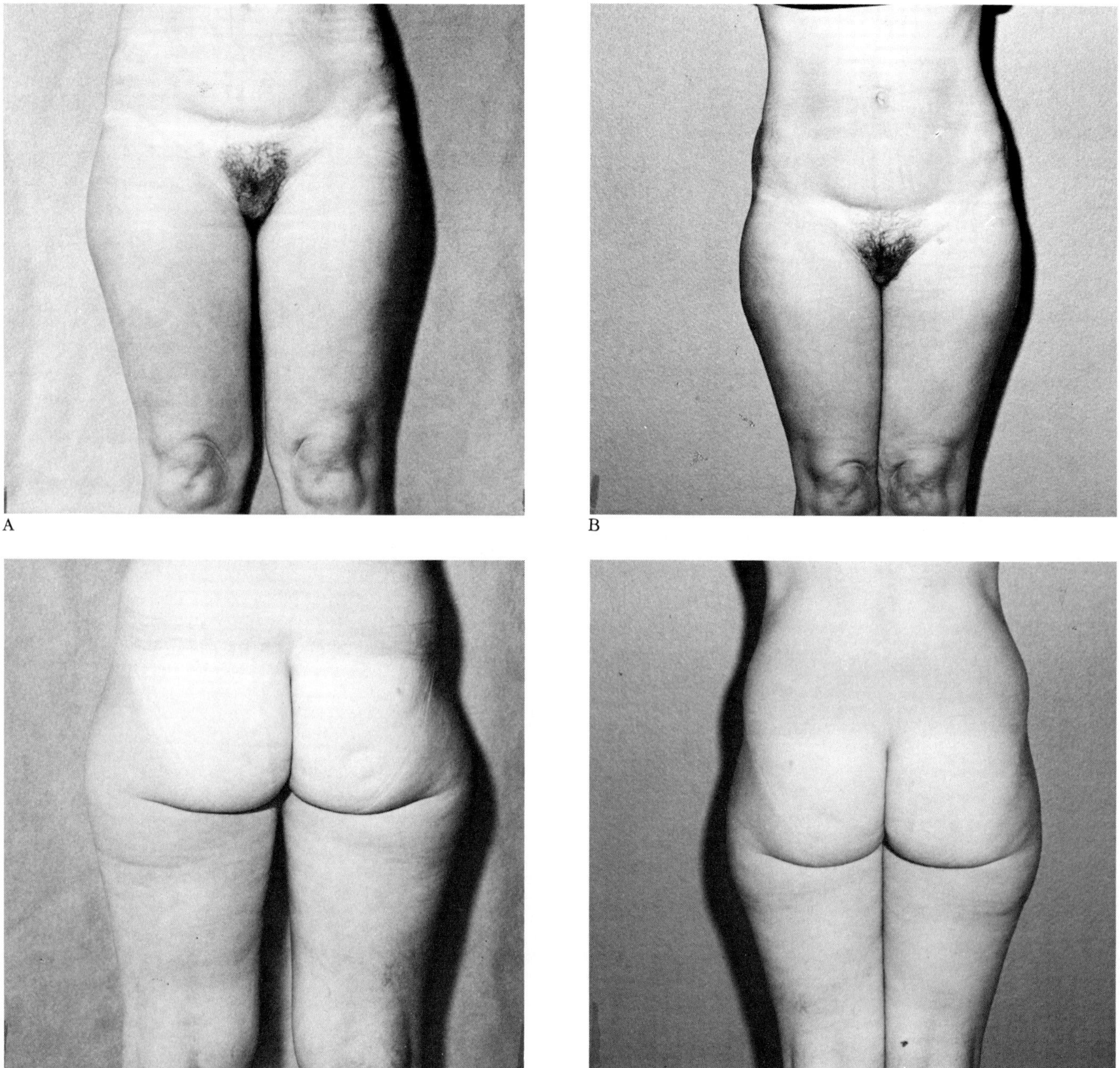

A B C D

Figure 27-7
A, C. Case operated on by infragluteal approach.
B, D. Postoperative view. Note the remodeled infragluteal fold.

POSTOPERATIVE CARE

Correct bandaging is just as important as a good surgical technique. We use two runs of 50% overlapping Elastoplast bandages directly on the skin with no interposed dressing material. The drain is pulled out directly through a cut in the bandage. Thus, it can be removed on the third day without changing the bandage. For the first 24 hours the whole leg is bandaged from the foot upward.

Patients are mobilized and discharged the first postoperative day. The bandages are removed at the earliest 2 weeks later. Professional activity (office work) can be assumed after 3 days. Sports are prohibited for 6 weeks unless the thighs are firmly bandaged during the exercise.

COMPLICATIONS

Although we do not administer antibiotics or anticoagulants, we have not had a significant infection, thrombosis, or embolism thus far. Also substantial blood loss does not occur, and no patient has had to have a transfusion. There was no significant difference between patients operated on under general anesthesia and those operated on with epidural anesthesia. In 87 cases of bilateral peritrochanteric localized fat excess subjected to an SAL procedure by the same surgeon (Kesselring), we found minor irregularities in 23 percent and sufficient irregularities in 20 percent to necessitate minor revisions, which were done under local anesthesia through a 1-cm local incision. Two cases of seroma formation healed without sequelae after puncture and fibrinogen glue instillation.

The only case in which we had a hematoma was a patient who insisted on having her bandages removed 8 hours after the operation, leading to the inevitable blood accumulation and hematoma organization. A secondary operation had to be performed to correct the resulting irregularities.

DISCUSSION

Suction-assisted lipectomy is a very valuable procedure for the elimination of undesired localized fat excess. The indications have to be critical and precise in order to obtain good results with predictable regularity.

The so-called tunneling procedure, lately recommended by Illouz and Fournier, might be of use in the abdomen, where numerous perforating vessels are present. Any bleeding into one or several of the tunnels would be difficult to drain (Fig. 27-8). In the lateral thigh region, it seems improbable that an even surface can be obtained with such a procedure.

The concept that "preserved connective tissue arcades aid in flap contraction and hemostasis" is not proved. We have certainly seen cases in which a "riding breeches deformity" has been transformed into a "saddlebag deformity," a problem due more to poor patient selection than bad surgical technique. It must be remembered that stretched slack skin will never adhere smoothly to a new contour after substantial fat removal, arcades or no arcades. To solve this problem, Meyer [9] proposes the application of fibrinogen glue, and current clinical trials are being evaluated.

We have not found any difference in bleeding between using a suction cannula with unsharpened orifice edges and using the Aspiradeps; avulsion of the fat lobules inevitably implies either tearing or cutting of their vascular pedicle. In either case, spontaneous hemostasis happens rapidly. The planing accuracy seems better with the cutting instrument. We do not recommend the infiltration of any agents preoperatively as this would distort the contour and make assessment difficult.

CONCLUSION

Suction-assisted lipectomy with the Aspiradeps is a valuable procedure for the removal of excessive localized fat mainly in the gluteoperitrochanteric region as well as in the abdominal, hip, and waist region. The application of this technique in other regions of the body will probably remain sporadic. Scrupulous indication, meticulous technique, and constant postoperative care are essential in order to obtain good results.

Figure 27-8
A, B. With good technique, postoperative compression and drainage, the layer resection does not produce seroma or readhesion. It seems to us the only means of creating a smooth fat removal that can be evaluated at the end of surgery. Creating multiple tunnels to allow structural collapse remains hypothetical.

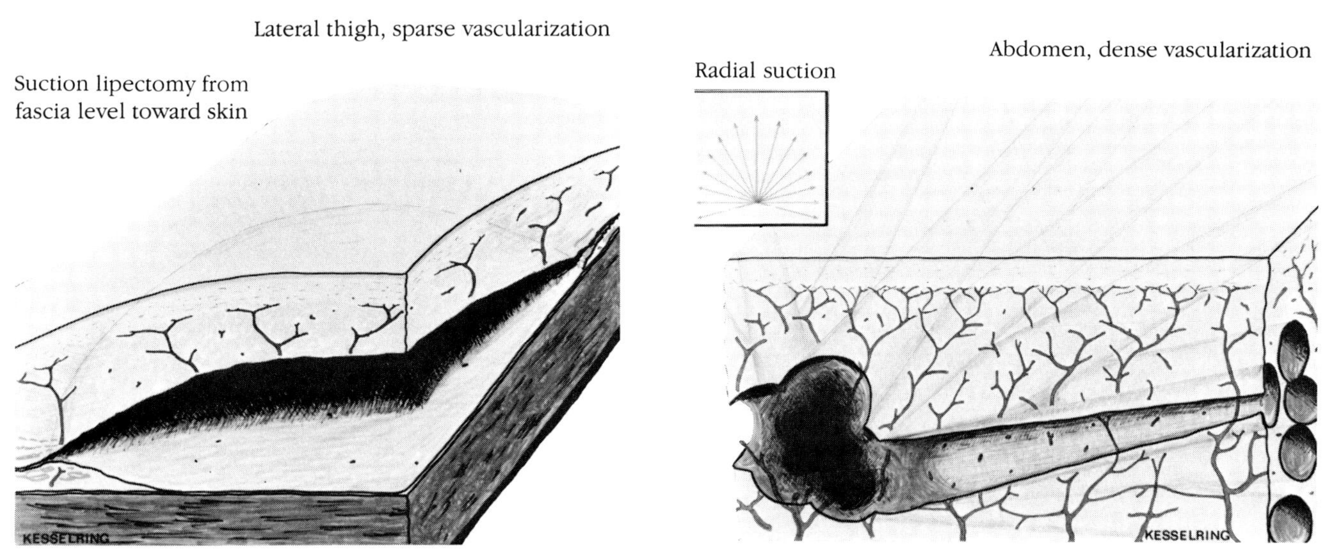

A. The layer technique

B. The tunneling technique

Collapsing Surgery and Body Sculpturing

Pierre F. Fournier
Yves-Gerard Illouz

In the early days of aesthetic plastic surgery, dermolipectomy was the only treatment for body sculpturing. It is a major surgical procedure with a morbidity that is not negligible. It results in a long scar of average to poor quality with occasional bulging above and below. More recently, closed techniques have been described. The uterine curet was first used. However, most of the practitioners quit because the results were disappointing. Then, in 1976 Arpad and George Fischer of Rome used a powerful suction machine connected with an electric cutting instrument, the Cellusactiotome. Next, a plane was made over the adiposity with another instrument, the planotome. The procedure was more or less modified later by different surgeons but differs very little from the original Fischer technique. These techniques have a wrong concept. A plane is created and then a cavity in one block. A sharp instrument is used. The procedure extensively damages the adipose tissue and can produce many complications, bleeding, hematoma, and lymphatic drainage. Normal healing may take a long time. The undesirable aesthetic results include skin irregularities and sagging of excess skin. These sharp techniques have had limited indications, except for trochanteric adiposities.

In 1977 a very different procedure was developed by Yves-Gerard Illouz, both in concept and in instruments used. It is a simple procedure, with minimal trauma for the adipose tissue, being both reliable and applicable to all body areas [4–6]. The idea is to leave as many connections between the deep fascia and the skin as possible, thereby avoiding damage to the blood and lymph vessels as well as sensory nerves [2, 3]. The main principles are as follows:

1. Only blunt instruments are used: blunt cannulas or lipodissectors, hollow or solid with blunt openings (Fig. 27-9).
2. "Tunnels" are created at different levels of the adiposity. To this end, to-and-fro movements (10–15) have to be made in each tunnel while the suction machine is working. A partial or "honeycombed lipectomy" is thus performed (Fig. 27-10). The lipodissector should never be used as a sickle or as a windshield wiper as this maneuver creates a wide plane of dissection or a cavity. It would therefore become the equivalent of the sharp technique with its attendant complications.
3. Minimal trauma ensues. In some cases, injecting a hypotonic solution at the beginning of the operation will help.
4. The dissection must be done in a plane deep to the adiposity. One or two centimeters of fat are left below the skin as it contains lymphatic vessels that are necessary for good tonicity and trophicity of the skin. Surface defects are also thus avoided.
5. The opening of the cannula should always be oriented downward; landmark on the handle of the cannula.
6. The incision should be distant from the adiposity for these reasons: to be concealed, to avoid scar contraction, and to create the tunnels more easily.
7. One has to use and not fight against skin contraction, a maneuver that is the reverse of what is required in most cases. After a honeycombed lipectomy, the fibrous tissue will shrink evenly and harmoniously if a deep and even resection was done.

Figure 27-9. Cannula or lipodissector. This instrument exists in different sizes and diameters. Lipodissectors are hollow or solid, straight or curved (Concorde shaped).

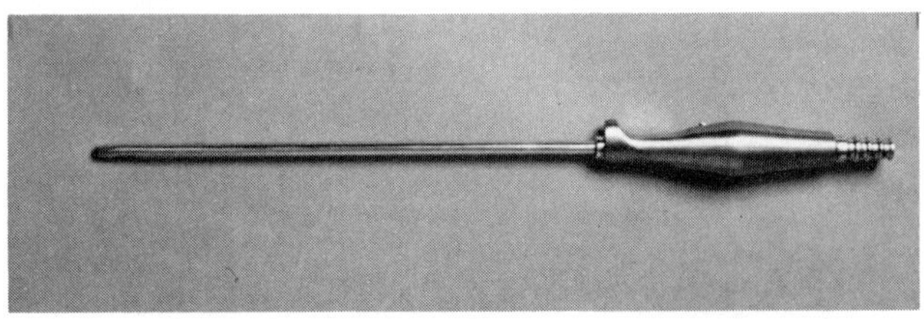

Figure 27-10. Principles of the procedure. A deep honeycombed lipectomy and a peripheral mesh (discontinuous) undermining is made (left) rather than a block lipectomy and a continuous undermining (right).

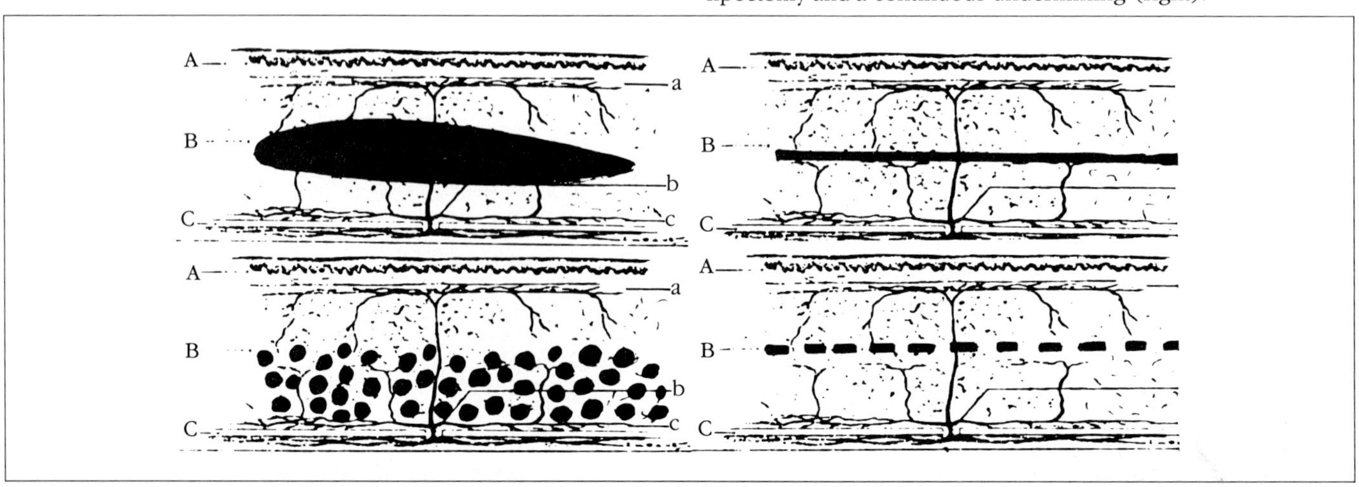

8. Not too much fat should be removed—somewhere between 100 and 150 cc, but no more.

These principles are essential for understanding the procedure's indications and contraindications. The authors have an experience of about 2000 patients, many with multiple indications.

INDICATIONS AND CONTRAINDICATIONS

All adiposities of the body surface can be treated. Several areas can be treated during the same session. The best cases are congenital lipodystrophies of the young female patient who has had previously unsuccessful medical or dietary treatment. That is to say, the ideal patients are those who would be rejected for a conventional dermolipectomy. Other cases, such as average or important adiposities, will be operated on according to the tonicity of the skin and could be treated if necessary in two or three stages. Certain patients will prefer to have skin irregularities or excess skin resulting from a minor procedure rather than undergo the alternative dermolipectomy with its long scar of poor quality and its major surgical characteristics. Male patients are good candidates because of their firm skin tonicity. Also, certain lipodystrophies are amenable, including lipomas, Dercum's disease, and Launois-Bensaude disease. We have obtained excellent results with these patients.

Generalized obesity is a contraindication. Obese patients are not good candidates, but they are treated in some clinics in several stages. A very large adiposity or a flabby skin is also a contraindication. A dermolipectomy should be done alone or combined with a liposuction.

PATIENT SELECTION

A very careful screening is essential. The ideal case is a young patient with firm skin and a limited regional adiposity. However, with experience, the surgeon who follows the principles of the technique—deep and even work, not too much removal, and peripheral mesh undermining—can benefit mature and older patients.

PATHOPHYSIOLOGY AND CLASSIFICATION

The adipocyte theory presumes that we are born with a fixed number of fat cells and only these cells are able to load fat. The adipocytes multiply and develop until puberty, but after puberty the number remains fixed. Thus, dietary restriction acts on the adipocytes to decrease their volume, but resumption of excess dietary intake increases cell volume rapidly. From experience with dermolipectomy patients, it was evident that subsequent weight gain was seen in other body regions but little in the operated area. Obviously, the number of adipocytes in this region had been excised. Similarly, after a liposuction, the results should be permanent in the treated part. Many cases of pregnancies have been observed after a liposuction and the operated areas were not significantly modified.

All parts of the body surface can be treated: trochanteric lipodystrophies, waist, buttocks (a new gluteal fold can be created), anterior and inner parts of the thighs, knees (medial and anterior parts), ankles, abdomen, false gynecomastia, arms (circumferential or posterior lipectomy), double chin, and cheeks in face-lifting (under direct vision).

SURGICAL TECHNIQUE

The adipose tissue in excess will be vacuumed out with a cannula connected to a powerful suction machine, following the aforementioned principles. A hypotonic solution will be used (wet technique). The solution, containing normal saline (100 ml), distilled water (20 ml), and hyaluronidase (100–1000 units according to firmness of the fat), is injected in combination with a local anesthetic. The amount varies according to the size of the adiposity—from 30 ml for a double chin to 80 ml for an average trochanteric lipodystrophy. No solution is used during the dry technique, which has a few advantages: time saved, less distortion of the tissues than after infiltration, and more exact evaluation of the fat removed. The adiposities are marked carefully with the patient in the standard position (Fig. 27-11). The adiposity is marked first. Then another marking is made 1.5 to 2.0 cm beyond the first one, and still another 8 to 10 cm outward for the peripheral mesh dissection. An estimation of the amount of adipose tissue should be made beforehand, and this is a matter of judgment and experience.

The anesthesia varies from local to regional block, or even general with or without intubation, prone or supine according to the adiposity to be treated and the surgeon's preference.

Incision

A 1-cm or less incision is made for introduction of the cannula some distance from the fat deposit to be treated. The cannula must be in intimate contact with the skin edge to create the required suction.

For trochanteric adiposities, buttocks, and hips the incision is placed in either the gluteal fold or the supratrochanteric area. For medial adiposities of the knees, it is in the inner part of the popliteal region. For the ankles, it is medial to the Achilles tendon. For the abdomen, it is either suprapubic or inside the umbilicus. For the arm, the axilla or near the elbow is commonly employed. For a double chin, the incision is lateral to the adiposity, in a fold or in the submental crease.

Dissection

The dissection is fan shaped from the incision and honeycombed (Fig. 27-12). One makes to-and-fro movements

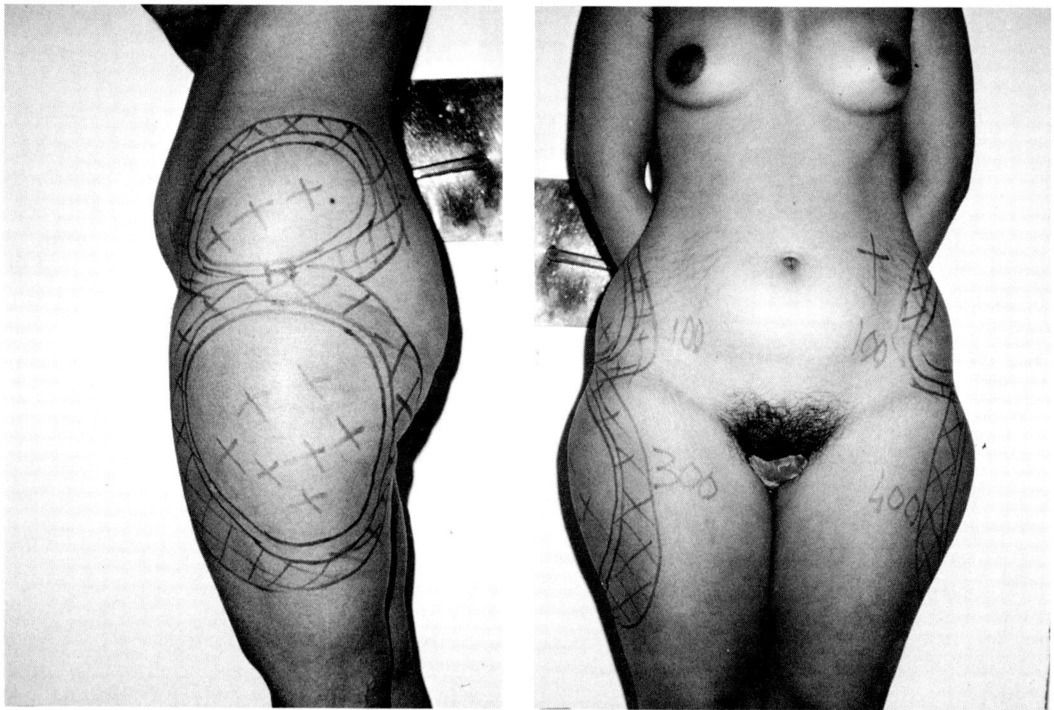

A B

Figure 27-11

A, B. The markings have to be done in the standing position, as does preestimation of the amount of adipose tissue to be removed (central area) and extent of peripheral mesh undermining (circular cross-hatching).

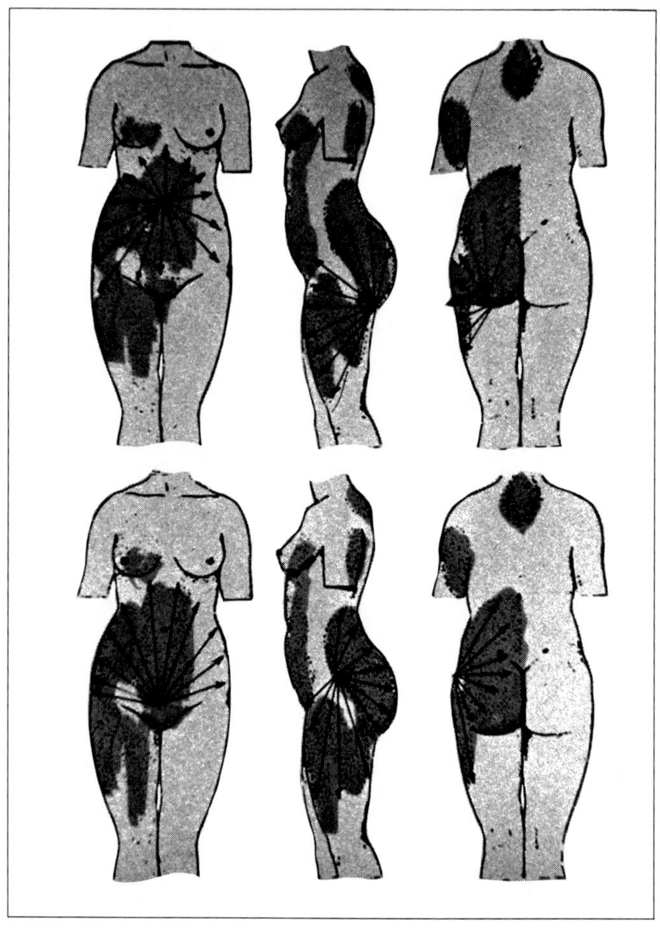

Figure 27-12. The dissection for the lipectomy is fan shaped from the site of the incision.

(10–15 in each tunnel). More tunnels are created at the higher level of the adiposity. The suction machine begins to work as soon as the first to-and-fro movement starts (Fig. 27-13A). The surgeon is in effect sucking out the fat while leaving undamaged vessels between the tunnels. These septa or columns of fat make the area more homogeneous and connect the deep and superficial planes. They also help in the resorption of the blood and lymph following the procedure.

Periodically, the suction is stopped to check the fluid in the tube. If excessive blood is seen, one switches sites and dissects elsewhere. The contents of the jar as well as the tube should be observed. The opening of the cannula is always turned downward except when a new gluteal fold is being created. The left hand should fold the skin to obtain a deep dissection, and one must be conscious that as in any reduction surgery the most important factor is not how much fat is removed but how much fat is left behind as well as its distribution.

After the honeycombed lipectomy is performed, a solid lipodissector is used to do a wide peripheral mesh undermining around the central resection (Fig. 27-13B). The fibrous bands tethering the skin to the deep fascia are ruptured. This maneuver facilitates easier contraction of excess skin. Skin irregularities are usually not observed after the operation. Occasionally they may be present, especially after trochanteric lipodystrophy, but they are far less significant than the preoperative deformity. If necessary, a counterincision can be made to do an effective mobilization of the peripheral skin (Fig. 27-14). Again, the lipodissector should not be used as a windshield wiper. Drainage is not done routinely. Only average or large adiposities are drained, although drainage is used if bleeding is persistent. We use a suction drain (Hemovac), removed after 1 or 2 days.

Figure 27-13
A. The cannula is connected to a powerful suction machine, which removes the adipose tissue.
B. The dissection for the peripheral mesh undermining is done with a straight or curved solid lipodissector.

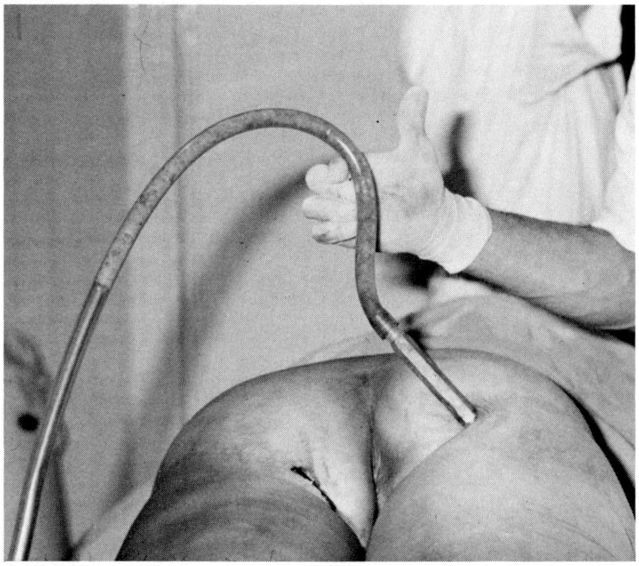

A

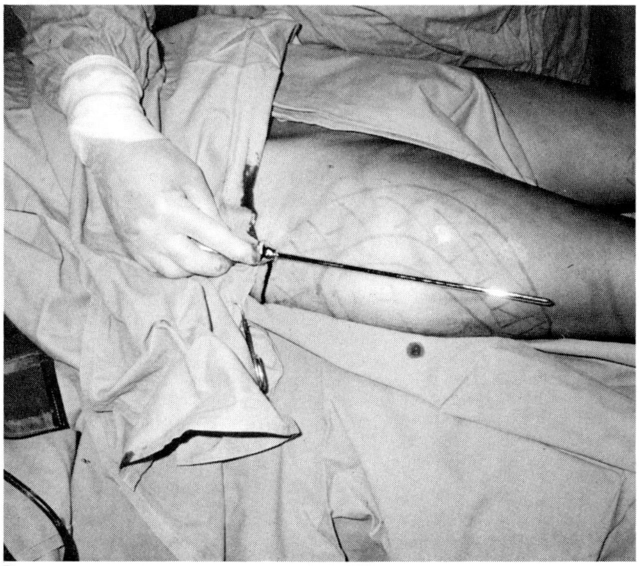

B

Dressing

The dressing is very important and should be done by the surgeon himself as in a rhinoplasty. Nonallergenic Elastoplast is used. The skin has to be redraped evenly. In trochanteric lipodystrophy, the skin is lifted first and the gluteal fold marked. The dressing acts as a splint and is removed after 1 week (Fig. 27-15). When the skin has been evenly redraped, the underlying honeycombed fat will also have been correctly positioned and will heal in the desired shape. The patient remains 2 days in hospital for large adiposities or when general anesthesia has been used. Edema, bruising, and dysesthesias are part of the operation and fade away in 2 to 3 weeks. Normal contour is obtained after 2 to 3 months (Figs. 27-16 and 27-17).

Figure 27-14. When necessary, a counterincision is made in a proper place to obtain a good result.

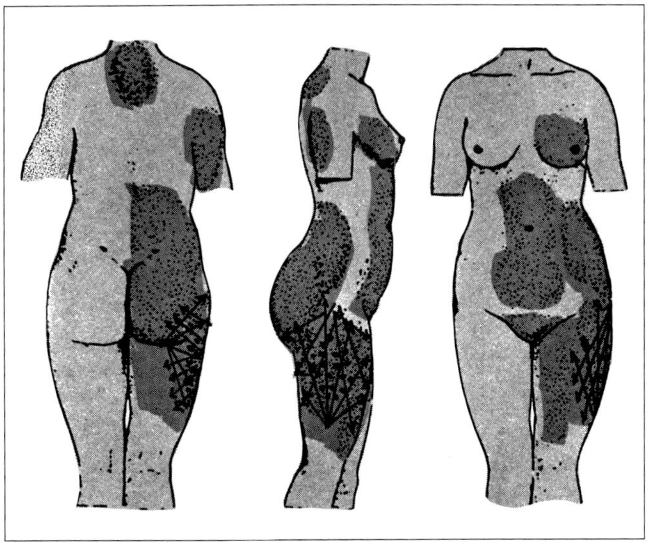

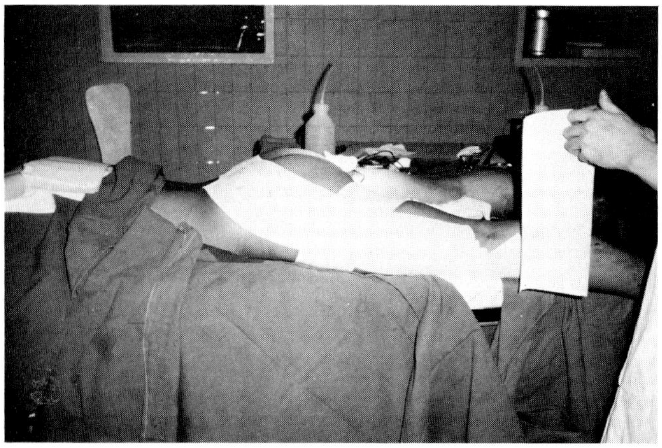

Figure 27-15. The dressing has to be an external splint after the skin has been redraped and molded. For a trochanteric lipodystrophy the skin has also to be lifted and the gluteal fold marked.

COMPLICATIONS

When the procedure is correctly performed, infection, hemorrhage, hematomas, seromas, and lymphatic drainage are not seen. Pain and discomfort are seldom encountered. Moderate inflammation does occur. Bulgings and depressions may be seen but fade away in 2 to 3 months. Most of the complications are of an aesthetic nature. Permanent bulgings and depressions are the hallmark of the untrained surgeon in this kind of technique. Asymmetric results may be noted in paired adiposities. Skin excess (checkerboardlike) or sagging of skin may be observed in patients over 35 years of age or after treatment of large adiposities or when no peripheral mesh undermining has been performed. No treatment of skin irregularities should be done before 6 months as they may diminish during this time. A touch-up is done with a small cannula (No. 6) on the bulging and a crisscross subcutaneous undermining. If the skin excess is large, a conventional dermolipectomy should be performed.

A fall in blood pressure and shock are possible in case of hasty or large resection of fat, especially when one is using the dry technique. The anesthesiologist should give fluids, plasma, or blood during the procedure and guide the surgeon according to the patient's condition.

Most complications are avoided by careful patient selection, deep and even work, wide peripheral mesh undermining, and good repositioning of the skin.

Figure 27-16
A, B. Trochanteric lipodystrophy—hips, buttocks, and gluteal fold; 600 cc removed on each side. One week after the operation.

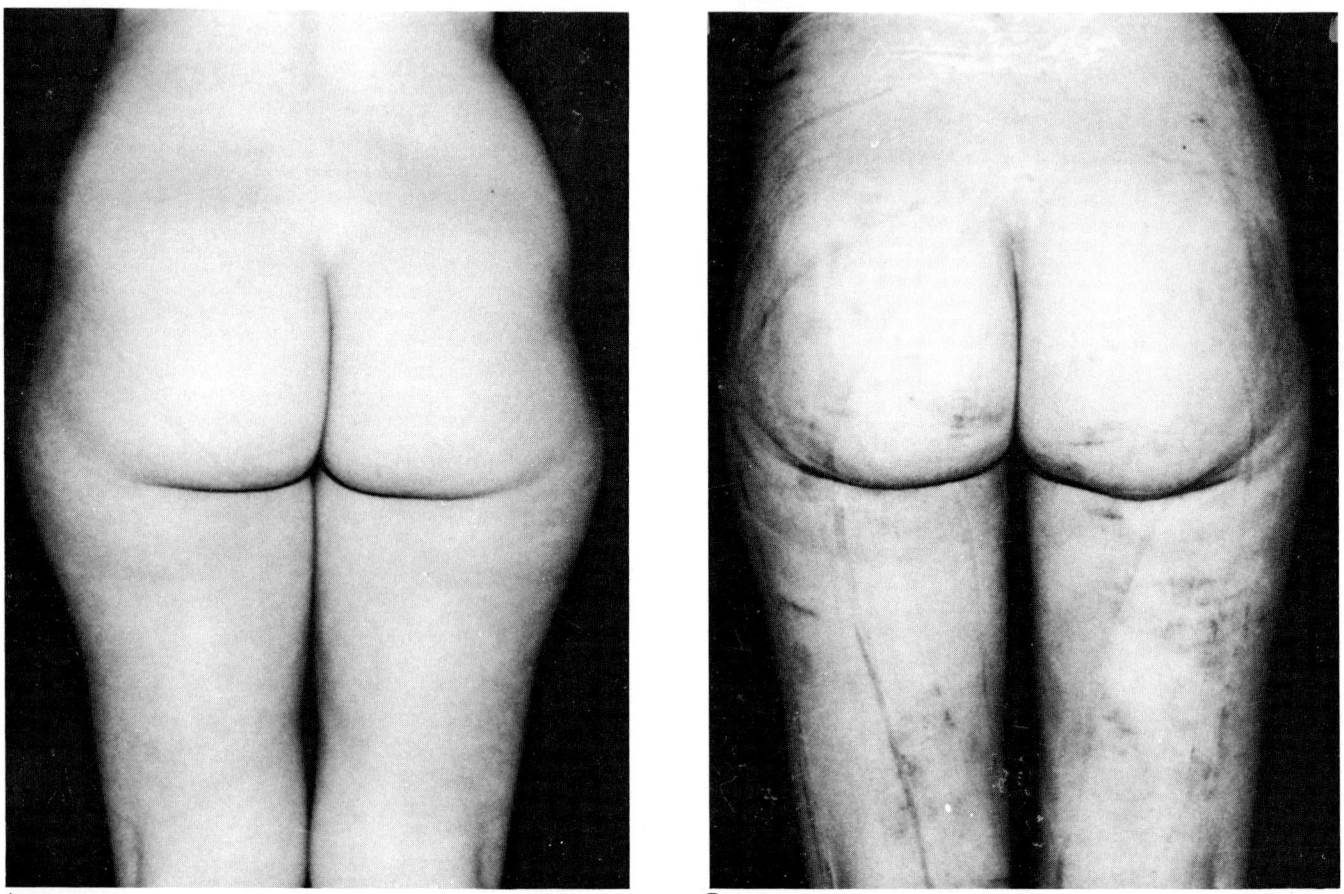

A B

DISADVANTAGES

This technique cannot be applied alone to large lipodystrophies with skin excess; a dermolipectomy should be done in those cases. However, it can be combined with a conventional dermolipectomy to obtain a better result as neighboring adiposities can be treated at the same time. In case of trochanteric lipodystrophy, after age 35 or when the quality of the skin is poor, skin irregularities have to be feared but can be avoided or decreased by a wide peripheral mesh undermining. For a few patients over 35, skin irregularities are preferred to a long, wide scar. Alternatively, a major operation can always be performed later if requested. With experience, mature or older patients can be treated satisfactorily, and in case of large adiposity a two- or three-stage procedure can be done.

ADVANTAGES

All parts of the body surface can be treated, as previously described. Circular fat removal is possible in the arm and the thigh with satisfactory results. The procedure is a simple closed one, and a normal life may be resumed shortly after the operation. It can be used as a "waiting procedure" in a diabetic patient or in a patient who wants another pregnancy in the near future. In such a case it would be hazardous or useless to perform an abdominoplasty. The operation can be used in combination with other procedures.

Defatting of the abdominal wall before an abdominoplasty can make surgery easier. The scar will be shorter as dog-ears are avoided. During all procedures, neighboring adiposities may be treated including hips during an abdominoplasty or axillary folds during a breast reduction. A tube flap can be defatted safely without risk of necrosis. In general surgery, the technique can be used to defat the operating area preoperatively if necessary—the abdomen before a gynecologic procedure or the knees or hips before orthopedic surgery. False genu valgum has already been successfully treated. However, the main advantage of this procedure is its permanent result. Recurrence has never been observed. Many patients have had pregnancies after the operation, and no relapses have been seen in the treated area, thus confirming the adipocyte theory. All these advantages led us to use this procedure as often as possible and to perform conventional dermolipectomy only in very large lipodystrophies.

SUMMARY

The technique of lipodissection as described by Illouz represents a major advance in the treatment of localized

Figure 27-17
A, B. Abdominal lipectomy and waist; 300 cc removed. One month after the operation.

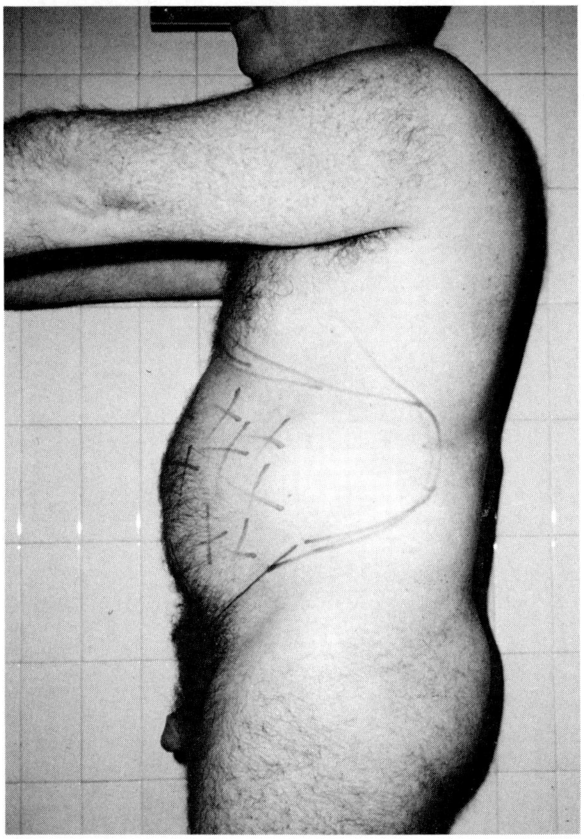

A

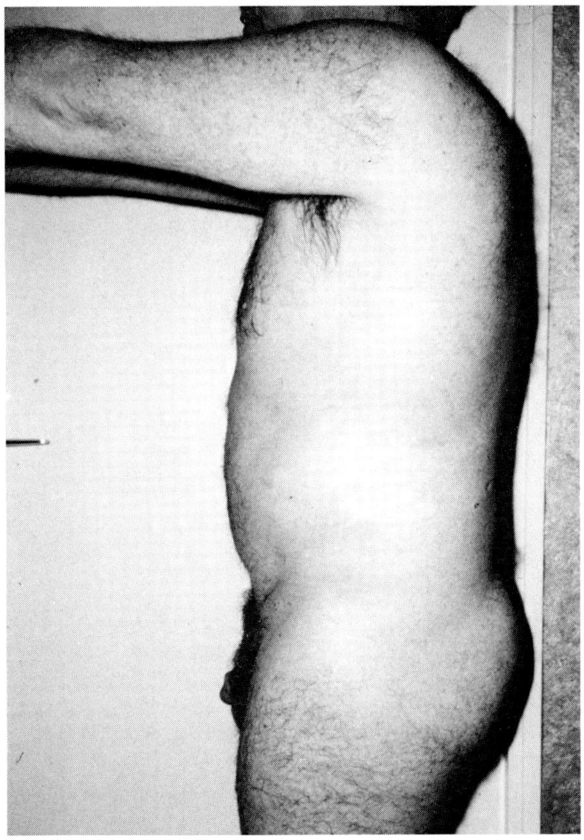

B

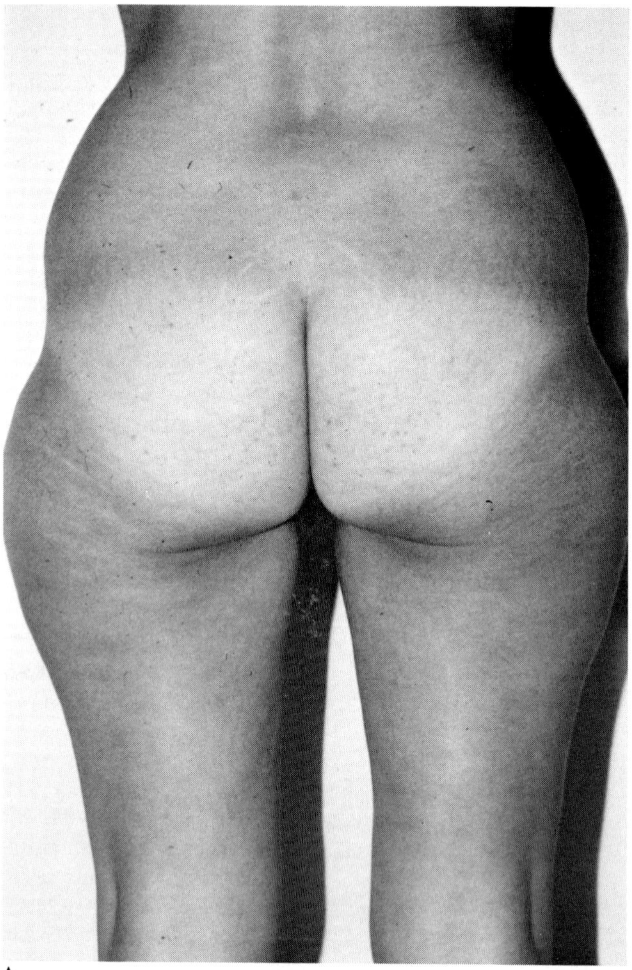

A

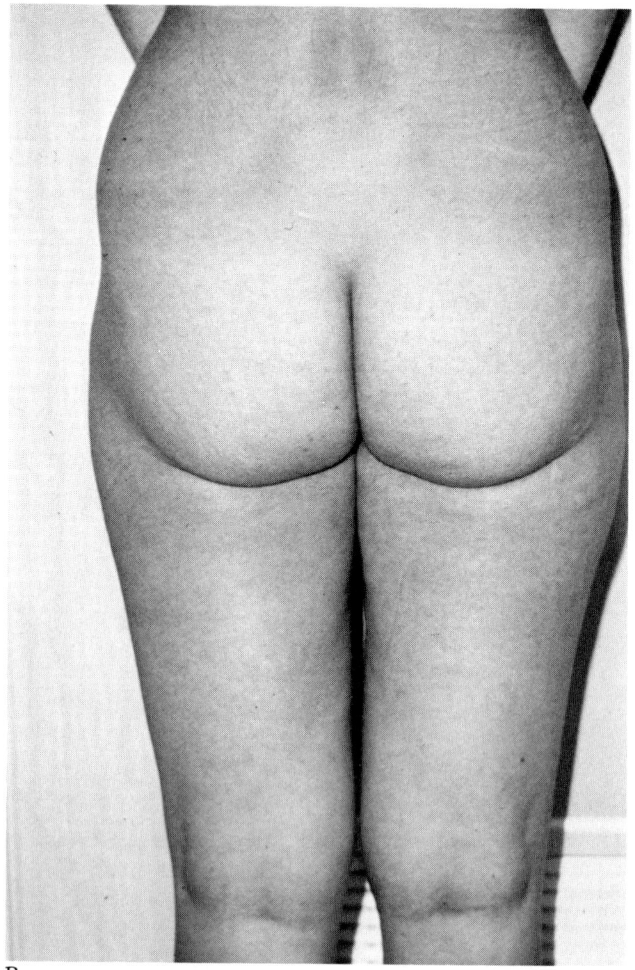

B

Figure 27-18
A. Patient with classic riding breeches deformity.
B. Result at 1 year following suction curettage.

adiposities. But it is not a panacea, and a careful screening of the patients is necessary if good results are to be obtained.

Since it is a real sculpture in vivo of the adipose tissue, the results improve with experience. This technique of honeycombed lipectomy with peripheral mesh dissection is far more reliable than the other technique of section curettage, with which it is often confused.

REFERENCES

1. Courtiss, E. Suction lipectomy: A retrospective analysis of 100 patients. *Plast. Reconstr. Surg.* 73:780, 1984.
2. Fournier, P. F., and Otteni, F. Traitement des Lipodystrophies Localisées par Aspiration. La Technique Seche. In S. A. Maloine (ed.), *Chirurgie Esthétique, 1981–1982.* Paris: Maloine, 1982. Pp. 59–78.
3. Fournier, P. F., and Otteni, F. M. Lipodissection in body sculpturing: The dry procedure. *Plast. Reconstr. Surg.* 72:598, 1983.
4. Illouz, Y.-G. Une nouvelle technique pour les lipodystrophies localisées. *Rev. Chir. Esthétique Langue Française* 6:3, 1980.
5. Illouz, Y.-G. Réflexions après 4 ans et demi d'expérience et 800 cas de ma technique de lipolyse. *Rev. Chir. Esthétique Langue Française* 6:9, 1981.
6. Illouz, Y.-G. Body contouring by lipolysis: A 5-year experience with over 3000 cases. *Plast. Reconstr. Surg.* 72:591, 1983.
7. Kesselring, U. K. Regional fat aspiration for body contouring. *Plast. Reconstr. Surg.* 72:610, 1983.
8. Kesselring, U. K., and Meyer, R. A suction curette for removal of excessive local deposits of subcutaneous fat. *Plast. Reconstr. Surg.* 62:305, 1978.
9. Meyer, R. Personal communication, 1982.
10. Schrudde, J. Lipexeresis in the Correction of Local Adiposity. Meeting of the International Society of Plastic Surgery, Rio de Janeiro, 1972.
11. Teimourian, B. Face and neck suction-assisted lipectomy associated with rhytidectomy. *Plast. Reconstr. Surg.* 72:627, 1983.

28. Upper Extremity

Paule Regnault
Rollin K. Daniel

Brachioplasty is a surgical procedure for reducing arm circumference and tissue redundancy. It corrects a significant source of embarrassment but leaves permanent scars. Surgical techniques have evolved from an elliptic excision to a more refined fishtail incision that is extended toward the elbow as required. Although the operation is conceptually simple, major complications can occur for the unwary. The present chapter discusses aesthetic procedures while modifications for the massive-weight-loss patient are discussed in the next chapter.

HISTORY

In the 1920s pioneering surgeons performed localized elliptic excisions of redundant arm tissues as an ancillary procedure for obese patients [16]. In 1973 Lewis [8] modernized the operation by combining a large excision with a proximal Z-plasty in the axilla to avoid scar contracture. For patients whose arm deformities continued into axillary webbing and thoracic folds, Pitanguy [11–13] extended the incision onto the thorax and into the inframammary fold. Baroudi [1] and Guerrero-Santos [5, 6] have reviewed the potential complications of brachioplasty. Recently, Regnault [14, 15] introduced a fishtail excision that permits definitive correction of more proximal deformities.

PATHOPHYSIOLOGY AND CLASSIFICATION

The youthful arm is considered an object of beauty and gracefulness throughout our culture. With advancing age, ptosis and wrinkling may cause severe embarrassment. As reviewed by Glanz and Gonzalez-Ulloa [3], aging results in loss of adipose tissue and stretching of the anchoring septa, producing a dramatic descent and flaccidity of the posterior arm. The ratio of the superior to the inferior arm segment is known as the coefficient of Hoyer, the inferior border of the medial humerus serving as the reference point. These authors found that the ratio was 1:1 in a 10-year-old child, but by age 70 had increased to 1.0:2.2 (Fig. 28-1). In thin individuals the basic deformity may be "crepiness" or wrinkling of the skin. For normal-weight patients, the primary concern is flaccidity and descent of the posterior border. In massive-weight-loss patients, the problem is redundancy and ptosis, which create a heavy hanging arm. Occasionally, obese patients will request debulking of tense fat arms. The severity of these conditions tends to evolve in a proximal to distal direction from axilla to elbow. Thus, it is possible to classify arm deformities as to their location: (1) *minor,* proximal third, (2)

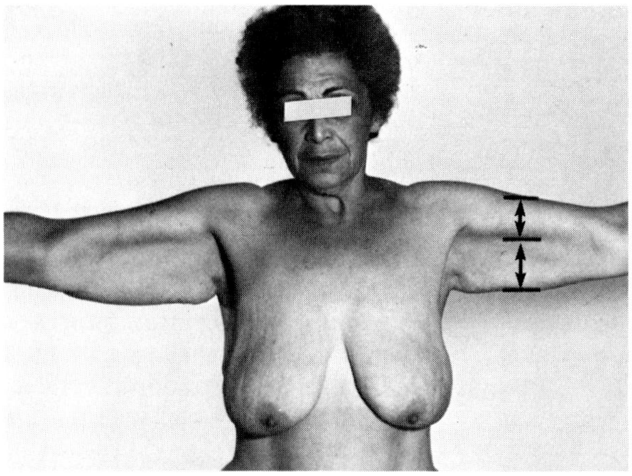

Figure 28-1. An older individual with flaccidity of the entire arm and a 1 : 3 coefficient of Hoyer on the right arm.

moderate, proximal and middle third, and (3) *major,* entire arm (Fig. 28-2). Surgically, the procedure is extended distally to remove the excess and may even eliminate bulging above the elbow.

CONSULTATION

Indications and Contraindications

Brachioplasty is indicated only for the highly motivated patient with a significant deformity. The procedure is excellent for eliminating excessive redundancy, especially if leisure-time activities are limited. If visible permanent scars are not acceptable to the patient, surgery should not be done. Some modification in dress is mandatory, i.e., no sleeveless dresses or halter tops. Active axillary hidradenitis is a contraindication to surgery. Brachioplasty is not done in postmastectomy patients and obese individuals with heavy thick arms. This latter group may be candidates for suction lipectomy.

Medical History

A detailed medical history is taken with emphasis on the upper extremity and torso. Specifically, one must inquire as to previous surgery, trauma, edema, breast diseases, axillary infections, and weight changes.

Motivation

Since acceptability of the final scars requires a *highly motivated* patient, one must determine why the patient wants the surgery and what results are expected. Also, one

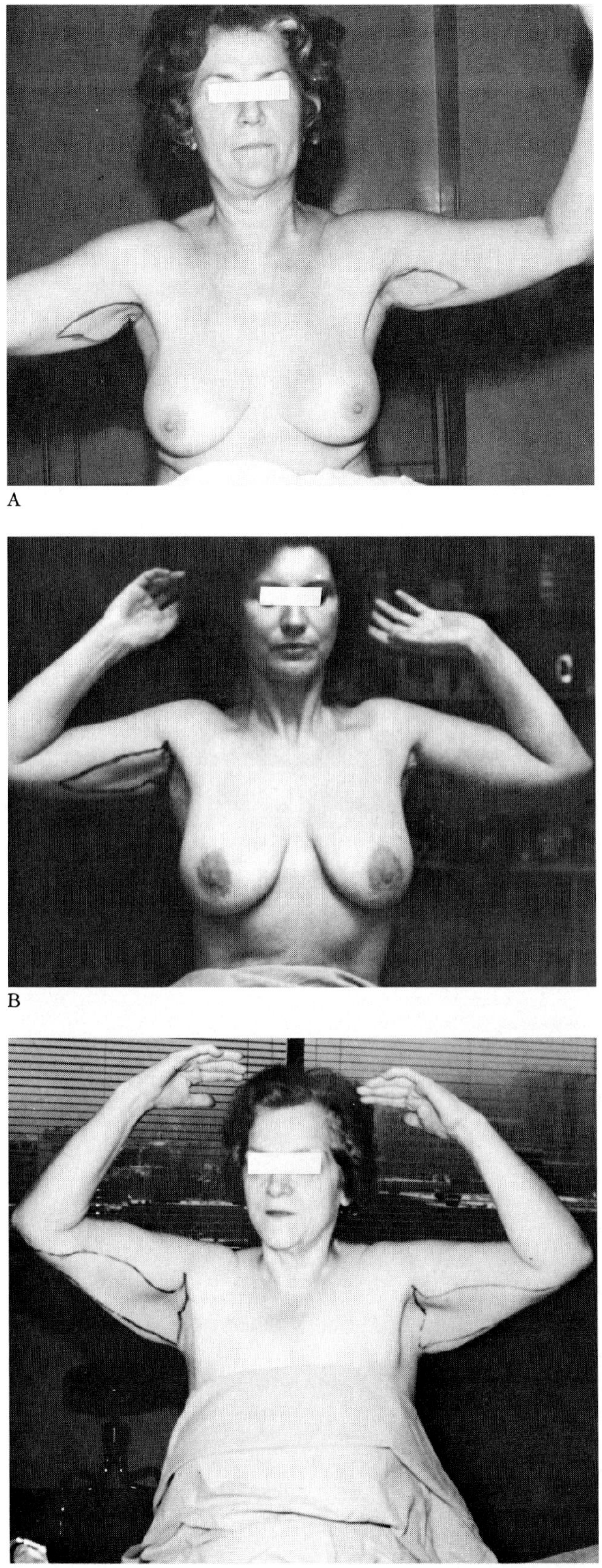

A

B

C

Figure 28-2. Classification of upper extremity deformities based on their location and requisite surgical technique.
A. Minor, proximal one-third.
B. Moderate, proximal and middle third. Note left arm was corrected 1 month previously.
C. Major, entire arm.

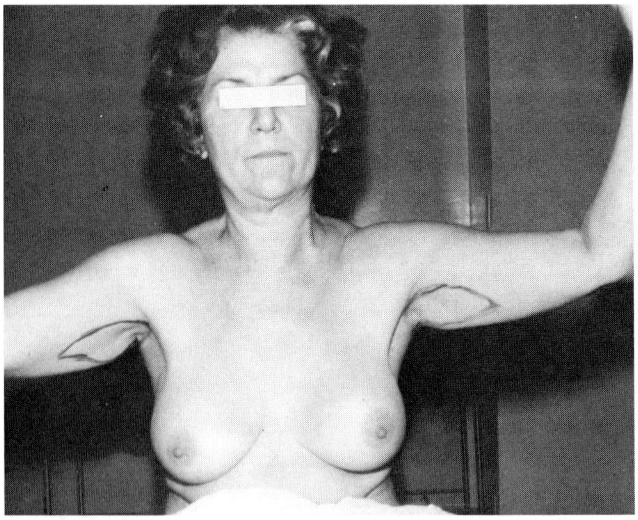

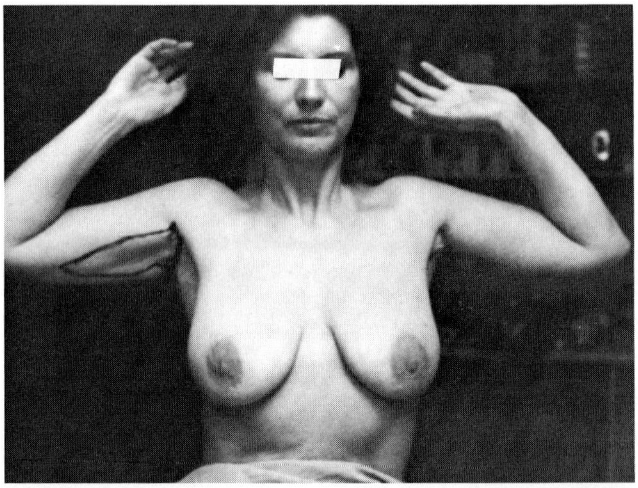

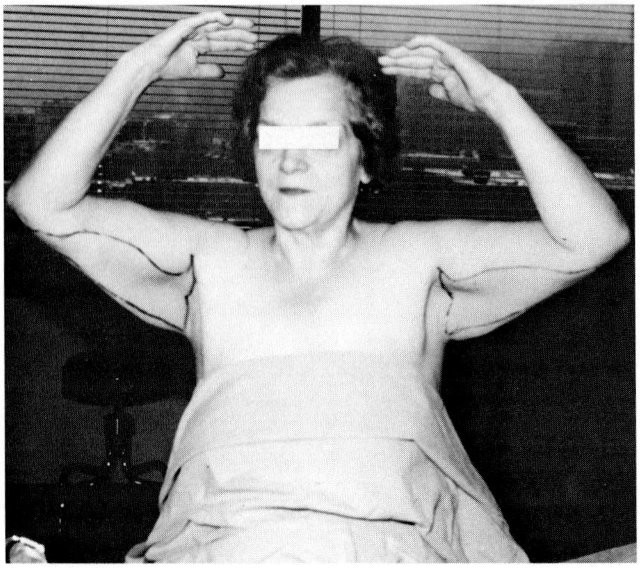

should determine whether the deformity is a personal dislike or a social embarrassment. When is it a problem? What is the routine and maximum degree of arm exposure? There is a great difference between the expectations of the older matron tennis player and those of the middle-aged moderately obese waitress. The former wants a perfect result with minimal scars on maximum exposure whereas the latter can cover the inevitable scars with sleeves of modest length.

Physical Examination

The patient should be examined nude from the waist up to facilitate exposure of the arms and the axillary continuation onto the trunk. The arms are abducted and the elbows flexed. The medial brachial sulcus is palpated and the location of the redundancy evaluated. Essentially, one must classify the type of deformity (redundancy or lipodystrophy), its severity (minor, moderate, or major), and the ease of surgical correction. Although one is able to pinch excess skin, one must determine the amount of resectable redundancy by rotating the inferior skin upward to the medial sulcus. Next, the entire extremity is examined for the presence of edema or previous trauma, and the axilla is checked for lymphadenopathy or acute infection. Finally, the patient is asked to show what is specifically disliked and what results are expected. At this point one should explain the surgical limitations and draw the anticipated scar on the patient's arm.

Aesthetic Goals

After the patient dresses, one should review the patient's complaint and deformity plus the proposed surgical technique. The objective is always tightening of the skin and excision of redundant soft tissues. In virtually every instance, the patient will express disappointment that the procedure leaves visible scars. Thus, a second consultation is often suggested. In contrast to the lower extremity, the surgeon must realize that skin redundancy is the primary problem and that volume alone is rarely the complaint. Thus, liposuction will serve as a useful adjunct, limiting the surgical excision, but will be the primary treatment modality in only those patients with firm, tense arms.

Informed Consent

It must be repeatedly emphasized to the patient that the deformity can be minimized but not completely eliminated, and that permanent scars will result. The expected sequence of wound healing is reviewed: an initial fine incision line, inflammation (the first month), hypertrophic scarring characterized by elevation and redness (3–9 months), and subsequent resolution to a white 5- to 10-mm-wide permanent scar (1 year). Also, minor scar revisions or contour corrections may be necessary, but not before 1 year. The routine complications of hematoma, edema, and minor skin slough should be noted as well as the anesthetic risks.

Patient Instructions

The patient is instructed to shower and scrub the axillae with pHisoHex for 2 days prior to surgery. Preparations should be made for limited arm movements postoperatively—no driving or heavy housecleaning. The axillae are showered the evening prior to surgery, and all medications for sleep and pain are taken as directed, including antibiotics. The patient is allowed to use the arms moderately at 1 week postoperatively and vigorously at 4 weeks (athletics).

ANATOMY

The upper extremity is composed of the axilla, arm, elbow, forearm, wrist, and hand. The axilla is bounded by an anterior fold (pectoralis major and minor muscles) and a posterior fold (subscapular, latissimus dorsi, and teres major muscles), which enclose its medial wall (ribs and serratus anterior muscle) and its lateral extension (biceps and coracobrachialis muscles). The skin and subcutaneous fat contain numerous hair follicles, apocrine sweat glands, and lymph glands. Within the subcutaneous fat course several significant sensory cutaneous nerves, including the costobrachial and medial brachial cutaneous. Deep to the fascia is the axillary neurovascular bundle. Anatomically, the arm begins at the lower border of the pectoralis major tendon and ends at the level of the medial epicondyle. Topographically, the arm may be divided into four *surfaces:* anterior, medial, posterior, and external. From a surgical viewpoint, the arm is divided into an anterior and posterior *compartment* at the medial and lateral biceps sulci, which are created by intermuscular fascial septa that penetrate from the deep fascia down to the humerus. The subcutaneous fat is thicker laterally and thinner medially. Since all incisions must be placed medially to minimize visibility, it is the medial subcutaneous structures that are at risk. As one progresses distally from the axilla, four sensory nerves pass from the deep fascia into the overlying skin: posterior cutaneous nerve of arm (axilla), costobrachial (axilla), medial cutaneous nerve of arm (upper third of arm), and medial cutaneous nerve of forearm (middle third of arm). In addition, the basilic vein is located subcutaneously as it ascends from the elbow before piercing the deep fascia midway up the arm. Although Franco [2] considers ligation of the basilic vein mandatory in brachioplasty, we disagree and advocate its careful preservation. The surgeon must also be aware of the parallel course of the medial cutaneous nerve of the forearm and the major lymphatic trunks, which accompany the basilic vein.

SURGICAL PRINCIPLES

The visibility of the arm and its longitudinal deformity force a different set of principles for upper extremity surgery as compared to that of the lower extremity. Numerous surgeons, including McCraw [9] and Musio [10], have attempted modified circular excisions in the axilla similar to a circular thigh-lift. However, the result is a highly visible scar and limited correction of the deformity. In contrast, an elliptic excision allows direct excision of the problem, and its medial placement reduces visibility.

Marking

Preoperative markings are the *critical factor* in determining correct location of the subsequent scar. With the patient sitting, the arms are abducted and the elbows flexed to 90 degrees for the drawings. Lewis [8], Baroudi [1], and Grazer and Klingbeil [4] have recommended an elliptic excision with the incision line placed 2 cm above a reference line connecting the axillary dome to the medial epicondyle. Unfortunately, this approach maximizes central excision without correcting the more severe proximal deformity or alleviating redundancy at the elbow (Fig. 28-3).

For this reason, we prefer a more flexible fishtail type of excision in which the incision line is located slightly above the medial brachial sulcus and the excision line parallels the posteromedial aspects of the arm. In contrast to Grazer and Klingbeil [4], who parallel the upper surface of the arm, we consider it important to follow the abnormal contour of the posterior arm to ensure its complete correction. Since the skin edges will be advanced from distal to proximal, we do not recommend preoperative transverse lines. Once the incision line is marked, with careful consideration of the axillary excess and the distal deformity, the amount of tissue to be excised is estimated by pinching and a proposed excision line is determined (Fig. 28-4A, B).

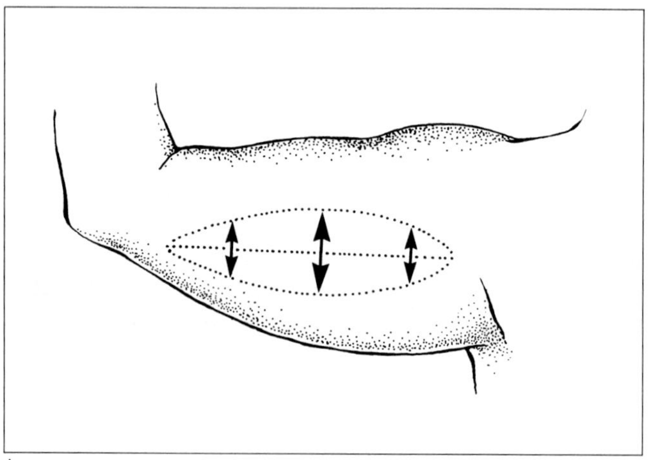
A

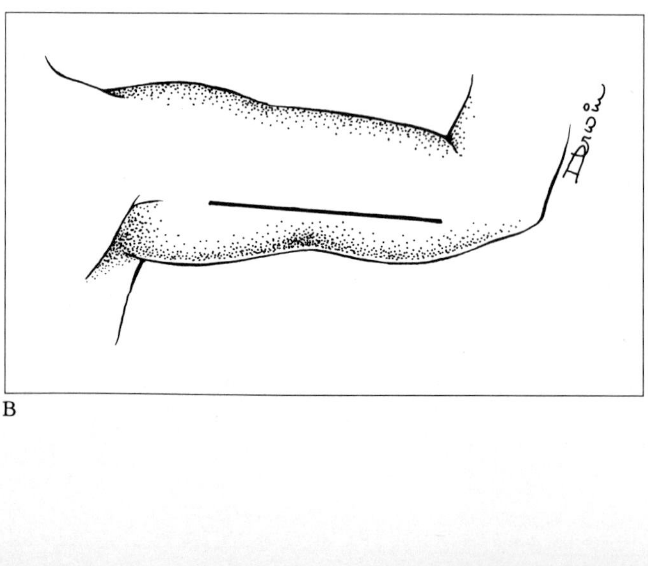
B

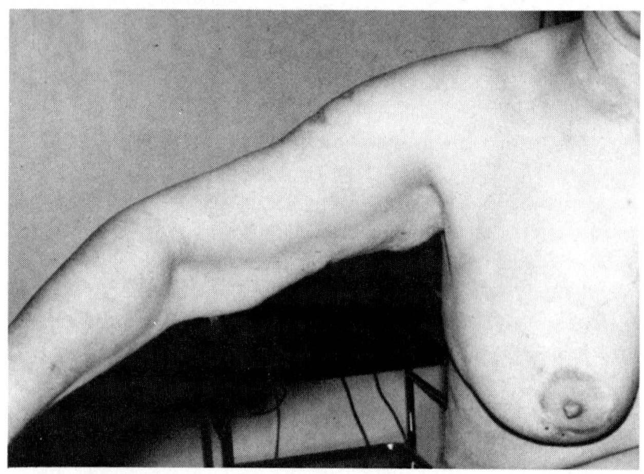
C

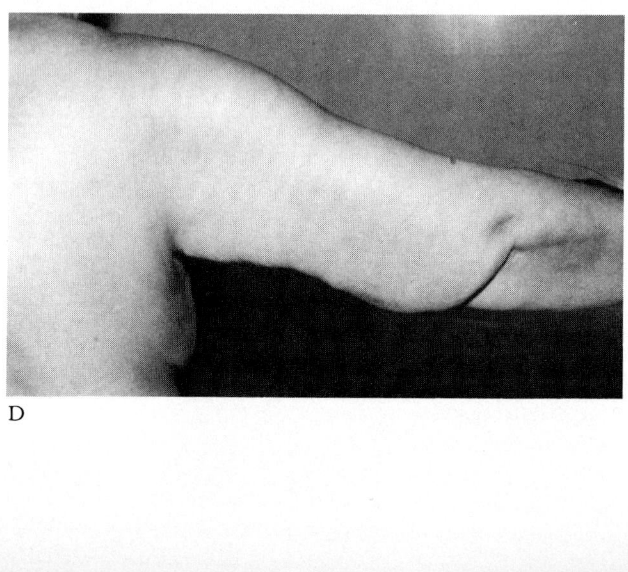
D

Figure 28-3
A, B. Standard elliptic excision results in maximum resection centrally but leaves redundancy in the proximal third and above the elbow.
C, D. Patient following elliptic excision done elsewhere demonstrating persistence of deformity at axilla and elbow.

Figure 28-4. Surgical technique for major brachioplasty.

A. Suspension of the arms.
B. Markings with proximal fishtail, an incision line passing along the medial sulcus curving above the elbow, and an excision line paralleling the posterior border of the arm. Closure is done with proximal traction bringing point A′ to A.
C. The incision is made and undermined down to the anticipated excision line.
D. Under tangential upward traction, the flap is split segmentally.
E. Subcuticular suture closure. Note fishtail closure.
F. Paper tape dressing. No drains are required.

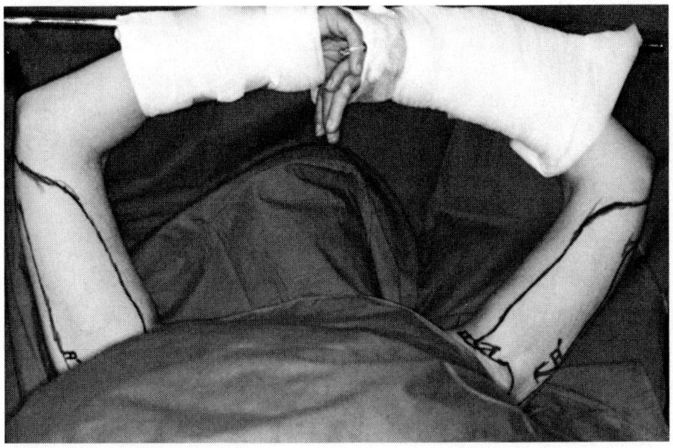

A

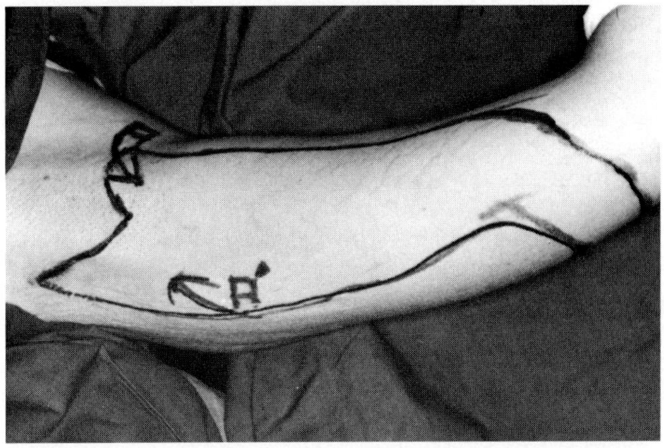

B

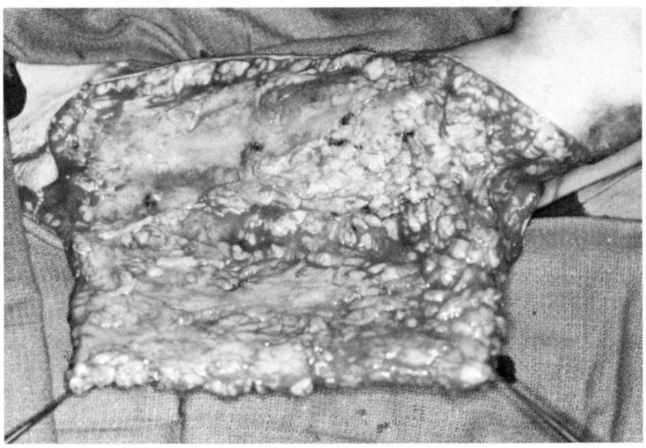

C

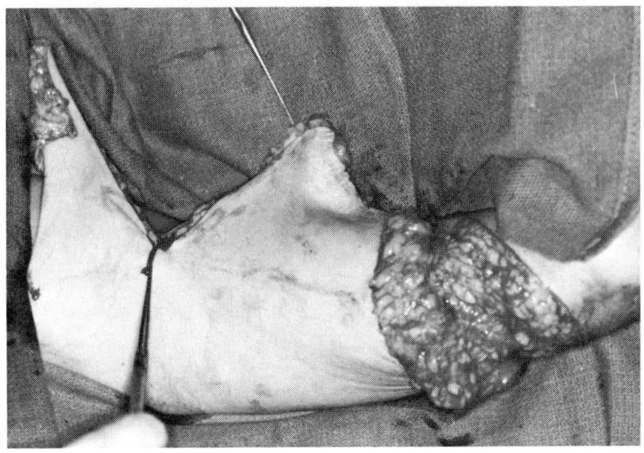

D

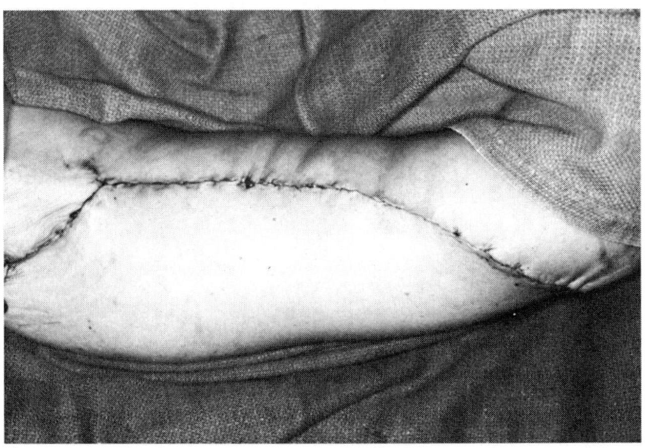

E

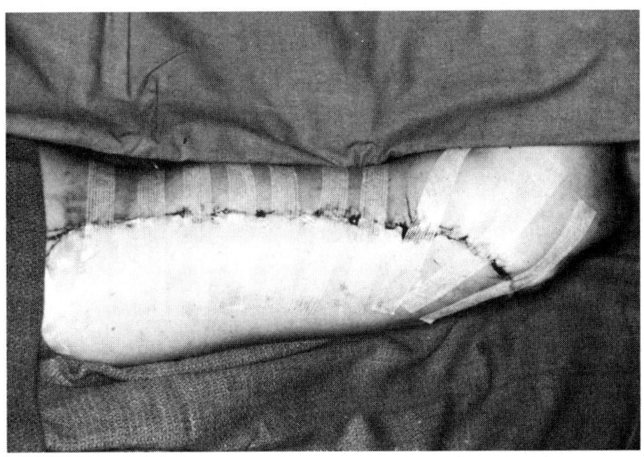

F

Preparation

If combined procedures are not being done, a local anesthetic consisting of dilute lidocaine (0.25%) and epinephrine (1 : 200,000) is used. The patient is placed supine with the arms abducted to the level of the head. Suspension of the arm above the head is done only in major brachioplasties.

Operation

The proximal medial incision is made first and carried down to the superficial fascia layer with preservation of major veins and cutaneous nerves. Dissection is extended to the proposed excision line (Fig. 28-4C). The skin elasticity and expected advancement are checked. Under proximal advancement, the flap is split segmentally and the excess resected. To ensure tightening of axillary redundancy, the inferior flap is advanced upward into the axilla (Fig. 28-4D). This combination of maximum proximal excision and proximal advancement on closure ensures correction of the deformity, in contrast to the classic ellipse, which often leaves proximal redundancies. Since undermining is negligible, drains are not required. A two-layer closure is done with 4-0 Vicryl, both interrupted subcutaneous sutures and a subcuticular running suture (Fig. 28-4E, F). As emphasized by Baroudi, the flap edges should not be sutured to the underlying fascia or visible depressions and irregularities will be created. The dressing consists only of adhesive tape.

SURGICAL TECHNIQUES

Brachioplasty

MINOR AND MODERATE BRACHIOPLASTY

In selecting the optimal procedure for the individual patient, one must determine the axillary deformity, distal extension, and location of maximum severity. If only the proximal one-half of the arm is involved, a minor brachioplasty is sufficient (Fig. 28-5). If the proximal and middle thirds of the arm are redundant, a moderate brachioplasty is required (Fig. 28-6). The extent of excision reflects the flaccidity of the arm and the anticipated advancement. Conservatism should be the rule. The medial incision line has a fishtail shape whereas the lateral extension is sharply tapered to avoid dog-ears. The central triangle that is left in the medial fishtail may preserve or remove the axillary hair depending on the patient's preference. The upper incision line is relatively straight whereas the posterior excision line follows the contour of the deformity. The dimensions of a minor brachioplasty average 10 × 4 cm whereas major brachioplasties may reach 20 × 7 cm.

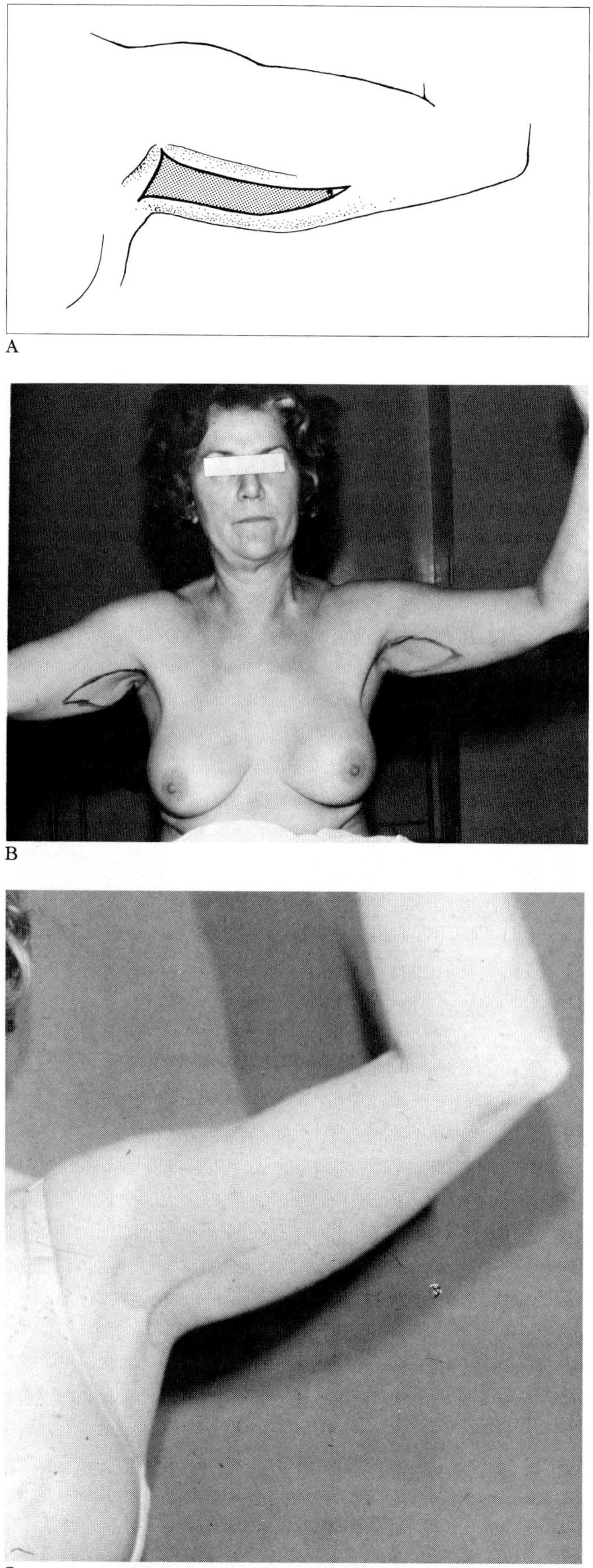

A

B

C

Figure 28-5. A minor brachioplasty.
A. Operative technique.
B. Deformity confined to proximal one-third.
C. Postoperative scar at 1 year.

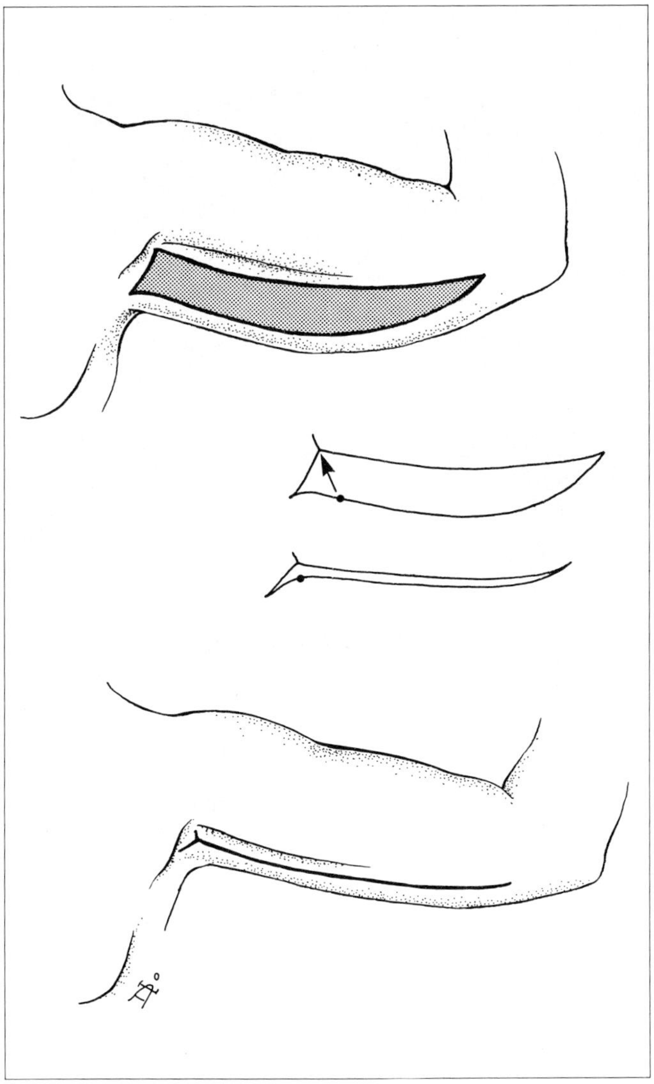

A

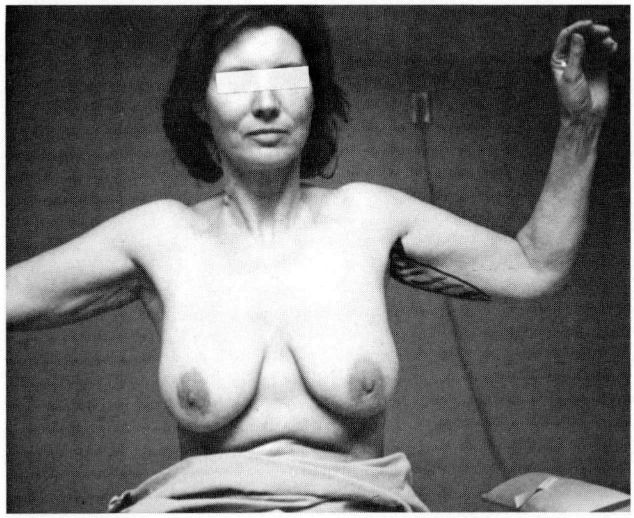

B

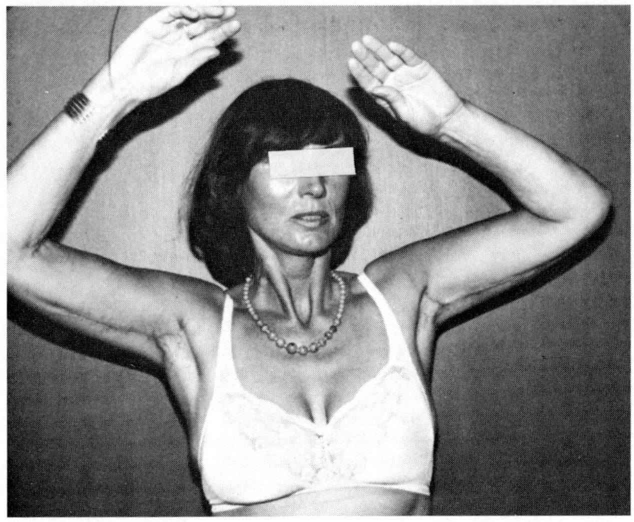

C

Figure 28-6. A moderate brachioplasty.
A. Operative technique.
B. Preoperative markings.
C. Postoperative result at 1 year.

The axillary and upper lines are incised and dissected down to the aponeurosis, which is carefully preserved. Dissection is continued down to the estimated excision line. With traction on the dissected flap, the adequacy of removal is verified, or modification is made to a line paralleling the preoperative marking. Meticulous hemostasis is essential. Maximum proximal traction is achieved by advancing a point on the lower flap to the upper portion of the fishtail. This point is selected by testing skin elasticity with a skin hook. A two-layer closure with absorbable sutures is done.

MAJOR BRACHIOPLASTY

If the entire arm is involved and skin redundancy above the elbow is a problem, a major brachioplasty is required. The markings are extended as a fusiform spiral turning posteriorly above the elbow (Fig. 28-7). The incision line is marked first and should turn posteriorly approximately 4 cm above the medial epicondyle, ending at least 2 cm above the olecranon in the extended position. The excision is approximately 30 cm in length, the width at the upper part approaches 4 to 8 cm, but the lower portion above the elbow rarely exceeds 2.5 cm. It is wise to check all markings with the arms by the side, as viewed from in front and behind. The entire operation is done with the elbow flexed to 90 degrees, thereby minimizing excessive skin resection. Closure is begun distally to avoid dog-ears. Localized excisions of skin redundancies at the elbow have been recommended by Kostianovsky [7], but the resulting scars would limit their value, especially if hypertrophy occurred.

Preaxilloplasty

Certain patients will complain of unsightly skin and fat excesses between the breast and the anterior shoulder. In

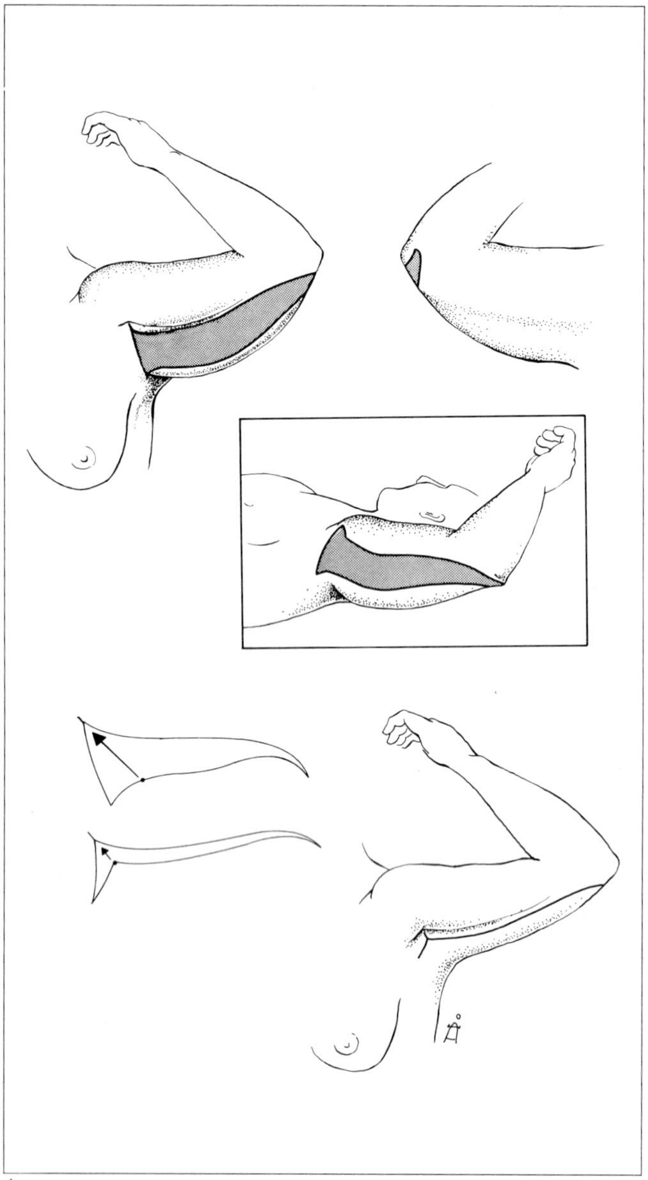

A

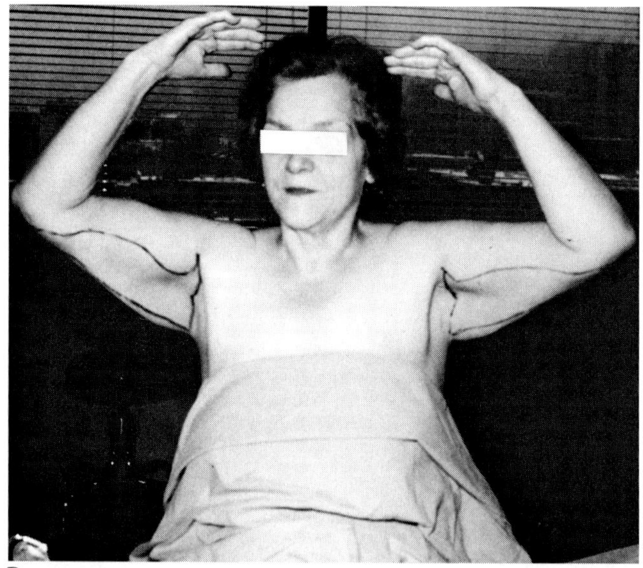

B

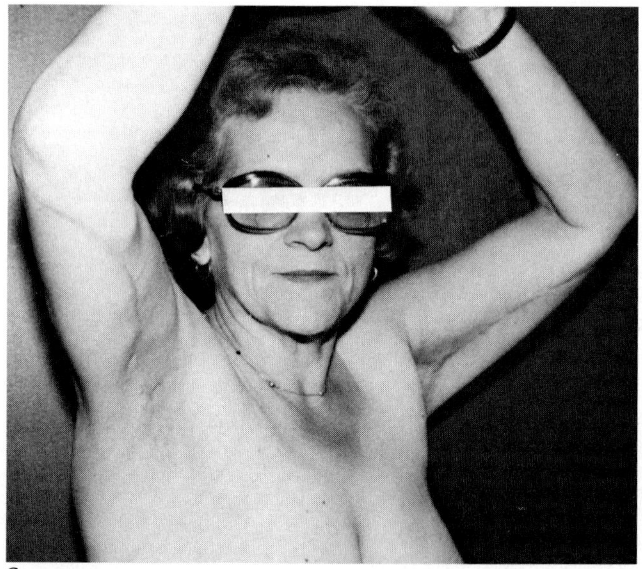

C

Figure 28-7. A major brachioplasty.
A. Operative technique.
B. Preoperative condition.
C. Postoperative result at 1 year. Note location of scar in the medial sulcus and in parallel creases above the elbow.

contrast to the typical axillary breast, this deformity is more diffuse and usually does not contain breast tissue. In younger patients, the tissue is quite firm and skin laxity is not significant. Following preoperative marking of the deformity in the standing patient, an M-excision is outlined in the axilla (Fig. 28-8). The intervening skin is undermined until the protuberant tissue is reached overlying the pectoralis major muscle. The deposit is excised with feathering of the edges, and then with tension on the skin. Any redundancy is excised, resulting in a zigzag closure. In severe cases, especially in older individuals and those who have undergone massive weight loss, a full-thickness direct excision is required. A superiorly curved crescent-shaped excision is used and so located that the final closure coincides with a natural fold in the sleeve-hole area (Fig. 28-9). The incision is done at the lower limit of the deformity and carried down to pectoralis major muscle. The fat is excised from the undersurface of the flap. Sufficient subcutaneous fat is left to avoid a postoperative depression. Then the redundancy is assessed, the flap split, and the tissue removed in a crescent shape. A small drain may be inserted and a two-layer closure done. Tapes cover the entire undermined area. The final scar follows a natural crease and is easily hidden by lingerie or sleeve holes of sleeveless dresses.

Hands

Occasionally, patients request correction of hand deformities that include wrinkling of the skin, "old-age" spots,

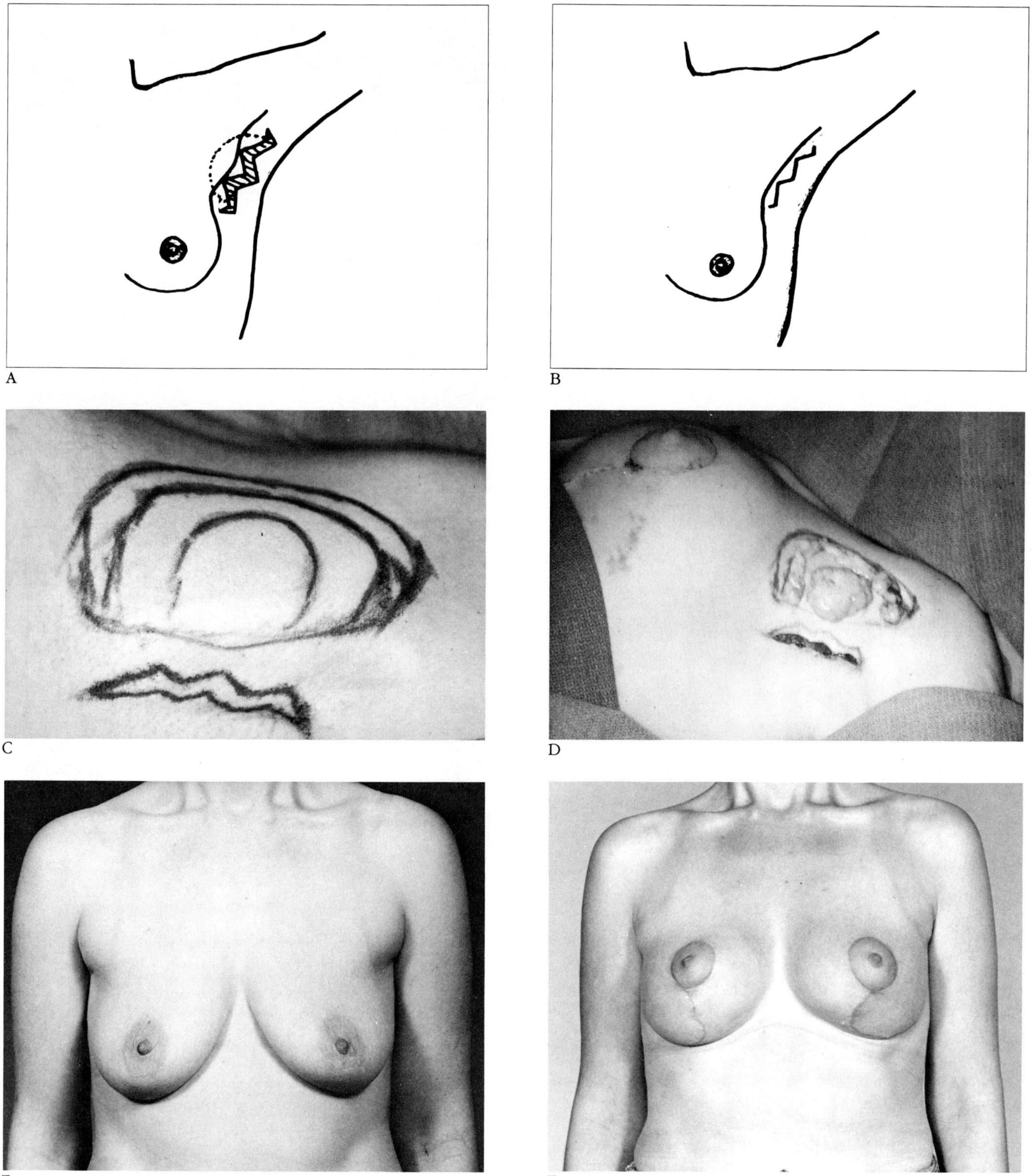

Figure 28-8. Technique for moderate preaxillary deformity in the younger patient.

A. Excision of redundant skin and undermining for removal of subcutaneous fat.
B. Zigzag closure located in the axilla.
C. Markings are made with patient standing. Central zone of maximum excision, then partial removal, and finally undermining.
D. Fat excision is followed by segmental skin splits to determine skin excess, usually 1 to 2 cm.
E. A 26-year-old person who requested mastopexy with augmentation as well as removal of preaxillary deformity.
F. Early postoperative result.

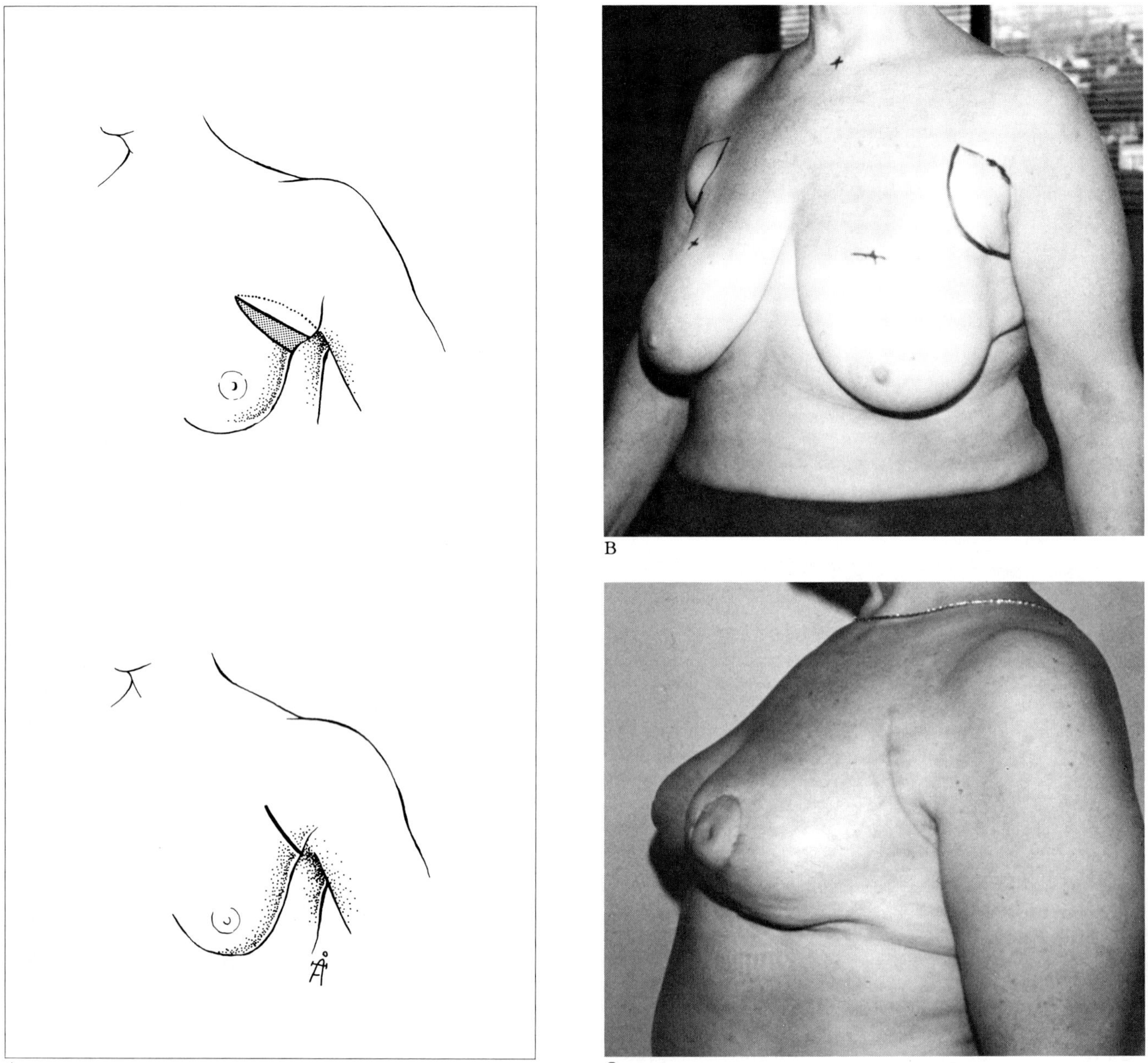

A

B

C

Figure 28-9. Severe preaxillary redundancy requiring direct excision.
A. Crescentic direct excision with undermining.
B. Preoperative condition. Note bulging above opposite breast.
C. Early postoperative result. Eventual fine scar will be covered by brassiere or swimsuit.

and tortuous visible veins. Pathologically, these changes represent direct damage to an increasingly atrophic skin with underlying dilated veins. Wrinkling can be corrected by excising excess skin via either a transverse wrist incision or an ulnar gull-wing incision at the juncture of dorsal and palmar skin. Lewis [8] considers ulnar rotation of the skin better than longitudinal traction but concludes that "resection of the skin of the hands is seldom indicated." Brown spots on the hand are usually senile lentigines and not senile keratoses. Although chemical peels can be effective, they cause visible scarring and a conspicuous transition zone at the nontreated forearms. Velazquez [17] has reported successful stripping of hand veins through small transverse incisions.

In general, we have not found aesthetic surgery of the hands to be worthwhile and refer the patients to dermatologists for treatment of pigmented lesions.

COMPLICATIONS

As always, complications can be minimized by careful patient selection, choice of the optimal operation, and constant attention to detail.

Intraoperative Complications

TIGHT CLOSURE
Tight closures are best avoided by sequential resection of the flap under gentle traction. If excessive tissue is removed, undermining and extension of the incision become necessary. Since the risk of hematoma and skin slough increases with undermining, hemostasis becomes even more important. As a last resort, one could insert a skin graft harvested from the resected specimen. Subsequent contracture and revision are better than an irreparable disaster.

Early Complications

SUTURE DEHISCENCE AND MARGINAL SKIN SLOUGH
These problems are often a consequence of excessive skin resection and subsequent tension on closure. If the resection is too great, undermining becomes necessary, increasing flap manipulation and risk of hematoma.

HEMATOMA AND SEROMA
If undermining is limited, hematomas are relatively rare, and simple postoperative elevation on two pillows will reduce their incidence. Seromas tend to occur in obese individuals and are drained as necessary.

Late Complications

VISIBLE SCARS
Although all brachioplasty incisions will be obvious with the arms elevated, scars that are visible on the posterior or anterior surface are unpleasant. Improper location is due to poor preoperative marking without reference to the medial brachial sulcus. One should always place the incision line slightly above the medial brachial sulcus and check to see whether the lines are visible from behind when the arms are down. Subsequent revision requiring appropriate rotation of the flaps is not possible before 1 year.

HYPERTROPHIC SCARS
Virtually all arm incisions undergo some degree of hypertrophy, and its severity appears to correlate with tension on closure and individual wound healing factors (Fig. 28-10). Scars are best in fair skin and older patients, worst in dark skin and younger patients. Also, brachioplasty for dermatochalasis gives better results than for lipectomy. In 25 percent of cases, triamcinolone is injected at 6 months to reduce scar hypertrophy. If scarring remains a distressing problem, a scar revision is recommended at 1 year.

EDEMA AND LYMPHEDEMA
Edema tends to be a problem following excess skin resection and tension on closure. Elevation and elastic compression may be required for several weeks. Severe swelling and persistent lymphedema may follow inadvertent resection of the axillary lymph nodes and ligation of the basilic vein with its associated lymphatics. This surgical error is avoided by careful dissection with preservation of all large veins and lymph nodes; it is better to leave a little fat than risk injury of vital structures.

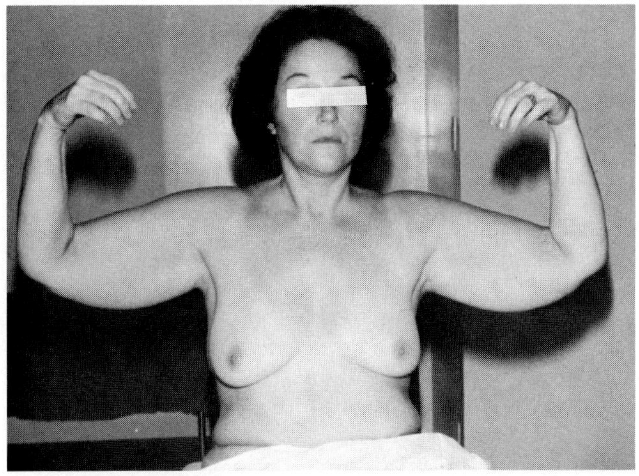

A

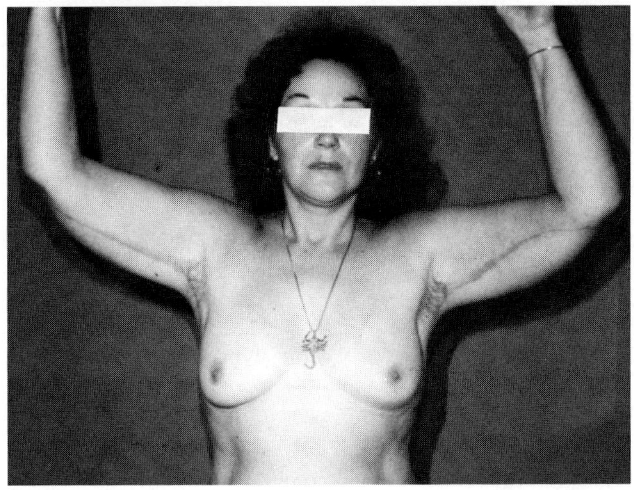

B

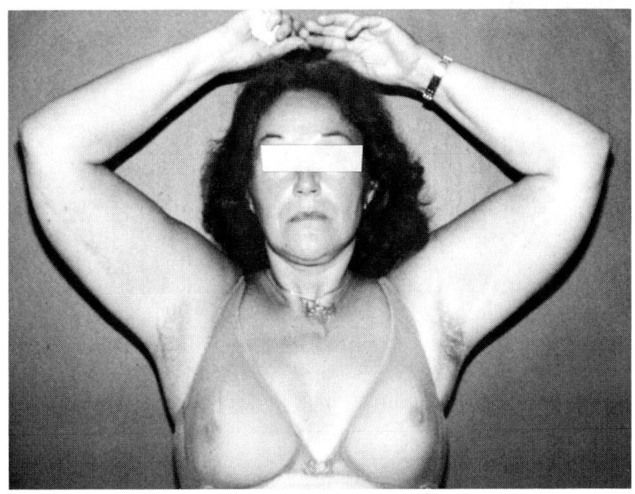

C

Figure 28-10
A. Preoperative condition consisting of disproportional adiposity and some flaccidity.
B. Hypertrophic scarring at 1 year.
C. Gradual fading of scars at 3 years, without further treatment.

NERVE INJURY
Division of cutaneous sensory nerves results in annoying numbness of the arm and occasionally painful neuromas. If a segment of nerve has been excised, thereby precluding end-to-end repair, the proximal nerve should be buried beneath the deep fascia.

CONTOUR DEFORMITIES
A tight closure will often produce transverse cutaneous folds centrally and dog-ears at either end. Constriction bands may occur beneath the cutaneous folds, leading to a permanent deformity. Daily massaging may reduce their visibility, although subsequent scar revision with undermining is often necessary. Additional contour deformities range from simple dog-ears to redundant tissue at either end; the former is a technical problem whereas the latter is a judgmental error indicating that a more extensive procedure should have been done.

RESULTS

Patient satisfaction and acceptance of the scar correlate with motivation and severity of the deformity. Since the scar is significant, the improvement obtained must be equally significant. Since the operation is undeniably effective, poor patient selection and inadequate preoperative counseling are the greatest source of dissatisfaction. One should avoid operating on overweight individuals with heavy tense arms; the resection will never be adequate, but the scar will always be apparent. Liposuction would appear ideal for these patients. Recurrence appears only after significant weight changes.

SECONDARY SURGERY

Secondary brachioplasty consists of either excision of redundancies (axilla, elbow) or scar revision. Persistence of the deformity follows either utilization of an elliptic excision or failure to do sufficient surgery; the former is avoided with the fishtail excision, the latter by preoperative counseling. Scar revisions are not undertaken before 1 year. It is essential to release all tension on the closure, and undermining may be necessary. Subsequent taping of the incision for up to 6 months is essential.

REFERENCES

1. Baroudi, R. Dermatolipectomy of the upper arm. *Clin. Plast. Surg.* 2:485, 1975.
2. Franco, T. Aesthetic Surgery of Upper and Lower Limbs. In J. F. Ely (ed.), *Transactions of the Seventh International Congress of Plastic and Reconstructive Surgery.* São Paolo: Cartgraf, 1980, P. 645.
3. Glanz, S., and Gonzalez-Ulloa, M. Aesthetic surgery of the arm. *Aesthetic Plast. Surg.* 5:1, 1981.
4. Grazer, F. M., and Klingbeil, J. R. *Body Images: A Surgical Perspective.* St. Louis: Mosby, 1980.
5. Guerrero-Santos, J. Arm-lift. In E. H. Courtiss (ed.), *Aesthetic Surgery: Trouble—How to Avoid It and How to Treat It.* St. Louis: Mosby, 1978.
6. Guerrero-Santos, J. Brachioplasty. *Aesthetic Plast. Surg.* 3:1, 1979.
7. Kostianovsky, A. S. Aesthetic surgery of the elbow. *Aesthetic Plast. Surg.* 5:163, 1981.
8. Lewis, J. R. *Atlas of Aesthetic Plastic Surgery.* Boston: Little, Brown, 1973.
9. McCraw, L. H. Surgical rehabilitation after massive weight reduction. *Plast. Reconstr. Surg.* 53:349, 1974.
10. Musio, L. Correction of Ptosis of the Upper Arm. In J. F. Ely (ed.), *Transactions of the Seventh International Congress of Plastic and Reconstructive Surgery.* São Paolo: Cartgraf, 1980, P. 659.
11. Pitanguy, I. Correction of lipodystrophy of the lateral thoracic aspect and inner side of the arm and elbow. *Clin. Plast. Surg.* 2:477, 1975.
12. Pitanguy, I. Dermolipectomy of the Abdominal Wall, Thigh, Buttocks, and Upper Extremity. In J. M. Converse (ed.), *Reconstructive Plastic Surgery* (2nd ed.). Philadelphia: Saunders, 1977.
13. Pitanguy, I. Aesthetic surgery of the upper and lower limbs. *Aesthetic Plast. Surg.* 4:363, 1980.
14. Regnault, P. Lipectomy. In W. C. Grabb and J. W. Smith (eds.), *Plastic Surgery.* Boston: Little, Brown, 1978. P. 838.
15. Regnault, P. Brachioplasty, Axilloplasty and Preaxilloplasty. In J. F. Ely (ed.), *Transactions of the Seventh International Congress of Plastic and Reconstructive Surgery.* São Paulo: Cartgraf, 1980. P. 639.
16. Thorek, M. Esthetic surgery of pendulous breast, abdomen and arms in females. *IMJ* 58:48, 1930.
17. Velazquez, J. M. Aesthetic surgery of the aging hand. *Aesthetic Plast. Surg.* 1:279, 1977.

29. Massive Weight Loss

Paule Regnault
Rollin K. Daniel

During the past decade, new surgical techniques for intestinal and gastric bypass have been developed for the treatment of morbid obesity. Massive weight loss is defined as a loss greater than 100 lb or an amount 100 percent above ideal weight. As a result, the aesthetic surgeon is seeing a greater number of patients who require total body contouring. Rather than applying conventional operations, the surgeon must select procedures modified specifically for the massive-weight-loss patient and devise a series of combined operations to achieve the optimal result (Fig. 29-1).

HISTORY

Since the early 1900s surgeons have been excising pendulous abdominal aprons and tightening baggy thighs in an attempt to eliminate obesity and its sequelae [20]. In a series of publications, Clarkson [4, 5] summarized these efforts and pleaded for a more radical approach. Recently, emphasis has shifted from excising the fat of the obese patient to body contouring of the near-normal-weight individual who has undergone a massive weight loss [11, 13, 18]. In 1972 McCraw [17] performed abdominoplasty, mastopexy, brachioplasty, and thigh-lift for a patient who had lost more than 200 lb. The dramatic result required several innovative modifications of then standard aesthetic procedures. McCraw's case report was followed by Zook's [26, 27] classic article emphasizing (1) careful planning to determine the type, number, combination, and sequence of the surgical procedures; (2) preoperative markings in the standing position; (3) long sinuous incisions to permit maximum resection; and (4) preservation of major veins and lymphatics. At the present time, the problem has changed from radical resection of obesity to radical reduction of the redundant skin envelope [23].

PATHOPHYSIOLOGY AND CLASSIFICATION

Morbid obesity may be defined as a weight of 100 lb or 100 percent over normal weight, whichever is less. The majority of patients become obese by the time they are adolescents, lose large amounts of weight by periodic dieting, but regain it on account of environmental stress [1, 2]. If external goals could be achieved (employment, increased social life) by altering body image, aesthetic surgery might aid in interrupting this cycle [15]. However, most patients remain obese unless weight loss is mandatory for medical reasons, usually cardiopulmonary incompetence, hypertension, or diabetes. The rapid reduction of weight following bypass surgery results in loss of fat tissue

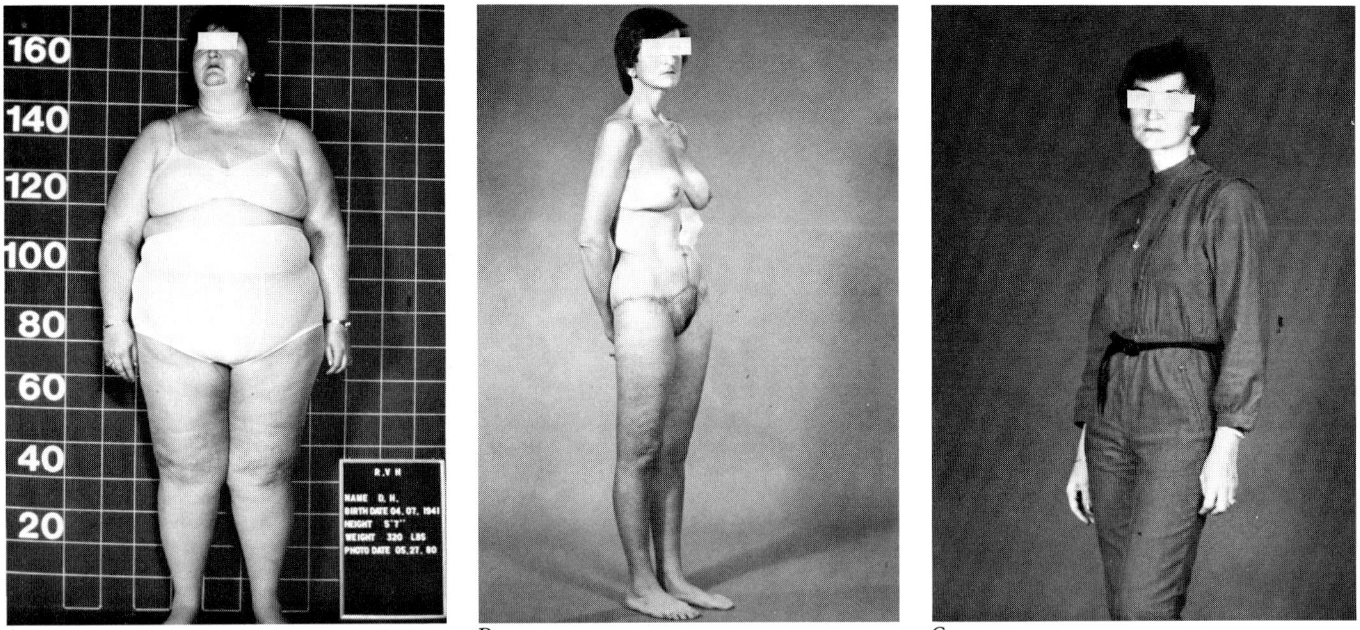

A B C

Figure 29-1. A 40-year-old patient with morbid obesity and subsequent correction. Her maximum-current-ideal weight ratio was 328 : 121 : 140.
A. Prior to gastroplasty.
B. Following multiple procedures including fleur-de-lis abdominoplasty, thigh lipectomy with vertical extension, breast augmentation, major brachioplasty, and rhytidectomy.
C. In standard clothing.

from abdominal viscera, regional deposits, and the subcutaneous layer [12]. Although the skin can contract, longstanding distention causes permanent changes to the dermis and elastic fibers [25]. It is our impression that the degree of skin redundancy is related to the amount and rapidity of weight loss and the patient's age. Since by definition all massive-weight-loss patients have shed more than 100 lb, the critical factor is the patient's age [6, 7]. For those under 30 years, correction of the abdomen and breasts is usually sufficient. In patients over 30 years, the entire body and all the limbs must be reduced. Conversely, one may classify the deformity as regionalized (breasts and abdomen) or generalized (total body). An additional parameter that has proved useful is the ratio of current weight to ideal weight. If the difference is greater than 20 percent, one can expect residual fat deposits leading to lipectomy rather than skin excision in the leaner patient. Emphasis should be placed not on the amount of weight loss but on the attainment of ideal weight as defined by insurance company tables (Table 29-1). To put correct weight in perspective, we use a three-part weight-listing system *(maximum — current — ideal).*

SURGICAL TREATMENT OF OBESITY

In 1963 Payne et al. [21] reported 10 cases of intestinal bypass for morbid obesity. The basic technique was a "14–4" bypass in which a 14-in. proximal segment of jejunum was sutured end-to-side to the distal 4 in. of the ileum. Although a mean weight loss of 123 lb was obtained in the first year, the associated problems of electrolyte imbalance, metabolic disturbances, and persistent diarrhea required a new procedure. Mason [16] devised the gastric bypass, in which a 15 to 30 percent fundic segment was sutured to the upper jejunum. Despite its effectiveness, the problems of anemia, peripheral neuritis, dumping syndrome, and reflex gastritis caused it to be modified. Eventually, a simple gastroplasty was devised that reduced the stomach to a 60-cc fundic pouch with a 12-mm channel [14]. Rather than a bypass of the intestine, the limiting factor is the volume that can be ingested and the amount required to satisfy the patient's desire to eat; thus, overindulgence is physically impossible.

In a series of 330 patients, the mean vital statistics revealed an age of 35, a 5 : 1 female predominance, and an excess weight of 150 lb. Following gastroplasty, the patient achieved 50 percent of ideal weight loss by 6 months with continued improvement for up to 2 years. Little change occurs beyond this point, and the new weight was maintained at 5 years after surgery. These results are in marked contrast to those of conservative medical regimens or jaw wiring, in which weight reduction is *not* maintained in 90 percent of morbidly obese patients.

What are the current indications and contraindications for intestinal bypass surgery? The physiologic criteria include (1) morbid obesity that has been present for 5 years and has not responded to a medical regimen, (2) an age between 15 and 50, and (3) absence of serious psychotic or medical diseases. At the present time, gastroplasty is the preferred procedure. In patients with reflex gastritis, gastric reduction plus bypass of the duodenum is done. The

Table 29-1. Desirable weights (weight in pounds according to frame — in indoor clothing)

Men of ages 25 and over	Height (with shoes on) 1-in. heels				
	Feet	Inches	Small frame	Medium frame **(key mean)**	Large frame
	5	2	112–120	118–129 **124**	126–141
	5	3	115–123	121–133 **127**	129–144
	5	4	118–126	124–136 **130**	132–148
	5	5	121–129	127–139 **133**	135–152
	5	6	124–133	130–143 **137**	138–156
	5	7	128–137	134–147 **141**	142–161
	5	8	132–141	138–152 **145**	147–166
	5	9	136–145	142–156 **149**	151–170
	5	10	140–150	146–160 **153**	155–174
	5	11	144–154	150–165 **158**	159–179
	6	0	148–158	154–170 **162**	164–184
	6	1	152–162	158–175 **167**	168–189
	6	2	156–167	162–180 **171**	173–194
	6	3	160–171	167–185 **176**	178–199
	6	4	164–175	172–190 **181**	182–204

Women of ages 25 and over	Height (with shoes on) 1-in. heels					
	Feet	Inches	Small frame	Medium frame **(key mean)**	Large frame	±10%
	4	10	92–98	96–107 **102**	104–119	
	4	11	94–101	98–110 **104**	106–122	
	5	0	96–104	101–113 **107**	109–125	
	5	1	99–107	104–116 **110**	112–128	99–121
	5	2	102–110	107–119 **113**	115–131	102–124
	5	3	105–113	110–122 **116**	118–134	104–128
	5	4	108–116	113–126 **120**	121–138	108–132
	5	5	111–119	116–130 **123**	125–142	111–135
	5	6	114–123	120–135 **128**	129–146	115–141
	5	7	118–127	124–139 **132**	133–150	119–145
	5	8	122–131	128–143 **136**	137–154	122–150
	5	9	126–135	132–147 **140**	141–158	126–154
	5	10	130–140	136–151 **144**	145–163	130–158
	5	11	134–144	140–155 **148**	149–168	133–163
	6	0	138–148	144–159 **152**	153–173	137–167

For women between 18 and 25, subtract 1 pound for each year under 25.

principal early complications are anastomotic leak and obstruction, with long-term sequelae including dumping syndrome and patient intolerance. Despite these risks, surgical treatment is now the best method of achieving massive weight loss, and the aesthetic surgeon is forced to devise ways of contouring excess skin rather than simply excising excess fat [3, 10].

CONSULTATION

The preoperative consultation must reveal the patient's physical and psychologic candidacy for multiple surgical procedures.

Indications and Contraindications

Total body contouring should be offered to patients undergoing surgical treatment for obesity. Following massive weight loss, the redundant skin envelope will cause personal hygiene problems, painful intertrigo, inability to dress normally, reduced physical activity, and psychologic stress. Surgery is not done before 1 year at a constant weight. Psychologically, the patient must be stable and willing to accept the need for multiple operations with significant scarring and potentially fatal complications.

Surgery is contraindicated in patients with serious medical problems, e.g., cardiorespiratory and diabetic conditions. It should be noted that significant weight loss frequently leads to amelioration of hypertension, diabetes, and respiratory problems. The presence of alcoholism or drug dependency should be discerned.

Medical History

A multisystem history is taken with particular emphasis on obesity and its complications. Also, the method of weight loss (medical or surgical) and its sequelae are important. Communication with the general surgeon who has treated the patient over a 2- to 3-year period is important for determining medical problems and candidacy for body contouring.

Motivation

Follow-up psychologic studies have shown that weight loss results in greater physical activity, with improvement in social life and employment opportunities. Thus, the patient's primary goal is to complete a weight-loss program and to get rid of the abhorred excess skin [8]. Although well aware of the extensive permanent scarring, the patient wants a better "shape" and the chance to wear more flattering clothes. However, one must be aware that many patients have unrealistic goals. A 40-year-old patient of one of the authors was obsessed with "finding a man" after completing her regimen. Her forceful personality, as manifested by her occupation as a bill collector, remained her primary negative factor despite a more pleasing shape. As the hoped-for goals fail to materialize, the patient can suffer significant depression and the surgeon can become an object of blame. A review of preoperative and postoperative psychiatric evaluations on patients undergoing intestinal bypass surgery indicates that, at 6 months, 45 percent had no change, 30 percent were improved, but 25 percent had deteriorated psychiatrically. However, the negative effects were not caused by surgery but rather stemmed from preexisting neurotic tendencies, continuing conflict situations, unanticipated events, and unachieved goals. Thus, the aesthetic surgeon must determine whether the patient's motivation is to complete a weight-loss program or to continue avoiding "life's problems."

Physical Examination

The patient is examined completely nude in the standing position. The degree of firm adiposity and skin redundancy is noted as well as the location of previous surgical scars. The overall torso configuration is assessed first: Is a waistline silhouette present or are multiple lateral "rolls" evident? The patient is examined anteriorly and posteriorly, with the arms raised to determine the best method of contour correction. Following torso and arm examination, the lower extremities are observed and the optimal procedure is selected—usually a circular thigh-lift with vertical extension. The breasts are then assessed. Next, the patient is evaluated in the recumbent position for abdominal hernias, intertrigo, skin ulceration, breast masses, etc.

If the patient decides to undergo surgery, a second series of detailed localized examinations will be necessary for each region, as described in previous chapters.

Aesthetic Goals

While the patient dresses, the surgeon should make a sketch of the patient and a proposed series of combined procedures. The patient's desires and condition are then reviewed. Frequently, the patient wants excision of the abdominal panniculus and tightening of the thighs. Surprisingly, the breasts are not a major concern in many patients. The patient must be willing to swap socially apparent deformities (skin redundancies) for privately visible deformities (scars). If the goal is to remove all traces of previous obesity, it cannot be achieved as extensive scars will always remain. The patient must be willing to accept a minimum of two or three hospitalizations scheduled several months apart. The surgeon should resist the inevitable pressure to do everything during one hospitalization. It is wise to remind patients that they did not become obese or lose their weight in one day. Each procedure is so extensive and the risks are so great that compounding their effect is foolish.

Informed Consent

It should be noted that gastroplasty is a relatively straightforward 2-hour operation done through a 20-cm midline incision with minimal blood loss and limited postoperative morbidity. In contrast, a torsoplasty or circular thigh-lift can be a major procedure of 3 to 5 hours' duration, with significant blood loss and life-threatening complications. The patient should be informed of the following:

1. As much excess skin and improvement in shape will be made as possible. However, the severity of the deformity precludes total correction.
2. The scars are extensive, are permanent, and do *not* fade to fine white lines because of tension and location near stretch points.
3. Delayed wound healing, marginal skin sloughs, and seromas are almost inevitable and are anticipated events.
4. Although rare, deep vein thrombosis and pulmonary embolus are significant risks, and every effort will be made to minimize them.

Preoperative Preparations

The aesthetic surgeon should contact the general surgeon or referring physician for additional information on the patient's emotional stability. A thorough physical examination and laboratory workup are necessary to rule out cardiopulmonary, metabolic, and blood problems. Although previous donations may permit autotransfusion, bank blood should be available. Photographs are taken. The junior author uses subcutaneous miniheparinization for all major procedures—5000 units preoperatively and then 5000 every 12 hours for 5 days.

SURGICAL PRINCIPLES AND TECHNIQUES

The fundamental principle of total body contouring is excision of as much redundant tissue as possible with minimal undermining and moderate tension. Incisions are placed to permit maximum excision, with scar visibility a secondary consideration, except in the extremities. It must be emphasized that these are mega-operations requiring preoperative nursing instruction, a two-team approach, and postoperative vigilance for major complications.

The critical decision is to determine the best method of torso contouring (Fig. 29-2). The three options are as follows:

1. The redundancy is predominantly anterior and can be excised directly with a standard or extended fleur-de-lis abdominal lipectomy.
2. An anterolateral deformity exists extending upward into the axilla, best corrected by a two-stage procedure consisting of an extended W-plasty followed by a "batwing" torso lipectomy incorporating a thoracobrachioplasty.
3. A circular deformity exists extending around to and including the back, thereby necessitating a limited or complete belt lipectomy. Further complicating the problem is the fact that many general surgeons do their own panniculectomy before referring the patient for "finishing touches." In most cases, the back has not been corrected and a secondary batwing torsoplasty is often necessary.

Once the optimal torso operation is determined, procedures are selected for breasts, upper extremities, and lower extremities. From our recent experience with 27 massive-weight-loss patients, it has become evident that one should correct the torso deformity first. If done correctly, a modified complete belt lipectomy can raise the buttocks and lateral and anterior thighs sufficiently to allow a medial thigh lipectomy with vertical extensions, thereby eliminating the need for a circular lift. Also, thoracobrachioplasties can influence the type of breast reduction or augmentation. In regard to the pubic area, a descending vertical component similar to a modified Weinhold is done to excise superior hooding; lateral folds are removed during medial thigh lipectomy. The use of skin staplers speeds wound closure and can reduce operative time by 50 percent albeit at the risk of some cross-hatching.

In general, it is best to offer a total approach, deciding which procedures are compatible and doing several on one admission rather than combining several procedures into one long operation. We often will do a brachioplasty, mastopexy, or rhytidectomy under local anesthesia during the patient's convalescence from thighplasty or torsoplasty. The results can be truly remarkable. Palmer et al. [19] reported 55 procedures on 38 patients with a mean weight loss of 61 kg. The operations performed included abdominoplasty (36) followed 6 months later by thighplasty (12), mammaplasty (3), or brachioplasty (4).

Which procedures can be combined? Any combination is acceptable except abdomen and thighs; the risk of complications and inability to achieve maximum lifting preclude their simultaneous execution (Fig. 29-3).

Torsoplasty

Correction of the torso depends on its location: anterior (fleur-de-lis), anterolateral (batwing), or circular (belt lipectomy). Approximately 85 percent of cases can be corrected by a fleur-de-lis resection that extends posteriorly.

EXTENDED FLEUR-DE-LIS

The basic principle remains direct excision of the anterior deformity, limited lateral undermining, medial advancement of the flaps, and resection of any epigastric deformity (Fig. 29-4). In massive-weight-loss patients one is able to excise far greater amounts of skin redundancy than in the moderately obese patients. Also, previous abdominal surgical incision facilitates patient acceptance of a vertical midline scar. The patient is placed in the prone position with the posterior deformity excised first, followed by the anterior resection.

BELT TORSOPLASTY

If the torso deformity is circular and the posterior redundancy cannot be eliminated by advancement into the axilla via a thoracobrachioplasty, a belt lipectomy is necessary. As originally proposed by Gonzalez-Ulloa [9] for the obese patient, the back incision often has delayed healing and produces a scar that undergoes hypertrophy and spreading. However, our modification for the massive-weight-loss patient has produced excellent results with acceptable scars. We reserve this procedure for the highly motivated patient with a severe deformity that cannot be corrected by any other method.

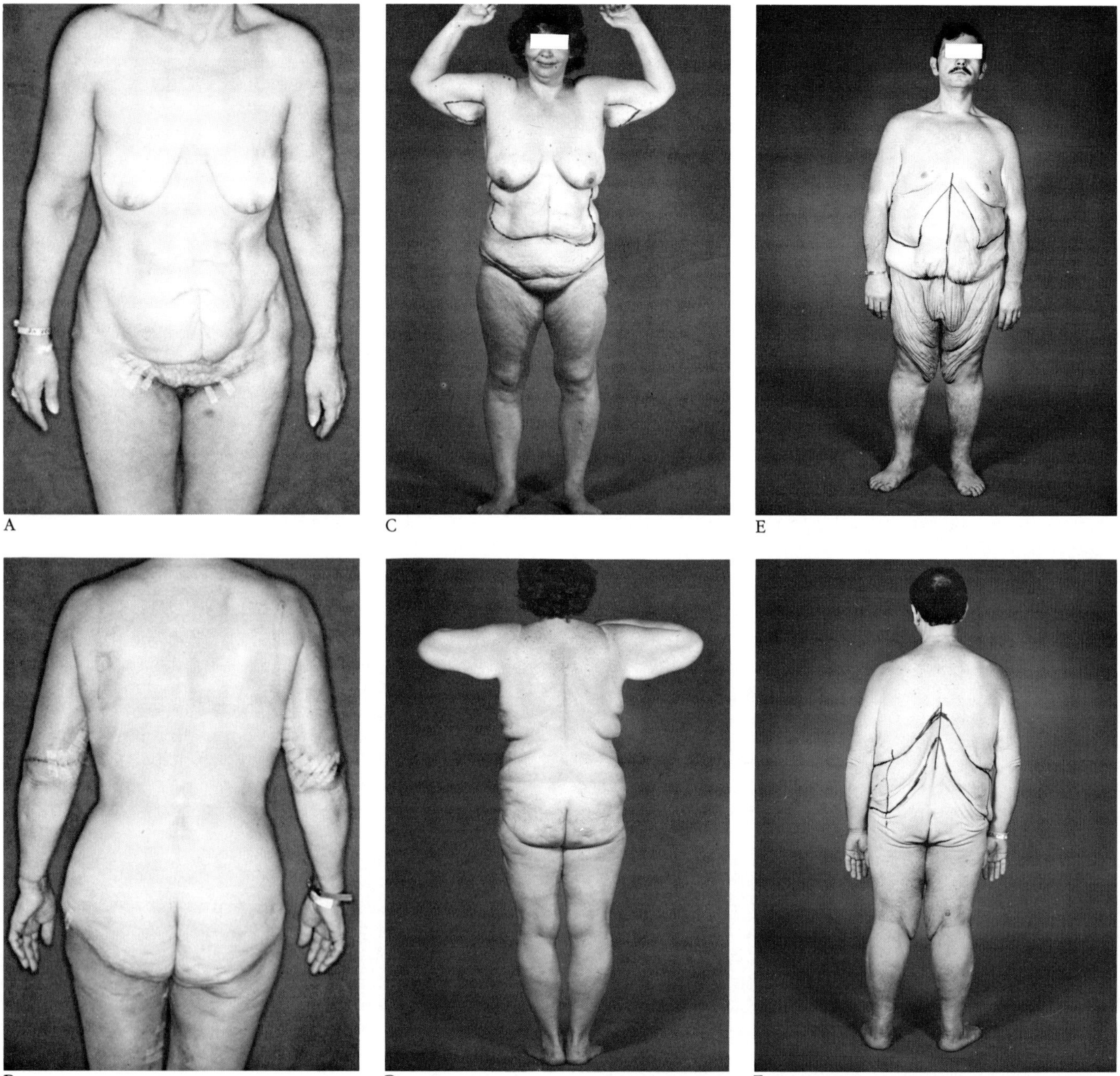

Figure 29-2. Location of torso obesity and maximum-current-ideal weight ratio.

A, B. Anterior deformity following a 100-lb weight loss with normal posterior silhouette and narrowing at the waistline. Fleur-de-lis torsoplasty is sufficient. Patient is 2 weeks after major brachioplasty and semicircular thigh-lift with vertical extensions (225 : 127 : 122).

C, D. Predominant anterior and lateral deformity. Combined abdominoplasty and batwing torsoplasty will correct the problem (295 : 185 : 142).

E, F. Circular deformity. A belt lipectomy is indicated (565 : 195 : 142).

Note significant differences in body fat distribution based on ratio of current to ideal weight.

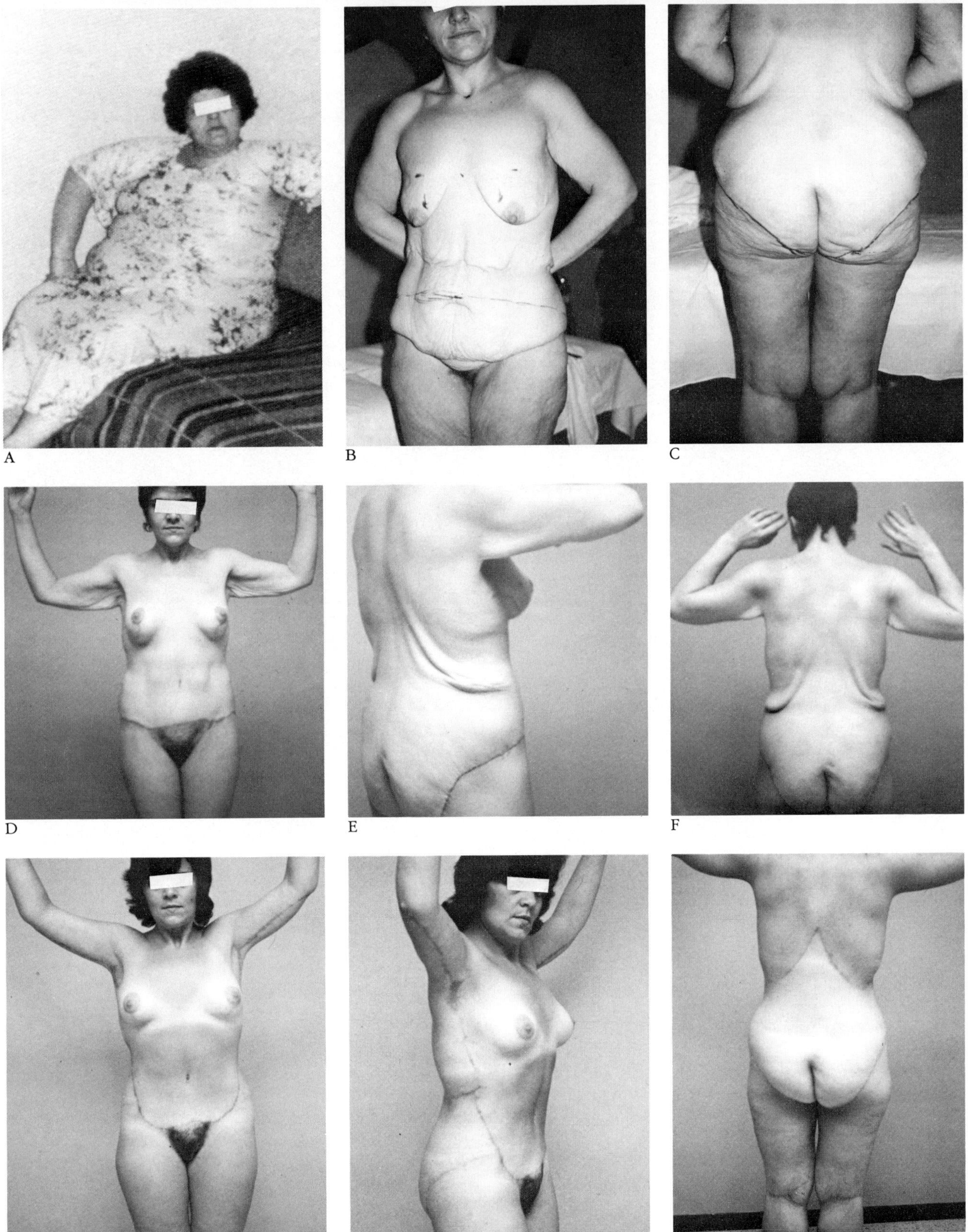

Figure 29-3. A total approach to correcting deformities associated in the massive-weight-loss patient.

A. Morbidly obese condition (220 : 140 : 116).

B. First operation consisted of an extended W-plasty and B-mastopexy with augmentation.

C. Second operation was a circular thigh-lift with vertical extension.

D–F. Result showing excellent correction but persistence of posterolateral torso folds and upper extremity laxity.

G–I. Final result following "batwing" thoracoplasty incorporating a major brachioplasty.

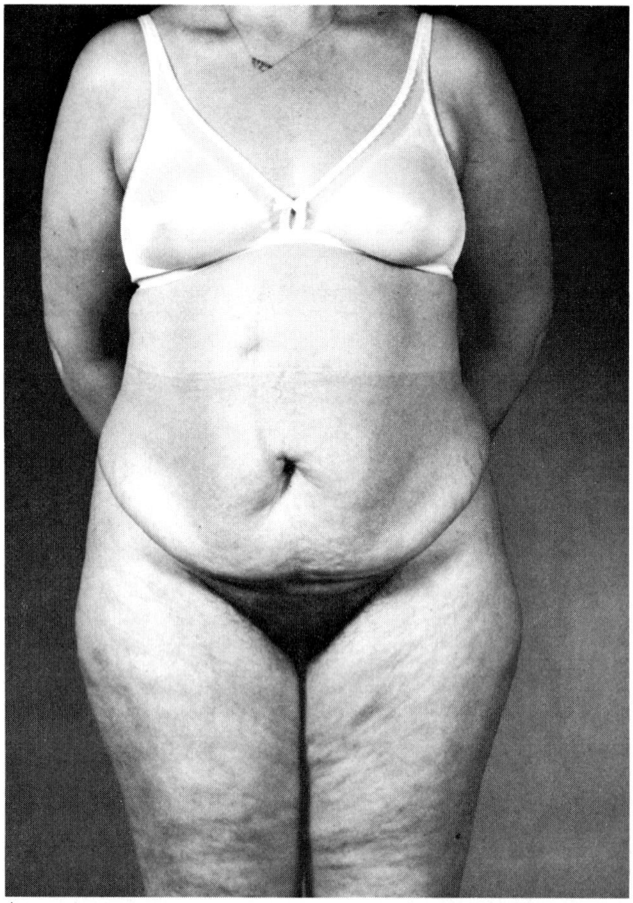

A

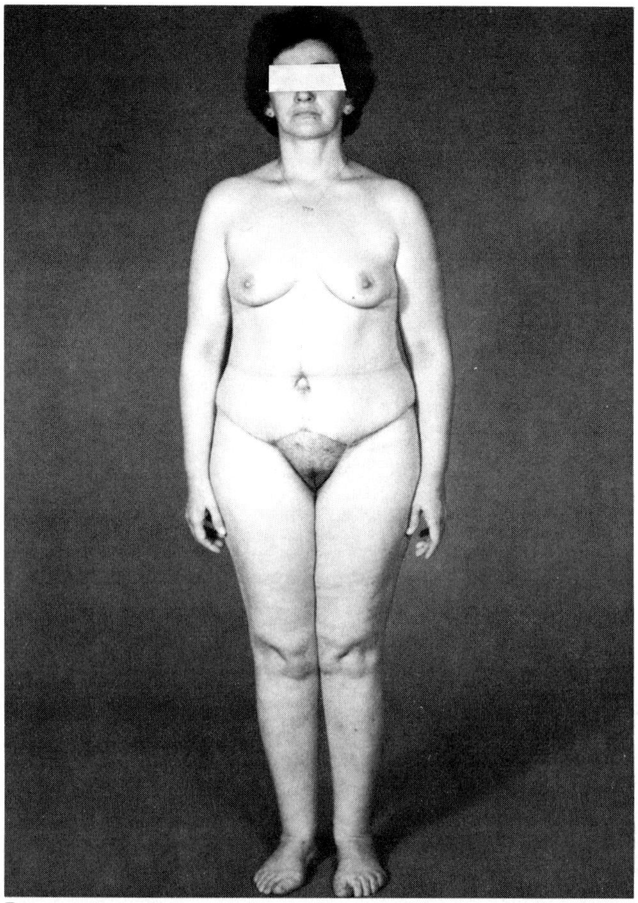

B

Figure 29-4
A. Patient following limited weight loss with right paramedian incision. Her maximum-current-ideal weight ratio was 210 : 155 : 136.
B. Result after a fleur-de-lis abdominal lipectomy.

Marking. In contrast to the belt lipectomy of Gonzalez-Ulloa [9], which was primarily a transverse excision for the moderately obese, this torsoplasty slopes superiorly to correct both the abdomen, the lateral rolls, and the back redundancy (Fig. 29-5). In certain cases a planned circular thigh-lift can be minimized as elevation of the ptotic buttocks is achieved. With the patient standing, the redundancy and elasticity are checked by grasping the tissue (Fig. 29-6). There are three objectives: (1) anteriorly, an abdominal lipectomy with limited undermining, transposition of the umbilicus, and plication of the muscles; (2) laterally, excision of the redundant rolls with sufficient mobilization to ensure elimination of transverse axillary rolls; and (3) posteriorly, excision of redundancy with accentuation of the waistline. Medially, the inferior incision line is similar to a W-plasty but laterally it remains beneath the abdominal pannus before sweeping superiorly. The excision line is determined by grasping the redundant tissue and estimating the maximum resection possible. To make certain that the axillary rolls are eliminated, one should usually see that the excision line approaches the level of the inframammary crease as it turns onto the back. The amount of excision posteriorly should be conservative, and crossing the midline is not required in all cases. Adjustments of the markings are often necessary to ensure maximum improvement. The midaxillary line is indicated as it represents the most lateral point of resection when the patient is prone. Since the redundant skin tends to "flow," careful positioning is required.

Operation. The patient is intubated, has a Foley catheter inserted, and is placed in the prone position. Prepping is carried as anteriorly as possible. The incision is made down to fascia, dissection is done along the aponeurosis, and the flap is elevated. The dissection is continued as anteriorly as possible, at least to the midaxillary line. With vertical traction posteriorly and angular traction laterally, the flap is split segmentally. Occasionally, some limited undermining and deep resection of adipose tissue may be necessary to eliminate the transverse axillary rolls [24]. Meticulous hemostasis is obtained, and then a two-layer closure is done. A sterile plastic drape is placed over the wound and the patient turned onto a second operating table. Following prep of the abdomen, the lower abdominoplasty incision is made and the deep dissection contin-

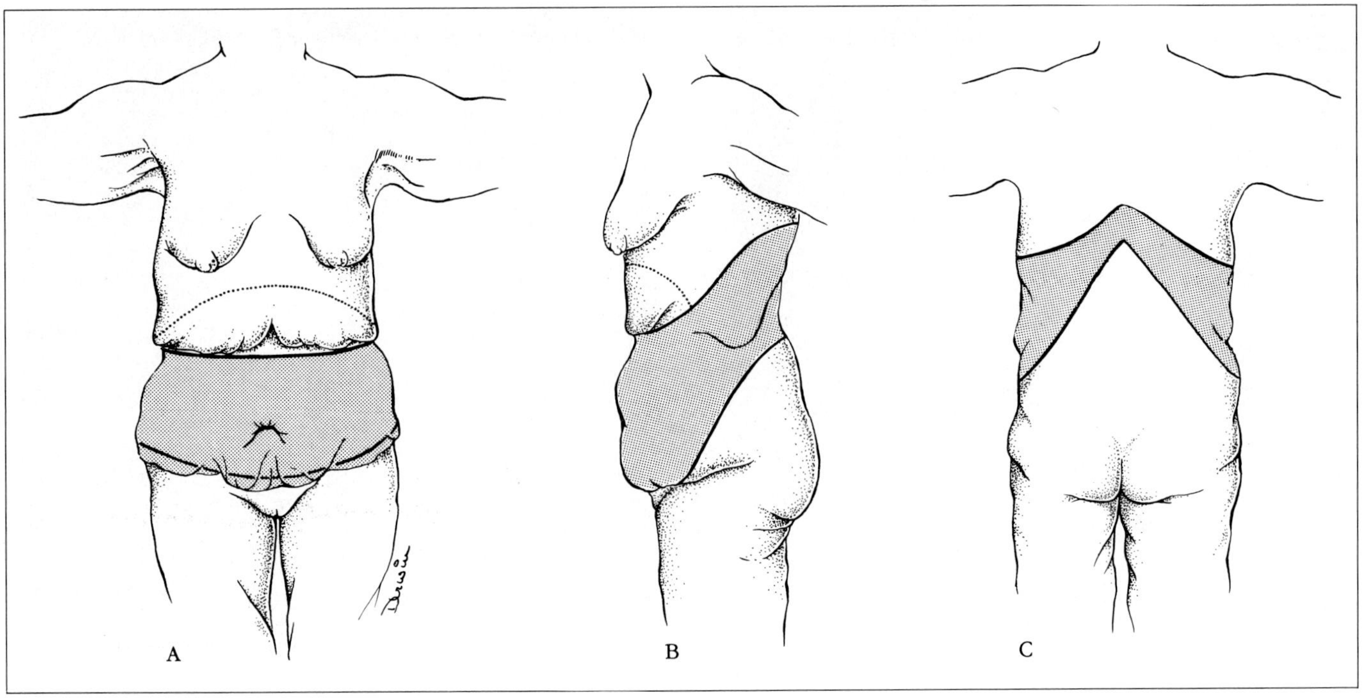

Figure 29-5
A–C. A circular sloping ring belt lipectomy.

ued up to the costal margin. Early splitting of the abdominal flap will facilitate exposure. In contrast to the medial advancement of the lateral flaps in a standard W-plasty, the traction should be vertical in the midline and transverse as one approaches the axillary line. Plication of the abdominal musculature is mandatory. Determination of excess tissue should be by manual approximation and *not* by flexing the operating table or vigorous traction on tissue clamps. After the excision is completed and the new umbilical location selected, the operating table is flexed. Large suction drains are inserted anteriorly. A two-layer closure is done.

BATWING TORSOPLASTY

If the torso deformity is primarily anterolateral rather than circular, the principal excision will extend from the iliac crest along the midaxillary line onto the arm. This technique is particularly valuable when the abdominal redundancy is limited or has been previously excised (Fig. 29-7). If a major abdominal deformity is present and correctable by an anterior approach, it should be dealt with first and the torsoplasty later. In certain patients with small ptotic breasts one can isolate the axillary skin onto the long thoracic vessel, deepithelialize the tissue, and pass it subcutaneously to augment the breasts.

Marking. The patient is examined in the standing position with the arms abducted and the elbows flexed. The ideal placement of the final scar is marked in the midaxillary line (Fig. 29-8). Then the amount of possible tissue excision is estimated and the borders are marked. As one progresses superiorly, the objectives are tightening of any abdominal redundancy, creation of a waistline silhouette, excision of lateral redundant rolls, especially in the breast area, and terminating in a major brachioplasty. The lines of traction required to achieve each of these objectives are marked.

Operation. The patient is placed in a lateral position with the arm freely draped and supported on an overhead arm board. The anterior incision is made down to fascia, and dissection continues posteriorly along the aponeurosis to the anticipated excision line. Undermining is restricted to the expected excision area. Moderate traction is placed on the elevated flap, which is then split segmentally along the premarked lines. Because of the hyperlaxity of the tissue, a greater tension on closure is tolerated than in the moderately obese patient. If the entire area cannot be excised, a new posterior excision line is marked paralleling the preoperative one. As emphasized by Zook [26], the tissue is so redundant that it will "flow" to the most dependent point, thus distorting the deformity and precluding a cut-as-you-go approach; the preoperative markings must be adhered to.

Following excision, meticulous hemostasis is obtained. A modified waistline plication of the external oblique muscle may be performed. The skin closure is done in two layers—a deep layer of interrupted 2-0 Vicryl and then a running subcuticular of 4-0 Vicryl. Drains are rarely required, and the dressing consists of paper tape. During the closure, a second operating table is prepared and a silastic foam mattress is covered with sterile drapes. The patient is then turned over, and a similar procedure is performed on the contralateral side.

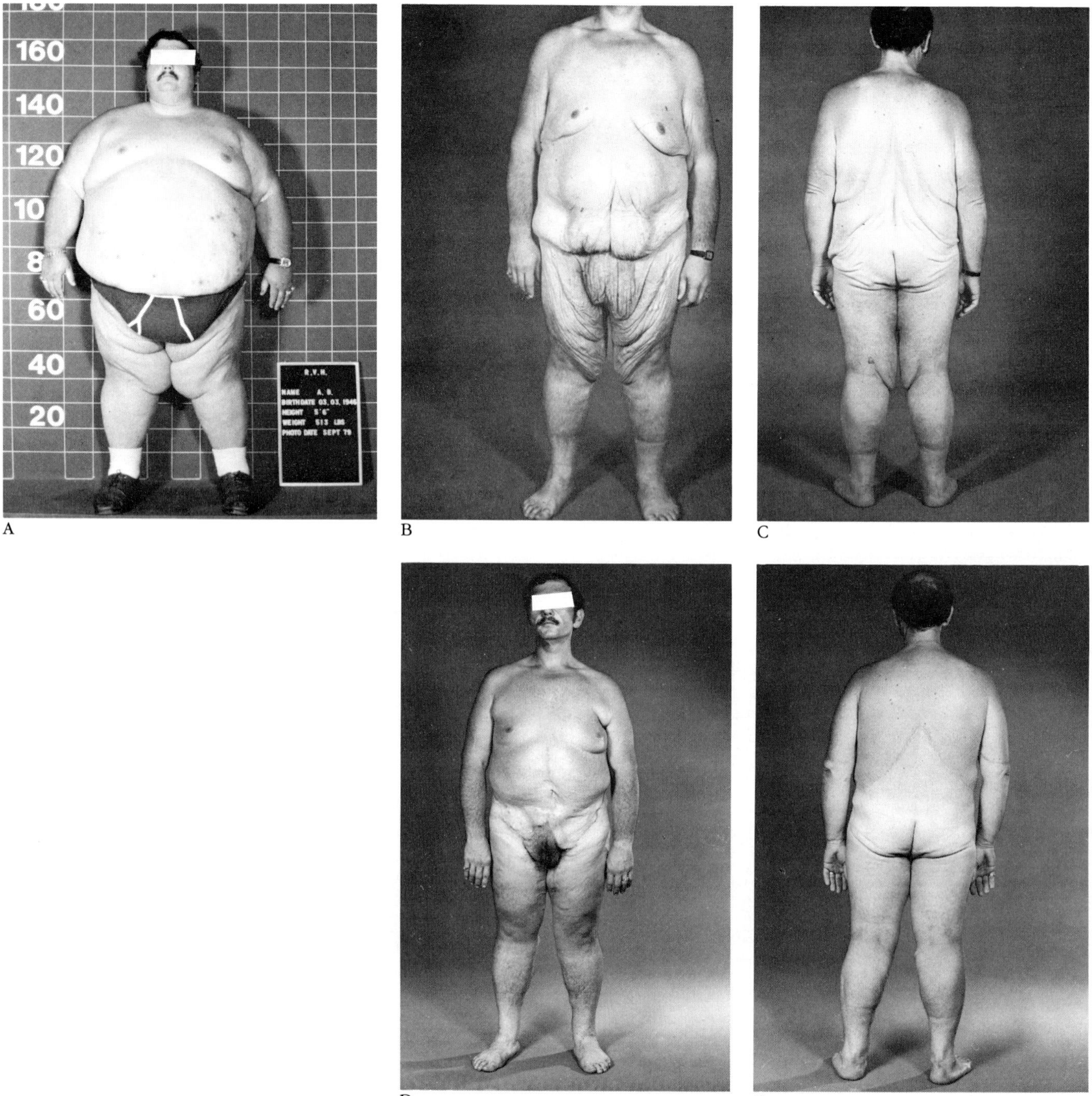

A B C D E

Figure 29-6
A. Morbid obesity.
B, C. Following weight loss (565 : 195 : 142).
D, E. Result following circular lipectomy and limited thigh-lift. Batwing torsoplasty and major brachioplasty are planned.

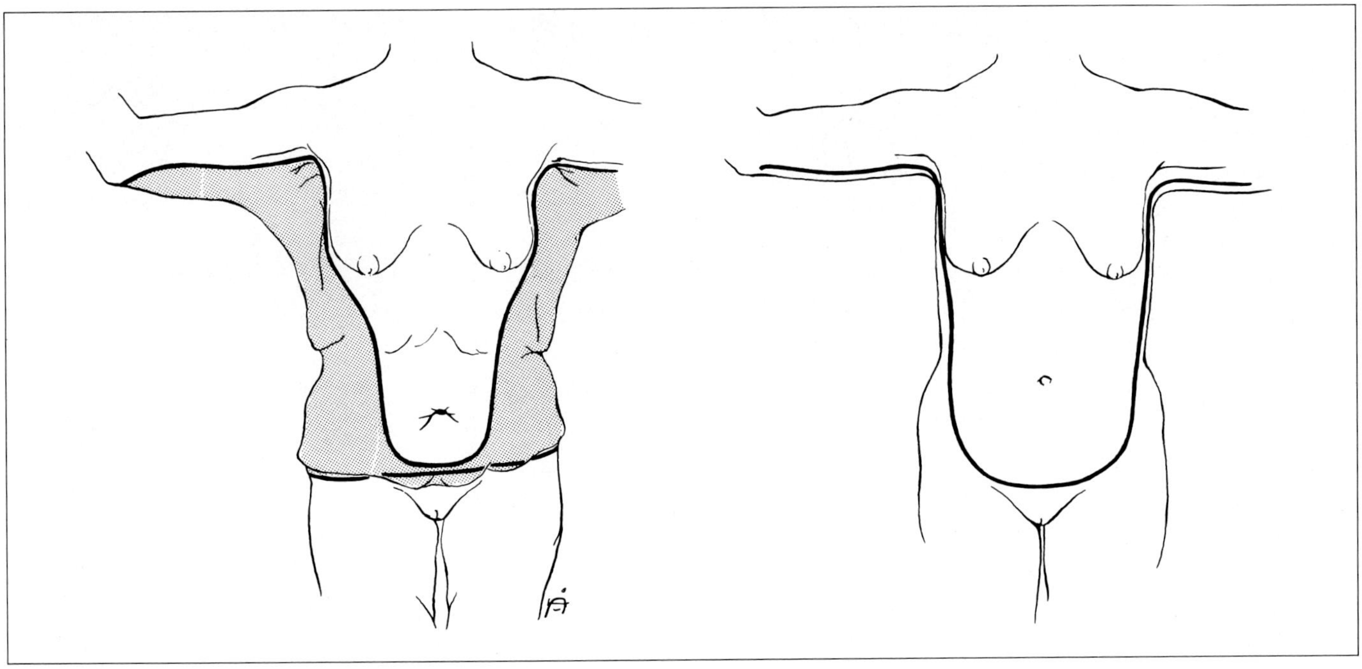

Figure 29-7. Batwing torsoplasty.

Lower Extremity

After massive weight loss, the redundant ptotic thighs are a social limitation and a personal hygiene problem. Correction necessitates a vertical excision plus a circular component ranging from medial to semicircular to complete (Fig. 29-9). Because of the weight loss, the trochanteric fat pad is rarely significant and the redundant buttock folds are minimized by the initial torsoplasty. Anteriorly, the upper incision line is often integrated with the panniculectomy or fleur-de-lis excision. Abnormal skin laxity requires the medial incision to be high enough to prevent subsequent descent and visibility. The vertical incision is placed along the posteromedial aspect of the thigh and turns transversely just above the popliteal fossa. Tightening of the thighs is achieved by direct excision of the transverse redundancy and upward traction on closure. As detailed elsewhere, the operation is begun anteriorly and the excess tissue elevated. The flap is split centrally and then excised as far as possible. The wounds are closed, and the patient is turned to allow completion of the circular excision and the vertical component. Undermining is not done.

Upper Extremity

THORACOBRACHIOPLASTY

In certain cases the upper extremity deformity stops at the axilla whereas in others it continues onto the thorax. If it is limited, a major brachioplasty with traction at the axilla is done (Fig. 29-10). If lateral folds are present along the upper thorax and contiguous with the breasts, a thoracobrachioplasty is recommended (Fig. 29-11). As originally proposed by Pitanguy [22], the incision descends along the posterior axillary line and then turns anteriorly to end in the inframammary sulcus. The amount of tissue to be excised is estimated and the excision line marked. Rather than a simple ellipse, the excision is planned to achieve maximum resection of the transverse folds and elevation of the tissue into the axilla, where a Z-plasty closure prevents longitudinal scar contracture (Fig. 29-12).

In accordance with the preoperative markings, the wound is infiltrated with dilute epinephrine solution (1 : 200,000) and the incision made down to fascia. The dissection continues along the aponeurosis until the posterior excision line is confirmed. Traction in an upward direction is placed on the posterior flap, and the two-layer closure progresses toward the axilla from both ends. A paper tape dressing is applied.

Breasts

In most cases the breasts are very ptotic, with thin skin and little firmness—the "flat pancake breast." Volume must be added to the breast to achieve any degree of upper quadrant fullness and projection. Correction requires a B-technique for major ptosis plus augmentation. The initial incisions are made, and the breast implant (165–350 cc), which has been selected preoperatively, is placed subpectorally. Since most of the patients are large, big implants are easily accommodated. The flaps are then mobilized, and any excess volume is excised from the inferior quadrants. A tight closure is necessary to ensure a supportive skin brassiere.

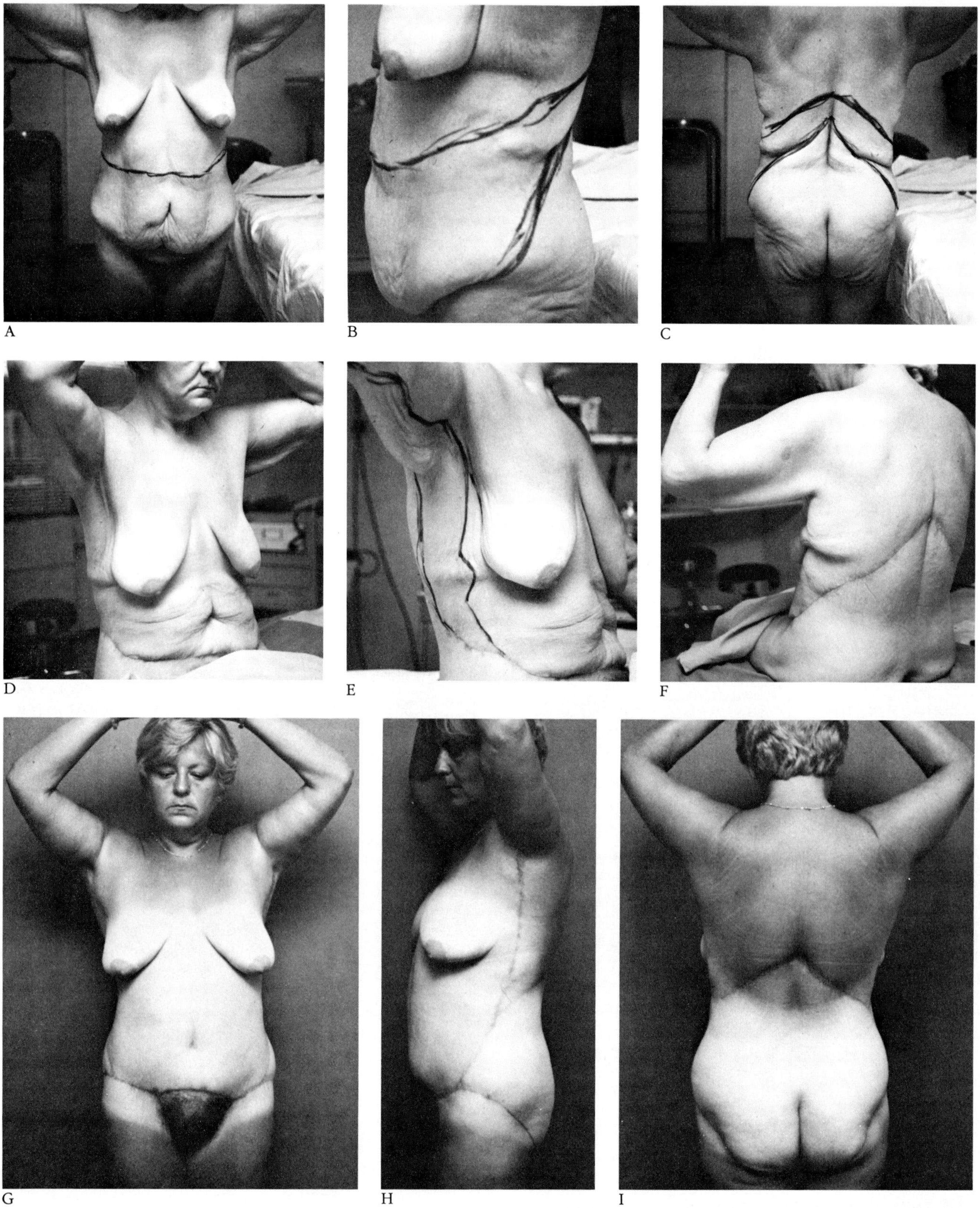

Figure 29-8

A–C. Patient with massive weight loss treated with an initial sloping ring belt lipectomy.

D–F. Outline for a batwing torsoplasty for correction of redundant upper abdominal laxity and upper extremity deformity.

G–I. Final result.

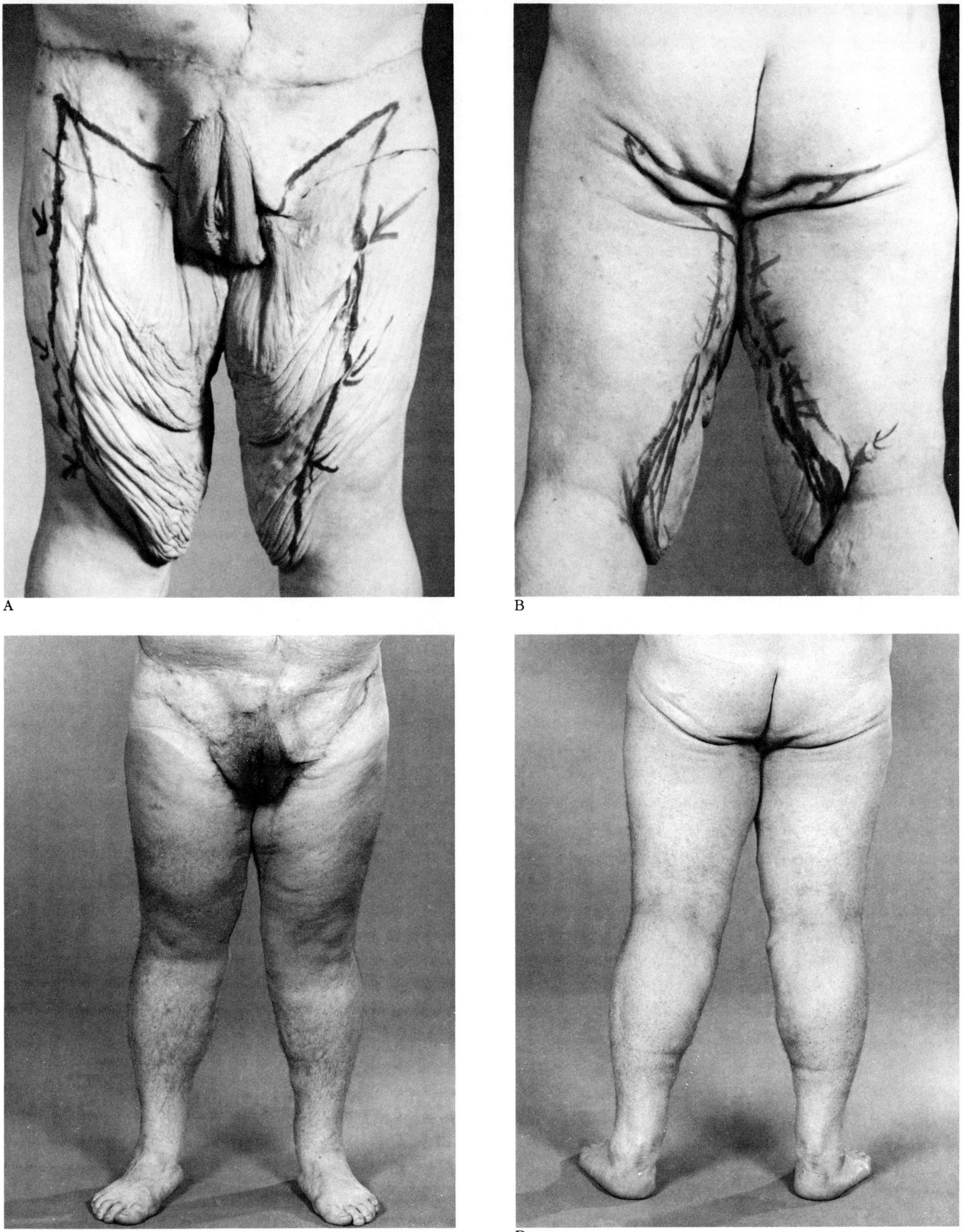

Figure 29-9

A, B. Redundancy of lower extremities in male patient requesting limited incisions.

C, D. Correction achieved with vertical excision and a short semicircular component.

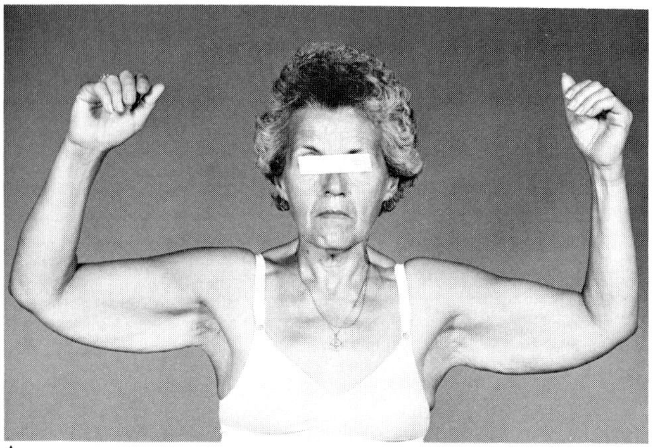

A

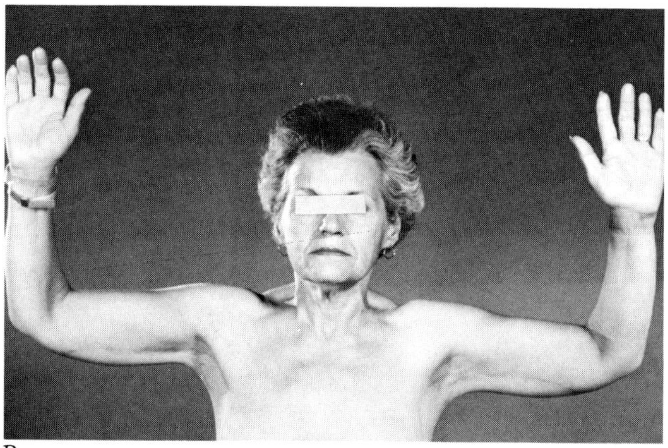

B

Figure 29-10
A. Marked arm flaccidity.
B. Correction achieved with a major brachioplasty.

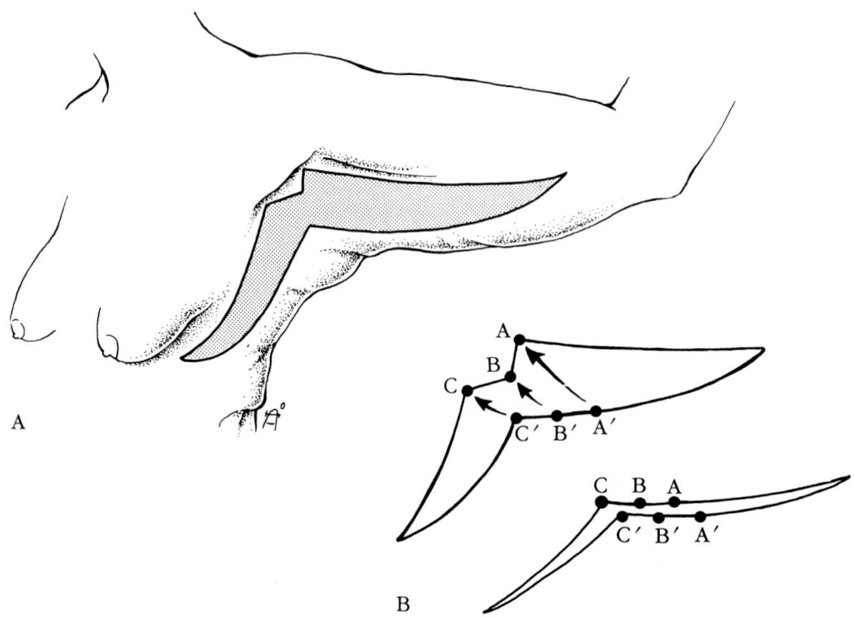

A

B

Figure 29-11
A, B. Thoracobrachioplasty.

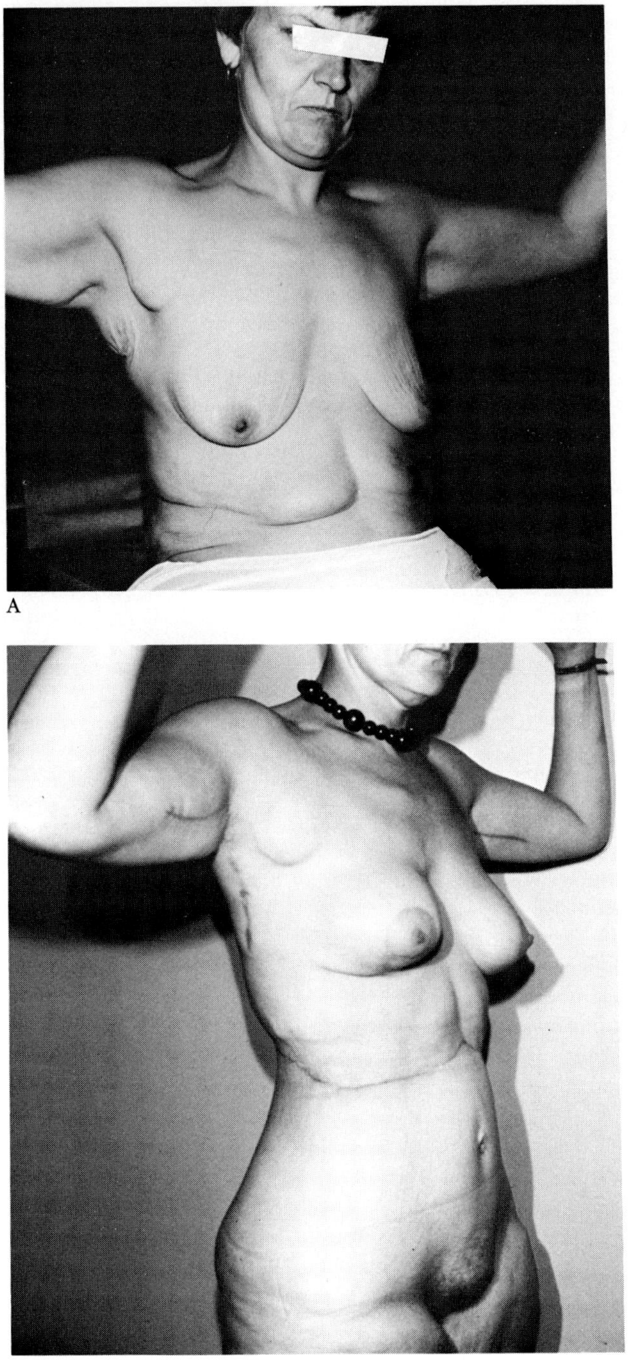

A

B

Figure 29-12

A. Patient requesting correction of upper extremity deformity as well as breast ptosis and upper abdominal redundancy.

B. Following thoracobrachioplasty, B-mastopexy with augmentation, and upper-level abdominoplasty.

As previously noted, transverse axillary folds do not represent a continuation of the breast. One should deal with these by direct excision via a thoracobrachioplasty or lateral torsoplasty, not by extending the breast incisions posteriorly. Later extensions of mammary incisions require patient repositioning and are rarely effective, and they do produce highly visible scars.

Rhytidectomy

The principal deformities are neck folds and sagging of the jowls. A submental incision is used to plicate the platysma, and then extensive undermining is done to allow removal of excess skin. The need for lipectomy is assessed directly but correlates with current ideal weight ratio. A tight closure is well tolerated, and the improvement is often dramatic.

COMPLICATIONS

Characteristic complications can be expected from each surgical procedure. However, the incidence is decreased because of limited undermining and skin extensibility. Importantly, hypertrophic scars occur infrequently, and patient acceptance is forthcoming. A subgroup forming an exception to this favorable situation is made up of patients who have undergone a massive weight loss but remain markedly overweight. Lipectomies rather than excision of skin redundancies are required, with their associated morbidity. If possible, one should perform only a panniculectomy, deferring additional body contouring until additional weight is lost.

RESULTS

In the short term, most patients are extremely pleased with their new contour, ease of purchasing clothes, and improved life-style. Since most bypass procedures are permanent, patients do not regain their weight, the obvious exception being the subgroup in whom the bypass was partially successful or subsequently failed. Long-term results will reflect the patient's psychologic adjustments and successful resolution of internal conflicts. It is tempting to speculate that body changes will be more permanent in females than males on account of social pressure.

SECONDARY SURGERY

Secondary procedures constitute limited revision (scars, dog-ears, bulges) of body contouring procedures or incorporation of previous panniculectomies into well-conceived torsoplasties. In most cases general surgeons will perform a transverse elliptic excision, stopping at the lateral limits of the operating table and sacrificing the umbilicus. The result is residual deformities in the epigastric region, flanks, and back. The solution is often an extended fleur-de-lis or belt torsoplasty, with umbilical reconstruction an appreciated addition.

REFERENCES

1. Bjorntorp, P. Effects of age, sex, and clinical conditions on adipose tissue cellularity in man. *Metabolism* 23:1091, 1974.
2. Bjorntorp, P., et al. Adipose tissue fat cell size and number in relation to metabolism in randomly selected middle-aged men and women. *Metabolism* 20:927, 1971.
3. Castle, H. E. Obesity and its surgical treatment by lipectomy. *Ann. Surg.* 54:706, 1911.
4. Clarkson, P. Lipodystrophies. *Plast. Reconstr. Surg.* 37:499, 1966.
5. Clarkson, P., and Jeffs, J. The Contribution of Plastic Surgery to the Treatment of Obesity. In T. Gibson (ed.), *Modern Trends in Plastic Surgery.* London: Butterworth, 1966.
6. Faust, I. M., Johnson, P. R., and Hirsch, J. Adipose tissue regeneration following lipectomy. *Science* 197:301, 1977.
7. Foged, J. Operative treatment of abdominal obesity especially pendulous abdomen. *Br. J. Plast. Surg.* 1:274, 1949.
8. Goin, J. M., and Goin, M. K. *Changing the Body: Psychological Effects of Plastic Surgery.* Baltimore: Williams & Wilkins, 1981.
9. Gonzalez-Ulloa, M. Belt lipectomy. *Br. J. Plast. Surg.* 13:179, 1960.
10. Jones, L. J., and Boines, G. J. Rehabilitation in obesity by lipectomy. *Del. Med. J.* 18:161, 1946.
11. Kamper, M. J., Galloway, D., and Ashley, F. Abdominal panniculectomy after massive weight loss. *Plast. Reconstr. Surg.* 50:441, 1972.
12. Knittle, J. L., and Ginsberg-Fellner, F. Effect of weight reduction on in vitro adipose tissue lipolysis and cellularity in obese adolescents and adults. *Diabetes* 21:754, 1972.
13. Larkin, C. N. Lipectomy for abdominal fat. *Conn. Med. J.* 7:706, 1950.
14. MacLean, L. D., Rhode, B. M., and Shizgal, H. M. Gastroplasty for obesity. *Surg. Gynecol. Obstet.* 153:200, 1981.
15. Mann, G. V. The influence of obesity on health. *N. Engl. J. Med.* 291:178, 1974.
16. Mason, J. K. Lipectomy: The surgical removal of excessive fat. *Postgrad. Med.* 32:381, 1962.
17. McCraw, L. H. Surgical rehabilitation after massive weight reduction. Case report. *Plast. Reconstr. Surg.* 53:349, 1974.
18. Meyerowitz, B. R., et al. From massive weight loss to abdominal panniculectomy. *R.N.* 37:1, 1974.
19. Palmer, B., et al. Skin reduction plasties following intestinal shunt operations for treatment of obesity. *Scand. J. Plast. Reconstr. Surg.* 9:47, 1975.
20. Passot, R. Correction Esthétique des Adiposités Localisées. In *Chirurgie Esthétique Pure.* Paris: Doin, 1931. Vol. 22.
21. Payne, J. H., et al. Metabolic observations in patients with jejunocolic shunt. *Am. J. Surg.* 106:273, 1963.
22. Pitanguy, I. Dermolipectomy of the Abdominal Wall, Thigh, Buttocks, and Upper Extremity. In J. M. Converse (ed.), *Reconstructive Plastic Surgery* (2nd ed.). Philadelphia: Saunders, 1977.
23. Regnault, P. Lipectomy. In W. C. Grabb and J. W. Smith (eds.), *Plastic Surgery.* Boston: Little, Brown, 1979.
24. Schwartz, A. W. Technique for excision of abdominal fat. *Br. J. Plast. Surg.* 27:44, 1974.
25. Sjostrom, L., et al. Cellularity in different regions of adipose tissue in young men and women. *Metabolism* 21:1143, 1972.
26. Zook, E. G. The massive weight loss patient. *Clin. Plast. Surg.* 2:457, 1975.
27. Zook, E. G. Thigh and Buttock Contouring. In E. H. Courtiss (ed.), *Male Aesthetic Surgery.* St. Louis: Mosby, 1982.

Appendix

PHOTOGRAPHIC CONSENT FORM USED BY THE AUTHOR

Photographic Consent

Patient: ______________________________

Date: ______________

In connection with the plastic surgical services which I am receiving from Dr. Morello, I consent that photographs may be taken of me or parts of my body, under the following conditions:

1. These photographs may be taken only with the consent of Dr. Morello and under such conditions and at such times as may be approved by him.
2. The photographs may be taken by Dr. Morello or by someone approved by him.
3. The photographs shall be used for medical records and if in the judgment of Dr. Morello, medical research, education, or science will be benefited by their use, such photographs and information relating to my case may be published and republished in medical journals or books or used for any other purpose he may deem proper in the interest of medical education, knowledge or research; provided, however, that it is specifically understood that I will not be identified by name.

Signed ______________________
(patient)

Witness ______________________

AMA STANDARD PHOTOGRAPHIC CONSENT FORM

Consent to Taking and Publication of Photographs

Patient ______________________________

Place ______________________________

Date ______________

In connection with the medical services which I am receiving from my physician, Dr. ______________, I consent that photographs may be taken of me or parts of my body, under the following conditions:

1. These photographs may be taken only with the consent of my physician and under such conditions and at such times as may be approved by him.
2. The photographs shall be taken by my physician or by a photographer approved by my physician.
3. The photographs shall be used for medical records and if in the judgment of my physician, medical research, education or science will be benefited by their use, such photographs and information relating to my case may be published and republished, either separately or in connection with each other, in professional journals or medical books, or used for any other purpose which he may deem proper in the interest of medical education, knowledge, or research; provided, however, that it is specifically understood that in any such publication or use I shall not be identified by name.
4. The aforementioned photographs may be modified or retouched in any way that my physician, in his discretion, may consider desirable.

Signed ______________________
(patient)

Witness ______________________

ASPRS PHOTOGRAPHIC CONSENT FORM

Patient Photographic Release Form

I hereby acknowledge that I have been advised by Dr. ______________ that photographs are to be taken of me or parts of my body which, together with details regarding medical services rendered to me, may be used by Dr. ______________ or the American Society of Plastic and Reconstructive Surgeons, Inc. (ASPRS) for public information purposes.

I hereby consent and agree that:

1. Photographs may be taken of me or parts of my body with the consent of Dr. ______________ and under such conditions and at such times as may be approved by Dr. ______________.
2. Such photographs shall be taken by Dr. ______________ or by a photographer approved by Dr. ______________ and may be modified or retouched in any way that Dr. ______________, in his/her discretion, deems desirable.
3. Such photographs and/or details regarding medical services that I have received may be shown, printed, or broadcast by Dr. ______________, or by the ASPRS, in any print or broadcast media, including but not necessarily limited to newspapers, pamphlets, educational films, and television, in order to inform the public about plastic surgery methods.
4. I release and discharge Dr. ______________ and the ASPRS, and all parties acting under their license and authority, from any and all claims or actions that I have or may have relating to such use and publication, and all rights, if any, that I may have in such photographs and details regarding medical services rendered me, including any claim for payment, in connection with any such use or publication.

I grant this consent as a voluntary contribution in the interest of public education, and my consent is subject only to the condition that I not be identified by name at any time during any use or publication by Dr. ______________ or by the ASPRS of these materials.

Dated: ______________________________ Patient ______________________________

____

Witness

____

Witness

(This form may be duplicated.)

Index

Index

Abdominoplasty, 617–638. *See also* Lipectomy, abdominal
- abnormal umbilicus with, 649
- aesthetic goals for, 621
- anatomy for, 622, 623
- with augmentation mammaplasty, 635, 636
- closure in, 627, 629, 632
- defined, 617
- early examples of, 8, 20
- hematoma and seroma with, 647
- history of, 617, 619
- incisions for, 617, 618, 619, 624, 625
- indications and contraindications for, 619, 621
- infection with, 647
- informed consent for, 621
- intraoperative complications, 647
- liposuction with, 680
- male, 632
- markings for, 624
- with mastopexy or breast reduction, 635, 637
- modifications for scars, 635, 638, 639
- motivation for, 621
- nerve injury with, 649
- pathophysiology and classification for, 619
- patient history for, 621
- persistent edema with, 649
- physical examination for, 621
- plication in, 624, 625
- preoperative preparations, 621–622
- preoperative screening for, 648–649
- resection in, 624, 627
- results of, 649
- scars with, 649
- secondary surgery to, 649, 650
- skin necrosis with, 647–648
- stitch and wound problems, 647
- thrombophlebitis and pulmonary embolus with, 648–649
- umbilicoplasty with, 627, 628, 630, 650, 651, 652
- undermining in, 624, 625
- W-plasty technique, 624, 625, 629–632, 633, 634

Acne scars
- chemical peeling for scars, 465, 473
- choice of treatment for, 494

Adipocyte theory, 687, 691

Adrenergic-blocking agents, preoperative use of, 78–79

Advisers, professional, 58

Aesthetic goals
- for abdominoplasty, 621
- for brachioplasty, 695
- for breast asymmetry treatment, 598
- for breast augmentation, 563
- for lower extremity dermolipectomy, 658–659
- after weight loss contouring, 708

Aesthetics, of rhinoplasty, 122–126

Aesthetic surgery
- characteristics of, 32–34
- defined, 31
- history of, 3–26

Aging, of face
- bone changes, 377–378
- causes of, 450

Ala
- collapsing, 210–211
- depressions on, 211

Alar lobule, anatomy of, 119–120

Alar rims
- alteration to, 180
- anatomy of, 175
- deformities of, 176

Aliphatics, preoperative use of, 77

Alopecia. *See* Hair loss

Alpha blocking agents, effects of, 78

Alphaprodine (Nisenti), 77

Analgesia
- for blepharoplasty, 359
- preoperative use of, 76–77

Anatomy
- of abdomen, 622, 623
- of arms, 695
- of breast, 500, 504–506
- of eyelids, 288, 347, 350–352
- of face, 372–374, 452–453
- of lower extremities, 659
- of nipple, 609
- of nose, 109, 110, 111
- for superficial fascia rhytidectomy, 422–423, 424, 425

Anesthesia
- for abdominoplasty, 630
- action and types of, 79–80
- for augmentation mammaplasty, 81
- for blepharoplasty, 81, 288–289, 322, 359
- for brachioplasty, 698
- for breast augmentation, 568, 569
- for chin advancement, 224
- for face-lifts, 80
- for forehead-lift, 311
- for male face-lift, 454–455
- for mastopexy, 546
- for otoplasty, 247, 253
- for rhinoplasty, 81, 126–127, 146, 161
- for superficial fascia rhytidectomy, 426

Ankle
- dermolipectomy on, 671
- liposuction on, 680

Anthelix (of ear)
- aesthetic goals for, 250
- evaluation of, 247, 248, 249
- historical treatment of, 252
- reconstruction of, 252, 253, 256, 257, 259, 264, 265

Antiadrenergics, preoperative use of, 78–79

Antibiotics, for lower extremity dermolipectomy, 664

Anticholinergics, preoperative use of, 78

Antihistamines, preoperative use of, 77
Aplasia
  and breast augmentation, 560
  defined, 595
Architect (for office construction), 46–47
Areola
  deformities of, 610, 613
  herniation of, 606
Arms. *See also* Brachioplasty
  anatomy of, 695
  liposuction on, 680
Aspiradeps, 681
Aspirin, contraindications for prior to surgery, 452
Atropine, preoperative use of, 76
Augmentation surgery. *See also* Breast augmentation substances used for, 22
Authorization forms, 452

B-technique
  mastopexy, 547, 548, 549
  reduction mammaplasty, 508–521
Bacitracin, for breast augmentation, 569
Banking, of cartilage and bone, 145
Barbiturates
  for blepharoplasty, 288, 289
  preoperative use of, 77
Basch procedure, 609
Benzodiazepine drugs, preoperative use of, 77
Beta-adrenergic–blocking agents, effects of, 78
Billing. *See* Cost accounting, for office surgery
Bleeding. *See also* Hemorrhage
  with breast augmentation, 582
  during rhytidectomy, 409
Blepharocanthoplasty, 299
Blepharochalasis, defined, 326
Blepharoplasty. *See also* Eyelids; Eyes
  aesthetic goals in, 328
  analgesia for, 359
  anatomy for, 288
  anesthesia for, 288–289, 332, 359
  chemical peel with, 341
  clinical examples, 362–367
  complications with, 293–294, 342–343
  contouring in, 359
  deformity classification, 326
  dressings for, 340, 362
  earliest, 15
  eyebrow-lift, 341
  festoons, 296, 298, 341
  with forehead-lift, 308, 309, 315, 318
  Gonzalez-Ulloa procedure, 299, 301
  history of, 287, 288, 325–326
  indications and contraindications for, 326
  instruments for, 359
  Kuhnt-Szymanowski procedure, 340–341
  in lateral region, 299
  lower lid correction, 291, 292, 358–359
  for male, 460, 462
Blepharoplasty—*Continued*
  markings for, 289, 332–333, 334, 359
  medications for, 81
  motivation for, 326, 353
  in older patient, 340, 358
  on Orientals, 356
  patient history for, 326, 353
  in periorbital region, 294–298
  photography for, 328
  physical examination for, 327, 353–354
  postoperative care, 293, 342–343
  ptosis correction, 341–342, 356
  results of, 343, 348, 349
  sequence in, 328
  standard, 335–340
  surgical principles for, 330–332
  surgical technique, 289, 290, 291, 359, 360, 361
  suturing for, 335, 359, 362
  tests for, 327–328
  timing of, 328
  on upper eyelid, 298–299, 354–358
    crow's feet excision, 354–355, 356
    preorbital resection, 354–355
    preseptal resection, 354
    pretarsal and preorbital smoothing, 355–356
    ptotic lid elevation, 356
    raising foundation, 354
    surgical fold security, 356–358
  in younger patient, 340
Blepharoptosis, test for, 328
Body contouring, total. *See* Weight loss, massive
Bone
  aging changes of facial, 377–378
  of nose, 110, 111–115
  postrhinoplasty deformities of, 214, 216
Brachioplasty, 693–704
  aesthetic goals for, 695
  anatomy for, 695
  anesthesia for, 698
  complications with, 702–704
  on hands, 700, 702
  history of, 693
  incisions for, 696–697, 698
  indications and contraindications for, 694
  informed consent for, 695
  major, 699, 700
  markings for, 696–697, 700
  minor and moderate, 698–699
  motivation for, 694–695
  pathophysiology and classification for, 693–694
  patient instructions for, 695
  patient's history for, 694
  physical examination for, 695
  postmassive weight loss, 715, 718, 719
  preaxilloplasty, 696–700, 701, 702
  procedure, 697, 698
  results of, 704
  scars with, 695, 703
  secondary surgery after, 704
Breast asymmetry treatment, 595–606
  aesthetic goals for, 598
Breast asymmetry treatment—*Continued*
  for breast and musculoskeletal deformities, 604
  complications with, 606
  history of, 595
  for hypertrophy and hypertrophy, 599, 603
  for hypertrophy and normal, 599, 602
  for hypoplasia and hypoplasia, 596, 598–599, 601
  for hypoplasia and normal, 596, 598, 600
  for hypoplasty and hypertrophy, 604
  indications and contraindications for, 597
  motivation for, 597–598
  pathophysiology and classification of, 595, 597
  patient history for, 597
  physical examination for, 598
  principles of surgery, 598
Breast augmentation, 559–593. *See also* Breast asymmetry treatment
  with abdominoplasty, 635, 636
  aesthetic goals for, 563
  anesthesia for, 569, 573
  capsular contraction from, 575, 576, 582, 585–586, 587, 588, 589
  capsulotomy for, 570, 571, 585, 586, 587
  erosion with, 585
  hemostasis for, 569
  history of, 559
  indications and contraindications for, 560
  informed consent for, 563–564
  inframammary approach, 564–568
  motivation for, 562
  partial retropectoral placement with, 564, 565, 566, 567, 568–569
  pathophysiology and classification for, 560, 561
  patient history for, 560
  periareolar approach, 565, 569–570
  physical examination for, 562–563
  prostheses for, 566
  prosthesis leakage with, 584–585
  results of, 586–587
  scars with, 564
  secondary surgery after, 587
  shape deformities with, 583
  TASPMA (transaxillary subpectoral mammary augmentation), 572–586
  with tuberous breast correction, 606
Breast reduction
  with abdominoplasty, 635
  aesthetic goals for, 504
  B-technique, 508–521
  complications with, 530–533
  excisional volume estimate, 500–501
  free nipple graft, 526–528
  glandular resection, 508
  history of, 499–500
  hypertrophy pathophysiology, 500–501, 502

Breast reduction—*Continued*
indications and contraindications for, 501
inferior pedicle technique, 522–526
informed consent for, 504
markings for, general, 506, 508
motivation for, 501–503
nipple transposition, 508
objectives of, 506, 508
patient history for, 501
physical examination for, 503–504
preoperative instructions, 504
ptotic breast, 506
results of, 533
secondary surgery, 534, 536
skin brassiere determination, 508
volume reduction, 528–529
Breasts
anatomy of, 500, 504–506, 539–540
axillary, 529–530
deformities of, 606–613
development of, 595
hypertrophy of, 500–501
implants, 543–544, 546. *See also* Protheses
liposuction on, 680
postmassive weight loss correction of, 715, 719
postreduction deformities of, 533
ptotic, 504, 506, 540, 557, 606
ptotic, mastopexy for, 539–558
size determination, 503–504
tuberous, 606, 607, 608
webbed, 529
Bupivacaine (Marcaine)
for face-lift, 454
metabolization of, 79
Buttocks
augmentation of, 662
deformities of, 661–662
liposuction on, 680
Butyrophenones, preoperative use of, 78
Bypass surgery, intestinal, 706–707

Calf
dermolipectomy on, 670
liposuction on, 680
Cameras, for clinical photography, 83, 85
Capsular contracture, with breast augmentation, 575, 576, 580, 582, 585–586
Capsulectomy, 587
Capsulotomy, 570, 571, 585, 586, 587
Carbolic acid, for chemical peeling, 463
Cartilage, crushing, for grafts, 194, 197
Cartilage, ear, in otoplasty, 251
Cartilage, nasal
alar, 114–118, 128
excessive resection of alar, 203
lower lateral, 174–175
overlapping, 185, 187, 190, 191
postrhinoplasty correction of, 209–212
quadrangular, 110
sesamoid, 114
Cartilaginous vault, of nose, anatomy of, 110, 111, 114–115
Cellulite
defined, 656
and surgical results, 658
Cellusactiotome, 686
Cephalosporin
for abdominoplasty, 630
with breast augmentation, 575–576
Cervicomental angle
creation of, 389, 390
improvement of, 398
normal versus obtuse, 377
Cheeks
collagen for furrows, 490–491
evaluation of, 275
liposuction on, 680
Cheiloplasty, augmentation, 484–485
Chemical face peeling, 341, 463–482
for chin wrinkles, 495
complications with, 476–477, 479
formula for, 466
histologic skin changes with, 476
history of, 463–464
information prior to procedure, 465–466
for lip wrinkles, 495
mask application and removal, 467, 468, 476
mixture application, 466–468
patient selection for, 464–465, 480
for pigmentation problems, 471–472
posttreatment care, 468–469
preparation for, 466
regional, 471
with rhytidectomy, 470–471
secondary procedure, 478, 479
sun exposure care, 469
systemic toxicity with, 476
terminology of, 463
thymol iodide powder application and removal, 468
Chin
anatomy of, 221–222
deviation classification and pathophysiology, 222
double, history of, 14, 15, 16
implant, 462
surgical procedures on, 398
witch's chin deformity, 401, 404
wrinkle treatment, 495
Chin, aesthetic procedures on, 221–244. *See also* Mentoplasty
advancement, 224, 225, 226, 227, 228, 239, 240
anesthesia for, 224
complications for, 240, 241, 242, 243, 244
sagittal
maximum, 234
minor, 230
moderate, 230–234
asymmetric deformities, 240
augmentation with alloplastics, 223, 224
combined, 240
consultation on, 223
history of, 221
reduction, 234
Chin, aesthetic procedures on—*Continued*
secondary surgery for, 244
vertical increase, 237, 238, 239
vertical shortening, 234, 235, 236, 237
Chloral hydrate, preoperative use of, 77, 80
Chlordiazepoxide hydrochloride (Librium), 77
Chloroprocaine (Nesacaine), action of, 79
Chlorpromazine (Thorazine)
for hypertension, 459
preoperative use of, 77–78
Chlorprothixine (Taractan), preoperative use of, 78
Circulatory system
of abdomen, 622
in breast, 504–505
in eye, 330
in forehead, 305–306
of lower extremities, 659
in nose, 120–121
Closure. *See also* Sutures
with breast reduction, 508
in lower extremity dermolipectomy, 661
for temple-lift, 394
Cocaine, for rhinoplasty, 126
Coefficient of Hoyer, 693
Collagen injection
for acne scars, 494
versus aesthetic surgery, 490–491
complications with, 490, 491
for contour irregularities, 460
for forehead creases, 490
for glabellar frown lines, 305
indications for, 489, 490
lesion selection, 490
long-term efficacy of, 491
method, 490
for neck creases, 490
patient selection for, 489
for periorbital wrinkles, 490
principles of, 489, 490
for solar exposure wrinkles, 494
Color coding, of charts, 54
Columella
aesthetics of, 122, 126
alterations to, 136
anatomy of, 116
deformities of, 176
hanging, 135, 179
hidden, 212, 213
recessed, 178–179
uncompensated short, 203
Communications, office, 54, 69
forms for, 54–58
Complications
with abdominoplasty, 647–649
with blepharoplasty, 293–294, 342–343
with brachioplasty, 702–704
with breast asymmetry treatment, 606
with breast augmentation, 575, 582–586
with breast reduction, 530–533

Complications — *Continued*
of chin advancements, 240–244
with collagen injections, 491
with dermolipectomy, 675–676
with forehead-lift, 320–322
with lipectomy, 435
with malar surgery, 283–284
with male face-lift, 459–460
with mastopexy, 555
with otoplasty, 267, 270, 272, 273
with platysma muscle resectioning, 411, 437, 438
with rhytidectomy, 379–380, 409–413
with suction lipectomy, 684–685, 690
with superficial fascia rhytidectomy, 429, 432–433
Concha, of ear
evaluation of, 249–250
historical treatment of, 252
positioning of, 253
reconstruction of, 253, 255
repositioning of, 258, 262, 263, 264, 265, 267
reduction of, 252, 258, 260, 261, 266, 267
Conjunctiva, anatomy of, 352
Consent, informed
for abdominoplasty, 621
for brachioplasty, 695
for breast augmentation, 563
for breast reduction, 504
for face-lift, 451–452
for forehead-lift, 310
forms for
ambulatory surgery, 70
photography, 723–724
for lower extremity dermolipectomy, 659
for mastopexy, 543
for postweight loss contouring, 708
for rhinoplasty, 108–109
for rhytidectomy, 379–380
Consultation, initial, 39
Consultation room, 49
Contour deformities
collagen for, 491, 493
after face-lift, 460
Contracts, for office construction, 46–47
Controlled substances, maintenance of, 59, 70
Corrugator muscle
anatomy of, 305
excision of, 315
resection of, 303, 304
Cosmetic surgery, defined, 31
Cost accounting, for office surgery, 72–73
Coumadin, for thrombophlebitis, 649
Crest, of nose
deformities of, 183, 184, 185
surgical techniques for, 185, 187, 188, 190
Crow's-feet
causes of, 352
choice of techniques for, 495
collagen injection for, 490
defined, 326
elimination of, 299, 300, 354–355, 356
Crow's-feet — *Continued*
Gonzalez-Ulloa procedure for, 299, 301
temple-lift for, 394, 395
Crus, of nose, 174–175
Crus, superior, 259, 266
Curet, uterine, 681
Cysts, postblepharoplasty, 294

Darwin's tubercle, 250, 253, 267, 268
Deformities, nasal
curved, 185, 187, 189
of nasal tip, 175–176
overlappings, 185, 187, 190, 191
saddlenose, 197, 198, 199
transnostril foreign body, 183, 184, 185
vertical crest, 183, 184, 185, 187, 188
Deformities, facial, classification of, 450
Depo-Medrol, 569
Dercum's disease, 687
Dermabrasion
for acne scars, 494
for solar exposure wrinkles, 494
Dermatochalasis, 326, 621
Dermolipectomy, abdominal. *See also* Abdominoplasty; Lipectomy, abdominal
defined, 617
history of, 617
Dermolipectomy, lower extremity, 655–678
aesthetic goals for, 658–659
anatomy for, 659
ankle, 671
buttock deformity, 661–662
calf, 670
circular thigh reduction, 666, 667, 671
classification and pathophysiology for, 656, 657
closure in, 661
complications with, 675–676
difficulties with, 658
generalized deformities, 662–663
gluteal depression, 667, 668, 669, 671, 676
history of, 655–656
incisions for, 659–660, 661, 664
indications and contraindications for, 658
informed consent for, 659
marking for, 664, 667, 673, 674
medial thigh deformity, 661
motivation for, 658
patient history for, 658
physical examination for, 658
popliteal area, 670, 675
preoperative preparations, 659, 664
resection in, 660
results of, 676
scars for, 659, 675
secondary surgery after, 676, 677
semicircular thigh resection, 663–665, 671
suction-assisted, 671. *See also* Lipectomy, suction
suspension in, 661
trochanteric deformities, 662–663, 667, 670, 671
trochanteric lipodystrophy, 676
Dermolipectomy, lower extremity — *Continued*
undermining in, 660
vertical extensions, 670–671, 672, 674
Diazepam (Valium)
for blepharoplasty, 289
for breast augmentation, 568, 569, 573
for chemical peel, 466
for face-lift, 454
with ketamine, 79–80
for preoperative anxiety, 80
preoperative use of, 77
for toxic reaction, 79
Dicloxacillin, for breast augmentation infection, 583
Dingman otoabrader, 253, 258
Diphenhydramine (Benadryl), preoperative use of, 77
Doctor-patient relationship, 34–35
Dome, of nasal tip
anatomy of, 174
defined, 115
Dopamine, preoperative use of, 78
Dorsum
aesthetics of, 122
anatomy of, 110
grafts to, 156
Dow-Corning breast prosthesis, 576, 577
Dressings
for abdominoplasty, 632
in B-technique reduction mammaplasty, 509
for blepharoplasty, 340, 362
for face-lift, 459
for forehead-lift, 315
for liposuction, 684, 689, 690
for lower extremity dermolipectomy, 664, 665
nasal packing, 191
for otoplasty, 267, 271
for rhinoplasty, 145–146
Drugs. *See* Anesthesia; *specific drugs*
for rhytidectomy, 390
Drugs, for outpatient surgery, 75–82
for augmentation mammoplasty, 81
for blepharoplasty, 81
for face-lifts, 80
local anesthetics, 79
prior to surgery, 76–79
for rhinoplasty, 81
Dry eye syndrome
postblepharoplasty, 293, 326
Schirmer test for, 327
Dye tests (for lacrimal drainage), 327–328

Ears. *See also* Otoplasty
aesthetics of, 250–251
protruding, early history of correction, 5
symmetry of, 251
Ebers papyrus, 463
Ecchymosis
with nasal tip rhinoplasty, 181
with rhinoplasty, 162
Ectropion, with blepharoplasty, 293
Edema
with abdominal lipectomy, 649
with brachioplasty, 703

Edema — *Continued*
with face-lift, 460
with lower extremity dermolipectomy, 675–676
with nasal tip rhinoplasty, 181
with rhinoplasty, 162
with rhytidectomy, 412
Egyptians, 463
Electrocardiogram (ECG) equipment, 81
Electrocautery equipment, 68
Electrocoagulation, with breast augmentation, 569
Electromyography (EMG), for paralysis from forehead-lift, 321
Endocrine, and breast hypertrophy, 500
Enophthalmos, with blepharoplasty, 294
Epinephrine
for blepharoplasty, 289, 291, 359
with blepharoplasty, 332
for brachioplasty, 698
for breast augmentation, 568, 569, 573
for face-lift, 454–455
for forehead-lift, 311
for hemostasis, 455, 508
for lower extremity dermolipectomy, 661
for mastopexy, 546
for otoplasty, 253
preoperative use of, 78
for rhytidectomy, 380, 426
for thoracobrachioplasty, 715
Epistaxis, postrhinoplasty, 161
Equipment
monitoring, 81
for surgery, 67–68
Escherichia coli, in wound infection, 433
Ethchlorvynol (Placidyl), preoperative use of, 77
Ethnoid plate, of nose, 110
Examination, physical
for abdominoplasty, 621
for blepharoplasty, 327, 353–354
for brachioplasty, 695
for breast augmentation, 562–563
for breast asymmetry correction, 598
for face-lift, 450–451
general, 39
for lower extremity dermolipectomy, 658
for mastopexy, 543
of nasal tip, 173–174
for reduction mammaplasty, 503–504
for rhinoplasty, 108
for rhytidectomy, 379
for weight loss contouring, 708
Examination rooms, design of, 47, 48, 49
Eye plasty, early history of, 8–9, 15–16, 17
Eyebrow-lift
with blepharoplasty, 341, 354
infrabrow, 320
with male face-lift, 460
supraciliary, 303, 304, 320
with temple-lift, 394
Eyebrows
anatomy of, 288
evaluation of, 307
placement of, 315
Eyebrows — *Continued*
post–forehead-lift complications, 322
ptosis, correction of, 453
transblepharoplasty suspension, 303
Eyelids. *See also* Blepharoplasty
anatomy of, 288, 306, 328–330, 347, 350–352
classification of deformities, 353
orbital fat of, 351
pathology of degeneration, 353
pathology of delamination, 353
pathology of displacement, 352
skin excision, with malar implant, 278
surgery on lower, 358–359
surgery on upper, 354–358
Eyes. *See also* Blepharoplasty
anatomy of, 328–330
sunken or hollow, 298

Face. *See also* Face-lift; Face-lift, male; Rhytidectomy
anatomy of, 372–374
anesthesia for, 426
deformity location, 378
liposuction on, 680
nerves of, 372–373
pathophysiology of deformities, 374–375, 377–378
rejuvenation techniques, 494–495
Face-lift. *See also* Rhytidectomy
for acne scars, 494
anatomy for, 452–453
early history of, 11–14, 16
expectations for, 450, 451
informed consent for, 451–452
medications for, 80
patient history for, 450, 452
patient selection for, 450, 451
physical examination for, 450–451
for solar exposure wrinkles, 494
terminology discussed, 449–450
Face-lift, male. *See also* Face-lift; Rhytidectomy
ancillary procedures, 460, 462
anesthesia for, 454–455
complications with, 459–460
dissection in, 455
drains in, 459
dressings for, 459
hemostasis for, 455
incisions for, 454, 455
lipectomy, 456–457, 458
marking for, 454
patient satisfaction in, 462
platysma muscle approximation in, 456
postoperative management of, 459
preparation for, 452
results of, 460
secondary surgery, 460
skin excision and closure in, 457, 458, 459
SMAS elevation in, 455–456, 457
technique selection for, 453–454
Facioplasty, defined, 449
Fasanella-Servat blepharoptosis procedure, 328, 342, 352
Fascia, of eye, 350
Fascia, superficial, of face
anatomy of, 422–423, 424
restored, 426
Fat
elimination in neck, 440
excision in rhytidectomy, 401
subcutaneous, in male face-lift, 457, 458
subcutaneous facial, 375, 453
submental, removal of, 442, 444
transplants, 20
Fees, 72, 452
Fentanyl (Sublimaze)
for face-lifts, 454
preoperative use of, 78, 80
Festoons, 296, 298, 341
Files, management of, 58, 69
Film, for clinical photography, 85
Flash units, for clinical photography, 85
Fluorescein dye test, 327
Flurazepam (Dalmane)
postoperative use of, 80
preoperative use of, 77
Follow-up, postsurgical, 43
Forehead
anatomy of, 305–306
collagen for wrinkles in, 490
deformity classification, pathophysiology, 306–307
rhytidectomy on, nerve damage with, 411
Forehead-lift
aesthetic goals for, 310
anesthesia for, 311
bicoronal, 303, 315, 316, 317, 318, 319
with blepharoplasty, 308, 309
chemical peel for, 305
combined, 315, 318
complications with, 320–322
consent for, 310
corrugator resection, 303, 304
for crow's-feet, 299
dissection in, 311, 312, 313
dressings for, 315
examination and evaluation for, 307
hairline, 303
history of, 302
indications for, 302
injection therapy, 305
on males, 318, 319, 320
markings for, 311
midforehead-lift, 303
motivation for, 307
muscle excision, 311, 313
patient history for, 307
postoperative management of, 315
preparations for, 310
skin excision and closure, 311, 312, 313, 315
supracilliary eyebrow-lift, 303, 304, 320
temporal lift, 303
transblepharoplasty eyebrow suspension, 303
wrinkle resection, 303, 305
Forms, printed, 54–58
action, 55
authorization, 452
consent, for photography, 98, 99

Forms, printed—*Continued*
  daily list, 55
  letter, 55
  report, 55, 56, 57, 58
  route slips, 55
  surgery schedule, 55
  telephone message, 55
Fracture, procedure
  defined, 138
  for rhinoplasty, 138
Freckles, chemical peeling for, 473
Frontalis muscle
  anatomy of, 305
  in forehead-lift, 311
Furnishings and decor of office, 50–53

Gastric bypass, 706
Gastroplasty, 706
Gender change, breast augmentation for, 560
Genioplasty. *See* Chin, aesthetic procedures on
Glabellar frown lines, 303, 305, 307
  choice of technique for, 495
  collagen injection for, 450
Gluteal depression
  correction of, 667, 668, 669, 671
  lateral, 676, 677
Glycopyrrolate (Robinul), preoperative use of, 78
Grafts. *See also* Implants; Prostheses
  to alar rims, 180
  autogenous, in rhinoplasty, 153, 156
  cartilage nose tip, 212
  dorsal, 156
  ear conchal cartilage, 176, 180
  malar, materials for, 276
  materials for, 158
  Meyer-Sheen lobular onlay, 212
  for nasolabial folds, 484
  nipple, 526–528
  Peck onlay cartilage, 130
  postoperative eyelid, 293
  reinserted inlay, in nose, 191, 193, 194, 196, 199
  for saddlenose, 207–208
  septal strut, 176
  Sheen tip, 130
  in supratip, of nose, 204, 156
  temporal fascial, 311

Hair follicle removal in males, 458, 459
Hair loss
  with forehead-lift, 321
  with male face-lift, 460
  with rhytidectomy, 379, 413
Hair pattern, 306
Haloperidol (Haldol), preoperative use of, 78
Hands, brachioplasty on, 700, 702
Helix, of ear, aesthetic goals for, 250
Hematoma
  with abdominal lipectomy, 647
  from blepharoplasty, 293, 294, 343
  with brachioplasty, 703
  with breast augmentation, 582
  with breast reduction, 530
Hematoma—*Continued*
  with face-lift, 460
  with forehead-lift, 320
  with lower extremity dermolipectomy, 675
  postrhinoplasty, 162
  prevention of, 459
  with rhytidectomy, 379, 409, 410, 411, 412
  with superficial fascia rhytidectomy, 432–433
Hemorrhage. *See also* Bleeding
  with nasal tip rhinoplasty, 181
  with rhinoplasty, 161
Hemostasis
  for breast augmentation, 569
  for breast reduction, 508
  for male face-lift, 455
  for mastopexy, 546
  for rhytidectomy, 383, 409
  for temple-lift, 394
Heparin, for thrombophlebitis, 649
Hernia
  with abdominoplasty, 645
  umbilical, 619
Heyer-Schulte prosthesis, 276, 575, 579, 580
History
  of abdominoplasty, 617, 619
  of blepharoplasty, 287, 288, 325–326
  of brachioplasty, 693
  of breast augmentation, 559
  of chemical peeling, 463–464
  of chin aesthetic surgery, 221
  of forehead-lift, 302
  of lower extremity dermolipectomy, 655–656
  of malar aesthetic surgery, 275–276
  of mastopexy, 539
  of obesity treatment, 705
  of otoplasty, 245, 252
  of reduction mammaplasty, 499–500
  of rhinoplasty, 101–102
  of rhytidectomy, 371–372
History, patient's
  for abdominoplasty, 621
  for blepharoplasty, 326
  for brachioplasty, 694
  for breast asymmetry correction, 597
  for breast augmentation, 560
  for breast reduction, 501
  for face-lift, 450
  for forehead-lift, 307
  for lower extremity dermolipectomy, 658
  for mastopexy, 540
  for rhinoplasty, 102–103
  for rhytidectomy, 379
  for weight loss contouring, 708
History-taking, 35
Hooding, temple-lift for, 394
Hump, nasal
  excessive removal of, 204, 206
  insufficient removal of, 201
  removal of, approaches to, 137–144
  resection of, extramucosal technique, 202–203
Hyaluronidase (Wydase, Alidase)
  for face-lift, 454–455
  for rhinoplasty, 127
Hydromorphine (Dilaudid), preoperative use of, 77
Hydroxyzine (Vistaril, Atarax), preoperative use of, 77, 80
Hyperkeratosis, chemical peeling for, 465
Hyperplasia, defined, 595, 596
Hyperthyroidism, lid retraction test with, 328
Hypertrophy
  defined, 595
  of nipple, 609–610, 612
  treatment of, 599, 603, 604
Hypoplasia
  breast augmentation for, 562
  correction of, 598–599, 600, 601
  defined, 595, 596

Immunoglobulin A, in nasal mucosa, 121
Implants, silastic, 223, 224. *See also* Grafts; Prostheses
Incisions
  for abdominoplasty, 624, 625
  bilateral intercartilaginous, nasal, 204
  for brachioplasty, 696–697, 698
  for breast augmentation, 564, 565
  on eyelids, 359, 360
  in forehead-lift, 311, 315, 316, 317, 318, 319, 320
  gull-wing, 181
  for liposuction, 687
  for lower extremity dermolipectomy, 659–660, 661
  for male face-lift, 454
  for nasal tip corrections, 209
  for rhinoplasty, 129, 146
  for rhytidectomy, 380, 381, 382, 383, 384
  for secondary rhytidectomy, 416
  spiral ("Chinese serpentine"), 187, 189
Infection
  with abdominal lipectomy, 647
  with lower extremity dermolipectomy, 675
  with nasal tip rhinoplasty, 181
  postrhinoplasty, 162
  postrhytidectomy, 411
  with reduction mammaplasty, 531
  with superficial fascia rhytidectomy, 433
Inferior pedicle technique (reduction mammaplasty), 522–526
Informing the patient, 40. *See also* Consent, informed
Inframammary crease, normal, 506
Infrapalpebral bulges, 296, 297, 298
Infrapalpebral depression, 294, 295, 296
Innovar, preoperative use of, 78
Insurance, office and practice, 58–59
Intercom system, office, 59
Intestinal bypass, 706–707
Intranasal lining, excessive resectioning of, 203
Intraorbital fat, herniation of, defined, 326
Isoproterenol (Isuprel), preoperative use of, 78

Jowls
formation of, 375
improvement of, 454

Kefzol, with lower extremity dermolipectomy, 664
Kenalog injection, 585, 587
Keratoconjunctivitis sicca. *See* Dry eye syndrome
Ketamine (Ketalar, Ketaject), for face-lifts, 454
Ketamine hydrochloride, preoperative use of, 79–80
Keystone area, defined, 111
Klebsiella, in wound infections, 433
Kuhnt-Szymanowski procedure, 335, 340–341

Labiomental folds, deepening of, 487, 488
Lacrimal system
dye tests of, 327–328
ptosis of gland, 298
in rhinoplasty, 162
Lagophthalmos, after blepharoplasty, 342
Latissimus muscle transfer, 604
Launois-Bensaude disease, 687
Lenses, for clinical photography, 83, 85
Levator action with ptosis, test for, 328
Levator aponeurosis, dissection of, 357
Levator palpebrae superioris, anatomy of, 351
Lid distension test, 327
Lidocaine (Xylocaine)
action of, 79
for blepharoplasty, 289, 291, 359
for brachioplasty, 698
for breast augmentation, 568, 569, 573
for face-lift, 454
for lower extremity dermolipectomy, 661
for mastopexy, 546
for ontoplasty, 253
Lighting
for clinical photography, 85–88
in operating room, 67
Lipectomy, abdominal, 638–647. *See also* Abdominoplasty
cervicofacial, 401
complications with, 435
history for, 617
incisions for, 617, 618
indications for, 619
lower medial obesity, fleur-de-lis operation, 644–645, 646, 647
on male, 456–457, 458
objectives and principles of, 440–441
surgical procedure for, 389–390, 391
technique for, 427, 428, 437
torso-obesity, belt lipectomy, 638, 640, 641
upper medial obesity, T-excision, 638, 642, 643
Lipectomy, suction, 679–692
after abdominoplasty, 649
advantages of, 681

Lipectomy, suction—*Continued*
with brachioplasty, 695, 704
complications with, 684–685
discussion of, 685
during lipectomy, 647
hip approach, 682, 683
Illouz tunneling procedure, 679–680, 685, 686–692
indications for, 681, 687
infragluteal approach, 682, 683, 684
instruments for, 681, 686
layer technique, 685
of lower extremities, general, 671
marking for, 682
postoperative care, 684
sites for, 682
wet technique, 687
Lipexeresis, defined, 671
Lipodissector, 686, 689
Lipodystrophy, trochanteric, 22, 23, 24
Lipoma, 375, 687
Lips
anatomy of, 119
rejuvenation of, 429, 442, 443, 453, 484–489, 491, 495
Lobule, of ear
aesthetic goals for, 250–251
control of, 253, 259
deformities of, with rhytidectomy, 412
historical treatment of, 252
Lobule, of nose
anatomy of, 110, 115–120
drooping, 180
Locator systems, 54
Log books, maintenance of, 69
Lorazepam (Ativan)
for blepharoplasty, 289
for breast augmentation, 569
preoperative use of, 77
Luedde exophthalmometer, 327
Lymphatics
of abdomen, 622, 623
of breast, 505
of lower extremities, 659
Lymphedema
with brachioplasty, 703
with lower extremity dermolipectomy, 676

Malar bags, 296, 298
Malar furrows, 328
Malar regions, aesthetic surgery on, 275–285
approaches to, 276–283
complications, 283–284
evaluation in, 275, 276
implants, 275–276
postoperative care, 283
zygoma reduction, 284
Males. *See also* Face-lift, males
abdominoplasty for, 632
aesthetic surgery on, 449–462
hair of, 452–453
skin of, 452
Malignancy, discovery of, with mammaplasty, 531

Mammaplasty. *See also Breast entries*
early history of, 6, 7, 15, 16, 19–22
Marcaine, for superficial fascia rhytidectomy, 426
Markings
for abdominoplasty, 624, 629
for blepharoplasty, 289, 332–333, 334, 359
for brachioplasty, 696–697
for breast reduction, 506, 508, 510, 511, 512, 513, 517, 522–523
for forehead-lift, 311
for liposuction, 682
for male face-lift, 454
for otoplasty, 253
for rhytidectomy, 380, 381
for semicircular thigh resection, 664, 667, 673, 674
for torsoplasty, 712, 713
Mastopexy. *See* Breasts, ptotic, mastopexy for
Medications
for abdominoplasty, 630
for blepharoplasty, 340
for breast augmentation, 569–570
for chemical peel, 466
Melonocervicoplasty, defined, 449
Meloplasty
defined, 449
procedure, 394, 396, 397
Mentoplasty
augmentation, 156–157
reduction, 157, 161
Meperidine (Demerol)
for breast augmentation, 573
preoperative use of, 77
Mepivacaine (Carbocaine), metabolization of, 79
Mesoridazine (Serenti), preoperative use of, 77
Microfibrillar collagen hemostat (Avitene), for hemostasis, 455
Milia
with chemical peeling, 477
postblepharoplasty, 294
Millard's composite alar flaps, 199
Miniheparin
for post–weight loss contouring, 708
for thrombophlebitis, 649
Morestin, Hippolyte, 449
early contributions to facial surgery by, 12
early contributions to mammaplasty by, 6
Morphine
for blepharoplasty, 288, 289, 359
for breast augmentation, 569
preoperative use of, 77
Morselizing devices, 681
Motivation
for abdominoplasty, 621
for blepharoplasty, 326–327, 353
for brachioplasty, 694–695
for breast asymmetry correction, 597–598
for breast augmentation, 562
for breast reduction, 501–503

Motivation — *Continued*
for forehead-lift, 307
for lower extremity dermolipectomy, 658
for mastopexy, 540
for rhinoplasty, 103, 104–107
for rhytidectomy, 379
for weight loss contouring, 708
Müller's muscle
anatomy of, 329–330, 351
test, 328
Multipurpose rooms, 49
Muramidase, in nasal mucosa, 121
Muscles
of abdomen, 622
of breast, 504
of chin, 222
excision of, in forehead-lift, 311
of eye, 329–330
of eyelid, 350–351
facial
deformities of, 377
frontal, 374, 425
platysmal, 373–374
of forehead, 305
of lower extremities, 659
Müller's, 328, 329–330, 351
nasal, 111, 112
orbicularis oculi, 288
Myocutaneous flap transfer, 604

Narcotics, preoperative use of, 76–77
Nares, 121
Nasal cavity, anatomy of, 120
Nasal valve, 120
Nasal vestibule, 120
Nasojugal furrows, 328
Nasolabial angle
demonstrated, 110
improvement of, 179–180
optimal, 175
Nasolabial folds
choice of technique for, 495
correction of, 453, 484, 485
face- and neck-lifting and, 450
in superficial fascia rhytidectomy, 429, 442, 443
Neck. *See also* Platysma muscle
collagen for wrinkles in, 490
liposuction on, 680
of male, 453, 454
platysma procedures, 401
preoperative warning on, 389
surgical procedures on, 398
youthful, defined, 377
Nerve damage
with abdominoplasty, 649
with brachioplasty, 704
with breast augmentation, 575, 583
with face-lift, 460
with forehead-lift, 320, 321
with mastopexy, 555
with reduction mammaplasty, 532
repair of severed nerve, 409
with rhytidectomy, 379, 411, 415, 441
with superficial fascia rhytidectomy, 429, 432, 433, 434, 435
Nerves
of abdomen, 622, 623
anesthetic effect on, 79
in arm, 695
auricular, 372
in breast, 505
in chin, 222
in eye, 330
facial, 372–373, 453
of forehead, 305
of lower extremities, 659
in nose, 121
Neuroleptanesthesia, defined, 78
Nipple. *See also Breast entries;* Nipple-areola complex
anatomy of, 609
free graft of, 526–528
herniation of areola, 606
hypertrophy of, 609–610, 612
inversion of, 609, 610, 611
normal form of, 505, 506
postreduction deformities of, 533
transposition, in reduction mammaplasty, 508
Nipple-areola complex (NAC). *See also* Nipple
deformities of, 609–613
malposition after reduction, 534
Nitroglycerin, preoperative use of, 80
Norepinephrine (Levophed), preoperative use of, 78
Nose. *See also* Rhinoplasty
aesthetics of, 122–126
alar rim deformities, 212, 213
anatomy of
blood supply, 120–121
bony vault, 111
cartilaginous vault, 110, 111, 114–115
lobule, 110, 115–120
muscles, 111, 112
nasal cavity, 120
nasal vestibule, 120
nerve supply, 121
septum, 114
soft tissue coverage, 111
early history of surgery on, 3–6, 11, 14, 16
hidden columella, 212, 213
physiology of, 121–122
pinched, 210
posttraumatic deformities of, 183–199
cartilage overlappings, 185
curved deformity, 185, 187, 189
hump resection, 191–197, 199
nasal splints, 191, 192
postoperative saddlenose, 197, 198, 199
stages of correction, 183
transnostril foreign body, 183, 184, 185
vertical crest, 183, 184, 185, 186, 187
septal perforations, 216
stenoses of the nares, 216–217
Nose, tip of
aesthetics of, 122, 129–130
Nose, tip of — *Continued*
alterations to
evaluation of, 135, 137
projection, 130, 131, 132, 133, 134, 135
rotation, 135
anatomy of, 110, 115–118, 129, 174–175
bifid or cleft, 210
collapsed, 211–212
correction of, 116
deformities of, classified, 175–176
examination of, 173–174
grafts to, 156
palpation of, 173
photography of, 174
postrhinoplasty supratip deformity, 201–204, 205
postrhinoplasty deformity, 209–212
rhinoplasty on
for alar rims, 180
for bulbous tip, 176
complications of, 181
for drooping lobule, 180
for nasolabial angle, 179–180
principles of, 115–117
for profile problems, 178
for projection problems, 176
for supratip fullness, 180–181
for wide tip, 178
surgical sequence on, 127
Nostrils
aesthetics of, 126
anatomy of, 119
base modifications, 145, 146
Nursing station, in office, 68

Obesity. *See also* Weight loss, massive
facial anatomy with, 423
morbid, defined, 705
pathophysiology and classification of, 619, 705–706
and thigh deformities, 656
treatment of
history of, 705
surgical, 706–707
weights, desirable, 707
Office
construction, 46
design
functional requirements, 47
materials and decor, 50–53
space requirements, 47–49
surgery suite. *See* Surgery, in office
traffic flow, 49–50
emergency systems, 59
insurance, 58
location choice, 45–46
management
communications, 54–58, 69
personnel, 58
records and files, 58, 69
rental versus ownership, 46
security, 59
settings, 34
Olfactory system, in rhinoplasty, 162
Operating table, choice of, 67

Orbicularis muscle, oculi
  adjustment of, 299
  anatomy of, 288, 329, 350
  resectioning of, 354
Ostectomy, of supraorbital ridges, 299
Osteotomy
  defined, 138
  double-level, 111
  lateral, 111
  for rhinoplasty, 137–138, 139, 140–144
  in sagittal advancement, 230
  techniques for, 148, 150, 152
Otoplasty. *See also* Ears
  aesthetic goals, 250–251
  anesthesia for, 247, 253
  anthelix reconstruction, 252, 253, 256, 257, 259, 264, 265, 267
  cartilage treatment in, 251
  closure and dressing in, 251, 267, 271
  combined deformities, 258, 264, 265, 266, 267, 270
  complications of, 267, 270, 272, 273
  conchal reduction, 252, 253, 258, 260, 261, 266, 267
  conchal repositioning, 253, 258, 262, 263, 264, 265, 267
  deformity evaluation for, 247, 248, 249–250
  history of, 245, 252
  lobule control, 253, 259
  marking for, 253
  patient selection for, 245, 247
  postoperative care, 267
  precautions in, 251
  preparation for, 253
  results of, 267
  secondary procedures, 270
  splinting with, 251, 252, 271
  superior crus reconstruction, 253, 259, 266
  surgical approach, 253, 255
  timing of, 247
Oxazepam (Serax), preoperative use of, 77
Oxygen, systems for, 81

Pachydermatochalasis, defined, 326
Pain
  with forehead-lift, 320–321
  postrhytidectomy, 413
Palpation, of nasal tip, 173
Panniculectomy, 617
Paraffin injections, 8–9, 10
Paraffinomas, with rhinoplasty, 162
Parrot's beak ("Polly beak"), 181, 203–204
Patient satisfaction, 40–42
  with abdominoplasty, 649
  males, 462
  with mastopexy, 555
  postrhytidectomy, 413
Patient selection, 35–38, 42
  for ambulatory surgery, 70
  for blepharoplasty, 326, 353
  for chemical peeling, 464–466
  for collagen injection, 489
Patient selection — *Continued*
  for face-lift, 450
  facilities and, 60
  for otoplasty, 245, 247
  for rhinoplasty, 103
Pectus excavatum deformity, 605, 606
Penicillin, with chin surgery, 230
Pentobarbital (Nembutal)
  for breast augmentation, 569, 573
  preoperative use of, 77
Periostitis, with rhinoplasty, 162
Perphenazine (Trilafon), preoperative use of, 77
Personnel, office
  education of, 71
  management, 58
  in surgery suite, 67
Phenergan, for blepharoplasty, 359
Phenobarbital (Luminal), preoperative use of, 77
Phenol
  characteristics of, 476
  for chemical peeling, 463, 466
Phenothiazine (Compazine)
  for blepharoplasty, 288
  for breast augmentation, 569
  preoperative use of, 77–78
Phentolamine, uses for, 78
Phlebitis, with breast augmentation, 583
Photography
  for blepharoplasty, 328
  for breast augmentation, 564
  camera equipment and film, 83, 85
  composition and shooting, 88–96, 97
  consent forms for, 723–724
  for forehead-lift, 310
  general, 39
  lights and lighting, 85–88
  for nasal tip surgery, 174
  privacy rights, 96, 98
  purpose of, 83
  for rhytidectomy, 380
  room for, 49
Piperazines, preoperative use of, 77
Piperidinediones (Nodular, Doriden), preoperative use of, 77
Piperidines, preoperative use of, 77
Planotome, 686
Platysma muscle
  closure of, in neck, 432
  deformities of, 377
  lateral modifications of, 389
  in lipectomy, 401
  medial approximation of, 388, 456
  nerve damage with, 411
  principles of surgery on, 383
  restored, 426
  transverse resection of, 427, 430, 437, 438, 439–440, 442
Poland syndrome, 595, 596, 597, 605
Popliteal area, 670, 675
Port-wine stains, 473
Practice analysis, 60
Preaxilloplasty, 699–700, 701, 702
Pregnancy
  and abdominal wall deformities, 619
  and breast hypertrophy, 500
Preoperative instructions, 452
Prilocaine (Citanest), metabolization of, 79
Privacy
  photography and, 96, 98
  provision for, 50
Procaine (Novocaine), action of, 79
Procerus, anatomy of, 305
Prochlorperazine (Compazine)
  with ambulatory surgery, 80
  preoperative use of, 77
Profileplasty. *See* Malar region, aesthetic surgery on
Progesterone, for breast hypertrophy, 500
Promazine (Sparine), preoperative use of, 77
Promethazine (Phenergan), preoperative use of, 77
Propoxyphene (Darvon), postoperative use of, 80
Propranolol (Inderal), uses and side effects of, 78–79
Prostheses. *See also* Grafts; Implants
  for breast augmentation, 566, 575, 576, 577, 586
  leakage of inflatable, 584–585
  malar, 275, 278
  migration of, in breast, 583
Pseudoptosis, of breast, 540, 547
Pseudosaddlenose, 207
Psychologic aspects
  of aesthetic surgery (general), 35–38
  of breast augmentation, 562
  fears of surgery, 75–76
  of massive weight loss, 708
  of reduction mammaplasty, 502–503
  of rhinoplasty, 103
Ptosis, breast. *See Breast entries*
Ptosis, eyebrow. *See* Eyebrows
Ptosis, of eyelid, 341–342, 356. *See also* Eyelids
Pulmonary embolus, with abdominal lipectomy, 648

Radix
  aesthetics of, 122
  anatomy of, 110
Records
  maintenance of, 58
  office, 58, 69
  of surgery, 69
Recovery room, in office, 68
Referrals
  dissatisfied patients, 41–42
  office location and, 46
Refusing a patient, 38
Reimbursement, 72, 452
Resection, in lower extremity dermolipectomy, 660
Resorption, in chin advancements, 242, 244
Respiration
  the nose in, 121–122
  and saddlenose, 206–207
Retrogenia. *See* Chin, aesthetic procedures on
Rhinitis, postrhinoplasty, 163

Rhinoplasty. *See also* Hump, nasal; Nose; Septum
  aesthetics of, 122–126
  anesthesia for, 126–127, 146
  assessment in, 102, 108
  closure in, 145
  complications of, 161–163
  consent for, 108–109
  dressings for, 145–146
  examination for, 108
  history of, 3–5, 6, 101–102
  history taking for, 102–103, 108–109
  incisions for, 129
  length changes, 135
  in males, 38
  medications for, 81
  motivation for, 103
  of nasal tip, 173–181. *See also* Nose, tip of
  nasolabial angle changes, 135
  nostril base modification for, 145, 146
  operative sequence for, 127, 129
  osteotomies for, 137–138, 139, 140, 141, 142, 143, 144
  pathophysiology and classification for, 102
  preparation for, 109, 126–127
  results of, 163
  secondary, 201–217
Rhytidectomy. *See also* Face; Face-lift; Face-lift, male
  aesthetic goals for, 379
  cervicofacial, 401
  with chemical peel, 465, 470–471
  classification of, 378
  combined procedures, 405
  complications of, 379, 380, 409–413, 415
  for crow's-feet, 299, 495
  defined, 371, 449
  excision and closure procedures, 390, 393
  with forehead-lift, 318
  hematomas with subcutaneous, 441
  hemostasis for, 383, 394, 409
  history of, 371–372
  incisions in, 380, 381, 382, 383, 384
  indications and contraindications for, 378
  informed consent for, 379–380
  for infrapalpebral bulges, 298
  length of effectiveness, 413, 415–416, 421
  lipectomy procedure, 389–390, 391, 401
  liposuction with, 680
  markings for, 380, 381
  meloplasty procedure, 394, 396, 397
  motivation for, 379
  neck and chin procedures, 398
  patient history for, 379
  photographs for, 380
  physical examination for, 379
  platysma procedures, 383, 388, 389
  post–massive weight loss, 719
  preoperative instructions, 380
Rhytidectomy—*Continued*
  preparation for, 380
  results of, 413, 415
  secondary, 415–416
  skin laxity and, 405
  SMAS procedure, 383, 385, 387, 388
  superficial fascia, 421–448
  temple-lift, 394, 395
  traction procedures, 390, 392
  undermining and dissection in, 383, 385
  upward traction in, 405, 406, 407, 408
Rhytidoplasty, defined, 449
Rhytidosis, periorbital, defined, 326. *See also* Crow's-feet
Riding breeches deformity
  aspects of, 657, 659
  liposuction for, 679–680

SMAS. *See* Superficial musculoaponeurotic system
Saddlenose, postoperative correction of, 197, 198, 199, 206–209
Sagittal advancement
  maximum, 234
  minor, 230
  moderate, 230, 231, 232, 233, 234
Salicyclic acid, for chemical peeling, 463
Scapha, of ear, 253
Scapha, reduction of, 267, 270
Scars
  with abdominal lipectomy, 649
  with brachioplasty, 695, 703
  with breast augmentation, 582, 583–584
  with chemical face peeling, 477, 479
  with "double eye" blepharoplasty, 366
  with forehead-lift, 321
  with lower extremity dermolipectomy, 659, 675
  with mastopexy, 555
  from otoplasty, 273
  postrhinoplasty, 163, 181
  postrhytidectomy, 412, 415
  with reduction mammaplasty, 531–532, 534
Scheduling surgery, 40
Schirmer tear test, 327
Schwager procedure, 609
Scoliosis, breast augmentation for, 578
Scopolamine, preoperative use of, 78
Secobarbital (Seconal), preoperative use of, 77
Secondary surgery
  for abdominoplasty, 649, 650, 651, 652
  after body contouring, 719
  after brachioplasty, 704
  face-lift, 460
  after lipectomy, 685
  after lower extremity dermolipectomy, 676, 677
  for ptotic breast, 555, 557
  rhytidectomy, 415–416
Security, of office, 59
Sedative hypnotics, preoperative use of, 77
Self-evaluation, surgeon's, 451
Sensation loss. *See* Nerve damage
Septorhinoplasty. *See also* Rhinoplasty
  surgical techniques for, 146, 148–149, 151, 152–153, 156
Septum, nasal
  anatomy of, 114, 116–117, 118, 120, 121, 175
  deformity correction, 144–145
  grafts to, 176
  perforation of, with rhinoplasty, 162
  perforations of, 216
  saddlenose, 197, 198, 199
Septum, orbital, anatomy of, 329, 350
Seroma
  with abdominal lipectomy, 647
  with brachioplasty, 703
Services, contracted, 58
Silicone
  for breast augmentation implants, 566
  for glabellar frown lines, 305
  for malar implants, 276
  for wrinkled upper lip, 485–486
Simons-Barraquer syndrome, 670
Sjögren's syndrome, postblepharoplasty, 293
Skin. *See also* Chemical face peeling
  of abdomen, 622
  of eye, 329, 350
  of face, 452
  of forehead, 305
  of lower extremities, 659
  of nose, 111
  in otoplasty, 251
  pigment changing techniques, 342
Skin problems
  with chemical peeling, 476–477, 479
  necrosis, 320, 411, 531, 647–648, 675
  of pigmentation, 413, 471–472, 494
  with rhinoplasty, 162
  severe laxity of, 405
  sloughing, 415, 460, 703
  wrinkle pathophysiology, 374–375
Smoking
  and skin problems, 460
  and thrombophlebitis, 648
Social aspects, of plastic surgery, 32–34
Solu-Medrol, in breast prostheses, 586
Spine, nasal, alterations to, 136
Splinting, for otoplasty, 251–252, 271
Splints, nasal, 191, 192
Squinch test, 298, 327
Staphylococcus aureus
  in breast augmentation infection, 531, 583
  in rhinoplasty infection, 162
  in wound infection, 433
Staphylococcus epidermidis, in breast augmentation infection, 596
Stenosis, postoperative, of nares, 216–217
Sterilization room, in office, 69
Steroid injection, in breast augmentation, 585
Stripper, fascial, 681
Suction equipment, choice of, 67
Suction lipectomy. *See* Lipectomy, suction
Sulcus, of ear, aesthetic goals for, 251

Sun exposure, postchemical peel, 469
Superficial musculoaponeurotic system (SMAS)
  anatomy of, 374, 422–423, 424, 425, 453
  defined, 371
  elevation of, 429, 439–440, 455–456, 457
  plications with meloplasty, 394
  restored, 426
  surgical procedures on, 383, 385, 387, 388
Supplies, for surgery suite, 69
Supraorbital nerve, anatomy of, 305
Supratip, of nose
  alteration to, 180–181
  secondary deformities to, 201–204, 205, 206, 207
Supratrochlear nerve, anatomy of, 305
Surgery, in office, 61–69, 71
  advantages and disadvantages of, 59–60
  costs. *See* Cost accounting, for office surgery
  decision about, 60–61
  discharge and follow-up, 71
  dress for, 71–72
  monitoring equipment for, 81
  patient flow, 70–71
  records, 69–70
  suite for, 61–72
  supplies for, 69
  support systems for, 81
Suspension, in lower extremity dermolipectomy, 661
Sutures
  for abdominoplasty, 632
  for blepharoplasty, 335, 359, 362
  in B-technique reduction mammaplasty, 509
  for face-lift, 459
  for forehead-lift, 315
  for mastopexy, 546
  for otoplasty, 251, 267
  for rhytidectomy, 390, 392, 393
  for superficial fascia rhytidectomy, 430–431
  transalar mattress, 210
  U, in nasal deformity correction, 187, 190, 191
Swelling. *See* Edema

Tarsal fixation techniques, cautionary on, 332, 340
Tarsal-orbital fascia, anatomy of, 329, 330, 352
Telangiectasia
  with chemical peel, 479
  chemical peeling for, 473
Telephone deformity, of ear, 250
Telephone system, office, 54
Temple-lift procedure, 394
Terminology
  of aesthetic surgery, 449–450
  of chemical face peeling, 463
Tests
  ophthalmologic, 327
  squinch, 298
Tetracaine (Pontocaine), action of, 79
Thighplasty, defined, 655
Thighs. *See also* Dermolipectomy, lower extremity
  aesthetic deformities of, 656
  anatomy of, 659
  early history of lifting, 17–18, 22, 24–25
  lipectomy, defined, 655
  liposuction on, indications for, 679–680
  medial deformity of, 661
  vertical excision, postmassive weight loss, 715, 717
Thioridazine (Mellaril), preoperative use of, 77
Thiothixene (Navane), preoperative use of, 78
Thioxanthenes, preoperative use of, 78
Thoracobrachioplasty, 715, 718, 719
Thorazine, for blepharoplasty, 359
Thrombin, for hemostasis, 455
Thrombophlebitis, with abdominoplasty, 648
Thymol iodide powder, 468
Tolazoline hydrochloride (Priscoline), effects of, 78
Torso, liposuction on, 680
Torsoplasty
  batwing, 710, 711, 713, 715
  belt lipectomy, 709, 710, 712–713, 714
  extended fleur-de-lis, 709, 710
  indications for, 619
Toxic reactions, to local anesthetics, 79
Tranquilizers, preoperative use of, 77
Transnostril foreign body
  described, 183, 184
  surgical techniques for, 185, 186
Transverse bar, in ear helix, 250, 262
Treacher Collins–Franceschetti syndrome, 234
Treacher Collins syndrome, 275
Triamcinolone, for hypertrophic scars, 649
Trichloracetic acid, for chemical peeling, 463
Trifluoperazine (Stelazine), preoperative use of, 77
Triflupromazine (Vesprin), preoperative use of, 77
Trochanter
  defatting of, 667, 670, 671
  deformities of, 662–663
  lipodystrophy of, 676
  liposuction for lipodystrophy of, 691
Turbinates, 121, 122
Two-layer shift, of Skoog, 421

Umbilicoplasty
  with abdominoplasty, 650, 651, 652
  procedure, 627, 628, 630
Umbilicus, abnormal, with lipectomy, 649
Undermining
  in lower extremity dermolipectomy, 660
  in rhytidectomy, 383, 385
  in secondary rhytidectomy, 416

Valium, with blepharoplasty, 335, 359
Valsalva maneuver, for venous pressure, 459
Vaseline injections, 8, 9
Vision loss, postblepharoplasty, 293
Vomer, of nose
  anatomy of, 110, 120
  resection of, 187
VOQ technique
  for large areola, 610
  in mastopexy, 544, 545, 546

W-plasty. *See* Abdominoplasty, W-plasty technique
Weight, desirable, 707
Weight loss, massive, 705–720. *See also* Obesity
  body contouring for, 707–708, 715, 718, 719–720
  surgery for, 706–707
  torsoplasty for, 709–713, 715
Workrooms in office, 68–69
Wound
  dehiscence, 411, 531, 703
  separation, 647, 675
Wrinkles
  causes of, 422–423
  fine, treatment of, 450
  pathophysiology and kinds of, 374–375
  post–forehead-lift, 322
  pretarsal and preorbital, 355–356
  resection of, 303, 305
  from solar exposure, 494
  on upper lip, 485–486

X-ray treatment, and chemical peel, 472–473
Xylocaine
  for blepharoplasty, 332
  for forehead-lift, 311
  for rhinoplasty, 126
  for rhytidectomy, 380

Z-plasty, 331
Zygoma, prominent, 284
Zygomaticofacial nerves, 305
Zygomaticofrontal nerves, 305
Zygomatic region, evaluation of, 275